Ramendra Pa

DEVELOPING SOLID ORAL DOSAGE FORMS: PHARMACEUTICAL THEORY AND PRACTICE

This work is dedicated to Drs R.D. Schoenwald, J. Keith Guillory, L.E. Matheson, E.L. Parrott, D.R. Flanagan, D.E. Wurster, P. Veng-Pedersen and the late D.J.W. Grant

By generously sharing their experience, time and wisdom, what they've taught us is well beyond what we learned in school

We are also forever indebted to our families for their love, understanding, and sacrifice

DEVELOPING SOLID ORAL DOSAGE FORMS: PHARMACEUTICAL THEORY AND PRACTICE

Executive editors

Yihong Qiu, Abbott Laboratories, IL, USA

Yisheng Chen, Novast Laboratories, Nantong, China

Geoff G. Z. Zhang, Abbott Laboratories, IL, USA

Associate editors

Lirong Liu, Pfizer Inc., NJ, USA

William R. Porter, Abbott Laboratories, IL, USA

AMSTERDAM • BOSTON • HEIDELBERG • LONDON • NEW YORK • OXFORD
PARIS • SAN DIEGO • SAN FRANCISCO • SINGAPORE • SYDNEY • TOKYO
Academic Press is an imprint of Elsevier

Academic Press is an imprint of Elsevier
30 Corporate Drive, Suite 400, Burlington, MA 01803, USA
32 Jamestown Road, London NW1 7BY, UK
525 B Street, Suite 1900, San Diego, CA 92101-4495, USA
360 Park Avenue South, New York, NY 10010-1710, USA

First edition 2009

Notice
No responsibility is assumed by the publisher for any injury and/or damage to persons or property as a matter of products liability, negligence or otherwise, or from any use or operation of any methods, products, instructions or ideas contained in the material herein.

Disclaimer
Medicine is an ever-changing field. Standard safety precautions must be followed, but as new research and clinical experience broaden our knowledge, changes in treatment and drug therapy may become necessary or appropriate. Readers are advised to check the most current product information provided by the manufacturer of each drug to be administered to verify the recommended dose, the method and duration of administrations, and contraindications. It is the responsibility of the treating physician, relying on experience and knowledge of the patient, to determine dosages and the best treatment for each individual patient. Neither the publisher nor the authors assume any liability for any injury and/or damage to persons or property arising from this publication.

Library of Congress Cataloging-in-Publication Data
A catalog record for this book is available from the Library of Congress

British Library Cataloguing in Publication Data
A catalogue record for this book is available from the British Library

ISBN: 978-0-444-53242-8

For information on all Academic Press publications
visit our website at www.Elsevierdirect.com

Typeset by Charon Tec Ltd., A Macmillan Company
www.macmillansolutions.com

Printed and bound in the United States of America

09 10 11 12 13 10 9 8 7 6 5 4 3 2 1

CONTENTS

List of Contributors   xxix
Foreword by J. Keith Guillory   xxxi

PART I

THEORIES AND TECHNIQUES IN THE CHARACTERIZATION OF DRUG SUBSTANCES AND EXCIPIENTS

1. Solubility of Pharmaceutical Solids
Venkatramana M. Rao, Ritesh Sanghvi and Haijian (Jim) Zhu

2. Crystalline and Amorphous Solids
Geoff G. Z. Zhang and Deliang Zhou

3. Analytical Techniques in Solid-state Characterization
Eric J. Munson

4. Salt Screening and Selection: New Challenges and Considerations in the Modern Pharmaceutical Research and Development Paradigm
Wei-Qin (Tony) Tong

5. Drug Stability and Degradation Studies
Deliang Zhou, William R. Porter and Geoff G.Z. Zhang

6. Excipient Compatibility

Ajit S. Narang, Venkatramana M. Rao and Krishnaswamy S. Raghavan

7. Theory of Diffusion and Pharmaceutical Applications

Yisheng Chen and Douglas R. Flanagan

8. Particle, Powder, and Compact Characterization
Gregory E. Amidon, Pamela J. Secreast and Deanna Mudie

9. Polymer Properties and Characterization
James E. Brady, Thomas Dürig and Sherwin S. Shang

10. Applied Statistics in Product Development
William R. Porter

PART II

BIOPHARMACEUTICAL AND PHARMACOKINETIC EVALUATIONS OF DRUG MOLECULES AND DOSAGE FORMS

11. Oral Absorption Basics: Pathways, Physico-chemical and Biological Factors Affecting Absorption
Zhongqiu Liu, Stephen Wang and Ming Hu

12. Oral Drug Absorption, Evaluation, and Prediction
Yongsheng Yang and Lawrence X. Yu

13. Fundamentals of Dissolution
Jianzhuo Wang and Douglas R. Flanagan

14. Dissolution Testing of Solid Products

Michelle Long and Yisheng Chen

15. Bioavailability and Bioequivalence

Hao Zhu, Honghui Zhou and Kathleen Seitz

16. *In Vivo* Evaluation of Oral Dosage Form Performance
Honghui Zhou and Kathleen Seitz

17. *In Vitro–In Vivo* Correlations: Fundamentals, Development Considerations, and Applications
Yihong Qiu

PART III

DESIGN, DEVELOPMENT, AND SCALE-UP OF FORMULATION AND PROCESS

18. Integration of Physical, Chemical, Mechanical, and Biopharmaceutical Properties in Solid Oral Dosage Form Development
Xiaorong He

19. Improving the Oral Absorption of Poorly Soluble Drugs Using SEDDS and S-SEDDS Formulations
Walt Morozowich and Ping Gao

20. Rational Design of Oral Modified-Release Drug Delivery Systems
Yihong Qiu

21. Development of Modified-Release Solid Oral Dosage Forms
Yihong Qiu and Guohua Zhang

22. Analytical Development and Validation for Solid Oral Dosage Forms
Xingchun (Frank)Fang, Geoff Carr and Ronald C. Freeze

23. Statistical Design and Analysis of Long-term Stability Studies for Drug Products
David LeBlond

27. Scale-up of Pharmaceutical Manufacturing Operations of Solid Dosage Forms
John Strong

28. Process Development, Optimization, and Scale-up: Powder Handling and Segregation Concerns
Thomas Baxter and James Prescott

29. Process Development and Scale-up of Wet Granulation by the High Shear Process

Lirong Liu, Michael Levin and Paul Sheskey

30. Process Development, Optimization, and Scale-up: Fluid-bed Granulation
Ken Yamamoto and Z. Jesse Shao

33. Development, Optimization, and Scale-up of Process Parameters: Pan Coating
Stuart Porter, Gary Sackett and Lirong Liu

34. Development, Optimization, and Scale-up of Process Parameters: Wurster Coating
David Jones

35. Process Analytical Technology in Solid Dosage Development and Manufacturing
Nancy E. Sever, Martin Warman, Sean Mackey, Walter Dziki and Min Jiang

PART IV

SELECTED TOPICS IN PRODUCT DEVELOPMENT

36. The Product Development Process
Lynn Van Campen

37. Product Registration and Drug Approval Process in the United States
Steven F. Hoff and Yisheng Chen

38. Modern Pharmaceutical Quality Regulations: Question-based Review
Wenlei Jiang and Lawrence X. Yu

39. Intellectual Property Law Primer
Joseph A. Fuchs

40. Product Lifecycle Management (LCM)
Erika A. Zannou, Ping Li and Wei-Qin (Tony) Tong

List of Contributors

Gregory E. Amidon (Chapter 8)
University of Michigan, Ann Arbor, MI, USA

Thomas Baxter (Chapter 28)
Jenike & Johanson Inc., Tyngsboro, MA, USA

James E. Brady (Chapter 9)
Aqualon Division, a Business Unit of
Hercules Inc., Wilmington, DE, USA

Geoff Carr (Chapter 22)
Patheon Inc., Ontario, Canada

Wei Chen (Chapters 25 & 26)
Eli Lilly and Company, Indianapolis, IN, USA

Yisheng Chen (Chapters 7, 14, 24 & 37)
Novast Laboratories (China) Ltd, Nantong, China

Tom Dürig (Chapter 9)
Aqualon Division, a Business Unit of Hercules
Inc., Wilmington, DE, USA

Walter Dziki (Chapter 35)
Abbott Laboratories, North Chicago, IL, USA

Xingchun (Frank) Fang (Chapter 22)
Novast Laboratories (China) Ltd., Nantong, China

Douglas R. Flanagan (Chapters 7 & 13)
University of Iowa, Iowa City, IA, USA

Ronald C. Freeze (Chapter 22)
Abbott Laboratories, Abbott Park, IL, USA

Joseph Fuchs (Chapter 39)
Rockey, Depke & Lyons, LLC, Chicago, IL, USA

Ping Gao (Chapter 19)
Abbott Laboratories, Chicago, IL, USA

Xiaorong He (Chapter 18)
Asymchem Laboratories, Morrisville, NC, USA

Steven F. Hoff (Chapter 37)
Abbott Laboratories, Abbott Park, IL, USA

Ming Hu (Chapter 11)
University of Houston, TX, USA

Richard Hwang (Chapters 25 & 26)
Pfizer Global R&D, Ann Arbor, MI, USA

Min Jiang (Chapter 35)
Abbott Laboratories, North Chicago, IL, USA

Wenlei Jiang (Chapter 38)
US Food and Drug Administration, Rockville,
MD, USA

David Jones (Chapter 34)
OWI-Consulting Inc, Ramsey, NJ, USA

David LeBlond (Chapter 23)
Abbott Laboratories, Wadsworth, IL, USA

Michael Levin (Chapters 29 & 32)
Metropolitan Computing Corporation (MCC),
East Hanover, NJ, USA

Ping Li (Chapter 40)
Novartis Pharmaceuticals Corporation, East Hanover,
NJ, USA

Lirong Liu (Chapters 29, 31, 32 & 33)
Pfizer Inc., Morris Plains, NJ, USA

Zhongqiu Liu (Chapter 11)
Southern Medical University, Guangzhou, China

Michelle Long (Chapter 14)
Abbott Laboratories, North Chicago, IL, USA

Sean Mackey (Chapter 35)
Abbott Laboratories, Abbott Park, IL, USA

Walt Morozowich (Chapter 19)
Prodrug and Formulation Consultant, Kalamazoo,
MI, USA

Deanna Mudie (Chapter 8)
University of Michigan, Ann Arbor, MI, USA

Eric Munson (Chapter 3)
University of Kansas, Lawrence, KS, USA

Ajit S. Narang (Chapter 6)
Bristol-Myers Squibb Co., New Brunswick, NJ, USA

Dale Natoli (Chapter 32)
Natoli Engineering Company, St. Charles, MO, USA

Brian Pack (Chapter 25)
Eli Lilly and Company, Indianapolis, IN, USA

Stuart Porter (Chapter 33)
International Specialty Products, Wayne, NJ, USA

William R. Porter (Chapters 5 & 10)
Abbott Laboratories, Abbott Park, IL, USA

James Prescott (Chapter 28)
Jenike & Johanson Inc., Tyngsboro, MA, USA

Yihong Qiu (Chapters 17, 20 & 21)
Abbott Laboratories, Abbott Park, IL, USA

Krishnaswamy S. Raghavan (Chapter 6)
Bristol-Myers Squibb Co., New Brunswick, NJ, USA

Venkatramana M. Rao (Chapters 1 & 6)
Bristol-Myers Squibb Co., New Brunswick, NJ, USA

Lisa Ray (Chapter 25)
Eli Lilly and Company, Indianapolis, IN, USA

Gary Sackett (Chapters 31 & 33)
Vector Corporation, Marion, IA, USA

Ritesh Sanghvi (Chapter 1)
Forest Laboratories Inc., Farmingdale, NY, USA

Pamela J. Secreast (Chapter 8)
Pharm Optima, Portage, MI, USA

Kathleen Seitz (Chapters 15 & 16)
Centocor Research & Development, Inc., Malvern, PA, USA

Nancy E. Sever (Chapter 35)
Abbott Laboratories, North Chicago, IL, USA

Sherwin Shang (Chapter 9)
Abbott Laboratories, North Chicago, IL, USA

Z. Jesse Shao (Chapter 30)
Arena Pharmaceuticals, Inc., San Diego, CA, USA

Paul Sheskey (Chapter 31)
The Dow Chemical Company, Midland, MI, USA

Timothy J. Smith (Chapter 31)
Vector Corporation, Marion, IA, USA

Suchinda Stithit (Chapters 25 & 26)
Century Pharmaceuticals, Indianapolis, IN, USA

John Strong (Chapter 27)
Abbott Laboratories, North Chicago, IL, USA

Wei-Qin (Tony) Tong (Chapters 4 & 40)
Teva Pharmaceuticals USA, Sellersville, PA, USA

Lev Tsygan (Chapter 32)
Metropolitan Computing Corporation (MCC),
East Hanover, NJ, USA

Lynn Van Campen (Chapter 36)
University of Wisconsin, Madison, WI, USA

Jianzhou (Jake) Wang (Chapter 13)
Gorbec Pharmaceutical Services, Durham, NC, USA

Stephen Wang (Chapter 11)
Schering-Plough, Kenilworth, NJ, USA

Martin Warman (Chapter 35)
Martin Warman Consultancy Ltd, Swalecliffe,
Kent, UK

Ken Yamamoto (Chapter 30)
Pfizer Global R&D, Groton, CT, USA

Yongsheng Yang (Chapter 12)
US Food and Drug Administration, Silver Spring, MD, USA

Lawrence X. Yu (Chapters 12 & 38)
US Food and Drug Administration, Rockville,
MD, USA

Erika A. Zannou (Chapter 40)
Novartis Pharmaceuticals Corporation, East Hanover,
NJ, USA

Geoff G. Z. Zhang (Chapters 2 & 5)
Abbott Laboratories, North Chicago, IL, USA

Guohua Zhang (Chapter 21)
Novast Laboratories (China) Ltd., Nantong, China

Jack Y. Zheng (Chapters 25 & 26)
Eli Lilly and Company, Indianapolis, IN, USA

Deliang Zhou (Chapters 2 & 5)
Abbott Laboratories, North Chicago, IL, USA

Honghui Zhou (Chapters 15 & 16)
Centocor Research & Development, Inc., Malvern, PA, USA

Haijian (Jim) Zhu (Chapter 1)
Forest Laboratories Inc., Farmingdale, NY, USA

Hao Zhu (Chapter 15)
Centocor Research & Development, Inc., Malvern, PA, USA

Foreword

Physical pharmacy, the application of physico-chemical principles to the solution of problems related to dosage forms is, as a discipline, rapidly disappearing from curricula in colleges of pharmacy. It is being replaced by an emphasis on communication skills and pharmacotherapeutics. Biopharmaceutics and pharmacokinetics, sciences that arose from the efforts of such early physical pharmacists as Sidney Riegelman, Milo Gibaldi, Gary Levy, John Wagner and Edward Garrett, are still considered essential, at least for the present. In graduate programs in pharmaceutics, physical pharmacy has taken a back seat to such fashionable and fundable areas as genetics and tissue scaffolding. Yet, the demand for the skills of the physical pharmacist remains strong in the pharmaceutical industry. That is why this textbook fills an important need.

Scientists entering the pharmaceutical industry today often lack the fundamental knowledge that is reflected in the chapters contained in this book. Many of the researchers entering industry have backgrounds in chemical engineering or organic chemistry. Their exposure to the principles of physical pharmacy is a deficit that must be overcome by on-the-job training and by extensive study. It is in the areas of preformulation, the development of new and sophisticated drug delivery systems, and the day-to-day work of optimizing the effects of new drug entities that this knowledge is most needed. There are, of course, many textbooks that deal with specific subjects important to the industrial pharmacist, focusing on tablets, capsules, disperse systems, parenterals, etc. However, there is a critical need for a comprehensive treatment of the science underlying each of these special areas, together with practical applications of the science that results in quality dosage forms. Questions related to solubility, dissolution, chemical and physical stability, interfacial phenomena, and the absorption and distribution of drug molecules are common to all. Consequently, a single textbook that brings together experts in all of these subjects can be an invaluable asset to the novice industrial scientist. Each chapter in this book contains a useful bibliography of references that can provide for ready access to current research in the field. We should be grateful that these authors have taken time from their busy schedules to share their knowledge and experience with all of us.

J. Keith Guillory, Ph.D.
Professor Emeritus
University of Iowa

THEORIES AND TECHNIQUES IN THE CHARACTERIZATION OF DRUG SUBSTANCES AND EXCIPIENTS

Solubility of Pharmaceutical Solids

Venkatramana M. Rao, Ritesh Sanghvi and Haijian (Jim) Zhu

1.1 INTRODUCTION

1.1.1 Implication of Solubility in Dosage Form Development

The solubility of a drug is one of its most important physico-chemical properties. The determination of drug solubility and ways to alter it, if necessary, are essential components of pharmaceutical development programs. The bioavailability of an orally administered drug depends primarily on its solubility in the gastrointestinal tract and its permeability across cell membranes. This forms the basis for the biopharmaceutical classification system (BCS).[1] Drug molecules are required to be present in a dissolved form, in order for them to be transported across biological membranes. Therefore, low aqueous solubility can either delay or limit drug absorption. Knowledge of the solubility of a drug is also important when direct administration into the blood stream is desired. Injectable formulations usually require a drug to be in solution for administration. In addition, a drug solution is preferred for conducting pharmacological, toxicological, and pharmacokinetic studies during the drug development stage. Thus, poor aqueous solubility not only limits a drug's biological application, but also challenges its pharmaceutical development. As a result, investigation into approaches for

solubility enhancement has been a regular feature of pharmaceutical research for several decades. The need for such approaches has been on a rise following the introduction of combinatorial chemistry and high throughput screening techniques to the drug discovery arena. The advent of these techniques, resulting in a rapid development of libraries of pharmaceutically active compounds, has led to a greater number of highly active compounds. At the same time, it has resulted in generation of a far higher percentage of extremely lipophilic and poorly water-soluble compounds adding more challenges to formulation development. It has been reported[2] that more than a third of the compounds registered by Pfizer in the late 1990s had solubilities that were lower than $5 \mu g/ml$.

While solubility enhancement remains one of the primary areas of focus during the drug development phase, there are several situations that may require solubility reduction. Development of sustained release products, taste masking, and enhancement of chemical stability are examples of such situations.

Knowledge of solubility also finds application in developing analytical methods for drugs. Reverse phase liquid chromatography is one of the most widely used techniques for pharmaceutical separation and analysis. Separation is based on the differential affinity of the solute towards the mobile phase and the stationary phase, which is a direct outcome of its solubility in these phases. The analysis of concentration using UV spectroscopy is also performed on drug solutions.

Based on the above discussion, it should be clear that solubility plays an important role in several avenues of pharmaceutical research. As a consequence, the determination of solubility remains one of the most commonly conducted experiments for any new compounds. While solubility experiments are sometimes perceived as trivial, accurate determination of solubility is a challenging exercise. A number of experimental variables may affect the solubility results, inducing high degrees of scatter in the data.[3] This builds a strong case for the applicability of tools for estimation of solubility based on theoretical calculations. While most of these calculation approaches are useful with respect to providing reasonable estimation and time saving, they can never completely replace the experimentally determined values.

This chapter is written with the intent of developing a thorough understanding of the concepts of solubility. The various physico-chemical forces and factors that determine the solubility of a solute in a solvent will be discussed in detail. The thermodynamics of solubilization and various theoretical models for its estimation have also been included. Considerable emphasis has been laid on the techniques used for solubility enhancement along with practically relevant examples. In addition, the various aspects of solubility determination experiments including challenges and strategies to overcome them are discussed.

1.1.2 Basic Concepts of Solubility and Dissolution

A true solution is a homogenous mixture of two or more components on a molecular level. Any sample collected from such a mixture will be representative of the entire bulk. In a two-component system, the component present in larger proportion is generally referred as the solvent, and the other as the solute.

When a solute is placed in contact with a solvent, mixing occurs due to the propensity of all molecules towards randomization, resulting in an increase in overall entropy of the system. The solute molecules start to break away from the surface and pass into the solvent system. The detached solute molecules are free to move randomly throughout the solvent bulk forming a uniform solution. Some of these solute molecules strike the bulk solute surface and redeposit on it. Initially, when the concentration of solute molecules is low in the solution, the number of molecules leaving the bulk solute surface is much higher. As the solvent bulk starts becoming saturated with the solute

molecules, the redeposition process starts to accelerate. Once sufficient solute molecules have populated the solvent bulk, the rate of molecules leaving becomes equal to the rate of redeposition (dynamic equilibrium). The concentration of the solute in the solvent at which this equilibrium is reached is defined as the thermodynamic solubility. The rate at which the equilibrium is achieved is the dissolution rate. Thus, solubility is an equilibrium concept, while dissolution is a kinetic phenomenon. Both are dependent on the experimental conditions, including temperature. The dissolution rate of a solute in a solvent is directly proportional to its solubility, as described by the Noyes–Whitney equation:[4,5]

$$\text{Dissolution rate} = \frac{dM}{dt} = \frac{DA}{h}(C_s - C_t) \quad (1.1)$$

where:
dM/dt is the rate of mass transfer
D is the diffusion coefficient (cm^2/sec)
A is the surface area of the drug (cm^2)
h is the static boundary layer (cm)
C_s is the saturation solubility of the drug
C_t is the concentration of the drug at time (t).

Solubility is expressed in units of concentration including percentage on a weight or volume basis, mole fraction, molarity, molality, parts, etc. The US Pharmacopeia and National Formulary describe solubility as the number of milliliters of solvent required to dissolve 1 gram of the solute.

It follows from the previous discussion that the equilibrium solubility of a solute will depend on its relative affinities towards solvent molecules and fellow solute molecules. Thus, the strength of molecular interactions, both inter and intra, affect solubility. While a detailed description of these interactions can be found in any physical chemistry book, they are discussed here briefly.

Ionic Interactions

Pure ionic interactions occur between two oppositely charged ions. Such interactions are relevant to pharmaceutical salts and ion pairs. An ion can also interact with a polar molecule (ion–dipole) or induce a dipolar character to a non-polar molecule (ion-induced dipole). When sodium chloride is dissolved in water, the free sodium and chloride ions interact with polar water molecules such that the positive head of water molecules interact with the chloride ions, while the negative head of water molecules interact with the sodium ions. By virtue of these interactions, pharmaceutical salts generally have a higher solubility than their free form. The strength of ionic interactions depends on the electrostatic charge density on the interacting ions, as well as the media properties, including dielectric constant and temperature.

van der Waals Interactions

Two molecules with permanent dipole moments can interact, when placed in sufficiently close proximity (dipole–dipole or Keesom interaction). The molecules will try to arrange in a manner to minimize the energy associated with them. Thus, the positive head of one molecule will position close to the negative head of the other molecule. The positioning, however, may not be ideal due to geometric constraints and random thermal motion of the participating molecules (entropic influence). As a consequence a situation arises where the participating molecules, on average, spend more time in an aligned position. Strongly polar molecules can induce polar attributes to non-polar molecules to result in dipole-induced dipole (Debye) interactions. The strength of van der Waals interactions is a direct outcome of the dipole moment and polarizability of the participating molecules, and is also affected by the media properties such as temperature.

Dispersion Interactions

Also known as London forces, dispersion interactions occur between any adjacent pair of atoms or molecules when they are present in sufficiently close proximity. These interactions account for the attractive forces between non-ionic and non-polar organic molecules, such as paraffin and many pharmaceutical drugs. The origin of these forces remains unclear, but it is believed that at any given instance molecules are present in a variety of distinct positions due to thermal oscillations. These positions give rise to a temporary molecular dissymmetry resulting in a dipole-type characteristic. This instantaneous dipole then induces polar character to the neighboring molecules and starts interacting with them.

Hydrogen Bonding

These interactions occur between hydrogen bond donating groups and strong electronegative atoms such as halogens, oxygen, and nitrogen. Hydrogen atoms become associated with electronegative atoms by virtue of electrostatics, and result in the formation of hydrogen bridges. These interactions are prevalent in aqueous and alcoholic systems. A large number of drugs are involved in either inter- or intra-molecular hydrogen bonding. The aqueous solubility of a drug is directly related to its hydrogen bonding capability. The higher water solubility of phenol, as compared to benzene and toluene, can be attributed to the former's hydrogen bonding nature. The evolving field of cocrystals is based on the hydrogen bond interactions between molecules of drug and the cocrystal former. The strength of hydrogen bond interactions depends upon the electronegativity of the participating atoms, as well as the temperature of the media. Since the requirement of ideal positioning is highest for hydrogen bonding interactions, they are more sensitive to temperature than other interactions.

1.2 THERMODYNAMICS OF SOLUTIONS

In order to grasp the concepts of solubility, it is essential to understand the basic thermodynamics of mixing. This section covers the various thermodynamic aspects that dictate the process of mixing.

1.2.1 Volume of Mixing

The volume of mixing, ΔV_{mix}, is the difference between the physical volume occupied by the mixture (V_{uv}) and the sum of physical volumes occupied by the solute (V_u) and solvent (V_v):

$$\Delta V_{mix} = V_{uv} - (V_u + V_v) \tag{1.2}$$

A negative volume of mixing is indicative of strong inter-molecular interactions between the solute and solvent molecules. Aqueous solutions of strong electrolytes have significantly large negative volumes of mixing, due to strong hydration of ions in the solution.[3] In the case of most pharmaceutically active compounds the volume of mixing is small and can be ignored.

1.2.2 Enthalpy of Mixing

The enthalpy of mixing, (ΔH_{mix}), is the difference between the sum of enthalpies of the solute (H_u), the solvent (H_v), and of the mixture, (H_{uv}):

$$\Delta H_{mix} = H_{uv} - (H_u + H_v) \tag{1.3}$$

From a strictly enthalpic standpoint, mixing is favored if ΔH_{mix} is negative. The excess enthalpy is liberated in the form of heat (exothermic process).

The energy of mixing (ΔE_{mix}) is related to the enthalpy of mixing as:

$$\Delta E_{mix} = \Delta H_{mix} - P \cdot \Delta V_{mix} \tag{1.4}$$

As previously mentioned, ΔV_{mix} is small, and therefore the values of ΔE_{mix} and ΔH_{mix} are close to one another.

1.2.3 Entropy of Mixing

The entropy of a pure system is a measure of the randomness of its molecules. Mathematically:

$$S = R \ln \Omega \tag{1.5}$$

where:

Ω is the number of ways molecules can be present in the system.

Since Ω is always equal to or greater than unity, entropy is either zero or positive. The entropy of a mixture, (ΔS_{mix}), is related to the number of ways the solute and solvent molecules can exist in pure forms, and in mixture:

$$\Delta S_{mix} = R \ln \left(\frac{\Omega_{mix}}{\Omega_u + \Omega_v} \right) \tag{1.6}$$

Generally, the molecules have more freedom to move around in a mixture, i.e., Ω_{mix} is greater than $\Omega_u + \Omega_v$. As a consequence ΔS_{mix} is usually positive. However, in rare situations where the molecules have less freedom in the mixture (solute molecules undergoing complexation-like interactions with solvent molecules),[6,7] ΔS_{mix} can be negative.

The entropy of mixing is related to the composition of the solution as:

$$\Delta S_{mix} = -R(X_u \ln X_u + X_v \ln X_v) \tag{1.7}$$

where:

X_u and X_v are the mole fractions of the solute and solvent, respectively, in the mixture.

In a two component system $X_v = 1 - X_u$; ΔS_{mix} can be written as:

$$\Delta S_{mix} = -R\left[X_u \ln X_u + (1 - X_u)\ln(1 - X_u) \right] \tag{1.8}$$

$$\Delta S_{mix} = -R\left[X_v \ln X_v + (1 - X_v)\ln(1 - X_v) \right] \tag{1.9}$$

It follows from Equation 1.7 that ΔS_{mix} will be highest for solutions containing equimolar amounts of solute and solvent molecules.

The slope of entropy of mixing as a function of solution composition is given by:

$$\begin{aligned}
\frac{\partial \Delta S_{mix}}{\partial X_u} &= -R \ln X_u + R \ln(1 - X_u) \\
&= -R \ln X_v + R \ln(1 - X_v)
\end{aligned} \tag{1.10}$$

It follows from Equation 1.10 that the slope will be highest in dilute solutions (when either X_u or X_v is small). Thus, the manifestation of entropy is highest in dilute solution, which explains why thermodynamically there is some miscibility between all systems.

1.2.4 Free Energy of Mixing

The free energy of mixing, ΔG_{mix}, determines the possibility and extent of two compounds mixing to form a solution. It combines the effects of enthalpy and entropy on mixing and is mathematically described as:

$$\Delta G_{mix} = \Delta H_{mix} - T \cdot \Delta S_{mix} \tag{1.11}$$

where:

T is the temperature in °Kelvin.

Like any thermodynamic process, mixing will occur if the free energy of mixing is negative. On the other hand, if the free energy of mixing is greater than zero there will be phase-separation. As mentioned in the previous section, solubility depends on the temperature of the system. It follows from Equation 1.11 that an increase in temperature will increase the effect of entropy, thus making mixing more favored. In addition, temperature may also affect ΔH_{mix}, particularly for hydrogen-bonded solvents such as water. It is well known that the strength of hydrogen bonding interactions is very sensitive to temperature. An increase in temperature makes the self-associated structure of water weaker. Since the self-associated structure of water is primarily responsible for poor aqueous solubility of non-polar solutes, including drugs, increasing the temperature thereby facilitates their solubility.

1.3 THEORETICAL ESTIMATION OF SOLUBILITY

While solutions of all states of matter (gas, liquid, and solid) exist in practice, the focus of this chapter will be on solutions comprising of liquid solvent, since these systems are most commonly encountered and have highest relevance in the pharmaceutical field. The backbone of the concepts discussed here may be applied to other systems, with some modifications.

1.3.1 Ideal Solutions

In an ideal solution the strength and density of interactions between the solute molecules and the solvent molecules are equal to that in the solution. In other words, the solute–solvent interactions are equal in magnitude to the solute–solute interactions and solvent–solvent interactions. Thus, the solute and solvent molecules have no preference in terms of interacting with other molecules present in the solutions. This results in the enthalpy (ΔH_{mix}^{ideal}) and volume of mixing (ΔV_{mix}^{ideal}) being 0. Such solutions rarely exist in practicality, but understanding the concept of ideal mixing provides a good platform to understand more complex systems. A solution comprising of solute and solvent bearing very close structural resemblance (in terms of functionality and size) may make nearly ideal solutions. A solution of water in heavy water nearly fits the description of an ideal solution.

The entropy of mixing of an ideal solution (ΔS_{mix}^{ideal}) is given by Equation 1.7. The partial molar entropy of mixing of the solute in a dilute solution is given by:

$$\Delta S_{mix}^{ideal}(u) = -R \ln X_u \qquad (1.12)$$

Since X_u is always less than 1, ΔS_{mix}^{ideal} is positive. The free energy of mixing for an ideal solution (ΔG_{mix}^{ideal}), which is the difference between the enthalpy and entropy of mixing, will therefore always be negative. Thus, in ideal solutions, a liquid solute will be miscible with the solvent in all proportions.

$$\Delta G_{mix}^{ideal}(u) = TR \ln X_u \qquad (1.13)$$

1.3.2 Effect of Crystallinity

In the case of an ideal solution of a crystalline solute, more considerations are required. As discussed above, the solute molecules have no preference in terms of interacting with other molecules in the solution. However, if the solute exists as a crystalline solid, the enthalpic component related to the crystallinity of the solute also warrants consideration. In other words, the liquid solute molecules are free to move around in the solution while the crystalline solute molecules have to be removed from the crystal lattice before they can start moving around. Mathematically, this can be stated as:

$$X_{solid}^{ideal}(u) = X_{liquid}^{ideal}(u) - Effect\ of\ Crystallinity \qquad (1.14)$$

The process is conceptually similar to melting of a solid, which is followed by dissolution of the liquid solute molecules, and is governed by the same interactions as melting.

The effect of crystallinity of a solid on its solubility is described by the Clausius–Clapyron equation:

$$R\ln X_u^{ideal} = \int_{T_m}^{T} \frac{-\Delta H_m^{(at\ T)}}{T^2} dT \qquad (1.15)$$

X_u^{ideal} represents the ideal solubility of the crystal and the effect of crystallinity on the solubility.

According to Kirchoff's law, the energy of an irreversible process is equal to the energy of a series of reversible processes between the same end points. Therefore, the irreversible enthalpy of melting at any temperature $T(\Delta H_m^T)$ can be described as the sum of the enthalpies for the following three reversible processes: heating the solid to its melting point, T_m (quantified by the heat capacity of the solid); melting the solid at its melting point (enthalpy of fusion); and cooling the liquid back down to T (quantified by the heat capacity of the liquid). The heat of melting at T, can thus be related to its value at the melting point as:

$$\Delta H_m^T = \Delta H_m^{Tm} + C_p^C(T_m - T) - C_p^L(T_m - T) \qquad (1.16)$$

C_p^C and C_p^L are the heat capacities of the crystal and liquid form, respectively.

Combining Equations 1.15 and 1.16, the effect of crystallinity can be calculated to be:

$$R\ln X_u^{ideal} = -\Delta H_m \frac{(T_m - T)}{T_m T} + \Delta C p_m \left[\frac{T_m - T}{T} - \ln \frac{T_m}{T} \right] \qquad (1.17)$$

where:

$\Delta C p_m$ is the heat capacity of melting.

According to the van't Hoff expression, the heat capacity of melting is close to zero. The Hildebrand[8] expression states that the heat capacity of melting is equal to the entropy of melting ($\Delta H_m / T_m$). This expression has been used by several workers including Prausnitz et al.,[9] Grant et al.,[10] and Mishra.[11] Later, Mishra and Yalkowsky[12] compared the mathematical significance of the two expressions and concluded that the results using either expression are close for solids melting below 600°K. Thus, Equation 1.17 can be simplified to the following form:

$$\log_{10}\left(X_u^{ideal}\right) = -\Delta H_m \frac{(T_m - T)}{2.303 R T_m T} \qquad (1.18)$$

Equation 1.18 may be further simplified by applying Walden's rule for entropy of melting. Walden[13] showed that the entropy of melting of coal tar derivatives, which can be assumed to represent organic solids like drugs, is constant at approximately 6.9R. Martin et al.,[14] Dannenfelser et al.,[15] and Jain et al.[16]

have successfully verified and extended the applicability of Walden's rule to several organic nonelectrolytes. Applying this approximation the effect of crystallinity on the solubility of crystalline solute at 25°C can be calculated by:

$$\log_{10}\left(X_u^{crystalline}\right) \approx -0.01(MP-25) \qquad (1.19)$$

where:

MP is the melting point of the solute expressed in °C.

The obvious interpretation of Equation 1.19 is that the effect of crystallinity will be greater for high melting solutes. It is intuitive that a high melting crystalline solid will offer greater resistance towards solubilization. It also follows that an increase in temperature will diminish the effect of crystallinity and therefore, result in increased solubility.

For liquid solutes, where there is a complete absence of crystallinity, Equation 1.19 should be omitted while calculating the solubility. The effect of crystallinity on solubility can be easily followed by referring to Figure 1.1.

1.3.3 Non-ideal Solutions

Nearly all solutions encountered in the pharmaceutical arena are not ideal. Non-ideal solutions or real solutions are formed when the affinity of solute molecules for each other is different than that towards the solvent molecules or *vice versa*. In either case, the enthalpy of mixing is not ideal. This results in a deviation from ideality that is related to the activity coefficient of the solute. The activity of a solute in a solution is equal to the product of its concentration and activity coefficient as:

$$\alpha_u = X_u \cdot \gamma_u \qquad (1.20)$$

where:

γ_u is the activity coefficient of the solute.

The mole fraction solubility of a crystalline solute in a non-ideal solution can be calculated by combining Equations 1.19 and 1.20:

$$\log_{10}\left(X_u^{real}\right) = -0.01(MP-25) - \log\gamma_u \qquad (1.21)$$

In the case of ideal solutions, γ_u is 1 and the solubility is ideal.

The mathematical meaning of γ_u is derived using various theories depending upon the type of solute and solvent molecules. Two of the most commonly accepted theories are regular solution theory and aqueous solution theory.

1.3.4 Regular Solution Theory

This theory is applicable largely to non-hydrogen bonding systems. According to the theory, γ_u is a function of following three steps in which mixing occurs:

1. Removal of a solute molecule from the solute surface. This involves breaking of solute–solute bonds, and the work required to accomplish this is given by W_{uu}.

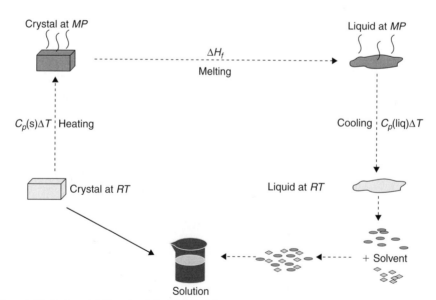

FIGURE 1.1   Role of crystallinity in solubility of solids. Modified from a presentation by Dr Kenneth Morris (Short Course on Solubility and Solubilization of Drugs, 2007)

2. Removal of a solvent molecule from bulk to create a cavity in which the solute molecule can fit. This involves breaking of solvent–solvent bonds and the work required for this is given by W_{vv}.

3. Insertion of the free solute molecule in the created cavity. This results in gain of work, which is given by W_{uv}. The cavity filling involves surfaces of both solute and solvent molecules, and that is why the total work gained is $2W_{uv}$.

The total work is therefore equal to $(W_{uu} + W_{vv} - 2W_{uv})$. The activity coefficient of a solute is related to this work by the following relationship:

$$\log_{10}(\gamma_u) = (W_{uu} + W_{vv} - 2W_{uv}) \cdot \frac{V_u \Phi_v^2}{2.303RT} \quad (1.22)$$

where:

V_u is the molar volume of the solute
Φ_v is the volume fraction of the solvent.

It is assumed that W_{uv} is the geometric mean of W_{uu} and W_{vv}. Upon applying this assumption, Equation 1.22 transforms to:

$$\log_{10}(\gamma_u) = \left(W_{uu} + W_{vv} - 2\sqrt{W_{uu} \cdot W_{vv}}\right) \cdot \frac{V_u \Phi_v^2}{2.303RT}$$

$$(1.23)$$

Equation 1.23 may be rewritten in the following form:

$$\log_{10}(\gamma_u) = \left(\sqrt{W_{uu}} - \sqrt{W_{vv}}\right)^2 \cdot \frac{V_u \Phi_v^2}{2.303RT} \quad (1.24)$$

The terms $\sqrt{W_{uu}}$ and $\sqrt{W_{vv}}$ are known as the solubility parameters of the solute (δ_u) and solvent (δ_v), respectively. Thus, Equation 1.24 becomes:

$$\log_{10}(\gamma_u) = (\delta_u - \delta_v)^2 \cdot \frac{V_u \Phi_v^2}{2.303RT} \quad (1.25)$$

The solubility parameter is a measure of the cohesive energy density (also referred as internal pressure) of a compound:

$$\delta = \sqrt{\frac{\Delta E_v}{V_m}} \quad (1.26)$$

ΔE_v and V_m are the enthalpy of vaporization and molar volume, respectively.

The solubility parameter is a measure of intermolecular interactions of a compound and can be used as a measure of polarity. Hildebrand and Scott[17] compiled solubility parameters for a number of compounds, and so did Hansen and Beerbower.[18] Hansen further extended the concept by ascribing contributions of the non-polar, polar, and hydrogen-bonding components of a molecule to the total solubility parameter.

Fedor[19] has proposed a scheme to estimate solubility parameters of liquid organic compounds based on a group contribution approach. Similarly, Sanghvi and Yalkowsky[20] have proposed a group contribution scheme to estimate the enthalpy of vaporization of organic compounds.

Equations 1.21 and 1.27 can be combined to calculate the solubility of a crystalline solute according to the regular solution theory:

$$\log_{10}\left(X_u^{regular}\right) = -0.01(MP - 25)$$

$$- (\delta_u - \delta_v)^2 \cdot \frac{V_u \Phi_v^2}{2.303RT} \quad (1.27)$$

It follows from Equation 1.27 that the solubility of a solute is a function of the difference in the cohesive energy densities of the solute and solvent. Thus, a liquid solute (no crystal term) with a molar volume of 100 ml will be completely miscible in a solvent if their solubility parameter difference is less than $7(J/cm^3)^{0.5}$.

The regular solution theory has been applied by several groups to successfully estimate the solubility of organic compounds in non-polar solvents. It appears that the geometric mean assumption does not seem to hold well for strongly hydrogen-bonded systems, limiting the applicability of the regular solution theory mainly to organic media. Martin et al.[21] proposed a correction factor to cater for the hydrogen-bonding interactions of the solvent. Similarly, the extended Hildebrand solubility approach[22] utilized an extra activity coefficient term to account for strong forces, including hydrogen bonding.

1.3.5 Aqueous Solution Theory

As discussed in the previous section, the regular solution theory is not applicable to hydrogen-bonding systems like water, since the geometric mean assumption is not valid in such systems. Yalkowsky et al.,[23,24,25] and later Amidon and Yalkowsky,[26] proposed that instead of using pressure–volume work to account for enthalpy of mixing, surface tension–area work should be considered. This theory is based on the concept that only the surface of the solute molecule is capable of interacting with solvent molecules. Thus, using surface area instead of volume work is more meaningful. The following equation was proposed to calculate the energy requirement for solubilization in an aqueous system:

$$\Delta E_u^{aqueous} = \Delta H_u^{aqueous} = (\gamma_w + \gamma_u - \gamma_{uw})A_u$$

$$= \sum \gamma_{uw}A_u \quad (1.28)$$

where:

γ_u and γ_w are the surface tensions of the pure solute and water, respectively

γ_{uw} is the solute–solvent interfacial tension

A_u is the surface area of the solute.

The entropy of mixing of aqueous systems is also non-ideal. The water molecules cluster around an organic solute to form a so-called "iceberg-like" structure. The aqueous solution theory accounts for this deviation by introducing a correction factor in the entropy term:

$$\Delta S_u^{aqueous} = \Delta S_u^{ideal} + \sum h_i A_u \qquad (1.29)$$

h_i is the contribution of the entropy of mixing per unit area due to "iceberg" formation at the molecular surface.

The free energy of mixing of aqueous solution is calculated using Equations 1.28 and 1.29:

$$\Delta G_u^{aqueous} = \sum \gamma_{uw} A_u - T\left(\sum h_i A_u + \Delta S_u^{ideal}\right) \quad (1.30)$$

This can be written as:

$$\begin{aligned} \Delta G_u^{aqueous} = \sum \gamma_{uw} A_u - T \sum h_i A_u \\ + T(RX_u \ln X_u + X_v \ln X_v) \end{aligned} \quad (1.31)$$

or:

$$\Delta G_u^{aqueous} = \sum g_u A_u + T(RX_u \ln X_u + X_v \ln X_v) \quad (1.32)$$

$g_u = -\gamma_{iw} A_i - T(h_i A_i)$ is the group contribution to the activity coefficient which caters to both the enthalpic and the entropic deviations to ideality.

The solubility of a crystalline solute in a hydrogen-bonding solvent can be calculated by combining Equations 1.21 and 1.32:

$$\log_{10}\left(X_u^{aqueous}\right) = -0.01(MP - 25) - \sum g_u A_u \quad (1.33)$$

Myrdal et al.[27,28,29,30] have developed a robust group contribution scheme, called the AQUAFAC approach, for estimation of the aqueous activity coefficient of organic compounds. Their work successfully demonstrates the applicability of aqueous solution theory.

1.3.6 The General Solubility Equation (GSE)

The general solubility equation utilizes the relation between the octanol–water partition coefficient of a solute and its water solubility, first proposed by Hansch et al.:[31]

$$\log_{10}(S_w) = -A \log_{10}(K_{ow}) + B \qquad (1.34)$$

K_{ow} is the octanol–water partition coefficient of a liquid solute, while A and B are solute specific constants.

The octanol–water partition coefficient is the ratio of the activities of the solute in octanol (a_o) and that in water (a_w). For dilute solutions where the activity coefficient is close to unity, K_{ow} can be approximated as:

$$K_{ow} = \frac{S_o}{S_w} \qquad (1.35)$$

S_o and S_w are the solubilities of the liquid solute in octanol and water, respectively.

$$\log_{10}(S_w) = \log_{10}(S_o) - \log_{10}(K_{ow}) \qquad (1.36)$$

Jain and Yalkowsky[32] proposed that $\log_{10}S_o$ can be replaced by 0.5 for solutes that are completely miscible with octanol. The explanation they provided is as follows.

The concentration of pure octanol is 6.3 molar. The saturated solution of a completely miscible solute of similar molar volume as octanol will contain 3.15 moles of the solute. Since the logarithm of 3.15 is about 0.5, Equation 1.36 can be modified in the following form to give the molar aqueous solubility of a liquid solute:

$$\log_{10}(S_w) = 0.5 - \log_{10}(K_{ow}) \qquad (1.37)$$

It has been discussed previously that, according to the regular solution theory, the miscibility of a solute with a solvent depends on the difference in their solubility parameters and molar volumes. Sepassi and Yalkowsky[33] have shown that in the case of octanol (solubility parameter of 21.1 $(J/cm^3)^{0.5}$ and molar volume of $158\,cm^3$), a liquid solute of molar volume $200\,cm^3$ will be completely miscible if its solubility parameter is between 15.2 and 27 $(J/cm^3)^{0.5}$. Since the solubility parameters of most drugs are in this range, their liquid forms are expected to be completely miscible in octanol.

Consistent with previous discussions, solute crystallinity should be to be taken into consideration while calculating the solubility of a crystalline solute. Thus, the solubility of a crystalline solute can be estimated using GSE by combining Equations 1.19 and 1.37:

$$\log_{10}(S_w) = 0.5 - \log_{10}(K_{ow}) - 0.01(MP - 0.5) \quad (1.38)$$

The GSE provides a very simple means of estimating aqueous solubility. Unlike the regular solution theory and aqueous solution theories, which require a number of empirically generated coefficients, GSE requires only two input parameters (melting point and octanol–water partition coefficient). The measurement of both the parameters is a routine part of the API characterization process. The value of $\log_{10}K_{ow}$ can also be estimated from the chemical structure by using one of several commercially available software packages (e.g., ClogP®, ACDlogPdB®, KowWin®). Machatha and Yalkowsky[34] compared these estimation schemes and concluded that ClogP® was the most accurate predictor of $\log_{10}K_{ow}$.

A variety of schemes for the prediction of melting points of organic compounds have been proposed. These have been reviewed by Katritzky et al.,[35] Dearden,[36] and Bergstrom et al.,[37] among others. Recently, Jain and Yalkowsky[38] have proposed a reasonably accurate group contribution scheme for melting point estimation using experimental data for over 2200 organic compounds, including a number of drugs.

The accuracy of GSE has been sufficiently demonstrated for several hundred non-ionizable organic compounds.[39,40,41,42] Recently,[43] the application of GSE has been extended to weak ionizable compounds by combining it with the Henderson–Hasselbalch equation.

Notice that, in Equations 1.37 and 1.38, the solubility is expressed in moles per liter. The constant (0.5) will change to 2.7 ($\log_{10}500$) if the solubility is expressed in grams per liter.

Besides the regular solution theory and aqueous solution theory, several other schemes have been proposed for the estimation of solubility. These have been reviewed extensively by Dearden,[44] and Jorgensen and Duffy.[45] Abraham and Li[46] have developed a model for estimating solubility based on specific solute–solvent interactions. The parameters used in the model include excess molar refraction, dipolarity, polarizability, hydrogen-bond acidity and basicity, and molecular volume of the solute. In addition, hydrogen-bonding terms are included to sophisticate the model. This model is very intuitive and simple to follow. However, the coefficients involved with each parameter have to be determined experimentally, and therefore using the model for drug molecules can be very cumbersome. Taskinen and Yliruusi[47] have compiled the various prediction schemes based on a neural network approach.

1.4 SOLUBILIZATION OF DRUG CANDIDATES

Solubility of drug candidates can be altered by modifying the crystal form or by changing solvent properties and conditions. As discussed in the previous sections, the equilibrium solubility is dependent on the properties and nature of interactions in solid state, as well as in solution state.

Polymorphs are two crystals that have the same chemical composition, but different arrangement of molecules or crystal packing. These differences in crystal packing may lead to differences in physico-chemical properties, including solubility. Solubility can also be altered by altering the chemical composition, as seen with salt formation, cocrystals or solid complexes. Another means of improving "apparent" solubility is by converting the crystalline drug into an amorphous state. In the solution state, solubility can be influenced by altering solution pH (for ionizable drugs) or use of additives such as complexing agents, surfactants, or cosolvents. Drug solubilization by pH control/salt formation, complexation/cocrystal formation, micellar solubilization by surfactants, and cosolvency will be discussed in the next sections. The remaining techniques are beyond the scope of this chapter.

1.4.1 Solubility Enhancement by pH Control and Salt Formation

A significant portion of drug candidates are weak acids, bases, and their salts.[48,49] As will be shown in the following sections, solubility of these compounds is dependent on the pH of the aqueous medium and the electrolytes in solution. The ionization equilibria and the intrinsic solubility of various unionized (free form) and ionized species (salt forms) determine the nature of dependency of drug solubility on pH.

Theoretical Expressions to Describe pH–Solubility Profiles

The pH–solubility profile of a monoprotic acid (HA) is obtained by superposition of the two distinct pH–solubility curves for the free form and the salt, with the constraint that the solubility of either species cannot be exceeded at a given pH (Figure 1.2). This profile is obtained by following the solubility of free acid (HA) in solutions containing different amounts of a base, e.g., MOH.

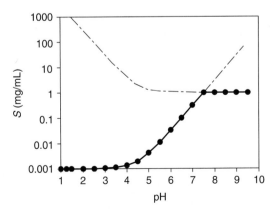

FIGURE 1.2 pH-solubility of free acid or its salt

The profile can be divided into two regions:[49] in Region I, the free acid is present as the excess solid in equilibrium with the solution. The total solubility is the sum of concentrations of unionized (free acid) and the dissociated form.

$$S_T = C_{HA} + C_{A^-} \qquad (1.39)$$

At equilibrium (saturation), the concentration of the free acid, C_{HA}, is equal to its intrinsic solubility (S_{HA}). The concentration of the dissociated form, C_{A^-}, is dependent on the free acid concentration, acid ionization constant, and pH.

$$C_{A^-} = C_{HA} \frac{K_a}{[H^+]} \qquad (1.40)$$

Thus, the total solubility of the free acid as a function of pH is given by the following equation:

$$S_T = C_{HA} + C_{A^-} = S_{HA} \cdot \left(1 + \frac{K_a}{[H^+]}\right) \qquad (1.41)$$

$$S_T = S_{HA} \cdot \left(1 + 10^{(pH - pK_a)}\right) \qquad (1.42)$$

In Region I, as the pH increases beyond the pK_a of the solute, the concentration of the ionized form increases, leading to an increase in the total solubility in an exponential fashion. This exponential increase in solubility occurs until a point (pH_{max}) where the maximum salt solubility is reached, and Region II of the pH–solubility profile begins. In Region II, the salt form is the excess solid in equilibrium with the solution. At equilibrium (saturation), the concentration of the dissociated form (salt), C_{A^-}, is equal to its intrinsic solubility (S_{A^-}). The concentration of the unionized form, C_{HA}, is defined by the ionization equilibrium and is dependent on the ionized form concentration (S_{A^-}) and the acid ionization constant, K_a.

$$S_T = C_{HA} + C_{A^-} = S_{A^-} \cdot \left(1 + \frac{[H^+]}{K_a}\right) \qquad (1.43)$$

The solubility of the salt, S_{A^-}, is dependent on the solubility product of the salt, K_{sp}, and the counterion concentration, M^+.

$$K_{sp} = S_{A^-} \cdot [M^+] \qquad (1.44)$$

In Region II of Figure 1.2 the solubility is constant, but this may not be the case when excess counterions (more than stoichiometric amounts) are present in solution as this will lead to suppression of the salt solubility (Equation 1.44). If the counterion M^+ is generated by a weak base, additional ionization equilibria between the charged and uncharged counterion need to be included in Equation 1.44. The ability of *in situ* salt formation would thus depend on the pK_a of the acid and pK_a of the conjugate acid of the base.

The above equations are expressed in terms of concentration, with the assumption that the activity coefficient for all the species is 1.0. This assumption may be reasonable for neutral species, but for charged species in solutions at high ionic strength, the activity coefficients are lower than 1.0. Therefore, assumption of activity coefficients being unity should be verified.[50] The expressions generated above are valid regardless of whether the excess solid that is added at the beginning of the experiment is free acid or salt form. The solubility at any given pH is therefore governed by pH, the intrinsic solubility of the free acid, the solubility product of the salt, and the concentration of the common ions. The various ionization and solid/liquid equilibria during solubilization of weak acid are shown in Scheme 1.1. It is imperative that the solid phase be analyzed after equilibration during solubility experiments, as the solid phase exists either as the free acid (AH) or its salt (A^-M^+), except at pH_{max}.

By analogy, the pH–solubility profile of a monobasic compound and its salt can be described by the following three equations:

In Region I, when pH > pH_{max}:

$$S_T = S_B \cdot (1 + 10^{(pK_a - pH)}) \qquad (1.45)$$

In Region II, when pH < pH_{max}:

$$S_T = S_{BH^+} \cdot (1 + 10^{(pH - pK_a)}) \qquad (1.46)$$

$$K_{sp} = S_{BH^+} \cdot [X^-] \qquad (1.47)$$

Figure 1.3 shows the pH–solubility profile of a freebase obtained by titrating with two different acids, HY and HX. The solubility curves generated in the two experiments (with different acids) show a similar exponential increase in solubility with pH in Region I (freebase is the solid phase). The solubility increases as the pH is lowered until pH_{max}, where the solubility product of the individual salt is limiting.

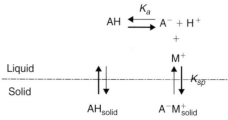

SCHEME 1.1 Ionization and solid–liquid equilibria. Drawn based on References 49, 51

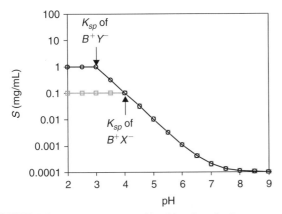

FIGURE 1.3 pH-solubility profile of free base in the presence of acids HX or HY

At equilibrium, at all the pH values (except at pH_{max}) only one solid phase (free base or salt) exists, irrespective of the nature of the starting solid material.[52] Therefore, it is important to confirm the identity of the form of the solid phase during solubility experiments. The ratio of the salt solubility and free form solubility drives the location of pH_{max}, which in turn defines the form of the solid phase at equilibrium. The location of pH_{max} is important, as it provides an indication of the relative physical stability of the free form versus salt forms in aqueous media and formulations. For example, it may be possible to make a salt of a very weak base (e.g., $pK_a \sim 2$–3), but when exposed to aqueous conditions in the pH range 1.0–9.0 that are relevant to physiology or formulations, the salt will likely be disproportionate to the free base. A thorough understanding of the pH–solubility profile of ionizable drugs is important for successful development of an ionizable drug candidate.

The discussion in this section has focused on the monoprotic acids and monobasic compounds. However, pH-dependency for other weak electrolytes such as zwitterions,[53] dibasic,[54] and diprotic drug candidates can easily be extended by using the same principles of mass balance, ionic equilibria, and the constraint that the solubility of any one of the species cannot be exceeded at a given pH.

1.4.2 Solubilization Using Complexation

For pharmaceutical systems, complexation may be defined as reversible non-covalent interaction between m molecules of drug with n molecules of a ligand species:[55]

$$m.D + n.L \xrightleftharpoons[]{K_{m:n}} D_m L_n$$

The equilibrium constant $K_{m:n}$ is sometimes known as the complexation or binding or stability constant.

$$K_{m:n} = \frac{[D_{m:n}]}{[D]^m \cdot [L]^n} \qquad (1.48)$$

It is possible for a drug to interact with the ligand to form more than one complex, each having a different stoichiometry, and each of these complexation reactions can be defined by the stoichiometry (m:n) and the equilibrium constant ($K_{m:n}$).

In the context of solubility and solubilization, complexation can best be studied using the phase solubility methods described by Higuchi and Connors,[56] and by Repta.[55] Based on the phase solubility diagram, i.e., dependence of solubility on ligand concentration, Higuchi and Connors suggested classifying complexation phenomena/complexes into the following two categories:

1. type A phase diagrams wherein the complex is soluble and does not precipitate irrespective of the ligand concentration;
2. type B phase diagrams wherein the complex precipitates when the ligand concentration reaches a critical value.

The type A phase diagrams are further classified into A_L, A_P and A_N, whereas type B phase diagrams are classified into B_I and B_S phase diagrams. The A_N, and B_I, type of phase diagrams are neither common, nor particularly useful from a solubilization perspective.

A_L-type Phase Diagrams

As shown in Figure 1.4, A_L-type systems show a linear increase in the drug solubility, S_T, as a function of the ligand concentration, L_T. Such an increase is seen when a soluble drug–ligand complex with a stoichiometry of m:1 is formed. The total drug solubility, S_T is given by:

$$S_T = [D] + m \cdot [D_m L] = S_0 + m \cdot [D_m L] \quad (1.49)$$

By applying mass balance on the ligand concentration, and using the definition of equilibrium constant, $K_{m:1}$, the following relationship between total drug solubility and total ligand concentration can be obtained:

$$S_T = S_0 + m \cdot \left(\frac{K_{m:1} \cdot [S_0]^m}{1 + K_{m:1} \cdot [S_0]^m} \right) \cdot L_T \quad (1.50)$$

It is noteworthy that an A_L-type phase diagram alone is not sufficient to define the stoichiometry of the soluble drug–ligand complex to be 1:1. As has been shown, total drug solubility linearly increases with total ligand concentration for m:1 drug–ligand complexes.

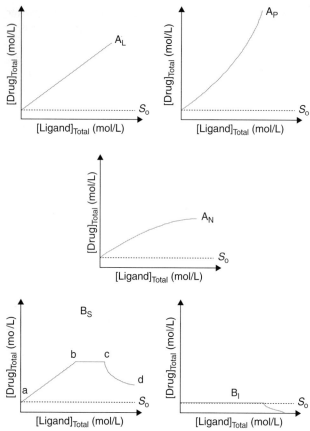

FIGURE 1.4 Drug–ligand phase solubility diagrams. Classified based on reference 56

In recent years, cyclodextrins have received considerable attention as ligands to solubilize hydrophobic drugs by forming inclusion complexes. For an inclusion complex with a stoichiometry of 1:1, the slope of the line from the A_L-type phase diagram can be used to estimate the equilibrium (binding) constant.

$$S_T = S_0 + \left(\frac{K_{1:1} \cdot S_0}{1 + K_{1:1} \cdot S_0} \right) \cdot CD_T \qquad (1.51)$$

$$K_{1:1} = \left(\frac{Slope}{(1 - Slope) \cdot S_0} \right) \qquad (1.52)$$

A_P-type Phase Diagrams

Formation of soluble complexes containing more than one molecule of ligand leads to positive deviation from linearity, and such phase diagrams are classified as A_P-type. Let us consider a drug–ligand system forming 1:1 and 1:2 complexes. The complexation equilibria can be written as follows:

$$D + L \underset{\phantom{K_{1:1}}}{\overset{K_{1:1}}{\rightleftharpoons}} DL$$

$$DL + L \underset{\phantom{K_{1:2}}}{\overset{K_{1:2}}{\rightleftharpoons}} DL$$

$$S_T = S_0 + K_{1:1} \cdot S_0 \cdot [L] + K_{1:2} \cdot K_{1:1} \cdot S_0 \cdot [L]^2 \qquad (1.53)$$

The free ligand concentration, [L] can be related to the total ligand concentration, $[L_T]$, using a mass balance equation for the ligand. Clearly, the total drug solubility will show positive deviation from linearity because, as the concentration of the ligand increases, the contribution of 1:2 complex formation increases. Dilution of drug–ligand systems forming higher-order complexes (A_P-type) may lead to precipitation of the drug, as the concentration of the drug after dilution may be higher than the solubility in the diluted solution.

B_S-type Phase Diagrams and Solid Complexes (Cocrystals)

A B_s-type phase diagram can be divided into three regions. In Region I (a–b), the drug solubility initially increases (linearly or non-linearly depending on the complex stoichiometry) with an increase in ligand concentration. Region II (b–c), representing the plateau portion, has both the complex and drug in the solid phase, and the total solubility is the sum of intrinsic solubility of the drug and that of the complex. Region III (c–d) begins when the ligand concentration becomes large enough to deplete the free drug concentration, thus decreasing the total drug solubility. At high ligand concentrations, complete removal of the free drug leading to a solid phase containing pure complex and the total drug concentration will be equal to the solubility of the complex.

Although drug–ligand solid complexes were reported in 1950s,[57,58] they have received considerable attention recently, but by a different name—cocrystals.[59,60,61] Recently, Nehl et al.[62] developed a theoretical framework for cocrystal (drug–ligand complex) phase solubility for cases where the drug and ligand form 1:1 complexes and/or 1:2 complexes.

The cocrystal solubility (drug concentration in solution with cocrystal as solid phase) can be described by the solubility product alone when the two components of the cocrystal do not interact in solution.

$$DL_{solid} \overset{K_{sp}}{\rightleftharpoons} D_{soln} + L_{soln}$$

$$K_{sp} = [D] \cdot [L] \qquad (1.54)$$

When the two components in solution also interact to form a 1:1 complex in solution, the total cocrystal solubility is dependent on the solubility product and the equilibrium (binding or complexation) constant.

$$D_{soln} + L_{soln} \underset{\longleftarrow}{\overset{K_{1:1}}{\longrightarrow}} DL_{soln}$$

$$K_{11} = \frac{[DL]}{[D] \cdot [L]} = \frac{[DL]}{K_{sp}} \quad (1.55)$$

The total solubility of the drug is given by:

$$S_T = [D]_T = [D]_{free} + [DL] = \frac{K_{sp}}{[L]} + K_{11} \cdot K_{sp} \quad (1.56)$$

The total drug solubility as a function of L_T can be modified to:

$$S_T = \frac{K_{sp}}{L_T - K_{11} \cdot K_{sp}} + K_{11} \cdot K_{sp} \quad (1.57)$$

The above equation describes the total drug solubility as a function of ligand concentration for a phase solubility system that contains pure 1:1 drug–ligand cocrystal in the solid phase, and a solution where 1:1 complex is formed. As predicted by Equation 1.57, the total solubility decreases as the ligand concentration is increased. For the case of carbamazepine/nicotinamide 1:1 cocrystal, Nehl et al.[62] showed that the total carbamazepine solubility decreased with an increase in nicotinamide concentration according to Equation 1.57. In the case where there is no interaction of the drug and ligand in solution, i.e., K_{11} is zero, the drug solubility is simply defined by the solubility product and ligand concentration in solution.

When studying the phase solubility of complexing agents, it is important to determine the nature of the solid phase along with the drug concentration in solution phase. Based on the experimentally determined solubility data, a phase diagram illustrating where drug, ligand, and cocrystal can exist or coexist in the solid phase must be constructed. Understanding the thermodynamic domains of the different forms (drug, ligand, and cocrystal) is essential in crystallization of the desired cocrystal, preventing undesirable phase transformations during crystallization and formulation of cocrystals.

1.4.3 Solubilization by Cosolvents

The use of cosolvents is well recognized in altering solubility of organic compounds. Despite the significant amount of work done by Yalkowsky[63] and coworkers, a comprehensive understanding of the theory of solubilization by cosolvents is lacking. Yalkowsky[63] presented some general features of cosolvents and solubilization by cosolvents. Cosolvents are partly polar, due to the presence of hydrogen bond donors and/or acceptors, thus ensuring miscibility with water. Cosolvents improve the solubility of drugs (nonpolar) because the small hydrocarbon regions of cosolvents reduce the ability of the water to squeeze out nonpolar solutes. The presence of cosolvents in aqueous medium leads to decreased solvent–solvent interactions, leading to reduction in properties (surface tension, dielectric constant, and solubility parameter) that are reflective of solvent polarity.

The solubility enhancement by a cosolvent is a function of both drug and cosolvent properties. The greatest enhancement in drug solubility is achieved by cosolvents or cosolvent–water mixtures with similar polarity to the drug. The addition of cosolvent can lead to increase or decrease in solubility, depending on the polarity of the drug candidate. Gould et al.[64] observed that the solubility of oxfenicine is decreased in the presence of ethanol. In some cases, a maximum in solubility is observed for an intermediate composition of cosolvent and water, rather than in pure solvents.

Yalkowsky and coworkers[65,66,67,68,69,70] presented a log–linear model to explain the solubility of nonpolar solutes in cosolvent systems. The mixed solvent is assumed to behave similarly to the weighted linear combination of the individual solvents. The general equation describing the solubilization by a cosolvent is defined by:

$$\log_{10}(S_{mix}) = \log_{10}(S_w) + \sigma \cdot f_c \quad (1.58)$$

S_{mix} is the solubility in the mixed solvent with f_c as the fractional cosolvent volume, S_w is the solubility in water, and σ is defined as the solubilizing power of the cosolvent. The above equation indicates that the solubility changes exponentially with cosolvent volume fraction. The logarithm of solubility increases linearly with the volume fraction of the cosolvent, and the slope of this line, σ, is dependent on the properties of both solute and the cosolvent.

$$\sigma = S \log_{10}(K_{ow}) + T \quad (1.59)$$

K_{ow} is the octanol–water partition coefficient and is related to the polarity of the drug molecule, whereas S and T are empirically-derived cosolvent-dependent constants. The S and T values have been estimated by Millard et al.[70] for a number of cosolvents.

The log–linear model is very useful as it allows estimation of solubilization of drugs in cosolvent systems, based on partition coefficient and the known values of S and T, for various pharmaceutically acceptable cosolvents.

Although the cosolvents enhance solubility of drug candidates by several orders of magnitude their use is limited, due to toxicity, especially at high concentrations. Due to the exponential dependence of drug solubility on volume fraction, dilution may lead to precipitation of drug, as the drug concentration after dilution may be higher than the solubility in the diluted solution.

1.4.4 Solubilization by Surfactants (Micellar Solubilization)

Surfactants are amphiphilic molecules that self-associate in solution and form aggregated structures known as micelles. The two most common models of micellization are the two-phase model and mass action model. From a solubilization perspective, drug molecules interact with micelles to form soluble drug "entities." In the two-phase model, the drug is assumed to be incorporated into the micelle, whereas in the mass action model the drug is assumed to reversibly bind to self-associated (micelles) surfactant aggregates.

The two-phase model, also known as the phase-separation model, assumes that above a critical concentration of surfactant molecules in aqueous solution, formation of micelles occurs. The micelles are considered to be a separate phase from the aqueous phase. It is assumed that micellization occurs only above the critical micellar concentration (CMC). Below the CMC, the total surfactant concentration is assumed to be the same as monomer (aqueous phase) surfactant concentration. Above the CMC, the free monomer (aqueous phase) surfactant concentration is assumed to be constant (equal to the CMC), and the micelle concentration can be obtained by subtracting the CMC from the total surfactant concentration.

Hydrophobic, non-polar drugs are thought be squeezed out of water into the hydrophobic regions of the micelles.[63] Since the interaction of drug molecules with surfactant monomers is assumed to be negligible, the solubility of the drug in aqueous solution at concentrations below the CMC is assumed to be the same as its intrinsic solubility, S_0. At surfactant concentrations above the CMC the total solubility of the drug, S_T, is given by the following equation:

$$S_T = S_0 + k(P_T - CMC) \qquad (1.60)$$

P_T is the total surfactant concentration drug, and k is a proportionality constant, known as the solubilizing capacity of the surfactant. The total solubility varies linearly with an increase in total surfactant concentration (micelle concentration). The non-linearity in solubility enhancement means that the solubilization capacity assumed to be a constant is, in reality, dependent on the surfactant concentration. This can be due to changes in micelle shape or aggregation numbers of the micelle.

Based on the mass action law model, self-association equilibrium between "n" surfactant monomers and the micelle is expressed as follows:

$$n.P_1 \xrightleftharpoons{\beta_n} P_n$$

The total surfactant concentration, P_T, can be defined by the following expression:

$$P_T = [P_1] + n \times [P_n] = [P_1] + n \times \beta_n \times [P_1]^n \qquad (1.61)$$

Drug solubilization in the surfactant solution can be depicted by multiple equilibria between the self-associated surfactant, P_n, and the drug.

$$i.D + P_n \xrightleftharpoons{k_i} D_i P_n$$

The saturation solubility of a drug in a surfactant solution is given as:

$$S_T = S_o + [P_n] \sum_{i=1}^{M} i \times k_i \times [S_o]^{i^n} \qquad (1.62)$$

It is difficult to estimate the individual equilibrium constants for the various species, and therefore the two-phase model is a more convenient and often sufficient way to describe the solubility of drugs in surfactant solutions.

1.4.5 Solubilization by Combination of Approaches

In the previous sections, the common techniques to improve solubility by pH control or by use of complexing agents, cosolvents, and surfactants have been discussed. However, it is common to find that a single approach of solubilization is not adequate to improve the aqueous solubility to the desirable extent. Generally, the combination of ionization with cosolvency, complexation or micellar solubilization leads to synergistic improvement in solubility of weak electrolytes. The combined effect of complexation and cosolvency, or complexation and micellar solubilization, on drug solubility can be variable. In the following sections, the theoretical framework describing drug solubilization by a combination of approaches is discussed.

Combined Effect of Ionization and Cosolvency

The total solubility of an ionizable drug in mixed solvent can be derived by writing the log–linear model for various drug species in solution. When considering a monoprotic weak acid or monobasic compound, the solubilization by cosolvency for the ionized and unionized drug moieties can be expressed using the log–linear model equations:[63]

$$\log_{10}\left(S_u^f\right) = \log_{10}(S_u) + \sigma_u \cdot f_c \qquad (1.63)$$

$$\log_{10}\left(S_i^f\right) = \log_{10}(S_i) + \sigma_i \cdot f_c \qquad (1.64)$$

S_u^f and S_i^f are the solubility of the unionized and ionized species, respectively, in the mixed solvent; S_u and S_i are solubility of the unionized and ionized species, respectively, in water; and σ_u and σ_i are solubilization power of the cosolvent for the unionized and ionized species. The total drug solubility is obtained by the sum of S_u^f and S_i^f, and is provided by the following equation:

$$S_T = S_u \cdot 10^{\sigma_u f_c} + S_i \cdot 10^{\sigma_i f_c} \qquad (1.65)$$

For a monoprotic weak acid:

$$S_T = S_0 \cdot 10^{\sigma_u f_c} + S_0 \cdot 10^{(\mathrm{pH} - \mathrm{p}K_a)} \cdot 10^{\sigma_i f_c} \qquad (1.66)$$

For a monobasic compound:

$$S_T = S_0 \cdot 10^{\sigma_u f_c} + S_0 \cdot 10^{(\mathrm{p}K_a - \mathrm{pH})} \cdot 10^{\sigma_i f_c} \qquad (1.67)$$

The solubilization capacity of the unionized species, σ_u, is typically found to be greater than that for the ionized species, σ_i, because the cosolvent can solubilize the unionized species (more polar) with greater efficiency than the ionized species (less polar). However, the decrease in solubilization capacity is more than compensated for by the increase in solubility of the ionized species, i.e., $S_i \gg S_u$. Therefore, it is possible that the combined effect of ionization and cosolvency is better than any single technique. The solubility of 2,2-diphenyl-4-piperidyl dioxolane hydrochloride salt in propylene glycol–water mixtures was better than the solubility of the free base in the mixed solvent or the hydrochloride salt in water.[71]

Combined Effect of Ionization and Micellization

The total solubility of a weak electrolyte undergoing ionization and micellization can be described by accounting for the free unionized drug, free ionized drug, micellized unionized drug, and micellized ionized drug.

$$S_T = S_u + S_i + k_u[P_T - \mathrm{CMC}] + k_i[P_T - \mathrm{CMC}] \qquad (1.68)$$

This equation is valid for surfactants that are either neutral or completely ionized in the pH range of interest. Li et al.[72] demonstrated that the falvopiridol (freebase with pK_a of 5.68) showed synergistic improvement in solubility due to the combined effect of lowering pH and use of polysorbate 20.

Combined Effect of Ionization and Complexation

The combined effect of ionization and complexation on drug solubility has been derived similarly to the above scenario of solubilization by ionization and micellization. The total drug solubility has been derived by different researchers[73,74,75] by considering the various species in solutions, i.e., free unionized drug, ionized drug, unionized drug–ligand complex, and ionized drug–ligand complex. Rao and Stella[76] derived an equivalent expression for the total solubility of a weak electrolyte undergoing 1:1 complexes with a ligand, based on apparent solubility and apparent binding constant at any given pH as:

$$S_T = S_{app} + \frac{K_{app} S_{app}}{1 + K_{app} S_{app}} L_T \qquad (1.69)$$

For monoprotic weak acids, K_{app} and S_{app} are defined as:

$$K_{app} = K^o \frac{[\mathrm{H}^+]}{K_a + [\mathrm{H}^+]} + K^- \frac{K_a}{K_a + [\mathrm{H}^+]} \qquad (1.70)$$

$$S_{app} = S_o \frac{K_a + [\mathrm{H}^+]}{[\mathrm{H}^+]} \qquad (1.71)$$

K_a is the ionization constant; K^o and K^- are the binding constants for the neutral drug–ligand complex and anionic drug–ligand complex, respectively. Similarly, for monobasic compounds,

$$K_{app} = K^o \frac{K_a}{K_a + [\mathrm{H}^+]} + K^+ \frac{[\mathrm{H}^+]}{K_a + [\mathrm{H}^+]} \qquad (1.72)$$

$$S_{app} = S_o \frac{K_a + [\mathrm{H}^+]}{K_a} \qquad (1.73)$$

K_a is the ionization constant; K^o and K^+ are the binding constants for the neutral drug–ligand complex and cationic drug–ligand complex, respectively. Rao and Stella[76] presented an interesting analysis of binding constant values for neutral versus ionized species (both acids and bases) with HP- and SBE-β-CD. They reported the ratio of $K^{charged}$ (K^+ or K^-) to K^o falls within two orders of magnitude, regardless of the type of cyclodextrins or drugs. However, S_{app} can vary over several orders of magnitude depending on the ionization type (acid or base), its pK_a, and the pH value. Although the variation of K_{app} and S_{app} with pH is in the opposite direction, the magnitude of increase in S_{app} far outweighs the decrease in K_{app} due to ionization, leading to a synergistic increase in total drug solubility, due to ionization and complexation.

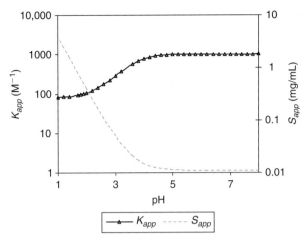

FIGURE 1.5 Variation of S_{app} and K_{app} as a function of pH for Thiazolobenzimidazole. The curves are reproduced based on equations in reference 77 and data from reference 74

Combined Effect of Cosolvency and Complexation

The combined effects of complexation and cosolvents on drug solubilization can be of synergistic or antagonistic nature. Some of the factors that need to be considered when using combinations of cosolvent and complexing agents are:

1. Due to solubilization by cosolvency, the free drug concentration available for complexation may be higher, leading to a synergistic improvement in solubility.
2. Formation of soluble drug–ligand–cosolvent ternary complexes leads to synergistic improvement in solubility.
3. Competition between the drug and cosolvent molecules for complexation with the ligand leads to a decrease in drug solubility.
4. Decrease in apparent binding constant for drug–ligand in cosolvent can occur.

Thus, the impact of combination of cosolvency and complexation on drug solubility needs to be evaluated on a case-by-case basis. Li et al.[77] provided a mathematical model for the total solubility by considering the free drug, drug–ligand complex and drug–solvent complex. The authors assumed that the solubilizing power of the cosolvent remains unchanged even in the presence of complexing agent; the decrease in binding constant can be empirically related to cosolvent concentration in an exponential fashion. They also assumed negligible complexation between cosolvent molecules and complexing agent. Fluasterone solubility increased linearly with HP-β-CD in all ethanol–water mixtures. In the absence of HP-β-CD, an exponential increase in solubility with percentage w/w

ethanol in line with the log–linear model discussed previously was observed. In the presence of HP-β-CD, the drug solubility first decreased, and then increased with an increase in percentage w/w ethanol. Using the mathematical models developed for this system, the authors were able to explain the experimental data.

Combined Effect of Complexation and Micellar Solubilization

Several interactions (equilibria) can coexist in solubility experiments in aqueous solutions containing complexing agent, surfactant, and drug. They include competitive complexation of drug and surfactant monomer with the complexing agent, equilibria between monomer and micelle, and solubilization of drug in the micelle. Yang et al.[78] presented experimental data and a semi-quantitative analysis of solubilization of NSC-639829 in aqueous solutions of SLS and (SBE)7M-β-CD. Rao and coworkers[79] presented a mathematical model to study the combined effect of micellar solubilization and complexation. This model assumes that ligand molecules or drug–ligand complexes do not interact with micelles, and higher order drug–ligand or surfactant monomer:ligand complexes are not formed. The phase-solubility profile in the presence of both complexing agent and surfactant are dependent on a number of factors. However, it is possible for one to predict this behavior, provided the binary interaction parameters between the drug, complexing agent and surfactant are known.

The first step in understanding the various equilibria is to determine P_f, the surfactant concentration that is unbound to the complexing agent. This requires solving the following quadratic equation:

$$K_P \times [P_f]^2 + (1 + K_P \times L_T + K_D \times S_0 - K_P \times P_T) \\ \times [P_f] - (P_T + P_T \times K_D \times S_0) = 0 \qquad (1.74)$$

K_P and K_D are 1:1 binding constants for surfactant monomer–ligand and drug–ligand, respectively.

If P_f is found to be lower than the known CMC value for the surfactant, the total drug solubility can be described as follows:

$$S_T = \left[D_f\right] + [D - CD] \\ = S_{oD-CD} + \frac{K_D \times S_0 \times L_T}{1 + K_P \times \left[P_f\right] + K_D \times S_0} \qquad (1.75)$$

According to the above equation, the total solubility will be lower in the presence of surfactant, due to competition between the drug and surfactant monomer for the complexing agent (Scheme 1.2A).

If P_f is greater than the known CMC value of the surfactant, the total solubility is defined as:

$$S_T = S_o + K_M \left(P_T - \text{CMC} - \frac{K_P \times \text{CMC} \times L_T}{1 + K_P \times \text{CMC} + K_D \times S_0} \right)$$
$$+ \frac{K_D \times S_0 \times L_T}{1 + K_P \times \text{CMC} + K_D \times S_0} \qquad (1.76)$$

According to the above equation, the combined solubility is less than the sum of the solubility values in the presence of individual additives, i.e., complexing agent or surfactant (Scheme 1.2B). It is also possible that the combined solubility is less than individual solubility values. Yang et al.[78] showed that for NSC-639829, the combined solubility in aqueous solutions containing both SLS and (SBE)7M-β-CD is less than the sum of the solubility values in aqueous solutions containing SLS or (SBE)7M-β-CD.

1.5 EXPERIMENTAL DETERMINATION OF SOLUBILITY

The importance of knowledge of solubility of a drug has been discussed earlier. As a consequence, the determination of solubility remains one of the most

SCHEME 1.2(A) Competitive complexation of drug and surfactant monomer to ligand (P_f < CMC). Redrawn based on Reference 79

SCHEME 1.2(B) Competitive complexation and drug solubilization into micellar phase (P_f > CMC). Redrawn based on Reference 79

routinely conducted experiments during the drug development stage. Although these experiments are commonly perceived as simple, accurate solubility determination may be far more challenging. Pontolillo and Eganhouse[80] have noted a scatter of five log units in the experimentally determined solubility of DDT. The AQUASOL database records a scatter of 10–30 times in the solubility of anthracene and fluoranthrene reported in literature. These observations showcase the fact that accurate determination of solubility is not trivial. Various aspects related to the solute and solvent of interest, experimental conditions, and the analytical techniques employed, play important roles in the determination of actual solubility. This section covers the various methods that have been conventionally employed for solubility determination. In addition, several factors that may affect the solubility and its measurement will be discussed.

All methods used for solubility determination primarily consist of two parts: saturating the solvent with the solute, and measuring the amount of solute present per unit of the solvent at that saturation state. In simple terms, the first part involves providing ample exposure of the solute to the solvent such that the dissolved solute molecules are in dynamic equilibrium with the undissolved molecules. A variety of analytical methods can then be used to measure the concentration of dissolved solute.

Before designing any solubility experiments, it is essential to identify whether the requirement is to determine thermodynamic equilibrium solubility or a kinetic dissolution rate. These concepts have been discussed in the previous section. The need to determine one over the other depends upon the application of the results obtained. If the goal is to prepare a liquid formulation, the equilibrium solubility information is more meaningful. However, dissolution rates are needed to access the release of drug from the formulation, and its subsequent absorption in the gastrointestinal tract.

The conventional approaches for measuring equilibrium solubility are based on the phase-solubility technique proposed by Higuchi and Connors.[56] An excess amount of the solute is placed with the solvent in a closed container, and shaken for a sufficient length of time. Immersing sealed containers in a constant temperature bath may be used to control the temperature of the system. Once equilibrated, the sample is phase-separated to remove undissolved solute, and analyzed quantitatively for dissolved solute content using nephlometry, UV absorbance or potentiometric measurements.[81,82] It is necessary to maintain the same temperature used for equilibration during the phase-separation process. The main disadvantage of this method is that it can be time-consuming, especially when there is a desire to run solubility experiments on a large number of compounds during the early discovery phase. Therefore, many variants of "kinetic solubility experiments" have been developed to rapidly screen a large number of compounds by either dissolving them in a solvent such as DMSO or using unidentified crystalline or amorphous phase. Various considerations are required while determining the solubility using this approach. Although the specific requirements can, and will, vary case-by-case, some general points are discussed here.

1.5.1 Stability of Solute and Solvent

It is essential that both the solute and solvent remain chemically and physically stable during the equilibration. The solute undergoing chemical degradation can result in more soluble or less soluble products, and provide misleading results. If the solvent is aqueous, hydrolysis of the solute may occur, generally resulting in the formation of more soluble degradation products. If the analytical method is not highly specific, such as UV-spectrophotometry, the measured solubility will be artificially higher than the actual solubility. The physical stability of both the solute and solvent must also be adequately considered. A hygroscopic solvent, like polyols, may pick up moisture during equilibration, which will result in a compositional change. For such solvents, care must be taken to protect against exposure to moisture. Similarly, while dealing with volatile solvents like low molecular weight alcohols, the container must be tightly closed to avoid solvent loss.

The physical form of the solute is an important determinant of its solubility. Polymorphic transitions, including conversion to or from hydrates/solvates, may occur during the equilibration process. Thus, it is essential to determine the form of the undissolved solute after equilibrium is achieved using a solid-state characterization technique like powder X-ray diffractometry. Determination of equilibrium solubility of a metastable form is difficult, due to conversion to the more stable form,[83] this is particularly the case for compounds that are anhydrates or lower-order hydrates that convert to the hydrate formed upon equilibration. The best one can do is to determine apparent solubility, often assumed to be the highest concentration observed during a solubility experiment.[84] Alternatively, the ratio of intrinsic dissolution rates for the two forms at identical hydrodynamic conditions, along with the solubility of the stable form, can be used to determine the solubility of the metastable form.[85]

On similar grounds, for ionizable solutes it must be determined whether the solute exists in the free form or as a salt. If the solubility is to be determined at a specific pH, adequate measures must be taken to maintain the pH in the desired range using buffers. The choice of buffer should be based on the pH-range desired and the selected buffer should have adequate buffer strength in that range. Monitoring and adjusting the pH of the system is essential, and the frequency of doing so strictly depends on the strength of the buffer used, ionic strength of the solute, and its dissolution rate. In addition to the pH, the ionic strength of the media also affects the equilibrium solubility, and must be maintained during the equilibration using common salts such as sodium or potassium chloride. The salt selected must not contain the same ion present in the solute to avoid common-ion effect.[86,87] Buffer components and salts used to adjust ionic strength may themselves form salts with ionizable drugs that have limited solubility. Thus, the identity of all insoluble residues must be confirmed, and the absence of buffer components or counterions of salts used to adjust ionic strength must be demonstrated.

1.5.2 Shakers and Containers

Proper wetting of the solute has to be ensured by choosing an appropriate shaker. The use of several types of shakers has been reported in the literature, including end-over-end shakers, wrist action shakers, magnetic stirrers, vortexers, etc. The selection of a shaker depends on the volume and viscosity of the solvent used. Generally, end-over-end shakers provide good solute–solvent exposure for small volumes (>20 ml) of solvents that have viscosity similar to that of water. Industrial-size shakers are available for manufacturing of solution formulations. The compatibility of the solute and the solvent with the container is essential. Glass is generally the material of choice, at least for small-scale experiments, as it is relatively chemically inert. Protection from light exposure for photo-labile systems can be achieved by either using amber vials or covering the container with an opaque material such as aluminum foil.

1.5.3 Presence of Excess Undissolved Solute

The presence of some undissolved solute during the entire length of equilibration is essential. However, a lot of undissolved solute must be avoided as there have been several reports claiming the dependence of the equilibrium solubility on the amount of excess solute present during equilibration. Wang et al.[88] noticed that the solubility of a diprotic weak base depended on the amount of hydrochloride salt added. More recently, Kawakami et al.[89] reported that when $40\mu g$ of indomethacin was added to 1 mL pH 5 or 6 citrate buffer, a much higher solubility was obtained compared to 5 mg added to the same solution, while a reverse trend was noticed in pH 6.5 and 7.0 phosphate buffer.

Supersaturation is another cause of imprecise solubility data. Ledwidge and Corrigan[83] reported that the self-association near pH$_{max}$ reduces the rate of nucleation of the final salt, and that when the free drug is used as the starting material higher levels of supersaturation are achieved.

Caution must be practiced if the solute contains soluble impurities. These impurities can influence the property of the media and, consequently, the solubility of the solute. They may also interfere with the technique used for solubility analysis. This is of particular concern if the analytical technique used is non-selective. The presence of impurities has been shown to impact the solubility of 7-(2-hydrocypropyltheophylline).[90]

1.5.4 Determination of Equilibrium

Information from prior experiments can be useful for gauging the time to achieve equilibrium. If no prior information is available, several samplings may be required to establish the time it takes to reach equilibrium. The periodicity of withdrawing sample depends on the dissolution rate of the solute. In order to minimize sampling, the interval can progressively be doubled. In other words, if the first sampling is performed two hours following the start of the experiment, the second sampling can be done after four hours, the third after eight hours, and so on. The sampling should be continued until the solubility for the last two sampling points is equal, indicating attainment of equilibrium. The last sampling point can be conservatively treated as the time required for the equilibration. While conducting this exercise it is important not to replace the solvent removed during sampling, as it will push the system away from equilibrium.

1.5.5 Phase-separation

Once the equilibrium between the dissolved and undissolved solute is achieved, the dissolved phase has to be separated and analyzed for solute concentration.

Several methods can be used to phase-separate the system. Filtration provides a convenient way to separate the dissolved phase and the undissolved solute. Appropriate filters can be chosen from a variety of configurations available to suit the need of the experiment. Commercial filters are available in a variety of size, pore dimensions, and membrane material. The compatibility of the filter with both the solute and solvent must be determined. Strongly organic solvent systems can leach out components from the filter membrane or its housing. On the other hand, some solutes can adsorb on the filter assembly, which can result in solubility artifacts. An example is amiodarone, which adsorbs onto some polyvinyl-based filters. As a general practice, the filter system must be "rinsed" by passing through the solution two to three times before collection. This ensures that the system is saturated with the solute and solvent prior to sampling, and will reduce artifacts.

Phase-separation can also be achieved by centrifugation. This technique is particularly useful if both the solute and the solvent are liquids. Following phase-separation, the clear supernatant is collected leaving behind the undissolved solute. Considerations must be made for possible compatibility issues of the solute or solvent with centrifuge tubes. Glass tubes are preferred whenever possible to minimize adsorption issues. Other factors include the speed and length of centrifugation, which depend on the properties of the solute and solvent.

Other methods for phase-separation include evaporative collection of solvent and selective adsorption of dissolved phase. These methods, although they can be useful in some situations, are less practical to carry out. Whichever method of phase-separation is used, control over temperature during the separation process is essential. Prolonged contact of undissolved solids with the supernatant saturated solution during the separation process at some temperature other than that at which equilibration was performed will likely result in under- or overestimation of solubility, depending on the temperature difference between the equilibration process and the phase-separation process.

1.5.6 Determination of Solute Content in the Dissolved Phase

Once the dissolved phase is separated, the solute concentration is determined analytically. Several techniques can be used including spectrophotometry, gravimetry, pH measurement, etc. Spectrophotometry is the most commonly employed technique based on its simplicity, accuracy, and chemical specificity. This technique is based on the well-known Beer's Law, according to which the absorbance of a chemical species is directly proportional to its concentration. A simple analysis can be performed by plotting a standard curve using known concentrations of the solute, followed by quantification of the unknown solute concentration in the solution. The solution may be diluted if needed, to fit in the concentration range of the standard curve.

In order to use this technique it is essential that the analyte molecules contain a chromophore, i.e., it is spectrally active in the UV or visible light region. If that is not the case, it can be chemically derivatized to make it spectrally active. The complexity of derivatization reactions depends upon the chemical structure of the solute, and in some cases may be a limiting factor.

It is a common practice to couple spectrophotometry with separation techniques, such as chromatography, to improve the specificity of the experiment. This approach is very useful in cases where either solvent or impurity/degradation products interfere with direct solute determination. It is particularly important at early stages of development, where solute purity may not be known.

Gravimetric analysis involves the determination of the weight of dissolved solute in a solution. This is primarily achieved either by solvent evaporation or solute precipitation using physical or chemical means. This approach is relatively simple, inexpensive, and does not require lengthy method-development steps. However, its broader application is marred by lack of sensitivity, selectivity, and practicality. Measurements of indirect properties, such as pH of the system or colligative properties that can yield information on the concentration of solute in a given solution have also been proposed.

1.5.7 Experimental Conditions

The external conditions in which the experiment is carried out can have a huge impact on the solubility results. The effect of temperature on solubility has been detailed in the discussion following Equation 1.11. Temperature may have a positive or a negative influence on the solubility depending upon the solute and solvent properties. Pressure significantly affects the solubility of gases, but generally has little influence on the solubility of liquids and solids. The presence of light may affect the chemical stability of photolabile solutes, and may artificially affect their solubility.

Besides the thermodynamically correct phase-solubility method, the solubility can be ball-parked by using the "synthetic" method. According to this method, a known amount of solute is added to a known amount of solvent, followed by a mixing step. If the solute dissolves completely, more is added and the process continues until a stage is reached after which the added solute does not dissolve. Alternatively, if the solute does not dissolve completely after the first round, more solvent is added, and the process continues until the solute dissolves completely. The approximate solubility can be calculated by the knowledge of the amount of solvent required to completely dissolve a known quantity of the solute. This method provides a simple means for approximate solubility determination. It is particularly useful for solutes available in limited amounts, as development of involved analytical method is not required. However, the approach lacks the sensitivity and selectivity of the phase-solubility approach.

References

1. Amidon, G.L., Lennernas, H., Shah, V.P. & Crison, J.R. (1995). Pharmaceutical Research 12, 413–420.
2. Gribbon, P. & Sewing, A. (2005). Drug Discovery Technologies 10, 17–22.
3. Deshwal, B.R., Lee, K.C. & Singh, K.C. (2006). Journal of Molecular Liquids 123, 38–42.
4. Noyes, A.A. & Whitney, W.R. (1897). Journal of the American Chemical Society 19, 930–934.
5. Hamlin, W.E., Northam, J.I. & Wagner, J.G. (1965). Journal of Pharmaceutical Sciences 54, 1651–1653.
6. Sanghvi, R. (2006). Drug solublization using N-methyl pyrrolidone: efficiency and mechanism, PhD Thesis. The University of Arizona.
7. Jain, P. & Yalkowsky, S.H. (2007). International Journal of Pharmaceutics 342, 1–5.
8. Hildebrand, J.H., Prausnitz, J.H. & Scott, R.L. (1970). *Regular and Related Solutions*. Van Nostrand Reinhold, New York.
9. Prausnitz, J.M., Lichtenhaler, R.L. & Gomez de Azevado, E. (1986). *Molecular Thermodynamics of Fluid Phase Equilibria*, 2nd edn. Prentice Hall, Englewood Cliffs, New Jersey.
10. Grant, D.J.W., Mendizadah, M., Chow, A.H.L. & Fairbrother, J.E. (1984). International Journal of Pharmaceutics 18, 25–38.
11. Mishra, D. S. (1988). Solubility of organic compounds in non-aqueous systems, PhD Thesis. The University of Arizona.
12. Mishra, D.S. & Yalkowsky, S.H. (1990). Industrial and Engineering Chemistry Research 29, 2278–2283.
13. Walden, P. (1908). Zeitschrift fur Angewandte Physik und Chemie 14, 713–728.
14. Martin, E., Yalkowsky, S.H. & Wells, J.E. (1979). Journal of Pharmaceutical Sciences 68, 565–568.
15. Dannenfelser, R.M. & Yalkowsky, S.H. (1996). Industrial and Engineering Chemistry Research 35, 1483–1486.
16. Jain, A., Yang, G. & Yalkowsky, S.H. (2004). Industrial and Engineering Chemistry Research 43, 4376–4379.
17. Hildebrand, J.H. & Scott, R.L. (1950). *The Solubility of Nonelectrolytes*. Rheinhold Publishing Corporation, New York.
18. Hansen, C.M. & Beerbower, A. (1971). *Encyclopedia of Chemical Technology*, 2nd edn. Wiley, New York.
19. Fedor, R. (1974). Polymer Engineering and Science 14(2), 147–154.

20. Sanghvi, R. & Yalkowsky, S.H. (2006). Industrial and Engineering Chemistry Research 45, 2856–2861.
21. Martin, A., Newburger, J. & Adeji, A.J. (1979). Journal of Pharmaceutical Sciences 68, iv.
22. Hildebrand, J.H., Prausnitz, J.M. & Scott, R. (1970). *Regular and Related Solutions*. Van Nostrand Reinhold, New York.
23. Yalkowsky, S.H., Flynn, G.L. & Amidon, G.L. (1972). Journal of Pharmaceutical Sciences 61, 983–984.
24. Yalkowsky, S.H., Amidon, G.L., Zografi, G. & Flynn, G.L. (1975). Journal of Pharmaceutical Sciences 64, 48–52.
25. Yalkowsky, S.H., Valvani, S.C. & Amidon, G.L. (1976). Journal of Pharmaceutical Sciences 65, 1488–1493.
26. Amidon, G.L., Yalkowsky, S.H. & Leung, S. (1974). Journal of Pharmaceutical Sciences 63, 1858–1866.
27. Myrdal, P.B., Ward, G.H., Dannenfelser, R.M., Mishra, D.S. & Yalkowsky, S.H. (1992). Chemosphere 24, 1047–1061.
28. Myrdal, P.B., Ward, G.H., Simamora, P. & Yalkowsky, S.H. (1993). SAR and QSAR in environmental research 1, 55–61.
29. Myrdal, P.B. & Yalkowsky, S.H. (1994). SAR and QSAR in environmental research 2, 17–28.
30. Myrdal, P.B., Manka, A. & Yalkowsky, S.H. (1995). Chemosphere 30, 1619–1637.
31. Hansch, C., Quinlan, J.E. & Lawrence, G.L. (1968). Journal of Organic Chemistry 33, 347–350.
32. Jain, N. & Yalkowsky, S.H. (2001). Journal of Pharmaceutical Sciences 90, 234–252.
33. Sepassi, K. & Yalkowsky, S. H. (2006). AAPS PharmSciTech 7(1), Article 26, http://www.aapspharmscitech.org.
34. Machatha, S.G. & Yalkowsky, S.H. (2005). International Journal of Pharmaceutics 294, 185–192.
35. Katritzky, A.R., Jain, R., Lomaka, A., Petrukhin, R., Maran, U. & Karelson, M. (2003). Crystal Growth & Design 1, 261–265.
36. Dearden, J.C. (2003). Environmental Toxicology & Chemistry 22, 1696–1709.
37. Bergstrom, C.A.S., Norinder, U., Luthman, K. & Artursson, P. (2003). Journal of Chemical Information and Computer Sciences 43, 1177–1185.
38. Jain, A., Yalkowsky, S.H. (2006). Journal of Pharmaceutical Sciences 95, 2562–2618.
39. Niimi, A. (1991). Water Research 25, 1515–1521.
40. Bruggemann, R. & Altschuh, J. (1991). QSAR Environ Toxicology 4, 41–58.
41. Ran, Y., Jain, N. & Yalkowsky, S.H. (2001). Journal of Chemical Information and Computer Sciences 41, 354–357.
42. Ran, Y., He, Y., Yang, G., Johnson, J.L.H. & Yalkowsky, S.H. (2002). Chemosphere 48, 487–509.
43. Jain, N., Yang, G., Machatha, S.G. & Yalkowsky, S.H. (2006). International Journal of Pharmaceutics 319, 169–171.
44. Dearden, J.C. (2006). Expert Opinion on Drug Discovery 1, 31–52.
45. Jorgensen, W.L. & Duffy, E.M. (2002). Advanced Drug Delivery Reviews 54, 355–366.
46. Abraham, M.H. & Le, J. (1999). Journal of Pharmaceutical Sciences 88, 868–880.
47. Taskinen, J. & Yliruusi, J. (2003). Advanced Drug Delivery Reviews 55, 1163–1183.
48. Gould, P.L. (1986). International Journal of Pharmaceutics 33, 201–217.
49. Serajuddin, A.T.M. & Pudipeddi, M. (2002). *Handbook of Pharmaceutical Salts*. Wiley-VCH, pp. 135–160.
50. Streng, W.H., His, S.K., Helms, P.E. & Tan, H.G.H. (1984). Journal of Pharmaceutical Sciences 73, 1679–1684.
51. Chowhan, Z.T. (1978). Journal of Pharmaceutical Sciences 67, 1257–1260.
52. Bogardus, J.B., Blackwood, R.K. (1979). Journal of Pharmaceutical Sciences 68, 188–194.
53. Maurin, M.B., Grant, D.J.W. & Stahl, P.H. (2002). *Handbook of Pharmaceutical Salts*. Wiley-VCH, pp. 9–18.
54. Serajuddin, A.T.M., Pudipeddi, M. (2002). *Handbook of Pharmaceutical Salts*. Wiley-VCH, pp. 135–160.
55. Repta, A.J. (1981). *Techniques of Solubilization of Drugs*. Marcel Dekker Inc., New York, pp. 135–158.
56. Higuchi, T., Connors, K.A. (1965). Advances in Analytical Chemistry, 117.
57. Higuchi, T., Lach, J. (1954). Journal of the American Pharmaceutical Association 43, 349.
58. Higuchi, T., Pitman, I.H. (1973). Journal of Pharmaceutical Sciences 62, 55.
59. Desiraju, G.R. (2003). Crystal Engineering Community 5, 466–467.
60. Dunitz, J.D. (2003). Crystal Engineering Community 5, 506.
61. Vishweshwar, P., McMahon, J.A., Bis, J.A. & Zaworotko, M.J. (2006). Journal of Pharmaceutical Sciences 95, 499–516.
62. Nehl, S.J., Rodriguez-Spong, B. & Rodriguez-Hornedo, N. (2006). Crystal Growth Design 592, 600.
63. Yalkowsky, S.H. (1999). *Solubility and Solubilization in Aqueous Media*. Oxford University Press, Oxford, UK.
64. Gould, P.L., Goodman, M. & Hanson, P.A. (1984). International Journal of Pharmaceutics 19, 149–159.
65. Yalkowsky, S.H., Amidon, G.L., Zografi, G. & Flynn, G.L. (1972). Journal of Pharmaceutical Sciences 61, 48–52.
66. Yalkowsky, S.H., Flynn, G.L. & Amidon, G.L. (1972). Journal of Pharmaceutical Sciences 61, 983–984.
67. Yalkowsky, S.H., Valvani, S.C. & Amidon, G.L. (1976). Journal of Pharmaceutical Sciences 65, 1488–1494.
68. Yalkowsky, S.H. Roseman, T.J. (1981). *Techniques of Solubilization of Drugs*. Marcel Dekker Inc., New York pp. 91–134.
69. Yalkowsky, S.H., Robino, J.T. (1983). Journal of Pharmaceutical Sciences 72, 1014–1017.
70. Millard, J.W., Alvarez-Nunez, F.A. & Yalkowsky, S.H. (2002). International Journal of Pharmaceutics 245, 153–166.
71. Kramer, S.F., Flynn, G.L. (1972). Journal of Pharmaceutical Sciences 61, 1896–1904.
72. Li, P., Tabibi, E. & Yalkowsky, S.H. (1999). Journal of Pharmaceutical Sciences 88, 945–947.
73. Tinwalla,, A.Y., Hoesterey, B.L., Xiang, T., Lim, K. & Anderson, B.D. (1993). Pharmaceutical Research 10, 1136–1143.
74. Johnson, M.D., Hoesterey, B.L. & Anderson, B.D. (1994). Journal of Pharmaceutical Sciences 83, 1142–1146.
75. Okimoto, K., Rajeswki, R.A., Uekama, K., Jona, J.A. & Stella, V.J. (1996). Pharmaceutical Research 13, 256–264.
76. Rao, V.M., Stella, V.J. (2003). Journal of Pharmaceutical Sciences 92, 927–932.
77. Yang, G., Jain, N. & Yalkowsky, S.H. (2004). International Journal of Pharmaceutics 269, 141–148.
78. Rao, V.M., Nerurkar, M., Pinnamaneni, S. & Raghavan, K. (2006). International Journal of Pharmaceutics 319, 98–106.
79. Pontolillo, J. & Eganhouse, E. US Geological Survey, Report 4201.
80. Glomme, A., Marz, J. & Dressman, J.B. (2005). Journal of Pharmaceutical Sciences 94, 1–16.
81. Fligge, T.A., Shuler, A. (2006). Journal of Pharmaceutical and Biomedical Analysis 42, 449–454.
82. Ledwidge, M.T., Corrigan, O.I. (1998). International Journal of Pharmaceutics 174, 187–200.
83. Khankari, R.K., Grant, D.J.W. (1995). Thermochimica Acta 248, 61–79.
84. Morris, K.R., Rodriguez-Hornedo, N. (1993). Encyclopedia of Pharmaceutical Technology 393.

85. Anderson, B. D. & Flora, K. P. (1996). *The Practice of Medicinal Chemistry*. pp.739–754.

86. Pudipeddi, M., Serajuddin, A.T.M., Grant, D.J.W. & Stahl, P.H. (2002). *Handbook of Pharmaceutical Salts*. Wiley-VCH, pp. 19–39.

87. Wang, Z., Burrell, L.S. & Lambert, W.J. (2002). Journal of Pharmaceutical Sciences 91, 1445–1455.

88. Kawakami, K., Miyoshi, K. & Ida, Y. (2005). Pharmacological Research 22, 1537–1543.

89. Tong, W. Q. (2007). Solvent Systems and Their Selection. In: *Pharmaceutics and Biopharmaceutics*, pp. 137–148.

Crystalline and Amorphous Solids

Geoff G. Z. Zhang and Deliang Zhou

2.1 INTRODUCTION

Of the several states of matter in which a substance can reside, the solid state is most commonly encountered and, therefore, the most important and relevant state for pharmaceutical development. Most of the pharmaceutical products on the market or formulations presently being developed are solid dosage forms. Even when a product is marketed or developed as a solution or a semi-solid formulation, a solid is usually selected and manufactured as an active pharmaceutical ingredient (API) for reasons such as the ability to crystallize and therefore to be purified, ease of handling, better chemical stability in comparison with liquids, etc. Therefore, understanding of various solid forms that may occur, as well as the rational selection of solid forms for development, is critical to the facile development of a particular chemical entity. Many books[1-7] and special journal issues[8-12] are devoted to this topic. This chapter, due to limitation of space, provides only a brief introduction to the fundamental principles and practical aspects of pharmaceutical solids. Interested readers are encouraged to read the books and reviews cited above.

2.2 DEFINITIONS AND CATEGORIZATION OF SOLIDS

The various types of pharmaceutical solids are shown in Figure 2.1. Solids can show differences externally or internally. External differences are referred to as the shape, or habit, or morphology of the particles, where the internal structures that make up the solid particles remain the same. Although important for pharmaceutical development, these are not discussed in this chapter. The focus of this chapter is on solids with distinct differences in their internal structure.

Based on the degree of long-range order/periodicity, solids are categorized into three groups. Amorphous phases are those solids that do not exhibit long-range order in any of the three physical dimensions. However, short-range order could exist for amorphous solids. Because of the importance of this class of solids to pharmaceutical development, it is discussed in detail in Section 2.7. If materials have long-range order in only one or two dimensions, they are liquid crystalline in nature. Liquid crystalline materials can be further categorized, based on the number of components contained therein, as is the case for crystalline solids. Since liquid crystals, with properties intermediate to conventional liquids and three-dimensional solids, are not frequently encountered, they will not be discussed in detail. The vast majority of pharmaceutical solids fall into the category of crystalline solids, because they exhibit long-range order in all three dimensions.

Crystalline solids can be further categorized into various sub-types based on the number of components that make up the solid internally, in a homogeneous fashion. The solid could be composed of the drug alone, or as adducts with one (binary), two (ternary), three (quaternary), etc. ... other chemical species. Although the number of other chemical species, apart from the drug itself, can increase without limit, it usually is a relatively low integer.

Developing Solid Oral Dosage Forms: Pharmaceutical Theory and Practice
ISBN: 978-0-444-53242-8

25

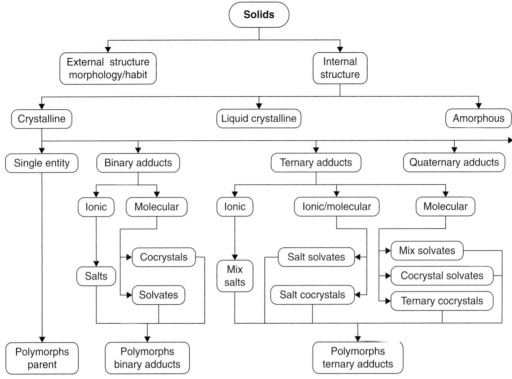

FIGURE 2.1   Categorization of pharmaceutical solids

When the overall chemical composition of solids is the same, they can nevertheless be different in internal structures. The ability of a substance to exist as two or more crystalline phases that have different arrangements and/or conformations of the molecules in a crystalline lattice is called polymorphism. These different solids are termed polymorphs. One point to emphasize is that, according to strict definition, different polymorphs are only different physically, not chemically. When these solids are melted or dissolved in solutions, they are exactly the same, both physically and chemically. However, in some special cases, the definition of polymorphism is extended slightly for convenience. There are many possible reasons for a substance to exhibit polymorphism and, sometimes, it may be difficult to pinpoint a single one. These reasons include packing; conformation (usually will exhibit different packing as well); hydrogen bonding pattern/motif; chirality, i.e., racemic compound versus racemic conglomerate (the definition is extended here because the racemic conglomerate is an equal molar physical mixture of the enantiomerically pure crystals, and therefore, is not a single phase); and tautomerism (the definition is, again, extended because different tautomers are chemically not equivalent). Polymorphism is relevant not only to solids composed of single components, but also to adducts of multiple components (binary, ternary, quaternary, etc. …). However, different polymorphs should have the same chemical composition, qualitatively and quantitatively, apart from the extension of definition mentioned above.

Adducts are formed where multiple chemical species are present in the crystalline lattices, again in a homogeneous fashion. Adducts can further be categorized based on the ionization states of these species: ionic, molecular or ionic/molecular. The same subcategorization described below applies to quaternary and higher adducts.

An ionic adduct is one that is made of ions only—cations and anions. For binary adducts, these are called salts. Various acids/bases can pair up to form different salts. The same acid/base pair can form salts of different stoichiometry. For ternary adducts these are called mixed salts, where one additional acid or base is involved in salt formation.

A molecular adduct is one that is made of neutral molecules. Depending on the physical state(s) of the additional component(s), it can be a solvate or a cocrystal. When this additional component is, in its pure form, a liquid at ambient conditions, the molecular adduct is called solvate. If the solvent is water, it is called hydrate. However, when the additional component is a solid at ambient conditions, the molecular adduct is called cocrystal. The boundary separating these two types of solids is somewhat arbitrary. Therefore, many published articles include solvates as cocrystals. However, there are distinct differences between the two types of solid adducts. In some situations, it may be helpful to distinguish them.

An ionic/molecular adduct is one that is made of both ionic and neutral molecules. This type of solid only exist for adducts having three or more components. One important thing to clarify here is that an acid or a base is not considered the same component as its ion. Thus a ternary ionic/molecular adduct is composed of one salt molecule (two components) and one neutral molecule. Again, based on the physical state of the neutral component, it could be a salt solvate or a salt cocrystal.

Unlike the previous categorization of solids,[13] this categorization system does not consider the structural details within the solids and, therefore, is widely applicable and is easier to use.

Cocrystal, although physically existed for quite some time and was formerly termed molecular complex, is a relatively new concept. Its definition has been a topic of discussion in recent years.[14–19] Based on these discussions, and the authors' personal viewpoint, cocrystal is here defined as "structurally homogeneous crystalline molecular adducts, made from components that are apparently neutral, that are by themselves solids at ambient conditions. The components are held together by interactions other than covalent or ionic bonds (hydrogen bonding, π–π, van der Waals, charge-transfer, halogen–halogen, etc.)."

Most adducts are stoichiometric in nature, i.e., there is a defined ratio between the components. However, some are nonstoichiometric,[20–25] for example cromolyn sodium and cefazolin sodium hydrates.[22,23]

In view of the importance of salts to pharmaceutical development, they will be discussed separately in Chapter 4. This chapter will include discussions on other crystalline solids, i.e., polymorphs, solvates/hydrates, cocrystals, and amorphous solids.

2.3 THERMODYNAMICS AND PHASE DIAGRAMS

Thermodynamics is one of the most important aspects in understanding pharmaceutical solids. Phase diagrams are usually constructed to express the thermodynamic relationships among various solid phases,

qualitatively or quantitatively. Depending on the types of solids, phase diagrams are constructed with respect to variables of different physical significance.

2.3.1 Polymorphs

Enantiotropy and Monotropy

When examining a pair of polymorphs, Polymorph I and Polymorph II, the stability relationship between the two polymorphs is determined **exclusively** by their free energy differences at different temperatures. The free energy of a particular solid is expressed in Equation 2.1:

$$G = H - TS \qquad (2.1)$$

where:
  G is the Gibbs free energy
  H is the enthalpy
  T is temperature
  S is the entropy.

Thus, the free energy for the transition from Polymorph I to Polymorph II:

$$\Delta G_{I \to II} = G_{II} - G_I = (H_{II} - TS_{II}) - (H_I - TS_I)$$
$$= \Delta H_{I \to II} - T \Delta S_{I \to II} \qquad (2.2)$$

$$\Delta H_{I \to II} = H_{II} - H_I \quad \text{and} \quad \Delta S_{I \to II} = S_{II} - S_I.$$

At any particular temperature, three different situations exist:

1. $\Delta G_{I \to II} < 0$: Polymorph II has lower free energy, and is therefore more stable than Polymorph I. The transition from Polymorph I to Polymorph II is a spontaneous process.
2. $\Delta G_{I \to II} > 0$: Polymorph II has higher free energy, and is therefore less stable than Polymorph I. The transition from Polymorph I to Polymorph II is not a spontaneous process. On the contrary, the transition from Polymorph II to Polymorph I is a spontaneous process.
3. $\Delta G_{I \to II} = 0$: Polymorph I and Polymorph II have the same free energy. Therefore, both polymorphs have equal stability. There will be no transition between the two polymorphs.

As shown in Equation 2.2, the free energy difference between the two polymorphs changes with temperature. The temperature at which the two polymorphs have equal stability is defined as the transition temperature (T_t).

If T_t is located below the melting points of both polymorphs, the two polymorphs are said to be enantiotropes, and the polymorphic system is said to exhibit enantiotropy or to be enantiotropic in nature. A representative phase diagram for an enantiotropic polymorphic system is shown in Figure 2.2(a). Below T_t, Polymorph I is more stable. Above T_t, Polymorph II is more stable. In this type of system the melting point of Polymorph I is lower than that of Polymorph II, although the melting point of Polymorph I may not be experimentally accessible because of facile solid–solid transition at lower temperatures.

If T_t is located above the melting points of both polymorphs, the two polymorphs are said to be monotropes, and the polymorphic system is said to exhibit monotropy or to be monotropic in nature. A representative phase diagram for a monotropic polymorphic system is shown in Figure 2.2(b). Throughout the temperature range, Polymorph I is more stable. Here, T_t is a hypothetical temperature, which is experimentally

not accessible. In this type of system the melting point of Polymorph I is higher than that of Polymorph II, although that of Polymorph II may not be experimentally accessible because of facile solid–solid transition at lower temperatures.

In constructing phase diagrams, the convention is to plot data for the stable phase using a solid line, and to use dotted lines to represent metastable phases, as shown in Figure 2.2.

Methods of Determining Stability Relationships Between Polymorphs

Many methods are available for determining stability relationships between polymorphs. Qualitative methods only determine the relationship with no precise knowledge of T_t. Quantitative methods, on the other hand, determine T_t first. The T_t is then compared to the melting points of each polymorphic form, and the stability relationship is thus defined. The relevant range of temperatures over which the stability relationship is of interest usually ranges from ambient temperatures to the melting point. However, in certain cases, the pertinent lower end of this range can extend below ambient temperatures, for instance, down to −50°C, which is relevant to freeze-drying processes.

Quantitative methods

Using heat of fusion data[26]   When heats of fusion can be experimentally determined, the stability relationship of the two polymorphs can be determined by calculating T_t and comparing this to the melting points. If T_t is lower than the lower melting point of the two polymorphs, the system is enantiotropic. If the calculated T_t is higher than the higher melting point of the two polymorphs, the system is monotropic.

Calculation of T_t begins with the design of a Hess cycle for the polymorphic transition, as shown in Figure 2.3, assuming that Polymorph II has a higher melting

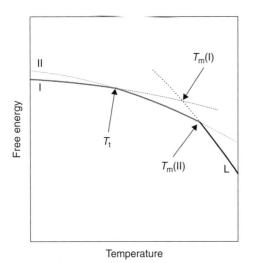

(a) Enantiotropy

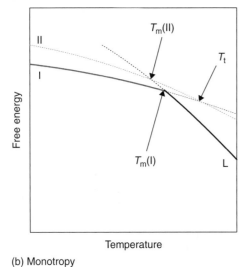

(b) Monotropy

FIGURE 2.2   Thermodynamic phase diagrams of polymorphs

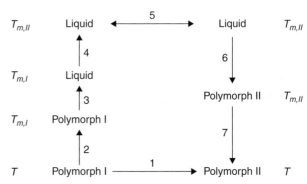

FIGURE 2.3   Hess cycle for polymorphic transition

TABLE 2.1 Thermodynamic quantities of individual processes in the Hess cycle of a polymorphic transition

Process	Nature of the process	ΔH	ΔS
1	Polymorph transition from I to II	$\Delta H_{I \to II}$	$\Delta S_{I \to II}$
2	Raise temperature of Polymorph I from T to its melting point	$\int_{T}^{T_{m,I}} C_{p,I}\, dT$	$\int_{T}^{T_{m,I}} \frac{C_{p,I}}{T}\, dT$
3	Melt Polymorph I to liquid at its melting point	$\Delta H_{m,I}$	$\Delta S_{m,I} = \frac{\Delta H_{m,I}}{T_{m,I}}$
4	Raise temperature of the liquid from melting point of Polymorph I to that of Polymorph II	$\int_{T_{m,I}}^{T_{m,II}} C_{p,L}\, dT$	$\int_{T_{m,I}}^{T_{m,II}} \frac{C_{p,L}}{T}\, dT$
5	Maintain the liquid at the melting point of Polymorph II	0	0
6	Crystallize Polymorph II from liquid at its melting point	$-\Delta H_{m,II}$	$-\Delta S_{m,II} = -\frac{\Delta H_{m,II}}{T_{m,II}}$
7	Lower temperature of Polymorph II to T from its melting point	$-\int_{T}^{T_{m,II}} C_{p,II}\, dT$	$-\int_{T}^{T_{m,II}} \frac{C_{p,II}}{T}\, dT$

point. Process 1 represents the polymorphic transition I → II at the temperature of interest. Alternatively, the same transition can be achieved by the series of Processes 2–7. The thermodynamic quantities, ΔH and ΔS, for each process are listed in Table 2.1.

Since Process 1 is equivalent to the sum of Processes 2–7, the enthalpy and entropy of Process 1 are the sums of the enthalpies and entropies of Processes 2–7 (Equation 2.3):

$$\Delta H_{I \to II} = \int_{T}^{T_{m,I}} C_{p,I}\, dT + \Delta H_{m,I} + \int_{T_{m,I}}^{T_{m,II}} C_{p,L}\, dT + 0$$

$$- \Delta H_{m,II} - \int_{T}^{T_{m,II}} C_{p,II}\, dT$$

$$= (\Delta H_{m,I} - \Delta H_{m,II}) - \int_{T}^{T_{m,I}} \Delta C_p\, dT$$

$$- \int_{T_{m,I}}^{T_{m,II}} (C_{p,II} - C_{p,L})\, dT$$

$$\approx (\Delta H_{m,I} - \Delta H_{m,II}) - \int_{T}^{T_{m,I}} \Delta C_p\, dT$$

$$\approx \Delta H_{m,I} - \Delta H_{m,II}$$

$$\Delta S_{I \to II} = \int_{T}^{T_{m,I}} \frac{C_{p,I}}{T}\, dT + \Delta S_{m,I} + \int_{T_{m,I}}^{T_{m,II}} \frac{C_{p,L}}{T}\, dT + 0$$

$$- \Delta S_{m,II} - \int_{T}^{T_{m,II}} \frac{C_{p,II}}{T}\, dT$$

$$= \left(\frac{\Delta H_{m,I}}{T_{m,I}} - \frac{\Delta H_{m,II}}{T_{m,II}} \right) - \int_{T}^{T_{m,I}} \frac{\Delta C_p}{T}\, dT$$

$$- \int_{T_{m,I}}^{T_{m,II}} \left(\frac{C_{p,II}}{T} - \frac{C_{p,L}}{T} \right) dT$$

$$\approx \left(\frac{\Delta H_{m,I}}{T_{m,I}} - \frac{\Delta H_{m,II}}{T_{m,II}} \right) - \int_{T}^{T_{m,I}} \frac{\Delta C_p}{T}\, dT$$

$$\approx \frac{\Delta H_{m,I}}{T_{m,I}} - \frac{\Delta H_{m,II}}{T_{m,II}} \tag{2.3}$$

The free energy of Process 1 can then be calculated from its enthalpy and entropy (Equation 2.4):

$$\Delta G_{I \to II} = \Delta H_{I \to II} - T \Delta S_{I \to II}$$

$$= (\Delta H_{m,I} - \Delta H_{m,II}) - \int_{T}^{T_{m,I}} \Delta C_p\, dT$$

$$- \int_{T_{m,I}}^{T_{m,II}} (C_{p,II} - C_{p,L})\, dT$$

$$- T \left(\frac{\Delta H_{m,I}}{T_{m,I}} - \frac{\Delta H_{m,II}}{T_{m,II}} \right) + T \int_{T}^{T_{m,I}} \frac{\Delta C_p}{T}\, dT$$

$$+ T \int_{T_{m,I}}^{T_{m,II}} \left(\frac{C_{p,II}}{T} - \frac{C_{p,L}}{T} \right) dT$$

$$= \left[\Delta H_{m,I}\left(1 - \frac{T}{T_{m,I}}\right) - \Delta H_{m,II}\left(1 - \frac{T}{T_{m,I}}\right)\right]$$

$$- \left(\int_{T}^{T_{m,I}} \Delta C_p \, dT - T\int_{T}^{T_{m,I}} \frac{\Delta C_p}{T} \, dT\right)$$

$$- \left[\int_{T_{m,I}}^{T_{m,II}} (C_{p,II} - C_{p,L})dT - T\int_{T_{m,I}}^{T_{m,II}} \left(\frac{C_{p,II}}{T} - \frac{C_{p,L}}{T}\right)dT\right]$$

$$\approx \left[\Delta H_{m,I}\left(1 - \frac{T}{T_{m,I}}\right) - \Delta H_{m,II}\left(1 - \frac{T}{T_{m,II}}\right)\right]$$

$$- \left(\int_{T}^{T_{m,I}} \Delta C_p \, dT - T\int_{T}^{T_{m,I}} \frac{\Delta C_p}{T} \, dT\right)$$

$$\approx \Delta H_{m,I}\left(1 - \frac{T}{T_{m,I}}\right) - \Delta H_{m,II}\left(1 - \frac{T}{T_{m,II}}\right) \quad (2.4)$$

In Equations 2.2, 2.3 and 2.4 the first approximation results from ignoring the heat capacity difference between Polymorph II and liquid, while the second approximation results from ignoring the heat capacity difference between Polymorph I and II.

Set $\Delta G_{I\rightarrow II}$ to zero, and the solution is the transition temperature. The caution to be exercised in this approach is that the solids of both polymorphs need to be highly crystalline; consequently, the melting points and heats of fusion can be accurately determined.

Using eutectic fusion data Calculation of T_t using heat of fusion data requires experimentally accessible data. Very often, compounds chemically decompose upon melting or physically transform before melting. In these cases, reliable heat of fusion data is not available. However, eutectic melting can be employed and eutectic melting data can be used to calculate the free energy difference between the polymorphs.[27] This method has been successfully applied to complicated polymorphic systems such as ROY,[28,29] chiral drugs such as tazofelone,[27,30] amino acids such as glycine,[27] and sugars such as D-mannitol.[27] Due to limitations of space and the complexity of derivation, interested readers are encouraged to study the original articles referenced above for derivations and applications.

Using solubility/intrinsic dissolution rate data The solubility of a solid is directly related to its free energy. If we define the standard state in solution as having an activity of one, which corresponds to the free energy

of zero, then the free energy of transfer from the standard state to Polymorph I is:

$$G_I - G_s = G_I = RT\ln a_I - RT\ln 1 = RT\ln a_I$$
$$= (H_I - H_s) - T(S_I - S_s) \quad (2.5)$$

The free energy of transfer from the standard state to Polymorph II is:

$$G_{II} - G_s = G_{II} = RT\ln a_{II} - RT\ln 1 = RT\ln a_{II}$$
$$= (H_{II} - H_s) - T(S_{II} - S_s) \quad (2.6)$$

Therefore, the free energy of transfer from Polymorph I to II is:

$$\Delta G_{I\rightarrow II} = G_{II} - G_I = (H_{II} - H_I) - T(S_{II} - S_I)$$
$$= \Delta H_{I\rightarrow II} - T\Delta S_{I\rightarrow II}$$
$$= RT\ln\left(\frac{a_{II}}{a_I}\right) = RT\ln\left(\frac{f_{II}}{f_I}\right)$$
$$= RT\ln\left(\frac{p_{II}}{p_I}\right) \approx RT\ln\left(\frac{m_{II}}{m_I}\right) \quad (2.7)$$

where:
  a is activity
  f is fugacity
  p is vapor pressure
  m is molal concentration.

The approximation is valid if Henry's law is obeyed. Application of the van't Hoff isochore gives:

$$\frac{d\ln a_I}{d(1/T)} = \frac{-(H_I - H_s)}{R} \approx \frac{d\ln m_I}{d(1/T)} \quad \text{and}$$

$$\frac{d\ln a_{II}}{d(1/T)} = \frac{-(H_{II} - H_s)}{R} \approx \frac{d\ln m_{II}}{d(1/T)} \quad (2.8)$$

From which it follows that:

$$\frac{d\ln\left(\frac{a_{II}}{a_I}\right)}{d(1/T)} = \frac{-(H_{II} - H_I)}{R} = \frac{-\Delta H_{I\rightarrow II}}{R}$$

$$= \frac{d\ln\left(\frac{f_{II}}{f_I}\right)}{d(1/T)} = \frac{d\ln\left(\frac{p_{II}}{p_I}\right)}{d(1/T)} \approx \frac{d\ln\left(\frac{m_{II}}{m_I}\right)}{d(1/T)} \quad (2.9)$$

When plotting the logarithms of the solubility values against reciprocal absolute temperature, a straight line should result if the solutions behave ideally. The temperature at which the two straight lines for the two polymorphs intersect corresponds to T_t. Alternatively, one could plot the logarithm of the solubility ratios against reciprocal absolute temperature. Again, a straight line should result. Extrapolation of this line to zero indicates the solubility ratio of the two poly-morphs is one, and the temperature corresponds to T_t.

When plotting solubility values against reciprocal temperature, weight-based concentration units, i.e., molal concentrations, are preferred over volume-based (molar) concentration units. This practice will elimi-nate errors due to thermal expansion of the solutions. However, there is minimum concern if the solubility ratios are being plotted, because the changes in volume cancel each other out.

If dissolution from the solid is solely diffusion controlled, there exists proportionality between the solubility and intrinsic dissolution rate (IDR) by the Noyes—Whitney equation.[31] One could measure the IDR at various temperatures for both polymorphs, analyze the data in the same way as that for solubility, and obtain the T_t. This method is particularly helpful when phase transitions occur readily, yet not instanta-neously. However, one should exercise caution when comparing dissolution rates of ionic or ionizable com-pounds in protic solvents, because many such dissolu-tion rates have significant contributions from reactive dissolution.

Using solubility/intrinsic dissolution rate and heat of solution data   The temperature dependence of solubility is related to the heat of solution, again for ideal solutions, as shown in Equation 2.8. If the solubility and the heat of solution are measured at one temperature, the entire solubility − temperature curve can be constructed. Comparing the curves for both polymorphs yields the T_t.

Alternatively, one can measure the solubility/IDR ratio at one temperature, which yields the free energy difference at that temperature. The enthalpy difference between the two polymorphs is the dif-ference in the heats of solution (which could also be measured by other means). A simple calculation will yield the T_t.

Qualitative methods

Using the definition   The stability relationship between the two polymorphs at one particular temperature can be determined by one of the techniques below.

1. The higher melting polymorph is more stable at higher temperatures;
2. When spontaneous transition is observed, the resulting polymorph is the more stable phase at the temperature where the transition is observed. The transition could be solid−solid transition isothermally or during heating, or solution-mediated in a non-solvate forming solvent;

3. The polymorph with lower solubility in a non-solvate forming solvent is more stable.

If the relationships that are determined at two differ-ent temperatures are the same, the polymorphic sys-tem is monotropic within this temperature range. On the other hand, if the determined relationships are different, then the system is enantiotropic within this temperature range. When an enantiotropic relation-ship is affirmed, the transition temperature is usually bracketed to a narrower range by determining the stability order at a series of temperatures.

Using the heat of fusion rule   To help decide the rela-tionship between two polymorphs, Burger and Ramberger[32,33] developed four thermodynamic rules. One of the two most useful, and reliable, rules is the heat of fusion rule:

> "If the higher melting form has the lower heat of fusion, the two forms are usually enantiotropic, otherwise they are monotropic."

Figure 2.4 illustrates the heat of fusion rule from a thermodynamic point of view. Several precautions should be taken in applying this rule:

1. be aware of the normal experimental errors in melting points and heats of fusion, especially when they are close for the two polymorphs;
2. use materials of high crystallinity and high purity. Solids of lower crystallinity usually have lower melting points and heats of fusion than those having high crystallinity. Melting point depression by impurities is a well-known phenomenon.

Using the heat of transition rule   Another useful and reliable rule, developed by Burger and Ramberger,[32,33] is the heat of transition rule for solid-state transitions, which states:

> "If an endothermic transition is observed at some tem-perature, it may be assumed that there is a transition point below it, i.e., the two forms are related enantiotropically. If an exothermic transition is observed at some temperature, it may be assumed that there is no transition point below it, i.e., the two forms are either related monotropically or the transition temperature is higher."

Again, Figure 2.4 illustrates the thermodynamic point of view. Several precautions should be taken in apply-ing this rule:

1. be aware that a crystallization exotherm from amorphous phase could be confused with a polymorphic transition. Therefore, materials of high crystallinity should be used in the study. It is a good practice to examine the solid phase after heating beyond the transition to ensure that the exotherm corresponds to a polymorphic transition;

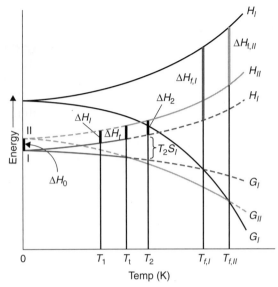

(a) Enantiotropy

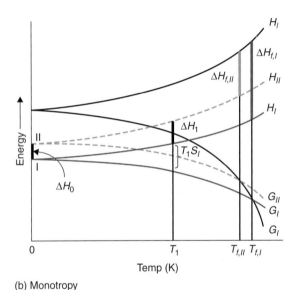

(b) Monotropy

FIGURE 2.4 Schematic illustration of Burger and Ramberger thermodynamic rules (replotted according to reference 33)

2. one can use the overall heat of transition when the polymorphic transition goes through melting and recrystallization. However, the heat of fusion of the recrystallized polymorph should be comparable to the reference material to ensure complete crystallization and thus the accuracy of the overall heat of transition.

2.3.2 Solvates/Hydrates

Of the many solvents that are incorporated into the crystal lattice, water is by far the most important for

pharmaceutical development. Therefore, all discussions and derivations in this section will use hydrates as examples. However, the principles described are the same and the equations derived can be easily converted and applied to solvates.

Anhydrate/Hydrate Equilibrium at Constant Temperature

The equilibrium between the anhydrate and hydrate of a drug (D) at a constant temperature and total pressure can be achieved by equilibrating through the vapor phase. The equilibrium is represented by Equation 2.10:

$$D \cdot nH_2O_{(solid)} \xrightarrow{\quad K_d \quad} D_{(solid)} + nH_2O_{(vapor)} \qquad (2.10)$$

where:

$D_{(solid)}$ is the anhydrate solid
$D \cdot nH_2O_{(solid)}$ is the hydrate solid
n is the stoichiometry of the hydrate
K_d is the hydration/dehydration equilibrium constant between the two solids.

The equilibrium constant can be described by Equation 2.11, and then simplified based on the assumption that water vapor acts as an ideal gas, and the activities of the solids are taken to be unity:

$$K_d^{vapor} = \frac{\left[a_{D_{(solid)}} \right]\left[a_{H_2O_{(vapor)}}^c \right]^n}{\left[a_{D \cdot nH_2O_{(solid)}} \right]} = \left[a_{H_2O_{(vapor)}}^c \right]^n$$

$$= [RH^c]^n = \left[\frac{p^c}{p^s} \right]^n \qquad (2.11)$$

In this equation, a is the activity, superscript c represents critical values, RH represents relative humidity, p^c represents the critical water vapor pressure, and p^s represents the saturated water vapor pressure at this temperature.

Three situations exist:

1. $p > p^c$; $RH > RH^c$; $a_{H_2O_{(vapor)}} > a_{H_2O_{(vapor)}}^c$: The hydrate is more stable than the anhydrate. The anhydrate will, therefore, spontaneously convert to the hydrate thermodynamically.
2. $p < p^c$; $RH < RH^c$; $a_{H_2O_{(vapor)}} < a_{H_2O_{(vapor)}}^c$: The anhydrate is more stable than the hydrate. The hydrate will, therefore, spontaneously convert to the anhydrate thermodynamically.
3. $p = p^c$; $RH = RH^c$; $a_{H_2O_{(vapor)}} = a_{H_2O_{(vapor)}}^c$: The hydrate and the anhydrate have equal stability, they will coexist thermodynamically. There will be no transformation in either direction.

A typical phase diagram for anhydrate/hydrate is shown in Figure 2.5. The curved portion, at high RHs, represents deliquescence and further dilution of the solution. Anhydrate/hydrate equilibration through the vapor phase is a slow process, and it can take weeks to months in order to achieve equilibrium. Therefore, studies are usually conducted to take advantage of the higher mobility in the solution state to attain equilibrium within a short period of time.[34,35] In these studies, water miscible organic solvents were employed to systematically modify the water activities in these solutions. Solids of anhydrate or hydrate, or mixtures of the two, were suspended in a series of the above solutions, and equilibrated at a defined temperature with agitation. The solids were recovered after certain times, much shorter than the times required for equilibration through the vapor phase, and examined by appropriate analytical techniques. The stability order at each individual water activity value was determined by the nature of the solid recovered. The critical water activity was then bracketed to a narrow range. Once developed, this method has been applied to many other anhydrate/hydrate systems with success.[36–41]

When an organic/water solution is in equilibrium with its vapor phase, the water activities in the solution and the vapor phases are the same. Therefore, it is common to further "equate" the water activity in solution to the relative humidity in the vapor phase. For example, 0.35 water activity is equivalent to 35% RH. The critical water activity values obtained from solution equilibration for anhydrate/hydrate systems are also "equated" to the critical relative humidity values obtained from the vapor phase equilibrium (RH^c). The reason why this can be done is demonstrated below.

In the case of solution phase equilibrium, water molecules released via dehydration are not present as

water vapor, instead they simply become part of the solution. Therefore, the equilibrium of interest, and the corresponding equilibrium constant are shown below in Equation 2.12 and Equation 2.13, respectively:

$$\text{D} \cdot n\text{H}_2\text{O}_{(solid)} \xleftrightarrow{\ K_d\ } \text{D}_{(solid)} + n\text{H}_2\text{O}_{(solution)} \quad (2.12)$$

$$K_d^{solution} = \frac{\left[a_{D_{(solid)}}\right]\left[a_{H_2O_{(solution)}}^c\right]^n}{\left[a_{D \cdot nH_2O_{(solid)}}\right]} = \left[a_{H_2O_{(solution)}}^c\right]^n \quad (2.13)$$

This equilibrium can be converted to the Equation 2.10 type of equilibrium, i.e., water as vapor through a further equilibrium of solution–vapor under constant water activity (Equation 2.14). However, the process of vaporization under constant water activity is at equilibrium, having ΔG of zero and K_{vap} of unity.

$$n\text{H}_2\text{O}_{(solution)} \xleftrightarrow{\ K_{vap}\ } n\text{H}_2\text{O}_{(vapor)} \quad (2.14)$$

Addition of Equations 2.12 and 2.14 affords Equation 2.10. Therefore, the equilibrium constant in Equation 2.10 is the product of those in Equations 2.12 and 2.14 (Equation 2.15):

$$K_d^{vapor} = K_{vap} \cdot K_d^{solution} = K_d^{solution} \quad (2.15)$$

Thus, the equilibrium constant obtained by equilibrating through the vapor phase is equal to that obtained through equilibrating through the solution phase. In the following section, superscripts and subscripts will not be used to differentiate the different routes of determination.

Temperature Dependence of Anhydrate/ Hydrate Equilibrium[42]

When temperature varies, the van't Hoff equation (also known as the van't Hoff isochore) which describes the temperature dependence of any equilibrium constant can be applied. This affords the determination of the temperature dependence of the critical water activity or relative humidity ($a_{H_2O}^c$ or RH^c), and the critical water vapor pressure (p^c), thus establishing the complete phase diagram with regard to both relative humidity (or water vapor pressure), and temperature. Applying the van't Hoff equation to the anhydrate/ hydrate equilibrium, Equation 2.16 is obtained:

$$\frac{d\ln K_d}{dT} = \frac{nd\ln(a_{H_2O}^c)}{dT} = \frac{nd\ln(\text{RH}^c)}{dT}$$
$$= \frac{nd\ln\left(\dfrac{p^c}{p^s}\right)}{dT} = \frac{\Delta H_d}{RT^2} \quad (2.16)$$

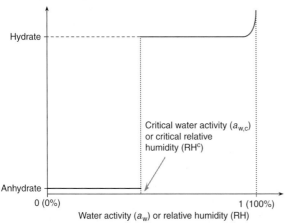

Identity of the crystal form/water content

Hydrate

Critical water activity ($a_{w,c}$) or critical relative humidity (RH^c)

Anhydrate

0 (0%)   1 (100%)

Water activity (a_w) or relative humidity (RH)

FIGURE 2.5 Thermodynamic phase diagram of anhydrate/hydrate pair

where ΔH_d is the dehydration enthalpy and R is the gas constant. Rearranging Equation 2.16 affords Equation 2.17:

$$d \ln K_d = d \ln(a_{H_2O}^c) = d \ln(RH^c) = d \ln \left(\frac{p^c}{p^s} \right)$$

$$= -\frac{\Delta H_d}{nR} d \ln \left(\frac{1}{T} \right) \qquad (2.17)$$

Assuming a constant dehydration enthalpy within the temperature range studied, the definite integral of this differential equation (Equation 2.17) between temperatures T_1 and T_2 is given by Equation 2.18:

$$\frac{\Delta H_d}{nR} \left(\frac{1}{T_1} - \frac{1}{T_2} \right) = \ln K_d^2 - \ln K_d^1$$

$$= \ln(a_{H_2O}^c)_2 - \ln(a_{H_2O}^c)_1$$

$$= \ln(RH^c)_2 - \ln(RH^c)_1$$

$$= \ln \left(\frac{p^c}{p^s} \right)_2 - \ln \left(\frac{p^c}{p^s} \right)_1 \qquad (2.18)$$

Since $\Delta G_d = \Delta H_d - T\Delta S_d$ and $\Delta G_d = -RT \ln K_d$, it follows that:

$$\ln K_d = \ln(a_{H_2O}^c) = \ln(RH^c) = \ln \left(\frac{p^c}{p^s} \right) = -\frac{\Delta H_d}{nRT} + \frac{\Delta S_d}{nR}$$

$$(2.19)$$

Here ΔS_d is the dehydration entropy. Therefore, a plot of the natural logarithm of K_d or $a_{H_2O}^c$, or RH^c, or p^c/p^s, versus the reciprocal temperature gives a straight line. The slope of the line is equal to $-\Delta H_d/nR$ and the intercept is equal to $\Delta S_d/nR$. Based on this set of equations, and the fact that dehydration is endothermic, it is apparent that the critical water activity or critical relative humidity increases upon raising the temperature. Therefore, it is desirable to keep hydrates in a cool, humid environment to avoid dehydration.

Another important parameter of the anhydrate/hydrate system is the critical temperature, T_c, which is defined as the temperature at which the critical water activity is unity or critical relative humidity is 100%. In other words, it is the higher limit of the temperature range where a hydrate is thermodynamically stable at some water activity or relative humidity. At temperatures higher than T_c, hydrate cannot be the stable phase. Applying this to Equation 2.18 affords Equation 2.20:

$$\ln K_d = \ln(a_{H_2O}^c) = \ln(RH^c) = \ln \left(\frac{p^c}{p^s} \right)$$

$$= \frac{\Delta H_d}{nRT_c} - \frac{\Delta H_d}{nRT} \qquad (2.20)$$

Comparing Equation 2.19 and Equation 2.20, it is apparent that $T_c = \Delta H_d / \Delta S_d$. Thus, T_c is characteristic of the anhydrate/hydrate system of interest.

In studying the physical stability of hydrates, p^c is frequently used. Therefore, it is useful to extend the above analysis beyond K_d, $a_{H_2O}^c$, RH^c, and p^c/p^s. Rearranging Equation 2.18 affords Equation 2.21:

$$\ln \frac{(p^c)_2}{(p^c)_1} - \ln \frac{(p^s)_2}{(p^s)_1} = \frac{\Delta H_d}{nR} \left(\frac{1}{T_1} - \frac{1}{T_2} \right) \qquad (2.21)$$

The temperature dependence of saturated water vapor pressure can be described by the well-known Clausius–Clapeyron equation (Equation 2.22):

$$\ln \frac{(p^s)_2}{(p^s)_1} = \frac{\Delta H_{vap}}{R} \left(\frac{1}{T_1} - \frac{1}{T_2} \right) \qquad (2.22)$$

Here ΔH_{vap} is the enthalpy of vaporization of water at the temperature of interest. Coupling Equation 2.21 and Equation 2.22 yields Equation 2.23:

$$\ln \frac{(p^c)_2}{(p^c)_1} = \left(\frac{\Delta H_d}{nR} + \frac{\Delta H_{vap}}{R} \right) \left(\frac{1}{T_1} - \frac{1}{T_2} \right) \qquad (2.23)$$

Equation 2.23 dictates that the plot of $\ln p^c$ against the reciprocal temperature will exhibit a greater slope than that of $\ln K_d$ ($\Delta H_d/nR + \Delta H_{vap}/R$ versus $\Delta H_d/nR$). This phenomenon was previously observed, yet not explained.[43]

2.3.3 Cocrystals

Since cocrystals differ from solvates only by the physical state of the pure components, the stability treatment is expected to be analogous to that for solvates. Indeed, an extension of the stability treatment was recently applied to cocrystals,[44] and is discussed below. The equilibrium among the drug (D), the cocrystal former (CCF), and the corresponding cocrystal (CC, i.e., D · nCCF) are shown in Equation 2.24. In this case, the CCF is assumed to come into intimate contact with the drug through a solution, however, the treatment is valid if the contact is achieved by other routes:

$$D_{solid} + nCCF_{solution} \xleftrightarrow{K_c} CC_{solid} \qquad (2.24)$$

Here n is the stoichiometry of the cocrystal and K_c is the cocrystal formation equilibrium constant. Analogous to the anhydrate/hydrate or non-solvate/solvate system, K_c can be expressed by the activities of the species involved in the equilibrium (Equation

2.25), and simplified based on the assumption that CCF molecules behave ideally in the solution, and the activities of the solids are taken to be unity.

$$K_c = \frac{\left[a_{CC_{(solid)}}\right]}{\left[a_{D_{(solid)}}\right]\left[a^c_{CCF_{(solution)}}\right]^n} = \left[a^c_{CCF_{(solution)}}\right]^{-n} \quad (2.25)$$

Here $a^c_{CCF_{(solution)}}$ is the critical CCF activity in solution (or expressed as $a_{CCF,c}$). As a first approximation, the activity of CCF in the solution equals the ratio of the concentration of the free CCF (uncomplexed with D) in solution, and the solubility of CCF in the absence of D in the same solvent. Again, there exist three situations:

1. $\left[a_{CCF_{(solution)}}\right] < \left[a^c_{CCF_{(solution)}}\right]$: D is favored over CC. CC will, therefore, spontaneously decompose to D thermodynamically.

2. $\left[a_{CCF_{(solution)}}\right] > \left[a^c_{CCF_{(solution)}}\right]$: CC is favored over D. CC will, therefore, spontaneously form from D and CCF thermodynamically.

3. $\left[a_{CCF_{(solution)}}\right] = \left[a^c_{CCF_{(solution)}}\right]$: D and CC have equal stability, they will coexist in a suspension of the CCF solution.

The same equations can be written if the drug is in solution and CCF and CC are in the solid state. This thermodynamic treatment can be easily extended to cocrystal systems with multiple stoichiometry. The phase diagrams are shown in Figure 2.6.

2.3.4 Amorphous Solids

If a crystalline solid is heated beyond its melting temperature and cooled back to its original temperature, and if sufficient time is not allowed for nucleation to occur, the liquid will become amorphous at temperatures below its melting point. That is, it will lose all long-range order. Initially, the supercooled liquid was able to adjust itself to the changing environment (temperature), giving off excess enthalpy, entropy, and volume, following the equilibrium line extended from the liquid state (Figure 2.7). The amorphous material in this temperature range is called a rubber or a supercooled liquid. However, at a certain lower temperature, due to the increased viscosity and decreased molecular mobility, the amorphous material will not be able to continue to follow the equilibrium line extended from the liquid state. Instead, it will deviate from the line, quenching the excess thermal motions that accommodate excess quantities such as free energy, enthalpy, entropy, and volume. The amorphous phase in this temperature range is called a glass.

This transition of states is called a glass transition, and the temperature at which this transition occurs is called the glass transition temperature (T_g). The glassy state is a kinetically frozen state, and is not thermodynamically stable. Therefore, a glass will relax gradually over time, releasing excess enthalpy, entropy, and volume to the environment so as to achieve a more stable state. This process is termed physical aging or annealing (Secion 2.7.1).

Theoretically, one could continue to extrapolate the liquid line beyond T_g. In doing so, it will eventually intersect the crystalline line, and pass beyond the line. This presents a conceptual contradiction, called the Kauzmann paradox,[45] which dictates that the disordered supercooled liquid has less entropy than the ordered crystal. The temperature at which this occurs is called the Kauzmann temperature (T_K). In reality, this entropy crisis is avoided through the intervening

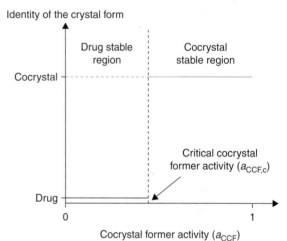

(a) With respect to the activity of the cocrystal former

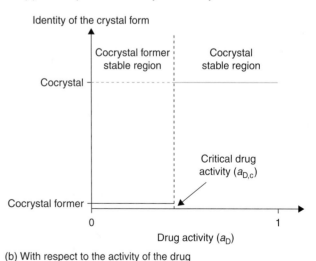

(b) With respect to the activity of the drug

FIGURE 2.6 Thermodynamic phase diagrams of cocrystals

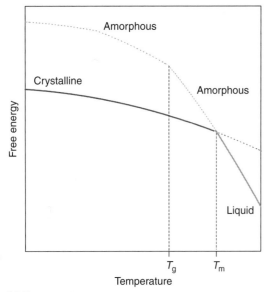

(a) Free energy

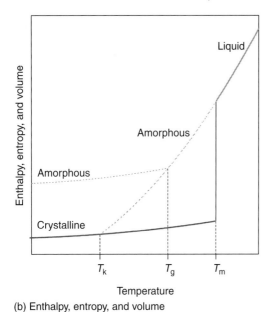

(b) Enthalpy, entropy, and volume

FIGURE 2.7　Phase diagrams of amorphous solids

thermodynamic properties such as volume, enthalpy, and entropy. However, the isobaric expansivity, α, isothermal compressibility, κ, and isobaric heat capacity, C_p, all show a step change around T_g, indicating a second-order phase transition according to the definition by Ehrenfest.[46]

The amorphous phase presents unique characteristics and challenges to pharmaceutical development, and is discussed in detail in Section 2.7.

2.4　PHARMACEUTICAL RELEVANCE AND IMPLICATIONS

As mentioned at the beginning of this chapter, crystalline solids are especially relevant to pharmaceutical development. Regardless of the types of formulations, APIs are mostly crystalline. The majority of APIs are polymorphs of the parents and salts.[47] A significant proportion of APIs are hydrates.[47] Solvates with various organic solvents are not usually used as APIs. However, they are frequently encountered in crystallization and characterization of pharmaceutical solids. Cocrystals, a re-emerging class of solids, have yet to be used intentionally in pharmaceutical products. However, they offer the potential to engineer properties of solids critical to pharmaceutical development. Although crystalline APIs are usually preferred during pharmaceutical development, varying degrees of amorphous contents can be generated inadvertently during pharmaceutical processing, such as milling, wet granulation, drying, and compaction (see Chapter 5). Many pharmaceutical excipients, such as naturally existing polymers, e.g., cellulose and starch; synthetic polymers, e.g., poly(methyl methacrylate), poly(acrylic acid), and poly(glycolic acid), as well as other chemically modified natural or synthetic polymers, are either amorphous or partially amorphous. Small amounts of amorphous content exist in almost every crystalline API. The presence of amorphous content in the API itself or other components of a drug product may have confounding impacts on the physico-chemical properties and ultimate performance of the drug product.

Owing to the differences in the internal structures [composition, dimensions, shape, symmetry, capacity (number of molecules), and void volumes of their unit cells for crystalline phases, and the lack of periodicity for the amorphous phases], various solids exhibit a variety of different properties. Over the years, these properties have been summarized for polymorphs,[48–51] but are properly applicable to all solids. These properties are listed in Table 2.2.

glass transition. Compared to its crystalline counterpart, the amorphous solid possesses excess thermodynamic quantities, including free energy, enthalpy, entropy, and volume (Figure 2.7). These excess quantities are termed "configurational" quantities. From the phase diagram (Figure 2.7) it is clear that, unlike the polymorphs, solvates, and cocrystals, amorphous phases are always metastable with respect to the crystalline phases, regardless of the environment (temperature, pressure, etc.). Unlike the first-order phase transitions, such as melting or vaporization, no discontinuity exists at the glass transition for

TABLE 2.2 Physical properties that differ among various solids[51]

1. Packing properties
   a. Molar volume and density
   b. Refractive index
   c. Conductivity, electrical and thermal
   d. Hygroscopicity
2. Thermodynamic properties
   a. Melting and sublimation temperatures
   b. Internal energy (i.e., structural energy)
   c. Enthalpy (i.e., heat content)
   d. Heat capacity
   e. Entropy
   f. Free energy and chemical potential
   g. Thermodynamic activity
   h. Vapor pressure
   i. Solubility
3. Spectroscopic properties
   a. Electronic transitions (i.e., ultraviolet—visible absorption spectra)
   b. Vibrational transitions (i.e., infrared absorption spectra and Raman spectra)
   c. Rotational transitions (i.e., far infrared or microwave absorption spectra)
   d. Nuclear spin transitions (i.e., nuclear resonance spectra)
4. Kinetic properties
   a. Dissolution rate
   b. Rates of solid-state reactions
   c. Stability
5. Surface properties
   a. Surface free energy
   b. Interfacial tensions
   c. Habit (i.e., shape)
6. Mechanical properties
   a. Hardness
   b. Tensile strength
   c. Compactibility, tableting
   d. Handling, flow, and blending

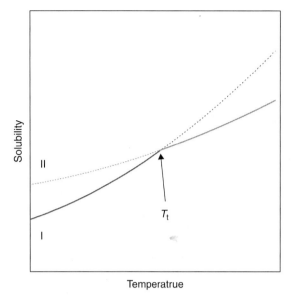

(a) Enantiotropy

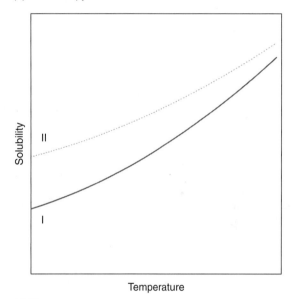

(b) Monotropy

FIGURE 2.8 Solubility values of polymorphs as a function of temperature

Many properties that differ among crystal forms provide the means to detect them, such as melting points and spectroscopic properties. Some properties are particularly important for pharmaceutical development, having significant impact on the performance and quality of drug products. They will be discussed in more detail in the following sections.

2.4.1 Solubility

As shown in Section 2.3.1, the solubility values of different polymorphs are directly related to their free energy. Therefore, different polymorphs will have different solubility in the same solvent, and the difference in the solubility will be a function of temperature (Figure 2.8). At one temperature (except for T_t), the metastable polymorph will be more soluble than the stable polymorph. It is this difference in solubility that is causing the difference in dissolution rates, and

driving the solution-mediated phase transformation (Section 2.5.3) for polymorphs. A survey of the solubility differences between polymorphic pairs has been conducted ($n = 81$).[52] The general trend reveals that the ratio of polymorph solubility is typically less than 2, although occasionally higher ratios can be observed.[52] Based on thermodynamics, the solubility ratio of the polymorphs is independent of the nature of the solvents, provided that Henry's law is obeyed (Section 2.3.1). In most dilute solutions, this is a valid statement.

Adducts (solvates, hydrates, and cocrystals), on the other hand, exhibit different solubility behavior. The solubility ratio, even the rank order, changes in solvents having different activity values. As in the case of polymorphs, this is also driven by thermodynamics. In pure organic solvents, where the activity of the solvent is nearly one, the solvate with the specific solvent will be the most stable phase, and have the lowest solubility. Other solid phases, such as polymorphs, hydrates, amorphous phases, and solvates with other organic solvents, will be metastable and have higher solubility values. Hydrates, as a special case of solvates, will have the same characteristics. In the same survey ($n = 24$),[52] a similar trend is observed for anhydrate/hydrate solubility ratios, although anhydrate/hydrate solubility ratios appear to be more spread out and higher than the typical ratio for polymorphs. The solubility of cocrystals is a function of the concentration of the cocrystal former.[53,54] The dependence is very much analogous to the solubility product (K_{sp}) for insoluble salts.

Thermodynamic analysis of amorphous phases indicates that it possesses higher free energy than its crystalline counterpart at all temperatures below the melting point. Therefore, amorphous materials will have higher solubility than crystalline solids at all temperatures (below the melting point) in any solvent.[55–59] This is of special interest to the delivery of poorly soluble drug molecules, and oral bioavailability enhancement.

2.4.2 Dissolution Rate and Bioavailability

As mentioned earlier, if dissolution from the solid is solely diffusion-controlled, proportionality exists between the solubility and dissolution rate by the Noyes–Whitney equation.[31] Thus, the differences in solubility translate directly to the differences in intrinsic dissolution rates among various solids. When particle size and distribution are similar, they also translate to the powder dissolution rates. Some of the classic examples include dissolution of the solid forms of succinylsulfathiazole[60] and iopanoic acid.[61] As generally understood, oral absorption is determined by the rate of dissolution of a dosage form in the gastrointestinal (GI) tract, and the rate of drug molecule permeation through the GI membrane. Drug absorption can be improved by rendering the drug amorphous for biopharmaceutical classification system (BCS) class II and IV compounds, where low solubility presents a significant barrier for oral absorption. Therefore, utilizing metastable solid forms, such as amorphous phases, and amorphous solid dispersions,[62–69] is a powerful tool in combating the poor ADME profiles of many modern drug candidates. Selecting the appropriate solid forms for development is thus critical to the facile development of high quality products.

One important consideration in this approach is that this solubility and dissolution enhancement is a transient effect. The higher concentrations achieved in the *in vitro* or *in vivo* dissolution media, beyond the equilibrium solubility, create driving forces for the nucleation and crystallization of the stable phases. Eventually, the stable phases will nucleate, and crystallize. However, certain time is required before the depletion of concentrations in solution. During this lag time, significant absorption could be accomplished. For some compounds, the extremely high permeability leads to the effective transport of the molecules through GI membrane. In these cases, the concentration build-up in the GI fluid will not occur.

2.4.3 Hygroscopicity

Moisture interacts with solids via four primary modes: adsorption, absorption, deliquescence, and lattice incorporation.[70,71] Water molecules can be adsorbed onto a solid surface by interacting with the molecules on the surface. Since water is a polar molecule capable of forming hydrogen bonding, polar moieties on the solid surface are important factors governing the affinity towards water adsorption. Particle size plays a role in moisture uptake by affecting the available surface area. Under normal conditions, water adsorption leads to monolayer formation, as well as a few additional molecular layers at higher relative humidity (RH). The solid–water interactions are the strongest between surface and water molecules in the monolayer, and become weaker with increasing distance from the surface. Therefore, water molecules in the adsorbed layers beyond the monolayer more resemble the bulk water, which may bear some importance to chemical instability.

A more significant mode of water–solid interactions is perhaps the absorption or sorption, which refers to the water molecules' penetration into the bulk solid, incorporation into the defects or amorphous regions, and formation of a solution. Due to the high free energy nature of the amorphous form, its affinity toward water molecules is much greater, resulting in much elevated moisture sorption. It has been shown that moisture adsorption can only account for a very insignificant portion of moisture content typically encountered in pharmaceutical solids (e.g., a few percent), for which the sorption mechanism is primarily responsible.[72] Deliquescence refers to the formation of a saturated solution around the solids when exceeding its critical RH. This mode of water–solid interaction is only important for relatively water-soluble compounds at high RH. Hydrates form when water molecules are incorporated into the crystal lattice. In this case, a critical water activity or relative humidity exists that governs the physical stability of the respective hydrate form (Section 2.3.2).

Moisture uptake can be greatly impacted by solid forms. Adsorption is a surface property therefore the surface of a solid form is a determining factor. In that sense, a more stable polymorph may not necessarily adsorb the least amount of moisture, what matters are the moieties which are exposed on the surface. However, the amorphous content or defects are the primary cause of the moisture uptake normally seen with pharmaceuticals, as discussed above, due to its high energetic nature, and a different mode of interaction. A small amount of amorphous content virtually exists for every crystalline API, and is likely exacerbated by API treatments such as milling, and by formulation processing such as wet granulation and drying. Therefore, its influence on moisture uptake and distribution, and subsequent product attributes, could be enormous.

2.4.4 Reactivity and Chemical Stability

Solid forms can impact reactivity and chemical stability of both API and drug in the finished product. The way in which solid forms influence their chemical stability is more apparent by examining the mechanisms of "solid-state" reactions.

Topochemical Reactions

The reactivity of a solid in a topochemical (or true solid-state) reaction is completely determined by its crystal lattice. This type of reaction is facilitated by proper positioning and orientation of the reacting moieties in the crystal lattices, and therefore requires minimum movement of the reacting molecules. Molecular packing in the crystal lattice is the primary factor dictating the rate of a topochemical reaction.

Solid forms are the best manifestation of topochemical reactions based on their very nature. Solid forms can determine end-reaction product. For example, 2-ethoxycinnamic acid showed polymorph-dependent photodimerization products.[73] The α polymorph formed a cis-dimer, the β polymorph formed a trans-dimer, while dimerization was not observed in solution. Solid forms can also determine whether a reaction can occur. For example, p-methylcinnamic acid undergoes photodimerization only with the β polymorph.[74] Its α polymorph is not reactive, because the distance separating the neighboring cinnamic acid double bonds is too long to allow for a [2 + 2] cyclization. For prednisolone and hydrocortisones, the reactivity towards O_2 was only observed in the

hexagonal solvates, where solvent channels were speculated to allow oxygen to access host molecules.[75,76] Increasing molecular mobility by destroying a crystalline order can actually slow down a topochemical reaction. For example, the rearrangement of methyl p-dimethylaminobezenesulfonate proceeded 25 times faster in solid-state than in the melt.[77,78]

Non-topochemical Reactions

Degradation of most pharmaceuticals is not topochemical in nature. These reactions require significant movement of the reacting molecules and are not true solid-state reactions. Nevertheless, these reactions are modulated by the physico-chemical and particle characteristics of the solids, such as crystallinity, moisture content, solubility, pH of the aqueous surface layer, particle size, melting temperature, etc., although it may be difficult to deconvolute the respective contributions.

Chemical stability of most pharmaceuticals is modulated by moisture. The earlier model proposed by Leeson–Mattocks[79] sheds some light on drug degradation, where a film of saturated solution was assumed to form around solid particles, although deliquescence is not generally expected below critical RH. The concepts of tightly bound (e.g., monolayer) and loosely bound (e.g., those beyond monolayer) moisture may also shed some light, despite their oversimplified nature. Probably the most significant is the moisture sorption into amorphous regions or defects, leading to significant increase in moisture uptake, as discussed previously.

Besides the topochemical reactions where crystal lattice dictates reactivity, solid forms can impact chemical stability by modifying the particular characteristics. First, the moieties exposed on crystal surfaces could be significantly different among different solid forms (or morphologies), which could either accelerate or inhibit a particular reaction. For example, the reactivity of flufenamic acid polymorphs with ammonia was related to accessibility of ammonium to host molecules on major faces, but not to the relative energetics of the polymorphs.[80] Secondly, the solid forms can differ in their aqueous solubility, as mentioned previously, which is certainly important for degradation through the Leeson–Mattocks model. Thirdly, moisture sorption could be drastically more significant for certain solid forms. Amorphous contents have higher affinity to water molecules, and form solutions with the latter. Since water is a great plasticizer, the water molecules absorbed into the amorphous regions can cause significant increase in molecular mobility, and are potentially harmful to chemical stability.[72,81] Certain higher energetic solid forms that may be used in pharmaceutical development, such as "desolvated solvate," tend to absorb more moisture and cause greater chemical degradation. Complete or partial phase transformations can occur inadvertently during manufacturing which can profoundly change chemical degradation in drug products.[82]

2.4.5 Mechanical Properties

In different solids, the molecules are arranged differently. The nature and extent of interactions among the molecules also varies among different solids. Intuitively, one would anticipate that these solids would respond differently under mechanical stresses. Under compression, plastic flow along slip planes has been well-documented as a mechanism for consolidation.[83] In the case of acetaminophen polymorphs, the stable polymorph (Form I, monoclinic) was found to be poorly compressible, requiring a significant amount of excipients to form tablets.[84–86] On the other hand, metastable polymorphs (Form II, orthorhombic) have been reported to have a higher cohesion index[87] and thus improved tableting properties. Careful analysis of crystal structure and face indexing[88] revealed that these crystals cleaved parallel to the {001} plane. This cleavage occurred due to a well-developed slip system, which is attributed to the presence of two-dimensional molecular sheets in Form II solids. These improved tableting properties of Form II were also confirmed by Heckel analysis, compressibility, and compactibility assessments.[89] Similarly, sulfamerazine metastable polymorph I has well-defined slip planes in its crystal lattice, thus exhibiting superior plasticity, and therefore greater compressibility and tabletability than the stable Polymorph II.[90] Water of crystallization in p-hydroxybenzoic acid monohydrate facilitates plastic deformation of the crystals, thereby enhancing their bonding strength, and forming stronger tablets than the anhydrate.[91]

2.5 TRANSFORMATIONS AMONG SOLIDS

As discussed in Section 2.3.1, polymorphic transformation is widely used in understanding polymorphic relationships. This section is focused on the various pathways for transformation between crystalline solid forms. Crystallization from amorphous materials, owing to its importance to pharmaceutical development, will be discussed separately in Section 2.7. In general, thermodynamics dictates the possibility of transformation between the various phases. Therefore, the discussion in Section 2.3 and an understanding of the particular system should be kept in mind.

Most of the transitions described below are second order transitions, i.e., they are kinetic in nature (except for melting). Therefore, the timescale of experiments can drastically change the pathways that a solid will take in transforming to the other forms. Sometimes, the resulting solid phase can also be different.

2.5.1 Induced by Heat

Molecular motions and mobility in solids generally increase when the temperature of the solid is raised. In addition, the free energy of the various phases changes with respect to temperature as determined by the thermodynamics. Therefore, heating is particularly effective in inducing phase transformations.

Polymorphic Transitions

As shown in Section 2.3.1, a pair of polymorphs can be related to each other either monotropically or enantiotropically. When heated, they exhibit different behavior upon undergoing transformations. Figure 2.9 illustrates all potential polymorphic transitions that can be observed when a polymorphic solid is heated in differential scanning calorimetry (DSC). The descriptions of the phase transitions are placed next to the thermal events in DSC traces, and explained in detail in Table 2.3. This table is arranged according to the polymorphic system, then the starting polymorph, and then the different possibilities of the transitions. Not all situations constitute polymorphic transition. When examining the thermal traces for polymorphic transitions, it is helpful to have the phase diagrams at hand (Figure 2.2).

Most of the transitions listed in Table 2.3 have been observed in real life, except for E II-3. In this case, Polymorph II converts via a solid–solid route to Polymorph I at a temperature below T_t. Unlike in E II-2, where the resulting Polymorph I converts back to Polymorph II when heated past T_t, Polymorph I melts without converting to Polymorph II. The reason that E II-3 is not observed is that the mobility of the solid is higher at higher temperatures; therefore, the kinetic resistance to polymorphic transitions is also likely to be less at higher temperatures.[50] For one pair of enantiotropic polymorphs, if the conversion in one direction is observed at lower temperatures, the likelihood of not observing the conversion in the other direction at higher temperatures is very low.

Experimentally, one could heat the solids to a temperature slightly above the transition, cool the solid back to ambient, reheat, and observe the reversibility of the transitions. Techniques like this have been used extensively to demonstrate the enantiotropic

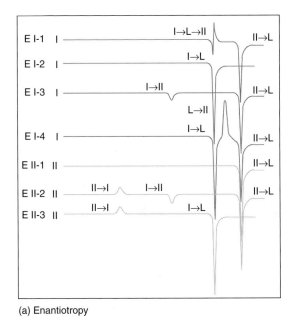

(a) Enantiotropy

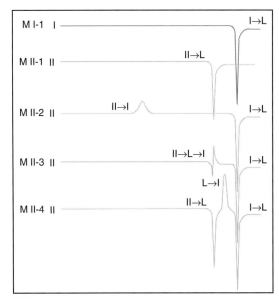

(b) Monotropy

FIGURE 2.9 Potential polymorphic transitions induced by heat

TABLE 2.3 Potential thermal events observed when heating a polymorphic solid

Thermal trace ID	Polymorphic system	Starting polymorph	Transitions (in the order of increasing temperature)
E I-1	Enantiotropic	I	Melting of I with concurrent recrystallization of II
			Melting of II
E I-2	Enantiotropic	I	Melting of I
E I-3	Enantiotropic	I	Solid-state conversion from I to II
			Melting of II
E I-4	Enantiotropic	I	Melting of I
			Recrystallization of II from liquid
			Melting of II
E II-1	Enantiotropic	II	Melting of II
E II-2	Enantiotropic	II	Solid-state conversion from II to I below T_t
			Solid-state conversion from I to II above T_t
			Melting of II
E II-3	Enantiotropic	II	Solid-state conversion from II to I below T_t
			Melting of I
M I-1	Monotropic	I	Melting of I
M II-1	Monotropic	II	Melting of II
M II-2	Monotropic	II	Solid-state conversion from II to I
			Melting of I
M II-3	Monotropic	II	Melting of II with concurrent recrystallization of I
			Melting of I
M II-4	Monotropic	II	Melting of II
			Recrystallization of I from liquid
			Melting of I

relationship between two polymorphs.[92–94] Due to differences in the mobility of solids at different temperatures, one can only draw positive conclusions, not negative ones. In other words, if reversibility of the transition is observed, it is conclusive for an enantiotropic relationship. However, when reversibility is experimentally not observed, one cannot conclude that the polymorphs are monotropically related.

For purposes of illustration, only dimorphic systems are described here. In reality, many polymorphic systems have three or more polymorphs. Therefore, the transformations upon heating could be much more complex than those demonstrated here. In complex cases several complementary analytical methods should be used together in order to understand the system.

Dehydration/Desolvation

The thermodynamic of solvates and hydrates (Section 2.3.2) dictates that they will be less stable at higher temperatures. Indeed, heating has been routinely applied to remove crystallization solvents that are incorporated into the lattice, i.e., desolvation. Thermogravimetric analysis (TGA) is one of the main characterization methods for solvates/hydrates. In principle, TGA monitors the weight change as a function of temperature. The total weight loss corresponds to the stoichiometry of the solvate/hydrate, while the temperature at which the weight loss begins is indicative of the physical stability of the solvate/hydrate.

The resulting solvent-free solids could be different when desolvating different solvates, or desolvating the same solvate under different conditions, or desolvating the same solvate under the same condition but different batches with different amounts of residue solvent.[95] Therefore, desolvation is one of the major approaches in polymorph screening to search for polymorphs.

Cocrystal Formation

Before the term cocrystal was created, this type of adducts was called solid-state molecular complexes. Many of them have been reported in the pharmaceutical literature. Very often the discoveries resulted from experiments to construct binary melting point phase diagrams. In the early days, thermomicroscopy was used. One would watch the solids as they were heated. Very often, after eutectic melting, the liquid would crystallize into a new solid which might correspond to a solid-state complex. Later on, the construction of phase diagrams shifted to DTA/DSC when they became widely available. The common practice was to melt the mixtures of solids first, cool and let them crystallize to ensure "perfect" thermal contact between the sample and the pans and intimate mixing of the two components, and then collect melting points during the second heating. This practice led to an even higher probability of the crystallization of complexes, because the liquid spent more time at higher temperatures and had more opportunity for crystallization.

2.5.2 Induced by Vapor

Since the vapor pressures of solids are usually very low, this section is more applicable to solvates/hydrates and less relevant to cocrystals. The thermodynamics of solvates clearly demonstrates that they are stable under a subset of conditions where the vapor pressure of the solvent in the environment is higher than some critical values. Under these conditions, the non-solvated crystal forms are metastable, and driving forces exist for converting them to the solvate forms. On the other hand, under the conditions where the vapor pressure is below this critical value, solvates are metastable, and driving forces exist for converting the solvates to the non-solvated forms.

Also demonstrated by thermodynamics, activities of the solvents are related to temperature. The same vapor pressure results in lower activities at higher temperatures. Thus, the desolvation phenomenon discussed in Section 2.5.1 is applicable here. However, what is different is the solvation/hydration phenomenon when non-solvated forms are exposed to a high solvent vapor pressure. Since exposure only to the organic solvent vapor is quite rare in pharmaceutical development, the discussions below will focus on the role of water vapor and hydrate formation.

Relative humidity can vary significantly from location to location, and from season to season. Therefore, the phase transition behavior of anhydrate/hydrate has been of particular interest in pharmaceutical development. The kinetic aspect of dehydration has also been studied extensively. From the thermodynamic point of view, when the RH of the environment is closer to RH^c the driving force for dehydration is lower. Therefore, the dehydration rate should decrease. This is, in fact, observed experimentally for the dehydration of amoxicillin trihydrate.[96] Isothermal dehydration rates were measured at a range of water vapor pressures at 68°C. Dehydration resulted in a poorly crystalline phase, and the phase boundary controlled kinetic model, under all conditions studied, best described the rates. When the rate constants are plotted against water vapor pressure, regardless of the size of the samples employed, straight lines result and both extrapolate to a common intercept (within experimental error) on the x-axis (Figure 2.10). This intercept corresponds to the RH^c.

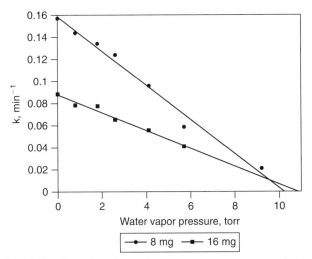

FIGURE 2.10 Plot of dehydration rate constant of amoxicillin trihydrate as a function of water vapor pressure[96]

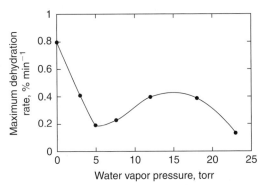

FIGURE 2.11 Maximum dehydration rate of carbamazepine dihydrate as a function of water vapor pressure at 44°C

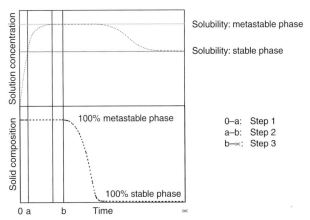

FIGURE 2.12 Concentrations in the solution and the solid compositions as a function of time during the solution-mediated phase transformation

In the case of carbamazepine dihydrate, however, the rate constant did not follow the same trend (Figure 2.11).[97] When dehydrating the hydrate at progressively higher water vapor pressures the rates decrease at first, pass through a minimum, then increase and pass through a maximum, and finally decrease again. This phenomenon is know as the Smith–Topley effect.[98–100] It has been observed in the dehydration of many other hydrates.[101–107] The cause of this "unusual" behavior is the existence of different dehydration products at low and high water vapor pressure. At extremely low water vapor pressure, the dehydrated phase is amorphous. The water of dehydration will have to diffuse through the amorphous matrix outside of each hydrate particle. However, slight increases in water vapor pressures result in the amorphous dehydrated phase undergoing transition to a crystalline phase, therefore creating channels for water to escape, thus facilitating dehydration. At even higher water vapor pressure, the driving force for dehydration starts to diminish, as in the case of amoxicillin trihydrate.

Exposing anhydrous solids to moisture to form hydrates usually requires excessively higher RH than the RH^c. The probable explanation is that the mechanism of transformation here is not solid−solid, but is instead a solution-mediated transformation. Therefore, bulk solution needs to be present for this mechanism to operate, which is only possible at very high relative humidity.

2.5.3 Induced by Solvents

When metastable solids are exposed to solvent, i.e., forming a suspension, conversion to the stable phase is facilitated due to the phenomenon called solution-mediated phase transformation (SMPT). The presence of the solvent does not change the thermodynamics and stability relationship, unless a solvate/hydrate forms with the solvent. However, owing to the much higher mobility in the solution state than in the solid, transformation to the stable phase is much faster. This process is analogous to the effect of catalysts for chemical reactions. Mechanistically, SMPT consists of three consecutive steps:[108–110]

1. initial dissolution of the metastable phase into the solution to reach and exceed the solubility of the stable phase;
2. nucleation of the stable phase;
3. crystal growth of the stable phase coupled with the continuous dissolution of the metastable phase.

The schematic representation of concentrations in the solution, as well as the solid compositions as a function of time is shown in Figure 2.12 for a typical SMPT process. Kinetically, each step is influenced by a number of factors. Some of the important ones are summarized in Table 2.4. For the overall SMPT process, Step 2 is usually the slowest, and therefore the

TABLE 2.4   Factors influencing the kinetics of the elementary steps of SMPT

SMPT step	Factors
1	Temperature (which in turn affects the solubility, diffusion coefficient, and viscosity of the medium);
	Agitation (which in turn affects the thickness of the diffusion layer);
	Initial solution concentration;
	Initial particle size and distribution (which in turn affects the initial surface area);
	Solid to solvent ratio;
	Solvent medium (which in turn affects the solubility and diffusion coefficient);
	Impurities or additives in the solution (e.g., polymers, which in turn affects the diffusion coefficient).
2	Temperature;
	Solubility ratio between the two phases;
	Solubility;
	Nature of the solvent;
	Agitation;
	Impurities or additives;
	Nature and quantity of the contact surfaces (for heterogeneous nucleation).
3	Dissolution component:
	Same as in Step 1, except that the concentration in the solution is higher than the solubility of the stable phase;
	Crystal growth component;
	Temperature;
	Solubility ratio between the two phases;
	Solubility;
	Nature of the solvent;
	Agitation;
	Available sites for growth;
	Number of nuclei;
	Presence of secondary nucleation;
	Surface roughness;
	Impurities or additives in the solution.

rate-determining step because it involves nucleation. For some fast-nucleating systems, the overall process could be dominated by Step 3. In this case, further differentiation can be made as to whether the process is dissolution or growth controlled.[108] However, differentiation was made based only on rates. Therefore, for the same system (same solid plus solvent), the controlling step could change by varying some of the experimental conditions (such as temperature, solid/solvent ratio, agitation, particle size, and distribution) and at different extents of transformation.

Many types of phase transitions have been observed for SMPT, these include:

1. amorphous to crystalline transition;
2. polymorphic transition;
3. interconversions among the parent and the adducts (ionic, molecular, ionic/molecular);
4. interconversions between the adducts.

The occurrences and utility of SMPT span a wide range of pharmaceutically relevant processes including solubility experiments, dissolution (*in vitro* and *in vivo*), API crystallization, polymorph/cocrystal screening and characterization, and pharmaceutical processing (such as wet granulation).

2.5.4 Induced by Mechanical Stresses

When mechanical stresses are applied to solids, they generate many defects. These imperfections create the necessary space and energy to initiate solid-state transitions, such as polymorphic conversion[110–112] and cocrystal formation from a mixture of the corresponding solids.[113,114] Extensive milling, however, often results in a loss of crystallinity, and conversion to amorphous material.

2.6 METHODS OF GENERATING SOLIDS

This section briefly summarizes the various methods to generate solids. All crystalline phases are generated by crystallization, where crystallization can occur from gas, liquid (neat or solution), and solid-states. Amorphous solids, on the other hand, are generated by the lack of crystallization processes. Hydrates/solvates are generated when crystallized from an environment with high and appropriate water/solvent activities. Ultimately, the driving force for crystallization is the difference in activity (chemical potential), which can be represented differently in gas (vapor pressure), liquid (concentration), and solid-state (free energy). Various methods are discussed in some detail below, and they are arranged according to the states of the media through which crystallization occurs: gas, liquid or solid states.

2.6.1 Through Gas

All liquids and solids have vapor pressures at a given temperature. The vapor pressure is a function of temperature, as described by the Clapeyron–Clausius equation. At higher temperatures, the vapor pressure is higher. Therefore, by heating a liquid or solid, one can achieve a certain vapor pressure (provided the substance does not decompose). When this vapor is in contact with a cooler surface, the material in the vapor phase will condense onto the cooler surface, thus generating crystalline polymorphs if nucleation occurs. If nucleation does not occur, the material will condense as amorphous phase (this is usually termed vapor deposition).

Heating is not the only method to generate supersaturation through vapor. It has been demonstrated that "reactions" in the vapor phase could effectively generate supersaturation, and crystallize adducts. One example is the formation of ephedrine free base racemic compound from two opposite enantiomers that are physically separated.[115]

This mode of crystallization is not usually used for hydrates and solvates.

2.6.2 Through Liquid

Through Neat Liquid

As shown in Section 2.5.1, polymorphs can be generated via crystallization from the neat liquid at high temperatures. They can also be generated at lower temperatures via crystallization from amorphous phases. The resulting polymorph is a result of the dynamic interplay between the nucleation and growth kinetics of the different polymorphs.

When exposed to moisture or organic solvent vapor, an amorphous phase will absorb solvent molecules from the vapor phase, leading to a reduced glass transition temperature and increased molecular mobility, and ultimately crystallization. This is further discussed in Section 2.7. Potentially hydrates and solvates can crystallize by this method.

Through Solution

Solvent evaporation

When evaporating solvent from a solution, the capacity that the solution can accommodate solute is reduced, thus supersaturation is eventually created. Upon nucleation, crystalline phases are generated. This evaporative crystallization can also be performed in a solution containing a mixture of solvents. In this case the more volatile solvent(s), ideally, is the good solvent for the solute. When activities of solvent or water are high during the crystallization process, the respective solvates or hydrates may be prepared. On the other hand, amorphous phases are generated if nucleation is sluggish or impaired.

Spray drying is on the extreme side of the rate of solvent removal. Usually, this process generates amorphous material because no time is given for nucleation to occur. However, crystalline phases have been generated via spray drying for some fast-nucleating systems.

Antisolvent addition

When an antisolvent (which does not provide solvency for the solute) is added to a solution, the composition of the solvent system changes. As a result the solubility of the solute consequently changes. The supersaturation necessary for nucleation can be generated in this fashion. Again, nucleation leads to crystalline solids, and the lack of nucleation leads to precipitation of amorphous materials.

The "vapor diffusion" method refers to placing a solution over the vapor of a volatile antisolvent. This method is, in fact, a combination of solvent evaporation and antisolvent addition methods. During the course of the process, the good solvent will evaporate from the solution. Meanwhile, the volatile antisolvent migrates to the solution via the vapor phase.

Reactive solvent addition

For ionizable compounds, pH adjustment in aqueous media is especially effective in creating supersaturation, because of the drastic differences in the solubility. The net effect is to increase the concentration of the less soluble unionized form. Again, nucleation leads to crystalline solids, and the lack of nucleation leads to precipitation of amorphous materials.

Temperature gradient

Most organic compounds have temperature dependent solubility; solubility is usually higher at higher temperatures. Therefore, cooling a saturated solution from higher temperatures will create supersaturation, generating crystalline phases upon nucleation.

Lyophilization is a common method of generating amorphous phases. It is a combination of temperature gradient and solvent evaporation methods. It usually begins with fast cooling of the solution to avoid nucleation. Crystallization of the solvents, and subsequent sublimation of solvent crystals, effectively remove the solvent from the system, leaving behind an amorphous solid.

Suspension method

As discussed in Section 2.5.3, the suspension method is particularly effective in generating more stable phases, polymorphs, solvates or hydrates. Recently, this method has also been extended to screen for cocrystals,[44,53,54] and has proven to be successful in screening for novel cocrystals.[116,117]

2.6.3 Through Solid

As shown in Section 2.4, solid-state phase transitions are one of the main methods used to generate various solid forms. Heating and cooling, varying relative humidity, and mechanical treatments often result in a change of solid form, thus making solid-state phase transition an attractive means of generating new solids.

2.7 AMORPHOUS DRUGS AND SOLID DISPERSIONS

As mentioned in Sections 2.3 and 2.4, an amorphous phase has higher free energy, enthalpy, and entropy than the crystalline counterpart, and thus finds application in improving oral bioavailability for BCS class II or IV compounds. However, its unique properties and metastable nature present significant challenges in commercial applications of this concept. In reality, there are only a handful of pharmaceutical products containing amorphous API that have been successfully marketed, despite several decades' efforts in research and development. As pointed out by Serajuddin,[118] the limited commercial success reflected challenges from manufacturing difficulties to stability problems. This section aims to briefly survey the fundamental properties of amorphous pharmaceuticals and their solid dispersions.

2.7.1 Characteristics of Amorphous Phases

Origin of the Glass Transition

A number of theories have been proposed to explain the origin of the glass transition and various properties of amorphous materials. The free volume theory and thermodynamic theory are among the most widely accepted.

Free volume theory[119–124] assumes that the volume of a liquid consists of the volume occupied by the constituent molecules, and the free volume in which molecules are free to move. The latter exists as voids between molecules, and provides the room for molecular diffusion. A void can open up due to thermal fluctuations, and thus allow a molecule to move through. The glass transition occurs when the free volume of the system falls below a critical value, and molecular motion by diffusion ceases compared to the experimental timescale.

Dolittle[125] proposed the following relationship between viscosity and free volume:

$$\eta = A \exp(b v_0 / v_f) \qquad (2.26)$$

Here v_0 is the molecular volume at $0\,K$, v_f is the free volume, and A, b are constants. Cohen and Turnbull[122] further related the molecular transport in glasses based on the free volume concept:

$$D = (1/3)(3 k_B T / m)^{1/2} \exp(-\gamma v^* / v_f) \qquad (2.27)$$

where D is the diffusivity, k_B is the Boltzmann constant, m is the molecular mass, and v^* is the critical free volume for molecular diffusion. The free volume theory provides a simple and plausible explanation, and is consistent with many experimental observations.

As mentioned previously, the glass transition exhibits the features of a second-order phase transition. Although the glass transition temperature does show kinetic characteristics, it has been suggested that a true second-order transition is masked. The Adam–Gibbs (AG)[126,127] model appears to be able to put together a rigorous explanation of the nature of glass transitions, and identifies the true second-order transition temperature with the Kauzmann temperature, thus avoiding the entropy crisis. It further relates the molecular relaxation time with the excess entropy of the amorphous phase or the configurational entropy, S_c:

$$\tau = \tau_0 \exp\left(\frac{C}{T S_C}\right) \qquad (2.28)$$

Here τ_0 is the relaxation time of molecules at an infinitely high temperature, which conceptually is the relaxation time of the unrestricted molecular relaxation.[128] The overall constant, C, is considered to be a material-dependent parameter which determines the magnitude of the temperature dependence of the relaxation time.

AG theory has been used extensively to explain the properties of the glassy state, and is more successful than the free volume theory in accounting for the pressure dependence of the glass-transition temperature.[129] However, it is not without criticism.[130,131]

Configurational Thermodynamic Quantities

The higher heat capacity, entropy, enthalpy, free energy, and other thermodynamic quantities of the amorphous state are due to additional modes of molecular motion in this state, including rotation and translation, which are collectively called configurations. Therefore, the excess thermodynamic functions are often called configurational quantities. It should be noted that anharmonic vibration might make a significant contribution to those quantities, as noticed by Goldstein[132] in the 1970s.

The configurational heat capacity, ΔC_p, entropy, ΔS, enthalpy, ΔH, and free energy, ΔG, can be calculated based on standard thermodynamic treatments:

$$\Delta C_p(T) = C_p^a(T) - C_p^x(T) \qquad (2.29)$$

$$\Delta H(T) = H^a(T) - H^x(T) = \Delta H_m + \int_{T_m}^{T} \Delta C_p\, dT \qquad (2.30)$$

$$\Delta S(T) = S^a(T) - S^x(T) = \Delta S_m + \int_{T_m}^{T} \frac{\Delta C_p}{T}\, dT \qquad (2.31)$$

$$\Delta G(T) = G^a(T) - G^x(T) = \Delta H(T) - T\Delta S(T) \qquad (2.32)$$

Here superscripts a, x, and m denote amorphous, crystalline, and melting, respectively.

Molecular Relaxation in the Amorphous State

A glass transition occurs when the timescale of molecular relaxation in the system crosses over the timescale of the observer. Therefore, the glass transition can be studied by changing the timescale of the system under study or the experimental probe. In that sense, the glass transition is purely a kinetic phenomenon, and the molecular relaxation time at the glass transition will apparently depend on the experimental conditions. For example, a fast heating or cooling rate corresponds to a shorter timescale of the probe, which causes the glass transition temperature to shift to a higher temperature (shorter timescale). Periodic perturbations can also be applied, such as in the case of dynamic mechanical analysis (DMA), temperature modulated differential scanning calorimetry (TMDSC), dielectric analysis, and rheometric analysis, where the frequency can be changed. Sometimes the comparison among different techniques is not straightforward. However, the average molecular relaxation time at T_g (onset) is approximately 100 seconds for typical DSC scans at 10°C/min.[133]

The temperature dependence of the molecular mobility in the metastable equilibrium supercooled liquid state is usually described by the Vogel–Tammann–Fulcher (VTF) equation,[134–136] as shown below, which can also be approximated by the Adam–Gibbs treatment.

$$\tau = \tau_0 \exp\left(\frac{DT_0}{T - T_0}\right) \qquad (2.33)$$

where T_0 is the temperature where molecular motion ceases (T_K), while D is a parameter signifying the temperature dependence of the relaxation time constant,

or strength of the glass-former. Angell classified glass-formers as either "strong" or "fragile."[137,138] A strong glass has less (lower activation energy) temperature dependence on molecular mobility near T_g than a fragile glass. Molecular mobility in strong glasses typically exhibits Arrhenius-like temperature dependence, while the Arrhenius plot for a fragile glass is significantly non-linear. A stronger glass is also indicated by smaller change in heat capacity at T_g than a fragile glass. The strength parameter D is higher for strong glasses (such as >100 for SiO_2). Most organic glass formers are fragile, generally with $D < 15$. Another useful parameter is the fragility parameter, m, which is related to D as follows:[139]

$$m = \frac{\Delta H}{2.303 R T_g} = \frac{DT_0}{2.303 T_g (1 - T_0/T_g)^2} \qquad (2.34)$$

ΔH is the apparent activation energy near T_g, which can be obtained through the heating rate dependence of the glass transition temperature.[140,141]

$$\Delta H = -R \frac{d \ln q}{d(1/T_g)} \qquad (2.35)$$

To an experimental observer, molecular motion appears to stop at $T < T_g$ because it takes longer than the timescale of the probe. However, molecular motion can be revealed at a longer timescale. An experimental glass is in a non-equilibrium state. When a glass is stored at temperatures below its T_g, this non-equilibrium state, coupled with mobility over a longer timescale, leads to the so-called "physical aging" or "annealing" phenomena. This is due to structural relaxation of the non-equilibrium glass towards the metastable equilibrium or supercooled liquid state, i.e., the ideal glass. A schematic representation of this structural relaxation is shown in Figure 2.13.

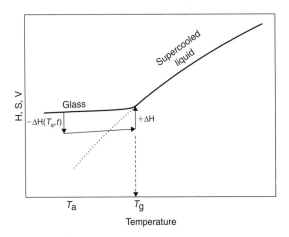

FIGURE 2.13 Schematic representation of the structural relaxation when a glass is annealed at temperature T_a for duration of t

According to the Adam–Gibbs theory on molecular relaxation in glass-forming liquids, these thermodynamic and dynamic properties are coupled. Therefore, during annealing as the excess enthalpy and entropy of the non-equilibrium glass decrease, the molecular mobility should also decrease. The rate and extent of this decrease in molecular mobility may be important to the physical stability of pharmaceutical glasses.[142]

Molecular relaxation time constant in the annealed glasses can be calculated using the AGV equation[133,143] via the concept of fictive temperature,[133,143–148] T_f:

$$\tau(T, T_f) = \tau_0 \exp\left(\frac{DT_0}{T - (T/T_f)T_0}\right) \qquad (2.36)$$

One feature of the structural relaxations in glasses is their non-linearity or non-exponentiality. To be brief, this refers to the non-constant relaxation time constant, which is due to the coupling between the relaxation time and configurational entropy or other quantities. Molecular mobility continuously decreases during the storage of pharmaceutical glasses.[142]

The nonlinearity produces so called memory effects; therefore history is an important factor in studying the structural relaxation in glasses. Non-linearity has been described using the stretched exponential KWW equation:

$$\phi(t) = \exp\left[-\left(\int_0^t \frac{dt'}{\tau(t')}\right)^\beta\right] \qquad (2.37)$$

Here, $\phi(t)$ is the fraction remaining at time t, and β is an empirical parameter indicating the distribution of relaxation time constants ($0 \leq \beta \leq 1$).

2.7.2 Characteristics of Amorphous Solid Dispersions

An amorphous solid dispersion refers to amorphous drug dispersed in a carrier or matrix in the solid state. Strictly speaking, the term dispersion itself implies phase immiscibility. However, in pharmaceutical literature, amorphous solid dispersions are loosely defined, and also include systems where the drug is dispersed in the matrix at the molecular level, i.e., solid solutions. The carriers usually consist of polymers and other "inert" excipients such as surfactants. These carriers could be either amorphous or crystalline themselves. However, amorphous carriers with complete phase miscibility in amorphous drugs offer the most advantages for pharmaceutical applications.

The presence of other components (e.g., polymeric carriers) will certainly modify the characteristics of the amorphous drug. Conceptually, two different scenarios could arise: amorphous drug–crystalline polymer, and amorphous drug–amorphous polymer. In the amorphous drug–crystalline polymer system, due to complete phase separation, most likely the properties of the system will be dominated by individual components, except that the interfacial interactions may change certain characteristics of the system (e.g., dissolution, aggregation, crystallization, etc.). The following discussion focuses on the other more common scenario: amorphous drug–amorphous carriers solid dispersions.

Thermodynamic Analyses and Phase Miscibility

Phase miscibility in amorphous solid dispersions is dictated by the thermodynamics of mixing. A decrease in free energy is a necessary condition to initiate mixing, however, it alone does not guarantee phase miscibility.

Entropy of mixing

Similar to mixing of small molecules, mixing of a polymer with a small molecule leads to an increase in entropy, and therefore favors mixing. However, unlike small molecular mixing, the position availability is limited for polymers due to restraint by the polymer chain, resulting in a smaller ΔS_{mix}. The entropy of mixing for a drug–polymer system can be treated by the Flory–Huggins lattice model:

$$\Delta S_{mix} = R(N_d \ln \phi_d + N_p \ln \phi_p) \qquad (2.38)$$

The subscripts d and p designate drug and polymer respectively, N is the number of sites occupied by drug or polymer, and ϕ is the volume fraction of drug or polymer in the mixture. In the lattice model treatment, the lattice site is usually defined by the volume of the small molecule. Each polymer molecule then occupies m such sites, where m is ratio of the molecular volume of the polymer to that of the drug.

Enthalpy of mixing

Similar to the treatment of regular solution theory, molecular interactions can be built into the lattice model. However, the original regular solution theory merely treated van der Waals interactions, which only accounted for positive deviations from Raoult's law. In the lattice model, specific interactions such as hydrogen bonding were also considered, which play an important role in dictating phase miscibility, and possibly, physical stability in amorphous solid dispersions. The enthalpy of mixing is often expressed as:

$$\Delta H_{mix} = RT(N_0 + mN_p)\chi\Phi_0\Phi_p \qquad (2.39)$$

where χ is called the Flory–Huggins parameter. $\chi\,kT$ represents the enthalpy change of introducing one solvent molecule to the polymer. Depending on the nature of polymer–drug interaction, the enthalpy of mixing can be positive (for example, in the case of only van der Waals interactions) or negative (for example, in the case of hydrogen bonding). Obviously, positive χ causes an increase in enthalpy and free energy, which disfavors mixing.

Free energy of mixing

Based on the Flory–Huggins model, the total free energy of mixing can be expressed as:

$$\Delta G_{mix} = RT\,[N_0 \ln \Phi_0 + N_p \ln \Phi_p \\ + (N_0 + mN_p)\chi\Phi_0\Phi_p] \qquad (2.40)$$

The entropy of mixing is the only term that always favors mixing. However, this term is much smaller than observed in mixing of small molecules, and cannot offset a large positive enthalpy of mixing.

Therefore, the free energy of mixing could be negative or positive depending on the sign and magnitude of the Flory–Huggins parameter. If the Flory–Huggins parameter is too large ($\chi > \chi_{crit}$), the free energy of mixing will be positive and no mixing is expected. Specific interactions such as hydrogen bonding make χ negative, thus phase miscibility may be favored.

$\Delta G_{mix} < 0$ alone does not necessarily imply a single phase. Figure 2.14 illustrates typical scenarios when mixing small drug molecules with amorphous polymeric carriers. In Figure 2.14a, $\Delta G_{mix} > 0$ for virtually all compositions; therefore mixing will not occur and the amorphous drug and polymer will stay in their own pure phases. (Strictly speaking, there will always be a certain extent of mixing. However, in reality the equilibrium phases can be considered as the same as each individual component.) Figure 2.14b represents partial miscibility. Phase miscibility occurs when $\phi_d < \phi_{d,1}$ or $\phi_d > \phi_{d,2}$. When $\phi_{d,1} < \phi_d < \phi_{d,2}$, the solid dispersion will be phase separated, however, not into their individual components, but into a

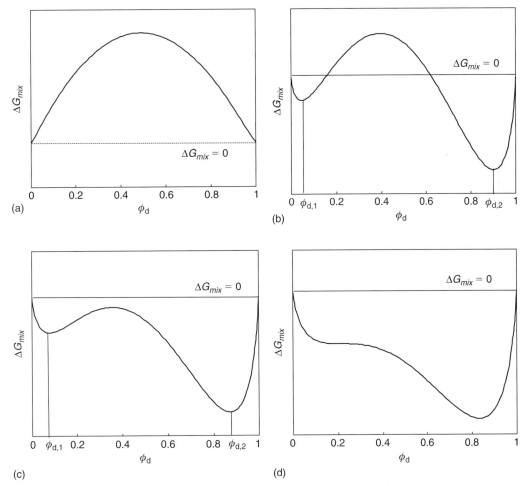

FIGURE 2.14 Schematic free energy of mixing (a) no mixing; (b) partial miscibility; (c) mixing but with phase separation at some compositions; and (d) complete miscibility

drug-rich phase ($\phi_{d,2}$), and a polymer-rich phase ($\phi_{d,1}$). In Figure 2.14c, $\Delta G_{mix} < 0$ for all compositions. However, any composition in the range $\phi_{d,1} < \phi_d < \phi_{d,2}$ will still decompose to two local minima represented by $\phi_{d,1}$ and $\phi_{d,2}$, similar to Figure 2.14b. Therefore, $\Delta G_{mix} < 0$ is only a necessary condition for complete phase miscibility. Figure 2.14d represents the complete phase miscibility.

Molecular Mobility in Amorphous Solid Dispersions

When a drug is molecularly dispersed in a polymer, its molecules experience an environment with both other drug molecules, and the polymer molecules. The same is true for the polymer. Molecular relaxation in such a dispersed matrix is therefore expected to reflect such an environment. The average mobility is usually intermediate between those of the pure components. Assuming additivity of free volumes of each component (ideal mixing), the T_g of an ideal binary mixture can be estimated using the Gordon–Taylor equation:[149,150]

$$T_{g,\,mix} = \frac{w_1 T_{g1} + K w_2 T_{g2}}{w_1 + K w_2} \quad (2.41)$$

Where w_1 and w_2 are the weight fractions of the components, and K is a constant which can be approximated by the ratio between the respective changes in heat capacity at T_g:

$$K = \Delta C_{p_2} / \Delta C_{p_1} \quad (2.42)$$

To the drug, the presence of the polymer usually causes an increase in T_g, which is often termed an antiplasticization effect. In addition, the presence of specific drug–polymer interactions can lead to an increase in T_g above that predicted. However, if the drug–polymer (adhesion) interaction is less than those in drug–drug or polymer–polymer (cohesion) pairs, then T_g is expected to be lower than predicted.

The change in molecular mobility in the amorphous phase by incorporating a second component is of practical relevance to pharmaceuticals other than amorphous solid dispersions. Moisture sorption is vastly increased in an amorphous phase compared to the corresponding crystalline phase. This can be explained by two reasons. The first is that an amorphous phase is more energetic, therefore increasing affinity between water and the drug molecules. The second reason is that by removing the crystal lattice, the previous barrier preventing water molecules from entering the crystal lattice vanishes, and water molecules are now able to access almost every host molecule. The latter reason is probably more important. Instead of moisture adsorption on the crystal surface, water molecules form a molecular dispersion with the drug, and the phenomenon is more appropriately called sorption. As predicted by the Gordon–Taylor equation, the consequence of moisture sorption into an amorphous phase is a drastically reduced T_g, and increased molecular mobility even for a small amount of moisture sorbed, due to the great plasticization effect of water which has a T_g of $-137°C$.

Solubility in Polymeric Matrix

It is apparent that a solid dispersion is metastable only when the drug loading exceeds the solubility limit. Therefore, the solubility of a crystalline drug in a polymeric matrix is of both theoretical and practical importance.

It has been challenging to determine drug solubility in amorphous solid dispersions experimentally, due to the highly viscous nature and slow kinetics of such systems. Theoretically, the solubility could be estimated once the Flory–Huggins interaction parameter becomes known. Methods to derive this parameter in polymer solutions include vapor pressure reduction, osmotic pressure, other solution techniques, as well as melting point depression. Most of these solution techniques are difficult to apply to drug–polymer systems. However, the melting point depression[151,152] can be well adapted to amorphous solid dispersions.[153] This approach is briefly described next.

When crystalline drug is in equilibrium with a polymer, the chemical potential of the crystalline drug equals that of the dissolved drug in the drug–polymer system. The chemical potential of the drug in solution can be derived based on the free energy of mixing:

$$\Delta \mu_d = \mu_d - \mu_d^0 = \left(\frac{\partial \Delta G_{mix}}{\partial N_d} \right)_{N_p, T, P}$$

$$= RT \left[\ln \Phi_d + \Phi_p \left(1 - \frac{1}{m} \right) + \chi \Phi_p^2 \right] \quad (2.43)$$

Here μ_d^0 is the chemical potential of the pure amorphous drug, which is the same as the molar free energy of the pure amorphous drug at the temperature of reduced melting point, T_m.

The molar free energy of pure amorphous drug can be related to that of the crystalline drug:

$$\mu_d^0(T_m) = G^a(T_m) = G^x(T_m) + \Delta H_m (1 - T_m / T_m^0)$$

$$+ \int_{T_m^0}^{T_m} \Delta C_p \, dT - T \int_{T_m^0}^{T_m} \frac{\Delta C_p}{T} \, dT \quad (2.44)$$

Here T_m^0 is the melting temperature of the pure crystalline drug, and $G^x(T_m)$ is the molar free energy of the crystalline drug at T_m, which is identical to its chemical potential, $\mu^x(T_m)$. The following relationship can then be obtained by equating the chemical potential of the drug in polymer, and that of the crystalline drug:

$$
-\frac{\Delta H_m}{R}\left(\frac{1}{T_m}-\frac{1}{T_m^0}\right)-\frac{1}{RT}\int_{T_m}^{T}\Delta C_p\,dT+\frac{1}{R}
$$
$$
\times\int_{T_m}^{T}\frac{\Delta C_p}{T}\,dT+=\ln\Phi_0+\left(1-\frac{1}{m}\right)\Phi_p+\chi\Phi_p^2 \quad (2.45)
$$

The χ parameter can then be estimated, based on the above equation using the melting-point depression data. A simplified equation has been used in the literature by ignoring the contribution from excess heat capacity:

$$
-\frac{\Delta H_m}{R}\left(\frac{1}{T_m}-\frac{1}{T_m^0}\right)=\ln\Phi_0+\left(1-\frac{1}{m}\right)\Phi_p+\chi\Phi_p^2 \quad (2.46)
$$

Once the χ parameter becomes known, one can estimate the solubility at lower temperatures. However, two points need to be made. First, the above equation only applies to systems where amorphous drug and amorphous polymer are in a single phase. As discussed in the previous section, the free energy of mixing will be further reduced if phase separation exists while $\Delta G_{mix} < 0$. Secondly, the solubility obtained from melting point depression corresponds to that in the rubbery state. However, amorphous solid dispersions are intended to be stored in the glassy state. Therefore, a large discrepancy might indeed be expected.

Solubilization certainly further reduces the driving force for crystallization of the amorphous drug. However, drug solubility in polymers at room temperature is generally quite small, therefore the tangible impact at normal storage temperatures is possibly limited.

2.7.3 Crystallization of Amorphous Drugs and Dispersions

Crystallization or physical instability is probably one of the greatest challenges for developing amorphous solid dispersions. Although there has been extensive research in this area, consensus has not been reached. Below is a brief summary on the current thinking on this subject.

Molecular Mobility

Molecular mobility plays a key role in physical and chemical stability in amorphous phases, and

its importance can be readily understood. For any physical or chemical process, the molecules involved must take appropriate positions and orientations, so that the process can proceed.[154] Therefore, molecular motions, such as translation and rotation, are essential in any physical or chemical change of the system. In solution or in the melt, molecular translation and rotation are usually faster than the physical or chemical change itself, so that the overall rate is independent of diffusion of the reactant or product. However, in the solid state, molecular diffusion is orders of magnitudes slower than in solution and, in most cases, can be comparable to, or even slower than, the rate of reaction. It is likely that molecular motion becomes partially or completely rate-limiting in solid-state reactions.

The partial correlation between molecular mobility and physical/chemical stability has been demonstrated for a number of pharmaceutical systems.[155–159] The crystallization rates of amorphous nifedipine in the presence of different excipients were correlated to the spin-lattice relaxation time of D_2O in these matrices.[155] Differences in crystallization rates of amorphous nifedipine, phenobarbital, and flopropione were attributed to their differences in molecular mobility.[156] In a follow-up study, the temperature dependence of physical stability of amorphous nifedipine and phenobarbital were correlated to a large extent to the temperature dependence of molecular relaxation time constant.[157] Physical stability of a lyophilized monoclonal antibody in sucrose and trehalose was correlated to molecular mobility measured by enthalpy relaxation, but not the glass transition temperature.[158] It was also shown that the fragility of the formulations played a role. Chemical degradation of amorphous quinapril hydrochloride demonstrated significant correlation with molecular relaxation time constant at temperatures below T_g.[159] Bimolecular reaction rates of acetyl transfer, and the Maillard reaction in lyophilized aspirin-sulfadiazine formulations, were concluded to be predictable based on molecular mobility.[160] While the chemical stability of lyophilized insulin showed correlation with the molecular mobility in trehalose formulation, the contribution of molecular mobility was found to be negligible in a PVP formulation.[161,162]

To maintain adequate physical stability, storage below T_g is apparently needed. However, unlike the metastable equilibrium supercooled state, molecular mobility in the glassy state is much higher, and is less dependent on temperature. Therefore, the advantage achieved by just storing an amorphous formulation at temperatures far below T_g is not as great as expected, based on that predicted using the VTF equation. Along the same lines, the suggestion of storage at the

Kauzmann temperature (typically $T_g - 50°C$, varying, however, depending on the fragility) will likely not provide the intended consequences because realistic glasses possess much higher mobility than ideal glasses, and molecular mobility at T_K is still significant. Nevertheless, raising the T_g of amorphous dispersions by incorporating a high T_g excipient is still a sound tactic, as implied by the Gordon–Taylor equation. However, the limitations of this approach need to be kept in mind. T_g is not necessarily a predictor for physical stability.[158] In addition, compromises may be necessary because a higher process temperature will usually be required for higher T_g formulations if the melt method is employed in manufacturing.

Rate of crystallization may also decouple from the viscosity of glasses. Hikima et al.[163] studied the o-terphenyl system, and observed that crystal growth increased abruptly near T_g and below, orders of magnitude faster than expected from diffusion-controlled growth. Most recently, Yu and coworkers identified a few pharmaceutical systems exhibiting similar behavior including indomethacin,[164] nifedipine,[165] and the ROY system.[166,167] Many questions still remain to be answered; however, this glass–crystal mode of crystal growth appeared to be related to the precursors present in liquid and crystal structure (polymorph).[166,167]

Free Energy Driving Force

In addition to the molecular mobility, the role of the free energy driving force has been historically discussed when dealing with crystallization from supercooled melts.[168] Mobility determines how fast a molecule can impinge the surface of a growing crystal. However, not every impingement leads to successful incorporation of the molecule. The probability of the molecule not coming back to the liquid phase is related to the free energy driving force: the higher the free energy difference, the more likely the molecule will stay in the crystal lattice. The relationship can be described as follows:[164]

$$u = (k/\eta)[1 - \exp(-\Delta G/RT)] \qquad (2.47)$$

Here η is the viscosity (proportional to molecular relaxation time constant), ΔG is the free energy driving force, R is gas constant, and k is a constant. While the viscosity of a supercooled liquid can be described by an empirical equation such as VTF, ΔG is approximately proportional to the degree of supercooling, $\Delta T = T_m - T$. Based on the above relationship, the temperature for the maximum crystallization rate falls between the glass transition temperature and the melting temperature, as depicted in Figure 2.15.

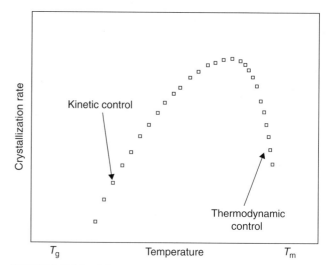

FIGURE 2.15 Schematic representation of crystallization rate from supercooled liquids

Configurational Entropy

Considering the metastable nature of an amorphous phase, i.e., $\Delta G = G^a - G^x > 0$, it is interesting that the amorphous phase has both higher enthalpy, and higher entropy. From the thermodynamic relationship $\Delta G = \Delta H - T\Delta S$, it can be concluded that the higher free energy of amorphous phase is due to the enthalpy factor, while the entropy term partially offsets the enthalpy term, which actually reduces the overall free energy. It is apparent that the free energy and the enthalpy of amorphous state facilitate reversion to the crystalline form. The entropy term appears to behave somewhat differently.

As discussed above, crystallization from supercooled melts are generally discussed in the context of molecular mobility, and free energy driving force. For crystallization near and below T_g, which is generally the case where physical stability of amorphous pharmaceuticals is concerned, crystallization is mainly dictated by molecular mobility. Indeed, molecular mobility is generally accepted as a principal factor governing the physical stability of amorphous phases.[62,170,171] One simple fact is that crystallization of amorphous phases proceeds much faster in the rubbery state compared to the glassy state. As briefly noted, molecular mobility has been correlated partially or fully to physical/chemical stability in a number of pharmaceutical systems.

Nevertheless, significant differences in crystallization behavior are observed across compounds, and these cannot be explained by mobility alone. For example, some amorphous phases crystallize almost immediately at the glass temperature (e.g., acetaminophen[172]), some crystallize below T_g in a relatively short time (e.g., griseofulvin,[173] nifedipine[156,157]), while others are quite stable. For some of the more stable amorphous phases, such as ritonavir,[172] crystallization in the glassy state is not observed, and it does not proceed at a significant rate above T_g without seeding. Because T_g corresponds to the temperature where the molecular relaxation time of the amorphous phase is equivalent to the experimental timescale, it is clear that the same molecular mobility results in different crystallization tendencies.

The authors have explored the physical stability of a diverse group of pharmaceutically relevant compounds, attempting to identify thermodynamic quantities contributing to crystallization tendency. Through this analysis it was concluded that the calorimetric configurational entropy also played an important role.[142,172]

In simple terms, configurational entropy is a measure of the difference in the number of configurations between the amorphous and crystalline phases. For molecules in the amorphous state to crystallize, the molecule has to pack into a defined crystal lattice with defined configuration or orientation. Therefore, the higher the configurational entropy, the lower the probability that the molecules will assume the desirable orientation for packing into the crystal lattice. Hence, a metastable amorphous compound with large configurational entropy tends to show greater physical stability. This is analogous to the common experience of chemists and biochemists that large molecules with numerous rotatable bonds are generally difficult to crystallize from solution. It has been hypothesized that configurational entropy serves as a thermodynamic measurement of the probability of nucleation, while the molecular mobility dictates the rate at which a molecule can change its configurations and serves as a kinetic measurement of nucleation. When these two quantities were evaluated with respect to molecular structure, it was possible to provide an assessment of physical stability. Therefore, in relative terms, small, rigid molecules will tend to crystallize more easily than large flexible compounds.

Recently, Ediger, Harrowell and Yu[174] surveyed the crystallization rates of a number of inorganic and organic systems, and identified a correlation between rate of crystallization and entropy difference. In light of this new development, it seems appropriate that roles of mobility, entropy, and free energy during crystallization can be discussed in the context of three consecutive events during crystallization: mobility determines the rate of molecule approaching a crystal surface; entropy relates to the probability of that approaching molecule having the desirable configurations; and the free energy dictates the probability of that molecule not

returning to the liquid phase. A more or less quantitative relationship may be represented as:

$$u = (k/\eta^\xi) \exp(-\Delta S/R)[1 - \exp(-\Delta G/RT)] \quad (2.48)$$

Here, ξ is a constant describing the extent of correlation between crystallization rate and diffusivity.

Crystallization Inhibition

Historically, polymers have been found to inhibit crystallization from solution. Among those pharmaceutically relevant ones, PVP has been extensively studied.[175–179] Other crystallization inhibitors include Pluronic F68,[180] cellulose derivatives,[181] and cyclodextrins.[182]

Polymeric carriers or other additives have also been shown to inhibit crystallization from amorphous solid dispersions. Thermodynamics dictates that amorphous drug would crystallize if given sufficient time. However, from the perspective of a formulation scientist, it is of great benefit if one can delay this crystallization process to obtain adequate shelf life. There are many examples of crystallization inhibition in amorphous solid dispersions,[183–189] however the mechanisms of such effects remain to be determined.

When dealing with solid dispersions, a key parameter is the molecular mobility or, approximately, the T_g. The antiplasticization effect of polymeric carriers is considered important, and could conceptually lead to a more stable amorphous phase than the drug itself. However, this factor alone is not entirely responsible for some experimental observations. For example, amorphous solid dispersions of felodipine with PVP, HPMCAS, and HPMC[189] showed similar stability profiles, while only its dispersion with PVP showed a significant increase in T_g for polymer loading up to 25%.

Specific interactions between drug and polymers were also considered to be important. For example, the inhibition of crystallization of amorphous indomethacin by PVP and PVP-co-PVA was ascribed to the hydrogen bonding interaction between the polymers and drug molecules.[184] PVP was found to inhibit crystallization of indomethacin more with larger particles than smaller ones,[185] and was consistent with the observation of predominantly surface nucleation. An ion–dipole interaction was proposed to be partially responsible for the crystallization inhibition in solid dispersions of PVP[186] and a developmental drug, which could not be attributed to mobility alone. The increase in physical stability of amorphous nifedipine in ethylcellulose and Eudragit RL® dispersions were also explained by the hydrogen bonding interaction between drug and the polymers.[187] Strong interactions were observed in acetaminophen/aminoacetanilide and PVP/polyacryric acid polymers, which led to improved physical stability[188] and correlated with the strength of the specific interaction.[190] However, the felodipine dispersions with PVP, HPMC, and HPMCAS showed similar inhibitory effect, although the hydrogen bonding strengths followed PVP > HPMC > HPMCAS.[189] The above findings may not appear to be consistent. The situation is quite complex with the presence of specific interactions. On the one hand, strong drug–polymer interactions lead to reduction in molecular mobility higher than predicted by free volume additivity alone. On the other hand, the presence of certain intermolecular structures between drug and polymer molecules due to specific interactions may create a kinetic barrier for the amorphous drug to crystallize. Additionally, specific interactions also decrease the free energy of the system. All the above factors appear to work towards stabilization, albeit maybe to different extents. However, it is difficult to delineate the individual contributions.

While it is important to maintain the physical stability of amorphous dispersions during storage, it is also useful to utilize similar concepts for solid dispersions during *in vivo* dissolution. The higher dissolution rate and apparent solubility of amorphous drug usually causes supersaturation during *in vivo* dissolution, and therefore may lead to precipitation in the GI tract and compromise oral bioavailability. If such a crystallization-inhibitory polymer is incorporated into the amorphous solid dispersion, then the *in vivo* precipitation may be delayed or completely eliminated, resulting in much improved oral absorption. It is ideal if the polymeric carrier can function as crystallization inhibitor, both during storage and during *in vivo* dissolution. However, the mechanisms may not be the same, and different inhibitors may indeed be necessary. A few examples have been reported. Various itraconazole solid dispersions were prepared by hot-melt extrusion, and compared with the commercial Sporanox® in a clinical study.[66] The bioavailability relative to Sporanox® was 102.9%, 77.0%, and 68% for the HPMC, Eudragit E 100, and Eudragit E 100-poly(vinylpyrrolidone-co-vinylacetate) solid dispersions, respectively, in opposite rank order of their *in vitro* dissolution data. The reason was speculated to be due to the crystallization-inhibitory role of HPMC during dissolution. Similarly, an *in vitro* dissolution study indicated that supersaturation was maintained for an amorphous solid dispersion of albendazole in hydroxypropyl methylcellulose phthalate (HP-55), but not with HPMC,[191] which lead to its higher *in vivo* performance in rabbits.[191]

2.8 SPECIAL TOPICS

2.8.1 Polymorph Screening and Stable Form Screening

Polymorph screening is a practice focusing on the discovery of crystalline solids, mostly polymorphs. However, it includes the search for hydrates/solvates as well. Historically, polymorph screening usually included the following approaches:

1. Recrystallization under various conditions: the crystallinity of the original solid is removed by dissolving in solutions or melting. Crystallinity is then regenerated under a variety of conditions (such as temperature, solvent, supersaturation, additives, etc.) to see whether it results in other crystal forms.
2. Examining the solid–solid transitions induced by heat, humidity, mechanical stresses, etc.

Although it is valuable to screen and discover all crystal forms for a particular compound, finding the most stable polymorph is practically the most important aspect in polymorph screening. A polymorph screening procedure that provides a greater probability of finding the stable polymorph was formulated.[192] The use of a suspension/slurry and the principle of solution-mediated phase transformation to facilitate this process was described in detail as follows:

1. Recrystallization:
   - use the available polymorph;
   - ensure complete dissolution of the solid, to eliminate any seeds of the original polymorph;
   - recrystallize at a low rate, either at a low cooling rate or at a low rate of solvent evaporation;
   - use a wide range of final temperatures. If cooling crystallization is employed, the induction time and the rate of transformation of the metastable phase to the stable phase may vary with temperature.
2. After recrystallization, add a small amount of the original polymorph to the suspension and stir for various times, and examine the solid phase regularly. The length of time depends on the compound of interest, and the longer the better, provided that it has satisfactory chemical stability in the solution. The minimum time recommended is seven days.
3. A range of solvents, with a variety of different characteristics such as hydrogen bonding, dielectric constant, solvency for the compound, should be employed.

This procedure improves the chance of finding the stable polymorph when a new pharmaceutical candidate is under investigation. Although slightly more time and effort are required, this procedure is technically easy and the outcome may easily outweigh the effort.

Recently, one variation of the above procedure, where initial crystallization was not performed, was reported being used in the routine early screening for stable phases.[193] Encouraging statistical data were reported by the authors:

> "Based on limited statistics ($n = 43$), approximately 26% of early discovery compounds (received as crystalline phases) converted to more stable polymorphs during the stable polymorph screen. To date, more stable polymorphs have not been observed for any of those 43 candidates that have advanced into development."

2.8.2 High Throughput Crystallization

Automation in crystallization has been on the rise in recent years, and has shown great promise in the areas of polymorph screening and crystal engineering, i.e., searching for cocrystals of better physico-chemical properties.[194–197] The advantages of robotic crystallization over conventional manual crystallization are several. First, the robot is designed to perform tasks in a parallel fashion; therefore, it is able to examine the various parameters quickly. Secondly, because of the rapidity, robotic crystallization is able to explore parameters influencing crystallization more thoroughly, leading to a better understanding. Thirdly, robotic crystallization requires less material. Fourthly, because of the thoroughness, robotic crystallization may produce crystal forms that are otherwise not accessible by conventional crystallization.

2.8.3 Miniaturization in Crystallization

Another trend in the crystallization of pharmaceutical materials is miniaturization. Reducing the material needed is essential for studies during early development, where the cost of API is extremely high and availability is scarce. Several studies were conducted using capillary tubes.[198–200] In addition to the benefit of reduced material consumption ($5-50\,\mu L$ of solution), in some cases, the authors reported the discovery of previous unknown polymorphs owing to crystallization in a confined space.

Most recently, microfluidics technology that is capable of scaling down further by 10- to 100-fold has been applied to crystallization. Although most of the current applications are toward the crystallization of proteins,[201–204] the extension to pharmaceutically relevant small molecules has already begun.[205–207]

References

1. Byrn, S.R., Pfeiffer, R.R. & Stowell, J.G. (1999). *Solid-State Chemistry of Drugs*, 2nd edn. SSCI, Inc, West Lafayette, IN.

2. Bernstein, J. (2002). *Polymorphism in Molecular Crystals*. Oxford University Press, Oxford, UK.

3. Brittain, H.G. (1999). Polymorphism in Pharmaceutical Solids. In: *Drugs Pharm. Sci.*, Vol. 95. Dekker, New York, NY.

4. Brittain, H.G. (1995). Physical Characterization of Pharmaceutical Solids. In: *Drugs Pharm. Sci.*, Vol. 70. Dekker, New York, NY.

5. Hilfiker, R. (2006). *Polymorphism: In the Pharmaceutical Industry*. Wiley-VCH Verlag GmbH & Co, KGaA, Weinheim, Germany.

6. Brittain, H.G. (2006). Spectroscopy of Pharmaceutical Solids. In: *Drugs Pharm. Sci.*, Vol. 160. Taylor & Francis, New York, NY.

7. Stahl, P.H. & Wermuth, C.G. (2002). *Handbook of pharmaceutical salts: Properties, selection, and use*. VHCA, Zürich, Switzerland and Wiley-VCH, Weinheim, Germany.

8. Suryanarayanan, R., & Byrn, S. R., (eds). (2001). Characterization of the solid state. Adv. Drug. Del. Rev. 48, 1–136.

9. Raw, A.S. & Yu, L.X. (eds). (2004). pharmaceutical solid polymorphism in drug development and regulation. Adv. Drug. Del. Rev. 56, 235–414.

10. Rogers, R.D. (ed.). (2004). Polymorphism in crystals. Cryst. Grow. Design 4, 1085–1441.

11. Rogers, R.D. (ed.). (2003). Polymorphism in crystals. Cryst. Grow. Design 3, 867–1040.

12. Matzger, A. J. (ed.), (2008). Facets of polymorphism in crystals. Cryst. Grow. Design 8, 2–161.

13. Haleblian, J.K. (1975). Characterization of habits and crystalline modification of solids and their pharmaceutical applications. J. Pharm. Sci. 64, 1269–1288.

14. Desiraju, G.R. (2003). Crystal and co-crystal. CrystEngComm. 5, 466–467.

15. Dunitz, J.D. (2003). Crystal and co-crystal: A second opinion. CrystEngComm. 5, 506.

16. Aakeröy, C.B. & Salmon, D.J. (2005). Building co-crystals with molecular sense and supramolecular sensibility. CrystEngComm. 7, 439–448.

17. Lara-Ochoa, F. & Espinosa-Perez, G. (2007). Crystals and patents. Cryst. Grow. Design 7, 1213–1215.

18. Bond, A.D. (2007). What is a co-crystal? CrystEngComm. 9, 833–834.

19. Lara-Ochoa, F. & Espinosa-Perez, G. (2007). Cocrystals definitions. Supramol. Chem. 19, 553–557.

20. Schmidt, A.C. & Schwarz, I. (2006). Solid-state characterization of non-stoichiometric hydrates of ester-type local anaesthetics. Int. J. Pharm. 320, 4–13.

21. Authelin, J.R. (2005). Thermodynamics of non-stoichiometric pharmaceutical hydrates. Int. J. Pharm. 303, 37–53.

22. Stephenson, G.A. & Diseroad, B.A. (2000). Structural relationship and desolvation behavior of cromolyn, cefazolin and fenoprofen sodium hydrates. Int. J. Pharm. 198, 167–177.

23. Chen, L.R., Young, V.G., Jr., Lechuga-Ballesteros, D. & Grant, D.J.W. (1999). Solid-state behavior of cromolyn sodium hydrates. J. Pharm. Sci. 88, 1191–1200.

24. Reutzel, S.M. & Russell, V.A. (1998). Origins of the unusual hygroscopicity observed in LY297802 tartrate. J. Pharm. Sci. 87, 1568–1571.

25. Variankaval, N., Wenslow, R., Murry, J., Hartman, R., Helmy, R., Kwong, E., Clas, S.D., Dalton, C. & Santos, I. (2006). Preparation and solid-state characterization of nonstoichiometric cocrystals of a phosphodiesterase-IV inhibitor and L-tartaric acid. Cryst. Grow. Design 6, 690–700.

26. Yu, L. (1995). Inferring thermodynamic stability relationship of polymorphs from melting data. J. Pharm. Sci. 84, 966–974.

27. Yu, L., Huang, J. & Jones, K.J. (2005). Measuring free-energy difference between crystal polymorphs through eutectic melting. J. Phys. Chem. B 109, 19915–19922.

28. Yu, L., Stephenson, G.A., Mitchell, C.A., Bunnell, C.A., Snorek, S.V., Bowyer, J.J., Borchardt, T.B., Stowell, J.G. & Byrn, S.R. (2000). Thermochemistry and conformational polymorphism of a hexamorphic crystal system. J. Am. Chem. Soc. 122, 585–591.

29. Chen, S., Guzei, I.A. & Yu, L. (2005). New polymorphs of ROY and new record for coexisting polymorphs of solved structures. J. Am. Chem. Soc. 127, 9881–9885.

30. Reutzel-Edens, S.M., Russell, V.A. & Yu, L. (2000). Molecular basis for the stability relationships between homochiral and racemic crystals of tazofelone: a spectroscopic, crystallographic, and thermodynamic investigation. Perkin 25, 913–924.

31. Noyes, A.A. & Whitney, W.R. (1897). The rate of solution of solid substances in their own solutions. J. Am. Chem. Soc. 19, 930–934.

32. Burger, A. & Ramberger, R. (1979). On the polymorphism of pharmaceuticals and other molecular crystals. I. Theory of thermodynamic rules. Mikrochimi. Acta [Wien] II, 259–271.

33. Burger, A. & Ramberger, R. (1979). On the polymorphism of pharmaceuticals and other molecular crystals. II. Applicability of thermodynamic rules. Mikrochimi. Acta [Wien] II, 273–316.

34. Zhu, H., Yuen, C. & Grant, D.J.W. (1996). Influence of water activity in organic solvent + water mixtures on the nature of the crystallizing drug phase. 1. Theophylline. Int. J. Pharm. 135, 151–160.

35. Zhu, H. & Grant, D.J.W. (1996). Influence of water activity in organic solvent + water mixtures on the nature of the crystallizing drug phase. 2. Ampicillin. Int. J. Pharm. 139, 33–43.

36. Khankari, R., Chen, L. & Grant, D.J.W. (1998). Physical characterization of nedocromil sodium hydrates. J. Pharm. Sci. 87, 1052–1061.

37. Bandyopadhyay, R., Erixon, K., Young, V.G. & Grant, D.J.W. (1998). *Effects of water activity on recrystallized L-lysine monohydrochloride*. World Congress on Particle Technology 3, Brighton, UK. July 6–9, pp. 1889–1909.

38. Beckmann, W. & Winter, G. (1999). Stability of the hydrate and anhydrate of pyrazzocarnil hydrochloride in water-ethanol mixtures and in moist air. 14th International Symposium on Industrial Crystallization, September 12–16. Cambridge, UK, pp. 236–245.

39. Wadso, L. & Markova, N. (2001). Comparison of three methods to find the vapor activity of a hydration step. Eur. J. Pharm. Biopharm. 51, 77–81.

40. Ticehurst, M.D., Storey, R.A. & Watt, C. (2002). Application of slurry bridging experiments at controlled water activities to predict the solid-state conversion between anhydrous and hydrated forms using theophylline as a model drug. Int. J. Pharm. 247, 1–10.

41. Sacchetti, M. (2004). Determining the relative physical stability of anhydrous and hydrous crystal forms of GW2016. Int. J. Pharm. 273, 195–202.

42. Han, J., Zhang, G.G.Z., Grant, D.J.W. & Suryanarayanan, R. Physical stability of pharmaceutical hydrates. In preparation.

43. Suzuki, E., Shimomura, K. & Sekiguchi, K. (1989). Thermochemical study of theophylline and its hydrate. Chem. Pharm. Bull. 37, 493–497.

44. Zhang, G.G.Z., Henry, R.F., Borchardt, T.B. & Lou, X. (2007). Efficient co-crystal screening using solution-mediated phase transformation. J. Pharm. Sci. 96, 990–995.

45. Kauzmann, W. (1948). The nature of the glassy state and the behavior of liquids at low temperatures. Chem. Rev. 43, 219–256.

46. Ehrenfest, P. (1933). Phase changes in the ordinary and extended sense classified according to the corresponding singularities of the thermodynamic potential. Proc. Acad. Sci. Amsterdam 36, 153–157.

47. The United States Pharmacopeia. (2007). 30th revision, United States Pharmacopeial Convention, Rockville, MD, USA.

48. Haleblian, J.K. & Mccrone, W. (1969). Pharmaceutical applications of polymorphism. J. Pharm. Sci. 58, 911–929.

49. Threlfall, T.L. (1995). Analysis of organic polymorphs. A review. Analyst (Cambridge, United Kingdom) 120, 2435–2460.

50. Giron, D. (1995). Thermal analysis and calorimetric methods in the characterization of polymorphs and solvates. Thermochim. Acta 248, 1–59.

51. Grant, D.J.W. (1999). Theory and origin of polymorphism. In: *Polymorphism in Pharmaceutical Solids*, H.G. Brittain (ed.) Marcel Dekker, New York, NY. pp. 1–33.

52. Pudipeddi, M. & Serajuddin, A.T.M. (2005). Trends in solubility of polymorphs. J. Pharm. Sci. 94, 929–939.

53. Nehm, S.J., Rodríguez-Spong, B. & Rodríguez-Hornedo, N. (2006). Phase solubility diagrams of cocrystals are explained by solubility product and solution complexation. Cryst. Grow. Design 6, 592–600.

54. Rodríguez-Hornedo, N., Nehm, S.J. & Seefeldt, K.F. (2006). Reaction crystallization of pharmaceutical molecular complexes. Molecular Pharmaceutics 3, 362–367.

55. Hancock, B.C. & Parks, M. (2000). What is the true solubility advantage for amorphous pharmaceuticals? Pharm. Res. 17, 397–403.

56. Imaizumi, H. (1980). Stability and several physical properties of amorphous and crystalline forms of indomethacin. Chem. Pharm. Bull. 28, 2565–2569.

57. Miyazaki, S., Hori, R. & Arita, T. (1975). Physico-chemical and gastro-intestinal absorption of some solid phases of tetracycline. Yakugaku Zasshi 95, 629–633.

58. Sato, T., Okada, A., Sekiguchi, K. & Tsuda, Y. (1981). Difference in physico-pharmaceutical properties between crystalline and non-crystalline 9,3″-diacetylmidecamycin. Chem. Pharm. Bull. 29, 2675–2682.

59. Mullins, J. & Macek, T. (1960). Some pharmaceutical properties of novobiocin. J. Am. Pharm. Ass. Sci. Ed. 49, 245–248.

60. Shefter, E. & Higuchi, T. (1963). Dissolution behavior of crystalline solvated and nonsolvated forms of some pharmaceuticals. J. Pharm. Sci. 52, 781–791.

61. Stagner, W. C. & Guillory, J. K. (1979). Physical characterization of solid iopanoic acid forms. 68, 1005–1009.

62. Hancock, B.C. & Zografi, G. (1997). Characteristics and significance of the amorphous state in pharmaceutical systems. J. Pharm. Sci. 86, 1–12.

63. Law, D., Krill, S.L., Schmitt, E.A., Fort, J.J., Qiu, Y., Wang, W. & Porter, W.R. (2001). Physicochemical considerations in the preparation of amorphous ritonavir-poly(ethylene glycol) 8000 solid dispersions. J. Pharm. Sci. 90, 1015–1025.

64. Law, D., Schmitt, E.A., Marsh, K.C., Everitt, E.A., Wang, W., Fort, J.J., Krill, S.L. & Qiu, Y. (2004). Ritonavir-PEG 8000 amorphous solid dispersions: *In vitro* and *in vivo* evaluations. J. Pharm. Sci. 93, 563–570.

65. Parke-Davis. (1999). Rezulin® [package insert].

66. Six, K., Daems, T., De Hoon, J., Van Hecken, A., Depre, M., Bouche, M.-P., Prinsen, P., Verreck, G., Peeters, J., Brewster, M.E. & Van Den Mooter, G. (2005). Clinical study of solid dispersions of itraconazole prepared by hot-stage extrusion. Eur. J. Pharm. Sci. 24, 179–186.

67. Yamashita, K., Nakate, T., Okimoto, K., Ohike, A., Tokunaga, Y., Ibuki, R., Higaki, K. & Kimura, T. (2003). Establishment of new preparation method for solid dispersion formulation of tacrolimus. Int. J. Pharm. 267, 79–91.

68. Breitenbach, J. (2006). Melt extrusion can bring new benefits to HIV therapy. Am. J. Drug Del. 4, 61–64.

69. Valeant Pharmaceuticals International. (2006). Cesamet® [package insert].

70. Zografi, G. (1988). States of water associated with solids. Drug Dev. Ind. Pharm. 14, 1905–1926.

71. Newman, A.W., Reutzel-Edens, S.M. & Zografi, G. (2007). Characterization of the "hygroscopic" properties of active pharmaceutical ingredients. J. Pharm. Sci. 97, 1047–1059.

72. Ahlneck, C. & Zografi, G. (1990). The molecular basis of moisture effects on the physical and chemical stability of drugs in the solid state. Int. J. Pharm. 62, 87–95.

73. Cohen, M.D. & Green, B.S. (1973). Organic chemistry in the solid state. Chem. Br. 9, 490–497.

74. Schmidt, G.M.J. (1964). Topochemistry. III. The crystal chemistry of some trans-cinnamic acids. J. Chem. Soc. 43, 2014–2021.

75. Byrn, S.R., Sutton, P.A., Tobias, B., Frye, J. & Main, P. (1988). Crystal structure, solid-state NMR spectra, and oxygen reactivity of five crystal forms of prednisolone tert-butylacetate. J. Am. Chem. Soc. 110, 1609–1614.

76. Byrn, S.R. & Kessler, D.W. (1987). The solid state reactivity of the crystal forms of hydrocortisone esters. Tetrahedron 43, 1335–1343.

77. Sukenik, C.N., Bonapace, J.A.P., Mandel, N.S., Lau, P.-Y., Wood, G. & Bergman, R.G. (1977). A kinetic and x-ray diffraction study of the solid state rearrangement of methyl p-dimethylaminobenzenesulfonate. Reaction rate enhancement due to proper orientation in a crystal. J. Am. Chem. Soc. 99, 851–858.

78. Sukenik, C.N., Bonopace, J.A., Mandel, N.S., Bergman, R.C., Lau, P.Y. & Wood, G. (1975). Enhancement of a chemical reaction rate by proper orientation of reacting molecules in the solid state. J. Am. Chem. Soc. 97, 5290–5291.

79. Leeson, L.J. & Mattocks, A.M. (1958). Decomposition of aspirin in the solid state. J. Am. Pharm. Ass. 47, 329–333.

80. Chen, X., Li, T., Morris, K.R. & Byrn, S.R. (2002). Crystal packing and chemical reactivity of two polymorphs of flufenamic acid with ammonia. Molecular Crystals and Liquid Crystals Science and Technology. Section A: Molecular Crystals and Liquid Crystals 381, 121–131.

81. Kontny, M.J., Grandolfi, G.P. & Zografi, G. (1987). Water vapor sorption of water-soluble substances: Studies of crystalline solids below their critical relative humidities. Pharm. Res. 4, 104–112.

82. Wardrop, J., Law, D., Qiu, Y., Engh, K., Faitsch, L. & Ling, C. (2006). Influence of solid phase and formulation processing on stability of Abbott-232 tablet formulations. J. Pharm. Sci. 95, 2380–2392.

83. Hess, H. (1978). Tablets under the microscope. Pharm. Tech. 2, 38–57.

84. Roberts, R.J. & Rowe, R.C. (1987). The Young's modulus of pharmaceutical materials. Int. J. Pharm. 37, 15–18.

85. Duncan-Hewitt, W.C. & Weatherly, G.C. (1990). Modeling the uniaxial compaction of pharmaceutical powders using the mechanical properties of single crystals. II: Brittle materials. J. Pharm. Sci. 79, 273–278.

86. Danielson, D.W., Morehead, W.T. & Rippie, E.C. (1983). Unloading and postcompression viscoelastic stress versus strain behavior of pharmaceutical solids. J. Pharm. Sci. 72, 342–345.

87. Martino, P.D., Guyot-Hermann, A.-M., Conflant, P., Drache, M. & Guyot, J.-C. (1996). A new pure paracetamol for direct compression: the orthorhombic form. Int. J. Pharm. 128, 1–8.

88. Nichols, G. & Frampton, C.S. (1998). Physicochemical characterization of the orthorhombic polymorph of paracetamol crystallized from solution. J. Pharm. Sci. 87, 684–693.

89. Joiris, E., Martino, P.D., Berneron, C., Guyot-Hermann, A.-M. & Guyot, J.-C. (1998). Compression behavior of orthorhombic paracetamol. Pharm. Res. 15, 1122–1130.

90. Sun, C. & Grant, D.J.W. (2001). Influence of crystal structure on the tableting properties of sulfamerazine polymorphs. Pharm. Res. 18, 274–280.

91. Sun, C. & Grant, D.J.W. (2004). Improved tableting properties of p-hydroxybenzoic acid by water of crystallization: A molecular insight. Pharm. Res. 21, 382–386.

92. Zhang, G.G.Z., Paspal, S.Y.L., Suryanarayanan, R. & Grant, D.J.W. (2003). Racemic species of sodium ibuprofen: Characterization and polymorphic relationships. J. Pharm. Sci. 92, 1356–1366.

93. Yada, S., Ohya, M., Ohuchi, Y., Hamaura, T., Wakiyama, N., Usui, F., Kusai, A. & Yamamoto, K. (2003). Solid phase transition of CS-891 enantiotropes during grinding. Int. J. Pharm. 255, 69–79.

94. Giordano, F., Rossi, A., Moyano, J.R., Gazzaniga, A., Massarotti, V., Bini, M., Capsoni, D., Peveri, T., Redenti, E., Carima, L., Alberi, M.D. & Zanol, M. (2001). Polymorphism of rac-5,6-diisobutyryloxy-2-methylamino-1,2,3,4-tetrahydronaphthalene hydrochloride (CHF 1035). I. Thermal, spectroscopic, and X-ray diffraction properties. J. Pharm. Sci. 90, 1154–1163.

95. Li, Y., Han, J., Zhang, G.G.Z., Grant, D.J.W. & Suryanarayanan, R. (2000). In situ dehydration of carbamazepine dihydrate: A novel technique to prepare amorphous anhydrous carbamazepine. Pharm. Dev. Technol. 5, 257–266.

96. Han, J. & Suryanarayanan, R. (1999). A method for the rapid evaluation of the physical stability of pharmaceutical hydrates. Thermochim. Acta 329, 163–170.

97. Han, J. & Suryanarayanan, R. (1998). Influence of environmental conditions on the kinetics and mechanism of dehydration of carbamazepine dehydrate. Pharm. Dev. Technol. 3, 587–596.

98. Topley, B. & Smith, M.L. (1931). Function of water vapor in the dissociation of a salt hydrate. Nature (London, United Kingdom) 128, 302.

99. Smith, M.L. & Topley, B. (1931). Rate of dissociation of salt hydrates-reaction CuSO4.5H2O = CuSO4 H2O + 4H2O. Proc. R. Soc. London A 134, 224–245.

100. Topley, B. & Smith, M.L. (1935). Kinetics of salt-hydrate dissociations: MnC2O4.2H2O = MnC2O4 + 2H2O. J. Chem. Soc., 321–325.

101. Garner, W.E. & Jennings, T.J. (1954). Nucleation phenomena arising during the dehydration of solid hydrates. Proc. R. Soc. London A 224, 460–471.

102. Garner, W.E. & Tanner, M.G. (1930). The dehydration of copper sulfate pentahydrate. J. Chem. Soc. 47–57.

103. Dollimore, D., Jones, T.E. & Spooner, P. (1970). Thermal decomposition of oxalates. XI. Dehydration of calcium oxalate monohydrate. J. Chem. Soc. Sec. A 17, 2809–2812.

104. Dollimore, D., Heal, G.R. & Mason, J. (1978). The thermal decomposition of oxalates. Part 14. Dehydration of magnesium oxalate dihydrate. Thermochim. Acta 24, 307–313.

105. Masuda, Y. & Nagagata, K. (1989). The effect of water vapor pressure on the kinetics of the thermal dehydration of zinc formate dihydrate. Thermochim. Acta 155, 255–261.

106. Masuda, Y. & Ito, Y. (1992). The effect of water vapor pressure on the thermal dehydration of yttrium formate dihydrate. J. Therm. Anal. 38, 1793–1799.

107. Seto, Y., Sato, H. & Masuda, Y. (2002). Effect of water vapor pressure on thermal dehydration of lithium sulfate monohydrate. Thermochim. Acta 388, 21–25.

108. Cardew, P.T. & Davey, R.J. (1985). The kinetics of solvent-mediated phase-transformations. Proc. R. Soc. London A 398, 415–428.

109. Rodríguez-Hornedo, N., Lechuga-Ballesteros, D. & Wu, H.J. (1992). Phase transition and heterogeneous/epitaxial nucleation of hydrated and anhydrous theophylline crystals. Int. J. Pharm. 85, 149–162.

110. Zhang, G. G. Z., Gu, C., Zell, M. T., Burkhardt, R. T., Munson, E. J. & Grant, D. J. W. (2002). Crystallization and transitions of sulfamerazine polymorphs. 91, 1089–1100.

111. Giordano, F., Bettinetti, G.P., Caramella, C. & Conte, U. (1977). Effects of grinding on the phase transitions of polymorphic modifications of sulfamethoxydiazine. Bollettino. Chimico. Farmaceutico. 116, 433–438.

112. Cheng, W.T., Lin, S.Y. & Li, M.J. (2007). Raman microspectroscopic mapping or thermal system used to investigate milling-induced solid-state conversion of famotidine polymorphs. J. Raman Spectrosc. 38, 1595–1601.

113. Etter, M.C., Reutzel, S.M. & Choo, C.G. (1993). Self-organization of adenine and thymine in the solid state. J. Am. Chem. Soc. 115, 4411–4412.

114. Kuroda, R., Imai, Y. & Tajima, N. (2002). Generation of a co-crystal phase with novel coloristic properties via solid state grinding procedures. ChemComm., 2848–2849.

115. Duddu, S.P. & Grant, D.J.W. (1992). Formation of the racemic compound of ephedrine base from a physical mixture of its enantiomers in the solid, liquid, solution, or vapor state. Pharm. Res. 9, 1083–1091.

116. Bucar, D.K., Henry, R.F., Lou, X., Borchardt, T.B., Macgillivray, L.R. & Zhang, G.G.Z. (2007). Novel co-crystals of caffeine and hydroxy-2-naphthoic acids: Unusual formation of the carboxylic acid dimer in the presence of a heterosynthon. Molecular Pharmaceutics 4, 339–346.

117. Bucar, D.K., Henry, R.F., Lou, X., Borchardt, T.B. & Zhang, G.G.Z. (2007). A "hidden" co-crystal of caffeine and adipic acid. Chem. Comm. 525–527.

118. Serajuddin, A.T.M. (1999). Solid dispersion of poorly water-soluble drugs: Early promises, subsequent problems, and recent breakthroughs. J. Pharm. Sci. 88, 1058–1066.

119. Fox, T.G. & Flory, P.J. (1950). Second order transition temperatures and related properties of polystyrene. 1: Influence of molecular weight. J. Appl. Phys. 21, 581–591.

120. Fox, T.G. & Flory, P.J. (1951). Further studies on the melt viscosity of polyisobutylene. J. Phys. Chem. 55, 221–234.

121. Fox, T.G. & Flory, P.J. (1954). The glass temperature and related properties of polystyrene—influence of molecular weight. J. Polym. Sci. 14, 315–319.

122. Cohen, M.H. & Turnbull, D. (1959). Molecular transport in liquids and glasses. J. Chem. Phys. 31, 1164–1169.

123. Turnbull, D. & Cohen, M.H. (1961). Free-volume model of amorphous phase glass transitions. J. Chem. Phys. 34, 120–125.

124. Turnbull, D. & Cohen, M.H. (1970). On free-volume model of liquid-glass transitions. J. Chem. Phys. 52, 3038–3041.

125. Doolittle, A.K. (1951). Studies in Newtonian flow. II. The dependence of the viscosity of liquids on free-space. J. Appl. Phys. 22, 1471–1475.

126. Gibbs, J.H. & Dimarzio, E.A. (1958). Nature of the glass transition and the glassy state. J. Chem. Phys. 28, 373–383.

127. Adam, G. & Gibbs, J.H. (1965). On the temperature dependence of cooperative relaxation properties in glass-forming liquids. J. Chem. Phys. 43, 139–146.

128. Angell, C.A. (1997). Why C1 = 16–17 in the WLF equation is physical—and the fragility of polymers. Polymer 38, 6261–6266.

129. Goldstein, M. (1973). Viscous liquids and the glass transition IV. Thermodynamic equations and the transition. J. Phys. Chem. 77, 667–673.

130. Johari, G.P. (2000). A resolution for the enigma of a liquid's configurational entropy-molecular kinetics relation. J. Chem. Phys. 112, 8958–8969.

131. Johari, G.P. (2002). The entropy loss on supercooling a liquid and anharmonic contributions. J. Chem. Phys. 116, 2043–2046.

132. Goldstein, M. (1976). Viscous liquids and the glass transition. V. Sources of the excess specific heat of the liquid. J. Chem. Phys. 64, 4767–4774.

133. Hodge, I.M. (1994). Enthalpy relaxation and recovery in amorphous materials. J. Non-Cryst. Solids 169, 211–266.

134. Vogel, H. (1921). Das Temperaturabhängigkeitsgesetz der Viskosität von Flüssigkeiten. Phys. Z. 22, 645–646.

135. Tammann, V.G. & Hesse, W. (1926). Die abhängigkeit der viscosität von der temperatur bei unterkühlten flüssigkeiten. Z. Anorg. Allg. Chem. 156, 245–257.

136. Fulcher, G.S. (1925). Analysis of recent measurements of the viscosity of glasses. J. Am. Ceram. Soc. 8, 339–355.

137. Angell, C.A. & Smith, D.L. (1982). Test of the entropy basis of the Vogel-Tammann-Fulcher equation. Dielectric relaxation of polyalcohols near Tg. J. Phys. Chem. 86, 3845–3852.

138. Angell, C.A. (1995). Formation of glasses from liquids and biopolymers. Science 267, 1924–1935.

139. Bohmer, R., Ngai, K.L., Angell, C.A. & Plazek, D.J. (1999). Nonexponential relaxations in strong and fragile glass formers. J. Chem. Phys. 99, 4201–4209.

140. Moynihan, C.T., Easteal, A.J. & Wilder, J. (1974). Dependence of the glass transition temperature on heating and cooling rate. J. Phys. Chem. 78, 2673–2677.

141. Moynihan, C.T., Lee, S.K., Tatsumisago, M. & Minami, T. (1996). Estimation of activation energies for structural relaxation and viscous flow from DTA and DSC experiments. Thermochim. Acta 280/281, 153–162.

142. Zhou, D., Grant, D.J.W., Zhang, G.G.Z., Law, D. & Schmitt, E.A. (2007). A calorimetric investigation of thermodynamic and molecular mobility contributions to the physical stability of two pharmaceutical glasses. J. Pharm. Sci. 96, 71–83.

143. Hodge, I.M. (1987). Effects of annealing and prior history on enthalpy relaxation in glassy polymers. 6. Adam-Gibbs formulation of nonlinearity. Macromolecules 20, 2897–2908.

144. Ritland, H.N. (1956). Limitations of the fictive temperature concept. J. Am. Ceram. Soc. 39, 403–406.

145. Tool, A.Q. (1946). Relation between inelastic deformability and thermal expansion of glass in its annealing range. J. Am. Ceram. Soc. 29, 240–253.

146. Tool, A.Q. & Eichlin, C.G. (1931). Variations caused in the heating curves of glass by heat treatment. J. Am. Ceram. Soc. 14, 276–308.

147. Narayanaswamy, O.S. (1971). A model of structural relaxation in glass. J. Am. Ceram. Soc. 54, 491–498.

148. Scherer, G.W. (1984). Use of the Adam-Gibbs equation in the analysis of structural relaxation. J. Am. Ceram. Soc. 67, 504–511.

149. Gordon, M. & Taylor, J.S. (1952). Ideal copolymers and the second-order transitions of synthetic rubbers 1: Non-crystalline copolymers. Journal of Applied Chemistry 2, 493–498.

150. Couchman, P.R. & Karasz, F.E. (1978). A classical thermodynamic discussion of the effect of composition on glass-transition temperatures. Macromolecules 11, 117–119.

151. Nishi, T. & Wang, T.T. (1975). Melting-point depression and kinetic effects of cooling on crystallization in poly(vinylidene fluoride) poly(methyl methacrylate) mixtures. Macromolecules 8, 905–915.

152. Hoei, Y., Yamaura, K. & Matsuzawa, S. (1992). A lattice treatment of crystalline solvent-amorphous polymer mixtures on melting-point depression. J. Phys. Chem. 96, 10584–10586.

153. Marsac, P.J., Shamblin, S.L. & Taylor, L.S. (2006). Theoretical and practical approaches for prediction of drug-polymer miscibility and solubility. Pharm. Res. 23, 2417–2426.

154. Zografi, G. (2000). The amorphous state. The 42nd Annual International Industrial Pharmaceutical Research and Development Conference, Madison, WI.

155. Aso, Y., Yoshioka, S. & Kojima, S. (1996). Relationship between water mobility, measured as nuclear magnetic relaxation time, and the crystallization rate of amorphous nifedipine in the presence of some pharmaceutical excipients. Chem. Pharm. Bull. 44, 1065–1067.

156. Aso, Y., Yoshioka, S. & Kojima, S. (2000). Relationship between the crystallization rate of amorphous nifedipine, phenobarbital, and flopropione, and their molecular mobility as measured by their enthalpy relaxation and 1H NMR relaxation times. J. Pharm. Sci. 89, 408–416.

157. Aso, Y., Yoshioka, S. & Kojima, S. (2001). Explanation of the crystallization rate of amorphous nifedipine and phenobarbital from their molecular mobility as measured by 13C nuclear magnetic resonance relaxation time and the relaxation time obtained from the heating rate dependence of the glass transition temperature. J. Pharm. Sci. 90, 798–806.

158. Duddu, S.P., Zhang, G. & Dal Monte, P.R. (1997). The relationship between protein aggregation and molecular mobility below the glass transition temperature of lyophilized formulations containing a monoclonal antibody. Pharm. Res. 14, 596–600.

159. Guo, Y., Byrn, S.R. & Zografi, G. (2000). Physical characteristics and chemical degradation of amorphous quinapril hydrochloride. J. Pharm. Sci. 89, 128–143.

160. Yoshioka, S., Aso, Y. & Kojima, S. (2004). Temperature—and glass transition temperature—dependence of bimolecular reaction rates in lyophilized formulations described by the Adam-Gibbs-Vogel equation. J. Pharm. Sci. 96, 1062–1069.

161. Yoshioka, S. & Aso, Y. (2005). A quantitative assessment of the significance of molecular mobility as a determinant for the stability of lyophilized insulin formulation. Pharm. Res. 22, 1358–1364.

162. Yoshioka, S., Aso, Y. & Miyazaki, T. (2006). Negligible contribution of molecular mobility to the degradation rate of insulin lyophilized with poly(vinylpyrrolidone). J. Pharm. Sci. 95, 939–943.

163. Hikima, T., Adachi, Y., Hanaya, M. & Oguni, M. (1995). Determination of potentially homogeneous-nucleation-based crystallization in o-terphenyl and an interpretation of the nucleation-enhancement mechanism. Phys. Rev. B 52, 3900–3908.

164. Wu, T. & Yu, L. (2006). Origin of enhanced crystal growth kinetics near Tg probed with indomethacin polymorphs. J. Phys. Chem. B 110, 15694–15699.

165. Ishida, H., Wu, T. & Yu, L. (2007). Sudden rise of crystal growth rate of nifedipine near Tg without and with polyvinylpyrrolidone. J. Pharm. Sci. 96, 1131–1138.

166. Sun, Y., Xi, H., Ediger, M.D. & Yu, L. (2008). Diffusionless crystal growth from glass has precursor in equilibrium liquid. J. Phys. Chem. B 112, 661–664.

167. Sun, Y., Xi, H., Chen, S., Ediger, M.D. & Yu, L. (2008). Crystallization near glass transition: transition from diffusion-controlled to diffusionless crystal growth studied with seven polymorphs. J. Phys. Chem. 112, 661–664.

168. Turnbull, D. & Fisher, J. C. (1949). Rate of nucleation in condensed systems. 17, 71–73.

169. Jolley, J.E. (1970). Microstructure of photographic gelatin binders. Photogr. Sci. Eng. 14, 169–177.

170. Hancock, B.C., Shamblin, S.L. & Zografi, G. (1995). Molecular mobility of amorphous pharmaceutical solids below their glass transition temperature. Pharm. Res. 12, 799–806.

171. Shamblin, S.L., Tang, X., Chang, L., Hancock, B.C. & Pikal, M.J. (1999). Characterization of the time scales of molecular motion in pharmaceutically important glasses. J. Phys. Chem. B 103, 4113–4121.

172. Zhou, D., Zhang, G.G.Z., Law, D., Grant, D.J.W. & Schmitt, E.A. (2002). Physical stability of amorphous pharmaceuticals: Importance of configurational thermodynamic quantities and molecular mobility. J. Pharm. Sci. 91, 1863–1872.

173. Zhou, D. (2003). Molecular Mobility, Physical Stability, and Transformation Kinetics of Amorphous and Hydrated Pharmaceuticals. Ph.D., University of Minnesota, Minneapolis.

174. Ediger, M.D., Harrowell, P. & Yu, L. (2008). Crystal growth kinetics exhibit a fragility-dependent decoupling from viscosity. J. Chem. Phys. 128, 034709.

175. Mehta, S. C. (1969). Mechanistic studies of linear single crystal growth rates of sulfathiazole and their inhibition by polyvinyl pyrrolidone. Preparation and dissolution of high-energy sulfathiazole polyvinyl pyrrolidone coprecipitates.

176. Simonelli, A.P., Mehta, S.C. & Higuchi, W.I. (1970). Inhibition of sulfathiazole crystal growth by polyvinylpyrrolidone. J. Pharm. Sci. 59, 633–638.

177. Sekikawa, H., Nakano, M. & Arita, T. (1978). Inhibitory effect of poly(vinylpyrrolidone) on the crystallization of drugs. Chem. Pharm. Bull. 26, 118–126.

178. Ziller, K.H. & Rupprecht, H. (1988). Control of crystal growth in drug suspensions. 1) Design of a control unit and application to acetaminophen suspensions. Drug Dev. Ind. Pharm. 14, 2341–2370.

179. Ma, X., Taw, J. & Chiang, C.-M. (1996). Control of drug crystallization in transdermal matrix system. Int. J. Pharm. 142, 115–119.

180. Ziller, K.H. & Rupprecht, H. (1990). Control of crystal growth in drug suspensions. III. Isothermal crystallization in the presence of polymers. PZ Wissenschaft 3, 147–152.

181. Wen, H., Morris, K.R. & Park, K. (2008). Synergic effects of polymeric additives on dissolution and crystallization of acetaminophen. Pharm. Res. 25, 349–358.

182. Uekama, K., Ikegami, K., Wang, Z., Horiuchi, Y. & Hirayama, F. (1992). Inhibitory effect of 2-hydroxypropyl-b-cyclodextrin on crystal growth of nifedipine during storage: superior dissolution and oral bioavailability compared with poly(vinylpyrrolidone) K-30. J. Pharm. Pharmacol. 44, 73–78.

183. Suzuki, H. & Sunada, H. (1998). Influence of water-soluble polymers on the dissolution of nifedipine solid dispersions with combined carriers. Chem. Pharm. Bull. 46, 482–487.

184. Matsumoto, T. & Zografi, G. (1999). Physical properties of solid molecular dispersions of indomethacin with poly(vinylpyrrolidone) and poly(vinylpyrrolidone-co-vinyl-acetate) in relation to indomethacin crystallization. Pharm. Res. 16, 1722–1728.

185. Crowley, K.J. & Zografi, G. (2003). The effect of low concentrations of molecularly dispersed poly(vinylpyrrolidone) on indomethacin crystallization from the amorphous state. Pharm. Res. 20, 1417–1422.

186. Khougaz, K. & Clas, S.-D. (2000). Crystallization inhibition in solid dispersions of MK-0591 and poly(vinylpyrrolidone) polymers. J. Pharm. Sci. 89, 1325–1334.

187. Huang, J., Wigent, R.J. & Schwartz, J.B. (2007). Drug-polymer interaction and its significance on the physical stability of nifedipine amorphous dispersion in microparticles of an ammonio methacrylate copolymer and ethylcellulose binary blend. J. Pharm. Sci. 97, 251–262.

188. Miyazaki, T., Yoshioka, S. & Aso, Y. (2006). Physical stability of amorphous acetanilide derivatives improved by polymer excipients. Chem. Pharm. Bull. 54, 1207–1210.

189. Konno, H. & Taylor, L.S. (2006). Influence of different polymers on the crystallization tendency of molecularly dispersed amorphous felodipine. J. Pharm. Sci. 95, 2692–2705.

190. Miyazaki, T., Yoshioka, S., Aso, Y. & Kojima, S. (2004). Ability of polyvinylpyrrolidone and polyacrylic acid to inhibit the crystallization of amorphous acetaminophen. J. Pharm. Sci. 93, 2710–2717.

191. Kohri, N., Yamayoshi, Y., Xin, H., Iseki, K., Sato, N., Todo, S. & Miyazaki, K. (1999). Improving the oral bioavailability of albendazole in rabbits by the solid dispersion technique. J. Pharm. Pharmacol. 51, 159–164.

192. Zhang, G.G.Z. (1998). Influences of Solvents on Properties, Structures, and Crystallization of Pharmaceutical Solids, Ph D Thesis. University of Minnesota, Minneapolis, MN.

193. Miller, J.M., Collman, B.M., Greene, L.R., Grant, D.J.W. & Blackburn, A.C. (2005). Identifying the stable polymorph early in the drug discovery-development process. Pharm. Dev. Technol. 10, 291–297.

194. Morissette, S.L., Almarsson, O., Peterson, M.L., Remenar, J.F., Read, M.J., Lemmo, A.V., Ellis, S., Cima, M.J. & Gardner, C.R. (2004). High-throughput crystallization: polymorphs, salts, co-crystals and solvates of pharmaceutical solids. Adv. Drug. Del. Rev. 56, 275–300.

195. Florence, A.J., Johnston, A., Price, S.L., Nowell, H., Kennedy, A. R. & Shankland, N. (2006). An automated parallel crystallisation search for predicted crystal structures and packing motifs of carbamazepine. J. Pharm. Sci. 95, 1918–1930.

196. Remenar, J.F., Macphee, J.M., Larson, B.K., Tyagi, V.A., Ho, J.H., Mcilroy, D.A., Hickey, M.B., Shaw, P.B. & Almarsson, O. (2003). Salt selection and simultaneous polymorphism assessment via high-throughput crystallization: the case of sertraline. Org. Proc. Res. Dev. 7, 990–996.

197. Peterson, M.L., Morissette, S.L., Mcnulty, C., Goldsweig, A., Shaw, P., Lequesne, M., Monagle, J., Encina, N., Marchionna, J., Johnson, A., Gonzalez-Zugasti, J., Lemmo, A.V., Ellis, S.J., Cima, M.J. & Almarsson, O. (2002). Iterative high-throughput polymorphism studies on acetaminophen and an experimentally derived structure for Form III. J. Am. Chem. Soc. 124, 10958–10959.

198. Chyall, L.J., Tower, J.M., Coates, D.A., Houston, T.L. & Childs, S.L. (2002). Polymorph generation in capillary spaces: The preparation and structural analysis of a metastable polymorph of nabumetone. Cryst. Grow. Design 2, 505–510.

199. Hilden, J.L., Reyes, C.E., Kelm, M.J., Tan, J.S., Stowell, J.G. & Morris, K.R. (2003). Capillary precipitation of a highly polymorphic organic compound. Cryst. Grow. Design 3, 921–926.

200. Childs, S.L., Chyall, L.J., Dunlap, J.T., Coates, D.A., Stahly, B.C. & Stahly, G.P. (2004). A Metastable polymorph of metformin hydrochloride: Isolation and characterization using capillary crystallization and thermal microscopy techniques. Cryst. Grow. Design 4, 441–449.

201. Li, L., Mustafi, D., Fu, Q., Tershko, V., Chen, D.L., Tice, J.D. & Ismagilov, R.F. (2006). Nanoliter microfluidic hybrid method for simultaneous screening and optimization validated with crystallization of membrane proteins. Proc. Natl. Acad. Sci. 103, 19243–19248.

202. Gerdts, C.J., Tereshko, V., Yadav, M.K., Dementieva, I., Collart, F., Joachimiak, A., Stevens, R.C., Kuhn, P., Kossiakoff, A. & Ismagilov, R.F. (2006). Time-controlled microfluidic seeding in nL-volume droplets to separate nucleation and growth stages of protein crystallization. Angew. Chem. Int. Ed. Engl. 45, 8156–8160.

203. Zheng, B., Tice, J.D., Roach, L.S. & Ismagilov, R.F. (2004). Crystal growth: A droplet-based, composite PDMS/glass capillary microfluidic system for evaluating protein crystallization conditions by microbatch and vapor-diffusion methods with on-chip X-ray diffraction. Angew. Chem. Int. Ed. Engl. 43, 2508–2511.

204. Talreja, S., Kenis P, J.A. & Zukoski, C.F. (2007). A kinetic model to simulate protein crystal growth in an evaporation-based crystallization platform. Langmuir 23, 4516–4522.

205. He, G., Bhamidi, V., Tan, R.B.H., Kenis, P.J.A. & Zukoski, C.F. (2006). Determination of critical supersaturation from micro-droplet evaporation experiments. Cryst. Grow. Design 6, 1175–1180.

206. He, G., Bhamidi, V., Wilson, S.R., Tan, R.B.H., Kenis, P.J.A. & Zukoski, C.F. (2006). Direct growth of g -glycine from neutral aqueous solutions by slow, evaporation-driven crystallization. Cryst. Grow. Design 6, 1746–1749.

207. Dombrowski, R.D., Litster, J.D., Wagner, N.J. & He, Y. (2007). Crystallization of alpha-lactose monohydrate in a drop-based microfluidic crystallizer. Chem. Eng. Sci. 62, 4802–4810.

3

Analytical Techniques in Solid-state Characterization

Eric J. Munson

3.1 INTRODUCTION

The characterization of pharmaceutical solids is very different from the characterization of pharmaceuticals in solution. The basic issues with pharmaceutical solids arise from the fact that the material is heterogeneous. In solution, most pharmaceutical systems can be characterized through a combination of high performance liquid chromatography (HPLC), solution nuclear magnetic resonance (NMR), and measurement of pH, in part because the systems are homogeneous. In the solid state the system is heterogeneous, and consists of particles of varying sizes and compositions. Moreover, many of the properties that are unique to the solid state, such as crystal form or drug–excipient interactions, disappear when the material goes into solution. Finally, the amount of information provided by various analytical techniques is usually much less than is provided by comparative techniques in solution. For this reason a combination of analytical techniques are usually used to study the material in the solid state.

Most of the analytical techniques used to characterize solids can be divided into two categories: bulk and molecular. Bulk techniques provide information about the state of the material, and rely upon global properties such as the thermodynamics or particle morphology of the system. Bulk techniques include differential scanning calorimetery (DSC), thermogravimetric analysis (TGA), and hot stage microscopy. These techniques provide information about the global state of the material. Molecular-level techniques, such as diffraction, and spectroscopic techniques, provide information

by probing the molecular-level interactions in the system. Although the techniques are divided into two categories, this does not mean that bulk techniques do not provide information about the molecular level interactions occurring in the solid, and *vice versa*. For example, DSC can be used to determine the solid form of the material, which is inherently a molecular-level interaction. Similarly, techniques such as powder X-ray diffraction (PXRD) and some spectroscopic techniques are sensitive to particle size and morphology.

The heterogeneous nature of the material imposes limits upon each of the analytical techniques used to probe the system. For example, many techniques can provide information about the pure form of an active pharmaceutical ingredient (API) or excipient, but have problems when an API is mixed with pharmaceutical excipients. For other techniques the time and amount of sample required to perform an analysis is an issue. This provides a balance in terms of using the techniques. For example, SSNMR is an excellent technique for the analysis of API in the presence of excipients, but often the time and amount of sample required makes it cost-prohibitive to use on a routine basis. This also requires an integrated approach to the use of multiple analytical instruments for the analysis of complex formulations.

The primary issues that need to be addressed in the characterization of a pharmaceutical solid include, but are not limited to, the following areas. For pure chemical materials these include: solid form identification (crystalline, amorphous, hydrates/solvates), quantitation of mixtures of forms, limit of detection of one or more forms in the presence of other forms, and

Developing Solid Oral Dosage Forms: Pharmaceutical Theory and Practice
ISBN: 978-0-444-53242-8

61

determination of particle size and morphology. In formulations the same areas apply, although the analysis of individual chemical species, such as an API in complex formulations, may be significantly more difficult. In addition, the extent of sample preparation must be considered, as well as the degree of data analysis required. Finally, the influence of sample form, such as particle size or shape, must be considered when performing the data interpretation. Some techniques, such as dynamic light scattering, only provide information about one particular aspect of the material, such as the particle size distribution. Other techniques, such as SSNMR, can provide information about a multitude of properties, including molecular structure and dynamics.

Each analytical technique can provide unique information about a drug substance or drug product, but the amount and quality of information is often dependent upon the level of expertise and experience of the user in obtaining and interpreting the data. Obtaining and interpreting a DSC thermogram or powder X-ray diffraction pattern is more difficult than obtaining and interpreting the data from a Karl Fischer titrimetry experiment. In the case of solid-state NMR spectroscopy the data acquisition and interpretation can be complicated, and can require a high degree of expertise, but the wide range of experiments and experimental variables means that the total information obtained can be much greater.

In this chapter many of the common analytical techniques used to characterize pharmaceutical solids will be discussed. Not all of the techniques will be discussed, nor will all of the applications. For each technique an introduction to the technique will be provided, followed by an evaluation of the use of that technique for characterizing pharmaceutical solids. At the end of the chapter some examples of the applications of the techniques will be provided.

3.2 REVIEW OF ANALYTICAL TECHNIQUES AND METHODS

Most, if not all, of the common analytical techniques have extensive literature review articles or books published about them, and it is not the purpose of this chapter to provide an additional review article. For this reason the focus is primarily on the basics of the technique, as well as how it may be applied to pharmaceutical solids. The purpose of this section is to provide some recent in-depth references for the topics addressed in this chapter. These references are found at the end of the chapter. The following sections are drawn primarily from these references.

Several books have descriptions of the analytical techniques used to characterize pharmaceutical solids. Byrn and coworkers have published a second edition to *Solid State Chemistry of Drugs*, and the first third of the book provides an introduction to most of the analytical techniques described here.[1] Brittain has edited several books that focus on polymorphism and methods to analyze polymorphs, including *Physical Characterization of Pharmaceutical Solids*[2] and more recently *Spectroscopy of Pharmaceutical Solids*.[3] Other books focused on pharmaceutical analysis or polymorphism in pharmaceuticals may also have selective sections that highlight the analytical techniques used to characterize pharmaceutical solids.

Review articles highlight the latest developments or application of techniques to pharmaceutical solids. A 2001 issue of *Advanced Drug Delivery Reviews* featured several articles related to characterization of the solid state.[4–6] A 2007 issue of the *Journal of Pharmacy and Pharmacology* also featured several articles that reviewed applications of spectroscopic techniques to pharmaceutical systems.[7–14] A recent review in the *Journal of Pharmaceutical Sciences* focused on the analytical techniques for the quantification of amorphous/crystalline phases in pharmaceutical solids.[15] *American Pharmaceutical Review* features many review articles of the analytical techniques described here, although often not at the depth found in a traditional review article. Giron has published a recent article in *American Pharmaceutical Review* on monitoring polymorphism of drugs.[16]

3.3 MICROSCOPIC METHODS

Microscopic methods can be divided into two categories. There are optical microscopy techniques that probe features on the order of a micron or larger, and electron microscopy techniques that study materials at sub-micron level. Some of the applications of microscopy include crystalline versus amorphous discrimination, monitoring of form changes with temperature, and particle size and morphology determination.

3.3.1 Optical Microscopy

Optical microscopy of pharmaceutical solids is usually combined with cross polarizers to analyze the birefringence of the material. Crystalline solids will usually display birefringence, which manifests itself in a particular pattern, as shown in Figure 3.1. Amorphous solids will usually not display birefringence.

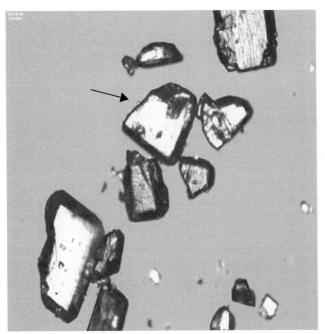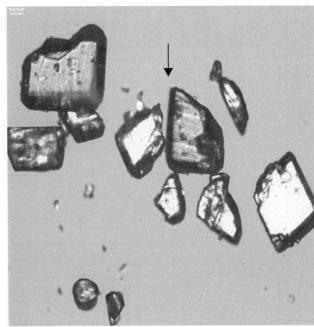

FIGURE 3.1 Optical microscopy of ascorbic acid crystals as taken through cross polarizers. The crystals on the left (a) have been reoriented by 90° compared to the crystals on the right (b). The change in the appearance of the crystals upon reorientation is characteristic of birefringence, and indicates in this case that the material is crystalline

This technique can be used to distinguish rapidly between the crystalline and amorphous forms of materials. This approach works best for pure materials, although it can also be used for formulations.

The combination of a hot-stage with cross polarizers is very powerful for monitoring the changes in pharmaceutical materials upon heating. When pharmaceutical materials are heated they may undergo physical or chemical changes that can be identified using microscopy. For example, crystals undergoing desolvation, especially channel solvates and hydrates, will release solvent(s) upon heating, which can be easily monitored during the hot-stage process. The resulting desolvated materials can remain relatively intact (desolvated solvate), become amorphous or recrystallize to a different crystalline form. Similarly, amorphous forms may recrystallize during heating. Finally, hot-stage microscopy can be useful in determining whether a reaction occurs entirely in the solid state or occurs through a melt.

A negative aspect of microscopy is that it does not provide chemical information about the species present in the sample. When a material changes form, it may also go through a chemical degradation process which microscopy cannot detect. This drawback can be overcome in part by combining microscopy techniques with a spectroscopic method, such as Raman spectroscopy.

There are few articles that focus primarily on optical microscopy, but microscopy techniques are commonly used in conjunction with other analytical techniques to study pharmaceutical solids.

3.3.2 Electron Microscopy

The wavelengths that are visible to the human eye limit the resolution obtained through optical microscopy to several hundred nanometers. An alternative is the use of electron microscopy, which can provide images with resolutions of a few nanometers. An example of the use of electron microscopy is shown in Figure 3.2. Crystalline lactose has a rectangular morphology consistent with crystalline material. Spray dried lactose is amorphous and appears as spherulites.

3.4 THERMAL ANALYSIS

Thermal analysis techniques are commonly used to characterize pharmaceutical solids. In general, thermal techniques rely upon the change in the properties of a material as it is heated. The advantage of most thermal techniques is that a very limited amount of sample (typically only a few milligrams) is required to acquire the data. A disadvantage of thermal methods is that

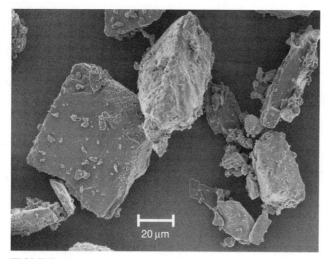
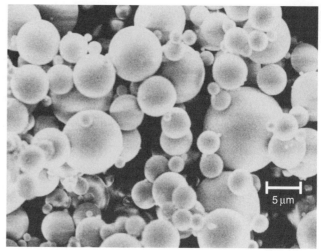

FIGURE 3.2   Electron microscopy of lactose. The electron micrograph on the left is of crystalline lactose. The micrograph on the right is of spray-dried lactose

the properties of the material that are being measured may be significantly different at higher temperatures compared to lower temperatures.

3.4.1 Differential Scanning Calorimetry

Differential scanning calorimetry (OSC) is one of the most common analytical techniques used to characterize pharmaceutical solids. In this technique, a sample and a reference are heated simultaneously while keeping them both at the same temperature. The amount of energy required to heat both the sample and the reference is monitored. The heat capacity of the sample remains relatively constant throughout the analysis, unless the material undergoes a form change, such as recrystallization or, in the case of an amorphous material, there is a glass transition that occurs. In this case, heat is produced by the sample (exothermic) when the material recrystallizes. Heat is absorbed by the sample (endothermic) when it melts. Solid–solid phase transitions may be either exothermic or endothermic. Specific rules have been developed that relate the heat of transition, as well as the heat of fusion, to the relative stability of polymorphic forms (see Chapter 2). DSC results are relatively easy to interpret for pure materials, and the instrument is relatively inexpensive and user-friendly compared with other analytical techniques such as powder x-ray diffraction (PXRD) and solid-state nuclear magnetic resonance spectroscopy (SSNMR).

DSC data can be acquired with either open or crimped pans. In an open-pan system, gases are allowed to escape through a pinhole or an incompletely sealed pan. In a closed-pan system, the pans are hermetically sealed to prevent solvent loss. The transition temperatures for events, such as desolvation, may be very different for an open- versus a closed-pan system, and it is important to know under which conditions the data were acquired, especially when comparing a DSC thermogram to thermogravimetric data.

Recent advances in the field include the use of modulated DSC (MDSC) and rapid-scan DSC. In MDSC it is possible to differentiate between the energy associated with reversible versus non-reversible transitions. In rapid-scan DSC, the sample temperature is heated much more quickly ($>100°C/min$) than is typical ($1-30°C/min$). The rapid temperature increase is more sensitive to specific transitions occurring in the sample, enabling lower limits of detection compared to a slower heating rate.

The following paragraphs describe some recent applications of DSC. The applications are representative of some of the current research in the field. The topics include quantitation of crystalline and amorphous fractions in drugs, characterization of solid dispersions, and estimation of physical stability of amorphous solid dispersions.

Recent work by Bruni and coworkers has shown that it is possible to quantify the amount of amorphous fraction of phenothiazine in a mixture of crystalline and partially amorphous sample.[17] The authors were able to determine the enthalpy change of the crystalline material, and use that value as a standard for 100% crystallized material. The material was made approximately 16% amorphous by ball milling the sample. Physical mixtures of the crystalline standard and the partially amorphous ball milled sample showed that there was excellent agreement between the predicted amorphous content and the amorphous content determined by DSC. This result complements earlier work by Lefort and coworkers, who studied ball milled trehalose using both solid-state NMR spectroscopy and DSC.[18] They found excellent agreement between DSC and solid-state NMR for physical mixtures of purely crystalline and purely amorphous trelahose. They then applied these techniques to samples that had been made partially amorphous using ball milling. The solid-state NMR spectra of the ball milled samples were very similar to the physical mixtures, allowing the authors to determine the amorphous content of the samples. The DSC results were less conclusive, and so the authors concluded that a technique that looks at local order (such as NMR) will be a successful method for the determination of the amorphous content of samples when techniques such as DSC might fail.

Sutariya and coworkers studied solid dispersions of rofecoxib using DSC and PXRD.[19] Formulations were prepared by spray drying (solid dispersion) or physically mixing either polyvinyl pyrrolidone (PVP):talc:drug (3:1:1) or hydroxypropyl methylcellulose (HPMC):talc:drug (4:1:1). They found that the physical mixtures had a much longer dissolution time compared to the solid dispersions, and that the PVP:talc:drug solid dispersion had a shorter dissolution time than the HPMC:talc:drug. DSC showed that the PVP:talc:drug formed a solid solution, whereas in the HPMC:talc:drug formulation the drug remained essentially crystalline. PXRD supported this conclusion. In a similar study, Yoshihashi and coworkers studied the physical stability of solid dispersions of either tolbutamide (TB) or flurbiprofen (FBP) in PVP using DSC and FTIR.[20] Samples containing various amounts of either TB or FBP were heated in the DSC to well above the melting point to eliminate any residual crystals. The samples were then cooled rapidly to a specified temperature, and the onset of crystallization monitored. The onset of crystallization was slowed by the presence of PVP for both drugs. FTIR showed that there was an interaction between the TB and PVP, but not for the FBP and PVP.

3.4.2 Thermogravimetric Analysis

In this technique a sample in an open pan is heated at a specific rate, and the weight gained or lost by the sample is monitored. The technique is primarily used to monitor loss of solvent or decomposition reactions. It is often used in conjunction with DSC to compare the enthalpy of transitions with the resulting weight gain or loss. The heating rate is typically comparable to that used for DSC.

3.4.3 Microcalorimetry

Isothermal microcalorimetry is slightly different from the above techniques in that the sample is kept at constant temperature. A change is induced in the sample, such as a crystallization of an amorphous material or a polymorphic or pseudopolymorphic transition, and the amount of heat gained or lost from the sample is monitored. Isothermal microcalorimetry has the advantage in that the sample is not heated, so the change is observed as it might typically occur at ambient conditions. It is also extremely sensitive to small changes in heat gained or lost, and is commonly used to detect small amounts of amorphous materials in the presence of crystalline material. A negative aspect of isothermal microcalorimetry is that it is not discriminatory, and therefore the exact nature of the transition must be known in order to interpret the data. This is an issue for complex formulations.

The methods described so far have focused on the characterization of the global properties of the material, rather than techniques that analyze the material at the molecular level. These include diffraction and spectroscopic techniques.

3.5 DIFFRACTION METHODS

3.5.1 Single-crystal X-ray Diffraction

Single-crystal XRD is one of the most powerful techniques to determine the structure of a molecule in a crystal. To acquire data from a single crystal, the sample is mounted and a narrow beam of X-rays is passed through it. The wavelength of the X-rays is on the order of the distance between the molecules in the crystal lattice, and the sample therefore acts like a diffraction grating. The diffraction occurs at angles corresponding to the Bragg equation: $n\lambda = 2d \sin \theta$, where λ corresponds to the wavelength of the X-rays, d corresponds to the spacing between reflection planes, and θ is the angle between the incoming X-ray and the reflection plane. The data corresponds to a two-dimensional pattern of spots that is related to the crystal lattice planes. The three-dimensional arrangement of atoms in the unit cell can be solved from this data. Single-crystal data provides information about molecular conformation and packing, hydrogen bonding networks, presence of channels, and solvent location. It has been one of the most definitive techniques used to determine polymorphism, as each crystal form must have differences in the conformation and/or arrangement of the molecules in the crystal lattice. The negative aspect of single-crystal XRD is that a crystal of sufficient size must be grown to be able to determine the crystal structure. This size has decreased dramatically with the use of synchrotron sources for X-rays, but it can still be an issue when the crystal form is generated using techniques not amenable to growing large crystals (such as grinding or lyophilization).

3.5.2 Powder X-ray Diffraction

PXRD is a common technique for the analysis of polymorphism in crystalline solids. The general principle behind PXRD and single-crystal XRD is the same, except that in PXRD the material is a powder. Instead of obtaining a two-dimensional pattern, the data corresponds to rings of greater and lesser intensity as it moves away from the center. The data can be represented as a one-dimensional powder pattern. The data is plotted as intensity versus 2θ angle. The diffraction pattern contains information about the unit cell parameters, which can be obtained by indexing the PXRD pattern. It is possible to determine the three-dimensional crystal structure from high-quality PXRD data using a process known as Rietveld Refinement. Powder X-ray diffraction has often been referred to as the "gold standard" for identification of polymorphs, because it is very sensitive to the unit cell parameters, which almost always vary between polymorphs. The intensity of peaks in a PXRD pattern can depend upon the particle size and morphology, which is often referred to as preferred orientation (Figure 3.3). This may cause some difficulty in interpretation of PXRD data. The diffraction pattern of an amorphous solid corresponds to a broad peak or peaks, often referred to as an amorphous halo because amorphous systems have little long-range order.

There have been several applications of PXRD to pharmaceutical solids. Some of the areas highlighted here include: quantitation of polymorphs in powders, quantitation of crystallinity in substantially amorphous materials, characterization of crystalline forms in intact film-coated tablets, compacts, and counterfeit products, and the determination of crystal structures from PXRD data.

Bansal and coworkers performed a comprehensive study of the capability of PXRD to quantify polymorphic forms of olanzapine (OLZ).[21] They prepared mixtures to show that PXRD could produce a linear calibration curve, and then showed that the corresponding correlation curve of predicted concentration versus actual concentration was linear, with a slope of approximately one and an intercept of zero. Topics such as accuracy, precision, limit of detection (LOD), and limit of quantification (LOQ) for this system were

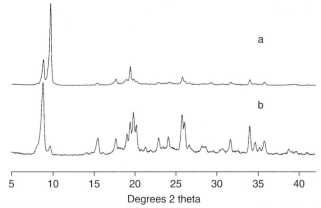

FIGURE 3.3 Powder X-ray diffraction patterns of lyophilized DL-proline. Both patterns correspond to the same crystalline forms, but the pattern in (a) reflects a greater degree of preferred orientation compared to (b)

addressed. In addition, the authors provide an extensive discussion of some of the potential errors associated with quantitative PXRD, including the effects of particle size and morphology, instrument reproducibility, sample positioning, and sample packing.

Yamada and Suryanarayanan studied the physical form of an anti-viral API in intact film-coated tablets using PXRD and microdiffractometry.[22] Microdiffractometry uses a focused X-ray beam that is focused on a small area of the sample, and a two-dimensional area detector for fast data acquisition. The API was known to have three polymorphs and a hemihydrate. Film-coated tablets were prepared containing approximately 15% API (w/w). Tablets containing each of the forms, as well as mixtures of the forms, were prepared. A peak or series of peaks could be identified which was unique to each form. Mixtures of one of the polymorphic forms and the hemihydrate were prepared to create an equation that can be used to quantify the amount of the hemihydrate in the tablet. They were able to determine that the film-coating process did not change the physical form in the tablet, nor did the form change upon stability testing.

Wildfong and coworkers used parallel-beam transmission PXRD to quantify solid-state phase transformations in powder compacts.[23] They used chlorpropamide as a model compound, since it has at least five different crystal forms. They found that concentrations of binary mixtures of two polymorphic forms could be determined using transmission PXRD, which has the advantage of not having to manipulate the samples for analysis.

Maurin and coworkers showed that PXRD is an effective technique for the detection of counterfeit drugs.[24] They used PXRD as a fast screening method for the identification of counterfeit Viagra® tablets.

It was shown that PXRD patterns of the counterfeit tablets could be readily distinguished from the genuine tablets. It was noted that the PXRD patterns were not suitable for trace analysis.

Suryanarayanan and coworkers used PXRD with synchrotron radiation and a two-dimensional area detector to detect crystallinity in pharmaceuticals that are primarily amorphous.[25] Synchrotron radiation, and a two-dimensional area detector, have both increased sensitivity and rapid data acquisition capability. This enables rapid detection of the onset of crystallization for amorphous sucrose. A LOD of 0.2% w/w was achieved for *in situ* monitoring of crystallization.

Shankland and coworkers used a combination of synchrotron and laboratory-based PXRD to obtain high-resolution data to determine the crystal structures of γ-carbamazepine (CBZ) and chlorothiazide N,N-dimethylformamide solvate (CT-DMF2).[26] Solving crystal structures from powder data is important when single crystals are not available. Shankland and coworkers were able to solve structures which contained four molecules in the asymmetric cell (CBZ), and two molecules in the asymmetric cell (CT-DMF2). This demonstrates that complex molecular structures can be determined from powders.

3.6 VIBRATIONAL SPECTROSCOPY

Vibrational spectroscopy techniques include infrared, Raman, and near-infrared spectroscopy. The infrared and Raman both encompass the wavelength range from $400-4000\,cm^{-1}$ and the near-infrared encompasses approximately $4000-14000\,cm^{-1}$ The difference between the infrared and near-infrared region is that the infrared corresponds to the fundamental vibrations of the molecular species, and therefore many of the regions in the spectrum can be assigned to specific functional groups. In near-infrared, the frequencies correspond to harmonics and overtones of the fundamental frequencies, and therefore the near-infrared spectrum is much more difficult to interpret. In Raman spectroscopy the sample is illuminated with a monochromatic light source, such as a laser, usually in the visible or near-infrared region. The Raman scattering of the light corresponds to shifting of the energy levels of the monochromatic source. The amount of shifting corresponds to the vibrational modes of the molecules. Because these techniques probe the fundamental vibrational frequencies of the molecules in the sample, there is some chemical information that can be obtained from the infrared spectrum. In the following section each of the techniques is described in greater detail.

3.6.1 Infrared Spectroscopy

Infrared spectroscopy works on the principle that a sample is irradiated with a broad spectrum of infrared light, of which a fraction of that light will be absorbed by the sample. Infrared spectra are acquired using either transmission or absorption mode, where the percent transmission is equal to:

$$\text{percent transmittance} = \frac{\text{Intensity absorbed}}{\text{Intensity of source}} \times 100$$

and the absorbance is given by:

$$\text{Absorbance} = \text{extinction coefficient} \times \text{path length} \times \text{concentration}$$

The absorption ranges for infrared spectroscopy can be divided into two sections. The region from $400-1000\,cm^{-1}$ is described as the fingerprint region of the spectrum, and is usually unique to a specific molecular compound. The region from $4000-1000\,cm^{-1}$ is defined for specific functional groups. For example, the carbon oxygen double bond, such as found in many carbonyl-containing functional groups such as ketones, aldehydes, esters, and carboxylic acids, absorbs at wavelengths around $1600-1800\,cm^{-1}$.

Infrared spectra are acquired using either a dispersive instrument or a Fourier transform instrument. Fourier transform instruments are constructed based upon an interferometer, where the infrared light from the source is split into two paths, one fixed and the other movable. As the movable path length varies, the intensity of the light will change as the source wavelengths add together either in phase or out of phase, which corresponds to constructive and destructive interference. This light then interacts with a sample, and passes to the detector. The Fourier transform of the resulting intensities acquired at various path lengths results in an infrared spectrum.

There are three common methods for preparing samples for infrared analysis. One method is to mix the sample with an alkali halide, such as KBr, forming a pellet through which infrared light may pass. The disadvantages of this approach include the tremendous amount of pressure that must be applied to the sample to form a pellet, which may cause form changes. Alternatively, the sample can be placed in a diffuse reflectance cell, in which the powder for analysis is placed in a sample cell, and infrared light impinges upon the sample. In attenuated total reflectance, the sample is placed on a crystal, and the infrared beam passes through the crystal. The sample interacts with the evanescent wave, which extends a few microns beyond the surface of the crystal.

Vibrational spectroscopic techniques are primarily used to characterize polymorphs and solvates/hydrates. Infrared spectroscopy is commonly used to provide information about the state of water in the material, and about hydrogen bonding in the system.

Kojima and coworkers studied both anhydrous and hydrate forms of ampicilline and nitrofurantoin using PXRD, TGA, and diffuse reflectance FTIR.[27] They found that diffuse reflectance FTIR was the most sensitive of the three techniques for determination of hydrate formation. Significant differences between the anhydrous and hydrated forms of ampicilline and nitrofurantoin were observed around $3500\,cm^{-1}$, corresponding to hydrogen bonding between water and the compounds. No peaks were observed for the anhydrous forms of these compounds. The authors were able to detect slight changes in the hydration state which were not detected using the other analytical techniques.

3.6.2 Raman Spectroscopy

In Raman spectroscopy the sample is typically illuminated with a laser. The light undergoes the Raman effect which means that a photon from the laser excites a ground state electron into a virtual state. The electron returns to the lower state, but in a higher vibrational level. The energy difference between the initial and scattered photon is known as Stokes scattering. Anti-Stokes scattering occurs when the incident photon starts from a higher vibrational state and relaxes to the lower final state, and is usually much weaker than Raman scattering.

There are several advantages for using Raman spectroscopy to study pharmaceutical solids. The techniques are relatively inexpensive compared to diffraction or SSNMR, and especially for Raman, can be used *in situ*. Another advantage of Raman spectroscopy is that they can be used in conjunction with a microscope to obtain chemical information about a small area of the sample. A chemical map of a tablet can be obtained by using a Raman microscope to scan the surface of the tablet. Additional information can be obtained by microtoming the sample. Raman spectroscopy can be used to identify and quantify polymorphic and pseudopolymorphic forms, providing there is sufficient resolution, and that there are available standards.

Vandenabeele and coworkers used Raman spectroscopy to study counterfeit Viagra® tablets.[28] They analyzed eighteen tablets which contained the API sildenafil in the tablet, but had different excipients. The Raman spectrum between 1150 and $700\,cm^{-1}$ could be used to help identify which tablets were genuine

and which were counterfeit. The authors were able to identify visually that three of the eighteen tablets were counterfeit. The Raman spectrum was able to identify nine additional tablets. The authors then combined principal components analysis with hierarchical cluster analysis to create an automated approach to differentiate between the genuine versus the counterfeit tablets.

Ribeiro-Claro and coworkers used Raman spectroscopy to monitor the transitions between hydrated and anhydrous forms of theophylline.[29] The authors acquired the Raman spectrum of theophylline hydrate (TPh) and anhydrate (TPa), and found unique regions of the spectrum for quantifying the forms. They were able to monitor the hydration of TPa and model it based upon the Avrami-Erofeev random nucleation equation.

3.6.3 Near-infrared

Near-infrared spectroscopy provides the least amount of interpretable information, because of the difficulty in assigning the peaks in the spectrum. However, it is very well suited to process control as it is robust and can penetrate further into the sample than infrared or Raman. The near-infrared spectrum can also provide information about particle size.

3.7 SOLID-STATE NUCLEAR MAGNETIC RESONANCE SPECTROSCOPY

SSNMR is an extremely powerful technique for the characterization of pharmaceutical solids. It is non-destructive and non-invasive, quantitative and selective, and can be used to study structure and dynamics. Despite the broad applications, there are several negative aspects of SSNMR, including the cost of instrumentation, the degree of expertise required to collect and analyze the data, the amount of sample required to perform an analysis, and the relatively low throughput.

The basic principles of Fourier transform NMR involve the excitation of nuclei using a broad radio-frequency pulse, followed by the receiving of the resulting signal (called the free induction decay or FID). The signal is in the time domain, so it is necessary to transform the data into the frequency domain using a Fourier transform. In solution NMR the data corresponds to the average conformation of the molecule because of rapid molecular tumbling. In SSNMR of small molecule crystalline and amorphous solids the molecules are in fixed conformations. This lack of motion means that the ^{1}H NMR spectrum contains peaks that are usually too broad to provide useful chemical shift information. For this reason, other nuclei such as ^{13}C, ^{15}N, and ^{19}F are more commonly studied in the solid state. In order to obtain a high-resolution SSNMR spectrum of these nuclei, the samples must be spun at high speeds at an angle of 54.7° with respect to the static magnetic field. This angle, known as the magic angle, effectively averages the orientational dependence of the chemical shift that exists in solids. The technique is referred to as magic-angle spinning (MAS). The strong coupling of abundant nuclei (such as ^{1}H) to dilute nuclei (such as ^{13}C) results in broad peaks for the dilute nuclei, unless high-power decoupling of the abundant nuclei is also used. The decoupling process is similar to that used in solution NMR, except that the power levels are much stronger because the magnitude of the coupling is much greater. Finally, a technique called cross polarization (CP) usually uses the magnetization of abundant nuclei such as ^{1}H to dilute nuclei such as ^{13}C. The advantage of using cross polarization is that the signal is increased by a factor of up to four for ^{1}H-^{13}C cross polarization, and that the relaxation time of ^{1}H nuclei are usually much faster than the ^{13}C, which means that more acquisitions can be taken per unit time.

Solution NMR is primarily used for structural determination, in part because the resulting frequency spectrum has peaks that can be related back to functional groups in the molecule, and also because advanced techniques such as two-dimensional NMR can be used to determine the connectivity of the functional groups. NMR techniques in the solid state have only recently approached the level of structural determination that is available in solution.

The main focus of SSNMR as it relates to solid oral dosage forms are those properties unique to the solid state. These include identification and quantitation of polymorphs and solvates in bulk drugs, as well as the characterization of the structure and mobility of API and excipients in formulations. Unlike PXRD, the peaks in an NMR spectrum can be assigned to specific functional groups. Since API and excipients usually have significantly different chemical functionalities, they appear in different regions of the spectrum. Excipients that do not have carbon (e.g., talc) do not contribute to the spectrum. Spectral editing techniques can be used to selectively study the API in a formulation by minimizing the contributions of excipients. SSNMR has emerged as a structural technique by combining advanced SSNMR experiments with theoretical predictions to rival crystallography as a method to determine the three-dimensional structure

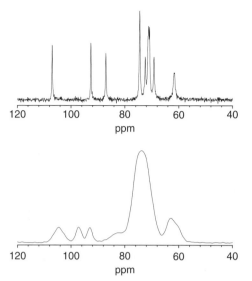

FIGURE 3.4 ^{13}C CPMAS NMR spectra of lactose. The spectrum above is of crystalline lactose. The spectrum below is of spray dried lactose

of molecules in a crystal lattice. Experiments can be performed at both high and low temperatures, which is extremely useful for investigating mobility.

The ^{13}C solid-state NMR spectra of the lactose samples shown in Figure 3.2 are shown in Figure 3.4. The spectrum of crystalline lactose has relatively sharp peaks, and the spectrum of amorphous lactose has peaks that are significantly broader. This agrees well with the micrographs shown in Figure 3.2.

There have been several reviews[14,30–35] and research articles[18,36–40] on the use of solid-state NMR spectroscopy to characterize pharmaceuticals. Two examples of the use of selective ^{13}C-labeling to selectively enhance peaks in the SSNMR spectrum are described below.

Peresypkin and coworkers used selectively ^{13}C-labeled butylated hydroxyl anisole (BHA) to determine its physical form in the presence of excipients.[41] They found that the BHA could exist in either a crystalline form, an amorphous form or in a liquid-like state. The state of BHA depended upon loading, and upon the type of excipient used. By using ^{13}C labeling the authors were able to determine the form of BHA even at loadings as low as 0.1% w/w.

Kellenbach and coworkers used selective ^{13}C labeling to enhance the sensitivity of studying polymorphism in low dose solid formulations.[42] A low-dose steroid drug with two known polymorphic forms was synthesized with ^{13}C labels in three sites in the molecule. They were able to determine the polymorphic form of the drug at 0.5% w/w. The authors noted that even lower levels were possible.

3.8 SORPTION TECHNIQUES

The knowledge of the sorption and desorption properties of water and organic solvents from pharmaceuticals is critical to understanding important areas such as drug stability. Stability studies are performed at specific temperature and relative humidity conditions, reflecting the importance of water sorption behavior on pharmaceutical systems. This section will primarily discuss water vapor sorption, as this is the most common and most important use of sorption technology, but other solvents may also be used.

The amount of water available for sorption is a function of water activity. Water activity (A_w) is defined as the vapor pressure of water (p) divided by the vapor pressure of pure water (p_o) at that temperature. Relative humidity (RH) is defined as the water activity times 100%. Since the vapor pressure of water is strongly dependent upon temperature, both temperature and relative humidity must be specified to determine the total amount of water available during the sorption/desorption process.

There are two general approaches to monitoring the properties of water sorption and desorption. The first is to place a series of samples into containers of various relative humidities, and allow the samples to come to equilibrium at that given temperature and RH. The RH is usually maintained by placing a saturated salt solution in the container. The water content of the sample is measured gravimetrically by comparing the sample weight before and after exposure to the specified conditions. Alternatively, the water content can be measured using Karl Fischer titrimetry. Multiple samples can be stored at the same relative humidity. The advantages of using saturated salt solutions are that the relative humidity remains approximately constant with respect to temperature, and that the cost of the equipment is relatively small. The disadvantages include: multiple sampling may be required to determine if the sample has reached equilibrium, and at least one analytical test (weighing or Karl Fischer titrimetry) must be performed for each sample at each relative humidity, which makes it extremely labor intensive.

The second approach is to automatically monitor the weight change as a function of relative humidity using a commercial water vapor sorption instrument. In this instrument the sample is placed in a chamber at a fixed temperature and RH, and the weight is monitored using a microbalance. The sample has reached equilibrium when the weight does not change. The temperature and/or RH are changed, and the weight of the sample is again monitored until it reaches the new equilibrium. On modern instruments the process

of monitoring weight and controlling temperature and RH is automated, which means that tens or hundreds of points can be acquired at various temperatures and relative humidities. The data is usually presented as a plot of relative humidity on the X-axis versus weight gain/loss on the Y-axis at a fixed temperature, where the weight displayed is the final weight at equilibrium.

Water vapor sorption techniques can provide information about the physical state of the sample, including differentiating between crystalline and amorphous compounds, and different crystalline forms. For amorphous compounds the weight of the sample may increase as the relative humidity increases, until the material begins to crystallize, at which time the weight may decrease, due to the crystalline form having lower water content than the amorphous form. For crystalline compounds the plot may contain discrete steps, as stoichiometric hydrates of the compound form with increasing RH. When non-stoichiometric hydrates are produced there may be no clear discrete steps. Water vapor sorption techniques can also be used to determine the RH at which the sample deliquesces or begins to form a liquid upon uptake of water. An example of the use of water vapor sorption is shown in Figure 3.5.

Taylor and coworkers investigated the water vapor sorption behavior of ranitidine HCl in which the deliquescence RH decreases in the presence of impurities.[43] Two polymorphic forms of ranitidine HCl had essentially the same water vapor sorption profiles, whereas the impure forms of the ranitidine HCl had much greater water sorption amounts at a specific RH compared to the pure forms. This suggests that a higher level of water uptake for impure materials could cause faster physical and chemical degradation.

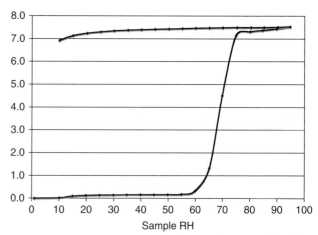

FIGURE 3.5 Water vapor sorption plot of a crystalline hydroscopic compound. The plot shows that the sample takes up about 7% water when exposed to a RH of >80%. The sample does not lose water as the RH is decreased. The data was acquired under isothermal conditions (~25°C)

3.9 OTHER TECHNIQUES

The techniques described in the previous sections usually provide complex information about the sample in terms of a spectrum or image. Temperature is often a variable that can be changed to provide additional information about the sample. For example, microscopy can provide information about the morphology and physical changes that might occur within samples, and can be used in conjunction with a hot stage to study desolvation reactions. Solid-state NMR provides information about structure, and can be combined with variable temperature to gain further insight into mobility. In general, these techniques primarily focus on the physical form of the material, i.e., whether it is crystalline or amorphous, and which particular crystalline form is present.

There are several other characteristics of powder pharmaceuticals which also must be determined, including particle size and morphology, electrostatic interactions, and surface properties (wettability, surface area, etc.). These techniques usually only provide one piece of information about the sample. Particle size/morphology characterization is very important, especially as it relates to the manufacturing process. Particle size is often determined by using light-scattering techniques and/or microscopy techniques. Since particle size and morphology can vary considerably with a sample, the techniques usually report an average particle size distribution. This distribution can vary depending upon the technique used to measure particle size. Surface properties, such as surface area, may also be significant to water uptake and stability.

3.10 CHARACTERIZATION OF SOLIDS USING COMPLEMENTARY ANALYTICAL TECHNIQUES

As was noted in the introduction, the heterogeneous nature of solids means that a wide range of analytical techniques should be used to fully characterize a solid pharmaceutical system. The complementary nature of the techniques means that each technique can provide a unique piece of information about the material or system. In general, the less that is known about the system means that more techniques will be required to fully characterize it. The techniques used to characterize drug substance may not be well-suited to study drug product. For example, DSC or TGA may not provide compound specific information because the transitions cannot be assigned to a specific chemical moiety. Many of the spectroscopic techniques, however, have individual peaks that may belong only to the drug substance being investigated. A carbonyl peak in an infrared or solid-state NMR spectrum may only belong to the drug substance, so any changes in that peak could be reasonably assigned to a change in the physical or chemical form of the compound instead of an excipient.

An example of the complementary nature of the techniques is shown in Figure 3.6. In this example the DSC thermograms, powder X-ray diffraction patterns, and solid-state NMR spectra of D-proline and DL-proline are shown. Proline is an amino acid which contains five carbons. The crystal structure of the pure enantiomer (either D or L) is different from that of the racemate. From an analytical view, some of the questions that might arise about these samples include:

1. are they crystalline or amorphous?
2. are they a pure crystalline form, or a mixture of forms?
3. is the DL-proline a racemic compound (a new crystal form containing both D and L enantiomers of proline) or a racemic conglomerate (a physical mixture of D and L crystal forms)?

Thermal analysis is useful to probe the thermodynamic properties of the two samples. In the case of D-proline (Figure 3.6a), a melting endotherm is observed at approximately 228°C. Although not shown, the heat of fusion could be calculated from the endotherm, providing additional information about the sample. This could be important for determining the monotropic versus enantiotropic relationship between any polymorphs that could be present. Above 230°C the compound begins to decompose. The DSC thermogram of DL-proline is shown in Figure 3.6b. Unlike D-proline, there is an endotherm at ~80°C, followed by two distinct endotherms between 215–220°C. The first endotherm is the result of either a polymorphic transition or a dehydration step. The two endotherms between 215–220°C are likely the result of the melting of two polymorphic forms of DL-proline. From the DSC the following conclusions could be drawn:

1. the D-proline sample appears to have only one form, with a melting point of ~228°C; and
2. the DL-proline sample contains more than one form, at least during the data acquisition.

The small endotherm for the D-proline at ~55°C is probably due to loss of residual water. The DL-proline sample is hydroscopic and contains a small amount of a monohydrate form. The evidence for the monohydrate form is found in the solid-state NMR spectrum (Figure 3.6f).

The powder X-ray diffraction patterns of the two forms are shown in Figure 3.6c, d. The peaks are very

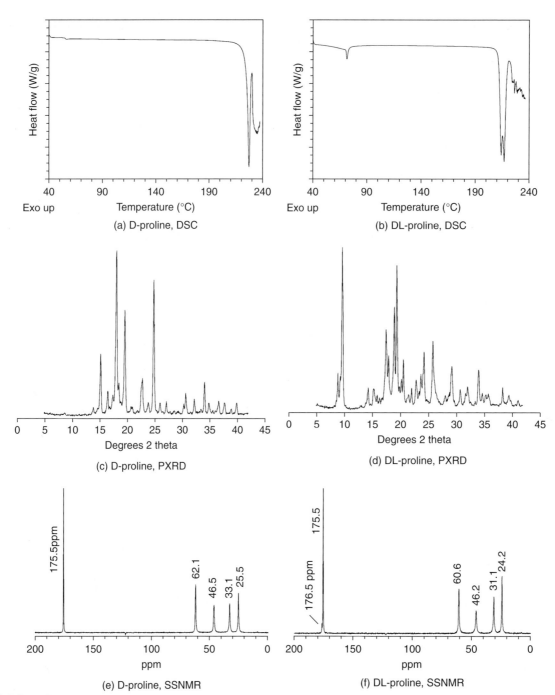

FIGURE 3.6 Differential scanning calorimetry (DSC) thermograms, powder X-ray diffraction patterns, and solid-state NMR spectra of D-proline and DL-proline

narrow, with no obvious indication of an amorphous halo, suggesting that the material is crystalline. As noted in the PXRD section, the patterns represent the unit cell parameters associated with these forms. The patterns are clearly different, as noted by the large peaks around 9−10° 2θ in the DL-proline, but absent in the D-proline pattern. Likewise, there is a large peak at ~25° 2θ in the D-proline that is absent in the DL-proline pattern. Care must be taken to avoid the possibility of preferred orientation as a possible artifact. This strongly suggests that this sample is not a racemic conglomerate, as noted above. Further data analysis of the PXRD patterns might allow the indexing of the pattern, which would provide information about the unit cell parameters. The data are probably not of sufficient quality for a full structure determination.

The ^{13}C CPMAS NMR spectra of D-proline and DL-proline are shown in Figure 3.6e, f. The D-proline spectrum has five peaks, indicative of five carbons in the molecule. Because there are only five peaks, this strongly suggests that there is one molecule in the asymmetric unit cell. All of the peaks in the spectrum can be assigned based upon their solution NMR resonances, as well as their anticipated chemical shifts based upon their functional groups. For example, the peak at 175 ppm corresponds to a carbonyl carbon, and the peaks below 70 ppm correspond to aliphatic carbons. The ability to assign specific peaks in the spectrum to particular functional groups is indicative of the difference between spectroscopic techniques and diffraction techniques. The DL-proline spectrum also has the similar type of spectrum. In general, chemical shifts should differ by no more than 10 ppm from their solution values. The spectra are different, in that several of the peaks have a chemical shift difference of up to 2 ppm. Chemical shifts are influenced by the packing and/or arrangement of the molecules in the crystal lattice, and the fact that there are differences indicate that the crystal forms are different, as supported by the DSC and PXRD data. The small peak at 176.5 ppm in the spectrum of DL-proline (Figure 3.6f) corresponds to the monohydrate form of DL-proline. In addition to the spectra shown here, relaxation measurements could be used to assess mobility of the proline carbons in the lattice. Line widths could also be compared to determine crystal quality. Finally, because ^{13}C is only ~1.1% natural abundance, selective ^{13}C labeling can be used to determine the location of ^{13}C-labeled L-proline in a sample composed primarily of D-proline.

Byrn and coworkers used a combination infrared spectroscopy, PXRD, and SSNMR to study the acid–base reaction between solid indomethacin and sodium bicarbonate.[36] Each of the analytical techniques was used to monitor the progress of the reaction. Infrared spectroscopy showed peaks which were between 3400 and 3600 cm^{-1} for the product sodium indomethacin trihydrate, which were not present for either of the reactants. Although both PXRD and SSNMR showed differences between a physical mixture of the reactants and the product, infrared was used to follow the reaction.

3.11 CONCLUSION

The purpose of this chapter is to provide an introduction to the most common analytical techniques used in solid-state characterization. The complicated nature of the solid state requires that a full suite of analytical tools be available to study the system, and the choice of the technique or techniques to use depends upon how much information is required about the system. In the characterization of a new pharmaceutical compound, most of the techniques described in this chapter would be used. Once a system has been fully characterized, a smaller subset of the techniques may be used to monitor features such as changes in physical form or particle size/morphology.

ACKNOWLEDGEMENTS

This work was supported in part by NSF CHE-0719464. The assistance of Robert Berendt, Eric Gorman, and Diana Sperger is gratefully recognized.

References

1. Byrn, S.R., Pfeiffer, R.R. & Stowell, J.G. (1999). *Solid State Chemistry of Drugs*, 2nd edn. SSCI, Inc., West Lafayette. p. 574.
2. Brittain, H.G. (1995). *Physical characterization of pharmaceutical solids*. Vol. 70. Marcel Dekker, New York, NY.
3. Brittain, H.G. (2006). *Spectroscopy of pharmaceutical solids*. Vol. 160. Taylor & Francis, New York, NY.
4. Yu, L. (2001). Amorphous pharmaceutical solids: Preparation, characterization and stabilization. Adv. Drug Delivery Rev. 48(1), 27–42.
5. Stephenson, G.A., Forbes, R.A. & Reutzel-Edens, S.M. (2001). Characterization of the solid state: quantitative issues. Adv. Drug Delivery Rev. 48(1), 67–90.
6. Bugay, D.E. (2001). Characterization of the solid-state: spectroscopic techniques. Adv. Drug Delivery Rev. 48(1), 43–65.
7. Zeitler, J.A., Taday, P.F., Newnham, D.A., Pepper, M., Gordon, K.C. & Rades, T. (2007). Terahertz pulsed spectroscopy and imaging in the pharmaceutical setting—a review. J. Pharm. Pharmacol. 59(2), 209–223.
8. Strachan, C.J., Rades, T., Gordon, K.C. & Rantanen, J. (2007). Raman spectroscopy for quantitative analysis of pharmaceutical solids. J. Pharm. Pharmacol. 59(2), 179–192.
9. Rasanen, E. & Sandler, N. (2007). Near-infrared spectroscopy in the development of solid dosage forms. J. Pharm. Pharmacol. 59(2), 147–159.
10. Rantanen, J. (2007). Process analytical applications of Raman spectroscopy. J. Pharm. Pharmacol. 59(2), 171–177.
11. Prestidge, C.A., Barnes, T.J. & Skinner, W. (2007). Time-of-flight secondary-ion mass spectrometry for the surface characterization of solid-state pharmaceuticals. J. Pharm. Pharmacol. 59(2), 251–259.
12. Lee, C.J., Strachan, C.J., Manson, P.J. & Rades, T. (2007). Characterization of the bulk properties of pharmaceutical solids using nonlinear optics—a review. J. Pharm. Pharmacol. 59(2), 241–250.
13. Jones, D.S. & Rades, T. (2007). Themed issue: Applications of novel spectroscopic techniques to pharmaceutical systems. J. Pharm. Pharmacol. 59(2), 145–146.
14. Harris, R.K. (2007). Applications of solid-state NMR to pharmaceutical polymorphism and related matters. J. Pharm. Pharmacol. 59(2), 225–239.
15. Shah, B., Kakumanu, V.K. & Bansal, A.K. (2006). Analytical techniques for quantification of amorphous/crystalline phases in pharmaceutical solids. J. Pharm. Sci. 95(8), 1641–1665.
16. Giron, D. (2008). Monitoring polymorphism of drugs, an on-going challenge: Part 1. Am. Pharm. Rev. 11(1), 66, 68–71.

17. Bruni, G., Milanese, C., Bellazzi, G., Berbenni, V., Cofrancesco, P., Marini, A. & Villa, M. (2007). Quantification of drug amorphous fraction by DSC. J. Therm. Anal. Calorim. 89(3), 761–766.

18. Lefort, R., De Gusseme, A., Willart, J.F., Danede, F. & Descamps, M. (2004). Solid state NMR and DSC methods for quantifying the amorphous content in solid dosage forms: An application to ball-milling of trehalose. Int. J. Pharm. 280(1–2), 209–219.

19. Mashru, R.C., Sutariya, V.B., Sankalia, M.G. & Yagnakumar, P. (2005). Characterization of solid dispersions of rofecoxib using differential scanning calorimeter. J. Therm. Anal. Calorim. 82(1), 167–170.

20. Yoshihashi, Y., Iijima, H., Yonemochi, E. & Terada, K. (2006). Estimation of physical stability of amorphous solid dispersion using differential scanning calorimetry. J. Therm. Anal. Calorim. 85(3), 689–692.

21. Tiwari, M., Chawla, G. & Bansal, A.K. (2007). Quantification of olanzapine polymorphs using powder X-ray diffraction technique. J. Pharm. Biomed. Anal. 43(3), 865–872.

22. Yamada, H. & Suryanarayanan, R. (2007). X-ray powder diffractometry of intact film coated tablets–an approach to monitor the physical form of the active pharmaceutical ingredient during processing and storage. J. Pharm. Sci. 96(8), 2029–2036.

23. Wildfong, P.L.D., Morley, N.A., Moore, M.D. & Morris, K.R. (2005). Quantitative determination of polymorphic composition in intact compacts by parallel-beam X-ray powder diffractometry. II. Data correction for analysis of phase transformations as a function of pressure. J. Pharm. Biomed. Anal. 39(1–2), 1–7.

24. Maurin, J.K., Plucinski, F., Mazurek, A.P. & Fijalek, Z. (2007). The usefulness of simple X-ray powder diffraction analysis for counterfeit control—The Viagra example. J. Pharm. Biomed. Anal. 43(4), 1514–1518.

25. Nunes, C., Mahendrasingam, A. & Suryanarayanan, R. (2005). Quantification of crystallinity in substantially amorphous materials by synchrotron X-ray powder diffractometry. Pharm. Res. 22(11), 1942–1953.

26. Fernandes, P., Shankland, K., Florence, A.J., Shankland, N. & Johnston, A. (2007). Solving molecular crystal structures from X-ray powder diffraction data: The challenges posed by gamma-carbamazepine and chlorothiazide N,N,-dimethylformamide (1/2) solvate. J. Pharm. Sci. 96(5), 1192–1202.

27. Kojima, T., Yamauchi, Y., Onoue, S. & Tsuda, Y. (2008). Evaluation of hydrate formation of a pharmaceutical solid by using diffuse reflectance infrared Fourier-transform spectroscopy. J. Pharm. Biomed. Anal. 46(4), 788–791.

28. de Veij, M., Deneckere, A., Vandenabeele, P., de Kaste, D. & Moens, L. (2008). Detection of counterfeit Viagra with Raman spectroscopy. J. Pharm. Biomed. Anal. 46(2), 303–309.

29. Amado, A.M., Nolasco, M.M. & Ribeiro-Claro, P.J.A. (2007). Probing pseudopolymorphic transitions in pharmaceutical solids using Raman spectroscopy: hydration and dehydration of theophylline. J. Pharm. Sci. 96(5), 1366–1379.

30. Berendt, R.T., Sperger, D.M., Munson, E.J. & Isbester, P.K. (2006). Solid-state NMR spectroscopy in pharmaceutical research and analysis. TrAC, Trends Anal. Chem. 25(10), 977–984.

31. Lubach, J.W. & Munson, E.J. (2006). Solid-state NMR spectroscopy. Polymorphism, 81–93.

32. Harris, R.K. (2006). NMR studies of organic polymorphs and solvates. Analyst (Cambridge, UK) 131(3), 351–373.

33. Tishmack, P.A., Bugay, D.E. & Byrn, S.R. (2003). Solid-state nuclear magnetic resonance spectroscopy-pharmaceutical applications. J. Pharm. Sci. 92(3), 441–474.

34. Bugay, D.E. (2002). Solid-state nuclear magnetic resonance spectroscopy. Drugs Pharm. Sci. (Handbook of Pharmaceutical Analysis), 117, 467–499.

35. Bugay, D.E. (1993). Solid-state nuclear magnetic resonance spectroscopy: Theory and pharmaceutical applications. Pharm. Res. 10(3), 317–327.

36. Chen, X., Griesser, U.J., Te, R.L., Pfeiffer, R.R., Morris, K.R., Stowell, J.G. & Byrn, S.R. (2005). Analysis of the acid-base reaction between solid indomethacin and sodium bicarbonate using infrared spectroscopy, X-ray powder diffraction, and solid-state nuclear magnetic resonance spectroscopy. J. Pharm. Biomed. Anal. 38(4), 670–677.

37. Sotthivirat, S., Lubach, J.W., Haslam, J.L., Munson, E.J. & Stella, V.J. (2007). Characterization of prednisolone in controlled porosity osmotic pump pellets using solid-state NMR spectroscopy. J. Pharm. Sci. 96(5), 1008–1017.

38. Lubach, J.W., Xu, D., Segmuller, B.E. & Munson, E.J. (2007). Investigation of the effects of pharmaceutical processing upon solid-state NMR relaxation times and implications to solid-state formulation stability. J. Pharm. Sci. 96(4), 777–787.

39. Barich, D.H., Davis, J.M., Schieber, L.J., Zell, M.T. & Munson, E.J. (2006). Investigation of solid-state NMR line widths of ibuprofen in drug formulations. J. Pharm. Sci. 95(7), 1586–1594.

40. Lubach, J.W., Padden, B.E., Winslow, S.L., Salsbury, J.S., Masters, D.B., Topp, E.M. & Munson, E.J. (2004). Solid-state NMR studies of pharmaceutical solids in polymer matrices. Anal. Bioanal. Chem. 378(6), 1504–1510.

41. Remenar, J.F., Wenslow, R., Ostovic, D. & Peresypkin, A. (2004). Solid-state nuclear magnetic resonance determination of the physical form of BHA on common pharmaceutical excipients. Pharm. Res. 21(1), 185–188.

42. Booy, K.-J., Wiegerinck, P., Vader, J., Kaspersen, F., Lambregts, D., Vromans, H. & Kellenbach, E. (2005). The use of ^{13}C labeling to enhance the sensitivity of ^{13}C solid-state CPMAS NMR to study polymorphism in low dose solid formulations. J. Pharm. Sci. 94(2), 458–463.

43. Guerrieri, P., Salameh, A.K. & Taylor, L.S. (2007). Effect of small levels of impurities on the water vapor sorption behavior of ranitidine HCl. Pharm. Res. 24(1), 147–156.

Salt Screening and Selection: New Challenges and Considerations in the Modern Pharmaceutical Research and Development Paradigm

Wei-Qin (Tony) Tong

4.1 INTRODUCTION

The pharmaceutical industry is facing unprecedented challenges as a result of increased economic and regulatory pressures in recent years. With a significant number of patents for blockbuster drugs expired or expiring in the next few years, pressure to rebuild drug pipelines is tremendous. While the advent of combinatorial chemistry, high-throughput screening, and other drug discovery innovations have resulted in many more hits and potential development candidates, properties of these development candidates are becoming less favorable for development.[1,2,3,4,5] To improve the properties of these new drug candidates, many pharmaceutical companies are putting "developability" of these new molecules as a selection criterion for drug candidates. There is now a greater collaboration between discovery and development scientists in evaluating such developability criteria as solubility, stability, permeability, and pharmacokinetics properties. This breakdown of barriers between discovery research and development represents a paradigm shift in the pharmaceutical R&D process.[5]

The solubility of an organic molecule is frequently enhanced more by an ionized functional group than by any other single means since the salt form of a drug is usually more soluble than the non-ionized form in an aqueous medium.[6] A salt form also can impact other physico-chemical properties of the drug substance, such as hygroscopicity, chemical stability, crystal form, and mechanical properties.[7] Since it can have such a profound impact on biopharmaceutical and pharmaceutical properties, an appropriate choice of the most desirable salt form is a critical step in the development process.

Over the last several decades, the process for salt selection has been well-established, and remained largely unchanged.[8] Because the decision for salt selection is equally driven by process, as well as by science, the R&D paradigm shift naturally calls for new considerations. First of all, since a salt can affect most physico-chemical properties of a drug candidate, the impact of salt on developability needs to be evaluated.[9] Secondly, since the development timeline is getting much shorter, the need to select the right salt the first time is becoming more important. Because of the poor biopharmaceutical properties of many new drug candidates, the need for special drug delivery systems is also increasing. Thus, the impact of choice of salt forms on the performance of drugs in these systems should be evaluated as part of the salt selection process.

The purpose of this chapter is to review salt screening and selection strategies, taking into account the new challenges and considerations of modern drug discovery and development processes. For completeness, some fundamental solubility theory pertinent to the salt selection decision is also briefly discussed. For the complete discussion of various salt forms currently in use in pharmaceutical products, the reader is directed to several excellent reviews.[8,10]

4.2 THEORETICAL CONSIDERATIONS

4.2.1 pH-Solubility Profiles and the Role of pK_a

The equilibrium for dissociation of the conjugate acid of a basic compound may be expressed by:

$$BH^+ + H_2O \overset{K'_a}{\rightleftharpoons} B + H_3O^+ \qquad (4.1)$$

HB^+ is the protonated species, B is the free base, and K'_a is the apparent dissociation constant of HB^+, which is defined as follows:

$$K'_a = \frac{[H_3O^+][B]}{[BH^+]} \qquad (4.2)$$

Generally, the relationships expressed in Equations 4.1 and 4.2 must be satisfied for all weak electrolytes in equilibrium, irrespective of pH and the degree of saturation. At any pH, the total concentration of a compound, S_T, is the sum of the individual concentrations of its respective species:

$$S_T = [BH^+] + [B] \qquad (4.3)$$

In a saturated solution of arbitrary pH, this total concentration, S_T, is the sum of the solubility of one of the species, and the concentration of the other necessary to satisfy mass balance. At low pH, where the solubility of BH^+ is limiting, the following relationship holds:

$$S_{T,pH\,<\,pH_{max}} = [BH^+]_s + [B] = [BH^+]_s \left(1 + \frac{K'_a}{[H_3O^+]}\right) \qquad (4.4)$$

pH_{max} refers to the pH of maximum solubility, and the subscript $pH < pH_{max}$ indicates that this equation is valid only for pH values less than pH_{max}. The subscript s indicates a saturated species. A similar equation can be written for solutions at pH values greater than pH_{max} where the free base solubility is limiting:

$$S_{T,pH\,>\,pH_{max}} = [BH^+] + [B]_s = [B]_s \left(1 + \frac{[H_3O^+]}{K'_a}\right) \qquad (4.5)$$

Each of these equations describes an independent curve that is limited by the solubility of one of the two species. The pH-solubility profile is non-uniformly continuous at the juncture of the respective solubility curves. This occurs at the precise pH where the species are simultaneously saturated, previously designated as the pH_{max}.[11]

In an uncomplicated system (such as described in Equation 4.1), the theoretical pH-solubility profile can be generated using Equations 4.4 and 4.5, given the solubility of the salt, the solubility of the free base, and the apparent dissociation constant. Figure 4.1 is the pH-solubility profile for the hydrochloride salt of a free base (B) constructed by assuming that the solubilities of the hydrochloride salt and the free base are $1\,mg/mL$ and $0.001\,mg/mL$, respectively, and that the pK'_a of the compound is equal to 6.5.

While the pK'_a does not determine the shape of the pH-solubility profile, it does fix the location of this profile on the pH coordinate. All other factors being equal, each upward or downward shift in the pK'_a is matched exactly by an upward or downward shift in pH_{max}. If the solubility of the free base is very small relative to that of the hydrochloride, the free base limiting curve (curve II) of the overall pH-solubility profile cuts deeply into the acidic pH range. Therefore, the solubility of the free base and the pK'_a basically determine the maximum pH at which formulation as a solution is possible, assuming the desired concentration exceeds the free base solubility. These effects are further illustrated in Figure 4.2.[12]

The pH-solubility profile of an acidic drug is the mirror image of the profile of a basic drug.[11,13]

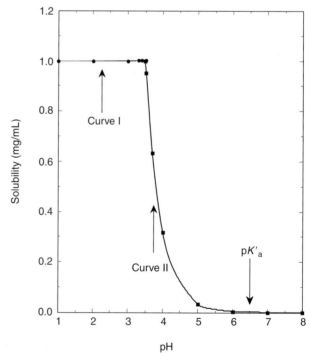

FIGURE 4.1 pH-solubility profile of an ideal compound BH^+Cl^-

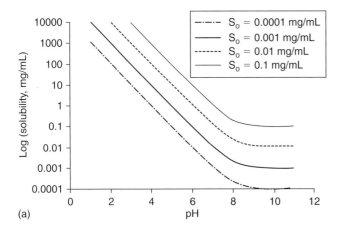

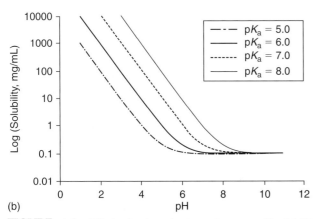

FIGURE 4.2 Effect of relevant parameters on pH-solubility curves: (a) effect of intrinsic solubility S_o; (b) effect of pK_a

4.2.2 Prediction of Salt Solubility and *In Situ* Salt Screening

Solubility prediction may be useful in early drug discovery phases when solubility measurement is not yet possible. The predicted solubility data may provide guidance in screening of computer designed combinatorial libraries and in lead optimization.

Unfortunately, despite all efforts in the last few decades, there is no simple reliable method yet for predicting solubility.[14] The available models are all for solubility prediction of non-electrolytes, and are not applicable to salts.

The solubility of the salt depends largely on the counterion. The hydrophobicity of the counterion and the melting point of the salt both play a role in the solubility of the salt form.[14,15] Since melting point data are difficult to obtain without making the actual salt, predicting salt solubility remains difficult.

One way to get a quick assessment of the solubilities of possible salts is to use an *in situ* screening method.[16] In this method the solubility of a basic drug is determined in the presence of various salt-forming

acids. Salt solubility is back-calculated knowing the initial amount of drug substance used in the solubility study, the acid concentration, and the final pH. This technique can quickly identify insoluble salts, and also gives some initial indication of the possibility for obtaining crystalline salts. Advances in automation make it possible to carry out screening in various recrystallization solvents, increasing the probability of identifying crystalline salts even more.

The solubility product and solubility of the salts formed *in situ* are calculated as follows. The amount of the compound precipitated, X_p, expressed as mg of the base form of the drug, can be calculated using:

$$X_p = X - S \cdot V \tag{4.6}$$

X (mg) is the amount of solid base added, S (mg/mL) is the solubility in the acid solution which is determined from solubility studies, and V (mL) is the volume of the solution. Assuming that the precipitate is composed only of the 1:1 salt, the concentration of the acid remaining in solution, $[A_S]$, can then be calculated:

$$[A_S] = [A] - \frac{X_P}{V \cdot MW} \tag{4.7}$$

[A] is the concentration of the acid used, and MW is the compound's molecular weight. Knowing the ionization constant of the acid, pK'_a, and the pH of the saturated solution, the concentration of the acid in its ionized form, $[A_{ionized}]$, can be calculated:

$$[A_{ionized}] = \frac{[A_S]}{1 + [H^+]/K'_a} \tag{4.8}$$

The molar concentration of the compound in solution is:

$$[S] = \frac{S(mg/mL)}{MW} \tag{4.9}$$

The K_{SP} of the salt can then be calculated:

$$K_{SP} = [S] \cdot [A_{ionized}] \tag{4.10}$$

Finally, the solubility of the salt, S_{salt} (mg/mL), is calculated as follows:

$$S_{salt} = (K_{SP})^{\frac{1}{2}} \cdot MW_S \tag{4.11}$$

MW_s is the molecular weight of the respective salt form of the drug.

4.2.3 Solubility and Dissolution Rate of Salts

Solubility determination of pharmaceutical salts is complicated for certain compounds, such as those with poor intrinsic solubility. Theoretically, after an excess amount of solid salt is equilibrated in water, the solution concentration at equilibrium should represent the solubility of the salt. However, this is only true if the pH of the saturated solution is below pH_{max}. For compounds with low intrinsic solubilities and weak basicity or acidity, their salts may convert to the unionized form in the solubility medium, depending on the final pH of the suspension. In such cases the measured solubility is only the solubility of the unionized form at those particular pH values. For example, the solubility of the phosphate salt of GW1818X was found to be 6.8 mg/mL when the solution pH was 5.0.[16] The pH_{max} is approximately 4 in this case. Analysis of the residual solid showed that the solution was in equilibrium with the free base, indicating that the solubility determined did not adequately represent the solubility of the salt. An additional complication is that the pH of the solubility sample may vary depending on the lots of drug substance used. This is because different lots of material may contain dissimilar amounts of residual acid, base or solvent impurities.

There are several ways to overcome this type of problem. One approach is to determine the solubility in a diluted acidic solution using the same acid that formed the salt with the base. The concentration of the acid solution needs to be such that the solution pH is lower than the pH_{max}. The solubility can then be estimated by correcting for the common ion effect from the acid used in the solubility study.[16] A second approach to ensure a lower solution pH than pH_{max} is to use a high ratio of drug to solvent.[17] However, this may not be possible for every compound.

When determining the solubility of salts in simulated gastric fluid, or media containing buffers, the salt may convert to the hydrochloride salt or the salt formed with one of the buffer species, depending on the relative solubility of the salts. If the simulated gastric fluid contains sodium chloride, the common ion effect of the chloride ion may significantly depress the solubility of a hydrochloride salt.

According to the modified Noyes–Whitney equation, the dissolution of a salt is proportional to both solubility and surface area:

$$\frac{dC}{dt} = \frac{DA}{hV}(C_s - C) \qquad (4.12)$$

where:
D is the diffusion coefficient
h is the thickness of the diffusion layer at the solid-liquid interface
A is the surface area of drug exposed to the dissolution media
V is the volume of the dissolution media
C_s is the concentration of a saturated solution of the solute in the dissolution medium at the experimental temperature

C is the concentration of drug in solution at time t.

The dissolution rate is given by dC/dt.

For the dissolution of salts, the pH of the diffusion layer is especially important. The solubility at this pH should be the one used in calculating the dissolution rate. Because of the self-buffering capability of salts at the diffusion layer, the dissolution of a soluble salt may be different from its unionized form. This is illustrated in Figure 4.3 where the hydrochloride salt dissolved faster at higher pH values, presumably due to the lower diffusion layer pH.[17] A practical method of estimating pH at the surface of a dissolving solid is by measuring the pH of a saturated solution of the drug substance in the particular aqueous medium.[18]

4.2.4 Dissolution of Salts in GI Fluids

In the stomach and intestine drug solubility can be enhanced by food and bile components such as bile salts, lecithin, and fatty acids. Depending on their properties, the degree of solubilization for different drugs varies. Factors that may affect the extent of solubilization include hydrophobicity (log P), molecular weight of the drug, and specific interactions between drug and bile salts.[19]

The solubility of a salt decreases if common ions, such as Cl^- and Na^+, are present, and since the dissolution rate is proportional to the solubility in the diffusion layer at the surface of the solid, any impact of a common ion on solubility would also influence dissolution rate.

Supersaturation in the intestinal fluid is an important property that can play a significant role in drug absorption. For compounds with poor intrinsic solubility in the intestinal fluid, solubility is often a

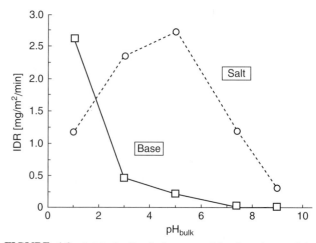

FIGURE 4.3 Intrinsic dissolution rate of bupivacaine, and its HCl salt, as a function of the pH of the dissolution medium

limiting factor for absorption. For many of these compounds it may not be possible to enhance the saturation solubility to the extent required such that the whole dose is dissolved in the GI fluid. In this case, creating or maintaining supersaturation in the intestinal fluid can be an effective way to enhance absorption of these compounds. For example, HPMC-AC has been shown to significantly enhance the absorption of several poorly soluble compounds.[20]

Depending on the properties of the salt and its corresponding base or acid, the fate of the salt in the GI tract may vary significantly. As illustrated in Figure 4.4, when the salt of the basic drug gets in the GI tract it may dissolve in the stomach and either remain in solution or

precipitate out as the free base when it gets emptied into the intestine. It may also convert to the hydrochloride salt if the hydrochloride salt is less soluble, especially with the influence of the common ion effect. In this case, the dissolution in the intestine is really the dissolution of the precipitated hydrochloride salt. To further complicate the situation, when salt conversion happens *in vivo*, the material can precipitate out as either crystalline or amorphous forms with different particle sizes. Dissolution of the salt of an acidic compound has its own complications. As shown in Figure 4.5, the salt is likely to convert to the free acid. When this happens, the liberated free acid may coat the surface of the remaining drug particles, causing dissolution to slow down.

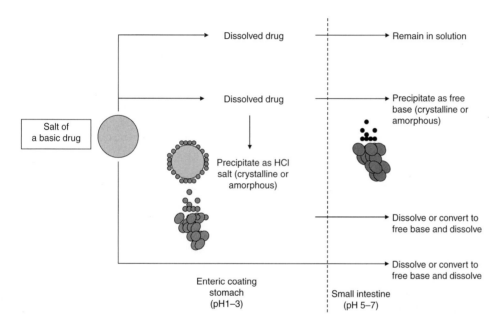

FIGURE 4.4 Dissolution process of the salt of a basic drug in the gastric and intestinal fluids

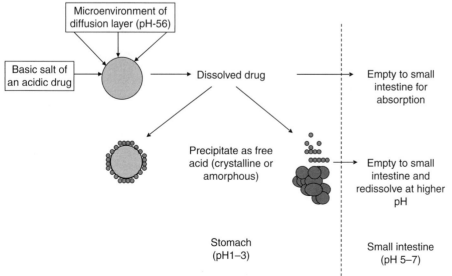

FIGURE 4.5 Dissolution process of the salt of an acidic drug in the gastric and intestinal fluids

TABLE 4.1 Compositions of FaSSIF and FeSSIF

	FaSSIF	FeSSIF
KH_2PO_4	0.39% (w/w)	
Acetic acid		0.865% (w/w)
Na taurocholate	3 mM	15 mM
Lecithin	0.75 mM	3.75 mM
KCl	0.77%	1.52% (w/w)
pH	6.5	5.0

To better predict the *in vivo* behavior of a salt, it is important to develop a good *in vitro* dissolution method taking into account the various possible conversions discussed above. Several dissolution systems that are shown to be able to better estimate or predict the supersaturation phenomenon have recently been reported.[21,22] To realistically estimate the impact of solubility on absorption, solubilities and degree of supersaturation in more physiologically relevant media should be determined. Two media that were developed based on literature and experimental data in dogs and humans have been used extensively in the industrial and academic research.[23] The compositions of these media, FaSSIF, simulating fasted state intestinal fluid, and FeSSIF, simulating fed-state intestinal fluid, are given in Table 4.1.

4.2.5 Impact of Salt Form on Other Solubilization Techniques

Because a salt has different physico-chemical properties compared to its unionized form, it is expected that it will behave differently in different solubilized systems. For example, a salt will frequently exhibit a lower complexation binding constant with cyclodextrins than a free base. However, since the solubilities of salts typically are higher, the salt may still have greater solubility in cyclodextrin solutions than the free base. In the case of sulfobutylether-β-cyclodextrins (SBE-β-CDs), because of the anionic sulfates in the substituents, their binding constants to certain molecules may be enhanced if the ionizable groups in these molecules are positively charged.[24]

Significantly different solubilities can also be expected for salts in solutions containing surfactants or in semi-polar non-aqueous solvents. Generally speaking, the addition of a cosolvent to an aqueous salt solution would be expected to reduce the solubility of the drug, due to reduction in the dielectric constant of the medium with a corresponding reduction

in the solvation of the ions. However, crystalline hydrate formation may increase solubility of certain salts in cosolvents.[25] For example, sodium sulfathiazole solubility almost doubles in 50% propylene glycol. Additionally, conversion of salts of weak bases to their free forms may not occur as readily in cosolvents compared to in water, due to the affect of cosolvents on the ionization constant of the free base.

Solubilization power, as measured by the percent solubility enhancement, may be lower for salts compared with their unionized forms, because the original solubility without solubilization components is higher; the final solubility of a salt in these systems may still be higher than the solubility of the unionized form. This is demonstrated by the solubility comparison for the hydrochloride salt and its free base of 2,2–Diphenyl-4–(2'-piperidyl)-1,3–dioxolane in propylene glycol (Figure 4.6).[11]

Salts will have different properties compared to their unionized forms in the amorphous form or in solid dispersion formulations. Their differences can result in different physical and chemical stability of the formulations containing amorphous drugs. This will be discussed in the next section.

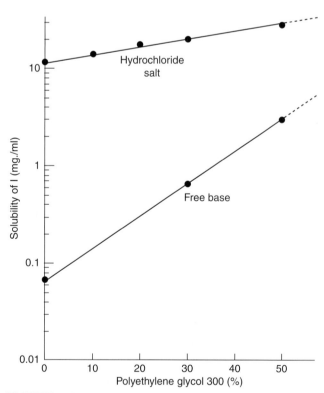

FIGURE 4.6 Solubilities of the hydrochloride salt and the free-base of 2,2-Diphenyl-4-(2'-piperidyl)-1,3-dioxolane in polyethylene glycol 300

4.2.6 Effect of Salts on Chemical Stability

The salt form may influence the chemical stability of the solid state. Two key contributors to the stability difference are:

1. interaction between the counter-ion and the molecule itself; and
2. pH differences in the microenvironment on the surface of drug substance.

The impact of microenvironment pH on chemical stability is more significant for those salts that have high aqueous solubility. The presence of excipients that can alter the microenvironment pH can make things even worse. Many salts of mineral acids are polar, leading to hygroscopicity and low microenvironmental pH; this can be disadvantageous for compounds that are readily hydrolyzed. However, salts formed with hydrophobic counterions may have low solubility and better stability, for example, the acyl sulfonate salt of xilobam is more stable than its sulfate salt.[28]

Since chemical reactivity in the solid state is correlated with the nature of crystalline modification, it is not uncommon to see a compound that has no stability issue in its thermodynamically stable form suddenly show a stability problem in a metastable form. The amorphous state is the most reactive, and can be a source for stability problems, especially for compounds that have an increased percentage of amorphous content upon process scale-up. Different salts will have different glass transition temperature (Tg), resulting in differences in physical and chemical stability.

4.2.7 Potential Disadvantages of Salts

Based on the theoretical considerations discussed above, there are clearly cases where a salt may not be a desirable choice for further development. Some of these undesirable properties include:

- common ion effect for compounds with poor solubility, such as an HCl salt;
- poor chemical stability in gastric fluid;
- poor solid-state stability at the microenvironment pH of the salt;
- precipitation of free acid/base form on the solid surface that reduces the dissolution rate of salts.

4.3 PRACTICAL CONSIDERATIONS

4.3.1 Drug Substance Considerations

Frequently, thermodynamically more stable forms are discovered after the process is scaled-up.

Comparing small-scale screening to large-scale production, two key differences that can significantly impact the nucleation process are the amount of impurities, and the time allowed for crystallization. As a general rule, small-scale screening should employ the purest material available (>99% pure). If the purity of the material is questionable, a purification process such as prep-scale LC should be carried out to improve the quality of the material.

4.3.2 Dosage Form Considerations

Many factors related to the dosage form should be considered when selecting a salt form. Considering all these factors will certainly reduce unnecessary complications later in the development process.

Oral Versus Parenteral Formulations

Ideally, the same salt should be selected for both parenteral and oral formulations. A particular salt form may have adequate solubility to give optimal oral bioavailability, yet not be soluble enough for a parenteral dosage form. In this case, selecting a salt form that has solubility high enough to meet the solubility requirements for parenteral formulation may be the determining factor in salt form selection. A simple *in situ* salt screening process may narrow down the choice to a smaller number of acceptable salt candidates. Of course, other physico-chemical properties must be adequate enough for oral dosage form development. In some cases, it may be necessary to use two different salt forms for oral and parenteral dosage forms, respectively.

Solution Versus Suspension

Sometimes it may be desirable to choose a less soluble salt for certain dosage forms, such as a suspension. For example, tetracycline is soluble and stable as the hydrochloride salt in a solution formulation. However, the calcium salt is the preferred choice for suspension formulation because its lower solubility overcomes the taste issue faced with a solution formulation.

High Dose Versus Low Dose

For many poorly soluble compounds, solubility and dissolution may not be the limiting factor to absorption when the doses are low. As the dose goes higher, solubility will become the limiting factor. Higher doses are always required for toxicological studies. When selecting a salt form for these compounds, it is important to understand from a pharmacokinetic (PK) point of view where this limitation may arise. This can be assessed by both *in vitro* methods such as simulation and prediction, and *in vivo* methods such as PK studies in animal species. If different salt forms are used for toxicology and clinical studies or a salt form is used for toxicology studies, but a neutral form is used for the clinical studies, how the salt form affects PK behavior and toxicity needs to be understood.

Immediate-release (IR) Versus Modified-release (MR)

A soluble salt may give a higher maximum concentration (C_{max}) compared to a less soluble salt form or the unionized form, and thus may not be desirable for certain indications. However, it may be more advantageous to choose a soluble salt, and control drug release using formulation means such as MR strategies. A compound needs to be sufficiently soluble over the wide range of physiological pH to avoid reduction in bioavailability when delivered in an MR dosage form (see discussion in Chapters 22 and 23).

Potential Combination Formulations

As combination products gain more popularity as a powerful product lifecycle management tool, considering potential combination products in which a drug may find use should not be ignored during salt selection. As discussed earlier, a salt may affect microenvironment pH and moisture migration, and may be chemically incompatible with other compounds. For example, when aspirin is combined with propoxyphene hydrochloride salt, its stability is significantly reduced. However, this incompatibility is avoided when propoxyphene napsylate is used instead in formulating the combination product.[28,29]

When two compounds are combined, their salts may also affect each other's solubility and dissolution rate, as a result of salt conversion and/or insoluble salt formation.

Solid Dispersion and Lipid-based Delivery Systems

Solid dispersions or high viscosity lipid-based formulations can be ideal environments for undesirable crystal growth. Solubility screening using these nonaqueous solvents should always include an examination of the residual solid to detect any potential crystal form conversion after adequate equilibration time. The effects of salts on the effectiveness of various solubilization techniques must also be taken into account.

4.3.3 Toxicity Considerations

The hydrochloride salt for basic compounds and the sodium salt for acidic compounds remain the most popular salts today, because the safety of these two salts has been well-demonstrated. If certain salt counterions not commonly in use need to be used, their intrinsic toxicity needs to be evaluated. For example, lithium cations at high doses may cause irreversible damage to the kidney; maleic acid has been reported to cause renal tubular lesions in the dog. Certain salts may cause local irritancy. For example, an irritant effect on the esophagus has been reported for highly soluble alprenplol hydrochloride, whereas less soluble alprenplol benzoate has no such irritant effect, believed to be related to the difference in solubility of the salts. The nitrate salt has been reported to cause ulceration and bleeding in the GI tract.[10]

Certain salt forming agents may interact with solvents used for crystallization, granulation or formulation, and form toxic reaction products. For example methanesulfonic acid used for forming mesylate salts, can interact with alcohols to form toxic esters. For this reason, mesylate salts are not very popular, despite the fact that the mesylate salt of many basic compounds is one of their more soluble salts.[10]

If a new counterion that has not previously been utilized in approved products has to be used, such a salt must be regarded as a new chemical entity with all the consequences for toxicological evaluation. Due to the difficulty in determining the causes of toxicity, safety assessment of other salts of the same active entity may be necessary. For this reason, unless there is a clear justification, salts previously used in approved products should be the first ones to be considered. Lists of commonly used salts are readily available in several recent reviews.[8,10,30]

4.3.4 Salt and Form Screening and Selection Strategies

To meet the challenges of the accelerated drug discovery and development process, salt and crystal form screening and selection strategies should balance resources and risks. The risks associated with salt and crystal form issues must be assessed as early as possible in the development process, so that the appropriate experiments can be completed in a timely fashion. Various considerations such as physico-chemical properties, biopharmaceutical properties, and the potential for scale-up should be considered as part of the screening and selection process.

Timing of Salt and Crystal form Screening and Selection

Although the choice of salt and crystal form can have a significant impact on the physico-chemical properties of drug candidates, the significance of this impact can differ from one molecule to another. For example, if the compound is very soluble and is chemically stable, then a salt or crystal form change may not significantly impact the performance of the final product. However, if the compound is chemically unstable, changing from a crystalline form to the amorphous form will have a detrimental effect, and may even result in product failure. Since resources and time to carry out salt and crystal form screening may be limited, assessing the risk associated with the individual development candidate will certainly help the scientist to focus efforts on where they are most needed.

Many poorly soluble compounds are high-risk drug candidates because their dissolution rate is often the rate-limiting step in the absorption of these compounds. The FDAs biopharmaceutical classification system defines low-solubility compounds as those whose equilibrium aqueous solubility in 250 mL of pH 1–7.5 aqueous solution is less than the amount contained in the tablet or capsule with the highest dosage prescribed.[31] Some compounds require development of dosage forms that can produce local supersaturation to enhance dissolution rate and absorption. Examples of such delivery systems include amorphous/solid dispersions, metastable polymorphs, and lipid-based formulations. These should certainly be considered as high-risk.

Compounds that are chemically unstable also should be classified as high-risk, since early selection of the proper salt and crystal form is crucial for the assessment of the potential for development. The successful development of these compounds will require proper control of the crystal form for the drug substance, and a thorough understanding of the effect of various formulation and process parameters on the crystal form and on stability. Typically, it is desirable to have salt and crystal form screening and selection completed prior to any GLP toxicology studies, since such studies are very expensive and time consuming.[9] However, for low-risk compounds, it may be feasible to delay selecting the final salt and crystal form until a later stage in development. For some projects, multiple candidates may be tried in human studies, even if only one candidate will be developed to a final product.

Keep in mind that salt screening and selection may not be the rate-limiting step for certain projects, even if they are completed in a later stage. The number of studies that need to be repeated will also depend on the properties of the compound and its salts.

Salt and Crystal form Screening and Selection Processes

Several strategies and decision trees for salt and crystal form selection processes have been proposed

recently.[32–37] Some strategies place the emphasis on processability and the ability to scale-up, while others focus on maximizing solubility, and on bioavailability enhancement. The choice of which strategy to employ may depend on who is driving the salt screening and selection process within the organization. Although ultimately a balance between process parameters, biopharmaceutical properties, and physico-chemical properties needs to be reached before a final decision can be made, a rational process/decision tree is still critical for saving time and resources.

Morris et al. developed a multi-tier approach where salts can be screened for their optimal physical form.[32] An updated version of this approach (Figure 4.1) was reported by Serajuddin and Pudipeddi.[35] In this approach, certain physico-chemical properties of salts are studied at each tier, and critical "Go/No Go" decisions are made based on the results of those studies (Figure 4.7).

Tong et al. proposed a process that is more applicable to poorly soluble compounds (Figure 4.8).[34,9] Since maximizing solubility and absorption is the key objective for poorly soluble compounds, this process uses an *in situ* salt screening method as the first step to screen out insoluble compounds. This approach eliminates the need to prepare those insoluble salts for further characterization. It is true that equilibrium solubility will differ depending on the form of the excess solid; however, if a salt already exhibits very poor solubility by the *in situ* screening method, it is reasonable to conclude that the solubility of the solid salt will most likely be even lower. For compounds that have very poor solubility as the hydrochloride salt, bioavailability of a more soluble salt should be evaluated with and without bypassing

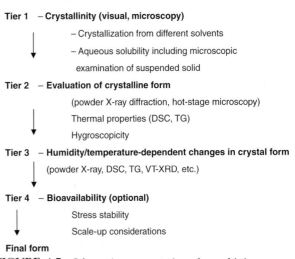

Tier 1 – **Crystallinity (visual, microscopy)**
    – Crystallization from different solvents
    – Aqueous solubility including microscopic examination of suspended solid

Tier 2 – **Evaluation of crystalline form**
    (powder X-ray diffraction, hot-stage microscopy)
    Thermal properties (DSC, TG)
    Hygroscopicity

Tier 3 – **Humidity/temperature-dependent changes in crystal form**
    (powder X-ray, DSC, TG, VT-XRD, etc.)

Tier 4 – **Bioavailability (optional)**
    Stress stability
    Scale-up considerations

Final form

FIGURE 4.7 Schematic representation of a multi-tier approach for the selection of optimal salt form for a drug

Tier 1 – Physical characterization of the unionized form
       – *In situ* salt screening to rank order solubility of potential salts

Tier 2 – *In vitro* testing:
       – Diluting the solution of the most soluble salt solution
         into simulated gastric fluid (SGF) and simulated intestinal fluid (SIF) to determine
         if the compound precipitates and in what form it precipitates
       – Intrinsic dissolution rates of the unionized form in SGF and SIF

Tier 3 – Animal PK studies:
       – Comparing the bioavailability of the solution of the most soluble salt with the
         suspension of the unionized form
       – If the hydrochloride salt is very insoluble or the compound is acid labile, test
         whether bypassing the stomach can improve bioavailability (intra-duodenal
         dosing or enteric coating)

Tier 4 – Preparation and characterization of top 2–3 salts:
       – Crystal form screening and characterization, chemical stability, solubility,
         processability

Tier 5 – Bioavailability confirmation if needed:
       – Suspension/capsule of the solid at projected clinical doses and toxicological
         doses

Final salt and crystal form

FIGURE 4.8 Salt selection decision tree for insoluble compounds

the stomach by using *MR* formulations. It is possible that the more soluble salt will have a higher dissolution rate due to differences in microenvironmental pH effects on particle surfaces. Bioavailability may be further improved by bypassing the stomach using an *MR* approach, thus reducing potential conversion to the hydrochloride salt. If other solubilization methods need to be combined with the salt form to maximize bioavailability enhancement, the solubility of various salts in different solubilizing agents needs to be studied. A process flow chart is shown in Figure 4.2. The key advantage of this approach is that it conserves resources and drug substance, by minimizing the number of pharmacokinetic studies required and the number of solid salts that must be prepared and characterized.

4.3.5 The Role of Automation and High Throughput Designs in Salt Screening

High throughput crystallization experiments with the free base in the presence of various salt forming agents can be a very effective way of identifying crystalline salts (Remenar et al., 2003). Several high throughput methods with automated or semi-automated sample handling, and characterization of salt and crystal forms, have been reported and are now commonly used across the industry. However, before engaging in massive screening, it is very important that the goals of the screening are identified, and the process of decision-making is defined. Lower throughput methods with more selective and targeted screening using more descriptive technologies may be just as effective in identifying the desirable salt and crystal form.

CASE STUDIES

Case Study #1: RPR111423

RPR 111423 is a very weak base with a pK_a of 4.25.[33] The strategy was to first carry out a comprehensive screening of various counter-ions and solvent matrix to identify two crystalline salts: monohydrochloride and a mesylate. The properties of these salts and the free base were then studied and compared.

The results showed that both salts significantly enhance solubility, but exist in 4–6 different polymorphs. They both readily convert to free base in water and intestinal fluids. The corresponding results for the free base indicated that it appeared to be the better candidate; it showed no evidence of polymorphism, and it was not hygroscopic. A subsequent study performed on samples of drug substance, and on simple capsule formulations, demonstrated that the dissolution rates of micronized free base were equivalent or superior to those of the salts under the same conditions. Thus, the free base was selected for further development.

A few key observations can be drawn from this case study. First of all, identifying what properties to modify by forming a salt prior to any salt screening can save time and resources: a salt may not always be needed. *In vitro* dissolution experiments and *in silico* simulation can be very useful tools to evaluate the need for a salt from a PK point of view. Additionally, a pharmacokinetic study in animals comparing a solution formulation to a suspension of the micronized free base at the projected clinical dose can provide further indication of whether a salt is needed. However, if the projected dose gets much higher for this compound, a salt would provide advantages. Sensitivity analysis using GastroPlus® software or estimation of the maximum absorbable dose can be good tools in understanding at what doses solubility and dissolution may become rate-limiting to absorption.

Case Study #2: RPR127963

RPR127963 is a crystalline, very weak base with a pK_a of 4.10.[33] The projected dose is up to 250 mg as an oral dosage form, and up to 50 mg/mL as an injectable form. A comprehensive evaluation of possible salts demonstrated that five crystalline salts (hydrochloride, mesylate, citrate, tartrate, and sulfate) could be readily produced. The properties of these salts and the free base were then studied and compared.

The free base was found to be low melting as an anhydrous solid, and formed multiple hydrates in the presence of water. The citrate, tartrate, and the hydrochloride salts were poorly soluble. The mesylate and the sulfate salts both had high melting points, excellent aqueous solubility, and were non-hygroscopic.

Additional studies showed that the sulfate salt had greater solubility in cosolvents. This would give the formulator a better chance of achieving a higher dose in an injectable formulation. Thus the sulfate salt was selected for further evaluation with the mesylate salt as the backup option.

This case demonstrated the importance of considering both oral and parenteral dosage forms in the salt selection process. Since several salts have poor aqueous solubility, an *in situ* salt screening would help identify these salts quickly without having to actually make these salts. Because of the potential for the toxic ester formation, exposure to alcohols in production of the mesylate salt should be avoided.

Case Study #3: L-649 923

L-649 923 as the free acid has stability challenges. It equilibrates rapidly with the less active cyclic γ-lactone in solution.[38] Four salts (sodium, ethylenediamine, calcium, and benzathine) were prepared and studied for their physico-chemical properties including solubility, intrinsic dissolution rate, crystallinity, hygroscopicity, thermal stability, photosensitivity, and drug-excipient compatibility.

The ethylenediamine salt was found to be crystalline, but was thermally unstable (20% loss after 40°C/2 weeks). The benzathine salt was also crystalline, but was poorly soluble and less bioavailable in animal studies. The sodium salt was amorphous and hygroscopic (picking up ~18% water at 76% RH). The amorphous calcium salt was chemically stable, not very hygroscopic (~1.2% water), but physically might not be stable. An analysis of the structure suggested that the compound would be difficult to crystallize, because it might be difficult for the two organic carboxylate anions of a racemate to form the required constrained crystal lattice network during the nucleation process. Based on these data, the amorphous calcium salt was selected for further development.

This case demonstrated the importance of considering the microenvironment pH of the solid to stabilize the drug product. Understanding degradation mechanisms should be the basis for selecting the right salt, and developing a chemically stable solid dosage form. As a general rule, for compounds that undergo moisture-induced degradation in acidic conditions, the following options should be considered:

- selecting a basic salt;
- minimizing the amount of free acid in the drug substance;
- ensuring basic microenvironment pH by adding an alkalizing agent to the formulation;
- avoiding an aqueous granulating process; and
- using excipients that have low water content.

4.4 CONCLUSIONS

Proper strategies for screening and selecting the appropriate salt and crystal form are essential for ensuring success in accelerating the process of drug discovery and development. The strategies selected should also balance and minimize resources and risks. Generally, the desired salt and crystal form should be identified early in the development process, typically prior to any GLP toxicology studies for compounds that carry high development risks. Salt and crystal form screening and selection should be an integrated process. When the appropriate screening strategies are employed, and various theoretical and practical considerations are taken, it is often possible to generate sufficient data so that the correct decision as to salt and crystal form selection can be made with a minimum amount of drug substance (1–10 g), and within a short period of time (4–8 weeks).

Bibliography

1. Curatolo, W. (1998). Physical chemical properties of oral drug candidates in the discovery and exploratory development settings. Pharmaceutical Science & Technology Today 1, 387–393.
2. Lipinski, C.A. (1997). Experimental and computational approaches to estimate solubility and permeability in drug discovery and development settings. Advanced Drug Development Review 23, 3–25.
3. Venkatesh, S. & Lipper, R.A. (2000). Role of the development scientist in compound lead selection and optimization. Journal of Pharmaceutical Sciences 89(2), 145–154.
4. Lipinski, C.A. (2002). Poor aqueous solubility—an industry wide problem in drug discovery. American Pharmaceutical Review 5(3), 82–85.

5. Borchardt, R.T., Edward, E.H., Lipinski, C.A., Thakker, D.R. & Wang, B.H. (2004). *Pharmaceutical Profiling in Drug Discovery for Lead Selection*. AAPS Press, Arlington, VA.

6. Neau, S.H. (2000). Solubility Theories. In: *Water-Insoluble Drug Formulation*, R. (ed) Liu,. Interpharm Press, Englewood, CO. pp. 6–22.

7. Davies, G. (2001). Changing the salt, changing the drug. The Pharmaceutical Journal 266, 322–323.

8. Bighley, L.D., Berge, S.M. & Monkhouse, D.C. (1995). Salt forms of drugs and absorption. In: *Encyclopedia of Pharmaceutical Technology*, J. Swarbrick, & J.C. Boylan (eds), Vol. 13. Marcel Dekker Inc., New York, NY. pp. 453–499.

9. Huang, L.F. & Tong, W.Q. (2004). Impact of solid state properties on developability assessment of drug candidates. Advanced Drug Delivery Reviews 56, 321–334.

10. Stahl, P.H. & Wermuth, C.G. (2002). Monographs on acids and bases. In: *Handbook of Pharmaceutical Salts, Properties, Selection, and Use*, P.H. Stahl, & C.G. Wermuth, (eds) Verlag Helvetica Chimica Acta, Zuruch and Wiley-VCH, Weinheim. pp. 265–327.

11. Kramer, S.E. & Flynn, G.L. (1972). Solubility of organic hydrochloride. Journal of Pharmaceutical Sciences 61(12), 1896–1904.

12. Li, S.F., Wong, S.M., Sethia, S., Almoazen, H., Joshi, Y. & Serajuddin, A.T.M. (2005). Investigation of solubility and dissolution of a free base and two different salt forms as a function of pH. Pharmaceutical Research 22(4), 628–635.

13. Serajuddin, A.T.M. (2007). Salt formation to improve drug solubility. Advanced Drug Delivery Reviews 59, 603–616.

14. Yalkowsky, S.H. & Banerjee, S. (1992). *Aqueous Solubility, Methods of Estimation for Organic Compounds*. Marcel Dekker, New York, NY.

15. Anderson, B.D. & Conradi, R.A. (1985). Predictive relationships in the water solubility of salts of nonsteroidal anti-inflammatory drug. Journal of Pharmaceutical Sciences 74, 815–820.

16. Tong, W.Q. & Whitesell, G. (1998). *In situ* salt screening—a useful technique for discovery support and preformulation studies. Pharmaceutical Development and Technology 3(2), 215–223.

17. Pudipeddi, M., Serajuddin, A.T.M., Grant, D.J.W. & Stahl, P.H. (2002). Solubility and dissolution of weak acids, bases and salts. In: *Handbook of Pharmaceutical Salts, Properties, Selection, and Use*, P.H. Stahl, & C.G. Wermuth (eds). Verlag Helvetica Chimica Acta, Zuruch and Wiley-VCH, Weinheim. pp. 19–39.

18. Sherif, I., Badawy, F. & Hussain, M.A. (2007). Microenvironmental pH modulation in solid dosage forms. Journal of Pharmaceutical Sciences 96(5), 948–959.

19. Horter, D. & Dressman, J.B. (1997). Influence of physicochemical properties on dissolution of drugs in the gastrointestinal tract. Advanced Drug Delivery Reviews 25, 3–14.

20. Shanker, R. (2005). Current concepts in the science of solid dispersions. 2nd Annual Simonelli Conference in Pharmaceutical Sciences, Long Island University.

21. Kostewicz, E.S., Wunderlich, M., Brauns, U., Becker, R., Bock, T. & Dressman, J.B. (2004). Predicting the precipitation of poorly soluble weak bases upon entry in the small intestine. Journal of Pharmacy and Pharmacology 56, 43–51.

22. Gu, C.H., Rao, D., Gandhi, R.B., Hilden, J. & Raghavan, K. (2005). Using a novel multicompartment dissolution system to predict the effect of gastric pH on the oral absorption of weak bases with poor intrinsic solubility. Journal of Pharmaceutical Sciences 94, 199–208.

23. Dressman, J.B. (2000). Dissolution testing of immediate-release products and its application to forcasting in vivo performance. In: *Oral Drug Absorption, Prediction and Assessment*, J.B. Dressman, & H. Lennernas (eds). Marcel Dekker Inc, New York, NY. pp. 155–181.

24. Thompson, D.O. (1997). Cyclodextrin-enabling excipients: their present and future use in pharmaceuticals. Critical Reviews in Therapeutic Drug Carrier Systems 14(1), 1–104.

25. Rubino, J.T. & Thomas, E. (1990). Influence of solvent composition on the solubilities and solid-state properties of the sodium salts of some drugs. International Journal of Pharmaceutics 65, 141–145.

26. Guillory, J.K. & Poust, R.I. (2002). Chemical kinetics and drug stability. In: *Modern Pharmaceutics, Drugs and the Pharmaceutical Sciences*, G.S. Banker, & C.T. Rhodes (eds), 4th ed. Marcel Dekker, New York, NY. pp. 139–166.

27. Yoshioka, S. & Stella, V.J. (2000). *Stability of Drugs and DosageForms*. Kluwer Academic Publishers, Plenum Publishers, New York, NY.

28. Walking, W.D., Reynolds, B.E., Fegely, C. & Janicki, C.A. (1983). Xilobam: Effect of salt form on pharmaceutical properties. Drug Development and Industrial Pharmacy 9(5), 809–919.

29. Kaul, A.F. & Harshfield, J.C. (1976). Stability of aspirin in combination with propoxyphene hydrochloride and propoxyphene napsylate. New England Journal of Medicine 294(16), 907.

30. USP. (2006). USP 29-NF24, US Pharmacopeial Convention, Rockville, MD.

31. Amidon, G.L., Lennernas, H., Shah, V.P. & Crison, J.R. (1995). A theoretical basis for a biopharmaceutic drug classification: The correlation of *in vitro* drug product dissolution and *in vivo* bioavailability. Pharmaceutical Research 12, 413–420.

32. Morris, K.R., Fakes, M.G., Thakur, A.B., Newman, A.W., Singh, A.K., Venit, J.J., Spagnuolo, C.J. & Serajuddin, A.T.M. (1994). An integrated approach to the selection of optimal salt form for a new drug candidate. International Journal of Pharmaceutics 105, 209–217.

33. Bastin, R.J., Bowker, M.J. & Slater, B.J. (2000). Salt selection and optimization procedures for pharmaceutical new chemical entities. Organic Process Research & Development 4(5), 427–435.

34. Tong, W.Q., Alva, G., Carlton, D., Viscomi, F., Adkison, K., Millar, A. & Dhingra, O. (1999). A strategic approach to the salt selection of an insoluble drug candidate. 13th AAPS Meeting. New Orleans, LA.

35. Serajuddin, A.T.M. & Puddipeddi, M. (2002). Salt-Selection Strategies. In: *Handbook of Pharmaceutical Salts*, P.H. Stahl, & C.G. Wermuth (eds). VHCA and Wiley-VCH, Weinheim. pp. 135–160.

36. Bowker, M.J. (2002). A procedure for salt selection and optimization. In: *Handbook of Pharmaceutical Salts*, P.H. Stahl, & C.G. Wermuth (eds) VHCA and Wiley-VCH, New York, NY. pp. 161–190.

37. Remenar, J.F., MacPhee, J.M., Larson, B.K., Tyagi, V.A., Ho, J.H., McIlroy, D.A., Hickey, M.B., Shaw, P.B. & Almarsson, O. (2003). Salt selection and simultaneous polymorphism assessment via high-throughput crystallization: The case of sertraline. Organic Process Research & Development 7(6), 990–996.

38. Cotton, M.L., Lamarche, P., Motola, S. & Vadas, E.B. (1994). L-649,923—the selection of an appropriate salt form and preparation of a stable oral formulation. International Journal of Pharmaceutics 109, 237–249.

Drug Stability and Degradation Studies

Deliang Zhou, William R. Porter and Geoff G.Z. Zhang

5.1 INTRODUCTION

Degradation studies are an important aspect of preformulation evaluation of the stability of drug candidates. These experiments aim to aid further formulation development by evaluating the intrinsic stability properties of a drug candidate in a timely manner by deliberate application of stress to cause degradation. To fulfill this purpose, preformulation scientists induce degradation of test materials by raising temperature, by increasing humidity when relevant (e.g., solid-state chemical and physical stability), by subjecting materials to sheer or compressive forces (e.g., solid-state physical stability), by exposing the test materials to various pH conditions or intensive UV-visible light (e.g., photostability) or by adding other reactants (e.g., acids, bases, peroxides). Forced degradation studies are sometimes described as stress testing, and are also performed to support analytical method development.

Preformulation degradation studies and forced degradation studies used to support analytical method development share many common features. Analytical chemists employ forced degradation studies as part of their program to develop stability-indicating analytical methods. Early drug degradation studies also serve to identify and prepare degradants that are likely to appear in the final drug product and limit its shelf life. In addition, these studies aid in the elucidation of degradation pathways, and the qualification of materials used in toxicology experiments. Forced degradation studies conducted to support analytical method development often put more emphasis on identifying the degradants. Preformulation degradation studies,

on the other hand, aim to predict the intrinsic stability of a drug candidate in order to anticipate problems that may arise down the development path. Cost savings can be realized if these activities can be coordinated.

Degradation studies can provide predictive information. Under certain circumstances, such as hydrolysis in solution, prediction of shelf life may be achieved with reasonable accuracy. However, in other cases, extrapolation of stability under stressed conditions (e.g., oxidative testing) to normal storage conditions is challenging. Stress testing is therefore a more qualitative than quantitative predictive tool; nevertheless, rank-order comparisons are often not only possible, but also useful for designing subsequent formulations. Early signs of instability of a drug candidate help to identify potential development issues, to foster development of potential stabilization strategies, and to suggest ways to optimize manufacturing processes.

This chapter will discuss the basic treatments of drug degradation studies, including kinetics, pathways, important factors, and typical practices for assessing both chemical and physical stability of pharmaceutical compounds.

5.2 CHEMICAL STABILITY

Chemical degradation probably represents the most important stability aspect of pharmaceuticals. Pharmaceutical scientists are responsible for examining the chemical stability of new drug candidates, for assessing the impact of stability issues on pharmaceutical development and processing, and for designing strategies to stabilize an unstable compound if necessary. They must understand the kinetics of chemical degradation, both in solution and in the solid state. They must also understand the commonly encountered degradation pathways of active pharmaceutical ingredients (API), and practical approaches for performing degradation studies.

5.2.1 Solution Kinetics

Chemical degradation reactions of pharmaceuticals follow the well-established treatments of chemical kinetics. A brief overview of chemical kinetics is presented next, followed by a discussion of catalysis and rate-pH profiles that are most relevant to degradation of pharmaceuticals.

5.2.2 Rate Equations

When a chemical reaction starts, the concentrations of reactants and products change with time until the reaction reaches completion or equilibrium. The concentrations of the reactants decrease, while those of the products increase over time. Therefore, the rate of a reaction can be represented either by the decreasing change in the concentration of a reactant or the increasing change in the concentration of a product with respect to time.

An arbitrary chemical reaction can be represented as:

$$a\text{A} + b\text{B} \rightarrow c\text{C} + d\text{D} \tag{5.1}$$

Here a, b, c, and d are the stoichiometric coefficients indicating the molar ratio of the reactants and products of the reaction. The rate of change of concentration of each species can differ, depending on the stoichiometric coefficients. Hence, a unified expression of the rate is preferred, which can be obtained via normalization:

$$\text{rate} = -\frac{1}{a}\frac{d[\text{A}]}{dt} = -\frac{1}{b}\frac{d[\text{B}]}{dt} = \frac{1}{c}\frac{d[\text{C}]}{dt} = \frac{1}{d}\frac{d[\text{D}]}{dt} \tag{5.2}$$

A negative sign is used for reactants so that the rate of a reaction is positive if it moves towards equilibrium or completion.

The rate of a reaction often depends on the concentrations of the reactants/products when other conditions are kept identical. Consider the hydrolytic reaction of ethyl acetate under alkaline conditions:

$$\text{CH}_3\text{COOC}_2\text{H}_5 + \text{OH}^- \rightarrow \text{CH}_3\text{COO}^- + \text{C}_2\text{H}_5\text{OH} \tag{5.3}$$

The rate of this reaction is proportional to the concentrations of each reactant species:

$$\begin{aligned}\text{rate} &= -\frac{d[\text{CH}_3\text{COOC}_2\text{H}_5]}{dt} = \frac{d[\text{C}_2\text{H}_5\text{OH}]}{dt} \\ &= k[\text{CH}_3\text{COOC}_2\text{H}_5][\text{OH}^-]\end{aligned} \tag{5.4}$$

Here k, the proportional constant, is called the specific rate constant, or briefly, the rate constant. This hydrolytic reaction is first order with respect to either ethyl acetate or hydroxide, and is an overall second-order reaction. The terms first order and second order will be defined below.

In general, the rate of the arbitrary reaction (Equation 5.1), may be written as:

$$\text{rate} = k[\text{A}]^\alpha [\text{B}]^\beta \tag{5.5}$$

Here α and β are the reaction order with respect to A and B, respectively. The order of the overall reaction is $n = \alpha + \beta$. This rate equation can be expanded to include more reactant/product species.

5.2.3 Elemental Reactions and Reaction Mechanism

The way a reaction equation is written merely represents the overall outcome of the reaction, and does not usually indicate how the actual reaction proceeds at a molecular level. For example, the reaction of hydrogen with bromine in the gas phase is usually written as:

$$\text{H}_2 + \text{Br}_2 = 2\text{HBr} \tag{5.6}$$

As written, it appears as if one H_2 molecule collides with one Br_2 molecule and generates two HBr molecules in one step. However, the reaction actually proceeds with a free radical chain mechanism, which consists of the following steps:

$$\text{Br}_2 \rightarrow 2\text{Br} \bullet \tag{5.7}$$

$$\text{H}_2 + \text{Br} \bullet \rightarrow \text{HBr} + \text{H}\bullet \tag{5.8}$$

$$\text{H}\bullet + \text{Br}_2 \rightarrow \text{HBr} + \text{Br}\bullet \tag{5.9}$$

As shown above, each step in a reaction scheme representing how the reactant molecules collide to form product(s) is called an elementary reaction. The reaction equation representing the overall outcomes is called the overall reaction. The number of molecules reacting in an elementary reaction is called the "molecularity" of that elementary reaction, and is a different concept from reaction order. An elementary reaction involving a single molecule is called unimolecular, while one that involves two molecules is called bimolecular, and so on. Processes involving three (termolecular) and more molecules in one step are rare.

An overall reaction may contain a number of elementary reactions. A complete scheme of these elementary reactions represents the actual path of a reaction, and is called the mechanism of the reaction. The beauty of the elementary reaction concept is that its rate follows the law of mass action. In simple words, the rate of an elementary reaction is directly proportional to the concentration of each reactant species involved in the elementary reaction, which is an outcome dependent upon the statistical aspects of the reaction. Therefore, the rate equation of an elementary reaction can be readily derived.

Among the elementary reactions comprising an overall reaction, one of these steps usually proceeds with the slowest rate. This slowest step is called the rate-determining step of a reaction and determines the rate of the overall reaction. Once the reaction mechanism is known, and the rate-determining step is identified, the expression of the overall rate of the reaction may also be readily derived.

5.2.4 Typical Simple Order Kinetics

Simple order reactions described in the following sections refer to reactions that are zero-, first-, and second-order. These reaction orders are commonly encountered in studies of the stability of pharmaceuticals. Their mathematical treatments are also relatively simple.

Zero-order Reactions

In zero-order reactions, the rate of the reaction does not depend on the concentration of the reactant; thus the rate is a constant:

$$\text{rate} = -\frac{d[A]}{dt} = k[A]^0 = k \qquad (5.10)$$

A is the reactant and k is the zero-order rate constant. In this case, the decrease in concentration of A is linear with time:

$$[A]_t = [A]_0 - kt \qquad (5.11)$$

$[A]_t$ is the concentration of A at time t, while $[A]_0$ is that at time zero, or the initial concentration.

First-order Reactions

First-order reactions appear to be the most commonly encountered in pharmaceutical stability studies.

The rate of a first-order reaction is proportional to the concentration of the reactant:

$$\text{rate} = -\frac{d[A]}{dt} = k[A] \qquad (5.12)$$

The concentration–time profile of the reactant for a first-order reaction follows an exponential decay to a limiting value, while that of the product follows an exponential increase to a (different) limiting value:

$$A \rightarrow C \qquad (5.13)$$

$$[A]_t = [A]_0 \exp(-kt) \qquad (5.14)$$

$$[C]_t = [A]_0[1 - \exp(-kt)] \qquad (5.15)$$

The half life, $t_{1/2}$, of the reaction is the time required for the reactant concentration to decrease to 50% of its original value; similarly, the times for the reactant concentration to decrease to 95% and 90% of its original values are designated as t_{95}, and t_{90}, respectively. These quantities can be obtained readily for a first-order reaction if the rate constant is known:

$$t_{1/2} = \frac{\ln 2}{k}; \quad t_{95} = \frac{\ln 0.95}{k}; \quad t_{90} = \frac{\ln 0.9}{k} \qquad (5.16)$$

A characteristic feature of first-order reactions is that the time required to lose the first 50% of the material ($t_{1/2}$) is the same as the time required to drop from 50% remaining to 25% remaining, from 25% remaining to 12.5% remaining, and so on.

Second-order Reactions

Many apparently first-order reactions observed for pharmaceuticals are actually second-order in reality. Usually two reactant molecules are required to collide to react. However, in practice, one reactant (e.g., water, hydrogen ion, hydroxyl ion, buffer species, etc.) may be in large excess so that its change in concentration is negligible, and an apparent first-order reaction is therefore observed.

For a second-order reaction where two reactants are involved:

$$A + B \rightarrow C \qquad (5.17)$$

The rate equation can be written as:

$$\text{rate} = -\frac{d[A]}{dt} = -\frac{d[B]}{dt} = k[A][B] \qquad (5.18)$$

The rate is first-order with respect to each reactant, but the overall reaction is second-order. The concentration–time profile of a second-order reaction can be represented as:

$$\frac{1}{[A]_0 - [B]_0}\left(\ln\frac{[A]_t}{[B]_t} - \ln\frac{[A]_0}{[B]_0}\right) = kt \qquad (5.19)$$

When the initial concentrations of A and B are identical, the concentration–time profile can be simplified as:

$$\frac{1}{[A]_t} - \frac{1}{[A]_0} = kt \qquad (5.20)$$

The $t_{1/2}$, t_{95}, and t_{90} values for a second-order reaction all depend upon the initial concentration of each species.

Figure 5.1 plots the reactant concentration–time profiles for theoretical zero-, first-, and second-order kinetics. Table 5.1 summarizes the rate equations, formula for calculating reactant concentration–time profiles, and half lives for the above simple order kinetics. The rate constants used to generate Figure 5.1 were assumed to be numerically identical in all cases. Identical initial reactant concentrations were assumed for the second-order reaction in both Figure 5.1 and Table 5.1.

Apparent (Pseudo-)Kinetic Orders

Zero-, first-, and second-order kinetics have been briefly discussed above; these models are likely to be the most frequently encountered in drug stability studies. In practice, only the concentration of the active pharmaceutical ingredient is usually monitored over time, while other reactants such as hydrogen ion, hydroxyl ion, and other buffer components are in large excess and are usually kept constant by methods such as pH-stating. Hence, a second-order overall reaction could appear to be a first-order reaction (with respect to drug concentration). The reaction is now said to be apparently first-order or pseudo-first-order. This is the case for most pharmaceutical hydrolytic reactions that are catalyzed by various species of buffers.

Apparent zero-order kinetics arise in situations when a source of the reactant exists that maintains the concentration of the reactant during the reaction. For example, the concentration of a drug in the solution phase of a suspended formulation is kept constant (at its solubility limit) if the dissolution rate of the drug from the solid phase is faster than the rate of degradation. Supposing that only the drug molecules in solution degrade significantly, the overall degradation kinetics would be apparently zero-order or pseudo-zero-order, although the actual kinetics may be first-order or apparently first-order in solution. Apparent zero-order kinetics may also arise in other situations, such as degradation in a surfactant solution where the

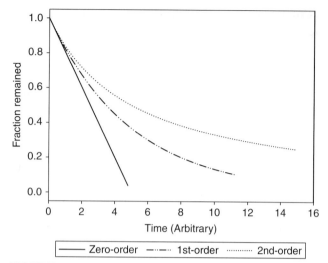

FIGURE 5.1 Reactant concentration–time profiles for theoretical zero-, first-, and second-order reactions

TABLE 5.1 Rate equations, reactant concentration–time profiles, and half lives for zero-, first-, and second-order reactions

Reaction order	Rate equation	Concentration–time profile	Half life
Zero-	$-\dfrac{d[A]}{dt} = k$	$[A]_t = [A]_0 - kt$	$t_{1/2} = \dfrac{[A]_0}{2k}$
First-	$-\dfrac{d[A]}{dt} = k[A]$	$[A]_t = [A]_0\exp(-kt)$	$t_{1/2} = \dfrac{\ln 2}{k}$
Second-	$-\dfrac{d[A]}{dt} = k[A]^2$	$\dfrac{1}{[A]_t} - \dfrac{1}{[A]_0} = kt$	$t_{1/2} = \dfrac{1}{k[A]_0}$

overall concentration of the surfactant is much higher than the critical micelle concentration (CMC), and degradation in the micellar phase is negligible. Finally, apparent zero-order kinetics occur when the extent of degradation is so small that the dependence of the reaction rate on the concentration of a reactant cannot be demonstrated because of experimental errors in measurement. Figure 5.1 shows that, assuming a reaction to proceed by a zero-order mechanism always predicts the greatest degree of decomposition as a function of time, other factors being kept equal. Thus, when the order of a reaction is in doubt, the conservative choice is to assume a zero-order kinetic model for the purpose of predicting the maximum amount of degradation that could be expected at some future time.

A distinction between true and apparent kinetic orders can be made by changing concentrations of other species (e.g., buffer concentration, pH or even different buffer components) or by changing the system so that the solubility of drug can be altered without changing the reaction mechanism.

5.2.5 Complex Reactions

Many reactions involve more than a single step, and are known as complex reactions. Depending on the reaction schemes, and the magnitude of respective rate constants, the overall kinetics may be approximated by zero-, first- or second-order rate equations. However, more often than not, the kinetic expressions are more complicated. Some commonly encountered complex reaction schemes are described next.

Reversible Reactions

Essentially, all reactions are reversible to some extent. However, the equilibrium constant may be so huge that the overall reaction can be treated as virtually one-directional. For the following simplest reversible reaction:

$$\text{A} \underset{k_{-1}}{\overset{k_1}{\rightleftharpoons}} \text{B} \qquad (5.21)$$

Here, k_1 and k_{-1} are the first-order rate constants for the forwarding and reversing reactions, respectively. The rate equation can be written as:

$$\text{rate} = -\frac{d[\text{A}]}{dt} = \frac{d[\text{B}]}{dt} = k_1[\text{A}] - k_{-1}[\text{B}] \qquad (5.22)$$

At equilibrium, the concentrations of species A and species B do not change any further because the rate of the forward reaction equals that of the reverse reaction:

$$\text{rate} = -\frac{d[\text{A}]}{dt} = \frac{d[\text{B}]}{dt} = k_1[\text{A}]_{\text{eq}} - k_{-1}[\text{B}]_{\text{eq}} = 0 \qquad (5.23)$$

The subscript "eq" designates quantities at equilibrium. Therefore:

$$K = \frac{[\text{B}]_{\text{eq}}}{[\text{A}]_{\text{eq}}} = \frac{k_1}{k_{-1}} \qquad (5.24)$$

K is the equilibrium constant, and is equal to the ratio between the rate constant of the forward reaction to that of the reverse reaction. Thus, Equation 5.24 provides a connection between the thermodynamic chemical equilibrium, and the kinetics of a reversible reaction. The concentration–time profile of a reversible first-order reaction can then be obtained:

$$\ln\left(\frac{[\text{A}]_0 - [\text{A}]_{\text{eq}}}{[\text{A}] - [\text{A}]_{\text{eq}}}\right) = (k_1 + k_{-1})t \qquad (5.25)$$

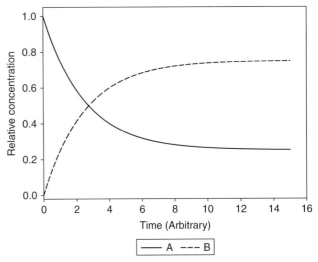

FIGURE 5.2 Concentration–time profiles for a theoretical reversible reaction

Figure 5.2 shows the time–concentration profiles for a theoretical reversible reaction assuming $K = 3$, $k_1 = 0.3$, and $k_{-1} = 0.1$.

Parallel Reactions

Sometimes more than one reaction pathway exists for degradation of a drug candidate. These pathways might lead to identical degradants or, more commonly, different degradants. Take for an example the following simplest parallel reaction:

$$\text{A} \overset{k_1}{\underset{k_2}{\underset{\searrow}{\nearrow}}} \begin{matrix} \text{B} \\ \text{C} \end{matrix} \qquad (5.26)$$

Here k_1 and k_2 are the first-order rate constants for reaction $\text{A} \rightarrow \text{B}$ and $\text{A} \rightarrow \text{C}$, respectively. The corresponding rate equation is:

$$\text{Rate} = -\frac{d[\text{A}]}{dt} = k_1[\text{A}] + k_2[\text{A}] = (k_1 + k_2)[\text{A}] = k_{\text{obs}}[\text{A}] \qquad (5.27)$$

Here $k_{\text{obs}} = k_1 + k_2$ is the observed apparent first-order rate constant. Mathematically, the concentration-time profiles can be obtained as follows:

$$[\text{A}]_t = [\text{A}]_0 \exp(-k_{\text{obs}}t) \qquad (5.28)$$

$$[\text{B}]_t = [\text{B}]_0 + \frac{k_1}{k_{\text{obs}}}[\text{A}]_0[1 - \exp(-k_{\text{obs}}t)] \qquad (5.29)$$

$$[\text{C}]_t = [\text{C}]_0 + \frac{k_2}{k_{\text{obs}}}[\text{A}]_0[1 - \exp(-k_{\text{obs}}t)] \qquad (5.30)$$

Figure 5.3 shows the concentration–time profile for a parallel reaction with $k_1 = 0.2$ and $k_2 = 0.1$.

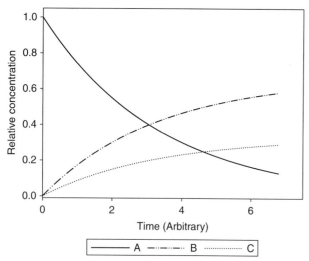

FIGURE 5.3   Concentration–time profiles for a theoretical parallel reaction

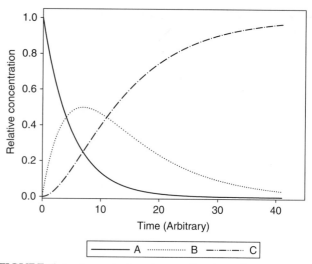

FIGURE 5.4   Concentration–time profiles for a theoretical consecutive reaction

Consecutive Reactions

Consecutive reactions involve an intermediate formed from the initial reactant that in turn is converted to the final product. For a simple first-order consecutive reaction from reactant A to product C via intermediate B:

$$A \xrightarrow{k_1} B \xrightarrow{k_2} C \tag{5.31}$$

The rate equations may be obtained as:

$$-\frac{d[A]}{dt} = k_1[A] \tag{5.32}$$

$$\frac{d[B]}{dt} = k_1[A] - k_2[B] \tag{5.33}$$

$$\frac{d[C]}{dt} = k_2[B] \tag{5.34}$$

The concentration–time profiles can be obtained by simultaneously solving the above differential equations:

$$[A] = [A]_0 \exp(-k_1 t) \tag{5.35}$$

$$[B] = \frac{k_1}{k_2 - k_1}[A]_0 \{\exp(-k_1 t) - \exp(-k_2 t)\} \tag{5.36}$$

$$[C] = [A]_0 + \frac{1}{k_1 - k_2}[A]_0 \{k_2 \exp(-k_1 t) - k_1 \exp(-k_2 t)\}$$
$$\tag{5.37}$$

The concentration–time profiles for a theoretical consecutive reaction are shown in Figure 5.4 for a

theoretical consecutive reaction $A \rightarrow B \rightarrow C$ with $k_1 = 0.2$, and $k_2 = 0.1$. Note that the time profile of the intermediate B shows a maximum.

5.2.6 Arrhenius Equation, Collision Theory, and Transition State Theory

The Arrhenius Equation

The rate of a reaction is usually affected by concentration, solvents, and catalysis and, very importantly, by temperature. The Q10 rule, attributed to pioneering physical chemist Jacobus H. van't Hoff, states that the velocity of a chemical reaction increases approximately two- to threefold for each 10°C rise in temperature. His student, Svante Arrhenius, expressed this more formally as:[1]

$$\frac{d \ln(k)}{dT} = \frac{E_a}{RT^2} \tag{5.38}$$

This can be integrated to give the exponential form:

$$\ln(k) = \ln(A) - \frac{E_a}{RT} \quad \text{or} \quad k = A \exp\left(-\frac{E_a}{RT}\right) \tag{5.39}$$

Here k is the rate constant, A is a constant known as the Arrhenius frequency factor (the limiting rate as the absolute temperature is increased to infinity), E_a is another constant called the activation energy, R is the universal gas constant, and T is the absolute temperature. The frequency factor determines the collision frequency between reacting molecules, while the activation energy is the energy barrier that the molecules must overcome in order to react and form product(s). Experimentally the frequency factor, and the activation energy, can be obtained respectively from the intercept and the slope of the Arrhenius plot of $\ln(k)$ *vs.* $1/T$.

Connors et al. pointed out that most drug degradations have activation energies of 12–24 kcal/mol;[2] however, higher activation energies have also been observed.[3] The Q10 rule assumes an activation energy of 13–20 kcal/mol; therefore, it provides a conservative estimate of the effect of temperature on drug degradation rates.

Classic Collision Theory of Reaction Rates

Reactant molecules must collide to react. However, not every collision leads to a successful reaction. The classical collision theory of reaction rates postulates that the reaction takes place only if the involved molecules exceed a certain minimum energy (the activation energy). Based on the above assumptions, an expression of the rate similar to the form in the Arrhenius equation can be derived.

The fraction of molecules with kinetic energies exceeding E_a can be derived using the Boltzmann distribution:

$$f(E_k > E_a) = \exp\left(-\frac{E_a}{RT}\right) \quad (5.40)$$

Here f is the fraction reacting (or probability of reaction), and E_k is the kinetic energy. Therefore, the rate can be expressed as:

$$\text{rate} = ZPC_{E_k > E_a} = ZPC_T \exp\left(-\frac{E_a}{RT}\right) \quad (5.41)$$

$C_{E_k > E_a}$ is the concentration of the reactant molecules with kinetic energy exceeding the activation energy, and C_T is the total reactant concentration. Z is the collision frequency, while P is the steric factor ($0 < P < 1$), because not every collision leads to a reaction. By comparison with the general rate law, one can immediately see that the expression of the rate constant, k, is similar to the Arrhenius equation:

$$k = ZP \exp\left(-\frac{E_a}{RT}\right) \quad (5.42)$$

ZP is identified with the Arrhenius frequency factor A, while E_a is the activation energy.

Transition State Theory

The classic collision theory assumes that the reaction is possible when reactant molecules with sufficient energies collide. It does not answer the question as to how they react. The transition state theory, developed around 1935 by Eyring and Polanyi et al.,[4] postulates that in addition to collision, a transition state (or activated complex) must exist in which the reacting molecules have an appropriate configurational geometry for the reaction to occur; furthermore, the transition state is in equilibrium with the reactants. In order for the activated complex to form, a certain energy barrier (the activation energy) needs to be overcome. Once the activated complex is formed it can decompose to products. In principle, the transition theory provides a means to calculate the rate of a reaction once certain properties of the activated complex, such as vibrational frequency, molecular mass, interatomic distances, etc., are known. This theory is also referred to as the absolute rate theory.

A simplified scheme can be represented as follows:

$$A + B \xrightleftharpoons{K^{\ddagger}} [A \cdots B]^{\ddagger} \longrightarrow C \quad (5.43)$$

The double dagger designates the transition state.

The transition state theory assumes that the decomposition of the activated complex is the rate-determining step of the reaction. Among all the molecular motions of the activated complex, there is one mode of vibration (frequency designated as ν) that will lead to the formation of the product. Combined with the equilibrium assumption, the rate of the reaction can be written as:

$$\text{Rate} = \frac{d[C]}{dt} = \nu[A \cdots B]^{\ddagger} = \nu K^{\ddagger}[A][B] \quad (5.44)$$

Thus, the rate constant of the reaction, k, has the form:

$$k = \nu K^{\ddagger} \quad (5.45)$$

Once the vibration frequency ν, and the equilibrium constant are known, the rate constant can be calculated. For example, the equilibrium constant can be obtained from statistical thermodynamic treatments of chemical equilibrium, while the frequency of the decomposition vibration can, as shown by Eyring, be approximated by:

$$\nu = \frac{k_B T}{h} \quad (5.46)$$

Here k_B is Boltzmann's constant, h is Plank's constant, and T is the absolute temperature. The final rate constant can be expressed as:

$$k = \frac{k_B T}{h} K^{\ddagger} = \frac{k_B T}{h} \exp\left(-\frac{\Delta G^{\ddagger}}{RT}\right)$$
$$= \frac{k_B T}{h} \exp\left(\frac{\Delta S^{\ddagger}}{R}\right) \exp\left(-\frac{\Delta H^{\ddagger}}{RT}\right) \quad (5.47)$$

$\Delta G^{\ddagger}$, $\Delta S^{\ddagger}$, and $\Delta H^{\ddagger}$ are the respective free energy, entropy, and enthalpy of activation. In comparison with the Arrhenius equation, it is immediately obvious that:

$$E_a = RT^2 \frac{d \ln k}{dT} = RT + \Delta U^{\ddagger}$$
$$= RT + \Delta H^{\ddagger} - \Delta(pV^{\ddagger}) \cong RT + \Delta H^{\ddagger} \quad (5.48)$$

$$A = \frac{k_B T}{h} \exp\left(\frac{\Delta S^{\ddagger}}{R}\right) \qquad (5.49)$$

$\Delta(pV^{\ddagger})$ is the change of pV when the activated complex is formed, and is negligible for most condensed phase reactions.

The transition state theory provides a better picture of chemical reactivity, and is still used today. It accounts for the influences on reaction rate by various factors, such as solvent, ionic strength, and dielectric constant. In general, enhancement of the reaction rate is expected if a factor stabilizes the transition state. However, sometimes changing one factor might also change the effects of other factors. Therefore, caution must be taken when such exercises are performed.

A schematic representation of the transition state theory is shown in Figure 5.5a. Figure 5.5b describes the situation where an intermediate exists. The intermediate is located at a local minimum on the potential energy surface, and in this case there are two separate activation energies.

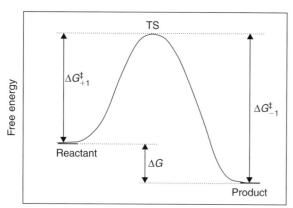

(a) Single-step reaction

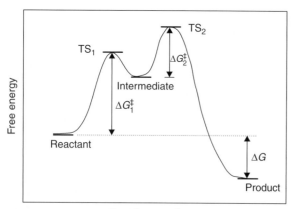

(b) Reaction with an intermediate

FIGURE 5.5 Schematic potential energy surface along the reaction coordinates

5.2.7 Catalysts and Catalysis

A catalyst is a substance that influences the rate of a reaction without itself being consumed. Positive catalysis increases the reaction rate, while negative catalysis reduces the reaction rate. However, positive catalysis is what is normally considered.

A catalyst changes the rate of a reaction by altering the free energy of activation (or activation energy) without altering the thermodynamic aspects of the reaction. In other words, the equilibrium of a reaction is not changed by the presence of a catalyst. A positive catalyst reduces the free energy of activation, while a negative catalyst increases it. Figure 5.6 describes the reaction coordinate with a positive catalyst.

The activation energy decreases in the presence of the catalyst; however the thermodynamics, as indicated by the ΔG of the reaction, are not altered.

Specific Acid–Base Catalysis

Hydrogen ions and/or hydroxyl ions are often involved directly in the degradation of pharmaceuticals. In many cases, the concentration of hydrogen ion or hydroxyl ion appears in the rate equation; the reaction is then said to be subject to specific acid–base catalysis.

For example, an ester drug is hydrolyzed in an acidic buffer; the second-order rate equation is:

$$\text{rate} = -\frac{d[D]}{dt} = k[H^+][D] \qquad (5.50)$$

Drug degradation studies are often carried out in buffered solutions where concentrations of hydrogen or hydroxyl ions are maintained as constant. In addition, the drug itself is usually the only species whose concentration is monitored over time. As a result, the

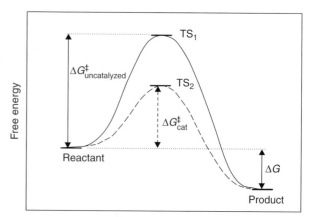

FIGURE 5.6 Schematic potential energy surfaces along a reaction coordinate with a positive catalyst

degradation kinetics is pseudo-first-order when the reaction is catalyzed by hydrogen or hydroxyl ions, with the apparent rate constant, k_{obs}:

$$k_{obs} = k[H^+] \quad \text{or} \quad \log k_{obs} = \log k - pH \quad (5.51)$$

For a reaction subject to specific acid catalysis, a plot of the logarithm of the apparent first-order rate constant with respect to pH gives a straight line of slope -1.

Similarly, for specific base catalysis, a plot of the logarithm of the apparent first-order rate constant versus pH gives a line of slope of $+1$:

$$k_{obs} = k[OH^-] \quad \text{or} \quad \log k_{obs} = \log k + pH \quad (5.52)$$

Hydrolysis of zileuton is subject to specific acid catalysis, but not base catalysis.[5,6] Hydrolysis of aspirin shows both specific acid- and specific base-catalysis.[7]

General Acid–Base Catalysis

General acid–base catalysis occurs when the buffering components catalyze a reaction. Either the acidic or basic components of the buffer, or both, can catalyze a reaction.

General acid–base catalysis often causes deviation of the rate-pH profile from the expected behavior. The exact magnitudes of general acid–base catalysis can often be obtained by varying buffer concentration while keeping the remaining conditions (ionic strength, pH, etc.) constant. A plot of the apparent first-order rate constant versus buffer concentration should be a straight line whose slope corresponds to the catalytic coefficient of the buffer at the studied pH. The intercept of this plot corresponds to the specific rate constant in the absence of general acid–base catalysis.

No distinction between the species responsible for general catalysis can be made by the above method. However, this could be achieved if the reaction is studied at different pH values with the same buffer species.

In general, the apparent first-order rate constant can be written as follows, taking into account both specific and general acid–base catalysis:

$$
\begin{aligned}
k_{obs} &= k_0 + k_H[H^+] + k_{OH}[OH^-] + k_1[\text{buffer species 1}] \\
&\quad + k_2[\text{buffer species 2}] + \cdots \\
&= k_0 + \sum_i k_i C_i \quad (5.53)
\end{aligned}
$$

Here k_0 is the intrinsic first-order rate constant in the absence of any catalysis, C_i is the concentration of species i, and k_i is the catalytic coefficient of species i.

The degradation of a number of pharmaceuticals has been shown to be subject to general acid–base

catalysis. Degradation of thiamine was found to be catalyzed by acetate ion, but not acetic acid, and is therefore an example of general base catalysis.[8] Citric acid, citrate ions, and phosphate ions all catalyze the decomposition of ampicillin, an example illustrating both general acid and general base catalysis.[9]

5.2.8 pH-rate Profiles

The pH-rate profile, or sometimes pH-stability profile or rate-pH profile, is the pH dependence of the specific rate constant of degradation of a compound, and is conveniently represented by a $\log(k)$ versus pH plot. pH-rate profiles provide insights on the catalytic nature of a reaction, and can help in developing more stable solution formulations and lyophilized products. pH-rate profiles also aid in the development of more stable conventional solid oral dosage forms (e.g., tablets), although solution stability information is not required to be as detailed in this case.

Many drug degradation reactions follow apparent first-order kinetics, and are subject to specific and/or general acid–base catalysis. The apparent first-order rate constants are what are usually plotted in a pH-rate profile. One should correct for general acid–base catalysis by buffer components by extrapolation to zero buffer concentration if the catalysis effect is significant.

Analysis of a pH-rate profile can be started by assuming all possible pathways, and writing down the corresponding rate equations (e.g., Equation 5.53). The presence or absence of a certain mechanism can then be verified by analyzing the kinetic data. A brief discussion of the more basic pH-rate profiles follows.

V-shaped, U-shaped, and other Truncated pH-rate Profiles

Specific acid and/or base catalysis is common in the degradation of carboxylic acid derivatives, such as esters, amides, substituted ureas, etc. In the absence of other more complicated mechanisms, the pseudo-first-order rate constant can be written as:

$$k_{obs} = k_H[H^+] + k_0 + k_{OH}[OH^-] \quad (5.54)$$

Here k_0 is the intrinsic apparent first-order rate constant, and k_H and k_{OH} are the catalytic coefficients for the hydrogen and hydroxyl ions, respectively. The resulting rate-pH profile plot consists of a straight line with slope of -1 in the acidic region, and another straight line with slope of $+1$ in the basic region (Figure 5.7a). Atropine[10,11] and diazepam[12] are example compounds having V-shaped pH-rate stability profiles. When k_0 is sufficiently large, the V-shaped pH-rate

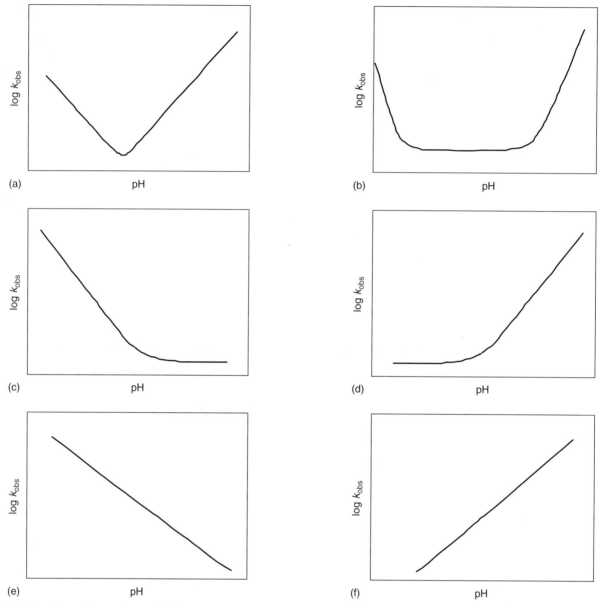

FIGURE 5.7   Schematic rate-pH profiles for reactions involving only a single reactive species with specific acid- and/or base-catalysis

profile may show a flat region and the resulting plot is U-shaped (see Figure 5.7b; hydrolysis of the β-lactam ring in cephalothin[13]).

Degradation of some drug substances may show only specific acid- or base-catalysis, but not both (e.g., hydrolysis of echothiophate[14]). The plot (Figure 5.7c or d) then either has a slope of −1 in the acidic region joined to a flat line extending into the basic region (specific acid catalysis) or a flat line in the acidic region joined to a line with slope +1 in the basic region (specific base catalysis). In some cases, only specific acid-catalysis or specific base-catalysis is observed; therefore the rate-pH profile consists of only a straight line (Figure 5.7e and f; e.g., lansoprazole[15]).

Figure 5.7 exhibits the above rate-pH profiles where only a single species is reactive with either specific acid- or base-catalysis, or both.

Sigmoidal pH-rate Profiles

Sigmoidal rate-pH profiles usually arise from the dissociation of the drug molecules. Many drug candidates are weak bases or weak acids. In the vicinity of pH = pK_a, the species distributions of a weak base or weak acid are sigmoidal when plotted as a function of pH. Therefore, if both the acidic and basic species of the compound can undergo degradation with differing rate constants, the rate-pH profile is expected to be sigmoidal. For example, for the decomposition of weak acid HA:

$$HA \xrightarrow{\quad k_{HA} \quad} product \qquad (5.55)$$

$$A^- \xrightarrow{\quad k_{A^-} \quad} product \qquad (5.56)$$

When the drug concentration is measured, a distinction between the ionized and unionized species is usually not made. The apparent rate of the reaction is:

$$rate = k_{HA}[HA] + k_{A^-}[A^-]$$

$$= \frac{k_{HA}[H^+] + k_{A^-}K_a}{K_a + [H^+]}\{HA\} \qquad (5.57)$$

K_a is the dissociation constant of HA, while $\{HA\}$ is the total concentration of HA. Therefore, a plot of the apparent rate constant is sigmoidal with respect to pH, so long as the rate constants are not identical. The rate constant of each species can be estimated from the limits of the apparent rate constant at low and high pH, and that $pK_a = pH$ at the inflection point of the sigmoidal pH-rate profile plot. If the change in rate is due to ionization at a single site, the sigmoidal curve will encompass slightly more than ± 1 pH units of the expected pK_a.

5-flurouracil is a weak diprotic acid, and has 2 ionization constants with $pK_1 = 7.3$ and $pK_2 = 11.3$. Among the three species, A^{2-} has the highest reactivity, while the neutral molecules H_2A and HA^- possess only slightly different rate constants. Therefore, the sigmoidal pH-rate profile[16] is rather obvious in the pH range 10.5–12.5 (Figure 5.8a). While the change in rate from pH 6 to pH 8 is only minor, the sigmoid shape can still be seen around the first pK_a.[16] Cycloserine is a zwitterion, with $pK_1 = 4.5$ (acid) and $pK_2 = 7.4$ (base). The three species have different reactivity, and follow the following order: $AH^{2+} > AH^{\pm} > A^-$. Therefore a broad sigmoidal pH-rate profile encompassing the pH range 3–9 (Figure 5.8b) was observed.[17] Degradation of barbital[18] and zileuton[6] also shows similar behavior.

Bell-shaped pH-rate Profiles

Bell-shaped pH-rate profiles show a minima or maxima. Different scenarios can lead to this kind of pH-rate profile. The most intuitive scenario arises from the existence of two ionizable functional groups in the molecule. For example, for a diprotic acid, H_2A, three species are in solution: H_2A, HA^-, and A^{2-}, where the concentration-pH profile of species HA^- is bell-shaped. Depending on whether the monoprotic species, HA^-, is the most or least reactive, the corresponding pH-rate profile could show either a

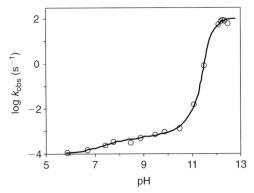

(a) 5-Fluorouracil

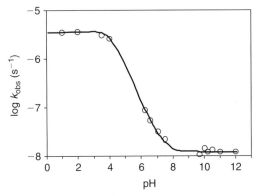

(b) Cycloserine at 25°C

FIGURE 5.8 Sigmoidal pH-rate profiles. Redrawn from references 16 and 17, respectively

maxima or a minima. Based on a similar argument, one can also show that the reaction between an acid and a base can lead to a bell-shaped pH-rate profile. In this case, the two ionizations are on different reactant molecules.

The third scenario occurs when ionization is combined with a change in the rate-determining step. For example, consider a consecutive reaction: $A \rightarrow B \rightarrow C$, where A is a monoprotic acid/base. The two species of reactant A may have very different reactivity with the rate-constant of step $B \rightarrow C$ falling somewhere in between. Therefore, in one pH region (below or above its pK_a), the step $A \rightarrow B$ is the slowest, whereas $B \rightarrow C$ becomes the rate-determining step over another pH range. A bell-shaped pH-rate profile then results, with one side of the bell corresponding to the ionization while the other corresponds to the switch of the rate-limiting step. Hydrolysis of hydrochlorothiazide[19,20] was proposed to be such a case (Figure 5.9). Its profile from pH 7 to 12 was probably caused by its two pK_a values of 8.6 and 9.9, respectively. However, the change from pH 7 to 2 could not be explained by ionization, and was hypothesized to be due to a switch of rate-determining step in the hydrolysis.

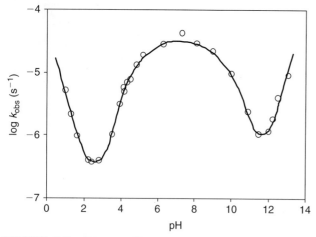

FIGURE 5.9   pH-rate profiles for hydrochlorothiazide at 60°C. Redrawn from reference 20

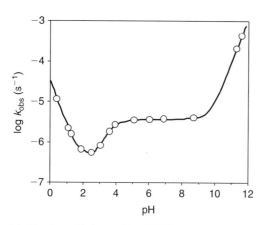

(a) pH-rate profile for aspirin at 25°C

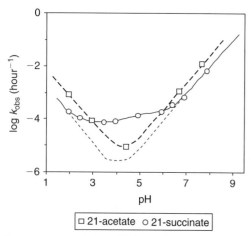

□ 21-acetate ○ 21-succinate

(b) pH-rate profiles for Methylprednisolone-21-acetate and Methylprednisolone-21-hemisuccinate at 25°C

FIGURE 5.10   Complex pH-rate profiles

More Complicated pH-rate Profiles

The presence of multiple ionization centers can complicate the analysis of a pH-rate profile (Figure 5.10a). However, their construction is based on similar principles. Depending on how far their pK_a values are isolated, some of the above-discussed features may not be fully developed in a particular pH-rate profile.

Additional features may be identified from a pH-rate profile. The pH-rate profile of aspirin shows evidence for specific acid-catalysis at pH <2 and specific base-catalysis at pH >10. The sigmoidal portion (pH 2–9) is due to the different reactivity of the neutral and ionized aspirin species.[7] The broad shoulder at pH 4.5–9 corresponds to the reactivity of ionized aspirin species with water, which is due to intramolecular catalysis:

Anderson et al.[21] studied the hydrolysis of methylprednisolone-21-esters in aqueous solutions. Hydrolysis of methylprednisolone-21-acetate (Figure 5.10b) showed a V-shaped pH-rate profile, indicating both specific acid- and specific base-catalysis. The structurally similar compound, methylprednisolone-21-succinate, however, showed quite a bit of deviation from that expected in the pH range 2 to 7. The higher reactivity in this pH range and deviation from the V-shaped pH-rate profile was again cause by intramolecular catalysis:

Information like this can not only provide significant insights on the stability itself, but is also helpful in designing a stable drug candidate.

5.2.9 Solid-state Reaction Kinetics

Solid dosage forms are the most common because they are easier to handle, more convenient to patients,

TABLE 5.2 Solid-state reaction mechanisms and their corresponding kinetic equations

Reaction mechanisms	Differential form $\frac{\partial \alpha}{\partial t} = k_T f(\alpha_{t,T})$	Integral form $g(\alpha_{t,T}) = k_T t$	Inverse integral form $\alpha_{t,T} = g^{-1}(k_T, t)$
Reaction order models:			
(F0) Zero-order	1	α	$k_T t$
(F1) First-order (Mampel)	$1 - \alpha$	$-\ln(1 - \alpha)$	$1 - e^{-k_T t}$
(F2) Second-order	$(1 - \alpha)^2$	$(1 - \alpha)^{-1} - 1$	$1 - (1 + k_T t)^{-1}$
(F3) Third-order	$(1 - \alpha)^3$	$\left(\frac{1}{2}\right)((1 - \alpha)^{-2} - 1)$	$1 - (1 + 2k_T t)^{-1/2}$
Nucleation models:			
(P2) Power law	$2\alpha^{1/2}$	$\alpha^{1/2}$	$k_T^2 t^2$
(P3) Power law	$3\alpha^{2/3}$	$\alpha^{1/3}$	$k_T^3 t^3$
(P4) Power law	$4\alpha^{3/4}$	$\alpha^{1/4}$	$k_T^4 t^4$
$\left(P\frac{3}{2}\right)$ Power law	$\frac{2}{3}\alpha^{-1/2}$	$\alpha^{3/2}$	$k_T^{2/3} t^{2/c}$
(A2) Avrami–Erofeev	$2(1 - \alpha)[-\ln(1 - \alpha)]^{1/2}$	$[-\ln(1 - \alpha)]^{1/2}$	$1 - e^{-k_T^2 t^2}$
(A3) Avrami–Erofeev	$3(1 - \alpha)[-\ln(1 - \alpha)]^{2/3}$	$[-\ln(1 - \alpha)]^{1/3}$	$1 - e^{-k_T^3 t^3}$
(A4) Avrami–Erofeev	$4(1 - \alpha)[-\ln(1 - \alpha)]^{3/4}$	$[-\ln(1 - \alpha)]^{1/4}$	$1 - e^{-k_T^4 t^4}$
(B1) Prout–Tompkins	$\alpha(1 - \alpha)$	$k_T t_{\frac{1}{2}} + \ln[\alpha/(1 - \alpha)]$	$\left(1 + e^{-k_T(t - t_{\frac{1}{2}})}\right)^{-1}$
Diffusion models:			
(D1) One dimensional	$1/2\alpha$	α^2	$k_T^{1/2} t^{1/2}$
(D2) Two dimensional	$[-\ln(1 - \alpha)]^{-1}$	$[(1 - \alpha)\ln(1 - \alpha)] + \alpha$	*
(D3) Three dimensional (Jander)	$\frac{3(1 - \alpha)^{1/2}}{2[1 - (1 - \alpha)^{1/3}]}$	$\left[1 - (1 - \alpha)^{1/3}\right]^2$	$1 - \left(1 - k_T^{1/2} t^{1/2}\right)^3$
(D4) Three dimensional (Ginstling-Brouhnshtein)	$\frac{3}{2}\left[(1 - \alpha)^{1/3} - 1\right]$	$1 - \frac{2\alpha}{3} - (1 - \alpha)^{2/3}$	*
Geometrical contraction models:			
(R1) Linear contraction	1	α	$k_T t$
(R2) Contracting cylinder	$2(1 - \alpha)^{1/2}$	$1 - (1 - \alpha)^{1/2}$	$1 - (1 - k_T t)^2$
(R3) Contracting sphere	$3(1 - \alpha)^{2/3}$	$1 - (1 - \alpha)^{1/3}$	$1 - (1 - k_T t)^3$

*No simple algebraic solution obtainable; solve by numerical approximation.

and do provide stability advantages in most cases. Degradation of an API in solid-state is more complicated than in solution, and a large part of its degradation behavior and kinetics can be attributed to the characteristics of its solid form.

5.2.10 Solid-state Kinetic Models

Various solid-state kinetic models have been discussed in literature, most of which have been applied to relatively simple systems, such as API crystals. These reaction models could be useful in elucidating the route and mechanism of solid-state reactions. The degradation kinetics of an API in a solid dosage form is even more complicated. However, zero- or first-order kinetics may be approximated for the first few percent of potency loss, which is most relevant for assessing the stability of a pharmaceutical product. Many so-called solid-state reactions might actually be moisture- or solution-mediated.

The concentration term in solid-state reactions is less clearly defined; therefore the extent of conversion, α, is predominately used. The quantity α is sometimes called the fractional conversion or fraction converted. Many different reaction mechanisms have been proposed to describe solid-state reactions, some of which are listed in Table 5.2. Models can be expressed in a differential form $f(\alpha_{t,T})$, as well as an integral form $g(\alpha_{t,T})$ or inverse integral form $g^{-1}(k_{t,T})$.

Reactions Involving Nucleation

Most solids contain defects. Defects are high-energy spots which can initiate physical and chemical changes, and play important roles when nucleation is the rate-limiting step of a reaction.

Avrami–Erofeev Equation

If the reaction involves random nucleation followed by the growth of nuclei of a defined dimensionality, the Avrami–Erofeev equation can be derived and may apply:[22,23,24,25,26]

$$[-\ln(1 - \alpha)]^{1/n} = kt \qquad (5.58)$$

Here n takes the value of 2, 3 or 4.

Avrami–Erofeev models have been observed for typical crystallization kinetics.

Prout–Tompkins Equation

The Prout–Tompkins equation[27] is derived based on the assumption of linearly growing nuclei that branch into chains:

$$\ln\left(\frac{\alpha}{1 - \alpha}\right) = k(t - t_{1/2}) \qquad (5.59)$$

Reaction kinetics of the type: solid $\rightarrow$ solid + gas often follow the Prout–Tompkins model.[28]

Reactions Controlled by Diffusion

In some solid-state reactions, reaction rates are controlled by diffusion of the reactants or products. This situation arises because mass transfer in the solid state is usually slow. Examples include curing of polymeric resins.

If the diffusion-controlled process is one-dimensional, then the one-dimensional equation may be derived:[29]

$$\alpha^2 = kt \qquad (5.60)$$

Similarly, the rate may be controlled by two-dimensional diffusion, as in a circular disc[30] or in a cylinder, or by three-dimensional diffusion as in a sphere.[31] The following equations can be derived for each case in turn:

$$(1 - \alpha)\ln(1 - \alpha) + \alpha = kt \qquad (5.61)$$

$$1 - \frac{2}{3}\alpha - (1 - \alpha)^{2/3} = kt \qquad (5.62)$$

A simplified three-dimensional diffusion equation was developed by Jander:[32]

$$[1 - (1 - \alpha)^{1/3}]^2 = kt \qquad (5.63)$$

Reactions Governed by Phase Boundaries

Some solid-state reactions involve two or more substances, where phase boundaries are formed between the reactants and the products. In some cases, the advance of the phase boundary so formed determines the rate of such a reaction. When the advance of the phase boundary is one-dimensional, then a zero-order reaction is obtained:

$$1 - \alpha = kt \qquad (5.64)$$

The two-dimensional phase boundary equation (contracting cylinder), and the three-dimensional phase boundary equation (contracting sphere) can be derived accordingly:[29]

$$1 - (1 - \alpha)^{1/n} = kt \qquad (5.65)$$

Here n takes the value of 2 and 3, respectively.

Higher (n-th) Order Reactions

These kinetic equations have similar formats as in solution kinetics. Most often, the first-order and second-order reactions are used. Higher orders are rare, and are difficult to interpret in solid-state reactions. In most cases, these equations provide an opportunity for curve-fitting rather than kinetic interpretation at the molecular level.

Bawn Kinetics

Sometimes the degradant is a liquid which serves as a solvent for the reactant: solid → liquid + gas. As a result, the reactant degrades both in the solid-state and in the solution state. When the kinetics in both phases is first-order, the Bawn kinetic model[28,33] may be appropriate:

$$\ln(1 + B\alpha) = Bk_s t \qquad (5.66)$$

Here k_s is the first-order rate constant in the solid-state, and B is the ratio between the first-order rate constant in solution state and that in solid-state. Bawn kinetics ceases to apply when the critical conversion is reached at which all of the remaining reactant dissolves.

Model-fitting versus Model-free Approaches

Conventionally, kinetic models in solid-state reactions are determined by a model-fitting approach, where the data are fitted to a number of reaction models, and the best model is then selected using statistical criteria. The process is often assisted by other experimental observations, such as microscopy. Difficulties arise for this model-fitting approach because solid-state reactions are usually more complex, and in many cases a change of reaction mechanism occurs during the course of the reaction. In addition, statistical distinction between models is not always achievable, such as in nonisothermal studies. A different methodology, called the model-free approach, has evolved within the last few decades and found application more recently in pharmaceutical systems.[34,35,36]

The idea of model-free approaches is evident upon transforming the basic kinetic equation:

$$\frac{d\alpha}{dt} = k(T)f(\alpha) = A\exp\left(-\frac{E_a}{RT}\right)f(\alpha) \qquad (5.67)$$

Here $d\alpha/dt$ is the instantaneous rate of a reaction, and $k(T)$ is the rate constant at temperature T, which is related to the activation energy E_a and frequency factor A through the Arrhenius relationship. The term $f(\alpha)$ represents the expression of the kinetic model (a function of the extent of conversion). For a reaction studied under a series of different conditions (e.g., different isothermal temperatures, different heating rates) the activation energy can be obtained at a specific extent of conversion, α_i, by transforming Equation 5.67 into:

$$\ln\left(\frac{d\alpha}{dt}\right)_{\alpha_i} = \ln[Af(\alpha)]_{\alpha_i} - \frac{E_{\alpha_i}}{RT_{\alpha_i}} \qquad (5.68)$$

It is not necessary to assume an explicit form of the reaction model $f(\alpha)$, because at the same conversion, $f(\alpha)$ is a constant number. The Kissenger[37] plot can be considered a special case of model-free kinetics.

In the model-free treatment, the activation energy is obtained as a function of the extent of conversion. If E_a is constant within experimental error with respect to the conversion, the reaction most likely follows a single kinetic model; otherwise a change of mechanisms is indicated. With this piece of information, construction of an underlying reaction model can be achieved for reactions following a single mechanism, while a change of mechanism can also be probed for reactions where E_a varies with conversion. Prediction using the model-free approach is also expected to be more accurate for complex solid-state reactions.

5.2.11 Physical Parameters Affecting Solid-state Kinetics

Solid-state reactions were hypothesized to consist of four general steps by Paul and Curtin:[38]

1. molecular loosening at the reaction site;
2. molecular change;
3. solid solution formation; and
4. separation of the product phase.

Similar steps have been suggested for physical transformations.[39] The four-step hypothesis can provide some insights to help us understand solid-state reactions.

Like reactions in the solution phase, temperature obviously influences the rate of a solid-state reaction, which can be usually be described by the Arrhenius relationship. Due to the constraint of the crystal lattice, solid-state reactions usually require a higher activation energy, compared to solution reactions. The applicability of the Arrhenius relationship to solid-state reactions has been debated, but has generally been observed over narrow temperature ranges. However, a change of temperature beyond that range could induce phase changes, which could alter the validity of the Arrhenius equation. For example, degradation of an amorphous pharmaceutical is not expected to follow the Arrhenius relationship when its glass transition temperature is crossed.[40] In addition, reaction mechanisms could change as temperature is changed.[41] Therefore, caution must be taken when the effect of temperature on solid-state degradation is studied. Some types of reaction are known not to follow the Arrhenius relationship. Free-radical oxidative degradation, both in solution and solid-state, is such an example, due to the autocatalytic nature of the process. Photolytic reactions are initiated by light absorption, and rarely depend on temperature. Indeed, some photochemical reactions can occur at temperatures near absolute zero.

If one envisions the first-step loosing of the molecules at the reaction sites, then the site of initiation of a solid-state reaction may have some "amorphous" characteristics. Hence, the degree of crystallinity of a solid phase is expected to affect the rate of a solid-state reaction. Solid-state reactions are enhanced by crystal disorder, which is related to the fact that amorphous regions have significantly higher molecular mobility, and hence higher reactivity, than crystalline regions. Even when the degree of crystallinity is not altered, a solid-state reaction can be enhanced by increasing its surface area (smaller particle size), and by increasing defects, because solid-state reactions are often initiated by defects at the surface of the material. It is not unusual that mechanical treatments such as milling exacerbate a stability problem by increasing the level of defects. However there are exceptions to the above generalization, which will be briefly touched on in topochemical reactions described below.

Moisture greatly influences solid-state reactions, which will also be discussed separately. Solid-state reactions can also be affected by other factors. For example, drug formulations may decompose faster in a tablet form than in the powder form, primarily due to more intimate contact.

5.2.12 The Role of Moisture

Water is ubiquitously present as atmospheric moisture, and has a profound effect on solid-state reactions. On the one hand, water can act as a reactant, and be involved in the reaction itself, such as in hydrolytic reactions. On the other hand, water is an excellent plasticizer; it increases molecular mobility of reactants and enhances drug degradation. In the worst case, water can form a saturated solution phase, and make the solid-state reaction solution mediated, which adversely affects stability to a great degree.

Various mechanisms exist for water molecules to interact with a solid. Water molecules can be incorporated into crystal lattice through hydrogen bonding and/or Van de Waals interactions. Generally, lattice water is not a cause of chemical instability. Some compounds rely on the interaction of water to form a stable crystal, thus improving their chemical stability. Water can also be adsorbed onto the surface as a monolayer and as multilayers. Water molecules in a monolayer may behave significantly differently than those in the second or third layers, the latter of which have

properties that presumably resemble bulk water. The concept of "bound" and "unbound" water has been suggested to explain solid–water interactions; however, it was found to be overly simplistic in some cases. "Bound" water was perceived to be unavailable for drug degradation, while "unbound water" was viewed as the major source of instability of pharmaceuticals. Various models have been applied to describe water–solid sorption, and some success has been achieved in describing the degradation kinetics resulting from such sorption. However, pharmaceutical solids usually contain various defects and, not uncommonly, various degrees of disordered, amorphous regions. Water molecules are preferentially absorbed into the interior of these regions. Because water is an efficient plasticizer, it significantly increases molecular mobility in the amorphous phase, which causes the drug degradation process to resemble more that occurring in the solution phase. Moisture adsorption onto crystal surfaces only accounts for insignificant amounts (on the order of 0.1% w/w) of total water content. Hence, the moisture level (a few percent) that is usually seen with bulk pharmaceuticals and formulations is primarily from absorption (into the interior), instead of adsorption (on the surface). In addition, at a relative humidity higher than some critical value, the drug or formulations containing the drug may undergo deliquescence, whereby drug degradation occurs primarily in the resulting solution phase (solution-mediated degradation). A more thorough discussion on water–solid interactions in pharmaceutical systems can be found elsewhere.[42]

The influence of moisture on degradation kinetics is complex, and various models have been proposed. The Leeson–Mattocks[43] model hypothesized that a saturated solution layer exists around solid particles, which sheds some light on the importance of moisture. However, very limited successes have been achieved on the quantitative aspect of moisture effects. Genton and Kesselring[44] initially showed the following equation held for nitrazepam degradation in solid-state:

$$\ln k = \ln A + \frac{E_a}{RT + B} \cdot RH \qquad (5.69)$$

Therefore, the Arrhenius relationship holds if RH is held constant. Furthermore, the logarithm of the rate constant changes linearly with relative humidity when temperature is held constant. This observation can be understood in the context that the relative humidity only affects molecular mobility in a reaction, but not the reaction pathways. Waterman et al.[45,46] have confirmed this relationship with a number of additional pharmaceutical systems. However, it should be emphasized that this relationship is not universal, and there are many exceptions.

5.2.13 Topochemical Reactions

A true solid-state reaction is a topochemical reaction. A true solid-state reaction can be identified if the reaction does not occur in solution or is much slower in solution or if the reaction products are different than those obtained in solution. True solid-state reactions depend highly on the molecular arrangements (conformations and configurations) or topologies in the solid-state. Therefore, the crystal structure of a solid phase determines its chemical reactivity. Different solid-state forms (polymorphs, solvates, salts, cocrystals) frequently exhibit different reactivity, and demonstrate true solid-state reactions.[47]

The first reported example for a topological thermal reaction is the rearrangement of methyl p-dimethylaminobenzenesulfonate to the p-trimethyl-ammoniumbenzenesulfonate zwitterion.[48,49] The molecules in monoclinic crystals are oriented almost ideally so as to facilitate reactions in the solid-state. On the contrary, the reaction rate is much slower (25 times) in its melt than in the solid-state. A pharmaceutical example is the deamidation of the asparagine residue of insulin;[50] in this case the amorphous state is far more stable than the crystalline state. However, a clear interpretation has not been provided, although it is reasonable to believe that the greater reaction rate observed with crystalline insulin should be related to the crystal packing. There are other examples provided in the text by Byrn[51] that different polymorphs lead to different reactivity; these provide other pharmaceutical examples of topochemical reactions.

5.3 COMMON PATHWAYS OF DRUG DEGRADATION

Despite the diversity of drug candidates, drug degradation follows some common pathways. By examining structural features of a drug molecule, possible degradation routes/products may be predicted to a certain extent, which may aid the design and execution of degradation studies.

Common mechanisms of drug degradation include thermolytic, oxidative, and photolytic. Thermolytic degradation refers to those that are driven by heat or high temperature, which normally follows the Arrhenius relationship. Any degradation mechanism can be considered "thermolytic," if high temperature enhances the rate, and "thermolytic" is a loose definition. Hydrolysis reactions form a subset of thermolytic degradation reactions, and are the most common drug degradation pathways; they will be discussed separately. Other thermolytic degradation pathways include ester/amide formation, rearrangement, isomerization/epimerization, cyclization, decarboxylation, hydration/dehydration, dimerization/polymerization, etc. Oxidation of drugs can proceed with different mechanisms: autoxidation, electrophilic/nucleophilic, and electron transfer reactions. Oxidative degradation reactions do not usually follow the Arrhenius relationship, due to their complex nature. Photolytic degradation can occur when drug or drug product is exposed to light. Photolytic degradation is initiated by light absorption; therefore temperature has a negligible effect. Photolytic degradation is not uncommon, but may be minimized during manufacturing, shipping, and storing of drug products by appropriate packaging.

5.3.1 Hydrolysis

Hydrolysis is by far the most commonly encountered drug degradation mechanism, both in solution and also in the solid state. Many drug molecules contain functional groups derived from relatively weakly bonding groups such as carboxylic acids. Hydrolysis of such derivatives is expected both in solution, and in the solid state, in the presence of water. In particular, the presence of hydrogen or hydroxyl ions likely catalyzes hydrolytic reactions. In the presence of relevant functional groups, such as alcohols, amines, esters, etc., either as solvent or solvent residuals, or more commonly, as excipients or impurities, the carboxylic acid derivatives can undergo certain types of reactions, such as alcoholysis and transesterification (e.g., aspirin-acetaminophen reaction[52]). These reactions follow similar mechanisms to hydrolysis, and will not be treated separately.

Hydrolysis of Carboxylic Acid Derivatives

Functional groups derived from carboxylic acid are common in pharmaceuticals. Examples include anhydrides, acyl halides, esters, amides, imides, lactams, lactones, and thiol esters. Esters (including lactones) and amides (including lactams) are among the most commonly seen. Carboxylic acid derivatives are usually prepared by a condensation reaction wherein the carboxylic acid is reacted with the corresponding functional group (alcohol, amine, etc.) with the expulsion of a molecule of water. Since this type of reaction is reversible, the reverse reaction can occur in the presence of added water:

$$R_1 \text{(C=O)} X + H_2O \longrightarrow R_1 \text{(C=O)} OH + HX \quad (5.70)$$

Here X = OCOR, Cl, OR, NR_2, SR. Sulfonates, sulfonamides, and other sulfonic acid derivatives follow similar pathways. Due to the greater electronegativity of oxygen atoms, the carbonyl group is polarized such that the oxygen atom carries a partial negative charge while the carbon atom carries a partial positive charge. As a result, the carbonyl group can be attacked nucleophilically (by attacking the carbon, using a nucleophile such as OH^-). The hydrolysis of carboxylic acid derivative usually proceeds with a tetrahedral intermediate, as shown below:

$$(5.71)$$

In the presence of hydrogen ion, the carbonyl oxygen is protonated, which enhances attack of the carbonyl carbon by weaker nucleophiles such as water. The above mechanism explains how the hydrolysis reaction can be catalyzed by either hydrogen or hydroxyl ions (specific acid–base catalysis), as well as by other nucleophiles (general acid–base catalysis).

Insights into the relative hydrolytic stability of carboxylic acid derivatives can be obtained in two aspects: nucleophilic attack of the carbonyl carbon, and relative leaving ability of the X group. Hydrolysis will be faster if the nucleophilic attack by X' is facilitated or if the leaving of X is facilitated, given that other conditions are similar. Electron-withdrawing groups in R_1 increase the electronegativity of the carbonyl group, thus promoting nucleophilic attack on the carbon; electron-withdrawing groups in X increase the basicity of X, stabilize X, and enhance the leaving ability of the X group. On the other hand, electron-donating groups will generally slow down hydrolysis. The effect of electron-withdrawing substituents on R_1 can be seen by comparing the relative hydrolysis rate of a series of substituted benzoate esters, while that of the leaving groups can been seen from the comparison of the hydrolysis rate of different carboxylic derivatives, such as anhydride, ester, amide, etc, which usually follows: acyl halide > carboxylic anhydride > ester > amide.

As a specific example, hydrolysis of phenol esters is much faster than that of corresponding alkyl esters, because the phenol anion is a much better leaving group. Because of this, phenol esters are generally more difficult to prepare than the corresponding alkyl esters. More detailed discussion on this topic can be found in a standard organic chemistry textbook, such as Carey.[53]

Hydrolysis of Acetals and Ketals

Acetals and ketals are relatively uncommon in pharmaceuticals however, they are present in some prodrugs. Acetals and ketals are formed by condensation reactions between alcohols and aldehydes, and alcohols and ketones, respectively, by removing a water molecule. Due to the unfavorable equilibrium in aqueous solution, and the relative facility of the hydrolysis reaction, they convert back to aldehydes and ketones quickly, particularly in acid solutions:

$$R_2C(OR')_2 + H_2O \xrightarrow{H^+} R_2C{=}O + 2R'OH \quad (5.72)$$

The mechanisms of these reactions are the reverse of the formation of the acetals and ketals, and are subject to specific acid catalysis, although general acid catalysis is observed in some cases.

Hydrolysis of other Carbonyl Derivatives

A few other types of carbonyl derivatives, such as imines, oximes, hydrazones, and semicarbazones, although not very commonly encountered in drug molecules, can undergo hydrolysis by reversal of the reactions leading to their formation:

$$R_2C{=}NR' + H_2O \rightarrow R_2C{=}O + R'NH_2 \quad (5.73)$$

$$R_2C{=}NOH + H_2O \rightarrow R_2C{=}O + HONH_2 \quad (5.74)$$

$$R_2C{=}NNHR' + H_2O \rightarrow R_2C{=}O + NH_2NHR' \quad (5.75)$$

$$R_2C{=}NN\overset{O}{\overset{\|}{H}}CNH_2 + H_2O \rightarrow R_2C{=}O + NH_2NH\overset{O}{\overset{\|}{}}CNH_2 \quad (5.76)$$

Hydrolysis of imines is the most facile of the reactions above, because the equilibrium constant of formation is unfavorable. On the other hand, oximes, hydrazones, and semicarbazones are usually more stable to hydrolysis, due to the fact that the equilibrium constants for formation are much higher, even in aqueous solutions. These hydrolysis reactions are usually catalyzed by both general acids and general bases. Switching of rate-determining steps has also been observed for hydrolysis of imines at different pH values.

Miscellaneous Hydrolysis Reactions

In general, both alkyl halides and aromatic halides are stable to hydrolysis. However, in certain situations, usually when activated by strong electron-withdrawing groups, halides can undergo hydrolysis. An example is chloramphenicol:[54]

$$(5.77)$$

The two chlorine atoms are connected to the alpha carbon of the carbonyl, which makes the alpha carbon more nucleophilic, and thus susceptible to hydrolysis.

Ethers hydrolyze to the corresponding alcohols via acidic catalysis. Aryl ethers are particularly unstable under mild acidic conditions, due to the stability of the oxyaryl cation intermediate. Thioethers undergo hydrolysis in a manner similar to ethers. Both ethers and thioethers are relatively stable at neutral or basic pH.

Sulfonamides and sulfonylureas are susceptible to acid hydrolysis. Sulfonamides hydrolyze to the corresponding sulfonic acid and amine, while sulfonylurea decomposes to the amine, carbon dioxide, and sulfonamide.

Carbamic esters hydrolyze to the corresponding carbamic acids, which in turn undergo decarboxylation, finally forming the amines.

Thiols can hydrolyze to the corresponding alcohols under both acidic and basic conditions.

Epoxides and aziridines are three-member rings, and contain significant strain. Both are susceptible to ring opening reactions via nucleophilic attack by water or other nucleophiles.

5.3.2 Oxidative Degradation

Oxidation presents an important drug degradation pathway, and is second only to hydrolysis. Although its significance to drug stability has been recognized, the study of oxidative stability has not been well-developed until more recently, partially due to its complicated nature. This section will briefly discuss the various mechanistic and kinetic aspects of oxidation.

Mechanisms of Oxidation

Under normal conditions the reaction between molecular oxygen and an organic molecule, although thermodynamically favorable, proceeds at an insignificant rate. The slow oxidation rate is due to the electronic configuration of molecular oxygen. The valence electrons of the O_2 molecule can be represented, according to molecular orbital theory, as:

$$(\sigma_{2s})^2(\sigma_{2s}^*)^2(\sigma_{2p_z})^2(\pi_{2p_x})^2(\pi_{2p_y})^2(\pi_{2p_y}^*)^1(\pi_{2p_z}^*)^1 \quad (5.78)$$

Here * designates an anti-bonding orbital. Ground state molecular oxygen has two unpaired spin electrons in its $\pi_{2p_y}^*$ and $\pi_{2p_z}^*$ orbitals, and is therefore in a triplet state. Most organic compounds, in contrast, are in a singlet ground state, with all spins paired. Direct reactions between singlet and triplet molecules violate the conservation law of spin angular momentum, and are not favorable. Therefore, for the direct reaction between oxygen and organic molecules to occur, one of the molecules needs to be excited to a state so that the spin states of both molecules match. Triplet ground state oxygen can be excited to the first excited singlet state (singlet oxygen) both chemically and photochemically. Oxidative reactions caused by singlet oxygen will be discussed briefly in the section on photolytic degradation pathways.

Oxidation of organic compounds occurs primarily via three mechanisms:

- nucleophilic/electrophilic processes;
- electron transfer reactions; and
- free radical processes (autoxidation).

Nucleophilic/electrophilic processes typically occur between peroxide and an organic reactant. For example, peroxide anion formed under basic conditions can attack drug molecules as a nucleophile. Under normal conditions, a drug will more likely be subject to electrophilic attack by unionized peroxide. Nucleophilic and electrophilic reactions typically follow Arrhenius behavior, and are accelerated at higher temperatures. However, when peroxides are heated, radical processes can be triggered, so non-Arrhenius behavior may be observed above a certain threshold.

In an electron-transfer process, an electron is transferred from a low electron affinity donor to an oxidizing species, which may be catalyzed by transition metals. Single-electron transfer reactions may exhibit Arrhenius behavior when the bond dissociation energy of the acceptor molecule is low, but breaking CH bonds requires so much energy that single-electron transfer reactions typically exhibit non-Arrhenius behavior.

The autoxidation process involves the initiation of free radicals, which propagate through reaction with oxygen and drug molecule to form oxidation products. Because of the complexity of the reaction mechanism, non-Arrhenius behavior may be observed. The three stages of autoxidation can be represented as:
Initiation:

$$In - In \rightarrow 2In \bullet \qquad (5.79)$$

$$In \bullet + RH \rightarrow In - H + R \bullet \qquad (5.80)$$

Propagation:

$$R \bullet + O_2 \rightarrow ROO \bullet \qquad (5.81)$$

$$ROO \bullet + RH \rightarrow ROOH + R \bullet \qquad (5.82)$$

Termination:

$$R \bullet + R \bullet \rightarrow R-R \qquad (5.83)$$

$$R \bullet + ROO \bullet \rightarrow ROOR \qquad (5.84)$$

$$RO \bullet + HO \bullet \rightarrow ROOH \qquad (5.85)$$

In the initiation stage, a pair of free radicals is generated. A variety of processes can generate free radical pairs by cleaving a chemical bond homolytically under the influence of heat or light. Several categories of organic compounds can be used to generate free radicals readily, such as azo compounds, acyl peroxides, alkyl peroxides, hydrogen peroxide, etc., some of which have been routinely used as free radical initiators in polymerization. For example, the initiation of radicals can be achieved using 2,2'-azobis(N,N'-dimethyleneisobutyramidine)dihydrochloride (AIBN):

$$(CH_3)_3C-N{=}N-C(CH_3)_3 \rightarrow 2(CH_3)_3C \bullet + N_2$$
$$(5.86)$$

The facile dissociation of azo compounds is not caused by the presence of a weak bond, as is the case with peroxides. Instead, the driving force for azo homolysis is the formation of the highly stable nitrogen molecule.

The two steps at the propagation stage are distinct. The first step, the reaction between the drug free radical with oxygen, is fast (on the order of 10^9 $M^{-1}s^{-1}$ at 300°K).[55] The second step, in which a hydroperoxide is formed and a drug free radical is regenerated, is 8–9 orders of magnitude slower, and is the rate-determining step. Therefore, the rate of autoxidation is generally unaffected by the oxygen concentration, unless the concentration of oxygen becomes significantly low.

The kinetics of autoxidation is complicated due to the multiple steps involved in the process. The reaction order with respect to substrate concentration varies in the range of zero to one. The most noticeable feature of autoxidation kinetics is the lag time, which corresponds to a stage of gradual build up of free radicals.

Besides catalyzing electron transfer processes, transition metals can also react with organic compounds or hydroperoxides to form free radicals:

$$M^{(n+1)+} + RH \rightarrow M^{n+} + R \bullet + H^+ \qquad (5.87)$$

$$M^{n+} + ROOH \rightarrow M^{(n+1)+} + RO \bullet + HO^- \qquad (5.88)$$

$$M^{(n+1)+} + ROOH \rightarrow M^{n+} + ROO \bullet + H^+ \qquad (5.89)$$

Typically, multiple mechanisms may occur simultaneously in an oxidative reaction, which introduces further complications.

Stabilization strategies can be developed based on the mechanisms of oxidative degradation for a particular compound.[56,57]

Prediction of Oxidative Stability

Oxidative stability of pharmaceuticals can be predicted to a certain extent by theoretical computations.[58] The susceptibility of an organic molecule to nucleophilic/electrophilic and electron transfer oxidative processes can be predicted using frontal molecular orbital (FMO) calculations. According to FMO theory, the site of reaction will occur between the lowest unoccupied molecular orbital (LUMO) of the electrophile and highest occupied molecular orbital (HOMO) of the nucleophile. Under normal conditions, the nucleophile is usually the organic compound. Therefore, properties of the HOMO of the organic reactant determine its propensity to be oxidized. Computing the HOMO of a reactant could thus yield useful information regarding the most susceptible sites for oxidation by nucleophilic/electrophilic and electron transfer processes.

For oxidative degradation via the free radical process, hydrogen abstraction is usually the rate-determining step for propagation. Therefore, stability of the corresponding free radicals should correlate with their susceptibility to autoxidation. Hence, a bond dissociation energy (BDE) calculation could provide insight regarding sites of potential autoxidation.

Functional Groups Susceptible to Oxidation

Amines are known to be prone to oxidation. Primary and secondary amines oxidize to hydroxylamines, which can dehydrate to imines or, after further oxidation, to oximes. Oxidation of aryl amines usually produces aryl hydroxylamines, which further oxidize to aryl nitroso compounds. Tertiary amines undergo oxidation, producing N-oxides, which are usually the final degradants. Protonation of the amine reduces its propensity to oxidation. However, protonation may not effectively protect against oxidation during long-term storage.

Nitriles are susceptible to oxidation by peroxides under slightly alkaline conditions. Acetonitrile is oxidized to unstable (and oxidizing) peroxycarboximidic acid; this has been known to enhance the susceptibility of organic compounds to oxidation by peroxide when acetonitrile is used as a co-solvent.[59]

Primarily, alcohols can be oxidized to the corresponding aldehydes, and then further to carboxylic acids. Phenols and other aryl hydroxyls are particularly susceptible to oxidation, due to the fact that conjugation in the aryl systems enhances the electron density on the oxygen atoms.

Pyrroles can be oxidized by peroxide to form pyrrolinones. Compounds containing unsaturated double bonds form epoxides by oxidation.

Thiol and thioethers are other examples of readily oxidizable organic functional groups. Thiols can oxidize to disulfide, sulfenic acid, sulfinic acid, and sulfonic acids under a variety of conditions, such as nucleophilic processes (peroxide), autoxidation, and electron-transfer reactions. Due to the affinity of thiols with transition metals, most thiols get oxidized via the metal-catalyzed electron-transfer process. Thioethers undergo oxidation to sulfoxides, and finally to sulfones, a process which may also be catalyzed by transition metals.

A methylene ($-CH_2-$) or methyne ($-CH-$ group is activated when the corresponding free radical formed by H-abstraction is stabilized by a neighboring group, such as carbonyl, carbon–carbon double bond, aromatic ring, or a heteroatom such as O, N, or S. The activated methylene or methyne group is a potential site of autoxidation, due to the stability of the free radical formed. These sites can be predicted using BDE calculation. Examples include phenylbutazone and benzyl alcohols.

5.3.3 Photochemical Degradation

Light

Light is a form of electromagnetic radiation, the energy of which is given by:

$$E = h\nu = \frac{hc}{\lambda} \qquad (5.90)$$

Here h is Plank's constant, c is the speed of light (3×10^8 m/s), ν is the frequency and λ is the wavelength. Hence, "red light" (700–800 nm) corresponds to an energy of 30–40 kcal/mol, while far ultraviolet light (~200 nm) corresponds to an energy of 140 kcal/mol. For comparison, the weakest single bonds commonly encountered in organic molecules have a strength of ~35 kcal/mol (such as an O—O bond), and the strongest single bonds have strengths of ~100 kcal/mol (e.g., a C—H bond). This simple comparison demonstrates that the energy of light is adequate to potentially lead to degradation of drug molecules if it is absorbed.

No photochemical reaction can occur unless light is absorbed (the Grotthuss–Draper law). The relevant radiation bands that are most likely to be problematic to pharmaceuticals are visible light ($\lambda \sim 400$–800 nm), and ultraviolet (UV) light ($\lambda \sim 200$–400 nm). Sunlight in the wavelength range of 200–290 nm is effectively absorbed by molecular oxygen and ozone in the upper atmosphere, and is therefore not considered to be important for photolytic degradation of drugs, although many organic substances do absorb strongly in this wavelength range.

Light Absorption, Excitation, and Photochemical Reactions

Accompanying the absorption of UV-visible light by a molecule is a change in its electronic configuration to an excited state. The electrons in the outermost shells of a molecule are the most susceptible ones, because these electrons are the least strongly bound to the molecule. From the point of view of FMO theory, electrons in the HOMO will be excited by absorption of light energy into its LUMO, where they possess higher potential energy that could cause photochemical degradation of the molecule.

Spin state is a characteristic feature for electron excitation, and plays an important role in photochemical reactions. Most organic molecules have a ground state HOMO with paired electrons, and are therefore in a singlet state (denoted as S_0, where the subscript 0 refers to the ground state). When one electron is excited from the HOMO to LUMO, its spin can be maintained (first excited singlet state, S_1) or flipped (first excited triplet state, T_1).

The excited electron can drop back to the ground state by giving up one photon; this is called a photophysical radiative process. The "allowed" singlet–singlet ($S_1 \rightarrow S_0$) emission is called fluorescence while the "forbidden" triplet–singlet ($T_1 \rightarrow S_0$) emission is called phosphorescence.

The excited electron can also drop back to the ground electronic state without emitting a photon by photophysical radiationless processes. In most cases, the excited electron falls back to the ground electronic state by releasing heat, which may result from collisions between excited molecules and other molecules (e.g., solvent molecules) in their environment. Transitions between states of the same spin (e.g., $S_1 \rightarrow S_0$ + heat) are "allowed" and this process is called internal conversion; transitions between states of different spins, such as $T_1 \rightarrow S_1$ + heat or $T_1 \rightarrow S_0$ + heat, are "forbidden" and are called intersystem crossing. The energy state diagram shown in Figure 5.11 describes these photophysical processes.

Not all atoms of a compound absorb UV-visible light, due to the mismatch of the energy of photon and the energetic gap between the ground and excited electronic states. A chromophore is defined as an atom or group of atoms that act as a unit in light absorption. Typical chromophores for organic substances include C=C, C=C, and aromatic groups.

Electronic excitation for C=C bonds involves $\pi \rightarrow \pi^*$ transitions between its electronic orbitals, while for C=C, $n \rightarrow \pi^*$ transitions are involved. Since the electronic occupancy of the excited state is different from that of the ground state, their properties are also different. For example, ethylene is planar in the ground state, while the excited state is twisted. Other properties, such as dipole moments and acid/base dissociation constants, are also changed in the excited state.

Molecules in excited states may undergo chemical reaction with themselves, due to their elevated energy state. The excited molecules may also jump back to ground state via photophysical radiationless routes. The electronic energy is converted to vibrational energy of the molecule in this case, which might be adequate to overcome the activation barrier in the ground state to bond dissociation and trigger chemical degradation.

From the photochemical point of view, most photodegradation reactions observed for pharmaceuticals tend to involve intermediates, and are not concerted in nature. The electronically excited state generated by stretching a σ-bond or twisting a π-bond can result in a "diradicaloid" structure where the two half-filled orbitals are nearly degenerate. The interaction of these two degenerated orbitals can then lead to the diradical singlet state, diradical triplet state, and two zwitterionic states (where one degenerated orbital is completely filled while the other is empty). The singlet π, π^* excited state, $S_1(\pi, \pi^*)$, has significant zwitterionic nature, and is expected to form a reactive intermediate via proton or electron transfer reactions, nucleophilic or electrophilic additions, or rearrangement. The triplet $T_1(\pi, \pi^*)$ state, on the other hand, is expected to generate diradical intermediates, and undergo primary photoreactions characteristic of radicals (e.g., H-abstraction, addition to unsaturated bonds, radicaloid rearrangements, hemolytic fragmentations). Both $S_1(n, \pi^*)$ and $T_1(n, \pi^*)$ are diradical in nature, and lead to qualitatively similar photochemical products. More detailed discussion of this topic can be found in the textbook by Turro.[60] Examples of photochemical degradation of drugs can be found in the text by Tønnesen.[61]

Photo-oxidation

Oxidation has frequently been observed in photochemical degradation reactions. Photo-oxidation can occur when excited triplet state molecules react directly with molecular oxygen, because an excited triplet state matches the ground spin state of molecular oxygen. In addition, another process appears to be important in which singlet oxygen is involved, called photosensitized oxidation. Photosensitization is a process whereby an initially light absorbing species (donor) transfers energy to and excites a second species (acceptor), provided that the acceptor has a low-lying triplet state. The donor could be a different species (such as a dye molecule), but could also be the drug molecule itself. The acceptor is also called a "quencher" because it quenches the excited state of the donor. Photosensitization allows a non-absorbing acceptor species to be excited in the presence of a light-absorbing donor molecule.

Two types of photo-oxidation exist. In Type I photo-oxidation, the donor transfers an electron or a proton to the acceptor (usually the drug), forming an anion or neutral radical, which rapidly reacts with molecular oxygen. A Type I process is also called an electron transfer or free radical process.

Type II photo-oxidation involves singlet oxygen. The first excited state of molecular oxygen, $^1\Delta$, lies

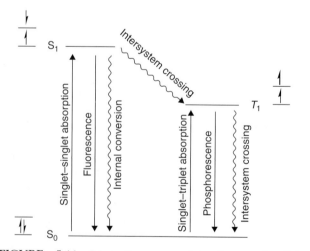

FIGURE 5.11 Schematic energy state diagram for light absorption

22.5 kJ/mol (1270 nm) above its ground state ($^3\Sigma$), which is of much lower energy than the triplet states of most organic molecules. Ground state molecular oxygen is generally an efficient quencher of the S_1 and T_1 states of organic molecules. The photosensitized singlet oxygen matches the spin states of a majority of organic molecules, which enhances their direct oxidation. Singlet oxygen can be generated using strongly light-absorbing dyes (e.g., Rose Bengal, methylene blue, etc.) via a photosensitization process.

5.3.4 Other Degradation Pathways

Hydration (addition of a molecule of water) can occur at a double bond, which is well-known in the case of fumaric acid.

Racemization of chiral centers can occur via formation of a planar intermediate, usually a cation, but a radical or anion intermediate can be involved as well.

Decarboxylation often occurs thermally for a β-keto carboxylic acid (e.g., norfloxacin[62]).

Amines are common functional groups in APIs, and are reactive in a variety of ways besides oxidation. Primary and secondary amines can react with counterions in a salt (e.g., maleic acid,[63] tartaric acid, etc.) or acids/acid derivatives in excipients (e.g., stearic acid or magnesium stearate[64]) to form the corresponding amides. Amines react readily with aldehydes (such as formaldehyde, which may present at low levels as a degradation product or impurity in excipients such as polyethylene oxide, polyethylene glycol, poloxamer, and carbohydrates) to form hemiaminals. The complex series of reactions between a primary or secondary amine and a reducing sugar causes color changes, and is well-known as the "Maillard browning reaction."

Other types of degradation reactions have also been observed, such as isomerization (fumaric acid ↔ maleic acid), rearrangements (cephalosporin), dimerization and polymerization (e.g., ampicillin and other ß-lactam antibiotics[65]), cyclization (e.g., aspartame,[66] moexipril[67]), and deamidation (e.g., asparagines residues in peptides and proteins).

5.4 EXPERIMENTAL APPROACHES TO STUDYING THE CHEMICAL DEGRADATION OF DRUGS

Drug degradation studies are a required component of stability testing conducted to support registration of new drug substances and drug products.[68]

However, the design and execution of accelerated stability testing methods, while well-established in many industries,[69] is still evolving within the pharmaceutical industry. In this section we survey current best practices.

5.4.1 Solution Thermal Degradation Studies

In conducting an accelerated thermal degradation study, the investigator typically exposes samples containing the test substance of interest to elevated temperature storage, and then measures the concentration or potency of the test substance remaining after various times. In the past, some methods for the interpretation of data obtained from such studies have focused primarily on the estimation and prediction of reaction rates; however, most users intend to employ these predicted rates to estimate concentrations or potencies at future times at temperatures not tested or to estimate the time until which the concentration or potency will remain within specified limits with a specified probability (shelf life prediction). Although methods that yield estimated rates may be used to obtain point estimates of concentrations, they are incapable of providing useful confidence interval estimates, so this review will focus on methods of obtaining and modeling accelerated degradation experimental data that yield concentration or shelf life estimates directly. Such methods require nonlinear modeling. Because modeling by nonlinear regression is more of an art than a science, previous experience in fitting nonlinear models is helpful.

Chemical kineticists have employed the Arrhenius model for years as a means to determine the energy of activation of a chemical reaction from the temperature dependence of the rate of reaction. Aside from a few studies on biologically derived pharmaceutical preparations,[70] only since the late 1940s did technologists[71–77] in the food and pharmaceutical industries begin to make use of the Arrhenius model to study degradation processes. In the mid-1950s, after introductory studies by Garrett, the use of the Arrhenius model to predict the shelf life of a pharmaceutical product at a lower temperature (e.g., room temperature) from the kinetics of its degradation studied at higher temperatures became common.[78–86] Prediction of shelf life became a primary focus of thermal stress degradation studies in both the pharmaceutical industry and the food industry, and, over the years, a number of investigators have sought to improve the statistical techniques used to treat the data so as to obtain better estimates of the precision with which shelf life could be predicted. In addition to the use of thermal stress degradation studies to predict shelf life, the time required to determine a reaction rate with a given precision can be reduced by determining the rate at an elevated temperature, where degradation occurs more quickly;[87] thus, Arrhenius models have attracted the interest of chemical engineers and physical chemists.

Early workers in the field of chemical kinetics relied upon graphical methods and simple numerical analysis techniques (such as point-by-point integration) to obtain estimates of the rates of chemical reactions and the effect of changing reaction temperature on these rates. Graphical techniques are important to visualize the data and to form initial judgments as to the overall quality of the data and relevance of the kinetic model; however, they are at best a crude way to obtain kinetic parameters, and are subject to bias on the part of the graphic artist in obtaining the "best" representation of the data. In addition, graphical methods offer no way to estimate the precision of fitted parameters. Numerical methods based upon point-by-point integration introduce an insidious form of serially correlated error into the final results, as each observation (except the first and last) is used twice. Typical kinetic experiments were run at only a few temperatures, one of which was usually close to ambient. Extraordinary measures to control temperature, and to select very precise analytical methods, are required to employ these methods effectively; in particular, measurement of the energy of activation of a reaction from determination of the rate at only two temperatures $\sim 10°C$ apart requires temperature control of $\pm 0.03°C$ and analytical precision of $\pm 0.1\%$ to obtain an error of $\pm 0.5\%$ in the energy of activation. These methods have been described in detail.[88]

The application of statistical methods, based on modeling by regression analysis to the evaluation of data obtained from accelerated chemical degradation studies in solution, was first applied to a study of the decomposition of a nitrogen-containing compound in 1954 by McBride and Villars.[89] These workers used a two-stage graphical approach, first estimating the rate constants at different temperatures, and then plotting the logarithms of the estimated rate constants versus reciprocal absolute temperature in a second step to obtain estimates of the Arrhenius model parameters. Garrett popularized this approach in the pharmaceutical industry.[90,91,92,93] The use of estimated reaction rates as if they were data reduces the large number of degrees of freedom inherent in the actual data to just a few degrees of freedom in the final model, enormously exaggerating the uncertainty with which interval predictions can be made outside of the time and temperature region studied. Since making such interval predictions is, perhaps, the most important purpose of conducting thermal stress degradation studies, the two-stage modeling approach is wholly unsatisfactory.[94]

Garrett and his followers usually made measurements at linearly spaced time intervals (e.g., daily) for a fixed duration (e.g., a month or two); measurements at the higher temperatures were terminated when the amount of drug remaining became too low to measure accurately. Most workers also made the same number of measurements at each temperature for each sampling time. This type of design can be called a "Garrett" design. It is not efficient.

Later, Tootill showed that a more efficient design consisted of obtaining measurements at roughly the same extent of decomposition.[95] Tootill was probably the first author to devise a method to use potency remaining at each time and temperature to directly fit an Arrhenius model to kinetic data; however, he did so by imposing strict design constraints. Tootill's 1961 design was actually an extension of the earlier design work of Box and Lucas,[96] who showed in 1959 that the most efficient design (when percent potency remaining could be measured, the reaction was known to be first order, and the Arrhenius model was known to be correct), was to measure the potency at such a time that 36.8% ($100\%/e$) of the substance remained at both the highest and lowest temperatures that could be studied; this design has properties that statisticians call d-optimal. Davies and coworkers[97,98] showed that the most efficient measurements for the estimation of reaction rates were only obtained after allowing the decomposition reaction to proceed for 1 to 2 half lives (50 to 75% decomposition), in agreement with the finding of Box and Lucas. This recommendation was based solely upon the statistical properties of the data, and ignored potential complications arising from changes in the major reaction pathway caused by the accumulation of degradation products as the reaction proceeds. Thus, Davies and Hudson[98] also recommended designs for which degradation was to be monitored until the same extent of degradation had occurred at each temperature, as previously recommended by Tootill,[95] and by Box and Lucas.[96] Subsequently, such designs will be referred to as "Box–Tootill–Davies" designs. These isoconversional designs are efficient.

Since rates are seldom measured directly, the Arrhenius model can be further integrated to yield, for pseudo-zero-order reactions:

$$P_{hij} = P_0 - t_{ij}Ae^{-\frac{E_a}{RT_j}} + e_{hij} \qquad (5.91)$$

For pseudo-first-order reactions:

$$P_{hij} = P_0 e^{-t_{ij}Ae^{-\frac{E_a}{RT_j}}} + e_{hij} \qquad (5.92)$$

Here P_{hij} is the hth measured potency at time t_{ij} and temperature T_j, P_0 is the estimated initial potency at time $t = 0$, and e_{hij} is the error in measuring P_{hij}. Carstensen and Su introduced this technique in the pharmaceutical field in 1971 as a method for directly fitting an Arrhenius model to potency data.[99] Nonlinear direct fitting of an Arrhenius model to concentration or potency data was further advanced by the work of Davies and Budgett,[100] who specifically addressed proper weighting of the data. Davies and Hudson later proposed standard methods for the statistical analysis of potency data obtained in the course of degradation studies based on this error analysis.[98] These authors reparameterized the Arrhenius models to explicitly account for the fact that it is the logarithm of estimated rate constants that is approximately normally distributed. Thus, for a pseudo-zero-order reaction:

$$P_{hij} = P_0 - t_{ij} e^{\ln(A) - \frac{E_a}{RT_j}} + e_{hij} \qquad (5.93)$$

For a pseudo-first-order reaction:

$$P_{hij} = P_0 e^{-t_{ij} e^{\ln(A) - \frac{E_a}{RT_j}}} + e_{hij} \qquad (5.94)$$

Instead of using the logarithm of the rate expected in the limit as the absolute temperature increases to infinity (the Arrhenius frequency factor A), the rate at any other temperature T can be used instead. Thus, one can substitute:

$$\ln(A) = \ln(k_{est}) + \frac{E_a}{RT_{est}} \qquad (5.95)$$

Furthermore, the rate at any particular temperature is inversely proportional to the time required to achieve a particular fractional degradation f. Thus, for a pseudo-zero-order reaction:

$$k_{T_{est}} = \frac{P_{t=0}(1 - f)}{t_{100f\%, T_{est}}} \qquad (5.96)$$

And for a pseudo-first-order reaction:

$$k_{T_{est}} = \frac{-\ln(f)}{t_{100f\%, T_{est}}} \qquad (5.97)$$

King et al.[101] independently recommended reparameterization with this additional substitution to estimate shelf life directly. Thus, for a pseudo-zero-order reaction, the Arrhenius model becomes:

$$P_{hij} = P_0 - (1 - f) P_0 t_{ij} e^{\frac{E_a}{R}\left(\frac{1}{T_{est}} - \frac{1}{T_j}\right) - \ln\left(t_{100f\%, T_{est}}\right)} + e_{hij}$$
$$(5.98)$$

And for a pseudo-first-order reaction, it becomes:

$$P_{hij} = P_0 e^{t_{ij} \ln(f) e^{\frac{E_a}{R}\left(\frac{1}{T_{est}} - \frac{1}{T_j}\right) - \ln\left(t_{100f\%, T_{est}}\right)}} + e_{hij} \qquad (5.99)$$

Here f is the fraction of undegraded drug remaining at time $t_{100f\%}$ at temperature T_{est}.

Simulation studies using a realistic assumed distribution of experimental errors in conjunction with a "Box–Tootill–Davies" design with $f_{min} = 0.8$ (corresponding to 20% degradation) give remarkably precise estimates of the logarithm of the projected shelf life when either of the above model equations are used. However, such a design is impractical to execute, since one might need to follow degradation at the lowest temperature included in the accelerated design for a period of time longer than needed to execute a real-time stability study at the temperature of interest T_{est}. Despite this shortcoming abbreviated studies, in which degradation is not allowed to proceed as far at the lower temperatures, can still give useful results, especially if one's interest is only in projecting whether the projected shelf life at T_{est} is greater than some required minimum (e.g., 2 years at $T_{est} = 25°C$).

It is convenient to design accelerated thermal degradation studies so that the temperatures used are selected from a series of equally spaced values on the reciprocal absolute temperature scale (e.g., 5, 15, 25, 37, 48, 61, 75, 90°C) at temperatures above the final temperature of interest T_{est}. Thus, to project the shelf life at 25°C, one might choose to use the three highest temperatures (e.g., 61, 75, 90°C). If we are only interested in determining whether or not a drug substance will be stable in solution for two years at 25°C, then even this much work is unnecessary. Assuming any reasonable range of expected activation energies, testing at only the two highest temperatures should provide an answer to our question. Of course, the further removed the actual temperatures selected are from the temperature of interest, the larger the error in prediction of the extrapolated value for the logarithm of the shelf life. Nevertheless, reasonable precision is still obtainable using this approach. It is feasible to design experiments that can be completed in a short period of time (weeks) to determine if the shelf life will be sufficiently long to permit commercial development of a solution dosage form with storage at either controlled room temperature or under refrigerated storage conditions. All that is needed to design an appropriate experiment is knowledge of the precision achievable by the analytical method that will be used to determine the fraction f remaining undegraded, the allowable extent of degradation f, and the desired storage temperature T_{est}. The design can be validated by simulation prior to execution, and the simulated results can be used to confirm that an adequate number of samples are taken at each temperature. Since most real degradation reactions are pseudo-first-order, sampling times at each temperature should increase exponentially (e.g., 0, 1, 2, 4, 7, 14, 28, … days) so that the change in the fraction remaining will be approximately constant between sampling times. Sufficient samples should be obtained at each temperature to estimate rate constants with equal precision. If one was confident of the order of the reaction, and anticipated degradation rates at each temperature, then the most efficient design would eliminate all intermediate time points, and simply measure the fraction present initially and after some fixed interval storage at each elevated temperature, reducing the analytical workload even further. However, thermal stress degradation studies are usually performed early in the development process, when little is known about the overall stability of the drug substance, so prudent experimenters will want to include samples at intermediate time points to ensure that sufficient usable data is obtained. A pilot experiment, with single samples taken at four temperatures selected from the list above on days 0, 1, 2, 4, and 7 (20 samples altogether), will often provide enough information to determine whether or not additional work is needed. Poorly stable materials can be rejected out of hand, and materials showing no degradation at even the highest temperature require no further study, since no practically achievable activation energy would be consistent with long-term instability if the Arrhenius model holds, and no degradation can be detected after a week of storage at more than 60°C above the intended real-time storage conditions.

Waterman and coworkers have recently extended this concept even further, to incorporate the effects of humidity (Equation 5.69).[102] These workers have demonstrated that, provided one can design experiments such that the same extent of decomposition is achieved under each of the conditions of temperature and humidity studied (so-called isoconversional conditions), one can estimate both the Arrhenius model parameters and the effect of humidity on the kinetics of decomposition of a drug, either as the API itself or as a component of a formulation, using a small number of measurements with good accuracy. This approach is especially useful for studying solid-state degradation, as isoconversional methods are independent of mechanism.

5.4.2 Solid-state Thermal Degradation Studies

The design of solid-state degradation studies is complicated by the fact that many solid-state degradation reactions do not follow Arrhenius kinetics outside a restricted range. Phase changes (glass transitions, crystalline melting, solvation/desolvation) are expected to radically alter degradation pathways. One must have a thorough understanding of the thermal behavior of the material to be studied prior to undertaking the design of a thermal stress degradation study of a solid material. In most cases, the objective of thermal stress studies on solids is to determine whether or not moisture will induce hydrolytic degradation. That being the case, the simplest approach is to just add water, stir, and heat.

Isothermal microcalorimetry can be used to study the potential reactivity of solids to water, either alone or in combination with excipients, in relatively short periods of time (days to weeks). Typically, a mixture of the solid(s) and 20% by weight added water is heated to 50–60°C, and monitored for thermal reactivity. Hydrolysis reactions are characteristically exothermic, and result in the generation of detectable heat signals within the first few days, even for slowly reacting substances. It is prudent to confirm degradation by chemical analysis of any mixture (e.g., by HPLC or LC/MS) that exhibits generation of heat. Isothermal microcalorimetry is a completely nonspecific technique that can be used to detect and monitor even the most complex reactions, such as the Maillard reaction between a primary or secondary amine drug and a reducing sugar such as glucose or lactose. This approach is most useful for establishing relative chemical reactivity, such as comparing different potential drug candidates as part of candidate lead selection or for selecting potential excipients to be used in formulation.

A less drastic measure is to store samples of solid materials under conditions of high humidity. Saturated solutions of NaCl maintain essentially 75% relative humidity over a wide range of temperatures, so it is possible to store samples in humidistats (sealed vessels containing a small amount of a saturated solution of NaCl in water) in ovens at different temperatures (e.g., 40, 60, 80°C), provided that no phase changes (such as melting, formation of hydrates, etc.) occur when the samples are heated. Dynamic moisture sorption gravimetric analysis and thermal gravimetric analysis can be used to confirm the absence of hydrate formation at the selected temperatures. Prudent experimenters, not having sufficient test material to perform a thorough characterization of its thermal properties, will opt to begin studies at a lower temperature (e.g., 40°C), and progress to studies at higher temperatures only if it is justifiable to do so when more material becomes available. The very first activity that should be undertaken in the characterization of any new drug substance is to set up a thermal stress degradation experiment for the solid drug substance. This should be started before any other work is undertaken, and only takes a few milligrams of material. Samples can be removed from thermal stress conditions at programed times, and stored at low temperature until an analytical method can be developed, assuming larger quantities of material can be obtained later. Often visual inspection will reveal stability problems, such as color changes, deliquescence, etc., that may dictate storage requirements for the substance being studied. The approach of Waterman and coworkers follows this strategy.[104]

5.4.3 Oxidative Degradation Studies

Oxidative degradation of drugs is usually caused by impurities (peroxide, transition metals, free radicals) present in the final products. Levels of these impurities are low, variable, and often difficult to control. Hence, oxidation screens are normally conducted in the presence of higher levels of oxidants, catalysts, and other probing reactants. Oxidative testing under these conditions is only prognostic, but not definitive in nature, and quantitative extrapolation to normal storage conditions is challenging and, in most cases, should be avoided. Hydroperoxides, the primary oxidative reagents, may further degrade at elevated temperatures. Therefore, most oxidative tests are carried out at relatively mild temperatures (e.g., ambient to 40°C).

As outlined in the section on oxidative degradation, three primary oxidative mechanisms exist: free radical autoxidation, nucleophilic/electrophilic processes, and electron transfer processes. A practical oxidative testing strategy should aim to pinpoint the intrinsic oxidative stability, and the possible oxidative mechanisms. Understanding of oxidative mechanisms allows for stabilization strategies to be developed. Identification of the primary/secondary oxidative degradants also aids elucidation of the degradation pathways.

A free radical initiator is frequently used to probe susceptibility of a compound to autoxidation. As mentioned previously, AIBN is a commonly used imitator for this purpose. Its homolytic decomposition half life in toluene is 10 hours at 65°C, and does not change significantly in different solvents. Tests can be made with molar ratios between AIBN and drug molecule ranging from 0.2 to 1.0. Experiments are often done at 40°C in order to preserve the primary degradants. However, AIBN is not water-soluble. Organic co-solvents, such as acetonitrile and lower alcohols, are necessary for most drug candidates with limited aqueous solubility. Each co-solvent may produce side reactions, and has its pros and cons. Water-soluble free

radical initiators are available, which have slightly different decomposition kinetics. Examples include 4,4′-azobis(4-cyanopentanoic acid) (ACVA), and 2,2′-azobis(2-amidinopropane)dihydrochloride (AAPH). Antioxidants known to act as free radical trapping agents can also be used to demonstrate radical oxidation in the absence of an added initiator by suppressing oxidation triggered by environmental stress.

Hydrogen peroxide, typically in the concentration range of 0.3% to 30%, is used to probe the electrophilic/nucleophilic oxidative stability of organic compounds at ambient temperature. Amines, thiols, thioethers, pyrroles, and indoles are functional groups that can be readily oxidized by peroxides. Baertschi[1] stated that, in his experience, a compound is particularly sensitive and could require special efforts for development if a 0.3% solution of hydrogen peroxide induces >20% degradation in 24 hours at room temperature. Alternatively, <5% degradation in 24 hours indicates a relatively stable compound that will likely not present significant challenges to development. Peroxides are present as impurities in many excipients, and some antioxidants are known to be particularly effective as suppressors of peroxide-mediate oxidation. Addition of such antioxidants can help to confirm that peroxide mediated oxidation is responsible for observed degradation.

Many so-called autoxidative degradations may actually be caused by catalysis due to heavy metals, which usually present at very low levels. This is particularly believed for thiols and thioethers, due to their strong interactions with transition metals. In addition, metal ions may react with peroxides, forming reactive hydroxyl radicals. Although levels of heavy metals are low in modern drug substances, their levels may be significant at the early stages. In addition, sensitivity towards metal catalyzed oxidation may be high for certain compounds. Therefore, a transition metal catalysis test still provides valuable information. Compounds that are highly sensitive to these tests may require special processing precautions to avoid metal contamination. Fe^{3+} and Cu^{2+} can be incorporated routinely in oxidative screening at ambient conditions. Chelating agents, such as EDTA, are particularly effective as suppressors of metal–ion catalyzed oxidation. If the addition of chelating agents reduces or prevents oxidative degradation in otherwise untreated samples, metal–ion catalysis due to low levels of contaminating metals is likely to be responsible for the degradation observed.

As an alternative, Tween® 80 (or another excipient containing polyoxyethylene moieties) in combination with Fe^{3+} or other transition metals (e.g., Mn^{3+}) can be used to screen the overall oxidative stability of a compound.[103] Exicipients containing polyoxyethylene moieties, such as Tweens and PEGs, always have low levels of peroxide contaminants. These peroxides react with Fe^{3+}, and produce peroxy radicals which cause escalation of free radical levels and further oxidation of the excipients. Therefore, the oxidative reaction mechanism in this system could be a combination of all three mechanisms.[104] The Tween test may well be suitable as a first line oxidative screen. Compounds resisting oxidation in this test could be considered as stable with respect to all three mechanisms of oxidation. For compounds that are susceptible to the Tween test, a further mechanism screen should be carried out using the individual tests.

Susceptibility to singlet oxygen can be tested as a supplement to the above oxidative screens, but it is usually not a routine test. A dye (e.g., Rose Bengal) can be selected to generate singlet oxygen under light exposure. However, appropriate controls should be applied because many organic compounds are themselves sensitive to photolytic degradation.

In addition to solution tests, a solid-state oxidative screen may provide useful information. Unlike the solution state, reactivity of molecules in the solid state is limited by their crystal packing, and is therefore controlled by their topochemistry. A particular solid form may be stable to oxidative degradation as a solid, even though when dissolved in solution it is not, which can provide criteria to select appropriate polymorphic and salt forms for development. The hydrogen peroxide solvate of urea serves as a convenient source of vapor phase hydrogen peroxide when gently heated, and may be used to supply hydrogen peroxide vapor exposure to solid samples in a manner analogous to the use of saturated salt solutions to supply water vapor at a constant relative humidity.

5.4.4 Photodegradation Studies

Photochemical instability is almost never a barrier to successful drug product development. Photochemically labile materials such as sodium nitroprusside are routinely manufactured, distributed, sold, and used to treat patients. The only issue to be resolved experimentally is whether or not protective packaging may be required, and whether or not protective lighting systems may be required in laboratory and manufacturing areas.

Photostability testing is required for regulatory approval, and a standard testing protocol for assessing photochemical stability has been established.[105] Pharmacopoeial methods for testing the light resistance properties of proposed packaging materials have also been established.

Commercially available test chambers equipped with an ICH Type I light source, such as a xenon arc lamp, are recommended for initial photochemical stress degradation studies. Chambers equipped with xenon sources typically irradiate samples with more than 2 × the required ICH dose of UV radiation when samples are exposed to 1 × the required ICH dose of visible light. Unless the test sample absorbs light in the visible region of the electromagnetic energy spectrum, setting the chamber to provide 1 × exposure to visible light should provide more than adequate radiation exposure.

In a typical experiment, replicate samples packaged in clear glass containers, clear glass containers wrapped in aluminum foil to exclude all light, and samples in representative colored glass (e.g., amber) containers are exposed to the Type I light source following the ICH test conditions. After the exposure has been completed (which may take a few hours, but typically less than one day, depending on the intensity of the xenon lamp radiation), the samples are assayed, and any degradation noted. Colored glass containers differ in light transmission properties, so the test should be performed with the least effective (generally the least intensely colored) container being considered. The test may need to be repeated with additional containers having lower specified light transmission.

For the purpose of evaluating laboratory and manufacturing lighting conditions, plastic filter material with defined light transmission properties can be used. A variety of fluorescent lamp tube shields are available commercially that meet this requirement. UV-filter tube shields made of polymethyl methacrylate are available with a cut-off frequency of 395 nm that effectively block all UV light; these are typically sold for use in museums, art galleries, and establishments selling textile products, where fading due to UV light exposure is a potential problem. So-called "gold" tube shields, designed for use in photolithography manufacturing facilities, effectively block both UV and blue light. Avoid the use of decorative tube shields sold for novelty lighting; many of these transmit some UV light even while blocking almost all blue, green, and yellow visible light. Prepare samples in clear glass containers; place some inside the selected filter tube. Wrap additional samples in aluminum foil to serve as controls. Expose all samples to a Type I light source until the requisite dose of radiation has been achieved. After the exposure has been completed, the samples are assayed. If samples exposed in the clear glass containers show evidence of degradation, but those packaged inside the plastic filter tubes do not, then the plastic filter tubes provide an adequate engineering control that will protect against degradation if installed on lighting fixtures used in production and laboratory areas.

To test for photochemical oxidation, sample containers can be purged with oxygen. Containers purged with an inert gas, such as nitrogen or argon, can serve as controls. A photosensitizing dye, such as Rose Bengal, can be added to test solutions.

Nearly all organic chemicals undergo photochemical degradation if exposed to high intensity short-wave UV light, such as may be obtained using a high-pressure mercury arc lamp. The degradation products so produced hardly ever reflect those obtained using longer wave UV or visible light radiation. The use of exotic light sources not likely to be encountered in normal handling and storage is not recommended.

5.5 PHYSICAL STABILITY AND PHASE TRANSFORMATIONS[106]

Physical stability refers to the ability of a solid phase to resist transformation under various conditions. Although in some cases tautomerism may be involved, this section encompasses phase transitions where the chemical entity of active pharmaceutical ingredient (API) remains the same.

As demonstrated in Chapter 2, various solid forms of a chemical entity may have different physico-chemical properties. Some of these properties are very relevant to pharmaceutical development, such as solubility/dissolution rate, hygroscopicity, melting point, chemical stability, etc. Extensive efforts are invested early on into the selection of an optimum solid form as an API for downstream development. The understanding of the physical stability of the selected API solid form is minimally necessary to realize the benefit of the selected solid form, to ensure the control during the manufacturing processes, and ultimately to ensure the quality of the finished products.

Transformations among solid forms, mainly as a pure substance, are discussed in detail in Chapter 2, where the applications of these transformations in understanding the interrelationships among the various forms are demonstrated. However, pharmaceutical products consist of many other ingredients, each serving its unique function. Many processing steps are therefore required to bring these ingredients together in a reproducible fashion to achieve certain quality attributes for the finished products. In light of the importance of phase transformations during pharmaceutical processing to preformulation/formulation

scientists and processing engineers, the discussions on physical stability in this chapter are biased toward the conditions encountered during pharmaceutical processing.

5.5.1 Types of Phase Transformations

Various solid forms exist for a certain chemical entity, as categorized in Chapter 2. Many possibilities exist for transformations among these forms. Some phase transformations are thermodynamically favored, and are therefore spontaneous. Some phase transformations are thermodynamically disfavored, occur only under stress, and require energy input from the environment. Many phase transformations proceed through a series of individual phase transformations induced by the changes in the environment. Table 5.3 lists the major types of phase transformations.

5.5.2 Mechanisms of Phase Transformations

The four underlying mechanisms for phase transformations, and the types of transitions for which these mechanisms could be operating, are listed in Table 5.4. Each of the mechanisms is discussed in further detail.

Solid-state Transitions

Some phase transitions occur in the solid state without passing through intervening transient liquid or vapor phases. Solid-state reactions have been described previously in Section 5.2.10 and can be mechanistically categorized into four classes: nucleation, geometrical contraction, diffusion, and reaction order models.[107,108,109,110,111,112] Each model includes several slightly different mechanisms. These mechanisms and their corresponding kinetic equations were summarized in Table 5.2. Recently, a model-free kinetic treatment has been applied to amorphous crystallization,[35] and to dehydration[36] of pharmaceuticals. This new approach is described in detail in Section 5.2.10.6. In summary, this approach provides flexibility in describing the kinetics, and therefore affords better predicting power. Moreover, this approach facilitates the elucidation of the reaction mechanisms, especially those complex ones. In general, the kinetics of phase transition via a solid-state mechanism is influenced by many factors such as the environment (temperature, pressure, relative humidity/partial pressure, etc.), the ideality of the solid phases (the presence and distribution of defects and strains), the physical characteristics of the

TABLE 5.3   Major types of phase transformations

Type	Explanation of phase transformation
A	*Polymorphic transition*: transition between the polymorphs. The crystalline phases include all types of crystalline solids. The composition of the solid remains the same
B	*Hydration/dehydration*: transition between anhydrates and hydrates or hydrates of different stoichiometry. The compositions of the solids differ by the number of water molecules
C	*Solvation/desolvation*: transition between solvent-free crystal forms and solvates, solvates of different stoichiometry or solvates of different nature (i.e., different solvents are incorporated into the crystalline lattice). The compositions of the solids differ by the nature and number of solvent molecules
D	*Salt/parent conversions or salt/salt exchange*: transition between the salts (ionic adducts), and the parent unionized compounds (free acids or free bases), between the salts of different stoichiometry or between the different salts. The compositions of the solids differ by the nature and number of counterions
E	*Cocrystal/parent conversions or cocrystal/cocrystal exchange*: transition between the cocrystals (molecular adducts), and the parent compound (unionized compounds or salts), between the cocrystals of different stoichiometry or between the different cocrystals. The compositions of the solids differ by the nature and number of cocrystal formers
F	*Amorphous crystallization/vitrification*: transition between crystalline and amorphous phases. The crystalline phases include all types of crystalline solids. Since the compositions of the amorphous phases are usually less well-defined, the compositions of the solids change in most cases

TABLE 5.4   Underlying mechanisms of phase transformations[106]

Mechanism	Types of phase transformations*
Solid-state	A−F
Melt	A, B and C (dehydration/desolvation only), D, E, F (vitrification only)
Solution	A−F
Solution-mediated	A−E, F (amorphous crystallization only); transitions occur only from the metastable phases to the stable phases under the defined conditions

*See Table 5.3 for definitions of types of phase transformations

solid particles (size and distribution, morphology), and the presence of impurities.

Melt Transitions

When a solid is heated above its melting point and subsequently cooled back to the ambient temperatures, the original solid phase may not be regenerated. Therefore, through this heating/cooling cycle, a phase transition may occur. Among the factors determining the final solid phase are the composition of the melt, relative rates of nucleation, crystal growth, and cooling. Impurities or excipients are also likely to affect the course of crystallization, and thereby the phase transformation. Formulations consist of many components, including API and excipients of different functions. Therefore, it is not only the melting of the API, but also the melting of the excipients that could give rise to phase transitions. In such multi-component and multi-phase systems, it is important to keep in mind phenomena such as melting point depression, eutectic formation among the various components, and the decrease in crystallinity (therefore the melting point) by some upstream pharmaceutical processing.

Solution Transitions

Very often the solid API will be dissolved, or partially dissolved, in a solvent (typically water) during processing. If subsequent solvent removal induces a transformation, this transformation mechanism is considered a solution mechanism. It is important to note that the transition can be from a metastable phase to the stable phases or *vice versa*. For instance, the drug may partially dissolve in water during wet granulation or it may completely dissolve in water during freeze-drying or spray drying. Once the solvent is removed, the solid drug will be regenerated from the solution. The regenerated solid may not be the same crystal form as the original phase, and it may consist of a mixture of phases. Thus, through solvent removal, a phase transition may occur. It is also important to realize that only the fraction of drug that is dissolved is capable of undergoing transformation through this mechanism.

The final solid may be a single phase or a mixture of amorphous and crystal forms, depending on the rate of solvent removal, the ease of nucleation and crystal growth of the possible crystal forms under the processing conditions, and the presence of other material in the solution. The undissolved solid drug may serve as seeds, and direct the crystallization toward the original crystal form. It may also, together with the insoluble excipients, provide surfaces for heterogeneous nucleation of a different phase. Soluble excipients may have profound effects on the nucleation and crystal growth of the drug, as many crystallization studies have demonstrated.[113]

Solution-mediated Transitions

As opposed to the solution mechanism, the solution-mediated mechanism only allows the transition from a metastable phase to the stable phases. This type of transformation is driven by the difference in solubility between the two phases. In contrast to the solution mechanism where transformation occurs during drying, the solution-mediated mechanism operates when the metastable phase is in contact with the saturated solution.

Three consecutive steps are involved in a solution-mediated transformation:[114,115,116]

1. initial dissolution of the metastable phase into the solution to reach and exceed the solubility of the stable phase;
2. nucleation of the stable phase;
3. crystal growth of the stable phase coupled with the continuous dissolution of the metastable phase.

Step (2) or (3) is usually the slowest step. When step (2) is rate-determining, any factor that affects nucleation will influence the overall transformation. These factors include speciation in solution, solubility and solubility difference between the phases, processing temperature, contact surfaces, agitation, and soluble excipients/impurities. When step (3) is the rate-controlling step, the kinetics of the conversion are determined by solubility difference, solid/solvent ratio, agitation, processing temperature, particle size of the original phase, and soluble excipients/impurities.

5.6 PHASE TRANSFORMATIONS DURING PHARMACEUTICAL PROCESSING[106]

5.6.1 Processes for Preparing Solid Dosage Forms and Associated Potential Phase Transformations

A comprehensive description of the processes used for preparing solid oral dosage forms can be found in many references and textbooks,[117,118,119] as well as Chapters 27–35 in this book. Commonly used methods and associated unit operations are summarized in Figure 5.12. The impact of these processes on solid phase transformations and associated challenges are discussed below.

Size Reduction

The first step during solid product processing often involves size reduction. Size reduction facilitates subsequent processing, and may enhance product performance (e.g., through improved morphology/flow properties, minimized segregation, enhanced uniformity, increased surface area, etc.). The principal means for accomplishing size reduction is by milling, which involves shearing/cutting, compressing, impacting or attrition of drug particles. Impact mills (e.g., hammer mills) and fluid-energy mills (e.g., jet mills) are widely utilized in the pharmaceutical industry. Other methods for size reduction, such as supercritical fluid technology,[120] are less frequently employed and will not be included in this discussion. Since impact milling typically imparts mechanical stress, and often generates heat, it may induce phase transitions, such as polymorphic transitions, dehydration/desolvation, or vitrification via solid-state or melt mechanisms. The rate and extent of these phase transitions will depend on characteristics of the original solid phase, the type of mill, and the milling conditions (such as the energy input). Digoxin, spironolactone, and estradiol are reported to undergo polymorphic transformations during the comminution process.[118] In most cases the drug substance is milled prior to being mixed with excipients, consequently the nature and extent of possible phase transformations can be detected more easily relative to the formulation.

Granulation/Size Enlargement

Before a powder can be compressed into a tablet or filled into a capsule, it must possess a number of physical characteristics including flowability, cohesiveness, compressibility, and lubrication. Since most pharmaceutical materials seldom possess all of these properties, granulation methods are frequently used to impart the required characteristics. Wet and dry granulations are the two most commonly used methods of preparing granules for tablet compression or capsule manufacture. Other granulation processes include spray drying and melt granulation, such as high shear melt pelletization, spray-congealing, and melt-extrusion.

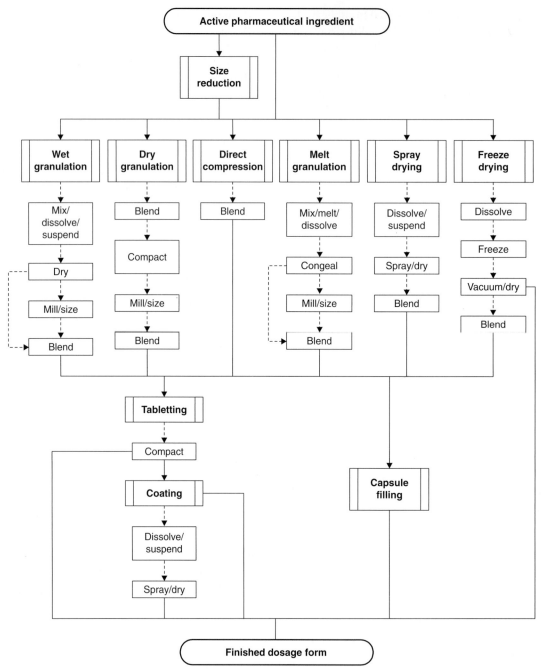

FIGURE 5.12   Common processes for preparing solid oral dosage forms[106]

Wet Granulation and Drying

Wet granulation is most widely used due to its versatility, and the greater probability that the resulting granules will meet the physical requirements for further processing. Wet granulation methods commonly used include low or high shear mixing, fluid-bed mixing and pelletization (e.g., extrusion/spherization).[117] Typical drying methods for the wet granules are tray drying, fluid-bed drying, and vacuum drying. Other methods include microwave drying, tunnel drying, and rotary current drying.[119] Although versatile, wet granulation is especially likely to induce phase transitions. The potential for phase transition of a substance will depend not only on its properties, but also on the conditions and the methods used for granulation and drying.

Conditions such as the amount of liquid used for granulation, the exposure time of the solid to the liquid, airflow, drying temperature, etc., vary with granulation and drying methods. The drug loading, solubility of the drug substance in the granulation liquid, and the procedure for incorporating the drug into the granules will determine whether the starting solid phase is partially or completely dissolved during the granulation process. The subsequent solvent removal rate, which also depends on the method used for granulation and drying, the nature and the concentration of the excipient dissolved, may influence the phase formed in the dried granules. Thus, in addition to the properties of the API and the composition of the formulation, the granulating and drying methods and conditions will determine whether solution or solution-mediated phase transformations, such as polymorphic conversion, hydration/dehydration, salt/parent conversion or salt/salt exchange, cocrystal/parent conversion or cocrystal/cocrystal exchange, and vitrification/crystallization will occur. If the drug is completely dissolved in the granulation fluid, the method of drying, and the type of excipients used, will determine whether transformation via the solution mechanism will occur. When less soluble drugs are suspended in the granulating fluid, a solution-mediated transformation may occur, leading to a phase transition from an anhydrous phase to a hydrate, from a salt/cocrystal to its parent, from an amorphous phase to its crystalline counterpart. The ability to detect phase transformations, and the number of analytical techniques that can be used for detection, will depend on the drug load in the granules and potential interference from the excipients.

Dry granulation

Dry granulation is typically used when the formulation ingredients are sensitive to moisture or when they are unable to withstand an elevated drying temperature. It is also used when the formulation ingredients have sufficient inherent binding or cohesive properties. Dry granulation is also referred to as precompression or as the double compression method.[117] Slugging and roller compaction are the two most commonly used dry granulation methods. The stresses applied during slugging may be lower than those applied by roller compaction because of the differences in dwell time. Since granulating solvent is not used during dry granulation, solution or solution-mediated phase transformations are eliminated, thus the probability of phase transitions with this granulation unit operation is reduced. However, the applied mechanical stresses during processing may lead to phase transformation via the solid-state or melt mechanisms. As is the case in the wet granulation process,

the ability to detect phase transformations, and the number of analytical techniques that can be used, will depend on the drug loading in the granules, and on the potential for interference from the excipients.

Melt granulation

The melt granulation process consists of partially or completely melting solid excipient(s), and then granulating with the API and other excipients, followed by reducing the mixture to granules by chilling and congealing. During this process, the API is subjected to heat, and may be partially or completely dissolved in the molten excipients. If the melting point is relatively low or the heating temperature is sufficiently high, the API may also melt during processing. Partially or completely melted API may also serve as a binder or congealing carrier. Subsequent cooling could induce phase transitions through the solid-state or melt mechanisms. In fact, this process is sometimes used by design for preparing crystalline or amorphous solid dispersions, thus taking advantage of phase transformation through the melt mechanism.

In a spray-congealing process, a low melting point carrier is employed to provide the fluidity necessary for spraying. At high temperatures, all or a fraction of the drug may be solubilized in the molten carrier. During spray-congealing, the hot droplets cool rapidly and solidify. Since rapid cooling/congealing is required for the formation of small particles with a narrow size distribution, it is possible that the drug may precipitate as an amorphous phase or as a metastable crystal form, following Ostwald's Rule of Stages.[121,122] In a high shear melt granulation, the temperature, extent and duration of heating, as well as the rate of cooling, are often significantly lower relative to the spray-congealing process. Thus, this process is less likely to initiate phase transitions. Similar to spray-congealing, the melt-extrusion process also requires complete melting of the carrier excipients. Although the rate of cooling is slower, this process is still likely to induce phase transitions.

Spray drying and freeze-drying

Spray drying produces powder particles that are homogenous, porous, and uniform in size and shape. The technique may also be used for encapsulating or coating drugs, to provide protection or release rate control. The process consists of bringing together a highly dispersed liquid and a sufficient volume of hot air to produce uniform droplets. Subsequent evaporation of the liquid leads to particle formation.[117] The feed liquid can be a solution, suspension or emulsion.

This process requires complete or partial dissolution of the drug in a solvent, and thus increases the likelihood for phase transitions involving solution mechanism. Solvent removal from droplets occurs in seconds, and this may lead to rapid crystallization of a metastable phase or to the formation of an amorphous phase through the solution mechanism.

Freeze-drying is often used to produce amorphous materials. In this case extremely low temperatures are used to limit molecular mobility, and to prevent nucleation of the drug and the excipients. The conditions for freeze-drying can have a major influence on the solid phase of the drug in the product. Although it is not a commonly used process for manufacturing solid oral dosage forms, freeze-drying has been used to prepare tablets for specific functions, e.g., Zydis® tablet for rapid dissolution.[123,124]

Granulation Milling/Sizing and Blending

A granulated solid is often subjected to milling, and at this stage the intensity and energy exerted on the API is generally lower than those exerted during initial particle size reduction. Although the risk of phase transition at this stage is less compared to that during API milling and granulation, the presence of excipients makes the detection of phase transitions difficult.

Prior to tablet compression or to encapsulation, granules are directly blended with lubricants and/or other excipients (e.g., lubricants, glidants, disintegrants) without modifying their physical properties. There is minimal risk of phase transitions occurring during the blending process.

Compression and Encapsulation

Lubricated granules are either compressed into tablets or filled into capsules. During tableting, granules may be subject to compression forces as high as 40 kN, with dwell times on the order of a few milliseconds. An energy impact of this magnitude may cause solid phase changes in either the API or the excipients via the solid-state mechanism. For example, caffeine, sulfabenzamide, and maprotiline hydrochloride have been reported to undergo polymorphic transformations during compression.[125] Phase transitions are seldom encountered during the capsule filling process because the solid is experiencing minimal thermal and mechanical perturbations.

Coating

When manufacturing finished tablet dosage forms, a film coating is often applied as an aqueous or solvent-based polymer system in coating pans or in a fluid-bed. The function of the coating may be to improve esthetics, provide taste masking or modify drug release. Less common coating techniques such as sugar coating, compression coating or microencapsulation will not be discussed here. The film coating process involves the application of a thin polymer-based coating solution to an appropriate substrate (tablets, granules or crystals) using a spray-atomization technique. To permit uniform distribution of the coating materials, and to prevent coating problems (picking, roughness or mottling), film coating parameters are optimized to create a balance between coating solution delivery rate and drying capacity. Rapid drying typically takes place during the application of the film coating. A highly efficient air exchange ensures that there is only a short time between the impingement of the coating liquid onto the tablet surface and the subsequent solvent evaporation. Thus the interaction between the core material and the coating liquid is generally minimal during film coating. In most cases it is unlikely that a phase transition will occur via the solution mechanism during film coating. When necessary, prior to application of the film coat, a polymer-based seal coat may be applied to the surfaces of the tablet cores first. This will prevent extended solid–liquid interactions during the subsequent film coating process.

For some modified release products, a portion of the total dose may be applied as a drug coating layer. This coat may provide immediate release for fast onset in a biphasic extended release system or it may provide immediate release in a pulsatile delivery system. The drug layer is typically applied by spraying a drug solution or a drug suspension onto the tablet surface, depending on the drug solubility and dose. Dissolving or suspending the drug in a liquid increases the potential for phase transitions to occur through the solution or solution-mediated mechanism. When a drug solution is used for coating, the probability that such operations will alter the solid phase of the drug is high, similar to that observed in the spray drying process that was discussed earlier. That is, rapid solvent removal in this coating process may lead to a transformation to a metastable crystal form or an amorphous phase in the drug layer via the solution mechanism. When a drug suspension is used for coating, if there is a more stable phase in aqueous medium, the probability that such operations will alter the solid phase of the drug through a solution-mediated mechanism is high. The anticipated risk is higher than that observed in the wet granulation process, and is a result of the following facts:

- The coating process is usually a much longer process than wet granulation.

- The suspension is usually made with drug particles that are very small (for better suspension, coating uniformity). This leads to faster dissolution to reach supersaturation and, therefore, more time for nucleation of the stable phase to occur.
- The suspension provides much higher specific solution medium, and is usually constantly stirred to ensure the uniformity of the suspension. If nucleation of the stable phase occurs, the conversion to the stable phase will proceed at a much faster rate.

5.6.2 Anticipating and Preventing Phase Transformations in Process Development

To anticipate and prevent solid phase transitions during manufacturing it is critical to have a thorough understanding of crystal forms and the amorphous phase of the API and excipients, as well as the interconversion mechanisms and processing options. This integrated knowledge is essential for the rational selection of the physical form of the API, the excipients, the manufacturing process, and for the selection of appropriate handling and storage conditions. In certain cases, even after the solid form and the preferred process are defined, it is advisable to monitor the crystal form of all incoming raw materials and the physical form(s) present in the final dosage unit. This monitoring is especially important in cases where dissolution or stability of the product is very sensitive to solid phase changes. The rigor used in monitoring will depend on the API, formulation, process, and analytical method. For a highly soluble, stable, and bioavailable molecule, the risk of process-induced phase change on stability and bioavailability may be relatively low. However, process-induced phase changes in the API and/or excipients may impact manufacturability or disintegration of the dosage form.

In selecting the crystal form of an API for development, the physico-chemical, biopharmaceutical, and processing properties must all be taken into consideration. In some cases it may be necessary to select an alternate crystal form in order to eliminate stability issues, dissolution rate differences or process-induced phase transitions. It is desirable to choose the crystal form that is least susceptible to phase transformations induced by heat, moisture, and mechanical stresses, provided that the biopharmaceutical and processing characteristics of the API are acceptable. Sometimes an alternate salt having fewer crystal forms may be chosen to minimize process-induced transitions. For example, the authors have encountered a scenario where a new salt form was selected following Phase I studies

due to clinical considerations. This change helped us to overcome manufacturing hurdles presented by the complexity of polymorphic phase transitions associated with the original salt form. This change in salt form drastically reduced the number of crystal forms (a single crystal form as opposed to seven processing relevant crystal forms for the original salt, and four processing relevant crystal forms for the parent). This new salt minimized the risk of phase transitions occurring during manufacturing, leading to greater processing flexibility in the development of a solid dosage form for Phase II clinical trials and beyond.

Phase transitions in crystalline excipients, and their impact on product performance, also cannot be ignored. For example, process-induced age-hardening in tablets may lead to a decrease in dissolution rates during storage of formulations containing a high level of crystalline excipients such as mannitol. If process-induced hardening is anticipated, variable product dissolution can be minimized through the use of intra- and extra-granular super disintegrants or by selecting alternative excipients.

In designing manufacturing processes for solid dosage forms, process-induced phase transformations can be anticipated based on preformulation studies. These transformations can be controlled and circumvented by selecting the appropriate process. If a solid phase is sensitive to moisture or to solvent, a dry or melt granulation may be used. If a drug substance undergoes an undesirable transition during milling or compression, melt granulation through melt-extrusion may be more desirable provided the drug is thermally stable. It may be possible to avoid milling the drug substance if particle size and shape can be controlled during crystallization. A capsule may be used in place of a tablet dosage form should compression be deemed undesirable. Polymorphic conversion during drying of an enantiotropic polymorph can be avoided by maintaining the drying temperature below the transition temperature. During film coating, solid–liquid interactions at the surface of moisture sensitive cores can be minimized or eliminated by first applying a seal coat that uses a solution of low viscosity at a slow spray rate. Alternatively, an organic solvent-based polymer system can be used for rapid solvent evaporation. These are just a few examples that illustrate how knowledge of solid-state properties of the API and excipients can be applied in formulation design and process selection. Rational formulation and process design can reduce the risk of "unpleasant surprises" in late stage development, and increase the efficiency during new product development. Ultimately, the quality of a solid product manufactured using the process of choice must be confirmed by real-time tests.

References

1. Arrhenius, S.A. (1889). Über die Reaktionsgeschwindigheit bei der Inversion von Rohrzucker durch Saüren. [On the reaction rate for the inversion of sucrose by acids] Z. Physik. Chem. 4, 226–248.

2. Connors, K.A., Amidon, G.L. & Stella, V.J. (1986). Chemical Stability of Pharmaceuticals. In: *A Handbook for Pharmacists*, 2nd edn. John Wiley & Sons, Inc., New York. p. 19.

3. Connors, K.A. (1990). *Chemical Kinetics: The Study of Reaction Rates in Solution*. Wiley-VCH Publishers, New York. p. 191.

4. Eyring, H. (1935). The activated complex and the absolute rate of chemical reactions. Chemical Reviews 17, 65–77.

5. Trivedi, J.S., Porter, W.R. & Fort, J.J. (1996). Solubility and stability characterization of zileuton in a ternary solvent system. European Journal of Pharmaceutical Sciences 4, 109–116.

6. Alvarez, F.J. & Slade, R.T. (1992). Kinetics and mechanism of degradation of Zileuton, a potent 5-lipoxygenase inhibitor. Pharmaceutical Research 9, 1465–1473.

7. Garrett, E.R. (1957). Prediction of stability in pharmaceutical preparations. IV. The interdependence of solubility and rate in saturated solutions of acylsalicylates. Journal of the American Pharmaceutical Association 46, 584–586.

8. Windheuser, J.J. & Higuchi, T. (1962). Kinetics of thiamine hydrolysis. Journal of Pharmaceutical Sciences 51, 354–364.

9. Hou, J.P. & Poole, J.W. (1969). Kinetics and mechanism of degradation of ampicillin in solution. Journal of Pharmaceutical Sciences 58, 447–454.

10. Zvirblis, P., Socholitsky, I. & Kondritzer, A.A. (1956). The kinetics of the hydrolysis of atropine. Journal of the American Pharmaceutical Association 45, 450–454.

11. Lund, W. & Waaler, T. (1968). The kinetics of atropine and apoatropine in aqueous solutions. Acta chemica Scandinavica 22, 3085–3097.

12. Mayer, W., Erbe, S., Wolf, G. & Voigt, R. (1974). Analysis and stability of certain 1,4-benzodiazepines of pharmaceutical interest. 2. Ring contraction in nordiazepam and clonazepam, pH dependence of the hydrolytic cleavage of the diazepam Faustan, and the use of kinetic methods to determine the stability behavior of diazepam in ampul solution. Die Pharmazie 29, 700–707.

13. Yamana, T. & Tsuji, A. (1976). Comparative stability of cephalosporins in aqueous solution: kinetics and mechanisms of degradation. Journal of Pharmaceutical Sciences 65, 1563–1574.

14. Hussain, A., Schurman, P., Peter, V. & Milosovich, G. (1968). Kinetics and mechanism of degradation of echothiophate iodide in aqueous solution. Journal of Pharmaceutical Sciences 57, 411–418.

15. Tabata, T., Makino, T., Kashihara, T., Hirai, S., Kitamori, N. & Toguchi, H. (1992). Stabilization of a new antiulcer drug (lansoprazole) in the solid dosage forms. Drug Development and Industrial Pharmacy 18, 1437–1447.

16. Garrett, E.R., Nestler, H.J. & Somodi, A. (1968). Kinetics and mechanisms of hydrolysis of 5-halouracils. The Journal of Organic Chemistry 33, 3460–3468.

17. Kondrat'eva, A.P., Bruns, B.P. & Libinson, G.S. (1971). Stability of D-cyclo-serine in aqueous solutions at low cncentrations. Khimiko-Farmatsevticheskii Zhurnal 5, 38–41.

18. Garrett, E.R., Bojarski, J.T. & Yakatan, G.J. (1971). Kinetics of hydrolysis of barbituric acid derivatives. Journal of Pharmaceutical Sciences 60, 1145–1154.

19. Mollica, J.A., Rehm, C.R. & Smith, J.B. (1969). Hydrolysis of hydrochlorothiazide. Journal of Pharmaceutical Sciences 58, 635–636.

20. Mollica, J.A., Rehm, C.R., Smith, J.B. & Govan, H.K. (1971). Hydrolysis of benzothiadiazines. Journal of Pharmaceutical Sciences 60, 1380–1384.

21. Anderson, B.D., Conradi, R.A. & Knuth, K.E. (1985). Strategies in the design of solution-stable, water-soluble prodrugs. I: A physical-organic approach to pro-moiety selection for 21-esters of corticosteroids. Journal of Pharmaceutical Sciences 74, 365–374.

22. Avrami, M. (1939). Kinetics of phase change. I. General theory. Journal of Chemical Physics 7, 1103–1112.

23. Avrami, M. (1940). Kinetics of phase change. II. Transformation-time relations for random distribution of nuclei. Journal of Chemical Physics 8, 212–224.

24. Avrami, M. (1941). Kinetics of phase change. III. Granulation, phase change, and microstructure. Journal of Chemical Physics 9, 177–184.

25. Erofeev, B.V. (1946). Generalized equation of chemical kinetics and its application in reactions involving solids. Compt. Rend. Acad. Sci. USSR 52, 511–514.

26. Johnson, W.A. & Mehl, R.F. (1939). Reaction kinetics in processes of nucleation and growth. Trans. Am. Inst. Min. Metall. Eng. 135, 416–442.

27. Prout, E.G. & Tompkins, F.C. (1944). Thermal decomposition of $KMnO_4$. Transactions of the Faraday Society 40, 448–498.

28. Carstensen, J.T. & Rhodes, C.T. (2000). *Drug Stability. Principles and Practices*, 3rd edn. Marcel Dekker, New York, NY. pp. 154–160.

29. Sharp, J.H., Brindley, G.W. & Achar, B.N.N. (1966). Numerical data for some commonly used solid-state reaction equations. Journal of the American Ceramic Society 49, 379–382.

30. Holt, J.B., Cutler, I.B. & Wadsworth, M.E. (1962). Rate of thermal dehydration of kaolinite in vacuum. Journal of the American Ceramic Society 45, 133–136.

31. Ginstling, A.M. & Brounshtein, B.I. (1950). The diffusion kinetics of reactions in spherical particles. Journal of Applied Chemistry of the USSR, English Translation 23, 1327–1338.

32. Jander, W. (1927). Reaktionen im festen zustande bei höheren temperaturen. I. Mitteilung. Reaktionsgeschwindigkeiten endotherm verlaufender Umsetzungen. Zeitschrift für Anorganische und Allgemeine Chemie 163, 1–30.

33. Bawn, C.H.E. (1955). Decomposition of organic solids. In: *Chemistry of the Solid State*, W.E. Garner, (ed.) Butterworths, London. Chapter 10.

34. Vyazovkin, S. (1997). Evaluation of activation energy of thermally stimulated solid-state reactions under arbitrary variation of temperature. Journal of Computational Chemistry 18, 393–402.

35. Zhou, D., Schmitt, E.A., Zhang, G.G., Law, D., Vyazovkin, S., Wight, C.A. & Grant, D.J.W. (2003). Crystallization kinetics of amorphous nifedipine studied by model-fitting and model-free approaches. Journal of Pharmaceutical Sciences 92, 1779–1792.

36. Zhou, D., Schmitt, E.A., Zhang, G.G.Z., Law, D., Wight, C.A., Vyazovkin, S. & Grant, D.J.W. (2003). Model-free treatment of the dehydration kinetics of nedocromil sodium trihydrate. Journal of Pharmaceutical Sciences 92, 1367–1376.

37. Kissinger, H.E. (1957). Reaction kinetics in differential thermal analysis. Analytical Chemistry 29, 1702–1706.

38. Paul, P.C. & Curtin, D.Y. (1973). Thermally induced organic reactions in the solid state. Accounts of Chemical Research 6, 217–225.

39. Byrn, S.R., Pfeiffer, R.R. & Stowell, J.G. (1999). *Solid-State Chemistry of Drugs*, 2nd edn. SSCI, Inc., West Layfayette, Indiana. pp. 259–260.

40. Duddu, S.P. & Monte, P.R.D. (1997). Effect of glass transition temperature on the stability of lyophilized formulations containing a chimeric therapeutic monoclonal antibody. Pharmaceutical Research 14, 591–595.

41. Olsen, B.A., Perry, F.M., Snorek, S.V. & Lewellen, P.L. (1997). Accelerated conditions for stability assessment of bulk and formulated cefaclor monohydrate. Pharmaceutical development and technology 2, 303–312.

42. Zografi, G. (1988). States of water associated with solids. Drug Development and Industrial Pharmacy 14, 1905–1926.

43. Leeson, L.J. & Mattocks, A.M. (1958). Decomposition of aspirin in the solid state. J. Am. Pharm. Ass. 47, 329–333.

44. Genton, D. & Kesselring, U.W. (1977). Effect of temperature and relative humidity on nitrazepam stability in solid state. Journal of Pharmaceutical Sciences 66, 676–680.

45. Waterman, K.C., Carella, A.J., Gumkowski, M.J., Lukulay, P., MacDonald, B.C., Roy, M.C. & Shamblin, S.L. (2007). Improved protocol and data analysis for accelerated shelf-life estimation of solid dosage forms. Pharmaceutical Research 24, 780–790.

46. Waterman, K.C. & Adami, R.C. (2005). Accelerated aging: Prediction of chemical stability of pharmaceuticals. International Journal of Pharmaceutics 293, 101–125.

47. Cohen, M.D. & Green, B.S. (1973). Organic chemistry in the solid state. Chemistry in Britain 9, 490–497, 517.

48. Sukenik, C.N., Bonopace, J.A., Mandel, N.S., Bergman, R.C., Lau, P.Y. & Wood, G. (1975). Enhancement of a chemical reaction rate by proper orientation of reacting molecules in the solid state. Journal of the American Chemical Society 97, 5290–5291.

49. Sukenik, C.N., Bonapace, J.A.P., Mandel, N.S., Lau, P.-Y., Wood, G. & Bergman, R.G. (1977). A kinetic and x-ray diffraction study of the solid state rearrangement of methyl p-dimethylaminobenzenesulfonate. Reaction rate enhancement due to proper orientation in a crystal. Journal of the American Chemical Society 99, 851–858.

50. Pikal, M.J. & Rigsbee, D.R. (1997). The stability of insulin in crystalline and amorphous solids: Observation of greater stability for the amorphous form. Pharmaceutical Research 14, 1379–1387.

51. Byrn, S.R., Pfeiffer, R.R. & Stowell, J.G. (1999). *Solid-State Chemistry of Drugs*, 2nd edn. SSCI, Inc., West Layfayette, Indiana. pp. 333–342.

52. Koshy, K.T. & Lach, J.L. (1961). Stability of aqueous solutions of N-acetyl-p-aminophenol. Journal of Pharmaceutical Sciences 50, 113–118.

53. Carey, F.A. & Sundberg, R.J. (1990). *Advanced Organic Chemistry. Part A: Structure and Mechanisms*, 3rd edn. Plenum Press, New York, NY.

54. Connors, K.A., Amidon, G.L. & Stella, V.J. (1986). Chemical Stability of Pharmaceuticals. In: *A Handbook for Pharmacists*, 2nd edn. John Wiley & Sons, Inc., New York. p. 64.

55. Boccardi, G. (2005). Oxidative Susceptibility Testing. In: *Pharmaceutical Stress Testing: Predicting Drug Degradation*, S.W. Baertschi, (ed.) Vol. 153. Taylor & Francis Group Boca Raton, Florida. p. 207.

56. Hovorka, S.W. & Schöneich, C. (2001). Oxidative degradation of pharmaceuticals: Theory, mechanisms and inhibition. Journal of Pharmaceutical Sciences 90, 253–269.

57. Waterman, K.C., Adami, R.C., Alsante, K.M., Hong, J., Landis, M.S., Lombardo, F. & Roberts, C.J. (2002). Stabilization of pharmaceuticals to oxidative degradation. Pharmaceutical Development and Technology 7, 1–32.

58. Reid, D.L., Calvitt, C.J., Zell, M.T., Miller, K.G. & Kingsmill, C.A. (2004). Early prediction of pharmaceutical oxidation pathways by computational chemistry and forced degradation. Pharmaceutical Research 21, 1708–1717.

59. Hovorka, S.W., Hageman, M.J. & Schöneich, C. (2002). Oxidative degradation of a sulfonamide-containing 5,6-Dihydro-4-Hydroxy-2-Pyrone in aqueous/organic cosolvent mixtures. Pharmaceutical Research 19, 538–545.

60. Turro, N.J. (1991). *Modern Molecular Photochemisty*. University Science Books, Sausalito, CA.

61. Tønnesen, H.H. (2004). *Photostability of Drugs and Drug Formulations*, 2nd edn. CRC Press, Boca Raton, Florida.

62. Florey, K. (1991). *Analytical Profiles of Drug Substances*. Academic Press, New York. p. 588.

63. Schildcrout, S.A., Risley, D.S. & Kleeman, R.L. (1993). Drug-excipient interactions of seproxetine maleate hemi-hydrate: isothermal stress methods. Drug Development and Industrial Pharmacy 19, 1113–1130.

64. Florey, K. (1991). *Analytical Profiles of Drug Substances*. Academic Press, New York. p. 557.

65. Larsen, C. & Bundgaard, H. (1978). Polymerization of penicillins. Journal of Chromatography 147, 143–150.

66. Leung, S.S. & Grant, D.J.W. (1997). Solid state stability studies of model dipeptides: Aspartame and aspartylphenylalanine. Journal of Pharmaceutical Sciences 86, 64–71.

67. Gu, L. & Strickley, R.G. (1987). Diketopiperazine formation, hydrolysis, and epimerization of the new dipeptide angiotensin-converting enzyme inhibitor RS-10085. Pharmaceutical Research 4, 392–397.

68. International Conference on Harmonisation of Technical Requirements for Registration of Pharmaceuticals for Human Use. (2003). *ICH Harmonised Tripartite Guideline Q1A(R2): Stability Testing of New Drug Substances and Products*.

69. Nelson, W. (1990). *Accelerated Testing: Statistical Models, Test Plans and Data Analysis*. John Wiley & Sons, New York.

70. Schou, S.A. (1960). Stability of medicaments. American Journal of Hospital Pharmacy 17, 5–17.

71. Oswin, C.R. (1945). Kinetics of package life. II. Temperature factor. Journal of the Society of Chemical Industry 64, 224–225.

72. Lauffer, M.A. (1946). Thermal destruction of influenza-A virus hemagglutinin. II The effect of pH. Archives of Biochemistry 9, 75.

73. Scott, E.M. & Lauffer, M.A. (1946). Thermal destruction of influenza-A virus hemagglutinin. III. The effect of urea. Archives of Biochemistry 11, 179.

74. Brodersen, R. (1947). Stability of penicillin G in aqueous solution as a function of hydrogen ion concentration and temperature. Acta Pharmacologica et Toxicologica 3, 345.

75. Jellinek, H. & Urwin, J.R. (1953). The hydrolysis of picolinamide and isonicotinamide in concentrated hydrochloric acid solutions. The Journal of Physical Chemistry 57, 900.

76. Blythe, R.H. (1954). *Shelf life and stability tests in drug packaging*. Glass Packer, August.

77. Garrett, E.R. (1954). Studies on the stability of fumagillin. III. Thermal degradation in the presence and absence of air. Journal of the American Pharmaceutical Association Scientific Edition 43, 539–543.

78. McBride, W.R. & Villars, D.S. (1954). An application of statistics to reaction kinetics. Analytical Chemistry 26, 901–904.

79. Garrett, E.R. & Carper, R.F. (1955). Predictions of stability in pharmaceutical preparations. I. Color stability in a liquid multisulfa preparation. Journal of the American Pharmaceutical Association Scientific Edition 44, 515–518.

80. Levy, G.B. (1955). Accelerated shelf testing. Drug and Cosmetic Industry 76, 472.

81. Youmans, R.A. & Maasen, G.C. (1955). Correlation of room temperature shelf aging with accelerated aging. Industrial & engineering chemistry research 47, 1487.

82. Huyberechts, S., Halleux, A. & Kruys, P. (1955). Une application de calcul statistique à la cinétique chimique. [An application of statistical calculus to chemical kinetics.] Bulletin des Societes Chimiques Belges 64, 203–209. .

83. Garrett, E.R. (1956). Prediction of stability in pharmaceutical preparations. II. Vitamin stability in liquid multivitamin preparations. Journal of American Pharmaceutical Association Scientific Edition 45, 171–178.

84. Garrett, E.R. (1956). Prediction of stability in pharmaceutical preparations. III. Comparison of vitamin stabilities in different multivitamin preparations. Journal of American Pharmaceutical Association Scientific Edition 45, 470–473.

85. Lachman, L. (1959). Prediction of the shelf life of parenteral solutions from accelerated stability studies. Bulletin of the Parenteral Drug Association 13, 8–24.

86. Garrett, E.R. (1962). Prediction of stability of drugs and pharmaceutical preparations. Journal of Pharmaceutical Sciences 51, 811–833.

87. Haynes, J.D., Carstensen, J.T., Callahan, J.C. & Card, R. (1959). Third Stevens Symposium on Statistical Methods in the Chemical Industry, 1, cited in Lachman L. Prediction of the shelf life of parenteral solutions from accelerated stability studies. Bulletin of the Parenteral Drug Association 13, 8–24.

88. Benson, S.W. (1960). *The Foundations of Chemical Kinetics.* Mcgraw-Hill Book Co., Inc., New York. pp. 75–93.

89. McBride, W.R. & Villars, D.S. (1954). An application of statistics to reaction kinetics. Analytical Chemistry 26, 901–904.

90. Garrett, E.R. (1954). Studies on the stability of fumagillin. III. Thermal degradation in the presence and absence of air. Journal of American Pharmaceutical Association Scientific Edition 43, 539–543.

91. Garrett, E.R. & Carper, R.F. (1955). Predictions of stability in pharmaceutical preparations. I. Color stability in a liquid multisulfa preparation. Journal of American Pharmaceutical Association Scientific Edition 44, 515–518.

92. Garrett, E.R. (1956). Prediction of stability in pharmaceutical preparations. II. Vitamin stability in liquid multivitamin preparations. Journal of American Pharmaceutical Association Scientific Edition 45, 171–178.

93. Garrett, E.R. (1956). Prediction of stability in pharmaceutical preparations. III. Comparison of vitamin stabilities in different multivitamin preparations. ournal of American Pharmaceutical Association Scientific Edition 45, 470–473.

94. Carstensen, J.T. (1995). *Drug Stability: Principles and Practices,* 2nd edn. revised and expanded. Marcel Dekker, Inc., New York. pp. 350–359.

95. Tootill, J.P.R. (1961). Slope-ratio design for accelerated storage tests. The Journal of Pharmacy and Pharmacology 13, 75T–86T.

96. Box, G.E.P. & Lucas, H.L. (1959). Design of experiments in non-linear situations. Biometrika 46, 77–90.

97. Davies, O.L. & Budgett, D.A. (1980). Accelerated storage tests on pharmaceutical products: effect of error structure of assay and errors in recorded temperature. The Journal of Pharmacy and Pharmacology 32, 155–159.

98. Davies, O.L. & Hudson, H.E. (1981). Stability of drugs: Accelerated storage tests. In: *Statistics in the Pharmaceutical Industry,* C.R. Buncher, & J.-Y. Tsay, (eds). Marcel Dekker, Inc., New York. pp. 355–395.

99. Carstensen, J.T. & Su, K.S.E. (1971). Statistical aspects of Arrhenius plotting. Bulletin of the Parenteral Drug Association 25, 287–302.

100. Davies, O.L. & Budgett, D.A. (1980). Accelerated storage tests on pharmaceutical products: effect of error structure of assay and errors in recorded temperature. The Journal of Pharmacy and Pharmacology 32, 155–159.

101. King, S.Y.P., Kung, M.S. & Fung, H.L. (1984). Statistical prediction of drug stability based on nonlinear parameter estimation. Journal of Pharmaceutical Sciences 73, 657–662.

102. Waterman, K.C., Carella, A.J., Gumkowski, M.J., Lukulay, P., MacDonald, B.C., Roy, M.C. & Shamblin, S.L. (2007). Improved protocol and data analysis for accelerated shelf-life estimation of solid dosage forms. Pharmaceutical Research 24(4), 780–790.

103. Baertschi, S.W. (2005). *Pharmaceutical Stress Testing. Predicting drug degradation.* Taylor & Francis Group, Boca Raton, Florida. p. 43.

104. Harmon, P.A., Kosuda, K., Nelson, E., Mowery, M. & Reed, R. A. (2006). A novel peroxy radical based oxidative stressing system for ranking the oxidizability of drug substances. Journal of Pharmaceutical Sciences 95, 2014–2028.

105. International Conference on Harmonisation of Technical Requirements for Registration of Pharmaceuticals for Human Use. (1996). ICH Harmonised Tripartite Guideline Q1B Stability Testing: Photostability Testing of New Drug Substances and Products.

106. Zhang, G.G.Z., Law, D., Schmitt, E.A. & Qui, Y. (2004). Phase transformation considerations during process development and manufacture of solid oral dosage forms. Advanced Drug Delivery Reviews 56, 371–390.

107. Garner, W.E. (1955). *Chemistry of the Solid State.* Academic Press, New York.

108. Van Campen, L. & Monkhouse, D.C. (1984). Solid-state reactions—theoretical and experimental aspects. Drug Development and Industrial Pharmacy 10, 1175–1276.

109. Byrn, S.R., Pfeiffer, R.R. & Stowell, J.G. (1999). *Solid-State Chemistry of Drugs,* 2nd edn. SSCI Inc., West Lafayette, IN.

110. Khawam, A. & Flanagan, D.R. (2006). Basics and applications of solid-state kinetics: A pharmaceutical perspective. Journal of Pharmaceutical Sciences 95, 472–498.

111. Vyazovkin, S. & Wight, C.A. (1997). Kinetics in solids. Annual review of physical chemistry 48, 125–149.

112. Brown, M.E., Dollimore, D. & Galwey, A.K. (1980). Reactions in the solid state. In: *Comprehensive Chemical Kinetics,* C.H. Bamford, & C.F.H. Tipper, (eds). Elsevier, Amsterdam. p. 340.

113. Mullin, J.W. (2001). *Crystallization,* 4th edn. Elsevier Butterworth-Heinemann, Oxford.

114. Cardew, P. T. & Davey, R. J. (1985). The kinetics of solvent-mediated phase-transformations. Proceedings of the Royal Society of London. Series A: Mathematical and Physical Engineering Sciences, 398, 415–428.

115. Rodríguez-Hornedo, N., Lechuga-Ballesteros, D. & Wu, H.J. (1992). Phase transition and heterogeneous/epitaxial nucleation of hydrated and anhydrous theophylline crystals. International Journal of Pharmaceutics 85, 149–162.

116. Zhang, G.G.Z., Gu, C., Zell, M.T., Burkhardt, R.T., Munson, E.J. & Grant, D.J.W. (2002). Crystallization and transitions of sulfamerazine polymorphs. Journal of Pharmaceutical Sciences 91, 1089–1100.

117. Rudnic, E. & Schwartz, J.B. (1990). Solid Oral Dosage Forms. *Remington's Pharmaceutical Sciences,* 18th edn. Mark Publishing, Easton, PA. pp. 1633–1647.

118. Lieberman, H.A., Lachman, L. & Schwartz, J.B. (1989). *Pharmaceutical Dosage Forms: Tablets,* 2nd edn. (revised and expanded), Vol. 1. Marcel Dekker, New York.

119. Lieberman, H.A., Lachman, L. & Schwartz, J.B. (1989). *Pharmaceutical Dosage Forms: Tablets,* 2nd edn. (revised and expanded), Vol. 2. Marcel Dekker, New York.

120. York, P. (1999). Strategies for particle design using supercritical fluid technologies. Pharmaceutical Science & Technology Today 2, 430–440.

121. Ostwald, W. (1897). The formation and changes of solids. Zeitschrift für Physikalische Chemie 22, 289–330.

122. Verma, A.R. & Krishna, P. (1966). *Polymorphism and Polytypism in Crystals.* Wiley, New York. pp. 15–30.

123. Seager, H. (1998). Drug-delivery products and the Zydis fast-dissolving dosage form. The Journal of Pharmacy and Pharmacology 50, 375–382.

124. Kearney, P. (2003). The Zydis oral fast-dissolving dosage form. Drugs and the Pharmaceutical Sciences 126, 191–201.

125. Chan, H.K. & Doelker, E. (1985). Polymorphic transformation of some drugs under compression. Drug development and industrial pharmacy 11, 315–332.

Excipient Compatibility

Ajit S. Narang, Venkatramana M. Rao and Krishnaswamy S. Raghavan

6.1 INTRODUCTION

The selection of excipients is vital in the design of a quality drug product. Excipients and their concentration in a formulation are selected based not only on their functionality, but also on the compatibility between the drug and excipients. An incompatibility may be defined as an undesirable drug interaction with one or more components of a formulation, resulting in changes in physical, chemical, microbiological or therapeutic properties of the dosage form. Excipient compatibility studies are conducted mainly to predict the potential incompatibility of the drug in the final dosage form. These studies also provide justification for selection of excipients, and their concentrations in the formulation as required in regulatory filings.

Excipient compatibility studies are often thought to be routine and cumbersome. However, these studies are important in the drug development process, as the knowledge gained from excipient compatibility studies is used to select the dosage form components, delineate stability profile of the drug, identify degradation products, and understand mechanisms of reactions. If the stability of the drug is found to be unsatisfactory, strategies to mitigate the instability of the drug can be adopted. Thus, methodical, carefully planned and executed compatibility studies can lead to savings in terms of resources and time delays associated with stability issues arising during late stage product development. The results from these studies can also be useful in determining the causes of stability issues if, and when, they surface at later stages in development.

Additionally, the regulatory expectations have increased significantly over time. This trend is expected to continue, as quality by design (QbD) initiatives continue to be advocated. Drug–excipient compatibility data is required to justify the selection of formulation components in development reports that go into filings. There has also been an increased regulatory focus on the critical quality attributes (CQA) of excipients and their control strategy, because of their impact on the drug product formulation and manufacturing process.

From a drug development process perspective, these studies are usually conducted after gaining some understanding of solution and solid-state stability characteristics of the drug substance (active pharmaceutical ingredient or API), but before the formulation development activities. An incompatibility in dosage form can result in any of the following changes:

- change in color/appearance;
- loss in mechanical properties (e.g., tablet hardness)
- changes to dissolution performance;
- physical form conversion;
- loss through sublimation;
- a decrease in potency; and
- increase in degradation products.

The focus of this chapter is on excipient compatibility as it relates to the physical and chemical stability of the drug in solid dosage forms. This chapter will summarize the common reasons for drug–excipient incompatibilities, and the current practices in excipient compatibility testing and data interpretation.

6.2 CHEMISTRY OF DRUG–EXCIPIENT INTERACTIONS

The most common reactions observed in pharmaceuticals are hydrolysis, dehydration, isomerization, elimination, cyclization, oxidation, photodegradation, and specific interactions with formulation components (excipients and their impurities). The main factors that affect these reactions are temperature, pH, moisture in solids, relative humidity of the environment, presence of catalysts, light, oxygen, physical form, and particle size of the drug and excipients.

A comprehensive discussion on chemistry of drug stability is out of the scope of this chapter. However, it is important to consider why excipient(s) may alter the stability of drug substances that are prone to certain types of degradation. Some of the common ways by which excipients may affect drug stability in the dosage form are by altering moisture content in the dosage form, changing microenvironmental pH in the dosage form, acting as general acid–base catalysts, directly reacting with drug or becoming a source of impurities that can either directly react with drug substances or participate as catalysts in the drug degradation. The excipients can also alter the physical and/or the chemical form of the drug through, for example, ion-exchange, transformation of polymorphs, and the formation of eutectic or solid solutions. The changes in physical or chemical state may in turn alter the chemical stability of the drug.

In the context of solid-state compatibility testing, two attributes of excipients are especially important to formulation stability and compatibility testing:

1. their ability to sorb water at variable humidity; and
2. the pH that the excipients impart.

6.2.1 Influence of Water and Microenvironmental pH

Most drugs and excipients contain water, which may be either bound or unbound. The bound water is the water of hydration or crystallization which is so tightly incorporated in the physical form of the material that it is practically immobile and is not available for reactions. This is exemplified by the stability of crystalline hydrates of hydrolytically unstable β-lactam antibiotics, wherein the water is incorporated in the crystalline matrix and is not available for reaction. As expected, the stability of these compounds is highly dependent on their crystalline state.[1] In contrast, unbound water usually exists in equilibrium with the atmosphere in an absorbed or adsorbed state

by the solid components, and has higher molecular mobility. The variation in the water content of an excipient with humidity reflects changes in the unbound water content.

The physical state of water in an excipient or the drug–excipient mixture determines its potential role in drug–excipient interactions. The water sorption–desorption properties of excipients are well-documented.[2,3] Presence of water in the solid-state systems has a significant impact on the stability, not only in causing the hydrolysis of drugs, e.g., of acetylsalicylic acid,[4] but also its participation as a reaction medium, and in increasing the plasticity and molecular mobility of the system. Excipients that strongly sorb water may prevent drug degradation by scavenging water in a closed system, e.g., colloidal silica[5] and silica gel.[6] Excipients with higher adsorption energy can decrease the reactivity of water in the system, compared with those with lower adsorption energy, as was shown in the case of nitrazepam (discussed in Section 6.2.3).[7] On the other hand, water in excipients such as microcrystalline cellulose are highly reactive, because it is weakly adsorbed.[8] This was the reason for the higher rate of hydrolytic degradation of aspirin in the presence of microcrystalline cellulose, versus microfine cellulose.[9] A study of water sorption–desorption of a system as a function of environmental humidity can indicate the strength of sorption of water, and its mobility within the system. The mobility of water molecules in a system can be directly measured by NMR and dielectric relaxation spectroscopy. Mobility of water in the system has been correlated to drug stability in drug–excipient mixtures in several cases, e.g., degradation of trichlormethiazide in gelatin gels,[10] and of cephalothin in its mixtures with microcrystalline cellulose.[11]

In addition, water activity is a direct indicator of the amount of free, mobile water in the system. Water activity is proportional to the relative humidity in a closed environment produced in equilibrium with the solid excipient or drug–excipient mixture. Several authors recommend use of water activity determination for drug product stability correlation over total moisture determination by Karl Fisher titrimetry, and/or water uptake by weight gain.[12] Thus, Burghart et al. correlated the water activity of solid oral dosage forms of levothyroxine and lyothyronine with their chemical stability.[12]

Unbound, weakly adsorbed water contributes to molecular mobility within the system, which is a prerequisite for chemical reactions. Sorbed water plasticizes amorphous solids by reducing the glass transition temperature, Tg.[14] The Tg of an amorphous solid represents transition from a highly rigid, less mobile, glassy state, to a rubbery, mobile state with higher free volume. Water sorption leading to reduction in Tg is known in excipients, such as starch, lactose, and cellulose,[13] and amorphous drugs such as indomethacin.[14] Molecular mobility of drugs and excipients in the solid state directly correlates with their reactivity.

The pH imparted by the excipient on the microenvironment of the solid state interfaces can have a significant impact on the chemical stability of the drug. For example, the degradation of a fluoropyridinyl drug in a capsule formulation was a function of the pH of the microenvironment, facilitating a nucleophilic substitution reaction whereby the fluorine substituent of the pyridine ring was replaced with hydroxyl groups.[15]

Excipients can have an acidic or basic surface pH, depending on their chemical nature and composition. For example, Glombitza et al. measured the surface pH using pH indicator dyes, and found that the surface of dicalcium phosphate was more acidic than that of microcrystalline cellulose.[16] For soluble excipients, the pH of the excipient solution is a simple indicator of the pH imparted by the excipients in solid state. For insoluble excipients, the pH of 5–20% excipient slurry in water could be used as an indirect indicator. The selection of excipients with compatible pH profiles, based on preformulation solubility and stability studies as a function of pH, is helpful in the design of excipient compatibility experiments. For example, acid labile drugs should not be combined with acidic excipients, such as hydroxypropyl methyl cellulose phthalate and HPMC acetate succinate. Similarly, magnesium stearate imparts a basic pH in its microenvironment, and may contribute to the instability of base-labile drugs. Stanisz found that the chemical stability of quinapril HCl in binary drug–excipient mixtures was significantly better with acidic excipients than basic magnesium stearate.[17] This study indicated that both the microenvironmental pH and humidity were significant factors in drug degradation. Thus, the presence of mobile water accelerates the surface pH effects of excipients by creating microenvironmental conditions of dissolved drug on the interacting surfaces.

Most drugs are salts of organic acids or bases which may exist as free acid or base forms at acidic or basic pH, respectively. Since a miniscule amount of drug may be dissolved in the free water, pH modifying excipients may result in the formation of the free acid–base form of the drug. If the free acid–base form is more unstable than the salt form, this would lead to enhanced degradation. It may also be volatile, and be lost by sublimation from the dosage form, leading to mass balance issues in terms of loss of drug not being accounted for by the presence of degradation products.[18]

6.2.2 Reactions with Excipients and their Impurities

Although generally considered inert, pharmaceutical excipients are organic compounds with functional groups that may undergo chemical reactions in the dosage form, especially with the reactive functional groups of the APIs. Furthermore, pharmaceutical excipients carry trace level reactive impurities that can either catalyze or directly participate in drug degradation.

A brief review of excipient synthesis, isolation, and/or purification can give vital clues about their potential impurities and other characteristics that may pose problems in the formulation. However, due to their proprietary nature, the availability of this information is difficult to come by, and restricted to informal vendor discussions and perusal of the patent databases in most cases. Several examples of the presence and implication of reactive impurities in pharmaceutical excipients are known in literature and can be used as a guiding reference (Table 6.1). Listed below are a few illustrative examples:

- Reactions of reducing sugars e.g., lactose, with primary and secondary amine drugs via Maillard reaction, followed by Amadori rearrangement to produce a multitude of colored products is well-known. The general mechanism of these reactions involves the reaction of the amine compound with the open form of the carbohydrate to form an imminium ion intermediate that can either close to a glycosamine compound or deprotonate to form the enol version of the rearrangement product[19] (Figure 6.1a).
- Even a non-reducing sugar can contain trace level(s) of reducing sugar. In the case of starch, the terminal glucose was reported to have reacted with hydralazine in the formulation (Figure 6.1b).[20]
- Formaldehyde and other aldehydes are known impurities in several excipients and packaging components. Formaldehyde is known to react with amine drugs to form N-formyl adducts (hemiaminals) that can further react to form dimer(s) (Figure 6.1c). Adefovir is known to react with formaldehyde to produce the reactive imine which can further undergo nucleophilic addition with another amine molecule to form a dimer.[21] Nassar et al. showed that BMS-204352 formed an adduct (hemiaminal) with formaldehyde impurity in the solubilizers, polysorbate 80 and PEG 300.[22] 5-hydroxylmethyl-2-furfuraldehyde, an impurity found in lactose, has been reported to react with haloperidol to form a condensation product (Figure 6.1d).[21]

TABLE 6.1 The method of manufacture of common pharmaceutical excipients and their potentially reactive impurities

Examples of excipients	Method of manufacture	Potentially reactive impurities	Examples of known incompatibilities
Lactose	Lactose is a natural disaccharide consisting of galactose and glucose and is present in the milk of most mammals. Commercially, lactose is produced from the whey of cows' milk, whey being the residual liquid of the milk following cheese and casein production. Cows' milk contains 4.4–5.2% lactose and it is 38% of the total solid content of milk.[2]	Lactose may contain glucose, furfuraldehyde, formic acid, acetic acid, and potentially other aldehydes.	Maillard reactions, Claissen–Schmidt condensation reaction of its impurity, 5-hydroxylmethyl-2-furfuraldehyde,[21] and catalysis of hydrolysis.[29]
Microcrystalline cellulose	Microcrystalline cellulose is manufactured by the controlled hydrolysis with dilute mineral acid solutions of α-cellulose, obtained as a pulp from fibrous plant materials. Following hydrolysis, the hydrocellulose is purified by filtration and the aqueous slurry is spray-dried to form dry, porous particles of a broad size distribution.[2]	The impurities in microcrystalline cellulose are glucose, formaldehyde, nitrates, and nitrites.	Water sorption resulting in increased hydrolysis,[9] Maillard reaction with residual glucose,[27] adsorption of basic drugs,[28] and non-specific incompatibilities due to hydrogen bonding capability.[15]
Povidone and crospovidone	Pyrrolidone is produced by reacting butyrolactone with ammonia. This is followed by a vinylation reaction in which pyrrolidone and acetylene are reacted under pressure. The monomer, vinylpyrrolidone, is then polymerized in the presence of a combination of catalysts to produce povidone. Water-insoluble cross-linked PVP (Crospovidone) is manufactured by a polymerization process where the cross-linking agent is generated *in situ*.[2]	Povidone and crospovidone contain significant levels of peroxides. Povidone may also contain formic acid and formaldehyde.[29]	Oxidation attributable to peroxides,[30] nucleophilic addition to amino acids and peptides,[31] and hydrolysis of sensitive drugs due to moisture.
Hydroxypropyl cellulose (HPC)	HPC is a water soluble cellulose ether produced by the reaction of cellulose with propylene oxide.[2]	HPC may contain significant levels of peroxides.	Oxidation of sensitive drugs due to residual peroxides.
Croscarmellose sodium	To produce croscarmellose sodium, alkali cellulose is prepared by steeping cellulose, obtained from wood pulp or cotton fibers, in sodium hydroxide solution. The alkali cellulose is then reacted with sodium monochloroacetate to obtain carboxymethylcellulose sodium. After the substitution reaction is completed, and all of the sodium hydroxide has been used, the excess sodium monochloroacetate slowly hydrolyzes to glycolic acid. The glycolic acid changes a few of the sodium carboxymethyl groups to the free acid, and catalyzes the formation of cross-links to produce croscarmellose sodium. The croscarmellose sodium is then extracted with aqueous alcohol, and any remaining sodium chloride or sodium glycolate removed. After purification, croscarmellose sodium of greater than 99.5% purity is obtained. The croscarmellose sodium may be milled to break the polymer fibers into shorter lengths, and hence improve its flow properties.[2]	Monochloroacetate, nitriles, and nitrates. Monochloroacetate can react with nucleophiles.	Weakly basic drugs can compete with the sodium counterion, thus getting adsorbed on the surface of the disintegrant particles.[35] Drug salt form conversion has also been reported.[32]
Sodium starch glycolate	Sodium starch glycolate is a substituted and cross-linked derivative of potato starch. Starch is carboxymethylated by reacting it with sodium chloroacetate in an alkaline medium, followed by neutralization with citric or some other acid. Cross-linking may be achieved by either physical methods or chemically by using reagents such as phosphorus oxytrichloride or sodium trimetaphosphate.	Monochloroacetate, nitriles, and nitrates are potentially reactive impurities.	Adsorption of weakly basic drugs and their salts due to electrostatic interactions.[33,34] In addition, the residual monochloroacetate may undergo S_N2 nucleophilic reactions.

Starch	Starch is composed of amylose and amylopectin, polymers of glucose connected by α 1,4 glycosidic linkages (in contrast to cellulose β 1,4 linkages). Amylopectin has occasional branch chains connected by α 1,6 glycosidic linkages. Starch is extracted from plant sources through a sequence of processing steps involving coarse milling, repeated water washing, wet sieving, and centrifugal separation. The wet starch obtained from these processes is dried and milled before use in pharmaceutical formulations. Pregelatinized starch is a starch that has been chemically and/or mechanically processed to rupture all or part of the starch granules, and so render the starch flowable and directly compressible. Partially pregelatinized grades are also commercially available.	Starch may contain formaldehyde, nitrites, and nitrates.	Terminal aldehydes in starch have been known to react with the hydrazine moiety of hydralazine HCl.[20] Starch may also be involved in moisture-mediated reactions, may adsorb drugs, and may react with formaldehyde resulting in reduced functionality as a disintegrant.[35,36]
Colloidal silicon dioxide		May contain heavy metal impurities.	May act as a Lewis acid under anhydrous conditions and may adsorb drugs.[39]
Stearic acid	Stearic acid is made via hydrolysis of fat by continuous exposure to a counter-current stream of high-temperature water and fat in a high-pressure chamber. The resultant mixture is purified by vacuum-steam distillation, and the distillates are then separated using selective solvents.		Stearic acid is incompatible with most metal hydroxides, and may be incompatible with oxidizing agents. Insoluble stearates are formed with many metals; ointment bases made with stearic acid may show evidence of drying out or lumpiness due to such a reaction when compounded with zinc or calcium salts. A number of differential scanning calorimetry studies have investigated the compatibility of stearic acid with drugs. Although such laboratory studies have suggested incompatibilities, e.g., naproxen, they may not necessarily be applicable to formulated products. Stearic acid has been reported to cause pitting in the film coating of tablets coated using an aqueous film coating technique; the pitting was found to be a function of the melting point of the stearic acid. Stearic acid could affect the hydrolysis rate of API if the degradation is pH dependent. It could also potentially react with an API containing a primary amine to form a stearoyl derivative.[37,38]

(Continued)

TABLE 6.1 (Continued)

Examples of excipients	Method of manufacture	Potentially reactive impurities	Examples of known incompatibilities
	Stearic acid may also be made via hydrogenation of cottonseed and other vegetable oils; by the hydrogenation and subsequent saponification of oleic acid followed by recrystallization from alcohol; and from edible fats and oils by boiling with NaOH, separating any glycerin and decomposing the resulting soap with sulfuric or hydrochloric acid. The stearic acid is then subsequently separated from any oleic acid by cold expression.		
Magnesium stearate	Magnesium stearate is prepared either by chemical reaction of aqueous solution of magnesium chloride with sodium stearate or by the interaction of magnesium oxide, hydroxide or carbonate with stearic acid at elevated temperatures. The raw materials used in manufacturing of magnesium stearate are refined fatty acids, which is a mixture of palmitic and stearic acid with certain specifications. A fatty acid splitting (hydrolysis) process takes place first, where glycerin and fatty acids are separated. The fatty acids are then further refined to yield tallow acid. Magnesium stearate can be prepared through two processes: 1. Fusion: simple acid base interaction between tallow acid and magnesium hydroxide; or 2. Saponification: tallow acid is saponified first with sodium hydroxide, making a sodium tallowate (salt), then magnesium sulfate is added to the sodium tallow solution, followed by pH adjustment, dilution with water, wash and dry.	Magnesium oxide is a known reactive impurity.	Magnesium stearate can form hydrates with water, and exists in four hydration states—mono-, di- and trihydrates.[39] MgO impurity is known to react with ibuprofen.[40] In addition, magnesium stearate provides a basic pH environment, and may accelerate hydrolytic degradation.[41] The magnesium metal may also cause chelation-induced degradation.[24]

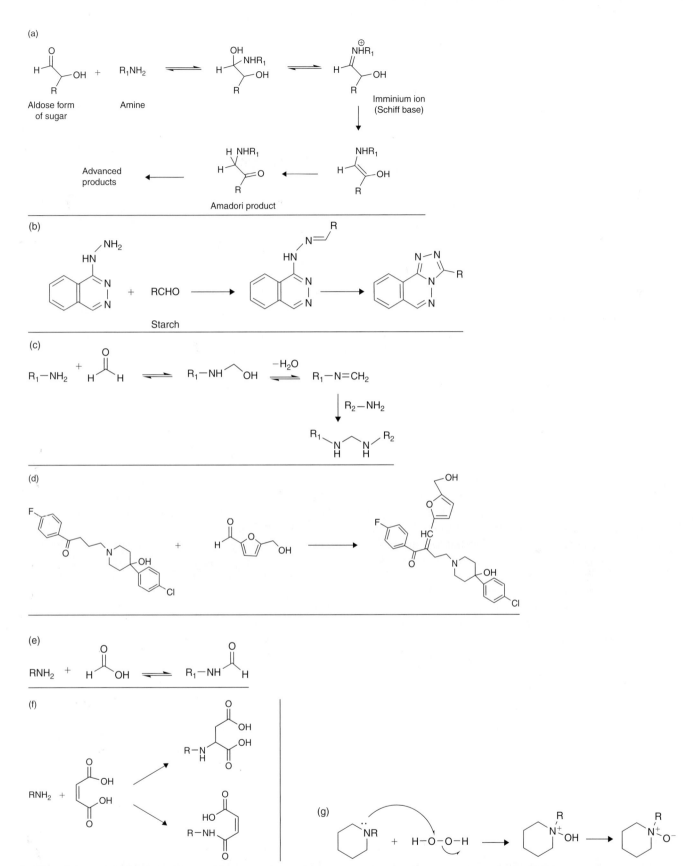

FIGURE 6.1 Examples of reactions of drugs with pharmaceutical excipients and their reactive impurities. (a) reaction of primary amine with a reducing sugar; (b) reaction of hydralazine with terminal aldehydes of starch residue; (c) reaction of an amine with formaldehyde; (d) reaction of haloperidol with the impurity 5-hydroxymethyl-2-furfuraldehyde (HMF) found in lactose; (e) addition of formic acid to an amine; (f) addition of amine to maleic acid; (g) formation of N-oxide from hydrogen peroxide impurity

- The formyl species could react with amines to form N-formamide (Figure 6.1e). For instance, Waterman et al. reported that varenicline, a secondary amine, can undergo N-methylation and N-formylation by reactive impurities (formyl and acetyl) found in the polymers used to manufacture osmotic tablets.[22] Formation of stearoyl derivative of norfloxacin is attributable to the stearate component of magnesium stearate. Similar to the mechanism shown in Figure 6.1e, it can be conceived that the secondary amine in norfloxacin would undergo nucleophilic addition to form the stearoyl amide. Seproxetine undergoes a Michael addition reaction with its counterion to form two addition products (Figure 6.1f).[23]
- The degradation of fosinopril sodium[24] in tablet formulations containing magnesium stearate was attributed to chelation by the magnesium ions.
- Drugs with alcohol groups can form esters with acids (e.g., formic acid) or undergo transesterification with esters (e.g., parabens). Similarly, acidic drugs can esterify with excipients containing alcohol groups such as PEGs.
- Trace levels of peroxides and metal ions in formulations are known to accelerate oxidation of drugs. Residual peroxides are also present in polyvinyl pyrrolidone (PVP), cross-linked PVP, and hydroxypropyl cellulose (HPC). Moreover, their content shows both batch-to-batch and manufacturer-to-manufacturer variation.[25] The peroxides can cause free radical initiated oxidation reactions, undergo nucleophilic addition reactions with tertiary amine to N-oxide, secondary amine to hydroxylamines, and sulfide to sulfoxide. For example, the hydroperoxide impurity in PVP has been shown to react with piperazine ring to form N-oxide (Figure 6.1g).
- Sodium glycolate is a residual reactant in the manufacture of the super-disintegrant, sodium starch glycolate, and has been known to cause degradation of drugs like duloxetine.[26]
- Silicon dioxide may contain significant levels of heavy metal impurities which may act as catalysts in certain oxidative degradation reactions.

6.2.3 Stabilizing Excipients

Although the thrust of compatibility studies is on the identification of potential or serious destabilizing aspects of drug–excipient interactions, excipients are often also utilized to improve formulation stability. For example, complexation with cyclodextrins has been shown to reduce drug instability in several cases.[44] Cyclodextrins complex with the labile drug inside their hydrophobic cavity, and shield it from common degradation mechanisms such as hydrolysis, oxidation, and photodegradation.

Stabilization of oxidation sensitive drugs by incorporation of antioxidants in the formulation is a well-known strategy. The chosen antioxidants could be water soluble (e.g., propyl gallate and ascorbic acid), or water insoluble (e.g., butylated hydroxy anisole (BHA), butylated hydroxy toluene (BHT) or α-tocopherol). The choice of antioxidants is based not only on their solubility properties, but also on mechanism of oxidation. Thus, compatibility studies often involve investigation of relative efficacy of different antioxidants in mitigating drug degradation.

In addition, the heavy metal catalyzed degradation reactions in formulations can often be mitigated by the use of chelating agents such as ethylene diamine tetraacetic acid (EDTA) or ethyleneglycol tetraacetic acid (EGTA). EGTA has a much higher affinity for calcium and magnesium ions than EDTA. For example, EDTA was used to mitigate oxidative degradation of dextromethorphan in its complexes with the ion exchange resin, divinyl benzene sulfonic acid.[42]

Stabilization of hydrolysis sensitive drugs intuitively disallows the selection of excipients with high residual moisture content and high water sorption capacity. Nonetheless, excipients with affinity for water might mitigate moisture sensitivity of the formulation by preferentially taking up the moisture permeating through the package during shelf life and accelerated storage. For example, edible silica gel, Syloid®, was used to stabilize extremely moisture-sensitive potassium clavulanate in oral solid dosage forms.[43] An interesting case was presented by Perrier and Kesselring of stabilization of nitrazepam in binary mixtures with excipients as a function of their nitrogen adsorption energy.[7] The authors assumed that the binding energy for water followed the same rank-order correlation as that of nitrogen. Use of excipients with higher binding energy was hypothesized to sequestrate any available moisture, and act as a stabilizer. Similarly, it can be hypothesized that the use of excipients that act as sorbents (e.g., microcrystalline cellulose and amorphous silica), might sequestrate reactive trace impurities (e.g., formaldehyde and formic acid) and volatile residues (e.g., methanol, ethanol, and isopropyl alcohol) from the formulation.[44] These strategies may be tested in applicable cases by spiking studies in the binary compatibility experiments or the use of mini-formulation designs that combine the offending and the protecting excipients.

Exposure to light can cause drug degradation by various mechanisms, such as addition reactions in unsaturated systems, polymerization, isomerization, photo-oxidation, and substitution reactions. The use of light-resistant packaging, e.g., amber glass and opaque high density polyethylene (HDPE) bottles, are standard practice for photo-labile drugs. In addition, to protect the drug during processing and packaging operations, light-resistant film coatings and the use of excipients such as cyclodextrins, dyes, and colored additives is often helpful. In addition, photolabile excipients can be used in the formulation of photosensitive drugs, just as antioxidants are used for oxidation sensitive drugs. In this case, substantial overlap of the ultra violet (UV) absorption spectrum of the excipient with the drug has been shown to improve the drug stability in several cases, e.g., stabilization of nifedipine by riboflavine or curcumin, and the stabilization of sulphisomidine using oxybenzone.[44]

6.3 CURRENT PRACTICES

Compatibility studies involve a series of activities designed to identify key drug–excipient incompatibilities, and their causes (Figure 6.2). Compatibility studies on new molecular entities invariably start with evaluation of existing information, and paper chemistry of the drug candidate to identify "soft spots" in the molecule. Presence of reactive or unstable functional groups, pKa value, and known reactivities of similar compounds provide useful information for the selection of excipients. In addition to the general literature, several computational programs have recently become available that can help predict potential degradation pathways of a drug candidate, e.g., CAMEO®, SPARTAN®, EPWIN®, and Pharm D³®. Many pharmaceutical companies also have internal databases

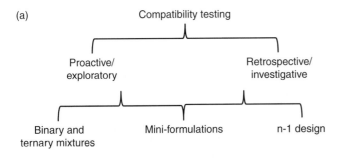

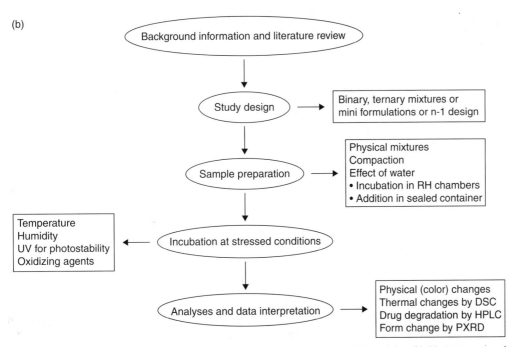

FIGURE 6.2 Typical modalities of compatibility testing (a) and the study execution (b). Various stages of the compatibility testing are highlighted in ovals, and the key decisions and variables involved in each stage are mentioned in square boxes

and software programs. Furthermore, preformulation studies on the physico-chemical characterization and forced degradation of the drug molecule are used to modulate the design of compatibility studies to detect the presence and extent of known reactivities.

Design of compatibility studies might involve the use of mixtures of drug with one or more excipients. These mixtures may be incubated at different stress conditions as physical mixtures *per se* or after compaction. Often water is added in these systems to evaluate its role in accelerating drug–excipient interactions. Addition of other ingredients, such as hydrogen peroxide to induce oxidative stress, is based on the background information of the molecule's sensitivities. The compatibility study samples are typically stored at elevated temperatures, and analyzed for physical and chemical changes in the drug at predetermined time intervals. In addition, binary mixtures of drug and excipients are analyzed by thermal methods such as differential scanning calorimetry (DSC), and isothermal microcalorimetry (IMC), for rapid assessment of potential incompatibilities. In short, compatibility studies involve several choices for each stage of testing depending on the drug candidate, available literature, and the goals of the study. The following sections will highlight the basis of some of these decisions.

6.3.1 Experimental Design

Compatibility studies are commonly carried out by accelerated stress testing, and evaluation of its effect on the binary or multicomponent drug–excipient mixtures. The design of experiments is governed by the potential formulation choices, and excipient preferences. These decisions are made in conjunction with all the other available preformulation data, API characteristics, and marketing preferences. These also determine the types of pharmaceutical excipients that are evaluated. For example, compatibility studies for a liquid formulation of an insoluble compound would differ widely, and include excipients such as surfactants and suspending agents, from the studies designed for a highly soluble compound.

Two- or Multi-component Systems

Proactive preformulation compatibility studies are traditionally carried out as binary or ternary systems. Binary mixtures of drug and common pharmaceutical excipients such as diluents or ternary mixtures of drug, a diluent, and excipients used in lower proportions such as disintegrants and lubricants, are incubated at accelerated conditions of temperature and humidity for extended periods of time, using drug alone and excipient alone as controls. Additional aggravating conditions, such as light and peroxides, are incorporated in the study design, depending on the characteristics of the drug molecule. Incompatibilities are physically identified by visual observation for color or physical form changes, and by spectroscopic and calorimetric methods, and are chemically quantified by analytical assays for drug content and impurities.

Binary design was used by Wyttenback et al. to study the excipient compatibility of acetylsalicylic acid or fluoxetine HCl in binary mixtures with 7 excipients using bi-level factors of temperature (40° and 50°C), humidity (10% and 75% RH), and time (1 and 4 weeks), leading to a total of 56 experimental runs for each drug.[45] The total impurity content of each run was measured by HPLC to determine the effect of each excipient on drug stability. In addition, they grouped together all excipients as a factor, and interpreted the data by analysis of variance using F-ratio to test whether the means of normally distributed populations are equal, and by the calculation of p-value. The data presented interesting insights into the relative stability of the two drug substances as a function of these factors and their interactions.

The n-1 Design and Mini-formulations

Compatibility studies are often aimed at solving formulation stability issues. In such cases studies are carried out with the exclusion of only one component in each sub-lot to identify the source of incompatibility. Often, mini-formulations are prepared with the exclusion of non-critical, quantitatively minor, and/or easily interchangeable ingredients, e.g., colors and flavors, from solutions and suspensions. Compatibility studies for the development of liquid formulations are invariably mini-formulation studies, since they require prior pH solubility and stability evaluation to use the appropriate buffer system in compatibility testing and base formulations.

The Plackett–Burman design may be used to design studies involving mini-formulations, although it is rarely used in practice. This design minimizes the number of experimental runs, and is capable of finding the excipients that cause major incompatibilities. It can examine n excipients in $n + 1$ experimental runs.[46] This design was utilized by Durig and Fassihi to investigate the compatibility of pyridoxal HCl with 11 excipients at two temperatures (25° and 55°C), and two humidity conditions (11% and 75% RH), using only 16 experimental runs.[47] In this study, they included eight experiments over the minimum required to study the effect of "pseudo-variables," to account for random experimental variation. This approach, however, does not take into account the variation in the concentration of excipients depending on the number of components present in the mixture.

6.3.2 Sample Preparation and Storage

Sample preparation for compatibility studies depends on the physical nature of the ingredients, and the conceptualization of the final formulation. Selection of appropriate drug to excipient ratios for binary compatibility studies is often carried out on the weight or molar basis of their expected usage in the final formulation. In the absence of a defined dose of the drug, as is often true of new molecules in the early stages of development, the worst case scenarios of least drug to excipient ratios are tested.

The least drug to excipient ratio is expected to provide the highest rate of possible drug–excipient interactions. For example, the amorphous calcium salt of the Merck compound L-649 923, a leukotriene D_4 antagonist, degraded by intramolecular esterification to form a γ-lactone. Its degradation rates were higher at lower drug doses, with both microcrystalline cellulose and pregelatinized starch as excipients.[48] These observations are in line with the hypothesis that reactions happen at the interface of the drug and the excipients. Higher rates of drug degradation with lower particle size excipients further support this hypothesis. Thus, hydrolysis of acetylsalicylic acid in tablets containing dibasic calcium phosphate dihydrate showed a rank order correlation with the particle size of the excipient.[49] Similarly, powdered magnesium stearate showed higher levels of drug degradation than its granular form.[41]

Sample Preparation

Binary mixture designs for solid-state samples often involve only physical mixing. Attention must be paid to the use of fine particles of both the drug and the excipient, and deagglomeration of either component, if needed. Often co-screening through a mesh is utilized to effect intimate mixing. Compaction of drug–excipient mixtures is carried out in solid-state compatibility testing. Milling and compaction of crystals can lead to the formation of an amorphous state.[50] Process stresses such as compaction, grinding, and drying may also lead to release of bound water from actives and excipients. For example, grinding was shown to dehydrate the crystal water of theophylline hydrate,[51] and affected the solid-state stability of

ampicillin trihydrate[52] and sodium prasterone sulfate.[53] Similarly, cefixime trihydrate showed reduction in crystallinity, and dehydration upon grinding in a ball mill.[54] Thus, compatibility studies involving grinding and compaction are helpful for moisture sensitive and low melting compounds, and also for drug substances for which milling is envisaged for particle size reduction.

Presence of water often accelerates degradation kinetics. In addition, sorbed moisture can accelerate isomerization and/or crystallization processes. One of the important goals of preformulation compatibility testing is to determine the feasibility of processing conditions, such as wet granulation and the moisture resistance need for packages. Thus, it becomes important to determine the case and extent of moisture sensitivity of the drug in the presence of excipients. To this end, water is often added to drug–excipient binary mixtures in closed systems to create a high relative humidity (RH) environment.[54] Alternatively, the compatibility mixtures are stored in open containers at different temperature and RH conditions. Care must be exercised in comparing the data across these designs, since potential volatilization and escape of reactive components in the open container storage conditions might give an indication of stability that may not hold true in the final dosage form.

Compatibility study experiments tend to be labor-intensive due to their exhaustive design. Automation of compatibility studies is often undertaken during the early development stages.[58] The automated systems can be used for determining drug solubility, forced degradation, and compatibility testing. Reactor blocks, consisting of an array of samples, can be prepared using automated liquid handlers and powder dispensers such as Gilson® and Autodose®, respectively. The blocks can be stored in different stressed conditions. Automated sampling at predetermined time points can be accomplished using robotic systems such as Jaba®. These operations may also be performed with fully automated systems such as the Symyx® Automated Forced Degradation System. This system can accurately weigh given quantities of excipients and actives in blocks of vials. The blocks are then robotically transferred to controlled environmental chambers, and removed at a predetermined time for analysis. The use of automated systems improves efficiency, and broadens the experimental space, thus allowing the execution of exhaustive, statistically robust experiments and generation of knowledge. This, when coupled with scientific rigor, could significantly reduce or even avoid the apperance of drug–excipient incompatibilities during later stages of drug product development.

The selection of accelerated environmental storage conditions for compatibility testing is based on the nature of the API, and the expected stresses during the storage of the finished dosage form. These include storage at elevated temperatures, higher humidities, and exposure to UV irradiation, peroxides, etc. While the International Council on Harmonization (ICH) and the regulatory authorities provide guidelines on the selection of accelerated storage conditions for the finished dosage form for confirmatory stability studies based on the target label storage requirements, the selection of accelerated conditions for compatibility studies is at the formulator's discretion.

Thermal Stresses

Isothermal stress testing (IST) or incubation of samples at constant higher temperatures as stress conditions is almost universal for compatibility studies. It is based on the underlying assumption that the kinetics of degradation reactions follows Arrhenius kinetics. Arrhenius equation states the reaction rate dependence on temperature:

$$k = A * e^{\frac{-Ea}{RT}}$$

where:

T is the temperature (in Kelvin)
R is the gas constant with a value of 8.314 $J/(K*mol)$
Ea is the activation energy in KJ/mol
k is the reaction rate constant
A is the Arrhenius constant.

The selection of higher temperatures is designed to accelerate reaction rates significantly, so that even relatively slow reactions become evident in a short period of time. For example, assuming the mean activation energy for solid-state reactions to be 105 kJ/mol,[55] the amount of drug degradation observed at 25°C in approximately 5 years would be evident in about 3 weeks at 60°C. Certain implicit assumptions of IST include:

- temperature independence of activation energy and reaction mechanism;
- absence of equilibrium or autocatalytic reactions;
- activation energies for different reactions of pharmaceutical relevance being in a relatively close range;
- stability of API *per se* under the stressed conditions.

The temperature is often maximized to increase reaction rate, and decrease testing time. However, care must be exercised in judicious selection of temperature, since above a certain temperature, the system may exceed the activation energies of alternative degradation pathways, thus resulting in non-representative data. A shift in the primary degradation processes is often indicated by the appearance of additional impurity peaks in the HPLC chromatogram. For example, while exploring accelerated degradation conditions for an experimental compound, Sims et al. observed that while incubation at temperatures up to 80°C resulted in the formation of the same impurities as at controlled room temperature and 60°C, samples stressed at 100°C showed many unrelated peaks.[56] Therefore, usually more than one stressed condition is chosen to determine if the degradation reactions observed at elevated temperatures might be the ones which have such high activation energies that they occur only under pharmaceutically irrelevant conditions.

Humidity and/or Water Content

The use of high moisture content for compatibility studies is intended to uncover not only the reactions in which water participates directly, e.g., hydrolysis, but also to investigate whether water increases reactivity in the solid state. Water adsorption on solid surfaces can enhance reactivity by acting as a medium or a plasticizer for the reacting species. Presence of water in the solid component mixtures provides the molecular mobility required for reactions to occur between the two solid components.

Water can be incorporated in the excipient compatibility samples in several ways:

1. preparation of a slurry or suspension;
2. addition of water, usually 20% of solids, in a closed system;[54] and
3. exposure of the system to controlled humidity conditions.

Each of these methods has advantages and disadvantages. While the slurry experiments do provide useful information for simulation of suspension dosage forms and rapid assessment of aqueous sensitivity of the drug substance, they often do not simulate conditions in solid dosage forms—which could be important to data interpretation in retrospective or investigational compatibility studies. The addition of a fixed proportion of water to the drug–excipient mixture in a closed system controls the initial amount of water in the system, and partly simulates wet granulation conditions. Nevertheless, water content in a sample changes depending on the water uptake kinetics and equilibrium moisture content of the sample at the storage temperature. Moreover, the same amount of water in the air results in lower relative humidity at elevated temperatures. In contrast, incubation of samples under controlled humidity conditions ensures consistent maintenance of equilibrium moisture levels in the solid system, thus enabling investigation of degradation reactions where water acts as a medium or just to increase the molecular mobility of reacting species.[56] However, the open container studies may lead to loss of reactive volatile impurities from the mixture, thus possibly altering the reaction pathways. In addition, storage of samples in constant humidity chambers (e.g., open-dish) can lead to increased induction times, thereby complicating kinetics as compared to water addition (or slurry experiments).

Given the pros and cons of each modality of testing, the formulation scientist must select appropriate conditions for each compatibility study design based upon the available preformulation data.

Mechanical Stress

Mechanical stress is often an unavoidable part of drug product processing conditions, e.g., milling and compaction. These stresses may lead to the formation of amorphous pockets of drug or crystal defects in the crystalline drug molecule or simply increase the intimacy and surface area of contact between the drug and the excipients in the mixture. Thus, mechanical stresses may lead to increased rates of degradation reactions. For example, milling of Procaine Penicillin G almost doubled its rate of degradation in compatibility studies with Emcompress® and Avicel®, as compared with the unmilled drug–excipient mixtures.[57] Similarly, Badawy et al. observed more than 3-fold higher hydrolytic degradation of an investigational compound DMP-754 in compacts with anhydrous lactose, as compared to uncompacted binary mixtures.[58]

In addition to chemical reactivity, compaction may also have an effect on the physical form of the drug. Thus, Guo et al. observed loss of crystallinity of quinapril hydrochloride, whose crystalline form exists as an acetonitrile (ACN) solvate, with ACN loosely incorporated in the crystal lattice channels. Loss of ACN was observed upon compaction, with concomitant loss of crystallinity, and increase of the cyclized degradant. This was attributed to the significantly lower activation energy for the cyclization reaction in the amorphous state than the crystalline state.[59]

Investigations of the effect of mechanical stresses are undertaken when instability is suspected in the investigational drug, e.g., in situations such as the use of a metastable polymorphic form or known chemical reactivities of the molecule. Simulation of mechanical

stresses in compatibility studies involves such procedures as grinding using a ball mill, and comilling of drug–excipient mixtures. In addition, Carver press for the preparation of compacts is often utilized to simulate the compaction during tableting and dry granulation processes.

Oxidative Stress

Oxidation is one of the most common causes of drug degradation in pharmaceutical systems. Oxidative degradation often presents unique patterns of drug degradation, for example, rapid growth of impurities following an induction period, and sensitivity to trace amounts of free radicals. If preformulation or API characterization studies reveal sensitivity to oxidation, the compatibility studies may be designed to comprehensively assess the extent of oxidation sensitivity, as well as to find ways to mitigate the same. These methodologies include, for example, one or more of the following:

- Spiking drug–excipient mixtures with different levels of oxidizing agents, such as hydrogen peroxide, metal impurities (copper and iron salts), or free radical initiators commensurate with the levels seen in excipients.[60]
- Comparing drug degradation in compatibility samples stored under air, oxygen, and nitrogen or argon in hermetically sealed containers.
- Incorporation of free-radical scavengers, and heavy metal chelating agents.[60]
- Packaging configurations that include the incorporation of oxygen scavenger inserts, and the minimum permeability materials of construction.[61]
- Use of different batches of excipients known to have residual peroxide content, e.g., polyvinyl pyrrolidone (PVP), cross-linked PVP, hydroxypropyl cellulose (HPC), polysorbate 80, and polyethylene glycol 400.[30]
- Studies with different antioxidants, e.g., butylated hydroxy anisole (BHA), butylated hydroxy toluene (BHT), α-tocopherol, propyl gallate, and ascorbic acid.[62]

For these studies sample preparation conditions, such as compaction, should be carefully controlled. Furthermore, peroxide impurities in excipients usually show batch-to-batch variation, thus necessitating the testing of batches with high and low level impurities. Spiking experiments are often carried out to quantify the acceptable limits of peroxide impurities in excipients, which may then be used to set incoming material specifications.[30]

6.3.3 Sample Analysis and Data Interpretation

The tests desired for a given set of compatibility studies, and the key outcomes measures depend not only on the envisaged final dosage form and product configuration, but also on the background data available on the chemistry and preformulation studies on the drug candidate. Most compatibility studies include visual inspection for any color changes, compact/tablet integrity and deliquescence, and quantitative chemical analysis for monitoring drug degradation. In addition, form changes of the active are monitored in samples of short-listed excipients.

Monitoring for Drug Degradation

Physical observation of stressed compatibility samples involves observation of changes in color, odor, deliquescence, powder/compact flow characteristics, etc. The inherent subjectivity in these observations is partly overcome by making rank-order correlations with control, refrigerated samples. Furthermore, UV-visible spectroscopy may be utilized to quantify changes in color. This method, however, suffers from the limitation that small changes in absorbance may not appear to be significantly different, and the degradant(s) may retain the chromophores of the drug, leading to negligible or no change in absorbance, even in the presence of degradation. Nevertheless, when significant differences are observed, these observations are often a good indicator of incompatibility between the components.

Several drugs show such evidence of discoloration as an indication of instability and/or incompatibility including, e.g., promethazine, phenylephrine, potassium clavulanate, cefuroxime axetil, and terbinafine. A common example is the discoloration, often browning, of formulations containing primary or secondary amines with reducing sugars such as lactose.[63] This is associated with Maillard reaction, whose end products can undergo Amadori rearrangement to form several colored intermediates and end products.[19]

HPLC with UV detection is by far the most commonly used method to quantify drug degradation by measuring drug potency, total impurities or the growth of a selected impurity over time and as a function of the storage conditions. Measurements of growth of single or all impurities are often preferred over the quantification of loss in potency. This is because a small change in a large number reduces the sensitivity in the interpretation of the data, e.g., a potency fall from 99.5% to 99.2% would likely be considered insignificant, but not an impurity level increase from 0.02% to 0.32%.

It is important that the sample extraction, along with the analytical methodology, is sound. Particular attention should also be paid to lack of mass balance issues, which can arise either due to poor extraction or retention of degradation products on the column, or due to reduction in response factor of the degradation products. When extraction problems are suspected, alternate solvents and agitation techniques should be utilized. To ensure that the column retention is not an issue, HPLC systems with a wide polarity range and longer run times can be employed. If the mass balance issue is severe, the relative response factors of drug and impurities may be assessed by taking the ratio of absorbance of the degraded sample to that of the initial (reference) sample measured by UV alone. This ratio should be identical to the ratio of total area counts for the degraded and initial sample, as determined by HPLC-UV. The main disadvantage of this method is that it is only useful when there is a severe mass balance issue. Although not used in routine analyses, alternative detectors such as evaporative light scattering detector (ELSD), mass spectrometry, corona charged aerosol detector (CAD), chemi-luminiescent nitrogen detector (CLND) or LC/NMR can be used when UV detection is not effective.

Thermal Methods

The use of quantitative, stability-indicating analytical methodology, such as HPLC may not be feasible during the early stages of drug development. In such cases, thermal methods may provide a quick, non-specific, and less labor intensive screening tool. However, it must be noted that results obtained from thermal methods are often not conclusive, and must be confirmed by another independent observation.

Thermal methods for compatibility testing rely on exothermic or endothermic energy changes in the sample. The most commonly applied thermal technique for compatibility studies is differential scanning calorimetry (DSC). It involves heating or cooling the sample in a controlled manner, and measuring the heat released or absorbed by the sample as the temperature of the sample and a reference standard are equally changed over time. Isothermal microcalorimetry (IMC), on the other hand, measures heat flow from the sample compared to a reference vessel, as the two are maintained at a constant temperature. IMC can be applied to detect extremely slow reactions so that drug–excipient mixtures can be monitored at room or low temperatures, and it is able to detect the reactions of "real life" significance.[64,65]

DSC analyses for compatibility evaluation involve recording the thermograms of the individual excipient, the drug, and their physical mixture at a standard heating rate, usually under a nitrogen atmosphere. A simple superimposition of these curves is then interpreted to determine whether the thermal properties of the mixture are a sum of the individual components, or an assumed fundamental property of non-interacting components. An interaction is, thus, identified as changes in the appearance or disappearance of a transition peak, and through changes in transition temperature, peak shape, and peak area. Nonetheless, caution should be exercised in interpreting the results of DSC for determining excipient compatibility, and it should be in conjunction with simultaneous application of other techniques such as infrared (IR) spectroscopy and isothermal stress testing (IST).

Verma and Garg presented an interesting case study where physical observations, IR spectroscopy, and IST were used in conjunction with DSC to determine excipient compatibility.[66] They recorded the DSC thermograms for the drug glipizide with the excipients microcrystalline cellulose (MCC), lactose, and TRIS buffer in 1:5, 1:5, and 1:1 drug to excipient ratios, respectively (Figure 6.3). In this study:

- The DSC thermogram of MCC showed a broad endotherm at 63.29°C attributed to the loss of adsorbed water, and glipizide showed a melting endotherm peak at 216.35°C. The physical mixture of the two excipients showed both the glipizide and the MCC endotherm peaks, indicating a lack of interaction. The IR spectrum of the physical mixture preserved the characteristic bands of glipizide, and did not show any new bands, confirming compatibility of glipizide with MCC.
- The thermogram of lactose showed endothermic peaks at 148.50°C (dehydration of bound water), 172.10°C (crystalline transition), 215.09°C (melting point), and a small peak at 221.02°C. The thermogram for the physical mixture did not show the drug melting peak, indicating interaction. The incompatibility was further confirmed with yellow discoloration of the blend upon heating.
- The thermogram of TRIS showed two endothermic peaks at 139.14°C (loss of adsorbed water) and 172.73°C (melting point). The wave-like endotherm at 300°C indicated decomposition of the TRIS buffer. In the physical mixture the TRIS buffer peak shifted to lower temperature (135.60°C), the drug peak was missing, and a broad hump was observed at 296.16°C. Although the missing drug peak indicated interaction, the IR spectrum of the physical mixture showed characteristic glipizide

bands, and no new peaks were observed indicating a lack of chemical interaction.

Thus, while the absence of drug peak in the physical mixture of drug–lactose was interpreted to indicate incompatibility, since it could be confirmed by a physical observation of color change; the absence of drug peak in the drug–TRIS buffer physical mixture was not interpreted as incompatibility, due to lack of any corroborating evidence by IR spectroscopy and other methods.

Isothermal microcalorimetry (IMC) can measure thermodynamic events in powder mixtures at real-time storage conditions, thus potentially pointing to the degradation reactions that are of relevance in the long term stability studies of the drug product. For example, it can pick up reactions that may lead to only 1–2% degradant accumulation over a year of storage at room temperature. The high sensitivity of this technique necessitates careful control of sample preparation, e.g., the uniformity of particle size of different samples, adequate mixing, and the effects of moisture. An example of the application of isothermal microcalorimetry is presented by Schmitt et al. who used this technique to study the compatibility of an experimental compound ABT-627 in binary mixtures with excipients.[66] They calculated the time average interaction power (P, μW) over an 8 hour period after the signal had reached an equilibrium value at isothermal conditions. The separate drug–excipient curves were used to construct a theoretical noninteraction curve, which was then subtracted from the actual mixture curve to obtain an interaction curve. They obtained a rank-order correlation between the calorimetric results and the results of area percent total degradant upon sample incubation at elevated temperatures for extended periods of time. The authors observed that apparent reaction enthalpies varied up to 3-fold within the same class of excipients. They recommend the use of this technique as a preliminary screen for excipients within a functional class for further investigation.

Another example of the application of IMC was presented by Selzer et al., who investigated drug–excipient mixtures as powders, granules, and compacts.[67,68] Exothermic heat flow at isothermal elevated temperature conditions was indicative of drug–excipient interaction. Higher heat flow in granulated and compacted samples indicated greater interaction, possibly due to higher surface area of contact between the drug and the excipient. The authors point out the confounding effects of interaction of crystallinity changes in the excipients, and physical events that can overlap with drug degradation curves and make the interpretation difficult.

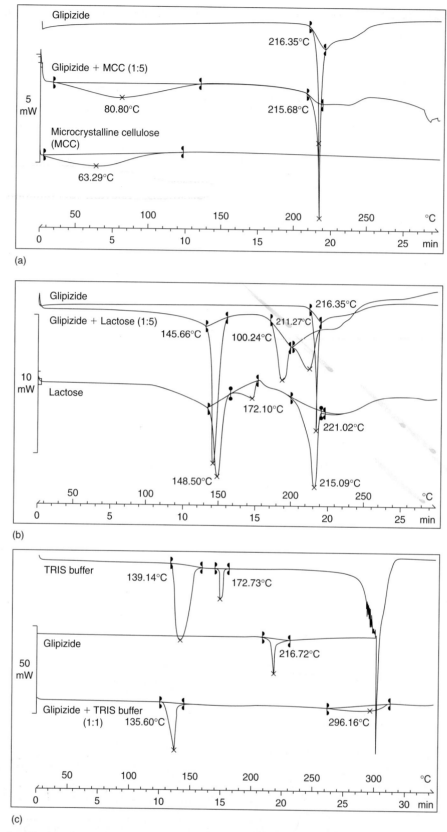

FIGURE 6.3 Example of application of DSC to excipient compatibility evaluation. (a) DSC thermograms of glipizide, MCC, and 1:5 glipizide-MCC mixture; (b) DSC thermograms of glipizide, lactose, and 1:5 glipizide-lactose mixture; (c) DSC thermograms of glipizide, TRIS, and 1:1 glipizide-TRIS mixture. Reproduced with permission from Verma and Garg[66]

Monitoring for Form Changes

The drug discovery and early stage development work is aimed at selecting not only the right molecule, but also its most preferred solid form. The physical form of the drug, polymorphic, and salt form has a significant impact on the physical, chemical, mechanical, and biopharmaceutical properties of the drug candidate. For example, a state with higher thermodynamic activity, e.g., the amorphous phase, generally has higher apparent solubility, diffusion-controlled dissolution rate, and also higher hygroscopicity and chemical reactivity. It also has a tendency to crystallize to a more stable form. The mechanisms underlying phase transformations have been discussed in literature.[69] It is important to ensure that dosage form composition and processing conditions do not alter or destabilize the physico-chemical form of the drug. It must be noted that although these investigations are not a routine part of compatibility testing they become very important if a metastable form is taken up for development or if there is data on the API stability that warrants monitoring for form changes.

Several analytical techniques can be utilized for the characterization of drug's form in the solid state, e.g., powder X-ray diffraction (PXRD), single crystal X-ray diffraction, infrared (IR) and near-infrared (NIR) spectroscopy, Raman spectroscopy, solid state nuclear magnetic resonance (ssNMR) spectroscopy, solvent sorption, polarized microscopy, and hot-stage microscopy. An example of the application of instrumental techniques to identify the impact of excipients on potential form change of the drug during wet processing was presented by Airaksinen et al. using nitrofurantoin as a model drug.[69] Nitrofurantoin exists in two anhydrous (designated α and β), and two monohydrous (designated I and II) forms. High humidity storage and processing conditions, e.g., wet granulation, may lead to the conversion of the anhydrous to the monohydrate form. The authors used PXRD and NIR spectroscopy to investigate form transformation of nitrofurantoin in physical mixtures with selected excipients. Their interpretation of PXRD data focused on the appearance of a peak specific to the monohydrate form that indicated form conversion. Similarly, NIR data was interpreted for the appearance of the absorption maxima for the water of crystallization in the monohydrate form. Such data sets help in establishing the rank-order relationships of the tendency of excipients to support or inhibit form conversion of the drug. The authors correlated the water sorption capacity and the amorphous/crystalline nature of the excipients with their role in moisture-induced form change of nitrofurantoin during processing. Their work demonstrates the utility of these techniques in investigating drug form changes as a part of the compatibility studies.

Kinetic Treatment of Compatibility Data

Kinetic analysis of excipient compatibility data can provide valuable insights into the reaction mechanisms, and help devise strategies to overcome stability issues. Unfortunately, the short duration of these studies prohibit a comprehensive kinetic evaluation. Furthermore, full kinetic treatment of data requires a rigorous experimental design involving multiple experimental and analytical runs, which are often limited by available resources and the urgency of these studies. In addition, it must be noted that the pharmaceutically relevant degradation profiles consist of only the initial stages of degradation, consisting of not more than a few percent formation of impurities, because of stringent shelf life product stability requirements. Generally, the loss in drug potency during excipient compatibility is minimal, and tracking loss of drug alone as a measure of compatibility can be misleading. The small loss in drug potency may be accompanied by the appearance of degradation products. The rate of appearance of degradation product(s) should be followed and fitted to kinetic model(s) that can best describe the degradation pathway.

A complete discussion on models describing kinetics of drug degradation is outside the scope of this chapter. It can be shown that, for the simplest cases of drug degradation following nth order (0, 1, 2, etc.) reaction, and assuming that the total loss in drug potency during the studies is minimal, the levels of drug product(s) increase linearly with time. Consider a drug, D, degrading to a product, P, with a rate constant, k. Let the order of the reaction be n. The rate expression for the loss of drug, and appearance of degradation product, can be expressed as follows:

$$\frac{d[D]}{dt} = -k \cdot [D]^n$$

$$\frac{d[P]}{dt} = k \cdot [D]^n \approx k \cdot [D_0]^n$$

This is, however, not the case when the reaction is reversible or one of the reactants (e.g., an impurity in excipient or water) is limiting or if the degradation product further degrades to other products. A common degradation pattern in pharmaceutical systems is rapid initial decay via first order kinetics, followed by leveling to a pseudo-equilibrium level.[70] This is observed when the reaction is dependent upon a depleting constituent of the system, such as water or small quantities of reactive impurities in the drug or excipients. Slowing of first-order decay kinetics to a pseudo-equilibrium level is also observed in solid–solid surface reactions, where impurity accumulation on the surface is responsible for the slowdown. First-order degradation kinetics with pseudo-equilibrium phenomena were reported by Carstensen for thiamine hydrochloride in microcrystalline cellulose,[71] and by Tardiff for the degradation of ascorbic acid.[72] Drug degradation can often lead to the formation of more than one impurity. Such cases necessitate the determination of reaction pathways, mechanisms, and kinetics to comprehend the overall profile of drug degradation. Drug reaction pathways can be diverse, and some of the examples include the zero-order degradation of aspirin in suspension;[73] first-order hydrolysis of triazolam;[74] second-order interaction of isoniazid with reducing sugars;[75] consecutive first-order degradation reactions of hydrocortisone hemisuccinate;[76] and the reversible and parallel degradation pathways of pilocarpine solution in the neutral pH region.[77]

Drug degradation pathways and patterns in the solid dosage forms and blends of powders are often different from those in the liquid state, mainly because of the heterogeneous nature of the systems. The heterogeneity of the solid state, as well as the changes in physical state of the drug and other components with time, leads to additional kinetic restrictions and modifications of reactions occurring in the solid state. Examples of such cases include: (a) diffusion controlled reactions, (b) solid-state reactions rate limited by the formation and growth of reaction nuclei, (c) reactions that form a liquid product, and (d) reactions limited by the amount of adsorbed water.

A diffusion-controlled reaction is modeled by a suspension of drug, D, undergoing an interfacial reaction with the reactant, A, in the liquid phase. In this case, the fraction of the drug that degrades, x, can be correlated with the growth of product phase layer with thickness y over the spherical drug particles of radius r over time, t using the following rate equations:

$$y^2 = 2k \cdot R \cdot ([A]_A - [A]_D) \cdot t$$

$$(1 - (1-x)^{1/3})^2 = \frac{2k \cdot R \cdot ([A]_A - [A]_D)}{r^2}$$

where:

R is the diffusion rate constant.

Note the correlation of increase in the thickness of product phase on the interface with the volume and surface area of the assumed spherical drug particles. This equation was proposed by Jander, and has been used to describe the thermal decomposition of mercuric oxalate, thiamine diphosphate, and propantheline bromide.[78]

Reactions of crystalline drug in the solid state can be limited to the imperfection sites or nuclei in the crystal. Solid-state reactions of this type limit the growth of impurity by the rate of formation and growth of nuclei sites. The initial rate of formation of degradation product, x, often the stage of reaction relevant to pharmaceutical systems, depends on the number of nuclei by the equation:

$$\frac{dx}{dt} = k \cdot N = k \cdot t^n$$

where:

N is the number of nuclei
n is a constant
k is the rate constant.

This equation was used to describe the initial hydrolysis rate of meclofenoxate hydrochloride,[79] propantheline bromide,[80] and aspirin.[81]

Reaction kinetics of solids leading to the formation of liquid products is complicated by reactions occurring in two media: the solid state and the liquid state. In this case, the overall reaction rate is obtained as a summation of the reaction rates in both states:

$$\frac{dx}{dt} = k_s \cdot (1 - x - Sx) + k_1 \cdot S \cdot x$$

where:

S is the solubility of the drug in the liquid state formed

k_1 and k_s are the rate constants in the solid and the solution states, respectively.

In this equation Sx, the product of fraction degraded and the solubility of drug in the liquid phase, represents the molecular fraction of drug in solution, and consequently $(1 - x - Sx)$ represents the fraction in the solid state. This equation can be integrated to its linear form:

$$\ln\left(1 + \frac{S \cdot (k_1 - k_s) - k_s}{k_s}\right) = (S \cdot (k_1 - k_s) - k_s) \cdot t$$

This equation, known as the Bawn equation, was used to describe the decarboxylation rate of benzoic acid and alkoxyfuroic acid derivatives.[83]

Another case of reactions in the solid state are the reactions occurring in the adsorbed moisture layer, which are limited by the amount of adsorbed water. Drug degradation in such cases can be described by the following apparent or real zero-order or first-order equations:

$$\frac{dx}{dt} = k \cdot V \cdot [D] \cdot [H_2O]$$

where:

V is the volume of adsorbed moisture
$[D]$ is the drug concentration
k is the reaction rate constant.

This model was used to explain the degradation of aspirin,[82] sulpyrine,[83] and 4–aminosalicylic acid.[84]

Solid-state reaction kinetics are inherently different from the kinetics of reactions in homogeneous phases, such as the solution state. For example, the reaction mechanism may not be the same throughout the reaction, as exemplified by Zhou et al. in the case of dehydration of nedocromil sodium trihydrate.[85] Also, the model-based approaches frequently fail to uniquely identify the best model that fits the data.[86] These considerations support the use of model-independent or model-free approaches, which enable the calculation of the reaction activation energy, E_a, without model assumptions.

Khawam and Flanagan presented an example of the complementary application of both model-dependent and model-free methods of analyses of solid-state reaction kinetics.[88] They applied these methods to the desolvation of sulfameter solvates with tetrahydrofuran, dioxolane, and dioxane, monitored by thermogravimetry. The authors noted that the application of the model-independent isoconversional analyses helped select the best model using the model-based approach, which otherwise was difficult, given the similar statistical fit parameters. The authors recommended application of the model-independent approach to evaluate fit using the model-based approach in order to select the reaction model that best fits the kinetic data. A detailed discussion of solid-state kinetics is beyond the scope of this chapter, and is discussed in a recent review by Khawam and Flanagan.[87]

6.4 CONCLUSIONS

Excipient compatibility studies are conducted with the primary goal of selecting dosage form components that are compatible with the drug. Methodically-conducted experiments also provide additional information on the stability profile of the drug, and identify degradation products and mechanisms. Furthermore, if the stability of the drug is found to be lacking, strategies to mitigate the instability of the drug can be adopted. The guidelines and principles presented in this chapter would be useful in appropriate design, conduct, and interpretation of compatibility studies to help accelerate formulation development activities and prevent or minimize surprises in drug development.

References

1. Hickey, M.B., et al. (2007). Hydrates and solid-state reactivity: A survey of b-lactam antibiotics. Journal of Pharmaceutical Sciences 96(5), 1090–1099.
2. Rowe, R.C. et al. (2003). *Handbook of Pharmaceutical Excipients*. APhA Publications.
3. Kontny, M.J. (1988). Distribution of water in solid pharmaceutical systems. Drug Development and Industrial Pharmacy 14(14), 1991–2027.
4. Patel, N.K., et al. (1988). The effect of selected direct compression excipients on the stability of aspirin as a model hydrolyzable drug. Drug Dev. Ind. Pharm. 14(1), 77–98.
5. Gore, A.Y. & Banker, G.S. (1979). Surface chemistry of colloidal silica and a possible application to stabilize aspirin in solid matrixes. Journal of Pharmaceutical Sciences 68(2), 197–202.
6. De Ritter, E., Magid, L., Osadca, M. & Rubin, S.H. (1970). Effect of silica gel on stability and biological availability of ascorbic acid. Journal of Pharmaceutical Sciences 59(2), 229–232.
7. Perrier, P.R. & Kesselring, U.W. (1983). Quantitative assessment of the effect of some excipients on nitrazepam stability in binary powder mixtures. Journal of Pharmaceutical Sciences 72(9), 1072–1074.
8. Fielden, K.E., Newton, J.M., O'Brien, P. & Rowe, R.C. (1988). Thermal studies on the interaction of water and microcrystalline cellulose. Journal of Pharmacy and Pharmacology 40(10), 674–678.
9. Ahlneck, C. & Alderborn, G. (1988). Solid state stability of acetylsalicylic acid in binary mixtures with microcrystalline and microfine cellulose. Acta Pharmaceutica Suecica 25(1), 41–52.
10. Yoshioka, S., Aso, Y. & Terao, T. (1992). Effect of water mobility on drug hydrolysis rates in gelatin gels. Pharmaceutical Research 9(5), 607–612.
11. Aso, Y., Sufang, T., Yoshioka, S. & Kojima, S. (1997). Amount of mobile water estimated from 2H spin-lattice relaxation time, and its effects on the stability of cephalothin in mixtures with pharmaceutical excipients. Drug Stability 1(4), 237–242.
12. Burghart, W., Burghart, K. & Raneburger, J. (2004). Solid formulation of levothyroxine and/or liothyronine salts containing controlled amount of water for stability. US Patent No. WO Patent Application Number 2 004 096 177.
13. Hancock, B.C. & Zografi, G. (1994). The relationship between the glass transition temperature and the water content of amorphous pharmaceutical solids. Pharmaceutical Research 11(4), 471–477.
14. Tong, P. & Zografi, G. (2004). Effects of water vapor absorption on the physical and chemical stability of amorphous sodium indomethacin. AAPS PharmSciTech 5(2). Article 26.
15. Chen, J.G., et al. (2000). Degradation of a fluoropyridinyl drug in capsule formulation: degradant identification, proposed degradation mechanism, and formulation optimization. Pharmaceutical Development and Technology 5(4), 561–570.
16. Glombitza, B.W., Oelkrug, D. & Schmidt, P.C. (1994). Surface acidity of solid pharmaceutical excipients. Part 1. Determination of the surface acidity. European Journal of Pharmaceutics and Biopharmaceutics 40(5), 289–293.
17. Stanisz, B. (2005). The influence of pharmaceutical excipients on quinapril hydrochloride stability. Acta Poloniae Pharmaceutica 62(3), 189–193.
18. Crowley, P. & Martini, L. (2001). Drug-excipient interactions. Pharmaceutical Technology Europe 13(3), 26–28. 30–32, 34.

19. Wirth, D.D., et al. (1998). Maillard reaction of lactose and fluoxetine hydrochloride, a secondary amine. Journal of Pharmaceutical Sciences 87(1), 31–39.

20. Lessen, T. & Zhao, D.C. (1996). Interactions between drug substances and excipients. 1. Fluorescence and HPLC studies of triazolophthalazine derivatives from hydralazine hydrochloride and starch. Journal of Pharmaceutical Sciences 85(3), 326–329.

21. Janicki, C.A. & Almond, H.R., Jr (1974). Reaction of haloperidol with 5-(hydroxymethyl)-2-furfuraldehyde, an impurity in anhydrous lactose. Journal of Pharmaceutical Sciences 63(1), 41–43.

22. Ahlneck, C. & Lundgren, P. (1985). Methods for the evaluation of solid state stability and compatibility between drug and excipient. Acta Pharmaceutica Suecica 22(6), 305–314.

23. Schildcrout, S.A., Risley, D.S. & Kleemann, R.L. (1993). Drug-excipient interactions of seproxetine maleate hemi-hydrate: isothermal stress methods. Drug Development and Industrial Pharmacy 19(10), 1113–1130.

24. Thakur, A.B., et al. (1993). Mechanism and kinetics of metal ion-mediated degradation of fosinopril sodium. Pharmaceutical Research 10(6), 800–809.

25. Huang, T., Garceau, M.E. & Gao, P. (2003). Liquid chromatographic determination of residual hydrogen peroxide in pharmaceutical excipients using platinum and wired enzyme electrodes. Journal of Pharmaceutical and Biomedical Analysis 31(6), 1203–1210.

26. Jansen, P.J., Oren, P.L., Kemp, C.A., Maple, S.R. & Baertschi, S.W. (1998). Characterization of impurities formed by interaction of duloxetine HCl with enteric polymers hydroxypropyl methylcellulose acetate succinate and hydroxypropyl methylcellulose phthalate. Journal of Pharmaceutical Sciences 87(1), 81–85.

27. George, R.C. (1994). Investigation into the yellowing on aging of Sabril tablet cores. Drug Development and Industrial Pharmacy 20(19), 3023–3032.

28. Rivera, S.L. & Ghodbane, S. (1994). In vitro adsorption-desorption of famotidine on microcrystalline cellulose. International Journal of Pharmaceutics 108(1), 31–38.

29. del Barrio, M.A., Hu, J., Zhou, P. & Cauchon, N. (2006). Simultaneous determination of formic acid and formaldehyde in pharmaceutical excipients using headspace GC/MS. Journal of Pharmaceutical and Biomedical Analysis 41(3), 738–743.

30. Hartauer, K.J., et al. (2000). Influence of peroxide impurities in povidone and crospovidone on the stability of raloxifene hydrochloride in tablets: Identification and control of an oxidative degradation product. Pharmaceutical Development and Technology 5(3), 303–310.

31. D'Souza, A.J., et al. (2003). Reaction of a peptide with polyvinylpyrrolidone in the solid state. Journal of Pharmaceutical Sciences 92(3), 585–593.

32. Rohrs, B.R., et al. (1999). Tablet dissolution affected by a moisture mediated solid-state interaction between drug and disintegrant. Pharmaceutical Research 16(12), 1850–1856.

33. Claudius, J.S. & Neau, S.H. (1998). The solution stability of vancomycin in the presence and absence of sodium carboxymethyl starch. International Journal of Pharmaceutics 168(1), 41–48.

34. Senderoff, R.I., Mahjour, M. & Radebaugh, G.W. (1982). Characterization of adsorption behavior by solid dosage form excipients in formulation development. International Journal of Pharmaceutics 83(1–3), 65–72.

35. Desai, D.S., Rubitski, B.A., Bergum, J.S. & Varia, S.A. (1994). Effects of different types of lactose and disintegrant on dissolution stability of hydrochlorothiazide capsule formulations. International Journal of Pharmaceutics 110(3), 257–265.

36. Al-Nimry, S.S., Assaf, S.M., Jalal, I.M. & Najib, N.M. (1997). Adsorption of ketotifen onto some pharmaceutical excipients. International Journal of Pharmaceutics 149(1), 115–121.

37. Botha, S.A. & Lotter, A.P. (1990). Compatibility study between naproxen and tablet excipients using differential scanning calorimetry. Drug Development and Industrial Pharmacy 16, 673–683.

38. Rowe, R.C. & Forse, S.F. (1983). Pitting: A defect on film coated tablets. International Journal of Pharmaceutics 17(2–3), 347–349.

39. Swaminathan, V. & Kildsig, D.O. (2001). An examination of the moisture sorption characteristics of commercial magnesium stearate. AAPS PharmSciTech 2(4), 28.

40. Kararli, T.T., Needham, T.E., Seul, C.J. & Finnegan, P.M. (1989). Solid-state interaction of magnesium oxide and ibuprofen to form a salt. Pharmaceutical Research 6(9), 804–808.

41. Ahlneck, C., Waltersson, J.-O. & P., L. (1987). Difference in effect of powdered and granular magnesium stearate on the solid state stability of acetylsalicylic acid. Acta Pharmaceutica Technologica 33(1), 21–26.

42. Eichman, M. L. (1999). Drug-resin complexes stabilized by chelating agents. US Patent Number 5 980 882.

43. Bax, R. P. (1998). Use of a combination of amoxycillin and clavulanate in the manufacture of a medicament for the treatment drug-resistant Streptococcus pneumoniae. US Patent Number 6 214 359.

44. Crowley, P.J. (1999). Excipients as stabilizers. Pharmaceutical Science & Technology Today 2(6), 237–243.

45. Wyttenbach, N., Birringer, C., Alsenz, J. & Kuentz, M. (2005). Drug-excipient compatibility testing using a high-throughput approach and statistical design. Pharmaceutical Development and Technology 10(4), 499–505.

46. Plackett, R.L. & Burman, J.P. (1946). The design of optimum multifactorial experiments. Biometrika 33, 305–325.

47. Durig, T. & Fassihi, A.R. (1993). Identification of stabilizing and destabilizing effects of excipient-drug interactions in solid-dosage form design. International Journal of Pharmaceutics 97, 161–170.

48. Cotton, M.L., Lamarche, P., Motola, S. & Vadas, E.B. (1994). L-649 923—The selection of an appropriate salt form and preparation of a stable oral formulation. International Journal of Pharmaceutics 109(3), 237–249.

49. Landin, M., et al. (1995). Chemical stability of acetylsalicylic acid in tablets prepared with different particle size fractions of a commercial brand of dicalcium phosphate dihydrate. International Journal of Pharmaceutics 123(1), 143–144.

50. Hancock, B.C. & Zografi, G. (1997). Characteristics and significance of the amorphous state in pharmaceutical systems. Journal of Pharmaceutical Sciences 86(1), 1–12.

51. Puttipipatkhachorn, S., Yonemochi, E., Oguchi, T., Yamamoto, K. & Nakai, Y. (1990). Effect of grinding on dehydration of crystal water of theophylline. Chemical & Pharmaceutical Bulletin 38(8), 2233–2236.

52. Takahashi, Y., Nakashima, K., Nakagawa, H. & Sugimoto, I. (1984). Effects of grinding and drying on the solid-state stability of ampicillin trihydrate. Chemical & Pharmaceutical Bulletin 32(12), 4963–4970.

53. Nakagawa, H., Takahashi, Y. & Sugimoto, I. (1982). The effects of grinding and drying on the solid state stability of sodium prasterone sulfate. Chemical & Pharmaceutical Bulletin 30(1), 242–248.

54. Serajuddin, A.T., Thakur, A.B., Ghoshal, R.N., Fakes, M.G., Ranadive, S.A., Morris, K.R. & Varia, S.A. (1999). Selection of solid dosage form composition through drug-excipient compatibility testing. Journal of Pharmaceutical Sciences 88(7), 696–704.

55. van Dooren, A.A. (1983). Design for drug-excipient interaction studies. Drug Development and Industrial Pharmacy 9(1&2) 43–55.

56. Sims, J.L., et al. (2003). A new approach to accelerated drug-excipient compatibility testing. Pharmaceutical Development and Technology 8(2), 119–126.

57. Waltersson, J.O. & Lundgren, P. (1985). The effect of mechanical comminution on drug stability. Acta Pharmaceutica Suecica 22(5), 291–300.

58. Badawy, S.I., Williams, R.C. & Gilbert, D.L. (1999). Chemical stability of an ester prodrug of a glycoprotein IIb/IIIa receptor antagonist in solid dosage forms. Journal of Pharmaceutical Sciences 88(4), 428–433.

59. Guo, Y., Byrn, S.R. & Zografi, G. (2000). Physical characteristics and chemical degradation of amorphous quinapril hydrochloride. Journal of Pharmaceutical Sciences 89(1), 128–143.

60. Hong, J., Lee, E., Carter, J.C., Masse, J.A. & Oksanen, D.A. (2004). Antioxidant-accelerated oxidative degradation: A case study of transition metal ion catalyzed oxidation in formulation. Pharmaceutical development and technology 9(2), 171–179.

61. Katsumoto, K., Ching, T.Y., Theard, L.P. & Current, S.P. (1997). Multi-component oxygen scavenger system useful in film packaging. US Patent No.

62. Huang, T., Gao, P. & Hageman, M.J. (2004). Rapid screening of antioxidants in pharmaceutical formulation development using cyclic voltammetry—potential and limitations. Current Drug Discovery Technologies 1(2), 173–179.

63. Castello, R.A. & Mattocks, A.M. (1962). Discoloration of tablets containing amines and lactose. Journal of Pharmaceutical Sciences 51, 106–108.

64. Cavatur, R., Vemuri, N.M. & Chrzan, Z. (2004). Use of isothermal microcalorimetry in pharmaceutical preformulation studies. Part III. Evaluation of excipient compatibility of a new chemical entity. Journal of Thermal Analysis and Calorimetry 78, 63–72.

65. Giron, D. (2002). Applications of thermal analysis and coupled techniques in pharmaceutical industry. Journal of Thermal Analysis and Calorimetry 68, 335–357.

66. Schmitt, E., Peck, K., Sun, Y. & Geoffroy, J. (2001). Rapid, practical, and predictive excipient compatibility screening using isothermal microcalorimetry. Thermochim Acta 380, 175–183.

67. Selzer, T., Radau, M. & Kreuter, J. (1999). The use of isothermal heat conduction microcalorimetry to evaluate drug stability in tablets. International Journal of Pharmaceutics 184(2), 199–206.

68. Selzer, T., Radau, M. & Kreuter, J. (1998). Use of isothermal heat conduction microcalorimetry to evaluate stability and excipient compatibility of a solid drug. International Journal of Pharmaceutics 171(2), 227–241.

69. Airaksinen, S., et al. (2005). Excipient selection can significantly affect solid-state phase transformation in formulation during wet granulation. AAPS PharmSciTech 6(2), E311–eE322.

70. Antipas, A.S. & Landis, M.S. (2005) In: Drugs and the Pharmaceutical Sciences. Taylor and Francis Group, LLC. pp. 419–458.

71. Carstensen, J.T., Osadca, M. & Rubin, S.H. (1969). Degradation mechanisms for water-soluble drugs in solid dosage forms. Journal of Pharmaceutical Sciences 58(5), 549–553.

72. Tardif, R. (1965). Reliability of accelerated storage tests to predict stability of vitamins (A, B-1, C) in tablets. Journal of Pharmaceutical Sciences 54, 281–284.

73. Blaug, S.M. & Wesolowski, J.W. (1959). The stability of acetylsalicylic acid in suspension. Journal of the American Pharmaceutical Association 48, 691–694.

74. Konishi, M., Hirai, K. & Mori, Y. (1982). Kinetics and mechanism of the equilibrium reaction of triazolam in aqueous solution. Journal of Pharmaceutical Sciences 71(12), 1328–1334.

75. Devani, M.B., Shishoo, C.J., Doshi, K.J. & Patel, H.B. (1985). Kinetic studies of the interaction between isoniazid and reducing sugars. Journal of Pharmaceutical Sciences 74(4), 427–432.

76. Mauger, J.W., Paruta, A.N. & Gerraughty, R.J. (1969). Consecutive first-order kinetic consideration of hydrocortisone hemisuccinate. Journal of Pharmaceutical Sciences 58(5), 574–578.

77. Yoshioka, S., Aso, Y., Shibazaki, T. & Uchiyama, M. (1986). Stability of pilocarpine ophthalmic formulations. Chemical & Pharmaceutical Bulletin 34(10), 4280–4286.

78. Yoshioka, S. & Stella, V.J. (2000). Stability of Drugs and Dosage Forms. Kluwer Academic, New York.

79. Yoshioka, S., Shibazaki, T. & Eijima, A. (1983). Stability of solid dosage forms. II. Hydrolysis of meclofenoxate hydrochloride in commercial tablets. Chemical & Pharmaceutical Bulletin 31, 2513–2517.

80. Yoshioka, S. & Uchiyama, M. (1986). Kinetics and mechanism of the solid-state decomposition of propantheline bromide. Journal of Pharmaceutical Sciences 75(1), 92–96.

81. Hasegawa, J., Hanano, M. & Awazu, S. (1975). Decomposition of acetylsalicylic acid and its derivatives in solid state. Chemical & Pharmaceutical Bulletin 23, 86–97.

82. Carstensen, J.T. & Attarchi, F. (1988). Decomposition of aspirin in the solid state in the presence of limited amounts of moisture II: Kinetics and salting-in of aspirin in aqueous acetic acid solutions. Journal of Pharmaceutical Sciences 77(4), 314–317.

83. Yoshioka, S., Ogata, H., Shibazaki, T. & Ejima, A. (1979). Stability of sulpyrine. V. Oxidation with molecular oxygen in the solid state. Chemical & Pharmaceutical Bulletin 27, 2363–2371.

84. Kornblum, S.S. & Sciarrone, B.J. (1964). Decarboxylation of P-Aminosalicylic acid in the solid state. Journal of Pharmaceutical Sciences 53, 935–941.

85. Zhou, D., et al. (2003). Model-free treatment of the dehydration kinetics of nedocromil sodium trihydrate. Journal of Pharmaceutical Sciences 92(7), 1367–1376.

86. Vyazovkin, S. & Wight, C.A. (1997). Kinetics in solids. Annual review of physical chemistry 48, 125–149.

87. Khawam, A. & Flanagan, D.R. (2006). Basics and applications of solid-state kinetics: a pharmaceutical perspective. Journal of Pharmaceutical Sciences 95(3), 472–498.

88. Khawam, A. & Flanagan, D.R. (2005). Complementary use of model-free and modelistic methods in the analysis of solid-state kinetics. The Journal of Physical Chemistry B 109(20), 10073–10080.

Theory of Diffusion and Pharmaceutical Applications

Yisheng Chen and Douglas Flanagan

7.1 INTRODUCTION

In nature, particularly in gas and liquid phases, molecules are frequently colliding with conservation of momentum. Collisions cause changes in the direction of movement of molecules or small particles, resulting in their random motion. Collisions between molecules and the walls of a container generate pressure in a gas or hydrostatic pressure in a liquid. Random motion of a particle caused by random bombardment by solvent (or gas) molecules due to thermal motion is well-known as Brownian motion. Diffusion is the process by which atoms, molecules or small particles are transported from a region of higher concentration to a region of lower concentration, due to random motion. Brownian motion or diffusion is a primary transport mechanism for small particles ($<0.1\,\mu$m) or molecules when the transport distance is small (i.e., less than a few millimeters). Over larger distances, diffusion is a slow process for material transfer, and other factors like convection are important to obtain significant transport of material in a reasonable time period (i.e., <1 day). In dissolution testing, diffusion and convection are combined processes that generate dissolved drug in solution.

The diffusion process is driven by entropy change, (i.e., $\Delta S > 0$ for diffusion). The process is an example of the second law of thermodynamics; no enthalpy is involved in the process (i.e., no heat or work is required). Diffusion is irreversible, because it can only occur in one direction—from high to low concentration.

The exact movement of any individual molecule (or small number of molecules) is completely random. The overall behavior (i.e., macroscopic) of a large population of molecules ($>10^6$) is quite predictable. Diffusion is a process of mass transport that involves the movement of one molecular species through another (i.e., drug in a gel). It occurs by random molecular motion from one point to another, and occurs in gas, liquid or solid states. Diffusion in liquid, gel or polymeric systems is of primary interest in the pharmaceutical sciences.

The subject of diffusion has been well studied, and a variety of models and their mathematical expressions related to pharmaceutical applications are available in the literature.[1,2,3,4,5,6] This chapter is intended to provide a review of the fundamental theory of diffusion, and approaches for the application of the theory to develop solutions for specific problems in pharmaceutical sciences.

7.1.1 Basic Equations of Diffusion

The two basic equations describing the diffusion process are the Fick's first and second laws.

Fick's first law: the rate of transfer (dQ/dt) of a diffusing substance through unit area (A) in one dimension (x) is proportional to the concentration gradient, $\partial C/\partial x$, as described in Equation 7.1:

$$J = \frac{dQ}{Adt} = -D\frac{\partial C}{\partial x} \qquad (7.1)$$

where:

J is the flux (rate of diffusion)

D is the diffusion coefficient

C is concentration

$\partial C / \partial x$ is the concentration gradient.

The negative sign indicates diffusion occurs in the direction from high concentration to low concentration.

Fick's second law: The rate of solute accumulation or concentration change, $(\partial C / \partial t)$, in an element volume, dV, is proportional to the flux gradient of the solute in the element, (dJ/dV). In other words, the rate of change of the number of molecules in the volume element equals the difference between the flux of molecules entering the element, and the flux of molecules leaving the element.

The mathematical form of Fick's second law can be developed from the first law by the following approach: molecules entering and leaving a volume element by diffusion can occur in three dimensions. The contribution of diffusion in one of the dimensions, x, to the concentration change in the volume element is depicted in Figure 7.1, where the surface area for diffusion remains constant along the diffusional path. By mass balance, the rate of change of molecules in the element can be described by Equation 7.2.

Thus the concentration change in this volume element can be formulated as the difference in fluxes into and out of the element, as shown below:

$$\frac{\partial C}{\partial t} dV = (J_{in} - J_{out}) dA \tag{7.2}$$

Utilizing the relationship of $dV = dA\,dx$, and replacing dx (in the flux expression) with ∂x, the rate of concentration change one-dimensional diffusion can be written as:

$$\frac{\partial C}{\partial t} = \frac{-\partial J}{\partial x} = D\frac{\partial^2 C}{\partial x^2} \tag{7.3}$$

Similar equations can be derived for diffusion in the other two dimensions, assuming that the diffusion coefficient in the volume element is constant. The rate of concentration changes can thus be written as the sum of contributions in three dimensions as:

$$\frac{\partial C}{\partial t} = D\frac{\partial^2 C}{\partial x^2} + D\frac{\partial^2 C}{\partial y^2} + D\frac{\partial^2 C}{\partial z^2} \tag{7.4}$$

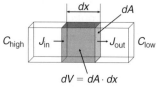

$$dV = dA \cdot dx$$

FIGURE 7.1 Volume element

The above equations are derived for the case where the surface area for diffusion remains constant. If the surface area for diffusion changes, such as the radial diffusion in a cylinder or in a sphere, the area changes must be taken into account. For diffusion in a sphere, Fick's second law is:

$$\frac{\partial C}{\partial t} = D\left(\frac{\partial^2 C}{\partial r^2} + \frac{2}{r}\frac{\partial C}{\partial r}\right) \tag{7.5}$$

For radial diffusion in a cylinder, Fick's second law can be expressed as:

$$\frac{\partial C}{\partial t} = D\left(\frac{\partial^2 C}{\partial r^2} + \frac{1}{r}\frac{\partial C}{\partial r}\right) \tag{7.6}$$

Diffusion can reach a steady state where concentration in a volume element does not change with time, but material still diffuses through the element. Using this criterion, the rate of change of the concentration gradient in the element at steady state according to Fick's second law is zero. For a one-dimensional system with constant surface area, the concentration gradient $(\partial C / \partial x)$ at steady state constant (the concentration profile) is linear with distance along the diffusional path in the system.

If one views Fick's first law as an equation for rate of mass transfer, then Fick's second law expresses the acceleration (or deceleration) of mass transfer.

7.1.2 Solutions for Diffusion Equations

The most fundamental diffusion equation, Fick's second law, is a partial differential equation. This equation must be solved for specific conditions before it can be used to solve practical problems. Mathematical solutions for actual systems can be obtained by taking the initial and boundary conditions of the real systems into consideration. Assuming the diffusion coefficient is a constant, solutions for many systems with different initial and boundary conditions have been derived, either as an error function (or a series of error functions) or as a Fourier series. These solutions can be found in the literature,[1–6] eliminating the need to derive them again. One can thus select the corresponding solution from the literature to fit the specific initial and boundary conditions for a particular system. These can be either infinite or finite systems, with or without perfect mixing (i.e., sink conditions) for the boundary conditions. A number of these cases will be presented and discussed below.

Diffusion from a Plane Source into an Infinite Medium

If a finite amount of solute, M, is deposited on an infinitely thin plane in the middle of an infinite tube of medium (i.e., water or gel), and the solute diffuses axially towards each end of the tube (i.e., one-dimensional diffusion) without mixing, as depicted in Figure 7.2, Equation 7.7 is the solution to Fick's second law for this one-dimensional system, assuming that the diffusion coefficient D is constant at constant temperature:

$$C(x,t) = \frac{M}{2\sqrt{\pi Dt}} \exp\left(\frac{-x^2}{4Dt}\right), \quad t > 0 \qquad (7.7)$$

As indicated in Figure 7.2, the concentration at $x = 0$ becomes smaller with time. At other points where $|x| > 0$, concentration increases with time when $\partial^2 C/\partial x^2 > 0$, and decreases when $\partial^2 C/\partial x^2 < 0$. The area under the concentration distribution curve is constant, because the entire initial mass, M, is retained. However, as t approaches infinity, C becomes infinitely small over all distance values.

Diffusion between Two Infinite Regions in Contact

This system consists of two regions in contact with one of the regions (i.e., $x > 0$) initially containing solute at concentration C_0, and the other region is free of solute (i.e., $C = 0$). Solute diffuses from the initially loaded region into the empty region without mixing. This system can be considered an extended version from the plane source system above by treating the system as containing an infinite number of plane sources of thickness, $\Delta\alpha$, each with an initial concentration, C_0, as shown in Figure 7.3.

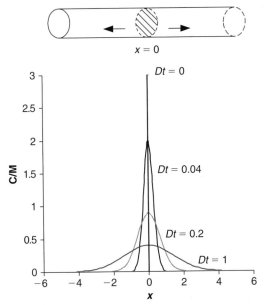

FIGURE 7.2 Plane-sourced one-dimensional diffusion system and the relative concentration profiles as a function of distance and time

The initial conditions are:

$$t = 0, C = 0 \text{ for } x < 0, \quad \text{and} \quad C = C_0 \text{ for } x > 0$$

Obviously, the amount of diffusing molecules in each segment is $C_0 \Delta\alpha$, and diffusion from each infinitely thin segment to the point, α, can be expressed by Equation 7.8:

$$C(x,t) = \frac{C_0 \Delta\alpha}{2\sqrt{\pi Dt}} \exp\left(-\frac{(x-\alpha)^2}{4Dt}\right) \qquad (7.8)$$

By superposition, diffusion from the entire region with initial distribution, C_0, can be obtained by integrating over all the infinitely small elements to obtain:

$$C(x,t) = \int_0^\infty \frac{C_0}{2\sqrt{\pi Dt}} \exp\left(-\frac{(x-\alpha)^2}{4Dt}\right) d\alpha \qquad (7.9)$$

Equation 7.9 can be rewritten in the form of an error function as:

$$C(x,t) = \frac{C_0}{2}\left[1 + erf\left(\frac{x}{2\sqrt{Dt}}\right)\right] \qquad (7.10)$$

Equation 7.10 shows that at the interface where $x = 0$, the concentration is constant at $C_0/2$.

The net amount of material transferred from the initially loaded region into the unloaded region (i.e., across $x = 0$) over time can be calculated using Equation 7.11.

$$Q_t = AC_0\sqrt{\frac{Dt}{\pi}} \qquad (7.11)$$

A is the cross-sectional surface area of the entire system. Note that Equations 7.10 and 7.11 are applicable for infinite regions in contact, or a short time approximation of finite systems with the same initial conditions as the infinite systems. As a short time solution it is assumed that the initially loaded region maintains C_0 at some distance from $x = 0$, and the initially unloaded region is still essentially free of solute at some distance from $x = 0$. The derivation of

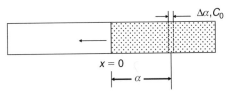

FIGURE 7.3 Infinitely extended region of uniform initial distribution

Equations 7.10 and 7.11, and properties of the error function are given in Appendix 7.4, Section 7.4.1.

Diffusion in Semi-Infinite Systems

If a semi-infinite polymeric gel or a large planar piece of biological tissue initially free of drug is in contact with a well-stirred saturated drug solution as depicted in Figure 7.4, the initial conditions are given by:

$$C = 0, \quad x > 0, \quad t = 0$$

$$C = C_s, \quad x = 0, \quad t > 0$$

C_s is the drug solubility at the interface of the solution and the gel or tissue surface.

Under the above conditions, the drug concentration profile that has diffused into the gel or tissue up to time t can be described by:

$$C(x, t) = C_s \left\{ 1 - erf\left(\frac{x}{2\sqrt{Dt}} \right) \right\} \quad (7.12)$$

The amount of drug that has diffused into the gel over time can be described by:

$$Q_t = 2AC_0 \sqrt{\frac{Dt}{\pi}} \quad (7.13)$$

Comparing Equations 7.11 and Equation 7.13, the rate of diffusion is doubled when half of the diffusion system is well mixed, and maintained at a constant concentration compared to the unstirred system, with all other conditions being the same.

In infinite and semi-finite systems, the concentration profiles are a function of diffusion distance and time; the thickness of the system does not affect the concentration profile until concentration profiles reach either boundary in the semi-infinite system.

Diffusion in Finite Planar Systems

When a planar gel of thickness $2h$, initially loaded with a solute at $C = C_0$, is placed into a well-stirred

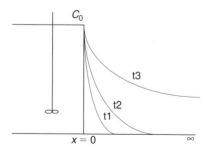

FIGURE 7.4   Diffusion in a semi-infinite system

medium maintained at a zero concentration, drug release occurs with an initial condition of:

$$C = C_0, \quad -h < x < h, \quad t = 0$$

and boundary conditions of:

$$C = 0, x = \pm h, t > 0, \text{ and } \frac{\partial C}{\partial x} = 0, x = 0, t > 0$$

For this finite system, the thickness of the gel does affect drug release. The complete solution for the concentration in the gel as a function of time and distance is:

$$C(x, t) = C_0 \left\{ 1 - \sum_{n=0}^{\infty} (-1)^n erfc\left(\frac{(2n+1)h - x}{2\sqrt{Dt}} \right) \right.$$
$$\left. - \sum_{n=0}^{\infty} (-1)^n erfc\left(\frac{(2n+1)h + x}{2\sqrt{Dt}} \right) \right\} \quad (7.14)$$

The amount of drug released from the gel over time is:

$$Q_t = 2AC_0 \sqrt{Dt} \left\{ \frac{1}{\sqrt{\pi}} + 2\sum_{n=1}^{\infty} (-1)^n \, ierfc\left(\frac{nh}{\sqrt{Dt}} \right) \right\} \quad (7.15)$$

For a small time, when $nh/\sqrt{Dt}$ is large, the *ierfc* terms become negligible, and Equation 7.15 can be simplified to Equation 7.13, which is useful for drug release not more than approximately 60%. This approximation can be understood by considering the fact that at earlier times the middle of the gel is still at C_0, thus the system can be viewed as being a semi-finite system. Therefore, Equation 7.15 can be reduced to Equation 7.13 for short time approximations, even though the systems differ in size.

Using the method of separation of variables (see Appendix 7.4, Section 7.4.2), the concentration in the finite planar systems can be expressed by a series of trigonometric distance and exponential time functions, known as Fourier series, as shown below:

$$C = \frac{4C_0}{\pi} \sum_{p=0}^{\infty} \frac{(-1)^p}{2p+1} \cos\frac{(2p+1)\pi x}{2h}$$
$$\times \exp\left(-\frac{(2p+1)^2 \pi^2 Dt}{4h^2} \right) \quad (7.16)$$

The amount of drug released from the gel is described by:

$$Q = \frac{8AC_0 h}{\pi^2}$$
$$\times \left\{ \frac{\pi^2}{8} - \sum_{p=0}^{\infty} \frac{1}{(2p+1)^2} \exp\left(-\frac{(2p+1)^2 \pi^2 Dt}{4h^2} \right) \right\} \quad (7.17)$$

Equation 7.17 is useful for drug release more than approximately 60%, and can be considered a useful long time solution. The Fourier series in this case is not a convenient short time solution because it requires too many terms to be calculated in the series to obtain accurate concentration profiles, but at longer times only a few terms (or possibly only the first term) are needed for accurate calculations.

Diffusion across a Planar Barrier

In membrane permeation studies, it is common to place a homogenous barrier membrane of thickness h between a donor solution and a receiver solution. The solutions on both sides are well mixed such that the concentration is maintained constant at C_0 in the donor solution, and at zero in the receiver solution (called "sink conditions"). Under these conditions, solute will diffuse from the donor solution through the barrier membrane, and pass into the receiver solution. The initial condition for this system is:

$$C = 0, \quad 0 < x < h, \quad t = 0$$

and the boundary conditions are:

$$C = C_0, x = 0, \quad \text{and} \quad C = 0, x = h, t > 0$$

Assuming a constant diffusion coefficient at constant temperature, the concentration profile of solute in the membrane can be found by separation of variables, and shown to be:

$$C = C_0 - \frac{xC_0}{h} - \frac{2C_0}{\pi} \sum_{n=1}^{\infty} \frac{1}{n} \sin \frac{n\pi x}{h} \exp\left(-\frac{n^2\pi^2 Dt}{h^2}\right)$$

(7.18)

At the early stage of diffusion when time is small, the concentration gradient is non-linear in the membrane, and changes with respect to time and distance. During this stage, sorption of solute by the membrane is the dominant process, because the rate of solute entering the membrane is much greater than the rate leaving the membrane on the receiver side. At longer times, as $t \to \infty$, the sorption by the membrane reaches a constant and the rate of solute entering the membrane is the same as that leaving the membrane. At this point, the solute concentration profile in the membrane becomes linear with distance, and does not change with time. This stage is commonly referred to as steady state.

Regardless of the time, the general equation for the amount of solute passing through unit surface area of membrane up to time t can be calculated by deriving the expression for the concentration gradient (dC/dx), and calculating the flux (J) at $x = h$, and then integrating the flux at this point over time. The resulting equation is:

$$Q = \frac{DC_0 t}{h} - \frac{hC_0}{6} - \frac{2hC_0}{\pi^2} \sum_{n=1}^{\infty} \frac{(-1)^2}{n^2} \exp\left(-\frac{n^2\pi^2 Dt}{h^2}\right)$$

(7.19)

As $t \to \infty$ as steady state is reached, the exponential term in Equation 7.19 becomes negligible, and the rate of solute diffusing through the membrane becomes constant with time, as described by the first two terms of Equation 7.19 shown below:

$$Q = \frac{DC_0}{h}\left(t - \frac{h^2}{6D}\right)$$

(7.20)

By extrapolating the linear profile back to $Q = 0$, an intercept on the time axis is obtained and is:

$$t_L = \frac{h^2}{6D}$$

(7.21)

t_L is commonly referred as the lag time. Steady state is reached asymptotically and is within ~99% of exact steady state at $t = 2.7\, t_L$, which can be used as a guiding line for membrane permeation studies to ensure that steady state is reached, if such a state is desired.

Equations 7.18–7.21 are in fact for a unique case in which the membrane is initially free of solute. In general, the membrane may initially contain solute at a concentration of C_i such that the initial conditions are:

$$C = C_i, \quad 0 < x < h, \quad t = 0$$

$$C = C_0, x = 0; \quad C = 0, x = h, t \geq 0$$

Crank[2] has shown that the general equation for the amount of solute that has diffused through a unit area of membrane is:

$$\begin{aligned} Q = {} & \frac{DC_0}{h}\left(t + \frac{C_i h^2}{2DC_0} - \frac{h^2}{6D}\right) \\ & - \frac{2hC_0}{\pi^2} \sum_{n=1}^{n=\infty} \frac{(-1)^n}{n^2} \exp\left(-\frac{n^2\pi^2 Dt}{h^2}\right) \\ & - \frac{4C_i h}{\pi^2} \sum_{m=0}^{m=\infty} \frac{1}{(2m+1)^2} \exp\left(\frac{-(2m+1)^2\pi^2 Dt}{h^2}\right) \end{aligned}$$

(7.22)

If $C_i = C_0$, as $t \to \infty$, Equation 7.22 approaches the linear function:

$$Q = \frac{DC_0}{h}\left(t + \frac{h^2}{3D}\right)$$

(7.23)

A burst time t_B (actually this is also a lag time) can be obtained by extrapolating the linear release profile to $Q = 0$,

$$t_B = \frac{-h^2}{3D} \tag{7.24}$$

Diffusion in a Sphere

Diffusion in a sphere is a three-dimensional process. The surface area for diffusion changes as mass diffuses radially. Taking this geometry into consideration, the differential equation for Fick's second law of diffusion in a sphere is:

$$\frac{\partial C}{\partial t} = D\left(\frac{\partial^2 C}{\partial r^2} + \frac{2}{r}\frac{\partial C}{\partial r}\right) \tag{7.25}$$

Setting $u = Cr$, it can be shown that:

$$\frac{\partial u}{\partial t} = r\frac{\partial C}{\partial t} \quad \left(\frac{\partial r}{\partial t} = 0\right),$$

$$\frac{\partial^2 u}{\partial r^2} = 2\frac{\partial C}{\partial r} + r\frac{\partial^2 C}{\partial r^2},$$

and Equation 7.25 can be written as:

$$\frac{\partial u}{\partial t} = D\frac{\partial^2 u}{\partial r^2} \tag{7.26}$$

This is exactly the same form as Equation 7.3 and can be solved in the same fashion as for one-dimensional planar diffusion.

For a homogeneous permeable sphere of radius R, initially free of solute and placed in a well stirred solution such that $C = C_0$ at $r = R$, the concentration profile in the sphere is given by:

$$C = C_0\left\{1 - \frac{2}{\pi}\sum_{n=1}^{\infty}\frac{R}{r}\frac{(-1)^{n+1}}{n}\sin\frac{n\pi r}{R}\exp\left(-\frac{n^2\pi^2 Dt}{R^2}\right)\right\} \tag{7.27}$$

The total amount of solute that has entered the sphere up to time t is:

$$Q = \frac{8R^3 C_0}{\pi}\left\{\frac{\pi^2}{6} - \sum_{n=1}^{\infty}\frac{1}{n^2}\exp\left(-\frac{n^2\pi^2 Dt}{R^2}\right)\right\} \tag{7.28}$$

Diffusion in a Cylinder

Assuming that axial diffusion through the two ends of a cylinder is negligible, radial diffusion in a cylinder is a two-dimensional diffusion system. The partial differential equation for this case has been given by Equation 7.6. Similar to the one-dimensional diffusion problems, solutions for radial diffusion in a cylinder can be derived using the error function or by separation of variables, which result in Bessel function solutions. Bessel function solutions may appear more complicated than those derived for the one-dimensional diffusion systems, but there are expressions available for numerous cylindrically symmetrical systems. Interested readers are referred to literature for the detailed mathematical treatments for general solutions. A simple case discussed here is the steady state radial diffusion through the wall of a hollow cylinder.

For outward diffusion through the wall of a hollow cylinder with inner radius a, and outer radius b, and with the concentration profile maintained constant at C_0 at $r = a$, and $C = 0$ at $r = b$, the steady state expression is:

$$D\left\{\frac{\partial^2 c}{\partial r^2} + \left(\frac{1}{r}\right)\frac{\partial c}{\partial r}\right\} = 0 \tag{7.29}$$

The general solution is:

$$C = A + B\ln r \tag{7.30}$$

From the boundary conditions, it can be determined that:

$$B = \frac{C_0}{\ln(a/b)}, \quad \text{and} \quad A = -\frac{C_0\ln b}{\ln(a/b)}$$

Therefore, the solution for $C(x, t)$ is:

$$C = \frac{C_0\ln(r/b)}{\ln(a/b)} \tag{7.31}$$

The quantity of drug released (Q) through $r = b$ into a perfect sink as a function of time is given by:

$$Q = \frac{ADC_0 t}{\ln(a/b)} \tag{7.32}$$

Equation 7.32 shows that, at steady state, the rate of diffusion through the wall of a hollow cylinder is constant, as expected, but the concentration profile as given by Equation 7.31 is non-linear.

Diffusion Combined with Other Processes

Diffusion and adsorption

Adsorption of diffusing molecules in some systems, such as in a reinforced polymer matrix or onto solids in suspensions, can occur during the diffusion process. For example, silicon dioxide or other fillers in reinforced polymeric membranes can adsorb the diffusant during membrane permeation. Adsorption leads to the immobilization of some of the diffusing substance, hence reducing the driving force and diffusion rate until adsorption reaches equilibrium with the free solute concentration at each position in the membrane.

Typically, the amount of substance immobilized by the adsorbent is determined by the adsorption isotherm, which is a function of the free concentration of the diffusant. To account for the adsorption, Fick's second law for one-dimensional diffusion is modified to give:

$$\frac{\partial C}{\partial t} = D \frac{\partial^2 C}{\partial x^2} - \frac{V_f}{\varepsilon} \frac{\partial A_d}{\partial t} \qquad (7.33)$$

Where A_f represents the sorption isotherm of the adsorbent, V_f is the volume fraction of adsorbent in the membrane, and ε is the porosity of the continuous polymeric phase.

In this case, the lag time for diffusion has been shown to be:

$$t_L = \frac{\tau^2 h^2}{6D} + \frac{1}{DC_0} \frac{V_f}{\varepsilon} \int_0^{\tau h} x A_f \, d_x \qquad (7.34)$$

h is the thickness of the membrane, and τ is the tortuosity due to the presence of the impermeable filler.

Equation 7.34 shows that lag time for membrane diffusion can be increased significantly, due to increasing tortuosity and adsorption by the filler. The effects of filler on lag time have also been verified by experimental results. Chen[7] studied the diffusion of 2-hydroxypyridine through polydimethylsiloxane (PDMS) membranes with different levels of silica filler. It was shown that lag time increased by ~10-fold by adding 23% silica filler into the PDMS membrane with thickness similar to the unfilled one. The lag time calculated agreed well with the predicted value from Equation 7.34. The filler effect on steady state flux, on the other hand, is substantially less than the effect on lag time. After adsorption reaches equilibrium at each point in the membrane, the steady state flux through the membrane containing 23% of the filler is ~50% of the unfilled one (Figure 7.5).

Diffusion and chemical reactions

If a chemical reaction occurs simultaneously with diffusion, the reaction reduces the free diffusant concentration. Similar to the adsorption problem, Fick's second law expression is reduced by the reaction rate R as described by:

$$\frac{\partial C}{\partial t} = D \frac{\partial^2 C}{\partial x^2} - R \qquad (7.35)$$

If the rate of reaction is simple (i.e., first-order) and is directly proportional to the rate of concentration change as a function of time ($R = k\partial C/\partial t$) the above equation can be rewritten as:

$$\frac{\partial C}{\partial t} = \frac{D}{1+k} \frac{\partial^2 C}{\partial x^2} = D' \frac{\partial^2 C}{\partial x^2} \qquad (7.36)$$

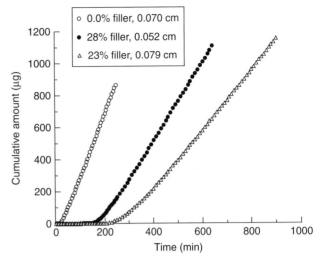

FIGURE 7.5 Flux of 2-hydroxypyridine through polydimethylsiloxane membranes with different levels of silica filler

D' is the reduced diffusion coefficient due to reaction. It can be seen from Equation 7.36 that the mathematical solution for diffusion coupled with a simple first-order reaction is the same as a simple diffusion process without reaction, except that the diffusion coefficient is reduced.

For reaction rates other than the above simple case, more complex solutions can be developed based on the applicable rate law, and the initial and boundary conditions for the diffusion–reaction process. Readers are referred to the literature[1-5] for details on more complicated diffusion–reaction problems.

7.2 THE DIFFUSION COEFFICIENT AND ITS DETERMINATION

From Fick's first law, the diffusion coefficient D can be defined as the rate of transfer of the diffusing substance across unit area and unitary concentration gradient of diffusing substance. From this definition, it can be shown that the diffusion coefficient has units of length^2/time, which is commonly expressed in cm^2/s. The diffusion coefficient is a property of a solute in a particular medium or matrix at constant temperature and pressure. It is dependent on temperature, viscosity, and the size of solute, as described by the Einstein equation:

$$D = \frac{k_B T}{6\pi\eta r} \qquad (7.37)$$

where:

k_B is Boltzmann's constant
T is the absolute temperature

η is the medium viscosity

r is the solute radius.

If all the values of the parameters on the right hand side of Equation 7.37 are known, the diffusion coefficient can be calculated.

For a given solute in a given medium, the dependency of the diffusion coefficient on temperature is described by:

$$D = D_0 \exp\left(-\frac{E_a}{RT}\right) \qquad (7.38)$$

D_0 is the hypothetical diffusion coefficient at infinite temperature and E_a is the activation energy of diffusion.

Assuming the diffusion coefficient is not affected by solute concentration the diffusion coefficient can be determined from steady state fluxes and/or lag times from a membrane permeation study or from release data of other well-defined systems at constant temperature. These methods are discussed below.

7.2.1 Steady State Flux Method

As discussed earlier, for membrane permeation with constant surface concentration, diffusion reaches steady state when the solute concentration profile in the membrane becomes linear with respect to distance. At steady state, the flux is proportional to the diffusion coefficient and concentration gradient as shown below:

$$J_{ss} = Dk\frac{\Delta C}{h} \qquad (7.39)$$

where:

J_{ss} is steady state flux

k is the partition coefficient

ΔC is the concentration difference between the donor and the receiver solutions.

If membrane permeation is conducted in aqueous solutions, the membrane may be covered by stagnant aqueous layers at the membrane–solution interface, either due to a significant partition rate into the membrane from the aqueous donor solution or by the poor hydrodynamics of mixing at the interface. Assuming that the thicknesses of the stagnant layers on both sides of the membrane are the same, a general flux equation is given by:

$$J_{ss} = \frac{\Delta C}{h_m/D_m k + 2h_a/D_a} = \frac{\Delta C}{(1/P_m) + (2/P_a)} \qquad (7.40)$$

The subscripts m and a indicate membrane and aqueous solutions, respectively, and P is the permeability coefficient.

Equation 7.40 shows that flux could be determined for the membrane with stagnant diffusion layers and depending on the properties of the membrane (i.e., thickness and partition coefficient) the aqueous diffusion layers may or may not contribute significantly to the overall flux. If $h_m/D_m k \gg 2h_a/D_a$, diffusion is controlled by the membrane. If $h_m/D_m k \ll 2h_a/D_a$, diffusion is controlled by the stagnant diffusion layers. It has been reported, under some common study conditions, the thickness of the stagnant aqueous diffusion layers are ~100 um. However, the thickness of these stagnant layers decreases as the agitation rate increases. If a membrane has sufficient thickness, and the study is conducted with a high stirring rate, the boundary layer effects may be negligible, although this assumption must be verified by experiment. Once proven that the boundary layer effects are negligible, the diffusion coefficient in a homogeneous polymer membrane can be calculated from the steady state flux data as shown below:

$$D_m = \frac{J_{ss}h}{k\Delta C} \qquad (7.41)$$

If the effect of the boundary layer effects is not negligible, additional experimentation must be conducted in order to obtain a reliable membrane diffusion coefficient. By determination of the total apparent permeability at constant temperature and constant stirring rate for membranes of different thickness,[8] the intrinsic membrane permeability can be calculated from the intercept of a graph of the reciprocal of apparent permeability coefficient P_{total} against the reciprocal of membrane thickness as described by:

$$\frac{1}{P_{\text{total}}} = \frac{1}{P_m} + \frac{2h_a}{D_a}\frac{1}{h_m} \qquad (7.42)$$

In order to obtain accurate diffusion coefficients, it is also important to carry out the membrane permeation experiment for a sufficiently large time to assure that a steady state is reached. As a general guide, flux data used for calculation should be determined at greater than 2.7 × lag time.

If the membrane is heterogeneous with impermeable inert domains, the measured value from steady state flux data is an apparent diffusion coefficient of the composite material. The fraction of the inert filler and the tortuosity must be accounted for to calculate an accurate diffusion coefficient of the continuous membrane phase according to:

$$D_{eff} = D\frac{V}{\tau} \qquad (7.43)$$

7.2.2 Lag Time Method

As discussed previously, when a membrane initially free of solute is used to conduct a permeation study with the concentration in the donor solution kept constant, and the receiver solution kept at zero concentration, the diffusion coefficient can be calculated from the lag time by:

$$D = \frac{h^2}{6t_L} \quad (7.44)$$

If the membrane contains inert fillers, the lag time is increased by the tortuosity, which must be taken into consideration for calculation of diffusion coefficient as:

$$D = \frac{\tau^2 h^2}{6t_L} \quad (7.45)$$

Care should be taken when a thin membrane is used to conduct a diffusion study in an aqueous solution. As discussed above, diffusion may be controlled by the aqueous boundary diffusion layer for some systems. In the extreme case when $h_m/D_m k \ll 2h_a/D_a$, the lag time is determined by the boundary layers as:

$$t_L = \frac{2h_a^2}{3D_a} \quad (7.46)$$

Obviously, the diffusion coefficient of the membrane could not be calculated from the lag time when the process is controlled by the stagnant layers.

If the membrane is initially equilibrated with the donor solution prior to initiation of the permeation study, there will be no lag time for permeation, but instead a negative burst time t_B, and the diffusion coefficient can be calculated from the burst time by:

$$D = \frac{-h^2}{3t_B} \quad (7.47)$$

When the membrane contains adsorptive fillers or some other domains capable of binding the diffusing substance, the lag time is the combined result of diffusion in the polymer, and adsorption or binding in the system; hence Equations 7.44–7.46 are no longer valid for calculation of diffusion coefficient. This is particularly important for biological membranes, because in many cases proteins in biological membranes can bind many kinds of organic compounds. For adsorptive and binding systems, the effects of adsorption or binding on the lag time, and hence on the diffusion coefficient, must be accounted for by using Equation 7.34 or modified versions of it.

If the adsorption isotherm of the filler is a simple linear equation as a function of the steady state concentration distribution (C_s) in the membrane as:

$$A_f = bC_s = bC_0 \left(1 - \frac{x}{h}\right) \quad (7.48)$$

then Equation 7.34 can be integrated. The result of the corrected lag time relationship with tortuosity and adsorption due to the presence of filler is given by:

$$t_L = \frac{\tau^2 h^2}{6D} \left(1 + b\frac{V_f}{\varepsilon}\right) \quad (7.49)$$

Thus, the diffusion coefficient can be expressed as:

$$D = \frac{\tau^2 h^2}{6t_L} \left(1 + b\frac{V_f}{\varepsilon}\right) \quad (7.50)$$

7.2.3 Sorption and Desorption Methods

Data from either absorption by the matrix or release/desorption from the matrix have frequently been used to determine the diffusion coefficient in polymer membranes. The exponential series given by Equation 7.17 can be used to determine the diffusion coefficients by curve fitting.

The short time approximation for Equation 7.15, as in Equation 7.13, is more convenient to use for the determination of the diffusion coefficient than from using both the initial sorption and desorption data. From the slope of the Qt versus $\sqrt{t}$ plot for the early release or sorption data, the diffusion coefficient can be calculated using Equation 7.51:

$$D = \frac{\pi k^2}{4C_0^2} \quad (7.51)$$

where:
k is the slope of the Qt versus $\sqrt{t}$ plot
C_0 is the initial concentration in the matrix in the case of release.

For a heterogeneous system with impermeable domains, Equation 7.51 must be corrected for porosity and tortuosity:

$$D = \frac{\tau\pi k^2}{4\varepsilon^2 C_0^2} \quad (7.52)$$

Theoretically, different methods should yield the same value for the same solute in the same polymer. However, if the polymer contains adsorptive domains, the results may not agree with each other, due to the difference in the free concentration of solute available for diffusion. This is due to the fact that adsorption or binding may be effective during the initial sorption study, but not during the early release stage. Therefore, it is important to understand and characterize the system before valid conclusions can be drawn.

7.3 PHARMACEUTICAL APPLICATIONS

7.3.1 Controlled Release

The study and design of different controlled release systems is probably the most important application of diffusion theory in pharmaceutical science. The critical part in such an application is modeling of the moving diffusion front in pharmaceutical systems. When a drug is completely dissolved in a homogeneous system, drug release into sink conditions can be described using the theoretical equations, such as Equations 7.17 or 7.28 discussed earlier, depending on the geometry of the system. When the system contains solid drug particles, the effects of excess solid drug substance sustaining the diffusion front, and hence the rate of drug release, must also be considered. The key approach to handle excess solid drug in the system is the application of diffusion theory in combination with the mass balance principle.

Release from Planar Matrix

For a planar matrix containing suspended drug particles, the release process can be described by the Higuchi equations.[9] The assumptions for drug release from this type of matrix system are:

1. drug loading is substantially higher than the solubility in the matrix;
2. a pseudo-steady state exists for drug release;
3. the drug particles are small compared to the average distance of diffusion;
4. drug releases into a sink condition; and
5. the diffusion rate out of the matrix is the rate-limiting step for drug release.

A schematic of drug release from a planar system containing suspended drug particles is shown in Figure 7.6.

By mass balance, the amount of drug released dQ from the depleted zone with thickness dh can be expressed as:

$$dQ = A\left(W - \frac{C_s}{2}\right)dh \qquad (7.53)$$

where:

A is the surface area
W stands for the total concentration of drug loading
C_s is the solubility in the matrix.

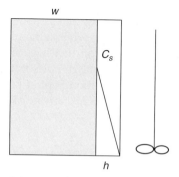

FIGURE 7.6   Schematic of drug release under sink condition for a planar matrix containing suspended drug particles

According to diffusion theory, the amount released during steady state can also be expressed by:

$$dQ = \frac{ADC_s}{h} dt \qquad (7.54)$$

Substituting Equation 7.54 into Equation 7.53, the thickness of the depleted zone h can be calculated by:

$$h = 2\sqrt{\frac{DC_s t}{2W - C_s}} \qquad (7.55)$$

Once the thickness is known, the amount of drug release over time can be calculated using:

$$Q = A\sqrt{(2W - C_s)DC_s t} \qquad (7.56)$$

When drug loading is substantially higher than solubility, Equation 7.56 is simplified to:

$$Q = A\sqrt{2WDC_s t} \qquad (7.57)$$

Equations 7.56 and 7.57 are the well-known Higuchi equations. These equations are applicable for drug release from a non-swelling or non-eroding matrix by diffusion uniformly through the matrix base.

For a hydrophilic drug loaded in a hydrophobic matrix system, diffusion through the matrix is not the main route for drug release. Instead, drug release mainly occurs by diffusion through the hydrophilic channels created after the drug particles dissolve and diffuse away from the matrix. In this case, the Higuchi equation is modified as:

$$Q = A\sqrt{2W \frac{\varepsilon D_a}{\tau} C_a t} \qquad (7.58)$$

where:

ε is the porosity
τ is the tortuosity
D_a and C_a are the diffusion coefficient and solubility in the aqueous medium respectively.

Release from a Spherical Matrix

Pharmaceutical dosage forms are rarely planar except for some patches for topical application. Solid dosage forms are more or less cylindrical or spherical. Drug release from the non-planar geometry of dosage forms is affected by the moving boundary, and the changing surface area for diffusion. The change in the surface area can be accounted for by using the geometric formula in the equation. Therefore, the approach of considering diffusion theory and mass balance simultaneously is applicable for finding the solution for drug release from suspended systems with different geometries. Higuchi's equation[10] for release from a spherical matrix bead of radius of r_0 suspended with drug particles at a concentration of W is derived as follows. All the assumptions for the planar matrix above are applied for this case. Assuming that $W \gg C_s$, by mass balance the quantity of drug released from the depleted layer is:

$$Q = Q_{r_0} - Q_r = \frac{4}{3}\pi W(r_0^3 - r^3)$$

$$\frac{dQ}{dt} = -4\pi r^2 W \frac{dr}{dt} \tag{7.59}$$

By diffusion theory, we know that flux at the diffusion front is:

$$\frac{dQ}{dt} = -AD\frac{dC}{dr} = -4\pi r^2 D\frac{dC}{dr} \tag{7.60}$$

There are too many unknown variables in Equation 7.60, and it must be simplified. The equation can be rearranged to:

$$\frac{dQ}{dt}\frac{dr}{r^2} = -4\pi D\,dC \tag{7.61}$$

Integration with respect to r and C leads to:

$$\frac{dQ}{dt} = \frac{4\pi DC_s}{\left(\dfrac{1}{r} - \dfrac{1}{r_0}\right)} \tag{7.62}$$

Substituting Equation 7.62 into Equation 7.59 and rearranging, one gets:

$$\left(\frac{r^2}{r_0} - r\right)W\,dr = DC_s\,dt \tag{7.63}$$

Equation 7.63 can be integrated to result in:

$$\frac{r^3}{3r_0} - \frac{r^2}{2} + \frac{r_0^2}{6} = \frac{DC_s}{W}t \tag{7.64}$$

The fraction F of drug release from the bead can thus be expressed as:

$$F = \frac{-DC_s}{Wr_0^2}t + \frac{3}{2}\left(1 - \frac{r^2}{r_0^2}\right) \tag{7.65}$$

Release from Matrixes of Other Geometries

The approach of combining diffusion theory with the mass balance principle is the key to developing solutions for controlled release systems. The approach can also be used to design new systems to achieve some desired release profiles. For example, Langer[11] developed a drug-loaded hemisphere with a dimple (empty inner hemisphere cocentered with the drug-loaded outer hemisphere) in the center of the planar surface of the hemisphere. The hemisphere was coated with an impermeable coating, except for the surface of the inner hemisphere dimple. Drug release occurs by inward diffusion through the dimple surface. The radial surface area at the diffusion front inside the drug-loaded hemisphere increases as the diffusion front advances. The increase of release surface area at the diffusion front compensates for the slowing effect of increasing diffusion distance, leading to a linear release profile. Langer showed that the mathematical solution by application of diffusion theory and the mass balance principle for the outward advancing diffusion radius r in the dimpled hemisphere system is:

$$\frac{r^3}{3r_0^3} - \frac{r^2}{2r_0^2} + \frac{1}{6} = \frac{DC_s}{Wr_0^2}t \tag{7.66}$$

where:
  r_0 is the radius of the dimple opening
  W is the drug loading in the matrix.

For $r \gg r_0$, the solution is:

$$\frac{r^3}{3} - \frac{r_0^3}{3} = \frac{DC_s}{Wr_0^2}t \tag{7.67}$$

The quantity of drug released over time is:

$$t = \frac{Q + \pi W r_0^3 - \frac{1}{2}(2\pi W r_0^3)^{1/3}(3Q + 2\pi W r_0^3)^{2/3}}{2\pi DC_s r_0} \tag{7.68}$$

Solutions for other systems, such as truncated cone, hollow cylinder or stadium-shaped matrix, etc., have also been developed. Results are available in literature.

7.3.2 Particle Dissolution

Diffusion theory has played a critical role in the study of the dissolution rate of solid particles. The difference in mathematical treatment for dissolution, compared with drug release, is that the diffusion path is assumed fixed for dissolution, while the diffusion path is increasing for drug release from matrixes.

Assumptions for application of diffusion theory for particle dissolution are that there is a stagnant diffusion layer surrounding the solid particles, and that the dissolution rate of the solid particles is controlled by diffusion of solute through the stagnant layer. Different assumptions about the thickness of the diffusion layer, and the concentration gradient of solute across the layer surrounding a mono dispersed spherical particle, lead to the development of different models for particle dissolution. These models are summarized in the following sections.

Cube Root Model

For large particles, the dissolution rate was found to be proportional to the difference between solubility and the bulk concentration of the solute, as described by the Noyes–Whitney equation:[12]

$$\frac{dQ}{dt} = k(C_s - C_b) \qquad (7.69)$$

where:

k is a proportionality constant
C_s is the solubility of the drug substance in the medium
C_b is the concentration in the bulk medium.

Subsequently, it was shown that proportionality constant k could be related to the thickness of the diffusion layer h surrounding the particle, the diffusion coefficient in the layer, and the surface area of the particle according to diffusion theory, assuming that the concentration gradient across the diffusion layer is linear. Therefore, the dissolution rate is determined by the diffusion rate through the layer, as described by the Nernst–Brunner model:[13]

$$\frac{dQ}{dt} = \frac{DA}{h}(C_s - C_b) \qquad (7.70)$$

When the bulk concentration is maintained at a sink condition, which is commonly assumed to be not more than 10% of the solubility, C_b can be ignored, and Equation 7.70 is simplified to:

$$\frac{dQ}{dt} = \frac{DA}{h}C_s \qquad (7.71)$$

For large particles, the diffusion layer on the particle surface can be approximated as planar when the thickness of the layer is substantially smaller than the particle diameter. Considering a spherical particle's surface area ($A = 4\pi r^2$), density (ρ), and the quantity ($Q = \rho V = 4\pi\rho r^3/3$), Hixson and Crowell[14] derived the remaining quantity of a particle during the dissolution process as:

$$Q^{1/3} = Q_0^{1/3} - k_{1/3}t \qquad (7.72)$$

$Q_0^{1/3}$ and $Q^{1/3}$ are the cube roots of the quantity of a spherical particle at time zero and at time t, and $k_{1/3}$ is the cube root rate constant, which is:

$$k_{1/3} = \left(\frac{\pi}{6\rho^2}\right)^{1/3}\frac{2DC_s}{h} \qquad (7.73)$$

The complete dissolution time of a spherical particle is:

$$t = \frac{r_0\rho h}{DC_s} \qquad (7.74)$$

Equation 7.72 is commonly referred to as the cube root equation, which is suitable for large particles whose diameter is substantially larger than the thickness of the diffusion layer.

Two-thirds Root Model

For a small and spherical particle, it can be assumed that the thickness of the diffusion layer is substantially greater than the particle radius, and is constant at all times. With these key assumptions, Higuchi and Hiestand[15] developed the relationship of particle radius with time as:

$$r^2 = r_0^2 - \frac{2DC_s}{\rho}t \qquad (7.75)$$

with the amount undissolved at time t being:

$$Q^{2/3} = Q_0^{2/3} - k_{2/3}t \qquad (7.76)$$

where $k_{2/3} = \left(\frac{4\pi}{3}\right)^{2/3}\frac{2DC_s}{\rho^{1/3}}$

The complete particle dissolution time according to this two-thirds root model is:

$$t = \frac{r_0^2\rho}{2DC_s} \qquad (7.77)$$

General Model

In recent years Wang and Flanagan have derived a general equation to unify previous models for dissolution of spherical particles.[16] In Wang and Flanagan's study, it was assumed that:

1. particles are spherical and dissolve isotropically;
2. the diffusion layer thickness is constant;
3. dissolution occurs in sink conditions;
4. the solid–liquid interface saturated concentration C_s and diffusion coefficient are constant; and
5. a pseudo-steady state exists.

The concentration gradient across the diffusion layer on the surface of the particle was determined to be:

$$\frac{\partial C}{\partial r} = -C_s \left(\frac{1}{a} + \frac{1}{h} \right) \qquad (7.78)$$

By diffusion theory and the mass balance principle, the general equation for particle dissolution is:

$$t = \frac{\rho h}{DC_s} \left(r_0 - r - h \ln \frac{h + r_0}{h + r} \right) \qquad (7.79)$$

And the complete particle dissolution time is:

$$t = \frac{\rho h}{DC_s} \left(r_0 - h \times \ln \frac{(h + r_0)}{h} \right) \qquad (7.80)$$

Wang and Flanagan have shown that for small particles the general equation is reduced to the two-thirds root model, and for large particles the equation is reduced to the cube root model.

One of the further applications of dissolution models in pharmaceutical science is the estimation of the complete particle dissolution time for poorly water-soluble compounds to guide product development. Assumptions for the following example are:

$D = 10^{-5} \, \text{cm}^2/\text{s}$, $C_s = 6 \, \mu\text{g/ml}$, $\rho = 1.4 \, \text{g/cm}^3$, $h = 50 \, \mu\text{m}$,

single spherical particle, sink condition, isotropic dissolution. Complete dissolution times for particles with varying diameters were calculated using equations for different models. The results are listed in Table 7.1. These indicate that for poorly soluble compounds, reducing particle size can decrease the dissolution time significantly. The table also shows that for small particles, the general model by Wang–Flanagan and the two-thirds root model by Higuchi–Hiestand produce similar results. For large particles, results of the Wang–Flanagan model are similar to the cube root model by Hixson and Crowell.

7.3.3 Packaging Study

Diffusion theory can also be applied to study the moisture uptake by solid pharmaceutical products

TABLE 7.1 Simulation of complete particle dissolution time

Diameter d (μm)	Complete dissolution time (hours) for a single particle		
	Flanagan Equation 7.80	Higuchi–Hiestand Equation 7.77	Hixson and Crowell Equation 7.74
1	0.01	0.01	1.6
10	0.8	0.8	16.2
20	2.9	3.2	32.4
40	10.3	13.0	64.8
100	49.7	81.0	162.0
1000	1231.8	8101.9	1620.4
5000	7464.8	202546.3	8101.9

during storage in sealed containers. Plastic containers are commonly used for packaging solid pharmaceutical products. These containers are permeable to moisture and other gases. The moisture permeating into the container is then absorbed by the product in the container via vapor phase transfer. Over time, the packaged product may absorb a sufficient quantity of moisture leading to a change of product quality. Moisture uptake by products due to moisture ingression has been shown to be predictable using diffusion theory and the mass balance principle.[17] Assuming that:

1. the moisture content of a product is a function of the equilibrium humidity;
2. moisture permeation through the container is the rate-limiting step;
3. the lag time for moisture diffusion through the container is negligible compared to the shelf life of the product; and
4. the moisture permeability of the container is constant at a given temperature.

Then the amount of moisture permeating into a container must be distributed to different components in the container as described by:

$$P(RH_{\text{out}} - RH)dt = \frac{d}{dRH} \left[\sum_{i=1}^{i=n} q_i f_i(RH) \right] dRH \qquad (7.81)$$

where:

P represents the apparent moisture permeability of the container

RH_{out} and RH represent the % relative humidity outside and inside the container

q_i and $f_i(RH)$ are the quantity and the moisture sorption isotherm of the ith component in the container, respectively.

Rearranging and integrating leads to the $t - RH$ profile inside the container as described by:

$$\int_0^t dt = \int_{RH_0}^{RH} \frac{(d/d_{RH})\left[\sum_{i=1}^{i=n} q_i f_i(RH)\right]}{P(RH_{out} - RH)} dRH \quad (7.82)$$

Once the $t - RH$ profile is calculated, the water content of drug product as a function of time can be estimated by substituting the RH at time t into the corresponding moisture isotherm of the product.

Equation 7.82 can be used as a tool to evaluate any packaging designs prior to conducting stability studies, or to evaluate the container equivalence for post approval container changes. Details for model development and application can be found in Chapter 24.

7.4 APPENDIX

7.4.1 The Error Function and Its Application

For diffusion in a system consisting of two infinite regions in contact with one region initially deposited with a solute at uniform concentration C_0 and the other region initially free of solute, the concentration profile of the solute in the system can be described by:

$$C(x, t) = \int_0^\infty \frac{C_0}{2\sqrt{\pi Dt}} \exp\left(-\frac{(x - \alpha)^2}{4Dt}\right) d\alpha \quad (A7.1)$$

By substitution of variables, namely:

$$\eta = \frac{(x - \alpha)}{2\sqrt{Dt}}, \quad d\eta = \frac{-d\alpha}{2\sqrt{Dt}} \quad (A7.2)$$

When $\alpha = 0$, $\eta = x/2\sqrt{Dt}$, and $\alpha = \infty$, $\eta = -\infty$, Equation A7.1 can be rewritten as:

$$C(x, t) = \frac{C_0}{\sqrt{\pi}} \int_{x/2\sqrt{Dt}}^{-\infty} \exp(-\eta^2) d\eta \quad (A7.3)$$

The error function is defined as:

$$erf(z) = \frac{2}{\sqrt{\pi}} \int_0^z \exp(-\eta^2) d\eta \quad (A7.4)$$

The properties of the error function are:

$$erf(0) = 0, \quad erf(\infty) = 1$$

$$erf(-z) = -erf(z),$$

$$erfc(z) = 1 - erf(z)$$

$$\frac{d}{dz}[erf(z)] = \frac{2}{\sqrt{\pi}} \exp(-z^2)$$

Using the form of the error function, Equation A7.3 can be rewritten as:

$$C(x, t) = \frac{C_0}{\sqrt{\pi}} \int_{x/2\sqrt{Dt}}^{-\infty} \exp\left(-\eta^2\right) d\eta$$

$$= \frac{C_0}{2}\left\{\frac{2}{\sqrt{\pi}}\left[\int_{x/2\sqrt{Dt}}^0 \exp(-\eta^2) d\eta + \int_0^{-\infty} \exp(-\eta^2) d\eta\right]\right\}$$

$$= \frac{C_0}{2}\left\{-erf\left(\frac{x}{2\sqrt{Dt}}\right) + erf(-\infty)\right\}$$

$$= \frac{-C_0}{2}\left\{erf\left(\frac{x}{2\sqrt{Dt}}\right) + 1\right\} \quad (A7.5)$$

Differentiation of Equation A7.5 leads to:

$$\frac{\partial C}{\partial x} = \frac{-C_0}{2\sqrt{\pi Dt}} \exp\left(-\frac{x^2}{4Dt}\right) \quad (A7.6)$$

According to Fick's first law, flux at the interface is:

$$J_{x=0} = \frac{dQ}{A\, dt} = -D\frac{\partial C}{\partial x_{x=0}} = \frac{C_0}{2}\sqrt{\frac{D}{\pi t}} \quad (A7.7)$$

The quantity of solute passing through the interface and released into the region initially free of solute can be determined by integration of Equation A7.7. The result is:

$$Q_t = \int_0^t AJ_{x=0}\, dt = \int_0^t \frac{AC_0}{2}\sqrt{\frac{D}{\pi t}} dt = AC_0\sqrt{\frac{D}{\pi t}} \quad (A7.8)$$

7.4.2 Derivation of Solution by Separation of Variables

Fick's second law for one-dimensional diffusion is

$$\frac{\partial C}{\partial t} = D\frac{\partial^2 C}{\partial x^2} \quad (A7.9)$$

Assuming that the two variables (time t and distance x) in the equation are separable such that:

$$C = X(x)T(t) \quad (A7.10)$$

Then $\dfrac{\partial C}{\partial t} = X \dfrac{\partial T}{\partial t}$, and $\dfrac{\partial^2 C}{\partial x^2} = T \dfrac{\partial^2 X}{\partial x^2}$

Fick's second law for one-dimensional diffusion can be written as:

$$X \frac{\partial T}{\partial t} = DT \frac{\partial^2 X}{\partial x^2} \qquad (A7.11)$$

This can be rewritten as:

$$\frac{\partial T}{T \partial t} = D \frac{\partial^2 X}{X \partial x^2} \qquad (A7.12)$$

Let $\qquad \dfrac{\partial T}{T \partial t} = -\lambda^2 D,$

Then the solution is $T = T_0 \exp\left(-\lambda^2 Dt\right)$

and $\qquad \dfrac{\partial^2 X}{X \partial x^2} = -\lambda^2$

Whose solution is $X = A \sin \lambda x + B \cos \lambda x$

Therefore the solution for Equation A7.10 is:

$$C = X(x)T(t) = (A \sin \lambda x + B \cos \lambda x) \exp\left(-\lambda^2 Dt\right)$$

$$(A7.13)$$

Since Equation A7.9 is a linear equation, the general solution is the sum of all solutions in the form of A7.13 expressed as:

$$C = \sum_{m=1}^{\infty} (A_m \sin \lambda_m x + B_m \cos \lambda_m x) \exp(-\lambda_m^2 Dt) \qquad (A7.14)$$

A_m, B_m, and λ_m are determined by the initial and boundary conditions. For drug release from a planar system with the initial condition being:

$$C = C_0, \quad -h < x < h, \quad t = 0,$$

and the boundary conditions being:

$$\frac{\partial C}{\partial x} = 0, \, x = 0, \, t > 0, \quad \text{and} \quad C = 0, \, x = +/- \, h, \, t > 0$$

It can be determined from the first boundary condition that the sine terms are not needed since:

$$\frac{\partial \sin x}{\partial x} = 1, \quad \text{and} \quad \frac{\partial \cos x}{\partial x} = 0 \text{ for } x = 0$$

Therefore, $A_m = 0$.

By taking $\lambda_m = (2m+1)\pi/2h)$, where m is any integer, both boundary conditions are satisfied by:

$$C = \sum_{p=0}^{\infty} B_m \cos \frac{(2m+1)\pi x}{2h} \exp\left(-\frac{(2m+1)^2 \pi^2 Dt}{4h^2}\right)$$

$$(A7.15)$$

And the initial condition is:

$$C_0 = \sum_{p=0}^{\infty} B_m \cos \frac{(2m+1)\pi x}{2h} \qquad (A7.16)$$

To find the values of B_m, both sides of the above equation are multiplied by $\left\{\cos[(2p+1)\pi x / 2h]\right\} dx$ and integrated from 0 to h as:

$$C_0 \int_0^h \cos \frac{(2p+1)\pi x}{2h} dx$$

$$= \int_0^h \sum_{p=0}^{\infty} B_m \cos \frac{(2p+1)\pi x}{2h} \cos \frac{(2m+1)\pi x}{2h} \qquad (A7.17a)$$

$$\frac{2hC_0}{\pi(2p+1)}\left(\sin \frac{(2p+1)\pi}{2}\right) = \frac{hB_m}{2}, \qquad (A7.17b)$$

for $p = m = 0,1,2,3,$etc

$$B_m = \frac{4C_0}{\pi} \frac{(-1)^p}{(2p+1)} \qquad (A7.18)$$

The complete solution for the problem discussed here is:

$$C = \frac{4C_0}{\pi} \sum_{p=0}^{\infty} \frac{(-1)^p}{(2p+1)} \cos \frac{(2p+1)\pi x}{2h}$$

$$\times \exp\left(-\frac{(2p+1)^2 \pi^2 Dt}{4h^2}\right) \qquad (A7.19)$$

The flux at $x = h$ is:

$$J_{x=h} = \frac{\partial Q}{A \partial t} = -D \frac{\partial C}{\partial x}$$

$$= \frac{2DC_0}{h} \sum_{p=0}^{\infty} \exp\left(-\frac{(2p+1)^2 \pi^2 Dt}{4h^2}\right) \qquad (A7.20)$$

And the amount of drug release over time is determined by integration of A7.20 as:

$$
Q = \frac{2ADC_0}{h} \int_0^t \sum_{p=0}^{\infty} \exp\left(-\frac{(2p+1)^2\pi^2 Dt}{4h^2}\right)
$$

$$
= \frac{8AhC_0}{\pi^2} \sum_{p=0}^{\infty} \frac{-1}{(2p+1)^2} \exp\left(-\frac{(2p+1)^2\pi^2 Dt}{4h^2}\right)\Bigg|_{t=0}^{t=t}
$$

$$
= \frac{8AC_0h}{\pi^2} \left\{ \sum_{p=0}^{\infty} \frac{1}{(2p+1)^2} - \sum_{p=0}^{\infty} \frac{1}{(2p+1)^2} \right.
$$

$$
\left. \times \exp\left(-\frac{(2p+1)^2\pi^2 Dt}{4h^2}\right) \right\}
$$

$$
= \frac{8AC_0h}{\pi^2} \left\{ \frac{\pi^2}{8} - \sum_{p=0}^{\infty} \frac{1}{(2p+1)^2} \right.
$$

$$
\left. \times \exp\left(-\frac{(2p+1)^2\pi^2 Dt}{4h^2}\right) \right\} \tag{A7.21}
$$

Since release occurs from both sides of the system, the total amount of drug release is:

$$
Q = 2AhC_0 \left(1 - \frac{8}{\pi^2}\right) \sum_{n=0}^{\infty} \frac{1}{(2n+1)^2}
$$

$$
\times \exp\left(\frac{-(2n+1)^2\pi^2 Dt}{4h^2}\right) \tag{A7.22}
$$

References

1. Jacobs, M.H. (1967). *Diffusion Process*. Springer-Verlag, Berlin.
2. Crank, J. (1986). *The Mathematics of Diffusion*, 2nd edn. Clarendon Press, Oxford.
3. Berg, C. (1983). *Random Walks in Biology*. Princeton.
4. Cussler, E.L. (1997). *Diffusion: Mass Transfer in Fluid Systems*. 2nd edn. Cambridge University Press, Cambridge.
5. Carslaw, H.S. & Jaeger, J.C. (1959). *Conduction of Heat in Solids*, 2nd edn. Oxford University Press, Oxford.
6. Flynn, L., Yalkowsky, S.H. & Roseman, T.J. (1974). Journal of Pharmaceutical Sciences 63, 479.
7. Chen, Y. (1994). PhD Thesis. The University of Iowa.
8. Hunke, A. & Matheson, L.E. (1981). Journal of Pharmaceutical Sciences 70, 1313.
9. Higuchi, T. (1961). Journal of Pharmaceutical Sciences 50, 874.
10. Higuchi, T. (1963). Journal of Pharmaceutical Sciences 52, 1145.
11. Langer, R., et al. (1983). Journal of Pharmaceutical Sciences 72, 17.
12. Nernst, W. (1897). J. Am. Chem. Soc. 19, 930.
13. Nernst, W. (1904). Z. Physik. Chem. 47, 52.
14. Hixson, A.W. & Crowell, J.H. (1931). Industrial & Engineering Chemistry Research 23, 923.
15. Higuchi, W.I. & Hiestand, E.N. (1963). Journal of Pharmaceutical Sciences 52, 67.
16. Huang, J. & Flanagan, D.R. (1999). Journal of Pharmaceutical Sciences 88, 731.
17. Chen, Y. & Li, Y. (2003). International Journal of Pharmaceutics 255, 217.

Particle, Powder, and Compact Characterization

Gregory E. Amidon, Pamela J. Secreast and Deanna Mudie

8.1 INTRODUCTION

As timelines become tighter, internal and external pressures abound for the pharmaceutical industry. The cost of drug development continues to rise at an alarming rate (with an average cost to market of $800 million per drug), making it imperative to develop drugs in more effective ways to reduce cost and time. Historically, early drug product development has focused on using design of experiments to manufacture numerous "kilogram size batches" to optimize the formulation, and gain a complete understanding of the manufacturing process. This method may produce a high-quality product, but requires the use of large quantities of expensive active pharmaceutical ingredient (API), and results in lengthy timelines.

Since most compounds do not make it through the development stages, a different approach is needed for product development. Recent efforts have focused on using material-sparing strategies to develop early solid dosage forms, such as powder-in-capsule and immediate release tablets. Formulations are developed by characterizating particle, powder, and compacts of API, excipients, and formulations at small scale (50–200 grams). Such characterization, coupled with some predictive tools, allows scientists to understand the important physical, chemical, and mechanical properties of materials to design robust formulations to formulate quickly, at a relatively low cost, and to achieve acceptable exposure in clinical studies. Some of the characterization methods discussed in this chapter are summarized in Table 8.1.

There are advantages and disadvantages to the material sparing paradigm. Using smaller amounts of material will result in a lower cost, but may increase the risk of working with a non-representative sample, which may result in errors. In order to reduce resource requirements, we have proposed strategies to decrease method development time and introduced general guidelines.

8.2 PARTICLE SIZE CHARACTERIZATION

Particle characterization is an important component of data driven formulation development on a material-sparing scale. Particle size, size distribution, shape, and texture can all have an impact on pharmaceutical processing and performance, hence consideration must be given to the impact of these parameters on the robustness of processing. This is true for API, excipients, and formulations (blends and granulations). When characterizing API, excipients or formulations, a representative sample must be obtained. The sample needs to be correctly and reproducibly prepared, and instrumental parameters must be correctly used for the analysis.[1] Each particle sizing method, replete with its own assumptions, will result in a unique measure of particle size and distribution, since a real sample exhibits a range of shapes and sizes whose complexity is compounded when analyzing multi-component systems such as formulations. Since no two methods of particle sizing will result in the same "numbers," it becomes important to distinguish

Developing Solid Oral Dosage Forms: Pharmaceutical Theory and Practice
ISBN: 978-0-444-53242-8

TABLE 8.1　Material-sparing characterization methods

Method	Measured parameters
Particle characterization	
Light microscopy	Size, shape, roughness, size range
Polarized light microscopy	Crystallinity
Scanning electron microscopy	Size, shape, roughness, size range
Sieving	Size, size distribution
Light diffraction particle size	Quantitative size, distribution, span
Powder characterization	
Helium pycnometry	True density
Bulk/tapped density	Bulk and tapped density, compressibility index
Shear cell	Powder flow parameters, flow function coefficient, unconfined yield strength, cohesion, effective angle of internal friction
Compact characterization	
Tablet compaction	Compaction pressure, solid fraction
Indentation test	Deformation pressure, elastic deformation
Tensile test	Tensile strength, compromised tensile strength
Tablet characterization	
Tabletability	Tensile strength—solid fraction relationship
Compactibility	Tensile strength—compression pressure relationship
Compressibility	Solid fraction—compression pressure relationship
Manufacturability	Tablet crushing force—compression force relationship

between different methods, and to use the same type of analysis when comparing lots of API, excipients or formulations, examining differences in performance that process changes make, etc. While many types of analyses for particle characterization are available and possible, this discussion will focus on those methods used in the material-sparing paradigm. Table 8.2 outlines the various techniques used for particle characterization in a material-sparing formulation development process. For those interested in more detailed information on particles size measurements, standard textbooks are recommended.[2]

Particle size measurements vary in difficulty depending on the shape of the particle. Spherical particles, for example, can be fully defined by their diameter. In reality, most particles are far from spherical; however, for certain analyses (such as laser light diffraction, discussed later in this chapter) a solid particle is considered to approximate a sphere. Since this measurement is based on a hypothetical, not actual, sphere and is only an approximation of the true particle shape, it is referred to as the equivalent spherical diameter of the particle.[3]

For other analyses of irregularly shaped particles (such as microscopic evaluation), information about both size and shape is needed. There are several different particle diameters that can be used in the evaluation of particle size; the most common of these are illustrated in Figure 8.1.[4] While length and width are diameters more often used in microscopic evaluation, the equivalent spherical diameter is widely used in laser light diffraction analyses. Another descriptor of particle diameter used in early formulation development is the sieve diameter, which is the width of the minimum square aperture through which a particle will pass.

Descriptors of particle shape include acicular, columnar, flake, plate, lath and equant, and should be included in the characterization of irregularly shaped particles. Degree of particle association (e.g., aggregate, agglomerate), and surface characteristics (e.g., cracked, smooth, porous), should also be noted.[4]

Since most APIs, excipients, and formulations are found in a range of sizes, size distribution of the materials must also be determined. When a bell-shaped curve resembling a normal distribution can describe particle size distribution, it can be described by the mean particle size and standard deviation. Again, however, many pharmaceutical powders do not fall into a bell-shaped distribution. Some are skewed toward the upper end of the particle size range. These powders are better described using a log-normal distribution that, when the data are plotted using a log scale for the size axis, resembles a normal distribution curve. When using a log-normal representation the geometric mean standard deviation, and geometric median particle size, are used to describe the distribution. Other pharmaceutical powders cannot be characterized by a single distribution, and may have bimodal or multimodal distributions. Cumulative frequency distribution curves may also be generated by adding percent frequency values to produce a cumulative percent frequency distribution. Sieving data is often presented in this manner.

8.2.1 Light Microscopy

Light microscopy is perhaps the ultimate material-sparing characterization technique, and forms the basis of the material-sparing approach as it pertains to particle characterization. With only a few milligrams of material, appearance, shape, extent of particle association,

TABLE 8.2   Summary of material-sparing particle characterization techniques

Method	Min, micron	Max, microns	Distribution	Shape	Texture	Grams	Crystallinity
Microscopy							
Light	1	1000	Yes	Yes	Yes	<0.1	**No**
Polarized	1	1000	Yes	Yes	Yes	<0.1	**Yes**
SEM	0.02	1000	Maybe	Yes	Yes	<0.1	**No**
Dynamic image analysis	1	10000	Yes	Yes	No	2–5	**No**
Light scattering							
Laser—wet	0.02	2000	Yes	No	No	1–2	No
Laser—dry	0.02	2000	Yes	No	No	1–2	No
Other							
Sieving	25–50	2000	Yes	No	No	3–5	No

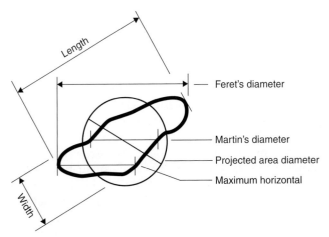

FIGURE 8.1   Particle shape parameters

and texture information may be quickly obtained. With a polarizing light microscope, extent of crystallinity may also be assessed. Particle size distributions (PSD) may be generated from microscopic evaluation, although it is a tedious and time-consuming process. Laser diffraction has become increasingly popular for PSD, and will be discussed later in the chapter. More recently, dynamic image analyzers have been developed which automate the analysis of particle size and shape by capturing images with a camera, transmitting them to a computer system, and then analyzing them electronically. Average particle size, size distribution, and shape information may be generated using this technique. Image analysis may be used for particles in the size range of 1 micron to 10 mm, but requires up to several grams of material depending on the difficulty of method development, and thus far has not been routinely used during the material-sparing formulation process.

For a compound light microscope, the type of microscope generally used, the practical size range is 1 micron to 1 millimeter. This type of microscope is used when fine detail must be resolved. The clarity or resolving power of the image depends on the sharpness of the image produced by the objective lens. Resolving power is defined as the smallest distance between two points such that the two points can be distinguished.[5] The sample is usually mounted in a medium that has sufficient contrast to the sample, and in which the sample is insoluble. The particles should all be in the same plane, be adequately separated from each other, and should represent the size and distribution of the entire sample population.

8.2.2 Scanning Electron Microscopy

Scanning electron microscopy (SEM) is another technique where only milligram quantities of material may be used to determine particle size, shape, and texture. In SEM a fine beam of electrons scan across the prepared sample in a series of parallel tracks. The electrons interact with the sample, and produce several different signals which can be detected and displayed on the screen of a cathode ray tube.[2] Particles less than 1 nm can be viewed, and since the depth of focus is so much greater than that of the light microscope, information on surface texture can be generated. SEM requires more time-consuming sample preparation than optical microscopy, and cannot distinguish between crystalline and non-crystalline materials. It is also more difficult to generate a particle size distribution using SEM since, while the information obtained is visual and descriptive, it is usually not quantitative since only a few particles are seen in the viewing field at one time. However, when SEM is used with other techniques such as laser diffraction, it can provide valuable additional information on particle texture, which may help to explain agglomeration or flow problems.

8.2.3 Sieving

Sieving is a simple method that is used for determining the particle size distribution of a powder. It is often the preferred method of choice for formulators, since it is a straightforward analysis that can be done during the formulation development process (after mixing or granulation of a formulation, for example). This technique is most often used for formulations or excipients since larger quantities are needed (3–5 grams is needed to perform an analysis using small-scale sonic sifting). API is not usually evaluated by sieving due to the particle size limitations, as well as the more irregular particle shapes. Sieving is most suitable for powders whose average particle size is greater than 25–50 microns.[1]

For material-sparing sieving, a sonic sifter using 3-inch sieves is employed. Sonic sieving combines two motions to separate the particles: a vertically oscillating air column to lift particles and carry them back against mesh openings at several thousand pulses per minute, and a repetitive tapping pulse to help reduce sieve blinding. Tapping also helps to deagglomerate samples with electrostatic, hygroscopic or other adhesion problems.[6] The raw data can be converted into a cumulative weight distribution, and the data presented as a percentage of the sample retained on each sieve (histogram) or a cumulative distribution as a function of sieve size. When data is plotted on a log–log plot (sieve size versus cumulative percent), unimodal versus polymodal distributions can also be determined. A detailed procedure for analytical sieving may be found in the USP general method <786 >, Method I (dry sieving).[7]

8.2.4 Light Diffraction

Laser light diffraction (LD) is becoming a preferred method for the determination of particle size distribution of pharmaceutical materials. This technique can be quite material sparing, using 1–3 grams of a material for a complete evaluation. Even less material may be used if combined with a microscopic or SEM evaluation to determine particle size, morphology, and fragility of the sample. There are several advantages to

LD methods. Analysis time is short, robust methods can be developed with a minimum of material, results are reproducible, calibration is not required, and a wide range of measurement is possible. LD technology is divided into two general methods. High angle light scattering is appropriate for very small (submicron) particles, and falls outside the scope of this discussion. Low angle light scattering is used for pharmaceutical materials in the micron size range or greater. Determination of particle size using low angle technology is only effective if one has a model to interpret it with. For particles much larger than the wavelength of light (~5 microns) any interaction with those particles causes the light to be scattered with only a small change in angle. This is known as Fraunhauer diffraction, and produces light intensity patterns that occur at regular intervals and are proportional to the particle diameter that produces this scatter. Fraunhauer diffraction-based instruments are applicable for particle size ranges of about 1–2000 microns, depending on the lens used.

Both wet and dry laser diffraction methods are possible, and are used in a material-sparing process. For dry dispersion LD, initial conditions such as pressure and lens size are determined by microscopy, with a short series of trial runs to assess correct pressure for dispersing particles without fracturing them and to confirm lens size. Too high a pressure may break down some fragile particles. With small tray accessories, these dry methods can use 500 mg or less for a complete analysis. Initial conditions for a wet method rely on a small set of standardized generic methods and microscopy. For wet methods it is important to choose a suspension medium where the sample has low solubility (hexane is often used) that will also disperse the sample adequately. Surfactants are occasionally used to facilitate dispersion and inhibit flocculation of the sample, but it is important to prevent particle dissolution in the surfactant solution. A filtered saturated solution can be used as the dispersing medium to effectively prevent particle dissolution in the medium. Sonication may be needed to break up aggregates, but fragility of the sample must be assessed since sonication may fracture individual particles and skew the results. Sample load is also important as a higher percentage of the sample in the dispersing solvent may cause aggregation.

Whether a wet or dry method is used during material-sparing formulation development depends on several factors, the most important of which are the properties of the material to be tested. Wet dispersion is frequently used for API characterization since it is a one-component system, easily screened for the appropriate non-soluble dispersant. Multi-component systems, such as mixes or granulations, are more amenable to dry dispersion techniques. There is no need to test the solubility of each component in the dispersant, since the dispersant for dry techniques is air. Dry dispersion techniques tend to be used when there is plenty of material available, since developing a method is straightforward with sufficient trial runs. Other factors that determine which method is utilized include operator experience, equipment availability, and personal preference.

8.2.5 Importance/Impact of Particle Size Characterization

Understanding a pharmaceutical powder's particle size, shape, and distribution is an important component of material-sparing formulation development. When working with the API, a few large or small particles in a batch can alter the final tablet's content uniformity (potency, segregation), dissolution profile, and/or processing (e.g., flow, compression pressure profile, and granulating properties if it is for dry granulation). Rohrs et al. have shown that, with only the predicted API dose and the geometric standard deviation, an estimate of the API particle size can be obtained that will have a 99% probability of passing USP Stage I content uniformity criteria. This is displayed graphically in Figure 8.2. It is useful for determining approximate figures for particle size requirements, including whether additional API processing such as milling is necessary.[8] API particle size and distribution data information can also help decide whether a direct compression formulation or dry granulation approach is most suitable. Examination of the API can also reveal inter- and intra-batch differences and/or trends. If, for example, the particle size distribution has changed from one batch of API to the next, this could significantly impact the processability of the final formulation.

Particle size and size distribution are also important, from a dosage form performance point of view, in that they are critical parameters in assuring that the desired dissolution rate is achieved for oral dosage forms. Several theoretical models for dissolution of powders have been developed.[9,10,11] Using a Noyes–Whitney type expression as a starting point, Higuchi and Hiestand,[10] as well as Hintz and Johnson,[11] derived expressions for dissolution of spherical particles as a function of time. While details are beyond the scope of this chapter, it is possible to predict the dissolution rate of poly-dispersed particle size distributions by summing up the predicted dissolution rate of individual size fractions of the powder. For example, using this approach, the predicted particle diameter

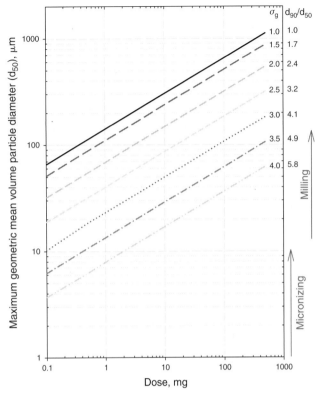

FIGURE 8.2 Content uniformity prediction as a function of particle size, distribution, and dose

necessary to achieve 80% dissolved in a USP dissolution apparatus in 30 minutes under sink conditions as a function of solubility and particle size distribution (sigma = geometric standard deviation of a log-normal distribution) is shown in Figure 8.3.[12] With this information, selection of an appropriate particle size and distribution needed to achieve the desired dissolution rate may be estimated.

Particle characterization of the in-process or final-formulation is also critical. Flow characteristics of formulations (which will be discussed later in the chapter) are based, among other factors, on shape, size, and size distribution of particles. Large, spherical particles flow better than smaller, irregularly shaped materials, for example.

8.3 POWDER CHARACTERIZATION

8.3.1 Density

True Density

The true density of a substance is the average mass of the particles divided by the solid volume, exclusive of all the voids that are not a fundamental part of the

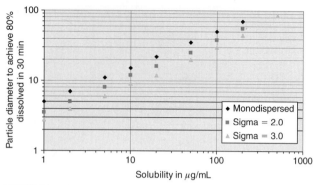

FIGURE 8.3 Predicted particle diameter necessary to achieve 80% dissolved in a USP dissolution apparatus in 30 minutes under sink conditions as a function of solubility and particle size distribution (sigma = geometric standard deviation of a log-normal distribution)

molecular packing arrangement; therefore, it should be independent of the method of determination.[13] There are three basic methods for determining true density:

- gas pycnometry or displacement;
- liquid displacement; and
- flotation in a liquid.

Gas pycnometry is used in the material-sparing paradigm for determination of true density as a small amount of material is used (usually 1–8 g), the method is easy, reproducible and reliable, and the method is non-destructive: that is the material may be reused after testing is complete.

The true density, ρ, can be calculated using Equation 8.1.

$$\rho = \frac{w}{V_p} \qquad (8.1)$$

where:

     w is the weight of the sample
     V_p is the powder volume.

Since the measured density is a volume-weighted average of the densities of all the individual powder particles, errors may be introduced if the gas sorbs onto the powder or if volatile contaminants escape from the powder during the measurement. Sorption may be prevented by using an appropriate gas, usually helium or nitrogen. Volatile components may be removed during purging of the sample, and sample weight is taken before and after purging to determine if volatile contaminants were removed. True density is an essential parameter for process development and solid dosage manufacturing. As discussed in more detail later in the chapter, true density is used to calculate solid fraction.

Bulk Density

Bulk density is the mass per unit volume of a loose powder bed. The unit volume includes the spaces between the particles, and the envelope volumes of the particles themselves. The method used to fill the material into that volume can affect the degree to which the powder is compressed, and can thus influence the bulk density value.[14,15] Bulk density can be calculated using Equation 8.2, where M = mass in grams and V_o = untapped apparent volume in milliliters.

$$\text{Bulk Density(g/mL)} = \frac{M}{V_o} \qquad (8.2)$$

The loose or "aerated" bulk density can be determined by allowing a defined amount of material to fill a container with a known volume under the influence of gravity.[17] The amount to which the particles collapse, and fill voids between the particles, will depend on a number of powder properties, including particle shape, particle size distribution, inter-particle friction, and cohesion.

Bulk density is typically measured by gently introducing a known sample mass into a graduated cylinder, and carefully leveling off the powder without compacting it. The untapped apparent volume is then read to the nearest graduated unit. As most pharmaceutical powders have densities in the range of 0.1–0.7 g/mL, a 25-mL graduated cylinder filled at least 60% full calls for a sample mass of approximately 2–11 g. (Since this test is non-destructive, the material may be reused.) USP requirements dictate a minimum graduated cylinder size of 25 mL.[17] However, if material is in short supply, a 10-mL graduated cylinder may be used. Although wall effects could be observed, this approach provides a reasonable estimate of the bulk density.

Bulk density is an essential parameter for process development and solid dosage manufacturing. It is used in determining the amount of powder that can fit in a space, such as a blender or a hopper on a tablet press or capsule filler. It is also used to determine the amount of powder that can be fitted into a capsule. Previous work has suggested that the effective bulk density of the same material will vary under different dynamics.[14,15]

Tapped Density

Tapped density of a powder is the ratio of the mass of the powder to the volume occupied by the powder after it has been tapped for a defined period of time.

The tapped density of a powder represents its random dense packing. Tapped density can be calculated using Equation 8.3, where M = mass in grams, and V_f = the tapped volume in milliliters.

$$\text{Tapped Density(g/mL)} = \frac{M}{V_f} \quad (8.3)$$

Tapped density values are generally higher for more regularly shaped particles (i.e., spheres), as compared to irregularly shaped particles such as needles. Particle size distribution has been shown to affect the packing properties of fine powders.[16] The packing properties of a powder can affect operations critical to solid dosage manufacturing, including bulk storage, feeding, and compaction.

Tapped density is measured by first gently introducing a known sample mass into a graduated cylinder and carefully leveling off the powder without compacting it. The cylinder is then mechanically tapped by raising the cylinder and allowing it to drop under its own weight using a suitable mechanical tapped density tester that provides a suitable fixed drop distance and nominal drop rate. There are two methods for measuring tapped density in the USP with different drop distance and drop rates.[17] The tap density of a number of pharmaceutical materials is shown in Figure 8.4.[18] As with bulk density measurements, a material-sparing approach can be undertaken by using a 10-mL graduated cylinder (1–4 gram sample requirement). This test is also non-destructive.

8.3.2 Flow

Flow assessment of active pharmaceutical ingredients (APIs), excipients, and formulations are routinely completed as part of solid dosage form development. Assessments must be made to ensure powder will flow adequately through processing equipment such as a roller compactor, hopper or tablet press. Poor flowability can lead to the inability to feed powder into the dies of a rotary tablet press, and can also cause tablet weight variation.

Due to the complexity of powder flow, and the factors that influence it, no single measure is currently adequate for defining flow. Unsurprisingly, many ways to measure flow currently exist, ranging from simple, qualitative methods, to more quantitative methods utilizing specialized technology. Factors such as the relative humidity of the environment, previous storage conditions, and degree of consolidation have a large impact on flowability, any of which can alter the test results.

The influence of physical and mechanical properties on powder flow is a subject of interest to formulation scientists. Factors such as particle size distribution and particle shape have been shown to influence flow.[19,20,21] Additional properties such as bulk and tapped density, bonding index, and internal friction coefficient are also thought to be contributors. An understanding of the effects of physical and mechanical properties on powder flowability can decrease the need to perform powder flowability analysis on some materials, resulting in significant time and resource savings.

An attempt has been made to model flowability based on physical and mechanical properties using complex methods such as artificial neural networks (ANNs), discrete element method (DEM), and constitutive models.[22,23,24] While these models have demonstrated a correlation between certain physical properties and the results of various methods for measuring flow, more work is required.

Compressibility Index and Hausner Ratio

The compressibility index (CI) is a measure of the propensity of a powder to consolidate.[25] As such, it is a measure of the relative importance of inter-particulate interactions. In a free-flowing powder, such interactions are generally less significant, and the bulk and tapped densities will be closer in value. For poorer flowing materials, there are frequently greater inter-particle interactions; bridging between particles often results in lower bulk density and a greater difference between the bulk and tapped densities. These differences in particle interactions are reflected in the CI. A general scale of powder flow using the CI is given in Table 8.3.[25] Compressibility index (CI) can be calculated as shown in Equation 8.4, where V_o = untapped apparent volume, V_f = tapped apparent volume.

$$\text{CI(\%)} = 100 \cdot \frac{(V_o - V_f)}{V_o} \quad (8.4)$$

Although this method cannot be used as a sole measure of powder flowability, it has the advantage of being simple to calculate, and it provides a quick comparison between API, excipients, and formulations. If bulk and tapped density measurements have already been performed, no additional material or experimentation is required to calculate the CI. CI has been correlated to manufacturing performance on machines such as capsule fillers. Podczeck et al. demonstrated a correlation between the minimum coefficient of fill weight variation and CI.[26]

The Hausner ratio (HR) is closely related to CI.[27] It can be calculated using Equation 8.5, where

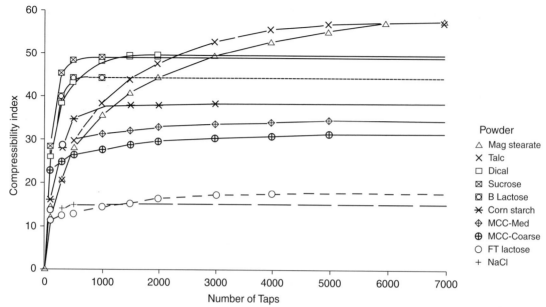

FIGURE 8.4   Influence of number of taps on the compressibility index

TABLE 8.3   Scale of flowability for compressibility index and Hausner ratio[31]

Flow character	Compressibility index	Hausner ratio
Excellent	≤10	1.00–1.11
Good	11–15	1.12–1.18
Fair	16–20	1.19–1.25
Passable	21–25	1.26–1.34
Poor	26–31	1.35–1.45
Very poor	32–37	1.46–1.59
Very, very poor	>38	>1.60

V_o = untapped apparent volume and V_f = tapped apparent volume.

$$Hausner\ Ratio = \frac{V_o}{V_f} \qquad (8.5)$$

Scales of flowability for compressibility index and Hausner ratio are included in Table 8.3.

Angle of Repose and Flow Through an Orifice

The angle of repose has long been used to characterize bulk solids.[28,29,30] Angle of repose is a characteristic related to inter-particulate friction or resistance to movement between particles. According to the USP, it is the constant, three-dimensional angle (relative to the horizontal base) assumed by a cone-like pile of material formed by any of several different methods.

Due to the high dependence of angle of repose measurements on testing conditions, angle of repose is not a very robust means of quantifying powder flow.[31]

Flow rate through an orifice is generally measured as the mass of material per unit time flowing from any of a number of types of containers (cylinders, funnels, hoppers). It is thought to be a more direct measure of flow than measurements such as angle of repose or Hausner ratio, because it more closely simulates flow of material from processing equipment such as from a tablet press hopper into a die. Measurement of the flow rate is heavily dependent on test set-up, such as orifice diameter.[32] Both angle of repose and flow-rate through an orifice methods require 5–70 grams of material, and therefore are not aligned with material-sparing strategies.

Shear Cell Methods

Shear cell methods measure flow on a more fundamental basis than the simple methods discussed above, providing more robust flow results. Shear cell methods allow the assessment of flow properties as a function of consolidation load and time, as well as powder–hopper material interactions.[33] Various types of shear cells exist, including rotational and translational cells.[34,35,36] While shear cell measurements are generally more time-consuming than the methods discussed above, they offer a higher degree of experimental control, leading to more reproducible results. They are used extensively in multiple industries, and significant advances in automation have occurred in the past five years.[37,38,39]

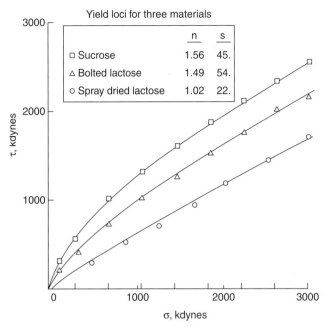

FIGURE 8.5 Yield loci for three materials

TABLE 8.4 Physical and mechanical properties and environmental factors influencing flowability

Physical and mechanical properties	Environmental effects
Particle size distribution	Consolidation load
Particle shape	Consolidation time
Bulk/tapped density	Shear effects (direction & rate)
Particle density	Particle/wall interactions
Moisture content	Air permeability
Crystallinity	Compressibility (a function of load and time)
Polymorphic form	Humidity/powder moisture content
Surface area	Packed density
Electrostatic charge	
Surface energy	
Elasticity	
Plasticity (ductility)	
Viscoelasticity	
Brittleness	

The shear cell analysis method is as follows: a bulk solid sample is carefully loaded into a container or "cell," taking care not to consolidate the powder during loading. The powder bed is typically preconsolidated at a defined load normal to the powder bed. As the load is applied, the powder bed is sheared until a uniform state of consolidation is reached (i.e., powder starts to "flow" and shear stress reaches a constant value). This value of the shear stress represents the shear strength of the powder at those conditions. Once preconsolidation is achieved, the normal load is reduced, and a normal load less than the preconsolidation load is applied. The bulk solid is sheared until the shear force goes through a maximum value and then begins to decrease. This maximum value represents the shear strength of the powder bed under those conditions. This process of preconsolidation, and subsequent consolidation at a reduced load, is repeated multiple times at different normal loads. This process is sometimes referred to as a yield locus test. A yield locus is constructed based on the shear data; it passes through the points defined by the shear and normal stress values during pre-shear and shear. Figure 8.5 shows the yield loci of three different materials, constructed using a simplified (translational) shear cell. The yield locus is characteristic of the physical and mechanical properties of the powder, as well as a number of environmental factors (a list of some of these factors is included in Table 8.4).

In addition to the yield locus, Mohr stress circles are constructed from the shear data to create graphical representations of the relationship between the normal and shear stresses. Mohr stress circles represent the stresses in cutting planes of a bulk solid, which are inclined through all possible angles. These stress circles are defined by Equation 8.6 and Equation 8.7, where σ_y is the stress acting on the element of bulk solid in the vertical direction, σ_x is the stress prevailing in the horizontal direction as a result of the vertical stress, and α is the angle defined by the cutting plane.

$$\sigma_n = \frac{(\sigma_y + \sigma_x)}{2} + \frac{(\sigma_y - \sigma_x)}{2} \cos(2\alpha) \qquad (8.6)$$

$$\tau = \left(\frac{\sigma_y - \sigma_x}{2}\right) \sin(2\alpha) \qquad (8.7)$$

A "small" Mohr stress circle is constructed tangential to the yield locus with its minor principle stress equal to zero. The "larger" Mohr stress circle is constructed tangential to the yield locus, and running through the pre-shear point. The larger Mohr stress circle represents the stress state in the bulk solid sample at steady state flow (i.e. the stress state at the end of pre-shear). These two Mohr stress circles help define the flow properties listed in Table 8.5.[40] An example of a yield locus and Mohr stress circles is shown in Figure 8.6. Some of the most commonly reported shear cell flow properties reported in

TABLE 8.5 Shear cell flow property names and definitions

Flow property	Definition
Major consolidation stress (σ_1)	Defined by the major principal stress of the larger Mohr stress circle.
Unconfined yield strength/stress (σ_c)	Defined by the major principle stress of the smaller Mohr stress circle. It is the stress at which the sample will break (flow) after a vertical stress has been applied to a consolidated sample.
Flow function coefficient (FFC)	The ratio of the major consolidation stress to the unconfined yield strength at a defined normal load.
Flow function	A flow function curve can be constructed by plotting the FFC values obtained by performing multiple yield locus tests at different preconsolidation normal loads.
Slope angle of the linearized yield locus (φ_{lin})	The angle defined by the linearized yield locus. The linearized yield locus is the line that is tangential to both Mohr stress circles.
Effective angle of internal friction (φ_e)	The angle defined by the line that runs through the origin of the diagram, and is tangent to the larger Mohr stress circle.
Angle of internal friction at steady state flow (φ_{sf})	The arctangent of the ratio of shear stress to normal stress of the preshear point (i.e., steady state flow). It characterizes the internal friction at steady state flow in the shear plane.
Cohesion (τ_c)	The shear stress at yield under zero normal stress, i.e. the intersection of the yield locus with the ordinate.

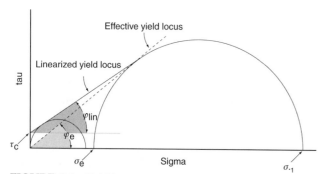

FIGURE 8.6   Yield locus and Mohr stress circle diagram

the literature are the angle of internal friction and the flow function.[41,42]

Because shear methods provide quantitative, reproducible results, the properties defined in Table 8.5 can be used to compare the flowability of different drug substances, excipients, and formulations. To properly compare data, the environmental factors listed in Table 8.4 should be kept constant. For example, Moreno-Atanasio et al. demonstrate an increase in the unconfined yield strength with an increase in preconsolidation stress using a uniaxial compression test. Shear cell methods are also used to characterize the performance of materials on equipment such as capsule-filling machines,[43] and tablet presses.[44] They are extensively used to design hoppers for feeding powders, and to study the effect of storage time on flowability.[45,46] Jenike developed a mathematical methodology for determining the minimum hopper angle and opening size for mass flow from conical and wedge shaped hoppers.[47]

Several different types of shear cell testers are available. The Schulze Ring Shear Tester is an annular or rotational shear tester. The bulk solid sample is contained in an annular shear cell containing a ring at the bottom and a baffled lid. Ring shear testers are considered to be relatively easy to operate, and provide good reproducibility.[40] A single yield locus test can be performed in approximately 30 minutes (of which the operator must be present about one third of the time). Multiple shear cell sizes are available. Depending on the particle size of the powder specimen a small, 10-mL shear cell can be used, allowing for a significant reduction in sample requirements. Medium and large shear cells are also available, which are able to accommodate samples with larger particle sizes. These cell sizes require sample volumes greater than approximately 31 mL and 73 mL, respectively.[48] A standard test method for using the Schulze Ring Shear Tester can be found in ASTM Method D 6773.[49]

The Jenike Shear Tester is a translational tester. The shear cell is cylindrical, and is split horizontally, forming a shear plane between the lower stationary base and the upper moveable portion. It consists of a closed ring at the bottom, a ring of the same diameter lying above the bottom ring, and a lid.[52] An advantage of the Jenike cell over the ring shear tester is that the powder bed is sheared more uniformly.[52] Disadvantages of the Jenike Shear Tester include the amount of material required, and the time required for a test. Depending on the powder, and the operator's skill, one to two hours per yield locus (during which the operator has to be present) are required. Results generated using the Jenike Shear Tester have been shown to correspond to those generated using the ring shear tester.[40] A standard test method for using the Jenike Shear Tester can be found in the ASTM Method D 6128.[50]

Additional Shear Testers

Schulze ring shear and Jenike shear cell testers are used extensively due to their commercial availability, though other shear cells are available. Plate or "simplified" shear cells have also been designed, which consist of a thin sandwich of powder between a lower stationary rough surface and an upper rough surface that is movable.[18,51] Uniaxial, biaxial, and triaxial testers have also been used for flow analysis, and have been discussed in the literature. The measurement principle of the uniaxial tester is similar to that of shear cells.[35,52]

Dynamic Test Methods

Avalanche testers assess the flowability of powders by measuring their avalanching behavior, which is related to powder cohesivity and flowability. Unlike shear cell methodology, this type of assessment is dynamic in nature,[53] which may be more applicable to low-shear processes such as blending, in which avalanching behavior of powder promotes mixing. Avalanche testing can be carried out in different types of equipment, including rotating drums and vibratory feeders.[54,55] Avalanche testing has been shown to distinguish between freely flowing powders, blends, and granulations.[56,57]

One of the most widely used rotating drum avalanche testers is the Aeroflow® (TSI, St. Paul, MN). Powder is filled into a transparent drum, which is then rotated at a fixed speed. The stress applied to the powder sample as a result of rotation causes the powder to shear, resulting in avalanche events.[58] The avalanche events are monitored by an optical sensor system. From the detector response data, a frequency or mass distribution of the avalanche events can be generated which can be used to determine various flowability parameters. Hancock et al. used the mean time to avalanche (mean of the distribution), and the coefficient of variation of the avalanche events, to characterize powder flow.[54]

One limitation of the avalanche tester is the qualitative nature of determining the regimes of avalanche flow in the rotating drum. Boothroyd et al. argued that the ideal flow regimes necessary for meaningful data analysis for pharmaceutical powders were the "rolling" and "cascading" regimes.[59] Another limitation of the system is the method development required prior to analysis. Rotational speed, measurement duration, and sample size must be optimized, as they have a great degree of influence over the measurement results.[54] A third limitation is the amount of material required, which limits the use of this technique in a material-sparing approach to formulation development. Hancock et al. proposed a sample size of 50 mL.[54]

Bhattachar et al. developed a vibratory feeder method for assessing avalanche behavior that requires a smaller sample size than for the Aeroflow® (1.2 g). Results compared to those generated using the Aeroflow®.[60] Despite the small sample size requirements this method is not widely used. The instrument is not commercially available, and has not been extensively tested.

8.4 COMPACT (MECHANICAL PROPERTY) CHARACTERIZATION

Many investigations have demonstrated the importance and impact of the physical and chemical properties of materials on powder processing. Physical properties such as particle size and shape clearly influence powder flow for example. The previous sections of this chapter provide some recommendations for how to proceed with characterization using limited quantities of materials. However, compact mechanical properties (i.e., those properties of a material under the influence of an applied stress) are also of great importance for solid dosage form development and manufacturing—particularly for tablet formulation. This section describes the importance of the mechanical properties of materials, as well as some basic principles and methodologies that can be used to investigate the influence of these properties on compaction. For the purposes of this discussion, physical properties are considered to be those properties that are "perceptible especially through the senses" (i.e., properties such as particle size, and shape). In contrast, mechanical properties are those properties of a material under an applied load: elasticity, plasticity, viscoelasticity, bonding, and brittleness.

Table 8.4 lists some of the physical and mechanical properties that influence powder properties and compaction. For example, surface energy and elastic deformation properties influence individual particle true areas of contact. Plastic deformation likely occurs to some extent in powder beds depending on the applied load, and almost certainly it occurs during the compaction of powders into tablets. Certainly at asperities, local regions of high pressure can lead to localized plastic yielding. Electrostatic forces can also play a role in powder flow, depending on the insulating characteristics of the material and environmental conditions. Particle size, shape, and size distribution have also been shown to influence flow and compaction. A number of environmental factors such as humidity, adsorbed impurities (air, water, etc.), consolidation load and time, direction and rate of shear, and storage container properties are also important. With so many variables, it is not surprising that a wide variety of methods have been developed to characterize materials. The focus of this chapter is on those useful methods that require limited amounts of material (bulk drug or formulation), and provide the most valuable information.

What holds particles together in a tablet? A detailed discussion is beyond the scope of this chapter, and excellent references are available in the literature.[61,62] However, it is important to realize that the forces that hold particles together in a tablet or powder bed are the very same forces discussed in detail in introductory physical chemistry texts. There is nothing magical about particle–particle interactions; the forces involved are London dispersion forces, dipole interactions, surface energy considerations, and hydrogen bonding. The consolidation of powders brings particles into close proximity, and these fundamental forces can begin to act effectively to produce strong particle–particle interactions (e.g., bonding). Particle rearrangement, elastic and plastic deformation of material can establish large areas of true contact between particles; if the resulting particle–particle bonds are strong, a strong and intact tablet is produced.

8.4.1 Important Mechanical Properties

Materials used in the pharmaceutical industry can be elastic, plastic, viscoelastic, hard, tough or brittle in the same sense that metals, plastics or wood are. The same concepts that mechanical engineers use to explain or characterize tensile, compressive or shear strength are relevant to pharmaceutical materials. These mechanical properties of materials can have a profound effect on solids processing.

The mechanical properties of a material play an important role in powder flow and compaction. These properties are critical properties that influence the true areas of contact between particles. Therefore, it is essential to characterize the properties. Reliable mechanical property information can be useful in helping to choose a processing method such as granulation or direct compression, selecting excipients with properties that will mask the poor properties of the drug or helping to document what went wrong, for example, when a tableting process is being scaled-up or when a new bulk drug process is being tested. Since all of these can influence the quality of the final product, it is to the formulator's advantage to understand the importance of the mechanical properties of the active and inactive ingredients, and to be able to quantify the properties.

Elastic Deformation

In general, during the initial stages of deformation, a material is deformed elastically. A change in shape caused by the applied stress is completely reversible, and the specimen will return to its original shape on release of the applied stress. During elastic deformation, the stress–strain relationship for a specimen is described by Hooke's law (Equation 8.8):

$$\sigma = E \cdot \varepsilon \tag{8.8}$$

where:

E is referred to as Young's modulus of elasticity
σ is the applied stress
ε is the strain $(\varepsilon = (1 - l_o)/l_o)$.

The region of elastic deformation of a specimen is shown graphically in Figure 8.6. The reader is directed to standard texts in material science and engineering for detailed discussions of elastic deformation. As long as the elastic limit is not exceeded only elastic deformation occurs.

The elastic properties of materials can be understood by considering the attractive and repulsive forces between atoms and molecules. Elastic strain results from a change in the intermolecular spacing and, at least for small deformations, is reversible.

Plastic Deformation

Plastic deformation is the permanent change in shape of a specimen due to applied stress. The onset of plastic deformation is seen as curvature in the stress–strain curve shown in Figure 8.7. Plastic deformation is important because it "allows" pharmaceutical excipients and drugs to establish large true areas of contact during compaction that can remain on decompression. In this way, strong tablets can be prepared.

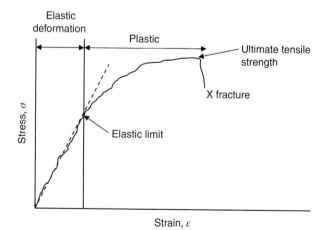

FIGURE 8.7   Stress–strain curve

Plastic deformation, unlike elastic deformation, is generally not accurately predicted from atomic or molecular properties. Rather, plastic deformation is often determined by the presence of crystal defects such as dislocations, grain boundaries, and slip planes within crystals. While it is not the purpose of this chapter to discuss this in detail, it is important to realize that dislocations and grain boundaries are influenced by factors such as the rate of crystallization, particle size, the presence of impurities, and the type of crystallization solvent used. Slip planes may exist within crystals due to molecular packing arrangements that result in weak interplanar forces. Processes that influence these (e.g., crystallization rate, solvent, temperature) can be expected to influence the plastic deformation properties of materials, and hence the processing properties. The reader is directed to standard texts in material science and engineering for detailed discussions of plastic deformation.

The plastic properties of a material are often determined by an indentation test.[63] Both static and dynamic test methods are available, but all generally determine the pressure necessary to cause permanent and non-recoverable deformation.

Brittle and Ductile Fracture

In addition to plastic deformation, materials may fail by either brittle fracture or ductile fracture; fracture being the separation of a body into two or more parts. Brittle fracture occurs by the rapid propagation of a crack throughout the specimen. Conversely, ductile fracture is characterized by extensive plastic deformation followed by fracture. Ductile failure is not typically seen with compacts of pharmaceutical materials. The characteristic snap of a tablet during hardness testing is indicative of brittle fracture.

Viscoelastic Properties

Viscoelastic properties can be important; viscoelasticity reflects the time-dependent nature of stress–strain. A basic understanding of viscoelasticity can be gained by considering processes that occur at a molecular level when a material is under stress. An applied stress, even when in the elastic region, effectively moves atoms or molecules from their equilibrium energy state. With time, the rearrangement of atoms or molecules can occur.

The stress–strain relationship can therefore depend on the time frame over which the test is conducted. In compacting tablets, for example, it is frequently noted that higher compaction forces are required to make a tablet with a given strength when the compaction speed is rapid. All pharmaceutical materials are viscoelastic; the degree to which their mechanical properties are influenced by rate depends on the material.

8.4.2 Overview of Methods

Characterizing mechanical properties has been an active area of pharmaceutical research for decades. The application of classic "engineering" methodologies to characterize pharmaceutical materials dates to the 1950s or before. With the advent of high-speed computer control, and monitoring of processes such as tablet compaction, the era of "dynamic" characterization of pharmaceutical materials was ushered in. Sophisticated instrumentation of rotary tablet presses and, in particular, the design of tablet compaction simulators with seemingly infinite control of the compaction process, has offered scientists an unprecedented opportunity to study the mechanics of materials at speeds representative of production tablet compaction. Yet, even today, both dynamic testing and the classic "quasi-static" engineering testing approaches offer opportunities to understand pharmaceutical materials. In this regard, dynamic and quasi-static testing are complementary tools. Both quasi-static and dynamic test methodologies will be discussed in the following sections. One key advantage of quasi-static testing is the ability to "independently" dissect out and investigate the various mechanical properties of a material. As stated previously, pharmaceutical materials can be elastic, plastic, viscoelastic, hard, tough or brittle. Ultimately, these individual components that cumulatively describe a pharmaceutical material determine its compaction properties in a dynamic compaction process.

The consolidation of powders into intact tablets is a process of reducing pores in a powder bed while creating interparticle bonds. During compression, materials experience complex stresses, the structure of the powder bed changes, and consolidation is brought about mainly by particle rearrangement, plastic deformation, and fragmentation.[64] The deformation of pharmaceutical materials is time dependent, and this dependency is related to the consolidation mechanism and dynamics of the consolidation process.[65,66,67,68,69] Under compression, for example, brittle materials are considered to consolidate predominantly by fragmentation; plastic materials deform by plastic flow. The time dependency of this process arises from stress relaxation for materials undergoing primarily plastic deformation. However, the compaction of brittle materials is often less influenced by speed, because fragmentation is rapidly achieved and prolonged exposure to the force has a limited effect on tablet properties.

Several researchers have previously identified the utility of solid fraction in describing tablet properties. Armstrong and Palfrey[70] concluded that differences in the tensile strength of tablets compressed at different speeds could be accounted for by differences in tablet porosity. Hancock and coworkers[71] found that tablet strength and disintegration time for tablets made on an eccentric press and a rotary press were comparable when considering a comparable solid fraction. Maarschalk and coworkers[72] found that tablet tensile strength of sorbitol as a function of tablet porosity was independent of compression speed. Finally, Tye and coworkers[64] extended this work to show that tablet solid fraction (SF) was the primary factor determining tablet strength for several pharmaceutical excipients (both brittle and ductile) over an extremely wide range of compaction speeds (dwell times from <10 msec to 90 sec).

The solid fraction (SF) of a compact can be calculated based on the true density (ρ_{true}) of the material (typically determined using pycnometry), the tablet volume (ν), and the tablet weight (Wt) (Equation 8.9):

$$SF = \frac{Wt}{\rho_{true} \cdot \nu} \qquad (8.9)$$

The relationship between the solid fraction, also referred to as relative density, and porosity (ε) is:

$$\varepsilon = 1 - SF \qquad (8.10)$$

8.4.3 Quasi-static Testing

Quasi-static testing typically applies variations of traditional engineering and material science testing methods to compacts (i.e., test specimens) of pharmaceutical materials. There are, for example, a number of variations of indentation, tensile, flexural, compression, and brittle fracture tests in the pharmaceutical literature.[73] The quantity of material required for testing varies from 1 to 100 grams. Methods for characterizing the elastic, plastic, and brittle properties of compacts of organic materials have, for example, been developed by Hiestand and coworkers.[74,75,76,77,78] These measures of tableting performance assess several key mechanical properties of compacted materials that have been shown to relate to tableting. Currently available methods typically require from 10 to 60 grams for complete mechanical property characterization using Hiestand's methods.

Test Specimen Preparation

It is important to properly prepare test specimens of pharmaceutical materials so quasi-static test results are not improperly influenced by "flaws" that may exist in the test specimen itself. Of the methods defined in the literature, the most refined method is to make square compacts using triaxial compression and decompression.[74] A split die (Figure 8.8) is used to make compacts that are substantially free of defects that may occur if a conventional compaction process were to be used. The split die permits triaxial decompression such that the pressure applied to all three axes is essentially equal during the decompression process.[74] This is achieved by computer control of the decompression process. The stresses in the compact are more uniformly relieved in three dimensions, and this minimizes the production and propagation of flaws within the compact.

Importance of the Solid Fraction

It is imperative to realize and address the fact that the mechanical properties of a compact are very much influenced by solid fraction. A change in solid fraction of 0.01 (i.e., a change in *SF* from 0.85 to 0.86) can result in a mechanical property change of 10% to 20%. For this reason, it is critical to compare the properties of a material at a "reference" solid fraction to ensure that one is "comparing apples to apples." Hiestand and coworkers[74] defined their reference solid fraction as 0.9 (i.e., porosity = 0.1 or 10%) while others have used a solid fraction of 0.85 or even extrapolated to a solid fraction of 1.0 (e.g., zero porosity). In comparing results from the literature, it is important to keep this in mind. It is recommended that a solid fraction in the range typical of tablet compaction be used. For compacts of organic materials, a reference solid fraction of 0.85 is in the midrange of those typically

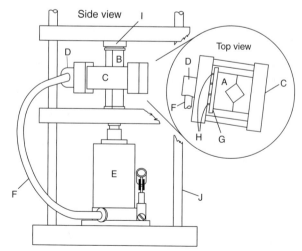

FIGURE 8.8   Schematic drawing of a simple triaxial press with a split die

observed. For inorganic materials (such as dicalcium phosphate) solid fractions in the 0.6 to 0.75 range are often observed for tablets. The wide range of mechanical properties observed means no ideal value can be identified for all materials.

Tensile Strength Determination

The tensile strength, σ_T, of a square test specimen provides extremely useful information. Several methods for determining it are available, and include traditional tablet hardness testing and transverse compression or square compacts. In transverse compression, specimens are compressed with platens 0.4 times the width of the compacts in the tensile testing apparatus.[74] The force necessary to cause tensile failure (tensile forces are maximum at the center of the tablet) is monitored by a load cell, and the magnitude of the force at fracture is determined. Testing of square compacts has advantages over the testing of circular compacts; however, circular compacts can be used. Conventional hardness testing of tablets can result in a measurement of tensile strength.[79] Similar results are obtained for round and square compacts when tensile failure is achieved. It is extremely important to compare measured properties such as tensile strength at the same solid fraction. Tensile strength values in excess of 1 MPa (typical range 0.1 to 4 MPa) are typically desired for tablets.

Pendulum Impact Device

A simple schematic of a pendulum impact device (PID) is given in Figure 8.9. This equipment permits the permanent deformation pressure of a compact of material to be determined under dynamic conditions.[74,75] Flat-faced, square tablets of the test substance are compressed at different compression pressures, and then subjected to impact with a stainless steel ball in the PID. The rebound height of the ball and the chordal radius of the dent are carefully measured, and used to calculate the permanent deformation pressure. In a simple sense, one is measuring the energy necessary to make the permanent deformation (the difference between the initial height of the ball and the rebound height). By measuring the volume of the dent, one can calculate the deformation pressure—the energy divided by the volume. The permanent deformation pressure is the pressure (i.e., stress) necessary to cause plastic deformation. This permanent deformation pressure, H, has been shown to be related to the yield pressure obtained using dynamic testing methods and Heckel analysis.[80] The dynamic hardness and tensile strength are shown in Figure 8.10 as a function of solid fraction for a common

pharmaceutical excipient. One can clearly see the impact of solid fraction on the measured mechanical properties.

Tableting Indices

Using the methodology described above, several indices of tableting performance have been developed by Hiestand and coworkers.[61,76] These indices provide relative measures of properties (i.e, dimensionless numbers) that reflect the performance of materials during processing.

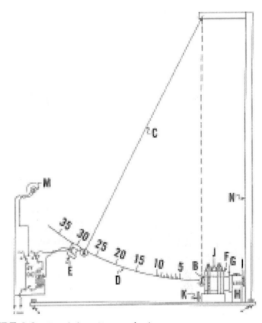

FIGURE 8.9 Pendulum impact device

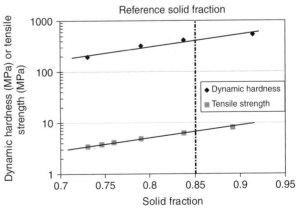

FIGURE 8.10 Dynamic hardness and tensile strength as a function of solid fraction

Bonding index

The purpose of the bonding index is to estimate the survival of strength during decompression;[76] it is defined in Equation 8.11:

$$BI = \frac{\sigma_T}{H} \qquad (8.11)$$

where:

σ_T is the tensile strength of the compact at a given solid fraction (typically 0.85 or 0.9 as defined by the user)

H is the permanent deformation pressure (i.e., hardness) of a compact at the same solid fraction.

The bonding index (BI) is, in essence, a measure of the ability of a material, on decompression, to maintain a high fraction of the bond that was created during compression. At maximum compression pressure, the bonded areas are at a maximum, because the true areas of contact are maximized. During decompression, some of that area and bond is "lost" due to elastic recovery. A high bonding index indicates that, relatively speaking, a larger portion of the strength remained intact after decompression. A low bonding index indicates that less of the strength remains. The term bonding index, then, is a good description since it, in effect, characterizes the tendency of the material to remain intact after it has been compressed. Tablets made of materials with poor bonding characteristics may be quite friable. Compacts made of materials with good bonding indices may, conversely, make strong tablets. A bonding index in excess of 0.01 (range 0.001 to 0.06) is typically desired.

Brittle fracture index

The brittle fracture index is a measure of the brittleness of a material. It is a measure of the ability of a compact to relieve stress around compact defects by plastic deformation. The brittle fracture index (BFI) is determined[74,75] by comparing the tensile strength of a compact, σ_T, with that of a compact with a small hole (stress concentrator) in it, σ_{To}, using the tensile test described above. A hole in the center of a compact weakens it. If a material is very brittle, theoretical considerations show that the tensile strength of a tablet with a hole in it will be about one-third that of a "defect free" tablet. If, however, the material can relieve stress, then the strength of the compact with a hole in it will approach that of a compact with no hole. The brittle fracture index is defined such that very brittle compacts have a *BFI* of 1, and very nonbrittle materials have a *BFI* close to 0; it is calculated in Equation 8.12.[74] *BFI* values less than 0.3 (range 0 to 1) are indicative of relatively nonbrittle materials.

$$BFI = 0.5 \cdot \left[\frac{\sigma_T}{\sigma_{To}} - 1 \right] \qquad (8.12)$$

Viscoelastic index

Hiestand and coworkers have further refined the concept of bonding index to include both a worst-case and a best-case bonding index.[76] The bonding index is determined under different experimental conditions: the rate at which the permanent dent is made in a compact is varied such that the viscoelastic properties of the material are assessed. If a material is very viscoelastic, there is substantial stress relaxation with time. It is reasonable to expect, then, that tablets that are slowly deformed during the determination of the hardness, H, may retain more of the bonded area than tablets that are rapidly deformed (i.e., as in the pendulum impact device), since some of the stresses developed during compaction will have a chance to be relieved. The dynamic bonding index (BI_d), sometimes called the worst case BI, is determined using a the pendulum impact device (PID) for measuring the indentation hardness (H_d), while the quasi-static bonding index (BI_{qs}), also sometimes referred to as the best case BI, is measured using a "quasi-static" or slow method for measuring indentation hardness (H_{qs}). The dynamic and quasi-static bonding index is calculated as previously described. The viscoelastic index (VE) is defined as the ratio of the dynamic to quasi-static indentation hardness:

$$VE = \frac{H_d}{H_{qs}} = \frac{BI_{qs}}{BI_d} \qquad (8.13)$$

Application of Quasi-static Testing to Formulation Development

The application of quasi-static testing methods and interpretation has been discussed extensively in the scientific literature. In addition to the pioneering work of Hiestand and coworkers,[61,62,63,74,75,76,77,78] additional research discussing the application of this methodology is available.[33,64,81,82,83,84,85,86,87,88,89,90] Benefits of a complete characterization of the mechanical properties of both the active ingredient and the excipients used in the formulation include:

- fundamental understanding of critical mechanical properties of the active ingredient and excipients;
- identification of mechanical property deficiencies and attributes;
- selection of excipients that can overcome deficiencies of active ingredient;

- identification of lot-to-lot variations in materials;
- identification of potential manufacturing problems associated with tableting process.

The reader is directed to the literature for a thorough discussion of the application of mechanical property characterization to formulation development. A fundamental understanding of the mechanical properties is essential to understanding compaction properties and the tableting process.[61,62,76,77,78,80] Development of mathematical models of mixtures has been used by Amidon,[91,92] and others,[88,87,93] to identify the type and quantity of excipient required to produce tablet formulations that have acceptable manufacturing properties. Figure 8.11 shows mechanical properties of binary mixtures of microcrystalline cellulose and lactose spray process.[91,92,96] From this figure, one can see that the mechanical properties of a mixture may be estimated knowing the mechanical properties of the two individual components. While the mechanical properties of mixtures are complicated,[94,95] estimating the properties of mixtures has been successfully used to identify suitable excipient types and quantities. A simplified equation for binary mixtures is given in Equation 8.14 or Equation 8.15:

$$\Phi_{mixture} = x(\Phi_A) + (1-x)(\Phi_B) \qquad (8.14)$$

$$\log(\Phi_{mixture}) = x \log(\Phi_A) + (1-x)\log(\Phi_B) \qquad (8.15)$$

where:

$\Phi_{mixture}$ is the mechanical property of interest for the mixture at the reference solid fraction

Φ_A, Φ_B are the properties of the pure components of the binary mixture at the same reference solid fraction

x is the fraction of component A.

While either equation may be used, experience has shown that the log-linear relationship shown in Equation 8.15 often produces better predictions for mixtures of common lactose-microcrystalline cellulose-based formulations. Further work is needed, however, to explore the science and predictability of mixtures.

For ternary mixtures, that is, for mixtures containing an active pharmaceutical ingredient as one component and a second "placebo" component containing two excipients, it is possible to estimate the mechanical properties of a mixture by extending this concept, as shown in Equation 8.16.

$$\log(\Phi_{Formulation}) = y \log(\Phi_{API}) + (1-y)$$
$$\cdot ([x]\log(\Phi_A) + [1-x]\log\Phi \qquad (8.16)$$

where:

y is the fraction of API in the blend

$(1-y)$ is the fraction of the blend that constitutes the placebo component.

While a simplification, this approach has been used to predict the properties of mixtures.[91,92,96] An example of the predicted mechanical properties of a ternary blend of API, and a placebo component consisting of microcrystalline cellulose and lactose spray process, is shown in Figure 8.12. A sound understanding of the mechanical properties of the individual components, and the range of desirable mechanical property values, allows for a rational selection of excipient types, grades and quantities.

8.4.4 Dynamic Testing

The most commonly used methods of studying the mechanical properties of solids under dynamic conditions include the use of the following instrumented equipment:

- Hydraulic press;
- Eccentric (single station) tablet press;
- Rotary tablet press;
- Compaction simulator;
- Compaction emulator (e.g., Presster™).

Accurate measurements of force and distance require careful construction of equipment and placement of instrumentation; several publications are available discussing these aspects.[97,98] Appropriate care is also needed during calibration, and for correction of measurements due to machine dimensional changes; tablet punches, for example, deform elastically and these changes should be considered.

While any of these instrumented presses may be used, the most commonly used for dynamic testing is the compaction simulator. The compaction simulator,[99] because of its sophisticated control and monitoring of the compaction process, generally offers the greatest flexibility in compression conditions. It is possible, for example, to carry out compression under constant velocity conditions for the compression and decompression phases (i.e., saw-tooth compression profile)—something not possible with other presses. Also of particular note is the demonstrated utility of a "linear" tablet press emulator (Presster™), that offers many of the advantages of a conventional compaction simulator in ease of use and experimental flexibility, as well as its ability to simulate virtually any commercially available rotary tablet press.[100] One limitation of the Presster™, though it may also be viewed as a benefit, is that it uses compression rolls of the same dimensions as those on a rotary tablet press, so compression profiles are limited to those described by conventional tablet press geometries of the tablet punch tooling as it moves under the compression rolls.

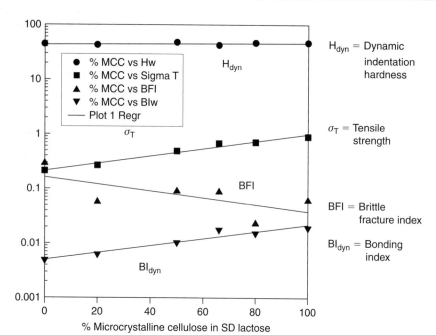

FIGURE 8.11   Mechanical properties of mixtures of microcrystalline cellulose and lactose spray process

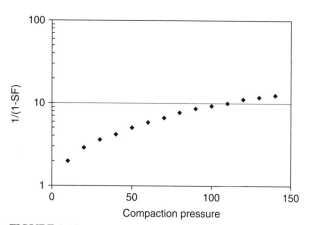

FIGURE 8.12   Heckel plot.

the dosage form are ultimately judged by the formulator, by quality assurance, and by the consumer.

A variety of pressure–porosity equations have been derived over the years.[101,102,103] The most commonly referenced of them is that of Heckel.[109] The Heckel equation (sometimes referred to as the Athy–Heckel equation) was derived assuming that the change in solid fraction (i.e., relative density) with compaction pressure is proportional to the porosity of the compact. Therefore, as porosity approaches zero, the change in solid fraction with compaction pressure, $d\rho/dP$, approaches zero. Therefore:

$$\frac{d\rho_r}{dP} \propto \varepsilon = (1 - \rho_r) \qquad (8.17)$$

And, integrating Equation 8.17, results in the classic Heckel equation:

$$\ln\left(\frac{1}{1 - \rho_r}\right) = kP + A \qquad (8.18)$$

where k is a measure of the plasticity of the material. It is related to the yield strength, Y, of a material by Equation 8.19.[104,109]

$$k = \frac{1}{3y} \qquad (8.19)$$

The constants in the Heckel plot are typically determined by regression analysis of the terminal linear portion of a plot of $\ln(1/(1 - \rho_r))$ versus P (see Figure 8.13). The yield strength, Y, of the material under the dynamic

With proper instrumentation, "in die" or "at pressure" measurements may be made during the compaction process. For example, the compaction pressure versus tablet porosity (compressibility) may be determined for a single tablet. This information, obtained under these dynamic testing conditions, can be used to generate an "in die" Heckel plot. Alternatively, measurements may be made on compacts after the tablet is removed from the die. These are "out of die" or "at zero pressure" measurements. Both in die and out of die methods have their advantages. Among the advantages of out of die measurements is that they represent the "final product" after decompression and ejection. The out of die properties are those by which

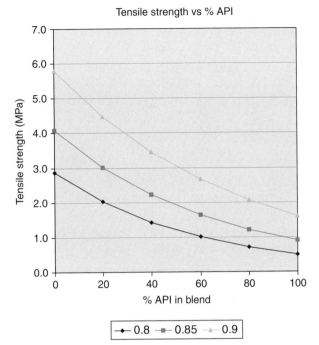

FIGURE 8.13 Predicted mechanical properties of a ternary blend of API, micro crystalline cellulose and lactose spray process.

conditions of the test is a measure of the deformability. In addition to yield strength, the shape of the Heckel plot has been used to distinguish volume reduction mechanisms.[105] Three types or families of curves are considered to reflect materials that undergo consolidation primarily by: (a) plastic deformation, (b) fragmentation, or (c) a variation of (a) which is plastic flow with no initial particle rearrangement.

Additional information regarding the compaction process may be obtained using dynamic testing conditions, including work of compaction, work recovered during decompression, work to overcome die wall friction, etc. A detailed discussion of these opportunities is beyond the scope of this chapter, and the reader is directed to the literature for further information. While very valuable as a research tool, the quantitative use of pressure–porosity measurements and analysis beyond the determination of yield pressure does not appear to be used routinely during formulation development and optimization.

Application of Dynamic Testing to Formulation Development

There are a number of reports of the use of dynamic testing of active ingredients and excipients in the literature. There are two key benefits of dynamic testing: (1) the properties can be determined under dynamic conditions representing those in a production environment; and (2) small quantities are typically

required (2–10 g). In contrast, disadvantages include the difficulty of factoring out the individual mechanical property "components" that, combined, determine how a material behaves during compaction.

The relationships between compaction pressure, tensile strength, and solid fraction are critical to understanding and characterizing the compaction process. The relationship between these three parameters is described as:

- Compactibility: relationship between tensile strength and solid fraction;
- Tabletability: relationship between tensile strength and compression pressure;
- Compressability: relationship between compaction pressure and solid fraction or porosity;
- Manufacturability: relationship between tablet crushing force and compression force.

Representative compactibility, tabletability, compressability, and manufacturability profiles for a compactable excipient are shown in Figures 8.14 through Figure 8.17. The compactibility, tabletability, and compressability profiles form the three faces of a three-dimensional plot as shown in Figure 8.18.[64] The Presster™ compaction emulator was used for these studies, although other properly instrumented presses can also be used. The compaction emulator was set up to emulate a Killian RST tablet machine (250 mm compression rolls) with a 27 msec dwell time (corresponding to 28 800 tablets/ hour) using 10 mm diameter flat-faced round punches with no precompression force.

Compactibility is the ability of a powder to be transformed into tablets with a resulting strength.[107] It is represented by a plot of tensile strength versus solid fraction. The compactibility is the most valuable of the three properties, since it reflects the two most important effects of applied pressure: tablet strength, and solid fraction. A representative compactibility profile of an excipient is shown in Figure 8.14. If one can achieve an acceptable tensile strength at an acceptable solid fraction with the application of pressure, a satisfactory tablet can be produced. Compactibility plots are largely independent of the process by which compacts are made, since only measured tablet properties (tensile strength and solid fraction) are involved. Compactibility plots are useful as a tool to compare formulations made on different equipment. If the formulations are the "same" then the "same" compactibility plots will be obtained.[64]

Tabletability is the capacity of a powder to be transformed into a tablet of specified strength under the effect of compaction pressure.[107] It is represented by a plot of tensile strength versus compaction pressure. Tabletability describes the effectiveness of the applied

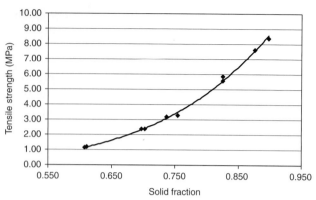

FIGURE 8.14 Compactability profile using a compaction emulator

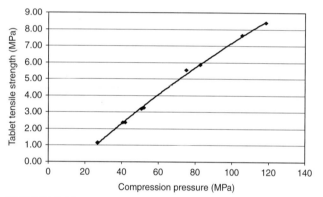

FIGURE 8.15 Tabletability profile using a compaction emulator

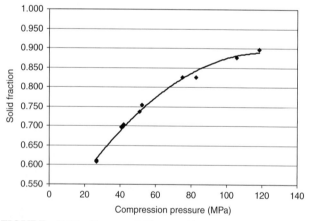

FIGURE 8.16 Compressibility profile using a compaction emulator

pressure in increasing the tensile strength of the tablet, and demonstrates the relationship between the cause (the compaction pressure), and the effect (the strength of the compact) (see Figure 8.15). Normally, a higher compaction pressure makes a stronger tablet. However, this relationship is often found to be speed

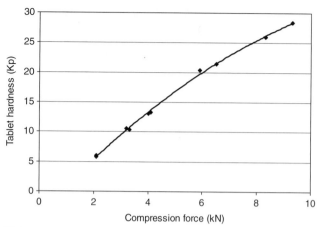

FIGURE 8.17 Manufacturability profile using a compaction emulator

dependent. Also, at high pressures, some materials may have lower tensile strength due to overcompaction.[106] Characterization of the tabletability provides excellent insight into the compaction process and mechanical properties of a material.

Compressability is the ability of a material to undergo a reduction in volume as a result of an applied pressure.[107,108] It is a measure of the ease with which a powder bed undergoes volume reduction under compaction pressure; it is represented by a plot showing the reduction of tablet porosity (i.e., the increase in solid fraction) with increasing compaction pressure (Figure 8.16). Compressability is often described by the Heckel equation.[109] Heckel plots, for example, have been widely used to assess the mechanism of deformation, and as a tool to estimate yield pressure. It is also well-known that tablet porosity is an important parameter, for example, in tablet disintegration and dissolution, since some porosity is often necessary to facilitate liquid penetration into tablets.[110,111]

Manufacturability, a plot closely related to tabletability, shows the relationship between the tablet crushing force (related to tensile strength), and compaction force (related to compression pressure). The manufacturability profile (Figure 8.17) is commonly considered by formulation scientists since it reflects the "measured" properties of a dosage form during manufacturing (tablet crushing strength and compression force). In general, however, pressure and tensile strength are preferred parameters to consider.

In summary, characterization of the compactibility, tabletability, compressability, and manufacturability of a formulation provides valuable information of the compaction process, and the prospects for a successful tableting process in manufacturing. Obtaining tablets with adequate tensile strength at a reasonable solid fraction with acceptable compression pressure is the

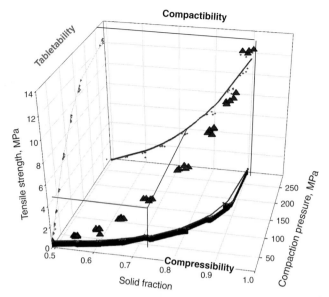

FIGURE 8.18 Three-dimensional tablet tensile strength, solid fraction, and compaction pressure curve

key to success. Robust formulations must not be on the "edge;" that is, they should provide the manufacturing scientist with the ability to adjust compression pressure to achieve the desired tensile strength and still maintain the solid fraction in a desirable range, such that the tablet performs as required.

8.5 CONCLUSIONS

As timelines become tighter and shortened, it has become more important than ever to quickly and efficiently characterize the critical properties of materials that will influence product development and performance. In this chapter, a discussion of those particle, powder, and compact properties that are most important in developing solid dosage forms has been discussed. The focus has been on methods that yield important information, yet require small quantities of materials. With a sound understanding of these properties, formulation development can proceed most efficiently and scientifically with greater success. Tomorrow's formulation and process scientists will require a sound understanding of these pharmaceutical material science principles, and must be able to apply them to the design and development of dosage forms in an efficient and scientifically rigorous way. The beauty of science is the knowledge and ability it gives us to reliably predict the future. As formulation and process scientists, the future we need to accurately predict is that of a consistent, reliable, manufacturable product that performs as expected.

References

1. Brittain, H. G. (2004). *Evaluation of the Particle Size Distribution of Pharmaceutical Solids. Profiles of Drug Substances, Excipients, and Related Methodology*, Vol. 31.
2. Allen, T. (1997). *Particle Size Measurement*, 5th edn. Vol. 1. Chapman & Hall, New York.
3. Stanforth, J. (2004). Particle-size Analysis, In: Pharmaceutics *The Science of Dosage Form Design*, M. Aulton (ed.). pp. 152–165.
4. US Pharmacopeia 27. (2006). US Pharmacopeial convention, Rockville, MD, pp. 2716–2717.
5. Newman, A. W. & Brittain, H. G. (1995). Particle Morphology: Optical and Electron Microscopies. In: *Physical Characterization of Pharmaceutical Solids*, H.G. Brittain, (ed.). Marcel Dekker, New York. pp. 127–156.
6. Operation and Maintenance Manual. (2004). Gilsonic Siever Model GA-8, Gilson Company, Inc., P.O. Box 200, Lewis Center, Ohio 43035-0200.
7. US Pharmacopeia 27. (2006). US Pharmacopeial convention, Rockville, MD. pp. 2720–2722.
8. Rohrs, B.R., Amidon, G.E., Meury, R.H., Secreast, P.J., King, H.M. & Skoug, C.J. (2006). Particle size limits to meet usp content uniformity criteria for tablets and capsules. Journal of Pharmaceutical Sciences 95(5), 1049–1059.
9. Dressman, J.B. & Fleisher, D. (1986). Mixing tank model for predicting dissolution rate control of oral absorption. Journal of Pharmaceutical Sciences 75, 109–116.
10. Higuchi, W.I. & Hiestand, E.N. (1963). Dissolution rates of finely divided drug powders I: Effect of a distribution of particle sizes in a diffusion-controlled process. Journal of Pharmaceutical Sciences 52, 167–171.
11. Hintz, R.J. & Johnson, K.C. (1988). The effect of particle size distribution on dissolution rate and oral absorption. International Journal of Pharmaceutics 51, 9–17.
12. Rohrs, B. R. & Amidon, G. E. (2005). Particle Engineering: A Formulator's Perspective. AAPS Arden House Conference. Harriman, New York.
13. US Pharmacopeia 27. (2006). US Pharmacopeial convention, Rockville, MD, pp. 2669–2670.
14. Mohanmmadi, M.S. & Harnby, N. (1997). Bulk density modeling as a means of typifying the microstructure and flow characteristics of cohesive powders. Powder Technology 92, 1–8.
15. Abdullah, E.C. & Geldart, D. (1999). The use of bulk density measurements as flowability indicators. Powder Technology 102, 151–165.
16. Suzuki, M., Sato, H., Hasegawa, M. & Hirota, M. (2001). Effect of size distribution on tapping properties of fine powder. Powder Technology 118, 53–57.
17. US Pharmacopeia 27. (2006). US Pharmacopeial convention, Rockville, MD, pp. 2638–2639.
18. Amidon, G.E. & Houghton, M.E. (1985). Powder flow testing in preformulation and formulation development. Pharm. Manuf. 2(7), 20–31.
19. Köhler, T. Influence of Particle Size Distribution on the Flow Behaviour of Fine Powders. Particle and Particle Systems Characterization, 8, 101–104.
20. Shinohara, K. (2000). Effect of particle shape on angle of internal friction by triaxial compression test. Powder Technology 107, 131–136.
21. Podczeck, F. (1996). The influence of particle size and shape on the angle of internal friction and the flow factor of unlubricated and lubricated powders. International Journal of Pharmaceutics 144, 187–194.
22. Kachrimanis, K., Karamyan, V. & Malamataris, S. (2003). Artificial neural networks (ANNs) and modeling of powder flow. International Journal of Pharmaceutics 250, 12–23.

23. Moreno-Atanasio, R., Antony, S.J. & Ghadiri, M. (2005). Analyis of flowability of cohesive powders using Distinct Element Method. Powder Technology 158, 51–57.

24. Tomas, R.J. (2001). Assessment of mechanical properties of cohesive particulate solids. Part 2: Powder flow criteria. Particulate Science and Technology 19, 111–129.

25. Carr, R.L. (1965). Classifying flow properties of solids. Chemical Engineering 72, 69–70.

26. Podczeck, F. & Newton, J.M. (1999). Powder filling into hard gelatine capsules on a tamp filling machine. International Journal of Pharmaceutics 185, 237–254.

27. Grey, R.O. & Beddow, J.K. (1969). On the Hausner Ratio and its relationship to some properties of metal powders. Powder Technology 2(6), 323–326.

28. Ho, R., Bagster, D.F. & Crooks, M.J. (1977). Flow studies on directly compressible tablet vehicles. Drug Development and Industrial Pharmacy 3, 475.

29. Nelson, E. (1955). Measurement of the repose angle of a tablet granulation. Journal of the American Pharmaceutical Association, Scientific Edition 44, 435.

30. Armstrong, N.A. & Griffiths, R.V. (1970). The effects of moisture on the flow properties and compression of phenacetin paracetomol and dextrose monohydrate. Pharmaceutica acta Helvetiae 45, 692.

31. US Pharmacopeia 27. (2006). US Pharmacopeial convention, Rockville, MD, pp. 3017–3020.

32. Khanam, J. & Nanda, A. (2005). Flow of granules through cylindrical hopper. Powder Technology 150, 30–35.

33. Amidon, G.E. (1995). Physical and mechanical property characterization of powders. In: *Physical Characterization of Pharmaceutical Solids*, H.G. Brittain, (ed.), Vol. 70. Dekker, New York. pp. 281–319.

34. Grossmann, J. & Tomas, J. (2006). Flow properties of cohesive powders tested by a press shear cell. Particulate Science and Technology 24, 353–367.

35. Schwedes, J. & Schulze, D. (1990). Measurement of flow properties of bulk solids. Powder Technology 61, 59–68.

36. Hiestand, E.N. & Wilcox, C.J. (1968). Some measurements of friction in simple powder beds. Journal of Pharmaceutical Sciences 57, 1421–1427.

37. Ho, R., Bagster, D.F. & Crooks, M.J. (1977). Flow studies on directly compressible tablet vehicles. Drug Development and Industrial Pharmacy 3, 475.

38. Marchall, K. & Sixsmith, D. (1976). The flow properties of microcrystalline cellulose powders. The Journal of Pharmacy and Pharmacology 28, 770.

39. Fizpatrick, J.J., Barringer, S.A. & Iqbal, T. (2004). Flow property measurement of food powders and sensitivity of Jenike's hopper design methodology to the measured values. Journal of Food Engineering 61, 399–405.

40. Schulze, D. "The behavior of powders and bulk solids," Fundamentals of Bulk Solid Mechanics, www.dietmar-schulze.de/grdle1.html.

41. Juliano, P., Muhunthan, B. & Barbosa-Canovas, G. (2006). Flow and shear descriptors of preconsolidated food powders. Journal of Food Engineering 72, 157–166.

42. Podczeck, F. & Mia, Y. (1996). The influence of particle size and shape on the angle of internal friction and the flow factor of unlubricated and lubricated powders. International Journal of Pharmaceutics 144(2), 187–194. 29 November.

43. Podczeck, F. & Newton, J.M. (2000). Powder and capsule filling properties of lubricated granulated cellulose powder. European Journal of Pharmaceutics and Biopharmaceutics 50, 373–377.

44. Nyqvist, H. (1982). Prediction of weight variation in tablet production from shear cell measurements. Acta pharmaceutica Suecica 19, 413–420.

45. Fitzpatrick, J.J., Barringer, S.A. & Iqbal, T. (2004). Flow property measurement of food powders and sensitivity of Jenike's hopper design methodology to the measured values. Journal of Food Engineering 61, 399–405.

46. Schulze, D. (1994). A new ring shear tester for flowability and time consolidation measurements. Proc. 1st International Particle Technology Forum, August. Denver/Colorado, USA, pp. 11–16.

47. Jenike, A. W. (1964). Storage and flow of solids. Bulletin 123. Engineering Experiment Station, University of Utah.

48. Dietmar Schulze. (2002–2004). Ring Shear Tester RST-XS Operating instructions.

49. ASTM International. Standard shear test method for bulk solids using the Schulze ring shear tester, D 6773–02.

50. ASTM International. Standard test method for shear testing of bulk solids using the Jenike shear cell, D 6128–00.

51. Hiestand, E. N. & Wells, J. E. (1977). A simplified shear cell apparatus and procedure. In: Proceedings of the International Powder and Bulk Solids Handling and Process Conference. Rosemont, IL, May, p. 244.

52. Schwedes, J. (2000). Testers for measuring flow properties of particulate solids. Powder Handling Process 12(4), 337–354.

53. Kaye, B.H. (1997). Characterizing the flowability of a powder using the concepts of fractal geometry and chaos theory. Particle and Particle Systems Characterization 14, 53–66.

54. Hancock, B.C. (2004). Development of a robust procedure for assessing powder flow using a commercial avalanche testing instrument. Journal of Pharmaceutical and Biomedical Analysis 35, 979–990.

55. Hickey, A.J. & Concessio, N.M. (1994). Flow properties of selected pharmaceutical powders from a vibrating spatula. Particle and Particle Systems Characterization 11, 457–462.

56. Rastogi, S. & Klinzing, G.E. (1994). Particle and Particle Systems Characterization 11, 453–456.

57. Doherty, R., Sahajpal, H., Poynter, R. & Lee, Y. (1999). The Journal of Pharmacy and Pharmacology 51, S323.

58. Boothroyd, E.M., Doherty, R.A., Poynter, R. & Ticehurst, M.D. (2000). Comparison of blend flow measured on the Aero-Flow™ with tablet weight uniformity. The Journal of Pharmacy and Pharmacology 52, 174.

59. Boothroyd, E.M., Doherty, R.A., Poynter, R. & Ticehurst, M. (2000). The Journal of Pharmacy and Pharmacology 52, 174S.

60. Bhattachar, S.N., Hedden, D.B., Olsofsky, A.M., Qu, X., Hsieh, W.Y. & Canter, K.G. (2004). Evaluation of the vibratory feeder method for assessment of powder flow properties. International Journal of Pharmaceutics 269, 385–392.

61. Hiestand, E.N. (2000). *Mechanics and Physical Principles for Powders and Compacts*. SSCI Inc, West Lafayette, IN.

62. Hiestand, E.N. (1996). Rationale for and the measurement of tableting indices. In: *Pharmaceutical Powder Compaction Technology*, G. Alderborn, & C. Nystrom, (eds), Vol. 71. Marcel Dekker, Inc, NewYork. pp. 219–244.

63. Hiestand, E.N., Bane, J.M., et al. (1971). Impact test for hardness of compressed powder compacts. Journal of Pharmaceutical Sciences 60(5), 758–763.

64. Tye, C.K., Sun, C. & Amidon, G.E. (2005). Evaluation of the effects of tableting speed on the relationships between compaction pressure, tablet tensile strength, and tablet solid fraction. Journal of Pharmaceutical Sciences 94(3), 465–472.

65. Rees, J.E. & Rue, P.J. (1978). Time-dependent deformation of some direct compression excipients. The Journal of Pharmacy and Pharmacology 30, 601–607.

66. David, S.T. & Augsburger, L.L. (1977). Plastic flow during compression of directly compressible fillers and its effect on tablet strength. Journal of Pharmaceutical Sciences 66(2), 155–159.

Polymer Properties and Characterization

James E. Brady, Thomas Dürig and Sherwin S. Shang

9.1 INTRODUCTION

The origin of the word polymer lies in the Greek *polu* for "many" and *meros* for "part:" consisting of many parts. The size and compositional and structural richness of polymers are all critical in determining the properties of the material, and the diversity of each trait is tied to the simple fact that the molecules each consist of "many parts." Polymeric materials are widely used in a broad range of pharmaceutical products, and constitute essential components of solid oral dosage forms. Therefore, it is important to understand the function of polymeric materials in the design and development of solid products and manufacturing processes.

Developing an understanding of the behavior of polymeric materials starts with the recognition that typical system variables such as basic physical properties, states or characteristics that are well-defined and discrete in number for small molecules, assume a continuous form with even the simplest of polymeric systems. Part of this is well appreciated by all. For example, pure small molecules have a distinct molecular weight with each molecule having the same nominal mass, neglecting, for the moment, the multiple natural isotopes possible for the atomic constituents. Polymers, on the other hand, are characterized by a diverse population in which there is a broad distribution of molar masses across the entire chain population. This is well-known and clearly understood since polymers are simply chains of many monomeric residues covalently linked together. It is less appreciated that other states which we routinely view as discrete, for example whether a molecule is

in solution or not, may also operationally assume some aspects of a continuous variable in polymeric systems. It is quite possible for extended segments of a polymer chain to effectively reside in bulk solution, while other parts still reside in a bulk polymer phase. Formally, the polymer is clearly not in formal solution. Yet the behavior of this system is clearly very different than another system, also not in formal solution, say an unswollen polymer sample sitting unsolvated immersed in a sea of solvent. Distributions in properties, states, and characteristics are what set the behavior of many polymers apart from small molecules in general. Coming to grips with the operational impact of this difference is the first step in productively using polymeric materials.

This chapter will emphasize some of the pragmatic consequences of continuous distributions in composition, molecular weight, and molecule state in the use of polymeric materials and the impact on their performance traits. While we will attempt to maintain a firm foot in fundamental science, each of the major subsections of this chapter could constitute a monograph in their own right. As such, the approach taken is to cover information that will be of immediate value to a user of polymeric excipients. This necessitates a very limited scope of coverage. In addition, we do not wish to become lost in sterile equations that only approximately describe the major features of polymeric systems, and often obscure important underlying operational principles. Where possible, we will appeal to experimental rather than theoretical examples to illustrate specific points. Our objective is to provide the user and formulator of polymeric materials an operational and pragmatic guide upon which to base

187

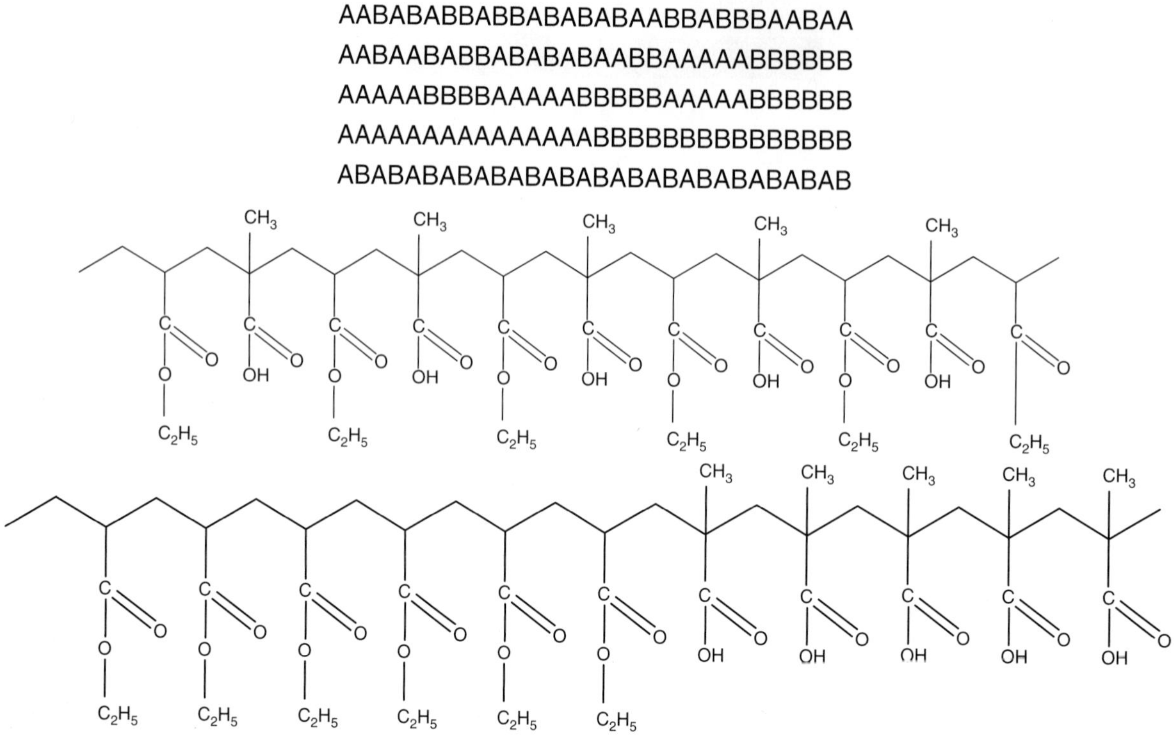

AABABABBABBABBABABABAABBABBBAABAA

AABAABABBABABABABAABBAAAAABBBBBB

AAAAABBBBAAAAABBBBBAAAAABBBBBB

AAAAAAAAAAAAAAAABBBBBBBBBBBBBBBB

ABABABABABABABABABABABABABABABAB

FIGURE 9.1   Examples of AB type copolymers in which the composition is the same (50:50 A:B), but the sequence of A and B monomers differ. Prototype copolymer structures shown top to bottom represent random, block graft, multiblock, diblock, and alternating AB copolymer systems. As a specific chemical example, consider the case of a 50:50 copolymer comprised of ethyl acrylate and acrylic acid as either an alternating, or diblock, architecture. The solution properties of these two materials, which have equal composition and molar mass, would be expected to be vastly different, as would solid state and melt properties

formulation decisions and understand the molecular origins of these performance metrics. Since the basic literature of polymer chemistry is readily available,[1-6] we will strive to not replicate that information here. Rather, this chapter should be viewed as an operational entry point into the practical utilization of polymeric materials.

In this chapter, we will consider basic structural issues surrounding polymeric materials. One general aspect to appreciate is that two samples with identical average molecular weight and composition may display very different behavior in specific applications. Since a polymer is comprised of chains of monomer units, the total number of monomers per chain (i.e., the molecular weight), the gross topology of the chain (linear versus branched), and the microstructural monomer sequence within and across the chains (i.e., block A–B copolymer versus random A–B copolymer versus a physical mixture of polymers A and B, see Figure 9.1) all impact the final properties of the material.

Determination of the average monomer composition and molecular weight of a polymeric sample are readily executed experiments using a variety of well-known techniques. Other attributes of polymeric materials, for example branching or large-scale composition

heterogeneity across chains, may require some level of experimental finesse, but can be addressed in broad terms. However, detailed questions regarding monomer sequencing within chains can be all but impenetrable in most instances, and often require appeal to indirect challenge/response experimental probes to even qualitatively characterize. This final detail is of significant importance in current research, since key performance properties can often be directly related to this elusive structural parameter.

9.1.1 Definition, Structure, and Nomenclature

The gross architecture of a polymer chain can be readily assessed by asking whether the chain or chain assembly can be mapped onto a 1- (linear), 2- (branched) or 3- (cross-linked network) dimensional object (Figure 9.2). In general terms, these distinctions reflect the natural spatial connectivity imparted by these chains when placed into a volume element, either in formal solution, a melt or the solid state.

How a polymeric chain mechanically couples to and transports within a medium comprised of either other polymeric materials or low molecular weight

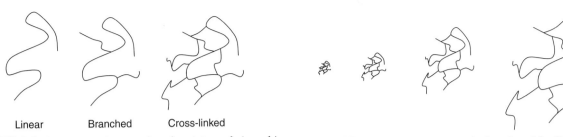

FIGURE 9.2 Diagrammatic examples of prototype chain architectures. A linear chain has been depicted as a random coil, although rigid or semi-rigid rods are also possible. The branched example is comprised of a main backbone with two extended long-chain branches, while more extensive branching and linking to other main backbones has been used to depict a typical cross-linked polymeric system

Linear   Branched   Cross-linked

FIGURE 9.3 Depending upon the length and flexibility of chain segments between covalent cross-links, a cross-inked polymer may be a very rigid and non-swelling solid (short, rigid segments between cross-links) or very highly swelling (low cross-link density between very flexible and solvent compatible segments) under the appropriate solvent conditions. In some cases, for example with a change of pH from highly acid to neutral or basic for a cross-linked polyacrylic acid system, conversion between collapsed and highly swollen states is readily and reversibly accomplished

solvent is determined in part by the gross topology of the chain system. Ultimately, the key physical attribute is the length, scale, and nature of connectivity between volume elements in solution, gel, melt or solid states, and how that connectivity propagates through space.

If one takes a linear chain and stretches it, a simple line is obtained. By the same token, the lowest dimensional object that a simple branched structure will yield under deformation, in the simplest case, is a two-dimensional planar object. A cross-linked network will yield a three-dimensional volume element under any applied deformation. In this sense, these three classes of chains are topologically and dimensionally distinct. As in any discussion involving polymeric species, the evolution between types is continuous rather than discrete, even when involving dimensional extent, simple characteristics, lengths, scales along principle axes are critical.

For example, as a simple linear chain is grafted with an increasingly long side chain in the midsection of the molecule, the evolution from a purely linear to a branched planar structure occurs in a continuous fashion. Likewise, as multiple chains having a two-dimensional architecture receive additional grafts on side chains, a similar transition from two- to three-dimensional character occurs. It is critical to appreciate that even aspects that appear firmly rooted in discrete representations, dimensionality in this example, may take on some attributes of a continuous variable if viewed from specific contexts.

The chain types shown in Figure 9.2 are assumed to represent covalently linked permanent structures. Polymeric materials of a given intrinsic topology may also assume a higher apparent dimensionality via dynamic self association. This association can involve either similar or compositionally distinct partners. Both types of examples exist in use, with self association of a hydrophobically modified polymer[7] reflecting the former case while the interaction of xanthan and locust bean gum

or sodium carboxymethyl cellulose and hydroxyethylcellulose are examples of the latter.[8] Finally, simple physical entanglements at high polymer concentrations can be viewed as a type of dynamic cross-link since many of the essential properties of cross-linked systems (structural robustness, high elasticity, slow transport of polymer and/or constituent polymer) will be achieved, particularly at relatively short timescales (minutes to hours).

Gross chain topology has an influence on the flow and mechanical properties of polymer melts and solutions, as well as over the timescales of structural relaxation. In general, as a system transitions from pure linear to highly cross-linked, the balance between the viscous and elastic nature of a solution or melt tends towards more elastic. This transition is similar in kind to that observed as the molecular weight of a polymer is increased. In terms of gross phenomenology, the basic causes are tied to similar origins, with the understanding that in a cross-linked or branched polymer sample permanent covalent linkages dominate the situations, while with high molecular weight linear polymers dynamic interchain entanglements, which can be akin to a transient cross-link, control system response.

In addition to extensively cross-linked pure polymer systems, an intermediate type of system is exemplified by cross-linked swellable microparticulates—the most common of these being provided by cross-linked acrylic acid based systems prepared in a microparticulate form. These are often used to control the flow properties of systems by simply encapsulating substantial fractions of the total system volume, but keeping it segregated into rather small length scale packets (see Figures 9.3 and 9.4). With large swelling ratios, relatively small amounts of particulate mass can basically encapsulate large volumes of liquid. This is often useful to build in a yield stress while

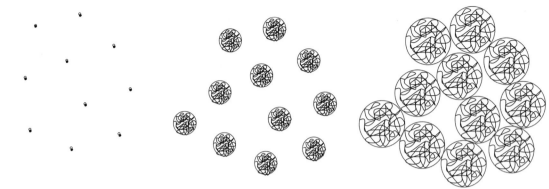

FIGURE 9.4　In addition to bulk cross-linked systems, the swelling of cross-linked microparticulate polymeric systems provides interesting opportunities for rheology control. As the particles swell, they first occupy a significant volume fraction of the dispersed phase and then reach a point at which all discrete swollen particles start to overlap and touch. Diameter ratios of 1:10:20, yielding a net 8000 fold volumetric swelling, is depicted above

maintaining a relatively low shear viscosity, since the propagation of shear forces is basically constrained to simple soft sphere hydrodynamic effects (versus chain entanglement for a molecular dissolved system), with a net length scale established by the dimensions of the swollen particle. In general, our attention below will be restricted to linear polymers, since they comprise the majority of systems of direct interest.

9.1.2　Types of Homopolymers and Copolymers

In dealing with polymeric materials, cautious delineation of whether a material is a homopolymer or a more complex copolymer is an extremely critical initial step in understanding the range of properties that can emerge in everyday use. In general, most of the polymeric materials that we deal with are much more profitably handled, and understood, if it is explicitly recognized that they are copolymeric in reality, and that the detailed sequence of the various residues is an important variable that can influence application properties in use. In some cases the distinctions are clear, in others they are not.

As a specific example of the potentially significant impact that sequence can have on a material, consider a simple AB copolymer which possesses equal molar amounts of A and B (Figure 9.1). For the same average chemical composition, molecular weight, and gross architecture, a significant range of structural archetypes can be prepared by manipulating only the sequence of the monomer units. That sequence can run from purely random, to somewhat blocky, to multiblock, to diblock, to purely alternating structures. If the monomer residues possess differing solution properties, for example consider a case in which one residue is relatively hydrophobic while the other

is very hydrophilic, sequence can have an overwhelming influence on properties such as solubility, phase behavior, and packing in the solid-state. As a specific case, consider poly(co-ethylacrylate-methacrylic acid) (Figure 9.1). The alternating and diblock architectures will yield vastly different physical properties (solubility, mechanical properties, etc.), and performance traits, despite the equivalence of molecular weight and average composition. Naturally, the argument can be extended to include a physical mixture of the two homopolymers which provide the same average molecular weight and composition values. Again, one has a system of near-identical molecular weight and composition, but the performance is anticipated to be distinctly different. In fact, the component polymers would likely be immiscible in the melt state, and prone to segregate if deposited from the solution state in, for example, a coating application.

As a second example, consider the simple case of sodium carboxymethylcellulose with an average degree of substitution of 1. In total, carboxymethyl substitution can occur at up to 3 hydroxyl positions on any anhydroglucose residue (Figure 9.5). In principle, a sodium carboxymethylcellulose chain can be comprised of unsubstituted anhydroglucose, have monosubstitution at either the 2, 3 or 6 hydroxyl positions, disubstitution at the 2/3, 2/6, or 3/6 positions or be a fully trisubstituted monomer. Even if the added detail of positional substitution is ignored and we consider only unsubstituted, mono-, di, and trisubstituted monomers as distinct entities, the system has to be considered as an ABCD copolymer. As noted above, the detailed sequence distribution of the A, B, C, and D monomer residues can have an impact on the final properties of the material if the intrinsic properties of those constituent monomers (polarity, hydrophobicity/hydrophilicity, charge state, propensity to participate

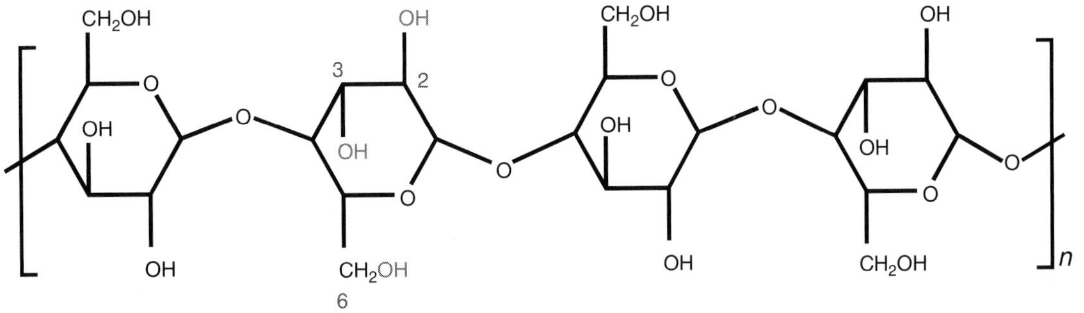

FIGURE 9.5 Basic structure of cellulose which is used as the starting material for any cellulosic derivative. Each anhydroglucose residue possesses three potentially reactive hydroxyl groups. These are indicated and numbered in the second residue according to the associated carbon on which they reside. For most reaction schemes, the 2 and 6 positions are more reactive than the 3 position

in interchain hydrogen bond association) differ significantly. Obviously, the solution and solid-state behavior of a neutral sugar (anhydroglucose) will be different from a trianion salt (sodium tricarboxymethyl anhydroglucose), due to the ionic charge and steric packing requirements of the latter and the facile possibility for hydrogen bond formation for the former.

As illustrated by the examples above, one expectation is that microstructural sequence variations will impact the local chemical nature of subsections within a polymer chain. In the case of poly(co-ethylacrylate-methacrylic acid) we see a transition from a nominally hydrophilic alternating copolymer to a system with distinct hydrophobic and hydrophilic blocks. In terms of expected solubility in water, the hydrophobic block will not find an aqueous environment amenable. Depending on the net balance of segment lengths and position along the backbone, this may manifest itself as anything from partial insolubility with a high propensity to swell, complete solubility with a tendency to adsorb onto surfaces, a tendency to self associate in solution or as gross insolubility in pure solvents with a decided need to employ binary solvent mixtures to achieve complete dissolution. A reality with polymeric materials is that all of these possibilities can, in principle, be expressed by materials of the same average composition via adjustment of molecular weight and chain microstructure sequence.

The case with synthetic copolymers is fairly obvious, and readily understood on the basis of the respective behavior of the constituent monomers. It is a less obvious situation with derivatized cellulosics, even though the underlying issues are identical and similar trait differences for nominally similar compositions are possible, although the underlying physical phenomena are somewhat distinct. With cellulosic derivatives, aside from the cases of cellulose esters

and ethyl cellulose, the possible constituent monomers are all fairly hydrophilic. However, similar issues remain and tend to be tied to the potential formation of hydrogen bonding junction zones in structurally regular domains of the material. These structurally regular domains can be due to short runs of contiguous unsubstituted anhydroglucose or uniformly substituted contiguous run lengths. In both cases the underlying feature is a structurally-regular domain than can be annealed into a highly ordered domain for which the primary events of dissolution (solvent penetration and separation of the packed chains) are kinetically disfavored due to cooperative multipoint hydrogen bond association.

This added level of complexity, which is intrinsic with derivatized cellulosic excipients but an important operational detail for any polymeric sample, needs to be appreciated in order to understand why materials that possess very similar average compositions can display rather different end use performance attributes in some applications.

9.2 COMMONLY USED CELLULOSE DERIVATIVES IN SOLID ORAL PRODUCTS

The basic architecture of the materials to be considered below is relatively simple linear polymers. This includes cellulosic derivatives and most major synthetic systems used in formulation. Aside from cross-linked cellulosics (e.g., croscarmellolose), most materials used are not branched/cross-linked as the native polymer chains. However, a number of materials do participate in reversible self association that can result in the formation of dynamically branched or cross-linked systems, and this secondary association equilibrium can exert an influence on the usage properties of the material.

Rather than develop a comprehensive treatment of the molecular properties of all the polymers used in formulating controlled release products, we will focus our attention on cellulose derivative chemistry. In broad strokes, the basic paradigms developed for cellulose derivatives will apply across the various chemical platforms available. A number of overviews of polysaccharide chemistry in general,[9] and cellulose derivatives in particular,[10] are readily available and despite their age remain worthwhile resources towards understanding key aspects of the chemistry.

As the name implies, cellulose derivatives are all based on cellulose provided by a variety of starting furnishes (wood pulp, chemical cotton). The starting polymer, cellulose, is a β 1–4 linked linear polymer of anhydroglucose. Due to the relatively stiff main chain backbone, the array of potential hydrogen bonding sites per monomer residue, and structural order inherent in the natural system, cellulose itself (Figure 9.5) is a largely intractable polymer. Dissolution of cellulose requires somewhat exotic solvent systems or *in situ* derivatization to cap self-associating hydroxyl groups.

The reaction chemistry used in the production of cellulosic derivatives[10] is based on removing that hydrogen bond mediated order from the system via activation with strong caustic, followed by reaction with various hydrophilic and/or hydrophobic substituents. This derivatization reaction introduces point packing defects along the main backbone, and prevents re-establishment of the higher level of order that was present in the native cellulose. The overall result is that the material is rendered soluble in a variety of solvents, with the preferred solvents being dependent on the substituents bound to the backbone. The overall molecular weight of the cellulose derivative is largely controlled by the specific selection of starting cellulose furnish for the higher molecular weight grades, with either *in situ* or post-derivatization oxidative or hydrolytic glycosidic chain scission being used to prepare the lower molecular weight members of a given chemical class.

Much of the solution chemistry of cellulose derivatives can be organized by understanding the interplay of the substituent as a defect in the native cellulose packing structure to increase solubility, with the use of substituent hydrophobicity and/or charge to tailor compatibility with nonaqueous or binary water/nonaqueous solvents.

Cellulose derivatives can be further classed according to whether or not the substituents can undergo a chain extension oligomerization (either in free solution or once grafted onto the cellulose backbone).

Hydroxypropyl and hydroxyethyl substituents are able to undergo chain extension, while carboxymethyl, methyl, and ethyl substituents effectively cap the reactive hydroxyl site when they are grafted onto the chain. In cases where the substituent is able to undergo chain extension, the degree of substitution (DS = number of substituent capped hydroxyls per anhydroglucose), and total molar substitution (MS = number of substituent moles per mole of anhydroglucose), will differ with MS ≥ DS. Note, for any cellulose derivative, DS ≤ 3 while the MS can be greater than 3, and is with, for example, hydroxypropylcellulose.

Cellulose derivatives are generally graded according to their viscosity under defined concentration conditions, which is ultimately tied to their molecular weight and substitution levels as expressed by the DS, MS or percent mass of grafted substituent. Note that in some cases (ethyl cellulose would be a specific example), the substituent used to quantify the mass loading of derivatizing reagent on the polymer, —OCH_2CH_3, reflects combination of the oxygen atom from the anhydroglucose with the ethyl group from the ethyl chloride used in the derivatization reaction.

Typical structures for the various common cellulose ethers are shown in Figures 9.6 to 9.12. As is apparent, these materials differ in the specific pendant groups, and their level bound to the same backbone. The situation with synthetic polymers is largely identical, except that it is generally the precise mixture of discretely different monomers that appear.

Table 9.1 provides typical data of the various grades of polymer available for each of the various chemical classes. A number of points quickly emerge. The range in average molecular weight represented in these polymers is extremely large—ranging from ~50 000 Daltons on the low side to 1 200 000 Daltons for the highest molecular weight materials available. This is a factor of 24 in net molecular weight. Owing to the variable content in residue formula weight provided by the pendant groups, direct comparison of the differences in degree of polymerization will differ slightly. In this case, net degrees of polymerization, basically the number of discrete monomer residues on average per chain, range from a low of roughly 215 for low molecular weight sodium carboxymethylcellulose to a high of about 4700 for the highest molecular weight grade of hydroxyethylcellulose. Again, the total dynamic range that chain length varies is by about a factor of 20.

The broad range in the average molecular weight or, equivalently, the degree of polymerization, tells only part of the story. These ranges reflect the wide variability in the population average values. Within a given population, in other words, for a given molecular

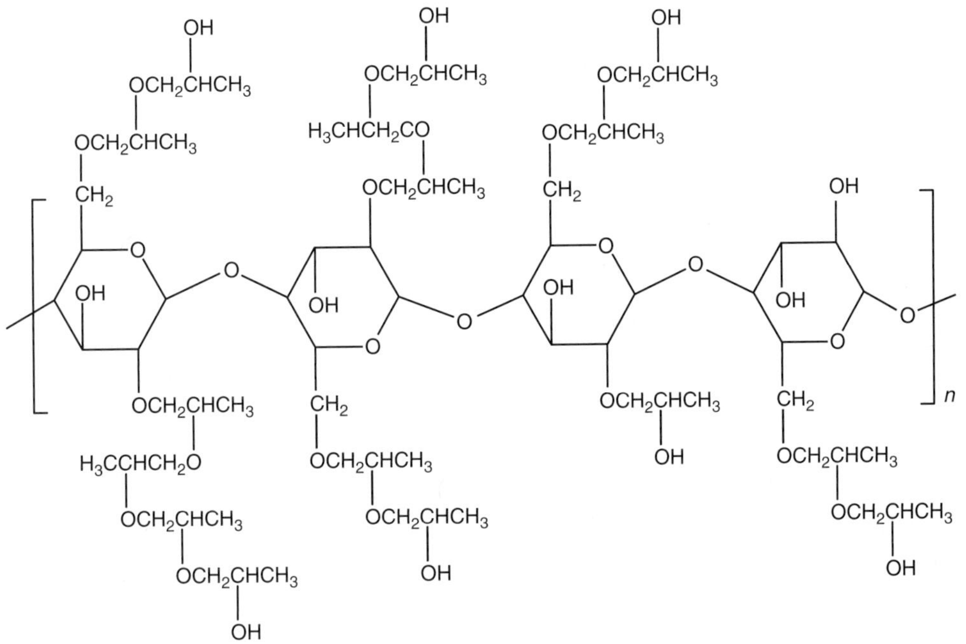

FIGURE 9.6 Typical structure for hydroxypropylcellulose. The net molar substitution in this example is 4.0. Note that there is a distribution in the hydroxypropyl chain length for the pendant groups added to the base cellulose polymer. The relatively high hydroxypropyl content yields a somewhat hydrophobic thermoplastic polymer which is sparingly soluble in hot water

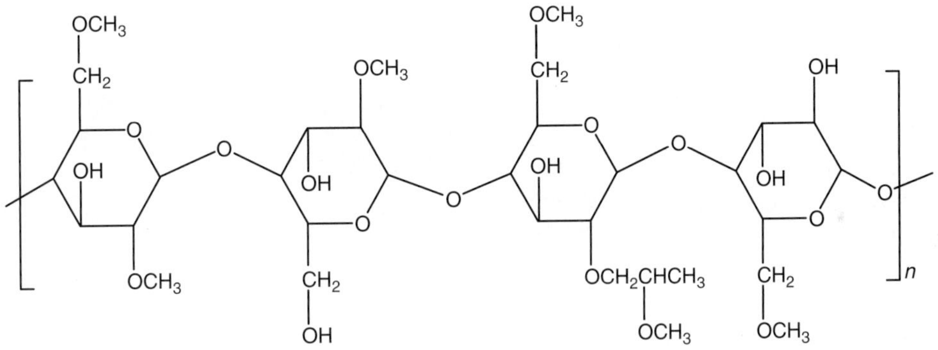

FIGURE 9.7 Typical structure for hydroxypropylmethylcellulose. This is an example of a mixed derivatized cellulosic containing both hydroxypropyl and methoxyl functionality. The specific system shown has a hydroxypropyl DS of 0.25 (~9.6 wt %) and methoxyl DS of 1.5 (~23 wt %). Due to the lower content of bound hydrophobic functionality relative to hydroxypropylcellulose shown in Figure 9.6, this material will generally display better water solubility at higher temperatures

weight, there is also a very disparate population of overall chain lengths present. For example, in a size exclusion chromatographic characterization of any of the high molecular weight cellulosics, the net range of molecular weights encompassed by the population of a given moderate- to high-molecular-weight sample will typically span a range from a few hundreds, to thousands, up to a few million. In other words, the net diversity in chain lengths is extremely broad, and easily spans a net range of 2–3 orders of magnitudes as the high and low molecular weight winds of the distribution are accounted. A typical example is shown in Figure 9.13. More typically, the polydispersity of a polymeric material is quantified by the ratio M_w/M_n. In cellulose deriviatives, depending on type and viscosity grade, this ratio can range from 3 to values of 20 or so. Once again, a fairly large number, yet relatively small when viewed across the complete assembly of chains.

To re-emphasize the points just made, while one must obviously speak in terms of population average quantities in examining polymers, these averages can suppress some of the range in values encompassed by the entire population.

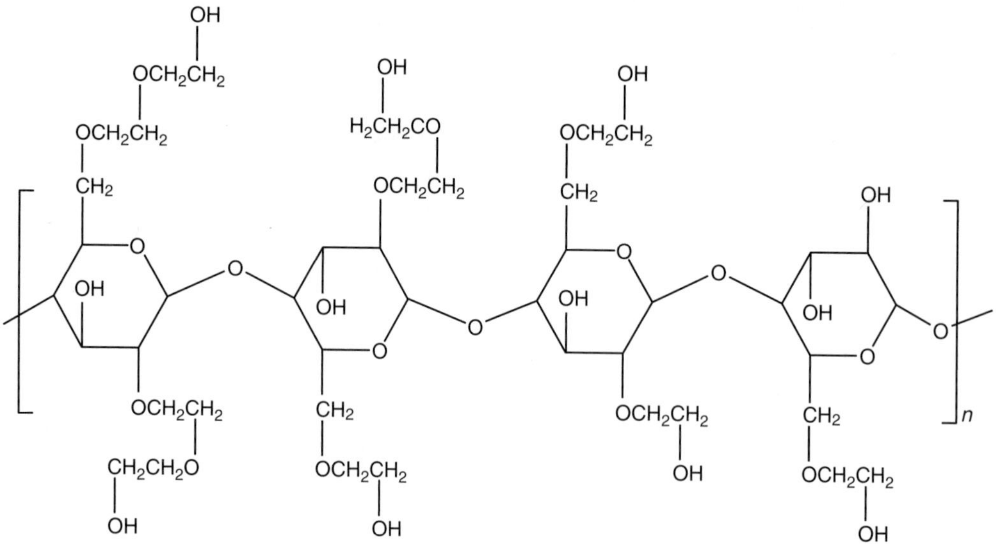

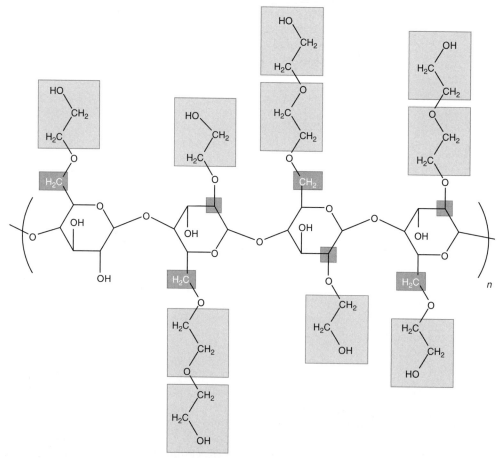

FIGURE 9.8 Typical structure for hydroxyethylcellulose. As with hydroxypropyl cellulose, a distribution in hydroxyethyl oligomer chain lengths exists. In this example, the hydroxyethylcellulose segment shown has a net molar substitution (MS) of 2.5, while the degree of substitution (DS) is 1.75 (=7/4)

FIGURE 9.9 An illustration of the difference between molar substitution (MS) and degree of substitution (DS) using hydroxyethylcellulose. In total, there are a maximum of three potentially reactive hydroxyl sites per anhydroglucose. In this example, substituted sites are indicated by the dark blocks, at the parent anhydroglucose carbon. Seven sites on four anhydroglucose rings are substituted, yielding a degree of substitution of 7/4 or 1.75. A total of 10 hydroxyethyl units are bound to the same four anhydroglucose units, yielding a molar substitution of 10/4 or 2.5

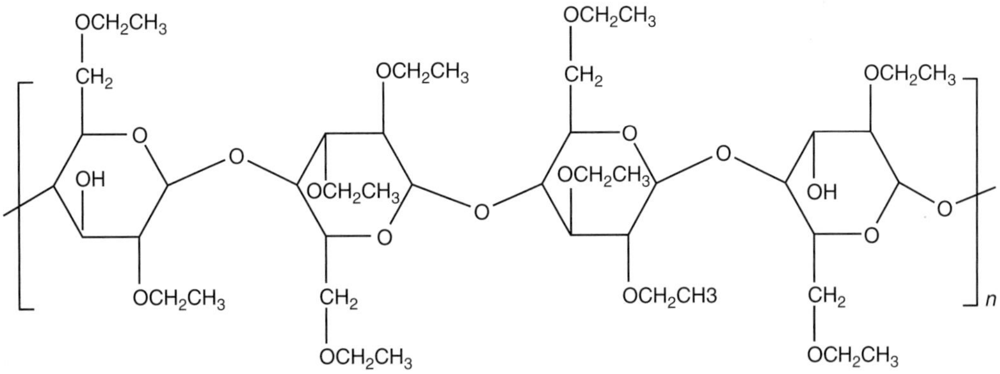

FIGURE 9.10 Typical structure for ethylcellulose with a net degree of substitution of 2.5. This corresponds to a wt % ethoxyl of 48.5, which is representative of an N or Standard grade of this material. If the net DS of the ethylcellulose is substantially increased to the order of 2.8, a largely insoluble material results, underscoring the interplay of solid state packing defects in modulating cellulose derivative solubility

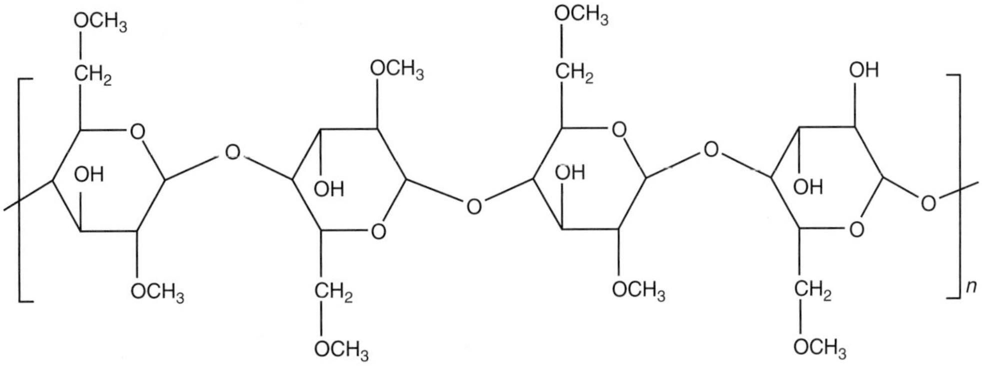

FIGURE 9.11 Typical structure for methylcellulose with a net degree of substitution of 1.75, which corresponds to a wt % methoxyl level of 29.1

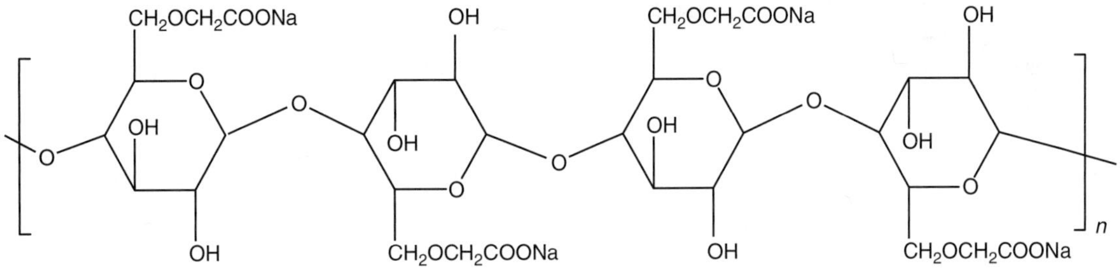

FIGURE 9.12 Representative structure of sodium carboxymethylcellulose. For graphic convenience, only substitution at the 6-position is explicitly shown. However, all three hydroxyl positions are available for substitution and a real polymer will be comprised of a mixture of primarily unsubstituted, monosubstituted or disubstituted monomer residues. This example is an idealized DS = 1 sodium carboxymethylcellulose

9.3 BASIC CONCEPTS AND CHARACTERIZATION OF POLYMERIC MATERIALS

Some specific example polymers were described above, as were some of the key traits used to characterize these polymers. In this section we'll delve somewhat deeper into the measurement of these traits, and the interrelationships between them.

At the most basic level, a polymeric material is defined by the average molecular weight distribution, and average composition. As has already been seen with molecular weight, the net range in molecular weight sampled is enormous. This can have important consequences. Traits that are dependent on properties

TABLE 9.1 Viscosity grade molecular weights for various cellulose derivatives

Viscosity grade (cP, at listed concentration)	Concentration (wt %)	Viscosity measurement conditions	Approximate molecular weight (Mw, Daltons)
Hydroxypropylcellulose (hydroxypropyl MS = 3.4–4.1)			
1500–3000	1	Brookfield (30 rpm/spindle 3)	1 150 000
4000–6500	2	Brookfield (60 rpm/spindle 4)	850 000
150–400	2	Brookfield (60 rpm/spindle 2)	370 000
150–400	5	Brookfield (60 rpm/spindle 2)	140 000
75–150	5	Brookfield (30 rpm/spindle 1)	95 000
300–600	10	Brookfield (30 rpm/spindle 2)	80 000
Hydroxyethylcellulose (hydroxyethyl MS = 2.5)			
3500–5500	1	Brookfield (30 rpm/spindle 4)	1 300 000
1000–2500	1	Brookfield (30 rpm/spindle 3)	1 000 000
4500–6500	2	Brookfield (60 rpm/spindle 4)	720 000
250–400	2	Brookfield (60 rpm/spindle 2)	300 000
75–150	5	Brookfield (30 rpm/spindle 1)	90 000
Hydroxypropylmethylcellulose (K type (19–24 wt % methoxyl), E type (28–30 wt % methoxyl), 7–12 wt % hydroxypropyl)			
~160 000–240 000	2	Ubbelohde, too high for reliable measurement	1 200 000
80 000–120 000	2	Ubbelohde	1 000 000
19 200–36 000	2	Ubbelohde	675 000
11 250–21 000	2	Ubbelohde	575 000
3000–5600	2	Ubbelohde	400 000
Sodium carboxymethylcellulose (nominal carboxymethyl DS levels of 0.7, 0.9, 1.2)			
1500–3000	1	Brookfield (30 rpm/spindle 3)	725 000
1500–3100	2	Brookfield (30 rpm/spindle 3)	395 000
400–800	2	Brookfield (30 rpm/spindle 2)	250 000
25–50	2	Brookfield (60 rpm/spindle 1)	90 500
50–200	4	Brookfield (60 rpm/spindle 2)	49 000
Ethyl cellulose (Standard or N type (48.0–49.5 wt % Ethoxyl), T type (49.6–51.0 wt % ethoxyl))[a]			
80–105	5	Ubbelohde 2C	215 000
40–52	5	Ubbelohde 2	160 000
18–24	5	Ubbelohde 2	140 000
12–16	5	Ubbelohde 1B	120 000
8–11	5	Ubbelohde 1B	75 000
6–8	5	Ubbelohde 1C	65 000

[a]Estimated, based on viscosity data

showing variation, take molecular weight as a specific example, may display particular sensitivity to specific portions of the molecular weight distribution. What this means is that those traits which are molecular-weight-dependent may differ between materials with nominally the same "average" molecular weights. A specific example would be the complete shear rate dependent flow curve of a blend of high and low molecular weight materials with that which is a pure intermediate molecular weight.

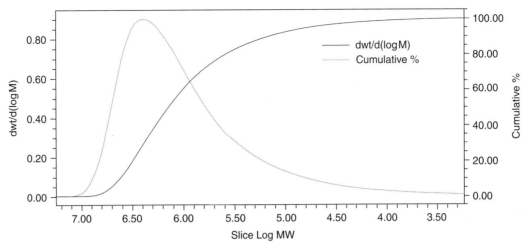

FIGURE 9.13 Representative molecular weight distribution profile of a high viscosity grade (1500–3000 cP, 1% solution in water) sample of hydroxypropylcellulose. The molecular weight scale calibration in this example refers to narrow distribution polyethylene oxide/polyethylene glycol. Note that in this example, the net range of material spans roughly 2000 to 10 000 000 Daltons from the start to the end of the complete molecular weight distribution. This is a fairly typical situation for high molecular weight polymers

9.3.1 Polymer Composition

At the crudest level, polymers are characterized by average composition variables that reflect either the total level of secondary substitution for derivatized systems (e.g., cellulose ethers) or the level of constituent monomers for a synthetic or natural copolymer system.

In general, cellulosic derivatives are compositionally characterized by the percent weight of functional group attached to the backbone, the degree of substitution (DS) per anhydroglucose or total molar substitution (MS) per anhydroglucose residue. These three modes of characterization are largely interchangeable with the preferred quantity often dependent on historical legacy and whether the substituent can form an oligomeric pendant group. In the latter case, the DS would not fully characterize the net amount of substituent on a chain.

It is important to recognize that the definition of operational "functional group" may include contributions from both the anhydroglucose residue and added functional reagent, leading to apparent percentage of weight function groups that may appear inordinately high. A good example of this would be ethyl cellulose, in which the average composition is typically expressed as the percentage of ethoxyl content. In this case, the ethyl portion of the ethoxyl group is derived from the derivatizing reagent (ethyl chloride) while the oxygen atom is provided by the anhydroglucose residue. For a typical N or Standard type ethylcellulose, a degree of substitution of 2.5 corresponds to a weight percentage of ethoxyl of 48.5. However, the actual percentage of mass imparted by the added

ethyl group is 31.3%, with the remainder contributed by the oxygen atom that is already a part of the main backbone polymer.

The second manner to characterize composition of cellulosics is to speak of the DS or degree of substitution. Each anhydroglucose residue along a cellulosic backbone possesses three reactive hydroxyl groups, located specifically at the C2, C3, and C6 positions. The average DS of a material quantifies the average number of hydroxyl groups that are derivatized per anhydroglucose. The maximum DS of any cellulosic material is 3, at which point all reactive hydroxyl functionality will have been consumed. The C2 and C6 positions are the most reactive sites, and will generally carry the bulk of the substituents.

When the derivatization reagent effectively caps the reactive hydroxyl functionality (e.g., methyl, ethyl or carboxymethyl functionality), the amount of bound functionality quantifies both the degree of hydroxyl substitution and total molar substitution. However, as already noted, if the substituent is able to oligomerize, as is the case with hydroxyethyl or hydroxypropyl substitution, the connection between degree of and molar substitution starts to diverge. Furthermore, in principle, the net molar substitution provided by an oligomerizing functional group is not bound to an upper limit determined by the number of backbone reactive sites, although steric constraints and reaction efficiency do provide a pragmatic limit. Of all available cellulosics, hydroxypropylcellulose is the most highly substituted system, with MS levels routinely in the vicinity of four.

In the case of synthetic copolymers, composition is typically determined by the average mole percent or weight percent of the various copolymer constituents, and/or the charge state for a titratable functionality. In general, this is controlled by the charge composition of the reaction mixture used to prepare the product.

In either case, there are a variety of experimental techniques that can be used to quantify the mean composition of the material. These techniques include direct functional group analysis, in the case of the derivatized cellulosics, while the average monomer composition is generally the target for synthetic copolymer systems. In part, this is related to the potential complexity with cellulosics that possess chain extended pendant groups.

One significant compositional difference between polymers and low molecular weight materials is that the detailed sequence distribution of the constituents at equivalent average compositions can have a significant impact on the final solution and solid-state properties of the polymer.

In contrast to the situation that exists with the determination of the average material composition, there is a dearth of direct experimental techniques which provide information on the sequence of monomers in a copolymer system. In general, one is left with fairly indirect experimental probes to assess monomer sequence.

In broad strokes, these indirect probes fall into two general classifications. First, there are the techniques that degrade the polymer to an oligomeric species, and then analyze the compositional heterogeneity of these oligomeric materials. While this approach provides insight into the compositional heterogeneity of the system, ascribing the difference observed between inter- and intra-chain sequence variations is sometimes quite ambiguous since one is unable to trace the fragments back to the originating polymers.

The second strategy is to examine the response of the system to applied challenges. Specific examples would include examining the solubility behavior in a variety of pure and mixed solvent systems, characterizing solubility as a function of temperature (cloud point) or using site-directed cleavage as an approach to probe specific structural motifs. An example of the latter would be enzymatic degradation which is selective to the presence of short runs of contiguous unsubstituted anhydroglucose. Both approaches have appeared in the literature.[11–15]

In each case an indirect response is used to provide qualitative insight into the presence or absence of specific run sequences. The utility of this approach is that it provides insight into the origins of observable performance differences between materials that have the same average composition and molecular weight. At this stage, the information derived from these types of measurements remains semi-quantitative.

9.3.2 Molecular Weight

Owing to the dispersity in chain lengths and potentially number of substituents per residue of an assembly of polymeric molecules, molecular weights must be discussed in terms of distribution averages. Three distinct types of averages are generally considered, the number, weight, and z-average molecular weights.

Defining relationships for these three quantities are as follows:

$$M_n = \frac{\sum_i n_i M_i}{\sum_i n_i} = \frac{\sum_i w_i}{\sum_i \frac{w_i}{M_i}}$$

$$M_w = \frac{\sum_i n_i M_i^2}{\sum_i n_i M_i} = \frac{\sum_i w_i M_i}{\sum_i w_i}$$

$$M_z = \frac{\sum_i n_i M_i^3}{\sum_i n_i M_i^2} = \frac{\sum_i w_i M_i^2}{\sum_i w_i M_i}$$

with

$$w_i = n_i M_i$$

where:

w_i is the mass of the fraction of polymer chains with molecular weight M_i
n_i is the number of these chains.

For a perfectly monodisperse polymer sample, $M_w = M_n$. One more frequently speaks of the population polydispersity or M_w/M_n, which is equal to 1.0 for a perfectly monodisperse sample since all the chains in that sample have precisely the same molecular weight. For the materials being discussed here, sample polydispersities will generally fall in the range of 10–20, dropping down to values of 3 or so for rather low molecular weight materials, and occasionally rising above 20 if the systems of differing viscosity grade have been blended. In understanding the performance of polymeric materials, high molecular weight polydispersity can often be a decided benefit. The most extreme example of this would be a synthetic polymer in which residual monomer serves as an integrated plasticizer of the polymeric solid to help control mechanical properties of the system. To varying extents, most low molecular weight constituents (including moisture and low molecular weight oligomers) can serve this type of role.

While the three molecular weight averages may appear to be a simple mathematical construct to characterize a polydisperse population, the origin of these relations reside in the different classical methods that one can employ to experimentally determine the absolute molecular weight of a polymer, and the distinct averaging schemes operative in these methods. The various techniques used to measure polymer molecular weight are well-described in the literature.[16–18]

Colligative property measurements of absolute molecular weight (vapor pressure lowering, boiling point elevation, osmotic pressure) are sensitive to the number average molecular weight. Techniques such as light scattering can, under certain circumstances, yield the weight average molecular weight. Finally, ultracentrifugation-based methods yield z-average molecular weight. In other words, the differing physical response for each of the measurement approaches provides intrinsically different forms of averaging within the polydisperse population. In addition to these absolute methods for determining molecular weight, any physical observable that possesses a molecular weight dependence—for example, solution viscosity at fixed concentration, can be used as an indirect proxy for a molecular weight determination with operational correlation methods providing the needed link to the actual molecular weight.

In recent years, size exclusion chromatography (SEC) has largely replaced these classical approaches for routine absolute molecular weight determination. SEC has a distinct advantage over the classical measurements in that it is able to provide direct information on the complete molecular weight distribution via a direct separation based on the hydrodynamic size of the molecules in solution. There are some additional pragmatic issues that potentially improve the robustness of the SEC based measurement including:

- Since a separation is performed, contamination of the sample with low molecular weight impurities has an inconsequential impact on the final result, since their contribution can be ignored at the data processing step.
- As a corollary, the sample concentration does not need to be accurately known in order to obtain a viable measurement. This can be of enormous help when dealing with in-process or formulated product samples.
- There are minimal sample requirements. Typical injected samples are 100–200 μl with a net concentration in the mg/ml range. This can be advantageous when sample is limited

(say in debugging processing details), but can have a negative side with respect to preparing a representative sample for analysis as the material is very heterogeneous. Naturally, subsampling of a large parent solution can readily address this issue.

The hydrodynamic size of a chain in solution, with fixed topology (i.e., linear or branched) will scale with molecular weight so the operational separation is effectively one of molecular weight, and provides for estimation of the various distribution quantities. Since the common detection schemes are generally concentration sensitive, the ith weight fraction (w_i) is the experimentally determined quantity, thus M_w is based on the actual analytical measurement results. In contrast, M_n and M_z rely on derived calculations from the acquired analytical with heavy weighting at either the low or high molecular weight wings of the distribution, which significantly lowers the precision of their determination. For a well-controlled and calibrated system, long-term variability of M_w determinations are generally better than ~5% relative with M_n, and M_z often ~10–15% precision. Note that these are rough results. Observed precision is composition dependent. Sample requirements, such as the need to employ a binary mobile phase to obtain a fully soluble form, can impact precision. Finally, shear forces in an analytical SEC column can be quite high. SEC system flow rates suitable for low and moderate molecular weight materials (1.0 ml/min for typical ~7–8 mm inner diameter SEC columns) may yield *in situ* shear degradation of the higher molecular weight grade materials available. The obvious approaches of either lowering the flow rate (to 0.25–0.50 ml/min) or using SEC packing materials with a larger particle size will remedy this problem.

By and large, routine SEC-based molecular weight determinations generally yield molecular weight averages that refer to chemically distinct narrow molecular weight distribution calibration standards used in calibrating the chromatographic system elution volume–molecular weight relationship. As such, reported molecular weights are often referred to as relative or equivalent molecular weights. Values provided by many laboratories adhere to this methodology. Finally, while most materials mentioned above (aside from sodium carboxymethylcellulose) are nominally nonionic, it is always strongly recommended that users employ some level of dissolved indifferent electrolyte in the SEC mobile phase. The reason for this is that even nominally nonionic polymers may possess low levels of carboxylate functionality due to adventitious oxidation events during preparation or aging. In the absence of screening indifferent electrolyte, chains that possess even a low level of charge may be electrostatically excluded from the internal pore volume of the packing material. In the absence of molecular weight sensitive detection, this occurrence can yield incorrect molecular weights, since the elution of the sample is now influenced by factors outside of size alone.

More recently, SEC separations have been combined with molecular weight sensitive detection schemes (online light scattering, online viscometry) to enable integrated development of operational absolute molecular weight–elution volume calibration of the system, and online determination of absolute molecular weight information. The potential compositional complexity of the copolymeric systems used as pharmaceutical excipients renders light scattering determinations of molecular weight rather more complex than simple characterization of typical synthetic homopolymer systems. While the absolute nature of light scattering molecular weight determinations are often touted, that ideal is often not completely realized with the complex copolymeric systems discussed here. Furthermore, absolute molecular weight determinations are quite dependent upon the determination of an accurate, specific refractive index increment (dn/dc). Inspection of the literature for tabulated values of this quantity often shows a wide range of values in rather similar solvent systems. Ultimately, the accuracy of absolute molecular weights often relies on the quality of this secondary quantity. Under well-controlled conditions using purified samples, dn/dc can be determined with high precision. The usual secondary issue associated with this is how strongly dn/dc varies with composition, and to what extent composition of the samples also varies.

While productive use of molecular weight sensitive detection rely on judicious understanding of all the factors required to generate quality data, one overriding value of the approach is that if adsorption of the analyte occurs on the stationary phase packing material, the result is unaffected to the degree that elution zones may overlap with genuinely low molecular weight material. In routine SEC which relies on the use of a secondary calibrant to allow creation of a MW/elution volume calibration curve, there is no direct indication if analyte is adsorbing to the stationary phase, and this will naturally have an enormous impact on any calculated results.

Although SEC is certainly one of the most used approaches to polymer molecular weight determination, the batch classical methods are still used.

Colligative property measurements include both vapor pressure and membrane osmometry. While both measurements rely on colligative effects, in a practical sense, they complement one another rather well.

Owing to the physical limitations of membranes, membrane osmometry is ill-suited for relatively low molecular weight polymers ($M_n < \sim 25\,000$ Dalton), and finds its main utility with relatively high molecular weight materials and, under carefully controlled conditions, polyelectrolytes. Since low molecular weight contaminants are able to equilibrate across the membrane, membrane osmometry is insensitive to low molecular weight contaminants. It is also insensitive to chemical heterogeneity, which is a major advantage in the analysis of copolymeric materials.

In contrast, vapor pressure osmometry tends to excel in the lower molecular weight region ($M_n < 20\,000$ Dalton) for which membrane osmometry is ill-suited. However, the technique is very sensitive to the presence of any low molecular weight impurities, which requires the use of highly purified samples, and is inapplicable to polyelectrolyte systems.

Although colligative property measurements have a well-founded physical basis, any methodology that allows an experimentalist to count molecules in an assembly can be used to provide an estimate of M_n. Other techniques that have seen utility in the literature include end group analysis, in which unique functionality or reactivity or end groups are used as a mechanism to count the total population of chains in a sample.

At the other end of the spectrum, analytical ultracentrifugation can be used to quantify the M_z of a sample population. While this technique has seen substantial use in the analysis of proteins and other biologically derived polymers, and has had a recent resurgence with the commercial rerelease of the BeckmanCoulter Optima XL-A series of instruments, it remains something of a niche technology, despite appreciable technical benefits (lack of a potentially adsorptive stationary phase as in SEC, wide range of solution conditions possible, ability to assess complicated equilibria, and ability to handle ultrahigh molecular weight and colloidal systems under conditions of very low sample shear).

The measurements of M_w averages tend to dominate molecular weight characterization of polymers. For the sake of this discussion, we will consider methods that directly measure M_w, together with methods such as viscometry which yield a response that generally tracks M_w.

For the determination of an absolute M_w, light scattering, either alone or in conjunction with size exclusion chromatography, is the primary experimental approach. The use of size exclusion chromatography with either narrow distribution molecular weight standards, or inline viscometric detection with universal calibration transformation, provides results that can range from a simple relative molecular weight, if the calibration standards are chemically distinct from the analyte, to near absolute M_w results.

Potential pitfalls of light scattering include the possible impact of dust or suspended precipitates for batch style measurements, association phenomena which result in inflation of the experimental results, the use of binary solvents to improve polymer solubility or lack of strict adherence to constraints required to guarantee that absolute results are obtained (chemical homogeneity of the chain populations, maintaining constant chemical potential of counterions for polyelectrolyte samples (often approximated by the use of "swamping" electrolyte in large relative excess), accurate values of dn/dc).

Pairing light scattering with a prior SEC separation adds substantial power to both techniques. While SEC provides a means to separate material according to its hydrodynamic volume in solution, it also provides an excellent means to filter the analytical sample to eliminate dust and other artifacts from the light scattering signal.

While the underlying fundamental physical quantity of interest is the molecular weight of a material, and most performance traits are related to the molecular weight, most materials are classified in a more operational manner via grade classification according to a viscosity measurement under specified conditions. Naturally, viscometry or rheology can be used as a method to quantify polymer molecular weight, as well as to provide other insights into the nature of the material.

Rheology is the study of the deformation and flow of material when subjected to an applied force.

The practical consequences of rheology play out in everyday experiences: in the kitchen as one thickens a water-based fluid with starch or forms a jelly through the use of gelatin dissolved at high temperature. In both extremes, the mechanical properties of the final preparation are manipulated through the judicious addition of a polymeric material. The science of rheology attempts to quantify the material changes exemplified by these systems. Detailed treatments of the complete scope of rheology are readily available.[19–22] Dealy has also prepared a convenient summary of official nomenclature and basic terms related to rheological science.[23]

In assessing the response of a material to an applied force, it is critical to appreciate that the applied force can span many orders of magnitude, ranging from simple gravity acting upon a particle suspended in a fluid medium to the very high shear rates experienced in high speed mixing or high deformation rates experienced in high speed conveyance and manufacture of solid products. Depending upon the particular details in manufacture and of usage, this entire range of shear or deformation rates may be sampled at various points in routine usage.

Rheology considers not only the viscous flow of liquids, but the elastic and plastic deformation of solids. In terms of the essential mechanics, the physical situations are quite similar (see Figure 9.14). Real materials possess both elastic and viscous traits, with the key feature being the timescale over which the shear force is applied relative to the intrinsic relaxation time for the material.

In most cases, the response of a system is quantified by measuring the shear stress (σ, Pa) that develops in a

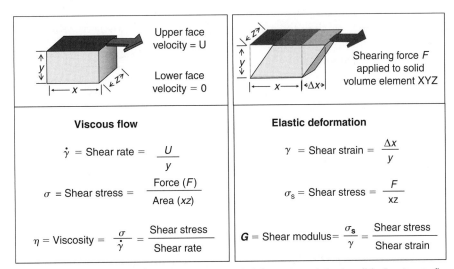

FIGURE 9.14 The basic mechanics of the flow of viscous liquids and deformation of elastic solids. In viscous flow the energy input into the system is dissipated, while it is stored in the pure elastic deformation of a solid. Real materials are viscoelastic in nature, displaying both viscous and elastic character, with the balance detemined by both the magnitude and duration of the applied force

system under the conditions of a controlled and specified shear rate ($\dot{\gamma}$, sec^{-1}) for viscous flow or shear strain (γ) for pure elastic deformation. Typically, one speaks of the viscosity (η) of a fluid, which is simply the ratio of the shear stress divided by the shear rate:

$$\eta = \frac{\sigma}{\dot{\gamma}}$$

or the shear modulus (G):

$$G = \frac{\sigma}{\gamma}$$

in the case of solids.

If we restrict our attention to liquid systems for the moment, in the simplest case, which experimentally applies to simple, low molecular weight, non-associating liquids, flow is directly proportional to the applied force. Equivalently, the ratio of the shear stress to applied shear rate is a constant independent of the applied shear rate (see Figure 9.15). Systems that behave in this fashion are termed Newtonian. Although it is not explicitly noted in the above, Newtonian fluids will also display a time invariant viscosity. If the shear rate is maintained constant over time, the temperature is maintained constant, and chemical degradation of the sample does not occur, the shear stress that results, and hence the measured viscosity, is also constant. Although most common Newtonian liquids are also low viscosity, these two traits are not inexorably tied together. For example, concentrated sucrose solutions possess substantial viscosity, and also exhibit Newtonian flow.

When a polymer is dissolved in a low molecular weight Newtonian solvent, the rheological response can become decidedly more complex. The most significant effect is that one observes that the solution viscosity is no longer independent of the applied shear rate under all conditions. One will generally observe that at vanishingly small shear rates, there will be a limited low shear Newtonian plateau over which the solution viscosity appears independent of the applied shear rate. As the applied shear rate is increased, one will enter a shear thinning regime in which the apparent viscosity drops as the shear rate is increased (see Figure 9.16). Finally, at very high shear rates one may observe re-establishment of a regime in which the apparent viscosity is again independent of the applied shear rate, yielding a limited high shear Newtonian plateau.

An example with actual data is provided in Figure 9.17. This profile shows the shear thinning behavior of various viscosity grades of 2.0 wt % Hypromellose in water. Note that even at rather low effective shear rates, achievement of a well-defined

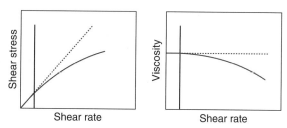

FIGURE 9.16 Most solutions of polymers exhibit some degree of non-Newtonian flow behavior. Simple shear thinning is the most straightforward case. In this example, the system is Newtonian until a critical shear rate is achieved. Above this critical shear rate the apparent viscosity drops with further increases in shear rate

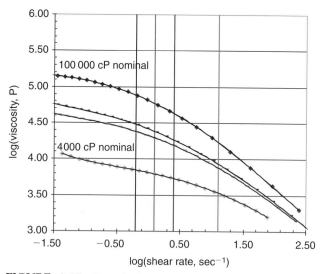

FIGURE 9.17 Typical shear thinning behavior exhibited by 2 wt % hypromellose solution in water. The minor apparent upturn in the apparent viscosity of the 4000 cP nominal viscosity sample is an instrumental artifact due to a low analytical signal. The vertical lines indicate (left to right) the effective shear rate applied in a Brookfield rotational viscometer equipped with a cylindrical fixture at 3, 6, 12, and 60 revolutions per minute (rpm)

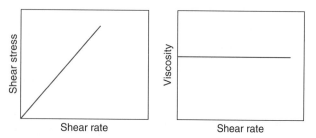

FIGURE 9.15 The simplest case for fluid flow is provided by a simple Newtonian liquid. In this case, the fluid viscosity is independent of the applied shear rate. Common low molecular weight unassociated liquids and solutions are Newtonian

low shear Newtonian plateau is not assured. Finally, the fairly strong shear rate dependence in the measured viscosity of a polymeric solution can have very practical consequences. As can be observed from the estimated shear rates for a determination of viscosity using a simple Brookfield rotational viscometer under rotational speeds commonly employed in laboratory work (3, 6, 12, and 60 rpm), for a shear thinning fluid, precise adherence to specified conditions is a clear requirement if intercomparison of results is desired. For example, the apparent viscosity of the 100 000 cP (grade designation based on 2% Ubbelohde viscosity using the USP methodology) would appear to be roughly 75 000 cP if measured at with a cylindrical spindle at 3 rpm, while the apparent viscosity is less than 20 000 cP if measured at 60 rpm. This is the reason that the shear rate of the measurement needs to be known in assessing viscometric results, particularly when the sample is in the semi-dilute regime (see below). Furthermore, while factors such as spindle rotation rates obviously impact the shear rate applied to a system, less obvious factors such as vessel size (if small relative to the rotational fixture in a Brookfield viscosity measurement) can also contribute to the actual shear rate applied to the sample.

In addition to the pronounced shear rate dependence in the apparent viscosity, the concentration dependence can be broken into two regimes for nonelectrolyte polymers, with some added complexities apparent in the case of polyelectrolytes. If one views the state of a discrete polymer chain as the concentration of a system is increased, the solvated chain will rotationally sweep out a distinct and large volume element of the solvent. In dilute solution, on average, all of the chains will be able to rotationally average their motions without any hindrance from neighboring polymer chains. However, as the concentration is increased, one will reach a point at which the rotationally averaged volume elements first touch, then overlap. Once these volume elements start to overlap, the chains start to entangle with one another. When this occurs, the concentration dependence of the apparent viscosity at constant shear rate increases substantially. This regime, under which polymer chains overlap and entangle with one another, is referred to as the semi-dilute concentration regime. If one were to examine the profile of apparent viscosity against concentration in log–log coordinates, two distinct power law regimes are generally apparent in the dilute and semi-dilute regimes. Power law exponents are generally close to 1 in the dilute regime, and increase to 3–4 as one transitions to the semi-dilute regime (see Figure 9.18). From a fundamental basis, characterization of the apparent viscosity dilute and semi-dilute regimes is best done using

results extrapolated to zero shear rate (i.e., reflective of the low shear Newtonian plateau). However, operationally, these analyses and general guides also apply with reasonable fidelity under conditions of finite shear. The distinction is important since most workers will have access to a Brookfield rotational viscometer to characterize these materials, with this style of measurement generally being practiced at effective shear rates well above that needed to observe the low shear Newtonian plateau.

In the case of polyelectrolyte, additional complications exist due to the strong dependence of the expansion of a solvated chain on the net ionic strength of a solution. Figure 9.19 depicts the dependence of the intrinsic viscosity of a sodium carboxymethylcellulose sample as a function of ionic strength in dilute solution. As one would anticipate, addition of indifferent electrolyte screens the repulsion of like charges along a polyelectrolyte backbone, allowing the chain to adopt a more relaxed random coil configuration in solution. The net result is a drop in viscosity in the system. As depicted in Figure 9.19, that drop in viscosity can be relatively large for modest changes in ionic strength.

In a solution with no added indifferent electrolyte, the general viscosity behavior of polyelectrolytes is similar to nonelectrolytes, with the added feature of the progressively increasing screening of bound charge sites yielding an apparent lowering of power law exponents in both the dilute and semi-dilute

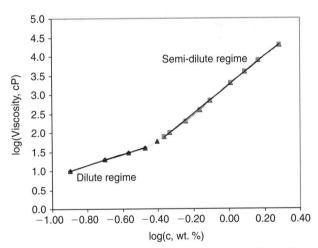

FIGURE 9.18 Example of the concentration dependence of viscosity for sodium carboxymethyl cellulose (DS ~ 0.7, 7H type) as concentration is varied from roughly 0.10 to 2.0 wt %. Clear distinction of the dilute and semi-dilute regimes is apparent. The solutions represented in this example were prepared using pure water as the solvent, hence the ionic strength of the solution is not held constant as the polymer concentration is increased. This results in a slight lowering of the power law slope in both the dilute and semi-dilute regimes

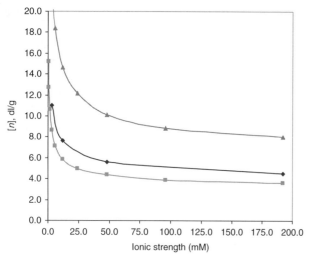

FIGURE 9.19 Impact of added electrolyte on the intrinsic viscosity of a typical polyelectrolyte, in this case sodium carboxymethylcellulose (NaCMC). (Original data from Pals, D. T. & Hermans, J. J. (1952). Rec. Trav. Chim. Pays-Bas, 71, 433–443.) At low ionic strength, the NaCMC chains adopt a relatively rigid rod-like conformation due to electrostatic repulsion between adjacent chain bound anionic charges. As the ionic strength is increased, this repulsive interaction is screened and the polymer adopts a less rigid conformation

regimes since the apparent ionic strength increases with polymer concentration. This complexity can be suppressed by the addition of an indifferent electrolyte to maintain a nearly constant net ionic strength in solution. Naturally, this can further suppress viscosity build in the system.

Finally, in addition to solution shear thinning due to alignment of chains by the applied shear field, the presence of labile association aggregates can yield a time dependent apparent viscosity that is dependent on the recent shear history of the sample (see Figure 9.20). This characteristic is termed thixotropy, and arises from the association-dissociation of aggregates which is much slower than the timescale of the measuring experiment.

Although relating solution rheology to molecular weight is best pursued using extrapolated zero shear values, the use of power law relationships in the semi-dilute concentration regime at finite shear typically yields operationally useful relationships for the quick estimation of molecular weight. Owing to pragmatic instrumental limitations, these experiments generally involve data acquired over a range of shear rates. This can lower the overall quality of the correlation, but it is still useful for routine estimates.

Power law relationships of the form:

$$\log(M_w) = a + b * \log\left(\frac{\eta}{c^{\alpha}}\right)$$

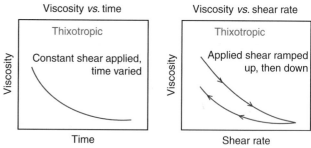

FIGURE 9.20 Polymeric systems in which reversible interpolymer association is possible display a characteristic known as thixotropy. Basically, the mechanical stress applied to the system causes reversible disassembly of the aggregate network. Under conditions of steady shear, this yields a slow decrease in the apparent viscosity over time. The extent of disassembly is dependent on the net force applied to the system, hence the drop in viscosity can occur from either a quiescent state or if a sheared system is subjected to a higher shear rate. By the same token, on a decrease in applied shear rate, the apparent viscosity exhibits recovery. The magnitude of the effect is generally quantified by measuring the disparity in flow curves obtained in a simple experiment in which the shear rate is ramped up then down with continuous recording of the viscosity

are often found to operationally model the data. In the equation above, M_w is the average molecular weight, while η is the solution viscosity at concentration c. The constants a, b, and α can be viewed simply as mathematical fitting constants, although α is related to the power law concentration exponent in the semi-dilute regime. An example of this treatment is shown in Figure 9.21 for three types of cellulosic derivative. The specific relationships shown are as follows:

Hydroxypropylcellulose

$$\log(M_w) = 5.08 + 0.305 * \log\left(\frac{\eta}{c^{3.2}}\right)$$

Hydroxyethylcellulose

$$\log(M_w) = 5.00 + 0.306 * \log\left(\frac{\eta}{c^{3.1}}\right)$$

Sodium carboxymethylcellulose

$$\log(M_w) = 4.78 + 0.356 * \log\left(\frac{\eta}{c^{3.1}}\right)$$

where:

M_w is the nominal material molecular weight
η is the solution Brookfield viscosity
c is weight percentage polymer concentration.

Naturally, these relations can be rearranged to yield initial estimates of the concentration of any specific grade of polymer required to achieve a target of viscosity.

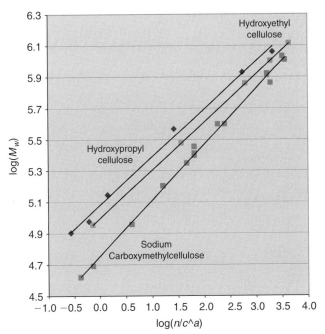

FIGURE 9.21 Polymer master viscosity/concentration/M_w profiles for cellulose ether excipients using Brookfield viscosity values at variable concentration and assuming a simple power law relationship. Separate curves for hydroxypropylcellulose, hydroxyethylcellulose, and sodium carboxymethylcellulose are shown. These curves span the entire product range viscosity for the derivative types shown and listed in Table 9.1

There are a few key points related to rheology and polymers that are worth noting:

1. Since the rheology of a polymer solution is molecular weight dependent, rheology/viscometry can be used as an indirect proxy to monitor molecular weight.
2. Although, strictly speaking, one should use the apparent viscosity extrapolated to zero shear in modeling the molecular weight dependence of polymer solution viscosity, reasonably good master curves obtained at finite shear rates and at variable concentration can be used to provide decent pragmatic estimates of the molecular weight of a polymer sample.
3. Owing to the very strong concentration dependence, the actual polymer concentration needs to be accurately known. Since the power law exponent of viscosity–concentration curves in the semi-dilute region have a log–log slope of 3–4, an x% error in specifying the concentration yields a 3x−4x% error in the calculated viscosity.
4. Solution viscometric experiments generally provide information related to the average M_w of a system. No information on the breadth of the molecular weight distribution is provided.

5. The magnitude of the exponent in the power law dependence in viscosity as a function of concentration, as seen in Figures 9.18 and 9.21, is the origin of typical "rules of thumb" used to estimate viscosity at different concentrations. For example, a doubling in weight percentage concentration often yields an increase in viscosity of roughly ten-fold, which follows directly from the type of power law behavior shown in Figure 9.18.

9.3.3 Polymers in Solution

Understanding the unique solution behavior of polymers mainly resides primarily in appreciating a few key points.

First, the high molecular weight of a polymeric solute significantly lowers the entropy of mixing for a polymer solvent binary system, lowering this component of the net free energy of solution. This was treated some time ago by Flory,[6] and more recently by Sanchez and Lacombe,[24–26] which captures the essential results.

At the most primitive level, taking a solution as a simple lattice model, we find:

$$\Delta S_{mix} = -R(n_1 \ln(\phi_1) + n_2 \ln(\phi_2))$$

or

$$\Delta S_{mix} = -R\left(\frac{\phi_1}{DP_1} \ln(\phi_1) + \frac{\phi_2}{DP_2} \ln(\phi_2)\right)$$

As is apparent from the inverse dependence of the premultiplier of each term on the degree of polymerization (DP) or, equivalently, molecular weight of the components in the mixture, if either one or both of these components is a high molecular weight material, the magnitude of the entropy is lowered as the molecular weight is increased. In broad strokes, as the molecular weight increases the free energy driving force for dissolution is lowered, since the gain in entropy by the polymer on dissolution is quite low.

One direct consequence of the lowered entropy of solution is that, in a chemically homogeneous system precipitation of a polymeric solute, as solvent conditions transition from good to poor, starts with the high molecular weight portion of the distribution and proceeds with decreasing molecular weight. This provides a relatively facile manner to perform crude molecular weight based preparative isolation. It also suggests that, for a partially soluble material (again, assumed to be chemically homogeneous) the undissolved fraction is typically enriched in the high molecular weight fraction.

Secondly, most polymers under consideration here are copolymeric materials, for which the various component monomers have rather different intrinsic solubility. For example, in the case of hydroxypropylcellulose, a single unsubstituted anhydroglucose moiety is quite hydrophilic, while a heavily hydroxypropylated anhydroglucose residue is rather hydrophobic. The constituent monomers in a real sample will span a wide range in hydrophobic nature, thus their distinct distribution across chains (inter-chain heterogeneity), and within chains (intra-chain heterogeneity). The net result is that at any specific solvent composition, a situation can arise in which subpopulations of entire chains may be soluble or insoluble or discrete subsections of single chains may be solvated or unsolvated.

Thirdly, the linear array of monomer groups provides a spatial template upon which relatively low energy intermolecular forces can operate in a cooperative fashion to yield fairly strong inter-chain associations. A specific example of this would be the inter-chain association of unsubstituted anhydroglucose runs in the sodium carboxymethylcellulose to yield textured solutions and thixotropic rheology.

With respect to gross solution behavior, the same basic rules that guide the dissolution of low molecular weight species also apply to polymers. As with low molecular weight materials, "like dissolves like." This is captured somewhat more quantitatively in the extended solubility parameter approach,[27–29] in which the cohesive energy of a material is divided into contributions arising from distinct types of intermolecular interactions (dispersive, polar, hydrogen bonding). While the usual admonishment that "like dissolves like" is somewhat more quantitatively expressed within the solubility parameter approach as a matching of the cohesive energy densities of the two materials (solubility is maximized when the cohesive energy densities of the solvent and solute are equal and decreases as they become increasingly disparate), the categorization of the extended solubility parameter approach places a rationale around the basic picture in terms of discrete interaction mechanisms that exist between molecules.

Unlike the situation with low molecular weight liquids, one cannot experimentally determine the molar energy of vaporization of polymers, and using the molar volume calculate a direct cohesive energy density ($\delta = (E_{vap}/V)^{0.5}$). However, one can perform challenge–response experiments to assess the solubility behavior of a polymer in a number of low molecular weight liquids (insoluble, partially soluble/swellable, soluble), and use those observations to construct solubility parameter based maps which can aid in the selection of optimum solvent systems for dissolving a polymeric material. As a specific example, consider

hydroxypropylcellulose.[30,31] Figure 9.22 contains the qualitative solution behavior of hydroxypropylcellulose in a variety of solvents presented as a two-dimensional solubility map in terms of the polar and hydrogen bond solubility parameters. As is apparent, there is a reasonably clear demarcation between the insoluble and partially or completely soluble regions. Note that the partially soluble and soluble regions exhibit substantial overlap. This is largely a consequence of the two-dimensional nature of the plot, which neglects the explicit contribution of dispersive interactions to solubility. The specific solvents for which hydroxypropylcellulose exhibits good solubility at low polar and/or hydrogen bond solubility parameters tend to be high refractive index liquids (aromatic or halogenated), which increases the dispersive contribution of the net solution energy.

The dissolution characteristics of the polymeric species become complicated when the constituent monomers have vastly different solvation requirements. In that case, the usual recommendation of "like dissolves like" may only apply to a portion of a given polymer chain. In this case, the use of binary and/or ternary solvent mixtures can often yield solutions not possible from any of the pure solvent components.

One other aspect of polymer solubility is the existence of upper and lower critical solution temperatures, referred to as UCST and LCST respectively, seen in aqueous solutions of many of these polymers.

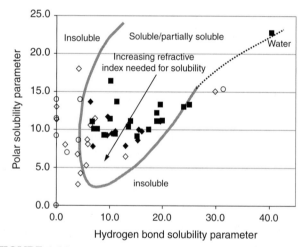

FIGURE 9.22 Solubility characteristics of hydroxypropyl cellulose as a function of polar and hydrogen bond solubility parameters. In this solubility map, the solid curve is soluble/insoluble phase boundary presented in reference 30. The dashed line is an interpolated boundary taking into account water solubility characteristics. Points shown represent the specific solvents listed in references 29–31 as yielding solutions , described as clear and smooth/soluble (■), moderately granular and/or hazy/partially soluble (◆) or insoluble (○), or uncharacterized systems of unknown solubility (◇).

The situation is diagrammatically shown in Figure 9.23. In the case of an LCST, the system splits into a two-phase system comprised of polymer rich and polymer lean compositions at high temperature. As the temperature is lowered, the composition of these two phases approaches one another, and then merges into a single phase at the LCST. Similar behavior occurs with the UCST, except that the transition from a two phase to a one phase system occurs as the temperature is raised.

In the current application settings, one typically observes an LCST from the perspective of a cloud point,

which is simply due to performing the experiment in reverse—starting with a homogeneous solution in the single phase region and raising the temperature until the solution splits into two phases. This occurs uniformly throughout the volume of solution, which typically yields small droplets of the polymer rich phase dispersed in the polymer lean phase. This generates a high level of scattered light, rendering the fluid opaque, and is the origin of the term "cloud point." Figure 9.24 provides an example of two chemically similar systems, hydroxypropylcellulose and hypromellose, both as 1% solutions in water. The substantial difference in cloud points is related to the substantially different hydrophobicity of these two materials. As is typical for marginally soluble hydrophobic materials, the addition of electrolyte will move the cloud point to lower temperature, as would an increase in the hydroxypropyl content of either system or the methoxyl level of the hypromellose sample.

9.3.4 Structure–Property Relationships

In polymer chemistry and materials engineering it is common to design novel materials and formulated systems with improved functional properties, based on detailed study and understanding of how the structure of a material impacts the physical and chemical properties that are critical to the end use. In the pharmaceutical industry it is common to apply this type of approach to the design of drug molecules. For example, quantitative structure–activity relationships are studied to enable the design of drug molecules with optimal therapeutic efficacy. A further

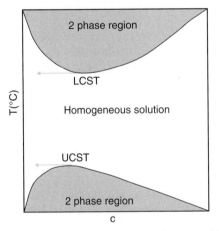

FIGURE 9.23 Schematic representation of upper and lower critical solution temperatures, UCST and LCST respectively. A UCST exists when a polymer transitions from partially soluble to soluble as temperature is raised, while an LCST occurs when a single homogeneous phase splits into two phases with the same increase in temperature. An LCST is often seen with relatively hydrophobic materials, while UCST behavior tends to be observed with systems involved in specific self-association phenomena

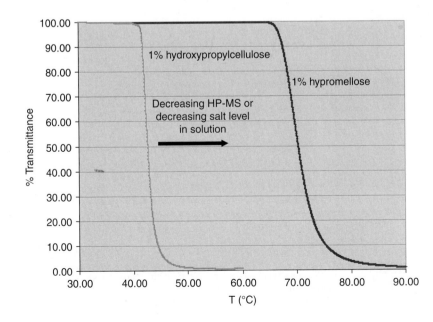

FIGURE 9.24 Cloud point curves for typical high viscosity grades of hydroxypropylcellulose and hypromellose (hydroxypropylmethyl cellulose). The major difference in cloud points between these two materials is reflective of the differing hydrophobicities (determined by a combination of hydroxypropyl and methoxyl groups for hypromellose). In addition to the native polymer composition, addition of indifferent electrolyte can lower the cloud point by a few degrees for typical physiologically relevant ionic strength

example is the optimization of drug solubility and stability through the selection of appropriate salt and crystal forms. Similarly, a good appreciation of structure–property relationships is also essential if formulators are to make rational, science-based choices when selecting polymers and other excipients as formulation components.

The following section will attempt to illustrate some of the major, generally applicable structure–property relationships that are of practical use, and specifically relevant to pharmaceutical polymers and their use in solid oral controlled release dosage forms. These include the impact of MW, substitution, and copolymerization on solution, gel, mechanical, and thermal properties. While the general principles are applicable across a wide range of polymers, many of the examples given here will focus on cellulose derivatives, the most commonly used class of polymers in modified release dosage form design.

Molecular Weight Effects

Effect of molecular weight on solution viscosity

Many polymer properties are molecular weight dependant, including solution and melt viscosity, glass transition temperatures, mechanical properties, and gel strength. Perhaps the most important and frequently applied structure property relationship is the correlation between dilute solution viscosity and molecular weight. As a longer polymer chain gyrates in solution it can be visualized to occupy a larger volume of the solvent, and collide and overlap more frequently with other long polymer chains, as compared to shorter polymer chains. The initial fundamental observation and prediction that solution viscosity is proportional to polymer molecular weight was made by Staudinger and Heuer.[32] For linear polymers the Mark–Houwink equation provides an empirical model for this is relationship:

$$\eta = KM^a$$

where:

η is the specific viscosity
M is the weight average molecular weight
K and a are polymer, solvent and temperature dependant.

Generally, a varies between 0.5 and 1. For poor solvents in which the polymer remains coiled, $a = 0.5$. For good solvents, a varies between 0.65 and 0.8. For stiff, asymmetrical molecules in good solvents, a may approach 1. It should be noted that the above discussion specifically applies to linear polymer molecules. Highly branched, bush shaped polymer structures

may have a large molecular weight, but occupy proportionally smaller volumes in their solvated state.

Effect of molecular weight on mechanical and thermoplastic properties

Many physical properties of amorphous polymers, including mechanical and thermoplastic properties, show a strong molecular weight dependence. Frequently, a general relationship applies where molecular weight changes in the lower middle molecular weight range result in large changes in the physical property of interest. However, as shown in Figure 9.25, after reaching a threshold level in molecular weight, further molecular weight increases result in only minor changes in the physical property of interest.

Often these phenomena can be explained on the basis of "chain end" concentration, i.e., lower molecular weight polymer chains are shorter, and thus for the same amount of material there is a proportionate increase in the number of molecules and thus chain ends. The chain ends tend to be associated with a greater degree of mobility and free volume as compared to the middle segments of a polymer chain. Lower molecular weight is generally associated with greater plasticity. In contrast, longer polymer chains (lower chain end concentration) are generally associated with increased elasticity and flexibility.

Mechanical strength of films　One of the most useful mechanical tests for polymeric and pharmaceutical materials in general is to determine its tensile strength and the accompanying stress–strain curve. This is generally done by using a mechanical testing machine,

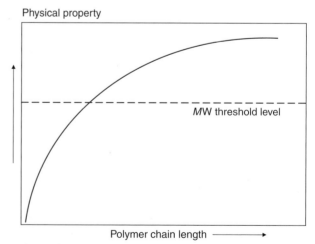

FIGURE 9.25 General relationship between polymer chain length (molecular weight) and physical properties such as tensile strength and T_g

and continuously measuring the force developed as the material is elongated at a constant rate of extension. Figure 9.26 illustrates a typical stress–strain curve. Important mechanical properties of a material include the modulus (slope of the initial curve) which is a measure of the material stiffness, yield stress, strength, ultimate strength, elongation at break, and toughness (area under the curve).

For practical purposes it is often useful to divide polymeric materials into five common classes depending on their stress–strain behavior. These common classes are illustrated in Table 9.2.

For polymer films, an increase in molecular weight tends to increase film tensile strength, elongation, and flexibility. This can be explained on the basis that longer polymer chains exhibit greater flexibility and elasticity. They can thus be extended further before rupture, as compared with short polymer chains. A general relationship describing this behavior is given by the following equation:

$$tensile\ strength = a - \frac{b}{M_n}$$

Where a is the tensile strength threshold, beyond which further molecular weight increases become ineffective, b is a material dependant constant, and M_n is number average molecular weight.[33] An example of this is given in Figure 9.27, which shows the viscosity (MW) dependence of ethylcellulose film properties.

Film strength is of significance in membrane reservoir controlled release dosage forms such as multiparticulates or tablets coated with ethylcellulose controlled release films. It has been shown that the drug release kinetics of such systems are directly proportional to the film strength and, by inference, polymer molecular weight (Figure 9.28). This is due to the fact that drug release from membrane–reservoir systems is osmotic pressure dependant. As the water enters the dosage forms via osmosis, and builds up hydrostatic pressure in the core, it increasingly exerts a stress on the membrane, until fissures and cracks open up resulting in release of drug due to osmotic pumping.[34-36]

Similar examples of increasing film strength with molecular weight are known for the majority of pharmaceutical polymers. A further example is the report by Prodduturi et al, describing the increased mechanical strength of drug loaded buccal films with increasing molecular weight of hydroxypropylcellulose used.[37]

Mechanical strength of tablets As previously indicated, longer polymer chains impart greater elasticity, while the greater chain-end concentration found with decreasing molecular weight results in greater plasticity and molecular mobility. For directly compressed tablets, lower polymer molecular weight therefore results in less post ejection elastic recovery, and greater permanent deformation. For example, low molecular weight hydroxypropylcellulose (HPC) grades have been reported to yield stronger tablets than high molecular weight HPC, due to greater plasticity and lower post-compaction ejection. However, this disadvantage of high molecular weight polymers can be partly neutralized by using fine particle size HPC (Figure 9.29).[38] Similar observations have also been made for ethyl cellulose matrix tablets.[39]

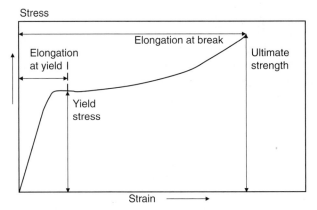

FIGURE 9.26 Typical tensile stress–strain curve for a polymer specimen tested in tension

TABLE 9.2 Common classes of materials based on their stress–strain curve characteristics (reference 33)

Class	Modulus	Yield stress	Ultimate strength	Elongation at break
Soft and weak	Low	Low	Low	Moderate
Soft and tough	Low	Low	Moderate	High
Hard and brittle	High	None	Moderate	Low
Hard and strong	High	High	High	Moderate
Hard and tough	High	High	High	High

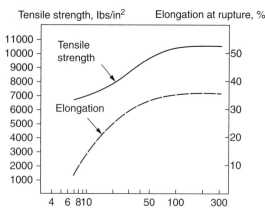

FIGURE 9.27 Ethylcellulose film properties as a function of solution viscosity (molecular weight). All solutions viscosity values reflect 5 wt. % ethylcellulose in a 80:20 blend of toluene:ethanol. (Courtesy of Aqualon Division, a Business Unit of Hercules Incorporated, Wilmington, DE)

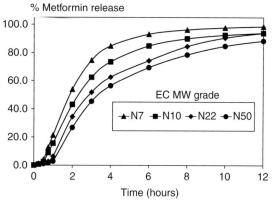

FIGURE 9.28 Drug release from metformin HCl pellets coated with various molecular weight grades of Aqualon® N Pharm ethylcellulose (EC)(34). N7, N10, N22, and N50 refers to different molecular weight grades with 7, 10, 22, and 50 cps solution viscosity (5 wt % solution in 80:20 toluene:ethanol) respectively

Glass transition temperature, melting point and melt index The glass transition temperature (T_g), melting point temperature, and melt index are fundamental characteristics related to thermoplastic behavior. Similar to mechanical properties, a negative inverse relationship has also been postulated for T_g and molecular weight:[41]

$$T_g = T_g^\infty - \frac{k}{M_n}$$

Where T_g^∞ is the glass transition at infinite molecular weight, and k is a constant. The greater flexibility and lower T_g of lower molecular weight polymers is attributed to the greater concentration and mobility of polymer chain ends versus the chain middle. Due to

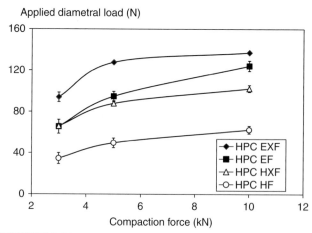

FIGURE 9.29 Compactability for various molecular weight and particle size types of hydroxypropylcellulose. Klucel® EXF Pharm HPC (80 kDA, 70 μm average particle size) Klucel® EF Pharm HPC (80 kDA molecular weight, 200 μm average particle size), Klucel® HXF Pharm HPC (1000 kDA molecular weight, 70 μm average particle size), Klucel® HF Pharm HPC (80 kDA, 200 μm average particle size). 300 mg pure polymer tablets were compressed on a Manesty Beta press using 7/16" round flat faced tooling

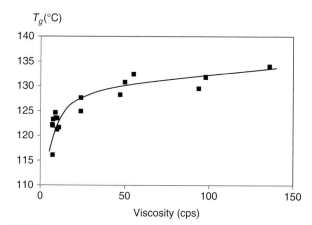

FIGURE 9.30 Glass transition temperature (T_g) as a function of solution viscosity (an indicator of molecular weight) for a series of Aqualon® Ethylcellulose polymers. In all cases, substitution was between 49.8 and 51 wt % ethoxyl content

their greater mobility, and the effective defect in material packing that they create, chain ends are associated with greater excess free volume. In a series of equally substituted polymers, lower molecular weight polymers will thus have a greater concentration of chain ends, resulting in greater excess free volume, greater molecular mobility, and lower T_g. Figure 9.30 shows the change in T_g as a function of solution viscosity (as an indirect proxy for molecular weight) for a series of ethylcellulose polymers.

T_g is an important fundamental property of amorphous and semicrystalline polymer systems, and is frequently correlated with properties such as plasticity and ductility, film forming ability, and stickiness.

TABLE 9.3 Factors affecting glass transition temperature (T_g) values

Molecular structural feature	Impact on T_g
Increased molecular weight	Higher
Increased symmetry	Higher
Increased length of flexible side chain	Lower
Addition of chain stiffening units	Higher
Addition of polar groups	Higher
Increased cross-link density	Higher

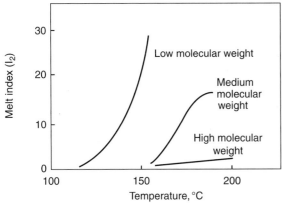

FIGURE 9.31 Melt index, I_2, as a function of temperature and Klucel® hydroxypropylcellulose molecular weight. The melt index is defined as the grams of molten material that is extruded under standard ASTM defined conditions in 10 minutes, at a given temperature and applied load

While polymer molecular weight is a major factor determining T_g values, numerous other structural factors will impact molecular rigidity and order, and, by implication, T_g. Some of these factors are summarized in Table 9.3.

Similarly to T_g, melting point temperatures and melt viscosity increase with increasing molecular weight. Operationally, polymer flow is typically characterized using a melt flow index, which is an inverse measure of melt viscosity. These properties are especially critical in modified release dosage form design in the context of thermal processing, such as melt extrusion, and injection molding. Frequently, higher melt flow index polymers are required for thermal processing in the range at or below 100°C, in order to avoid thermal degradation of drug and acceptable throughput rates. Figure 9.31 shows the variation of melt flow indices for different molecular weight grades of hydroxypropylcellulose, a thermoplastic polymer which is commonly used in melt extrusion processes, such as the manufacture of oral film strips, and other extruded drug delivery devices.

Effect of molecular weight on gel strength

The relationship between gel strength and polymer molecular weight is of particular importance in the field of modified release dosage form design. For hydrophilic matrix tablets, the gel strength will determine the erodibility of the matrix system. Erosion can be described as polymer dissolution or the disentanglement of polymer chains from the gel surface and transfer of the polymer to the bulk solution. Erosion can be used to the formulator's advantage when designing a delivery system for insoluble drugs. Here, erosion is the main mechanism facilitating transfer of the insoluble drug out of the tablet matrix and into the dissolution medium. However, poor release characteristics such as variable burst release and dose dumping may be expected for a highly soluble drug that is formulated in a highly erodible dosage form.

For hydrophilic polymers such as hypromellose and hydroxypropylcellulose compressed into matrix tablets, the disentanglement concentration of the polymer follows a nonlinear, inverse relationship with molecular weight.[42] Furthermore, polymer matrix erosion rate has also been shown to vary with molecular weight in a non-linear, inverse manner:[43]

$$erosion\ rate = kM_n^{-a}$$

It should be noted that the opposite relationship applies to matrix swelling, i.e., swellability increases with molecular weight up to a limiting threshold level. The rate and extent of polymer matrix swelling, erosion, and the drug solubility and concentration are the dominant compositional factors determining drug release kinetics from matrix tablet systems. Figures 9.32, 9.33 and 9.34 show the impact of polymer molecular weight on matrix tablet erosion and swelling and drug release for a typical sparingly soluble compound, nifedipine.

Side-chain Substitution Effects

The structure of the side-chain substituents on the polymer backbone is a major compositional factor impacting polymer functionality. Important aspects of substitution are the chemical structure of the substituents, the extent of backbone substitution, and the uniformity of substitution. In this section we will mainly focus on the impact of substituent type and the extent of substitution on the functionality in modified release systems.

Side-chain structure (substituent type)

Effect of side-chain structure on polymer solubility In most cases, substitution of less polar groups for hydrogens or hydroxyls on a polymer chain leads to reduction in

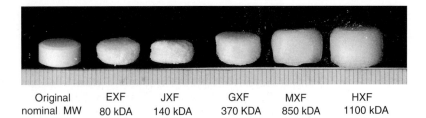

| Original | EXF | JXF | GXF | MXF | HXF |
| nominal MW | 80 kDA | 140 kDA | 370 KDA | 850 kDA | 1100 kDA |

FIGURE 9.32 Effect of Klucel® Pharm HPC molecular weight grade on erosion and swelling behavior of nifedipine matrix tablets subjected to dissolution testing for 4 hours. Formulation: 20% nifedipine, 30% HPC, 49.5% microcrystalline cellulose and 0.5% magnesium stearate

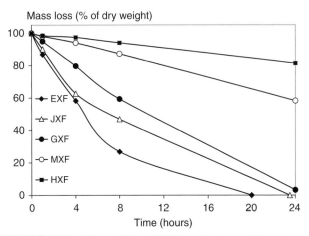

FIGURE 9.33 Effect of Klucel® HPC molecular weight grade on matrix erosion. Nominal molecular weights for Klucel® EXF, JXF, GXF, MXF and HXF Pharm HPC are 80, 140, 370, 850, and 1100 kDA, respectively. Formulation: 20% nifedipine, 30% HPC, 49.5% MCC, and 0.5% magnesium stearate

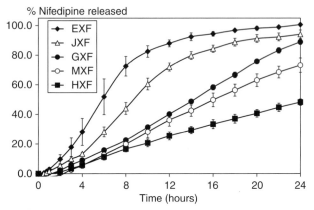

FIGURE 9.34 Effect of Klucel® HPC molecular weight grade on nifedipine dissolution. Nominal molecular weights for Klucel® EXF, JXF, GXF, MXF, and HXF Pharm HPC are 80, 140, 370, 850, and 1100 kDA, respectively. Formulation: 20% nifedipine, 30% HPC, 49.5% MCC, and 0.5% magnesium stearate

TABLE 9.4 Solubility parameters for a series of cellulose ethers and other materials of interest

Polymer or drug molecule	Average solubility parameter,* δ (MPa¹ᐟ²)
EC (2.7 DS)	19.2
HPC (3.8 MS)	23.2
HPMC (1.9 MS)	23.6
HEC (2.5 MS)	25.0
NaCMC (0.7 DS)	28.9
Cellulose	31.1
PVA	30.2
PEO	19.3
Metformin HCl (highly water soluble drug)	27.2
Itraconazole (low water soluble drug)	19.5

*calculated as the average of the Hildebrand, Hansen, Fedors, and van Krevelen solubility parameters

crystallinity and, usually, also a reduction in melting points. Such changes are thus generally expected to improve thermoplasticity and polymer solubility. A good example is presented by cellulose, a naturally occurring polymer comprised of anhydroglucose units. Native cellulose has considerable microcrystalline character. When the free hydroxyls on the anydroglucose backbone are substituted with hydroxyalkyl side chains, e.g. hydroxypropyl or hydroxyethyl groups, the crystallinity of the resultant hydroxypropyl or hydroxyethyl cellulose is below the limit of reliable quantification (<10%). Moreover, unlike microcrystalline cellulose, the derivatized cellulose ethers are freely gelling and soluble in water. Polymer water solubility can be further enhanced by deliberate inclusion of highly polar, ionizable substituents. Sodium carboxymethylcellulose (Na CMC) is an example of this.

Unlike small drug molecules, it is not useful to describe the solubility of a polymer in a given solvent system in terms of saturation concentration values (e.g., g/ml). Among the more useful methods, solubility parameters can be used to evaluate the solubility and compatibility between a polymer and solvent or other additives with solvent-like properties.

Additionally, for water solubility, equilibrium moisture content (hygroscopicity) and cloud point are useful indirect measures of water solubility. The solubility parameters for a series of differently substituted cellulose ether molecules and other materials of interest to formulators are shown in Table 9.4.

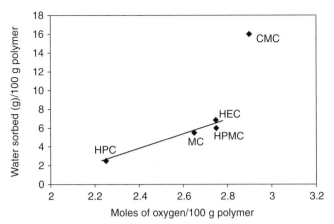

FIGURE 9.35 Effect of oxygen content on the equilibrium moisture content of a series of cellulose derivatives (hydroxypropylcellulose (HPC), methylcellulose (MC), hydroxypropylmethylcellulose (HPMC), hydroxyethylcellulose (HEC), sodium carboxymethylcellulose (CMC)). Adapted from Klug[44]

For many polymers including cellulose, the relationship between water solubility and the nature of the side chain or substituent chemistry can be understood in terms of hydrogen bonding between the hydrogen atoms of water, and the polar oxygen atoms present in the polymer backbone and on the side chains. Studying a series of alkali celluloses of similar molecular weight, Klug[44] showed that polymer hydrophilicity increases as the oxygen content of the derivatized cellulose increases, due to either the type or the extent of substitution. Sodium carboxymethylcellulose is an exception, due to its ionic character. The increased hydrophilicity impacts numerous important properties such as hygroscopicity, cloud point, matrix tablet swelling ability, and matrix gel strength. The general relationship is shown in Figure 9.35.

Effect of side-chain structure on gel strength, swelling and erosion in matrix systems From Figure 9.35 it can be seen that the differently substituted cellulose derivatives can be ranked in the following order of ascending hydrophilicity: HPC < MC < HPMC < HEC and CMC. The difference in hydrophilicity due to substitution on the polymer backbone is particularly important for the functionality of hydrophilic matrix systems. As shown in Figure 9.36, polymer hydrophilicity, in combination with molecular weight, has a major impact on matrix swelling and erosion behavior. For medium and low soluble drugs these factors are the main determinants of release mechanism and release kinetics (Figure 9.37).

Effect of side-chain structure on mechanical properties The nature of the side chain substituent type also significantly impacts mechanical and thermoplastic properties.

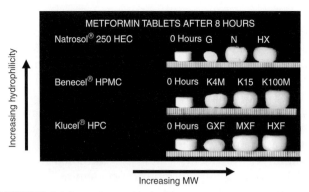

FIGURE 9.36 Matrix tablet swelling and erosion behavior as a function of hydrophilicity (cellulose ether substitution) and molecular weight

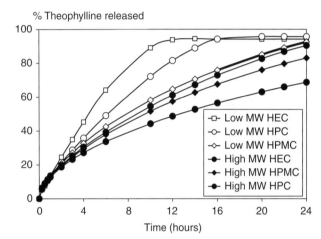

FIGURE 9.37 Drug release from matrix tablets as a function of cellulose ether chemistry and molecular weight

HPC and ethylcellulose (EC) are significantly more thermoplastic than HPMC and HEC. The compactibility of matrix forming cellulose ethers has been reported to increase in the following rank order: HEC < HPMC < HPC.[45]

Extent of side-chain substitution

In addition to the identity of the side-chain structure, the amount of side-chain substitution on the polymer backbone can also exert a significant effect on physical and chemical properties of the polymer.

Effect of extent of substitution on solubility

When highly polar hydroxyl groups on crystalline cellulose are substituted with hydroxyalkyl groups to manufacture HPC or HEC, water solubility initially increases due to a reduction in crystallinity and hydrogen bonding between the cellulose backbone chains. However, as the amount of hydroxyalkyl substitution continues to increase, the polymer becomes increasingly hydrophobic. As shown in Figure 9.38, the equilibrium moisture content steadily decreases as molar substitution increases from 2.0 to 5.0 for both HEC and HPC. A similar relationship has also been demonstrated for the cloud point.[44] An exception to this behavior are polymers with ionic groups in their side chains. In this case, increasing the level of highly polar substituents will increase water solubility. For example, when the degree of substitution for sodium carboxymethylcellulose is increased from 0.7 to 1.2, the equilibrium moisture content at 50% relative humidity increases from 13 to 18%.[44]

Effect of extent of substitution on mechanical properties

In addition to increased hydrophobicity, an increase in the amount of less polar substituents generally also results in an increase in polymer plasticity. As shown in Figure 9.39, in the case of tensile film strength,

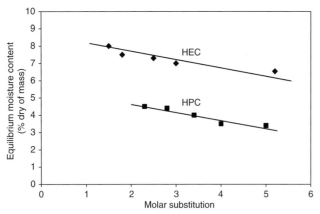

FIGURE 9.38 Effect of substitution level on the equilibrium moisture content of hydroxypropyl and hydroxyethyl cellulose at 50% relative humidity. Adapted from reference 44

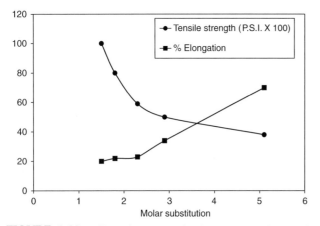

FIGURE 9.39 Effect of amount of substitution on the tensile strength and percentage elongation of a hydroxyethylcellulose film at constant thickness, 50% relative humidity and 25°C. Adapted from reference 44

this manifests in lower ultimate tensile strength, but greater elongation and film flexibility. In contrast, increasing the amount of highly polar, ionic side-chains tends to result in an increased T_g, a markedly less thermoplastic material. As a result, films will tend to exhibit relatively high tensile strength, but will be very brittle and inflexible, with minimal elongation at break. Sodium carboxymethylcellulose shows this behavior, and as a result requires high levels of added plasticizer if useful, defect-free films, suitable for tablet or particle coating are to be achieved.

For polymers compressed into tablets, increasing the number of non-polar substituents generally results in increased plasticity, lower elastic recovery after compression and ejection, and consequently denser compacts with higher diametral crushing strength (tensile failure). Similarly, decreasing the number of more polar substituents will have the same effect. The compaction behavior of a series of hypromellose and methylcellulose grades with varying levels of methoxyl (less polar, hydrophobic, susbtituent) and hydroxypropyl (more polar, more hydrophilic substituent) groups illustrates this.[15] As can be seen in Table 9.5, as the percentage of methoxyl in the polymer increases, and the percentage of hydroxylpropyl decreases, for a series of similar viscosity polymers, the tablet strength significantly increases.

An additional example of the significant effect that an increase in the number of non polar substituents can have is provided by ethylcellulose (EC). It has been reported that higher compactability of EC was associated with high ethoxyl content and low molecular weight (low viscosity) (Figure 9.40).

High substitution and low molecular weight was also correlated with significantly higher crystallinity and higher melting points, while the amorphous regions had lower glass transition temperatures (Table 9.6). Compaction simulator studies showed that the net effect of this unique solid-state structure is a marked reduction in post-compaction elastic recovery of the polymer (Figure 9.41). Less energy of compaction

TABLE 9.5 Tablet tensile strength for a series of hypromellose and methylcellulose samples of similar viscosity when compressed at 15 kN (46)

Polymer type	Methoxy %	Hydroxy propyl %	Tensile strength (MPa)
HPMC 2208	10–24	4–12	1.5
HPMC 2910	28–30	7–12	1.6
HPMC 2906	27–30	4–7.5	2.8
MC	27.5–31.5	0	3.5

was therefore lost due to post-compaction axial expansion, resulting in denser compacts with lower porosity. This had a significant effect on drug diffusion from non-swelling, porosity-controlled matrix tablets. Additionally, the reduced viscoelasticity resulted in lower strain rate sensitivity (10% versus typically 20–25% for other EC types).

Copolymerization

Thermal properties of copolymers

When the monomers of two crystalline homopolymers are combined, the degree of crystallinity and the melting point are usually depressed. The following relationship frequently applies:

$$\frac{1}{T_m} = \frac{1}{T_m^0} - \frac{R}{\Delta H_m} \ln(n)$$

where:

n is the mole fraction of crystalline constituent
T_m is the melting point of the copolymer

T_m^0 is the melting point of the pure homopolymer
ΔH_m is the heat of fusion.[2]

In contrast, the glass transition temperature, T_g, of random copolymers usually falls into the range between that of the two corresponding homopolymers. This difference between how T_m and T_g of a copolymer is affected can be attributed to the fact that crystal structure disruption is not relevant to T_g of the amorphous polymer domains. Frequently, a simple weight average mixing rule of the following type can be applied to get an approximate idea of the resultant T_g of the copolymer:

$$a_1 w_1 (T_g - T_{g1}) + a_2 w_2 (T_g - T_{g2}) = 0$$

where:

T_{g1} and T_{g2} refers to the individual homopolymers
w_1 and w_2 are weight fractions of monomers 1 and 2
a_1 and a_2 depend on monomer type.[48]

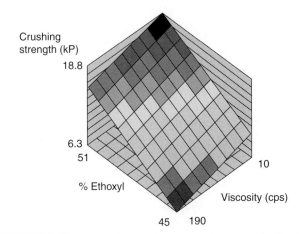

FIGURE 9.40 Effect of ethoxyl content and viscosity (molecular weight) on compactibility of ethylcellulose (EC). Maximum tablet strength is achieved for high ethoxyl, low viscosity EC

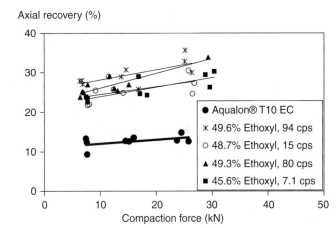

FIGURE 9.41 Effect of ethoxyl content and viscosity on post-compaction axial recovery. High ethoxyl, low viscosity Aqualon® T10 EC has the lowest axial recovery

TABLE 9.6 Effect of ethoxyl content and viscosity on selected solid state properties of ethylcellulose

Ethoxyl (wt %)	Viscosity (cps)	Crystallinity (%)	Melting point (°C)	T_g (°C)	Crushing force (kP)*
50.4	9	24.6	257.0	122.1	20.9
50.8	9	28.5	261.1	124.6	18.8
50.0	50	15.3	246.6	130.7	14.6
49.6	94	17.8	261.0	129.5	16.1
48.0	10	9.1	210.0	131.0	14.7
48.5	94	7.9	224.3	133.5	11.5
47.5	10	8.2	178.6	135.1	12.3

*275 mg pure ethylcellulose tablets compressed on a Betapress at 25 kN

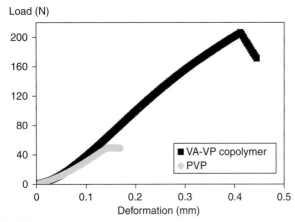

FIGURE 9.42 Load–deformation plots for the pure polymer tablets of povidone ($T_g \sim 161°C$ and copovidone ($T_g \sim 101°C$) subjected to diametral compression

Mechanical properties of copolymers

As a comonomer is added to a crystalline polymer, crystallinity, T_g, and T_m are usually decreased, with a resultant increase in copolymer plasticity and flexibility. Therefore, copolymers are frequently better film-formers and tablet-binders than the initial homopolymer. Povidone (polyvinyl-2-pyrrolidone, PVP) and copovidone, the 6:4 random copolymer of vinyl pyrrolidone and vinyl acetate (VP–VA copolymer) present a common pharmaceutical example. PVP, although frequently used as a tablet binder, is relatively stiff, brittle, and hygroscopic. The brittleness and stiffness is reflected in the relatively high T_g of approximately 163°C. In contrast VP–VA copolymer has a significantly lower T_g of approximately 101°C, is a lot more flexible and plastic, and has lower moisture uptake than PVP. This results in a significantly improved compactibility, as seen in Figure 9.42.

9.4 CONCLUSION

In many respects polymeric materials have a pre-eminent position among excipients, as they form the backbone of modern pharmaceutical practice and modified release technologies in particular. With the exception of a few technologies, the majority of modified and controlled release technologies rely on the unique properties of polymers to achieve drug release control through a variety of mechanisms. These may include dissolved drug diffusion through water insoluble, polymeric film coatings or diffusion and erosion from water soluble, hydrogel forming polymeric systems. Some of the obvious, inherent properties of polymers which continue to enable the development of new technologies include their large molecular weight, which facilitates entanglement and network formation, thus allowing diffusion control. Also important is the availability of large numbers of different polymers which are generally regarded as safe, and which have good processing and manufacturing properties such as solubility in aqueous systems and common non-aqueous solvents, good stability, good plastic deformation and compaction properties, and excellent film forming properties.

As highlighted in this chapter, the key to understanding and productively using polymeric materials in solid dosage form design and general industrial practice is to appreciate their unique properties as compared to well-defined, discrete small molecules. In particular, unlike small molecules with well-defined and discrete structure, state and properties, polymers are best viewed in terms of a continuum and distribution of structural and physical property characteristics and states. Furthermore while structure–property relationships are frequently complex and multi-factorial, we hope to have conveyed that even with the application of only a small set of relatively simple rules and principles it is possible to make more rational and science-based decisions with regard to polymer selection to achieve desired effects and robust systems. This is particularly important in the context of the current industry focus on "Quality by Design," and the fact that polymeric materials frequently comprise a significantly greater proportion of the modern dosage form than does the drug. Looking to the future it is clear that polymers will continue to be a tool in the development of controlled release dosage forms.

References

1. Mark, J., Ngai, K., Graessley, W., Mandlkern, L., Samulski, E., Koenig, J. & Wignall, G. (2004). *Physical Properties of Polymers*, 3rd edn. Cambridge University Press, UK.
2. Sperling, L.H. (2005). *Introduction to Physical Polymer Science*, 4th edn. Wiley-Interscience, New York.
3. Ferry, J.D. (1980). *Viscoelastic Properties of Polymers*, 3rd edn. Wiley-Interscience, New York.
4. Odian, G. (2004). *Principles of Polymerization*, 4th edn. Wiley-Interscience, New York.
5. Tanford, C. (1961). *Physical Chemistry of Macromolecules*. John Wiley & Sons, New York.
6. Flory, P.J. (1953). *Principles of Polymer Chemistry*. Cornell University Press, Ithaca.
7. Landoll, L.M. (1982). Nonionic polymer surfactants. J. Polymer Science, Polymer Chem ed. 20, 443–455.
8. Casas, J.A. & García-Ochoa, F. (1999). Viscosity of solutions of xanthan/locust bean gum mixtures. J. Science Food Agriculture 79, 25–31.
9. BeMiller, J.N. & Whistler, R.L. (eds). (1993). *Industrial Gums—Polysaccharides and Their Derivatives*, 3rd edn. Academic Press, New York.
10. Ott, E., Spurlin, H. M. & Grafflin, M. W. (eds Parts I-III), Bikales, N. M & Segal, L. (eds Parts IV, V). (1954). *Cellulose and*

Cellulose Derivatives, Vol. V, High Polymers. Wiley Interscience, New York.

11. Momcilovic, D., Schagerlo1, H., Ro1me, D., Jo1rnten-Karlsson, M., Karlsson, K.-E., Wittgren, B., Tjerneld, F., Wahlund, K-G. & Brinkmalm, G. (2005). Derivatization using dimethylamine for tandem mass spectrometric structure analysis of enzymatically and acidically depolymerized methyl cellulose. Analyt. Chem. 77, 2948–2959.

12. Richardson, S., Andersson, T., Brinkmalm, G. & Wittgren, B. (2003). Analytical approaches to improved characterization of substitution in hydroxypropyl cellulose. Analyt. Chem. 75, 6077–6083.

13. Schagerlo, H., Richardson, S., Momcilovic, D., Brinkmalm, G., Wittgren, B. & Tjerneld, F. (2006). Characterization of chemical substitution of hydroxypropyl cellulose using enzymatic degradation. Biomacromolecules 7, 80–85.

14. Schagerlo, H., Johansson, M., Richardson, S., Brinkmalm, G., Wittgren, B. & Tjerneld, F. (2006). Substituent distribution and clouding behavior of hydroxypropyl methyl cellulose analyzed using enzymatic degradation. Biomacromolecules 7, 3474–3481.

15. Wittgren, B. (2004). Wood Material Research—Importance for Industry. Presentation at the Opening Seminar, Wood Material Science Research Programme; Tuesday, April 6, Marina Congress Center. Katajanokanlaituri 6, Helsinki, Finland.

16. Barth, H.G. & Mays, J.W. (eds). (1991). *Modern Methods of Polymer Characterization*. Wiley-Interscience, New York.

17. Cooper, A.R. (1989). Determination of Molecular Weight. In: *Chemical Analysis, A Series of Monographs on Analytical Chemistry and Its Applications*, (eds)., Vol. 103. Wiley-Interscience, New York.

18. Mori, S. & Barth, H.G. (1999). *Size Exclusion Chromatography*. Springer-Verlag, New York.

19. Macosko, C. (1994). *Rheology, Principles, Measurements and Applications*. VCH, New York.

20. Barnes, H.A., Hutton, J.F. & Walters, K. (1989). *An Introduction to Rheology*. Elsevier, Amsterdam.

21. Lapasin, R. & Pricl, S. (1995). *Rheology of Industrial Polysaccharides*. Chapman and Hall, London.

22. Morrison, F.A. (2001). *Understanding Rheology*. Oxford University Press, Oxford.

23. Dealy, J.M. (1995). Official nomenclature for material functions describing the response of a viscoelastic fluid to various shearing and extensional deformations. J. Rheology 39, 253–265.

24. Sanchez, I.C. & Lacombe, R.H. (1976). An elementary molecular theory of classical fluids: Pure fluids. J. Phys. Chem. 80, 2352–2362.

25. Lacombe, R.H. & Sanchez, I.C. (1976). Statistical thermodynamics of fluid mixtures. J. Phys. Chem. 80, 2568–2580.

26. Sanchez, I.C. & Lacombe, R.H. (1978). Statistical thermodynamics of polymer solutions. Macromolecules 11, 1145–1156.

27. Hildebrand, J.H., Prausnitz, J.M. & Scott, R.L. (1970). *Regular and Related Solutions*. Van Nostrand Reinhold, New York.

28. Hansen, C.M. (1969). The universality of the solubility parameter concept. I & E C Product Research and Development 8, 2–11.

29. Barton, A.F.M. (1988). *CRC Handbook of Solubility Parameters and Other Cohesion Parameters*. 4th CRC Press, Boca Raton, FL.

30. Archer, W.L. (1991). Determination of Hansen solubility parameters for selected cellulose ether derivatives. Ind. Eng. Chem. Res. 30, 2292–2298.

31. Klucel® Hydroxypropylcellulose: Physical and Chemical Properties. Hercules Incorporated, Aqualon Division, Wilmington DE (250–2F, rev. 10–01 500).

32. Staudinger, H. & Heuer, W. (1930). Highly polymerized compounds. XXXIII. A relationship between the viscosity and the molecular weight of polystyrenes (translated). Ber. Bunsenges Phys. Chem., 63B, 222–234.

33. Billmeyer, F.W. (1984). *Textbook of Polymer Science*, 3rd edn. John Wiley & Sons, New York. pp. 242–357.

34. Dürig, T. et al. (2005). Fundamental studies on modified release pellest coated with ethylcellulose. Aqualon Pharmaceutical Technology Report, PTR-33.

35. Hjartstam, J., Borg, K. & Lindstedt, B. (1990). The effect of tensile stress on the permeability of free films of ethylcellulose containing hydroxypropylmethyl cellulose. Int. J. Pharm. 61, 101–107.

36. Rowe, R.C. (1986). The effect of the molecular weight of ethyl cellulose on the drug release properties of mixed films of ethyl cellulose and hydroxypropyl methylcellulose. Int J. Pharm 29, 37–41.

37. Prodduturi, S., Manek, V., Kolling, W.M., Stodghill, S.P. & Repka, M.A. (2004). Water vapor sorption of hot melt extruded hydroxypropyl cellulose films: Effect on physico-mechanical properties, release characteristics and stability. J. Pharm. Sci. 93, 3047–3056.

38. Picker-Freyer, K. M. & Dürig, T. (2007). Physical mechanical and tablet formation properties of hydroxypropylcellulose: In pure form and in mixtures. AAPS PharmSciTech, 8, Article 92, http://www.aapspharmscitech.org

39. Katikaneni, P.R., Upadrashta, S.M., Rowlings, C.E., Neau, S.H. & Hileman, G.A. (1995). Consolidation of ethylcellulose: effect of particle size, press speed and lubricants. Int. J. Pharm. 117, 13–21.

40. Skinner, G. W., Harcum, W. W., Lusvardi, K. M., Lau, S-F. & Dürig, T. (2003). Evaluation of hydroxypropylcellulose as a direct compression binder. Aqualon Pharmaceutical Technology Report, PTR-25.

41. Fox, T.G. & Flory, P.J. (1950). Second-order transition temperatures and related properties of polystyrene. I, Influence of polymer molecular weight. J. Appl. Phys. 21, 581–591.

42. Ju, R.T.C., Nixon, P.R. & Patel, M.V. (1995). Drug release from hydrophilic matrices. I. New scaling laws predicting polymer and drug release based on the polymer disentanglement concentration and the diffusion layer. J. Pharm. Sci. 84, 1455–1463.

43. Reynolds, T.D., Gehrke, S.H., Hussain, A.S. & Shenouda, L. S. (1998). Polymer erosion and drug release characterization of hydroxypropyl methylcellulose matrices. J. Pharm.Sci. 87, 1115–1123.

44. Klug, E.D. (1971). Some properties of water soluble hydroxyalkyl celluloses and their derivatives. J. Polym. Sci., Part C 36, 491–508.

45. Baumgartner, S., Smid-Korbar, J., Vrecer, F. & Kristl, J. (1998). Physical and technological parameters influencing floating properties of matrix tablets based on cellulose ethers. S.T.P. Pharm.Sci. 8, 285–290.

46. Rajabi-Siahboomi, A.R. & Nokhodchi, A. (1999). Compression properties of methylcellulose and hydroxypropylmethylcellulose polymers. Pharm. Pharmacol. Commun. 5, 67–71.

47. Durig, T. et al. (2007). Importance of structure-function relationships and particle size distribution in optimizing powder flow and compactibility of directly compressible ethylcellulose. Aqualon Pharmaceutical Technology Report, PTR-38.

48. Wood, L.A. (1958). Glass transition temperatures of copolymers. J. Polym. Sci. 28, 319–330.

Applied Statistics in Product Development

William R. Porter

10.1 INTRODUCTION

What is meant by statistics? The collection, classification, presentation, and interpretation of facts, especially numerical facts concerning governmental affairs and the community, became known over time as the field of statistics. By the 1600s in Europe, various thinkers began to link the descriptive compilation of numerical data in government and business with the emerging fields of probability theory in mathematics, and error analysis in physics and astronomy; they proposed that inferences about future events could be drawn from the numerical data previously collected. The discovery of the normal probability distribution in the early 1800s, the concept of the arithmetic mean as the "best" value to represent a data set, and the variance (or its square root, the standard deviation) to represent the dispersion around this "best" value are intimately linked. French mathematician Pierre Simon Laplace posited the arithmetic mean as the "best" value at the end of the 1700s; he invented the method of least squares and demonstrated that the variance, a measure of dispersion, was minimized when the arithmetic mean was used as the "best" value. German polymath Carl Friedrich Gauss then discovered the normal probability distribution, and showed that it had the properties needed to support this line of reasoning. Although his initial argument was circular, eventually he and Laplace developed the mathematical tools to establish the validity of the normal probability distribution. These historic developments, and others equally important, can be found in sources listed in the bibliography at the end of this chapter.

Statistics is more than just a branch of mathematics; it has become the science of summarizing and describing particular data in a sample from a larger population so that wider inferences can be made about the population itself. Although mathematicians have contributed greatly to the development of the theoretical underpinnings of statistics, scientists and engineers working in various fields of study in which statistical tools find use have contributed many important practical applications.

10.1.1 Statistics: A Tool for Decision Making and Risk Assessment

We all make measurements and use them to make decisions. Whenever we use numbers to make decisions, we run the risk of making a mistake, because all numbers are more or less unreliable.

> There is no true value of anything. There is, instead, a figure that is produced by application of a master or ideal method of counting or measurement. This figure may be accepted as a standard until the method of measurement is supplanted by experts in the subject matter with some other method and some other figure.
>
> W. Edwards Deming[1]

If you measure something, you can be certain of only one thing: your measurement is wrong. If what you measured is important enough, then sooner or later some other person will come along and measure it more accurately and more precisely than you did. You can only take comfort in the fact that he or she will also be wrong, though perhaps not quite so wrong as you

Developing Solid Oral Dosage Forms: Pharmaceutical Theory and Practice
ISBN: 978-0-444-53242-8

were. The question is: even though you are wrong, is your measurement close enough to the "true" value to serve as a basis for taking action? And also, what is the risk that your value isn't good enough?

Whenever we use measurement data to make decisions, we are using statistical techniques of data summarization and presentation, and statistical methods for making inferences about the real world from measurements we have made, even if we may not consciously be aware of this. Some of us use statistical techniques and methods better than others. Those who do, frequently get their products to market first. A thorough presentation of the concepts and tools of statistics needed by scientists and engineers working on pharmaceutical product development would fill a book by itself; indeed, it would fill many books. Fortunately, some of these books have been written, although the application of statistical reasoning to pharmaceutical product development is still a rapidly evolving field of study. The intent of this chapter is to review basic concepts of statistical thinking, and to point the reader to more detailed and exhaustive sources for further study in the accompanying bibliography.

10.1.2 Sources of Uncertainty

Since every measurement is wrong, we should ask how wrong it is. Uncertainties in measurements are of three kinds: those due to outright blunders, those due to assignable (and controllable) causes, and those due to natural (and uncontrollable) random fluctuations. At the very core of modern theories of physics we learn that nature itself is unpredictable and random at the atomic scale. Random variation permeates the universe, and can never be eliminated. However, variation due to assignable causes is another matter. A major goal of statistically designed research and development programs is to ferret out these assignable causes of variation, and remove or control them. To err is human; mistakes happen. Statistical tricks, such as randomization of processing activities that occur naturally in a time sequence, and the use of so-called robust methods, can help to identify particularly mistake-prone activities.

10.1.3 Natural (Random) Variation

When scientists go into the laboratory to perform an experiment that has previously been done, they expect to get "essentially the same" results. When engineers take a reading from an instrument monitoring an ongoing well-established process, they expect to get "essentially the same" reading. If the scientists got exactly the same result or the engineers got exactly the same instrument reading, we would be suspicious. Indeed, if the scientists or engineers continued to get exactly the same result, we would conclude that either the measurement tools they are using are too crude for the job at hand or they are committing fraud. They are either incompetents or criminals. This is not the case for people engaged in numerical data collection in other fields, such as accounting, in which the objects to be measured are countable, artificial, human constructs. The amount of money in a bank account at a particular time is, or should be, an exact value. It should not matter who counts the money; the result should be the same. Indeed, if two accountants didn't find exactly the same bank balance, we would be suspicious. At least one of them must be incompetent or a criminal. Nature doesn't work that way. Natural things vary, and they vary randomly. It is this very randomness in the way measurements of natural phenomena exhibit variation that allows us to make predications, because random phenomena can be modeled mathematically. Of course, the predictions we make based on randomness are not exact; rather, they have a certain probability associated with them. Whenever we make a decision based upon numerical data obtained from nature, we run the risk of making a wrong decision. Probability theory helps us to quantify this risk.

In mathematics, the variation exhibited naturally is often called "error." This is an unfortunate choice, since in the English language, as well as many others, the word "error" is associated in popular usage with malfeasance. Mathematics distinguishes between "errors" and "mistakes." People never make errors; people make mistakes. Errors happen; mistakes are caused. In mathematical statistics, an error is just the difference between an actual and expected value. Although the difference between the theoretical, ideal "true" or expected value and what is measured (the actual, concrete "true" or observed value) may be called the error of the measurement, this usage does not imply that the difference is a deliberate mistake. Both the predicted and observed values are "true" in a sense, even though they differ.

One philosophy of statistical reasoning considers a particular instance of measurement as just one of series of potential measurements that may have been made in the past or could possibly be made in the future. In this view, measurements we take will vary about some expected ideal value. In the long run, if we take a sufficiently large number of repeated measurements, our actual values will tend to cluster around this expected value, with some predictable random variation.

Another philosophy of statistical reasoning considers a particular measurement as a confirmation of some previously held point of view; each time we repeat the measurement (or reconfirm the projection we had previously made) we narrow and refine our beliefs. In this view, measurements we take will converge around some refined value, again with some predictable random variation. In either case, random variation is unavoidable, not correctable, but describable and useable to infer probabilities.

Scientists and engineers should be careful when communicating with others; you will need to explain to them that when you speak about random errors, you are not talking about mistakes. Rather, you are speaking about quantifiable natural variation that can be used to estimate the risk of making incorrect decisions. Random "error" is something that can be measured. It is, indeed, the measure of worthiness or reliability of the measurement with which it is associated. Measurements without an associated estimate of their variability are completely useless.

10.1.4 Systematic Error (Bias) and Blunders

However, there are other sources of variation that are not random. Diverse environmental and procedural factors can conspire to shift the measured value we obtain away from the ideal value that we would obtain in the absence of these factors. These systematic deviations from the ideal value really are "errors" in the popular sense. They are mistakes, although often unintentional. These "errors" are avoidable or at least correctable. These mistakes differ from outright blunders, because they occur consistently, are reproducible, change in magnitude in predictable ways, and affect every measurement. Much of the literature of statistics is devoted to devising strategies for the avoidance of this type of "error," which we call bias. Although common sense can provide much insight into the avoidance and elimination of bias, statistical methods can be used to quantify bias, and provide the means to design experiments to systematically eliminate bias. Much of what follows in this chapter is devoted to achieving precisely this goal.

Blunders, on the other hand, occur erratically, are not reproducible, vary enormously and unpredictably in magnitude, and affect very few measurements. Some effort has been made by statisticians to develop tools for identifying these types of error, which we call outliers. Although statistical methods can be used to identify outliers, common sense and an understanding of human psychology are required to design processes to reduce and minimize the effects of blunders.

10.2 EXPLORING DATA: TYPES OF DATA

There are only three kinds of mathematical data: nominal, ordinal and numerical. For each type of data different statistical techniques and methods of evaluation have been devised. Nominal data consist of counts of objects in categories (e.g., the number of ewes in a flock of sheep). Ordinal data consist of the rankings of elements within a set (e.g., the order of students in a class by performance). Numerical data are, of course, what we normally think of when we speak of measurements: a real number associated with the result of the measurement process. Simply keeping these distinctions in mind can eliminate much of the confusion that naïve students of statistics experience. Generally speaking, methods appropriate for handling numerical data are those that have been most thoroughly studied and developed. Being able to obtain a numerical measurement gives you the most flexibility in terms of presenting and interpreting the results. However, many scientists and engineers are surprised to learn that statistical methods based on ranking procedures can be nearly as powerful as those based on numerical results. This can come in handy sometimes, when the absolute numerical value of a measurement is in doubt but its ranking among similar measurements is not. On the other hand, procedures based on counts in categories are not nearly so satisfying. Much information is lost when a set of numerical results are converted into a count of those measurements that meet a specification, and those that do not. Although such categorization schemes may be convenient, especially when communicating results to a non-technical audience, the information becomes almost useless for further analysis and interpretation.

10.2.1 Nominal (Categorical) Data

Nominal data are obtained by conducting a census or survey. You line up all the objects that you are interested in, sort them into groups ("classes" or "categories") based on some selection criterion ("attribute") of your choice, and count them. The measurement is, in this case, a property of the group as a whole, and not the individual members of the group. The measurement is frequently reported as a ratio or percentage: 57 out of 90 sheep are black; 43% of voters support my candidate, 25% support her opponent, 12% are undecided, and 20% declined to answer. Nominal data abounds in political, economic, and sociological studies; it is frequently encountered in clinical research, but is less commonly used by researchers in the physical sciences. You will encounter nominal data in the simplest type of quality assurance work: sampling by attributes. Anybody can always impose a nominal classification scheme arbitrarily on any data set, so well-established statistical techniques for data collection and display, and methods for drawing inferences from such data, can always be used by merely reducing the data at hand to counts in categories. This universality of applicability is countered by a serious defect: getting other people to agree to accept your quirky classification scheme may require considerable negotiating skills. Categories are nearly always arbitrary; nature has few natural boundaries. Be wary of using categorical methods yourself, and be skeptical about conclusions drawn by others based on categorical data. Often you will find it to be true that the classification scheme used was chosen in such a way as to confirm the prejudices of the person who devised it. To counter this, it is best to get all parties who will be impacted by decisions made on the basis of nominal data to agree on a set of rules for performing the classification before any data are actually collected. In practice, this is a difficult task; at least some parties will have preconceived notions of what the data can be expected to look like, and will argue for classification rules that they believe will most benefit themselves. For these reasons, this chapter will gloss over techniques and methods that rely on nominal data. However, there are some nominal classification schemes that rely upon categories derived from numerical results obtained from the data themselves, so they have some value. For example, one can count the number of successive measurement values collected on one day that are larger than the average of the measurements collected on the previous day. If this run of numbers above the previous average is sufficiently large, the probability that today's data has an average no larger than yesterday's average can be computed using the laws of probability. Or, manufacturers and regulatory authorities could agree to abide by a classification scheme set by a pharmacopeia that involves comparing a measured numerical value to a predetermined standard value; units whose measured values exceeded the agreed-upon limit might be classified as unacceptable. The fraction of nonconforming units then tells you something about the overall quality of the material. However, other types of data which provide information about the individual members of a group, instead of just properties of the group as a whole, are intrinsically more powerful.

10.2.2 Ordinal Data

Ordinal data are actually rarely obtained in practice in pharmaceutical process research and development. To truly collect ordinal data, one has to compare each and every member of the group of objects being ranked with every other member of the group. Simplistically, this would require making $n(n - 1)/2$ comparisons; this is tedious unless the total number of members in the group is small. It is simple to arrange a set of objects in order of mass using a two-pan balance, for example. Merely compare pairs of objects in the group to determine which is the less massive of the two, and then systematically compare this object with each of the other objects in the group, always retaining the least massive object on a balance pan. Once an exhaustive comparison of all the objects has been made, set aside the least massive object that was found, and then repeat the entire procedure using the rest of the group. Mathematicians call this approach to ranking the "bubble" sort. Although the simplest of sorting algorithms to implement, it is also the least efficient way to compare objects. Mathematicians have developed more efficient sorting algorithms to perform this type of operation on larger data sets, but even so, the procedure is tedious if a physical comparison has to be done for each pair of items.

Chemists and engineers rarely perform rankings by direct comparison. However, it is trivially simple to convert numerical data into rankings using computerized sorting with an efficient sorting algorithm (so that each item needs to be physically measured only once), and sometimes an analysis of the data using ranking methods will lead to a different conclusion (perhaps a more conservative one) about the risk associated with the interpretation of the data. There was a period of time, before computers became inexpensive and ubiquitous, when ranking methods were actively developed as an alternative to numerical techniques as a way to save money on computation; now their value lies mainly in the fact that they require making fewer assumptions about the data. Although these methods will not be discussed extensively in this chapter, you should be aware that they exist, that they are frequently nearly as powerful as numerical methods, that they require fewer assumptions to be made about the frequency distribution associated with the data, and that they can serve as a quick alternate approach to provide confirmation of a more sophisticated and complicated analysis based on numerical results.

Ranking methods might be more appropriate to use when the amount of data actually available is quite small, and you really have little confidence in assumptions about the nature of the variability seen in the data set; at least you will be spared making a rash prediction that is utterly dependent upon assumptions about the data that may later be found unsupportable. Ranking methods are also used extensively in conjunction with numerical methods when certain assumptions about the data required to support a traditional numerical analysis cannot be met (such as, for example, the assumptions that deviations from the fitted model are normally distributed). Methods based on rankings are less sensitive to outliers than completely numerical methods. These methods are frequently lumped together with some methods appropriate for nominal data analysis under the topic of "nonparametric statistics."

10.2.3 Numerical Data

Numerical data are what we, as scientists and engineers, are accustomed to working with. We use a device with a measurement scale, typically graduated in equal intervals, to obtained so-called interval scale numerical data. Objects measured on such a scale are larger or smaller than other objects by some additive factor. Such data can include both positive and negative real numbers, since the zero point of an interval scale can be arbitrarily chosen. Time, for example, is measured on an interval scale.

Other numerical data are measured on a so-called ratio scale. Objects measured on such a scale are proportionally larger or smaller than other objects by some multiplicative factor. Such data can include only positive real numbers, since the zero point of a ratio scale is fixed absolutely. Temperature, for example, is measured on a ratio scale. Obviously, if one takes the logarithm of a ratio scale measurement, the resulting value can be displayed on an interval scale.

Although some people make much ado about the difference between interval scale and ratio scale numerical data, most applied scientists and engineers tend to ignore this distinction, sometimes at their peril. Statistical methods for numerical data almost invariably have been designed for interval scale measurements; when negative numbers are physically meaningless, trouble can ensue. Sometimes it is prudent to use logarithms to avoid this problem; sometimes it is more bother than it is worth. Just be careful, and treat negative results with caution. Ask yourself, is this physically meaningful?

10.2.4 Continuously Variable Data and Digitization Pitfalls

Another potential problem in the collection and analysis of numerical data are that the statistical methods applied to numerical data assume that the numbers are elements of the set of what mathematicians call "real" numbers. They are not quantized. There are no gaps between real numbers. Pick any two real numbers and there is always another real number halfway between them. The set of real numbers is continuous and smooth. However, we have no way to express real numbers in written form using numerals. We can only express numbers in writing by truncating them to some agreed number of digits. Digital data are "integral" numbers; they consist of members of the set of integers, multiplied by some power of ten. There are gaps of finite size between any two digital measurements. Digital data are discontinuous and granular. This is a real problem (pun intended). Fortunately, with sufficiently sensitive measuring tools (that is, tools which produce sufficiently small granularity), this is a problem that can be reduced to the extent that it has no practical consequences, simply by increasing the number of digits retained in the written data so that the distance between possible successive values is too small to affect any decisions we make based upon the data. A large part of measurement science is devoted to the issues caused by insufficiently small granularity in digital data.

Related to this digitization problem is a "zero" problem. Since most physical measurements have a true zero point, there is some region of measurement space close to this zero point where measurement is actually physically impossible. This becomes especially critical when one encounters signal averaging. If you record the same analog signal source over and over again, and add all the recorded data together, the noise will tend to cancel out, since the noise is equally likely to be greater than or less than the baseline detector response level. Signals, which always deviate from the baseline response in the same direction, will add together to produce a net signal that is the sum of all the tiny individual signals: $0.001 + 0.001 + 0.001 + 0.001 + 0.001 + 0.001 + 0.001 + 0.001 + 0.001 + 0.001 = 0.010$. If you digitize the signal before performing the addition, and each miniscule signal is below the threshold value that the instrument uses to differentiate a signal from noise (say, 0.002), you get an entirely different result: $0.001 + 0.001 + 0.001 + 0.001 + 0.001 + 0.001 + 0.001 + 0.001 + 0.001 + 0.001 = 0.000$. Digitization can (and frequently does) result in loss of information. Thus, the degree of granularity of the data becomes critical to success.

Rounding of data is another potential problem. We were all taught in school to round numbers, and carry only the significant digits in calculations. Rounded numbers are digital data with even larger granularity (and therefore less information) than the original data. Rounding is obviously going to exacerbate digitization issues. Numerical data should never be rounded at intermediate stages of analysis, but only when the results are finally presented. There are procedures for rounding numbers that maximally preserve the information content of the data which will be demonstrated once we have discussed other critical concepts.

10.3 EXPLORING DATA: GRAPHICAL TECHNIQUES

First, plot the data. Few humans can make any sense of a bunch of numbers in a table. Even if you can, your boss or your colleagues or your customer cannot. Draw a picture. This is always the first step in the analysis of data.

Frequently, you will see graphs in the popular press or on the Internet with cute little pictures lined up like ducks in a row to represent some data. Avoid cuteness; it distorts and confuses. When plotting data, aim for simplicity. The less ink used to plot the data, without sacrificing necessary detail, the better. See the bibliography for books on how to graph data. Communicating numerical information with pictures is part art, part science. Simple is beautiful and truthful; needlessly complex is ugly and misleading. As Albert Einstein reportedly said, "Everything should be made as simple as possible, but not simpler."

10.3.1 Graphing Nominal Data

A number of different ways have been proposed to plot nominal data. Bar charts and pie charts are the most popular.

10.3.2 Bar Charts

Bar charts are a good way to display counts-in-categories. The bars can be either vertical or horizontal; it's a matter of taste and tradition. Stacked bars can be used to show how fractions of total response vary when the same set of responses is measured under different conditions.

In Figure 10.1, the number of failures of a filter unit occurring per year is plotted on the Y-axis versus the location of the units on the X-axis. A more useful plot is a Pareto plot, in which the data are sorted from lowest failure rate to highest failure rate. This makes visual estimation of the differences easier, and clearly shows which site has the worst performance (see Figure 10.2).

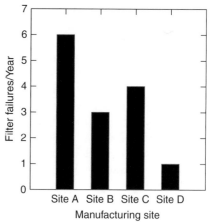

FIGURE 10.1   Example of a bar chart

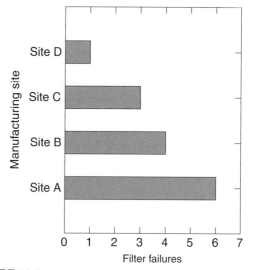

FIGURE 10.2   Example of a pareto chart

10.3.3 Pie Charts

Unless you need to display the fraction of different responses to a single experimental condition where the fractions vary widely in magnitude, a bar chart is generally easier to read and make visual comparisons than a pie chart. Figure 10.3 shows the same filter failure data plotted as a pie chart.

10.3.4 Graphing Univariate Numerical Data

Univariate data consist of a set of measurements of the same property collected under a fixed set of conditions. If the measurements exhibit sufficiently small granularity, the resulting data will scatter smoothly around some central value. A graphical display of the data should help the reader visualize both the

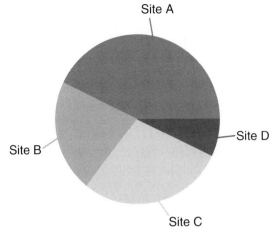

FIGURE 10.3   Example of a pie chart

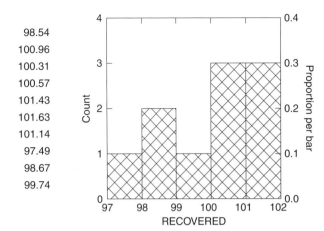

FIGURE 10.4   Example of a histogram

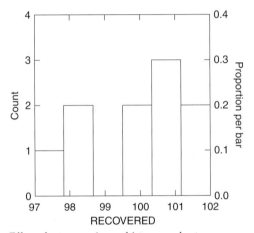

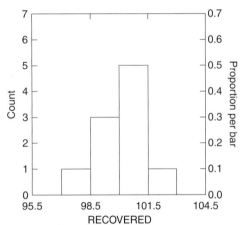

FIGURE 10.5   Effect of category size on histogram chart

approximate location of the central value, and dispersion of the data. The amount of dispersion controls the scale of the graph.

10.3.5 Histograms

A histogram is a sophisticated type of bar chart in which the categories are ranked classifications of the numerical data. The idea behind the histogram is to increase the coarseness of the granularity of the data, to reduce its complexity and achieve a simpler display. The concept is based on the observation that if we round data to sufficiently few significant digits, we can lump similar values together into well-defined categories. When the data to be displayed are continuously variable numerical measurements, some arbitrary system of dividing the range of the scale into an equal number of categories must be devised to create this deliberate distortion. Unless different people agree

to a set of rules for doing this, each person will draw a different histogram. The set of ten values on the left side of Figure 10.4 are plotted as a histogram consisting of five categories on the right side of Figure 10.4. In this case, the category boundaries are set at integer values of the measured response on the X-axis, and the number of measurements with values greater than or equal to the lower category boundary but less than the upper category boundary, are plotted on the Y-axis, as shown in Figure 10.4.

Figure 10.5 shows the same data plotted with the width of the bars changed to 0.8 measurement units (left), and to 1.5 measurement units (right).

As you can see, the plot can be arbitrarily manipulated to change its appearance by simply changing the width and number of categories used to deliberately distort the data. This type of plot can be very deceptive. Which is the best plot? Histograms are popular in textbooks because of their long historical usage. Much better graphical display techniques have been developed for depicting univariate data that are rule-based, so that every person who plots the data according to the agreed-upon rules will generate an identical plot, given the same set of data to work with.

10.3.6 Quantile Plots

Quantile plots (also known as cumulative distribution plots) are a better way of illustrating the distribution of a variable than histograms. The quantile of a sample is simply the data point corresponding to a given fraction of the data. With ten data points in a sample, the data themselves are plotted on the X-axis, and the corresponding quantiles (in this case, the midpoints of the intervals 0.0–0.1, 0.1–0.2, etc.) are plotted on the Y-axis, as shown in Figure 10.6.

If the data represents samples from a "normally distributed" population (about which more will be said later) then the plot should be roughly S-shaped (ogee-shaped). With such a small sample, nothing much can be said about the distribution of these measurements. Quantile plots are much more useful for displaying properties of the distribution of points in larger samples (>100 points).

10.3.7 Box Plots

Box plots reveal elements that control the shape of the distribution of measurements in a sample. The plot itself is based upon ordinal properties of the data. A rectangle is drawn with boundaries that enclose the middle 50% of the data (that is, from the twenty-fifth percentile to the seventy-fifth percentile). The box is divided with a line at the fiftieth percentile of the data (the median value, defined below). Lines ("whiskers") extend from either end of the box to reach the data most distant

from the fiftieth percentile that are still within 1.5 × the interquartile range (the distance between the twenty-fifth and seventy-fifth percentiles); these two boundary points are called the "inner fence." Additional boundary points are plotted at 3 × the interquartile range from the twenty-fifth or seventy-fifth percentiles; these additional boundary points are called the "outer fence." Experimental points between the inner and outer fences are plotted using asterisks, while experimental points outside the outer fences are plotted using open circles. In this way, aberrant data points are emphasized and easily classified as merely unlikely (asterisks) or highly improbable (circles). Box plots can be generated using relatively small data sets, so they provide an excellent tool for visually depicting the location of the central value and spread associated with the distribution of measurements in a sample, as shown in Figure 10.7.

The box plot of the ten data points used previously to generate the various histograms and the quantile plot reveal that the data in the sample all lie within the inner fences, and that the values are scattered lopsidedly about the central value, approximately 100.4. Of the various plots that can be used to depict the central value and spread of the relatively small samples frequently encountered in pharmaceutical product development, the box plot is probably the most useful.

10.3.8 Graphing Bivariate Data

Frequently, the same kind of continuously variable measurements are collected under different sets of circumstances. If these circumstances can be defined as different categories, then we need to plot the categories on one axis (usually the X-axis), and the continuously variable data on another axis (typically the Y-axis). In some cases, the categories have a natural ranking (such as when data are collected on successive days) or the categories can be ranked by some other defining characteristic (the amount of an added excipient, for example). In such cases, the order of plotting the categorical data may be important. Finally, in some cases the defining characteristic for each data set may itself be a continuously variable value, such that each experimental measurement is obtained at a different value of the characteristic circumstance, such as temperature or the concentration of some other

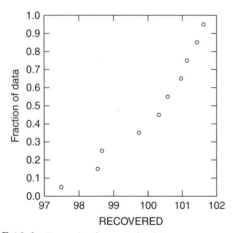

FIGURE 10.6   Example of a quantile plot

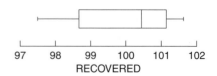

FIGURE 10.7   Example of a box plot

ingredient. Different types of graphical displays work best in each of these cases.

10.3.9 One Variable Nominal: Bar Graphs, Dot Plots, and Line Plots

When one variable is nominal (categorical) and the other is a continuously variable numerical measurement, then graphs similar in style to the bar graph used to plot counts in categories can be modified to depict the central value and a measure of dispersion for each set of numerical measurements (see Figure 10.8).

It is difficult to see, but the error bar for the data set labeled "RECOVERED_2" is somewhat larger than the other three error bars. Although bar graphs are commonly used to depict this type of data, dot plots

or dot plots with connecting lines may be more useful (see Figure 10.9).

The dot plot is the least cluttered, and has the advantage of more clearly depicting and emphasizing the spread of the data. Now the larger error bar for the "RECOVERED_2" data set is more clearly visible. A connecting line makes it easier to compare the relative magnitudes of the central values. All three of these plots are intended to visually convey exactly the same information. Do they?

10.3.10 One Variable Nominal: Box Plots

If it is important to reveal greater details about the spread of the data, then multiple box plots can be used when the X-axis variable is nominal, as shown in Figure 10.10.

One advantage of the box plot in this example is that it gives a better picture of the spread of the data, and can reveal aberrant points. In this case, the data set for "RECOVERED_2" is shown to have a single aberrant measurement between the inner and outer lower fences. The rest of the data seems to be distributed in much the same manner as the other data sets. This plot illustrates the point that outlying values can greatly distort the appearance of conventionally drawn plots; the box plot is relatively immune to such distortion.

10.3.11 Both Variables Numeric and Random: Quantile–Quantile Plots

A version of the quantile plot is useful for comparing two sets of continuously variable numerical data collected under different circumstances. This type

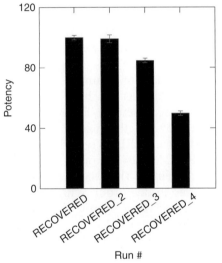

FIGURE 10.8   Example of a bar graph for numerical data

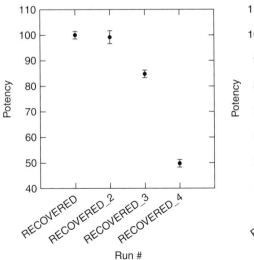

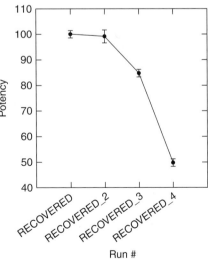

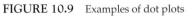

FIGURE 10.9   Examples of dot plots

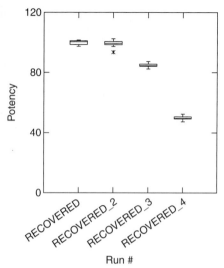

FIGURE 10.10   Example of multiple box plots

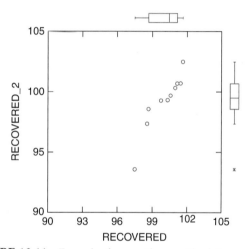

FIGURE 10.11   Example of a quantile–quantile plot

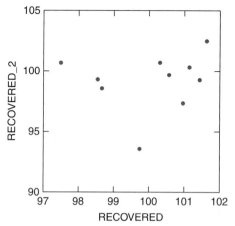

FIGURE 10.12   Example of a bivariate scatterplot

10.3.12 Both Variables Numeric: Scatterplots

When two continuously variable sets of numerical data are to be compared, the traditional way to do this is simply to plot the data using an XY-coordinate system. This works, for example, when each measurement in one data set can be associated with one, and only one, measurement in the second data set. Suppose, for example, that we want to compare the data in the "RECOVERED" set with the data in the "RECOVERED_2" set by the order in which the assay results were obtained. That is, we pair the results for the first sample in one group with the results of the first sample in the other group, and so on. What we see is shown in Figure 10.12.

The aberrant point in the "RECOVERED_2" data set is actually matched to a value in the "RECOVERED" data set that is close to the central value for that data set. There doesn't seem to be any correlation between order of sample analysis and the results observed.

More commonly, we plot some measured value of interest against some known, pre-selected value of some other variable: in this example, we plot the measured response in the "RECOVERED_2" data set versus the concentration of an excipient used to make the trial formulation, as shown in Figure 10.13.

Because of the aberrant data point in this set of measurements, there is a suggestion that the highest concentration of EXCIPIENT_A may be problematic. However, we already know that this single datum seems to be problematic itself.

10.3.13 Multivariate Data

Product development is a complex process. Frequently, scientists and engineers want to compare

of plot is especially helpful in revealing differences between two groups of data when combined with box plots for each data set taken individually, as shown in Figure 10.11.

In this example, the quantiles of the "RECOVERED" data set are plotted on the X-axis, and the quantiles of the "RECOVERED_2" data set are plotted on the Y-axis. Box plots have been added to each axis; the aberrant point in the "RECOVERED_2" data set is clearly revealed. Such plots are especially useful for troubleshooting purposes, as problematic data are easily identified. Note that the quantile plot does not presuppose that there is any connection between the first measurement in one data set and the first measurement in the second data set.

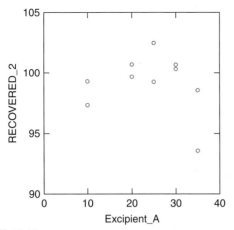

FIGURE 10.13 Another scatterplot example

if they were nominal for the purpose of constructing a scatterplot matrix. This is illustrated for the "RECOVERED," "RECOVERED_2," "RECOVERED_ 3," and "RECOVERED_4" data sets in the array below. Each is plotted as a function of "EXCIPIENT_A" concentration, and arranged in order of execution of the experiments (see Figure 10.14).

Inspection of the entire collection of graphs suggests that the concentration of "EXCIPIENT_A" has no particular effect on the recovered drug activity. These plots were generated using conventional software, and were simply shrunk to fit on one page.

more than two variables at a time, but we are limited to plotting in two dimensions on paper. Even on a computer screen, where animation can be used to enhance perception, plotting data in more than three dimensions is an impossible task. Although many clever graphical techniques have been attempted to get around these limitations, there remains only one method that doesn't require elaborate drafting or computer software: scatterplot matrices.

10.3.14 Scatterplot Matrices

Scatterplot matrices are simply arrays of scatterplots in which each scatterplot is arranged in a row or column of an array corresponding to a different value of a nominal factor. It is possible to construct a rectangular array of scatterplots to represent the effects of two nominal, and one continuously variable, factors on a continuously variable response. Since many experiments are performed using experimentally controlled factors at fixed and equal intervals, even if these factors themselves are measurable on a continuous scale, the fact that we have selected equally-spaced steps for our experiment allows us to treat such factors as

10.4 DATA DISTRIBUTIONS

By now it should have become apparent that sets of repeated measurements of the same process obtained under selected experimental conditions typically show apparently random scatter around some central value. The shape of these distributions is difficult to determine from small samples such as we normally obtain in the laboratory, but mathematical statisticians have demonstrated that certain well-characterized probability distributions can frequently be used to model, with good approximation, the actual experimentally obtained distributions for different types of measurement data. We will consider only a few of the most common by way of illustration.

10.4.1 Binomial Distribution

A favorite of teachers of statistics, the binomial distribution governs the probable outcome of an event with only two possible outcomes, such a flipping a coin. We know from experience that if we flip a "fair" coin, it is as likely to land heads-up as it is to land tails-up. From this knowledge we can predict the odds of getting two heads in a row or one head and one tail if we flip the coin twice. (An aside: Question: How do you know a coin is "fair?" Answer: You flip it a lot

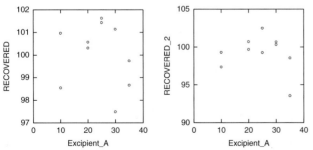
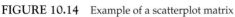
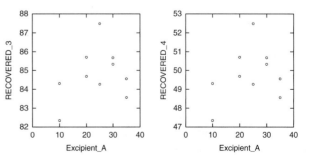

FIGURE 10.14 Example of a scatterplot matrix

of times and see if, in the long run, you get as many heads as tails. If you already know that heads and tails are about equally likely by experiment, then it is fair to say the coin is approximately "fair." If I tell you the coin is "fair," and I won't let you test it yourself, don't bet on the outcome of my next toss of the coin.)

There is an extension of the binomial distribution for cases in which more than two outcomes can be obtained, such as rolling dice. The salient feature of this, and related probability distributions, is that they apply to nominal data, that is, counts in categories. If you have census-type data, then the binomial distribution or one of its cousins is likely to describe the probabilities of the various outcomes you will observe.

10.4.2 Poisson Distribution

The Poisson distribution is used to model the probability of rare, but countable, events. It is an approximation to the binomial distribution when the total sample size is large, and the number of items in the sample exhibiting the property of interest is a very small fraction of the total. You may encounter it in circumstances where a small number of countable events are measured as part of a time series. Radioisotope disintegrations or the number of defective tablets in a shipping carton are examples of data that typically behave approximately as if they followed a Poisson distribution.

10.4.3 Normal (Gaussian) Distribution

The famous bell-shaped curve we all learned about in school theoretically describes the probability distribution associated with a population of measured values obtained using a continuously variable numerical measurement scale that has certain ideal properties. The name of Gauss has become associated with this distribution, although Laplace did related work contemporaneously. Both were concerned with the problem of obtaining the "best" representation of a series of supposedly identical measurements, a problem that bedeviled astronomers trying to establish the orbits of heavenly bodies or physicists attempting to measure natural phenomena such as barometric pressure based upon sometimes-crude measurements. The normal (or Gaussian) probability curve is a mathematical idealization of the types of distributions of errors empirically found to be associated with various kinds of measurement processes.

Keep in mind that no actual collection of measurement data, even data collected under the most careful and meticulous conditions, has ever been demonstrated to be "normally distributed," any more than any real coin that can be tossed has ever been shown to be "fair" in the sense defined previously. These simplistic mathematical abstractions are useful approximations to what we actually encounter in nature. As statistician George Box said, "All models are wrong, but some are useful." The overwhelming majority of techniques and methods of inference found in statistics textbooks are utterly dependent upon the assumption that the data set you are working with is a random sample from some normally distributed population of random variables. Since the assumption of a normal distribution is critical to many statistical inferences, one should always question how badly the actually observed distribution of measurement errors would have to deviate from assumed normality to invalidate the inferences made—then see if it does!

10.4.4 Other Useful Distributions

Many other probability distributions are encountered in statistical work, such as Student's t-distribution, which is related to Fisher's F-distribution, which in turn is related to the χ^2 distribution, all of which are important in describing the properties of measures of variability associated with samples taken from a population that exhibits a normal probability distribution. There are many others of importance to statistical inference. Read about them in the books listed in the bibliography. And remember that they, too, are simplistic mathematical constructs that only approximate the behavior of real data.

10.5 LOCATION: CENTRAL TENDENCIES

Most distributions, experimental or theoretical, that are of interest to scientists and engineers are unimodal; that is, they are characterized by having a single most probable value. Be aware, though, that sometimes bimodal or multimodal distributions are encountered in experimental work. This is frequently the case when particle size distributions are measured in the laboratory. Although the bulk of the material may consist of particles whose size does tend to vary around some central value, with some typical degree of dispersion, we often find that the material is contaminated by dust ("fines"), and lumps of agglomerated material that are both atypical of the rest of the particle size distribution. Multimodal behavior is usually considered to be undesirable, and evidence that some problem has occurred that requires correction.

10.5.1 Data for Central Value and Dispersion Examples

To illustrate techniques for summarizing data, consider the following example.

> An analytical chemist assays a control sample by HPLC in order to determine if the chromatography system is suitable for use for analyzing experimental samples. The following data are obtained:

Peak area, mV-sec
9850.484709
10043.677788
9695.965881
9992.653704
9568.279745

These data will be used to illustrate calculations of "best" estimates of the central value (location) and dispersion (scale) of the data.

10.5.2 Arithmetic Mean

The arithmetic mean of a set of data are simply the average value, which is obtained by adding all the individual measurements in the data set, and then dividing this sum by the total number of measurements used to compute the sum. Every data set has a mean. Statisticians typically indicate a sample mean symbolically using an italic roman letter with a horizontal bar over it:

$$\overline{x} = \frac{\sum\limits_{i=n}^{i=n} x_i}{n}$$

Using the sample data set, we find:

$\overline{x} = 9830.2123654$ (without any rounding)

Probability distributions also have means. If the entire population of measurements can be counted, then the arithmetic mean is calculated in the same way as illustrated above. However, you cannot actually compute the mean of a probability distribution such as the normal (Gaussian) distribution, because the distribution is hypothetical and based upon the notion that it represents an infinite population of random values. Statisticians usually use greek letters to represent the characteristic parameters of probability distributions or ideal populations.

The mean of any theoretically discrete distribution with N members of the population is:

$$\mu = \frac{\sum\limits_{i=1}^{i=N} x_i}{N}$$

The mean of any theoretically continuous distribution is simply the limit, as the sample size is increased to infinity, of the sum of all the measured values divided by the number of all the measured values:

$$\mu = \lim_{n\to\infty} \left(\frac{\sum\limits_{i=n}^{i=n} x_i}{n} \right)$$

The arithmetic mean of a set of measurements has certain desirable properties: it is an unbiased estimate of the mean of the population of measurements from which the present data set can be considered to be a sample; it has the minimum variance of any such estimate, and, if the frequency distribution associated with that population were a normal probability distribution, the sample mean would also be the maximum likelihood estimate of the population mean.

Other types of means, such as weighted means, geometric means, and harmonic means are sometimes encountered; see the books in the bibliography for more information.

10.5.3 Median

We have already encountered the median in the construction of box plots; it is the fiftieth percentile of the distribution of values in a set of measurements. If the data set contains an odd number of elements, the median is the middle value when the data are ranked from smallest to largest. If the data set contains an even number of elements, the median is the average of the two middle-most values when the data are ranked from smallest to largest. The calculation of the median is unaffected by aberrant values in the data set. The mean, on the other hand, can be heavily biased if even one of the measured values used to estimate it is seriously biased. The median is said to be a "robust" estimate of the central value of a symmetric distribution. When you encounter a new set of measurement data about which you know very little, it is prudent to use the median to estimate the central value. This is why the box plot is so useful for plotting new and unfamiliar data sets. You are less likely to be misled. There is no consensus symbolism for the median; spell it out or define your own symbol (although many authors use an italic roman letter with a tilde over it). Using the sample data set, we find:

median = $\tilde{x}$ = 9850.484709 (without any rounding)

10.6 DISPERSION

The dispersion of measured values around this central value is just as important as the central value of a unimodal distribution. Several different kinds of measures of dispersion are commonly encountered.

10.6.1 Range

The range is simply the difference between the highest measured value and the lowest measured value in a set of measurements. This measure of dispersion is most easily computed when the set of measurements is small enough that you can pick out the minimum and maximum by visual inspection. Of course, for larger data sets, a computer can easily find these two values, and compute the range for you. Since the range is so easily obtained, it plays an important role in the application of statistics to quality control. The range is exceptionally sensitive to aberrant data, since such data tend to be either the minimum or maximum value in a data set. There is no consensus symbolism for the range; although the symbol R appears frequently, spell it out or define your own symbol. Using the sample data set, we find:

range (R) = 475.398043 (without any rounding)

The range is an essentially useless measure of dispersion for a population; in particular, if the frequency distribution associated with the population is the normal probability distribution, the range in that case would be infinite.

10.6.2 Interquartile Range and Median Absolute Deviation from the Median

We have already seen the interquartile range used as a measure of dispersion in the construction of box plots. Like the median, the interquartile range is relatively insensitive to aberrant data. However, there is another measure of dispersion that can be obtained from numerical data that is even less sensitive to aberrant data, namely the median absolute deviation from the median. This takes a bit of calculation, and

so would normally be calculated using a computer. First, obtain the median by ranking all of the data. Next, calculate the absolute value of the difference between each other member of the data set and the median value. Now find the median of all these absolute values of differences. The result is the median absolute deviation from the median. This is just as robust an estimate of dispersion as the median itself is a robust estimate of the central value, so the pair are often used as surrogates for the mean and standard deviation (described below) when there are questions about whether or not some of the data may be aberrant. There is no consensus symbolism for the interquartile range or the median absolute deviation from the median, although MAD is frequently used: spell them out or define your own symbols.

interquartile range = 296.687823 (without any rounding)

median absolute deviation from the median (MAD) = 154.518828 (without rounding)

10.6.3 Variance and Standard Deviation

The traditional measure of dispersion is obtained from the variance, which is the adjusted average of the squares of the deviations of the individual measurements in a set of measurements from their arithmetic mean. The square root of this number is called the standard deviation, usually represented by an italic roman letter, such as s:

$$s^2 = \frac{\sum_{i=1}^{i=n}(x_i - \bar{x})^2}{n-1} = \frac{\sum_{i=1}^{i=n}x_i^2 - \frac{\left(\sum_{i=1}^{i=n}x_i\right)^2}{n}}{n-1}$$

$$= \frac{n\sum_{i=1}^{i=n}x_i^2 - \left(\sum_{i=1}^{i=n}x_i\right)^2}{n(n-1)}$$

$$s = \sqrt{s^2}$$

Using the sample data set, we find:

s^2 = 39749.1148125907103 (without any rounding)

s = 199.371800 (rounded to the same number decimal places as the original data)

The variance, as calculated above, is the appropriate algorithm to use when computing the variance of a set of measures that is a subset of a larger population of measurements. If that larger population is countable (finite in number), then the variance of the population is calculated by replacing the quantity $(n-1)$ with n everywhere it occurs. Consult the books listed in the bibliography to learn more about this. This can be an issue in practice, because some computer and pocket calculator algorithms calculate the variance using the correct denominator for samples, while others use the correct denominator for finite populations. Microsoft Excel, for example, has worksheet functions that will calculate either value; you have to choose the correct function to use. This is a case where you simply must read the manuals or help files for any software you may use to perform statistical calculations, in order to find out which algorithm is being used. A greek letter, such as σ, usually represents the population standard deviation:

$$\sigma^2 = \frac{\sum_{i=1}^{i=N}(x_i - \mu)^2}{N} \text{ (for countable populations)}$$

$$\sigma^2 = \lim_{n \to \infty}\left(\frac{\sum_{i=1}^{i=n}(x_i - \mu)^2}{n}\right) \text{ (for infinite populations)}$$

$$\sigma = \sqrt{\sigma^2}$$

The variance (and standard deviation) can be calculated for any sample data set, and is a property of any population. Note that several different algorithms are shown above for calculating the sample variance. The first version requires that a table of all the values be created, so that the individual differences from the mean can be calculated first, then squared, summed, and divided by one less than the total count. The second and third algorithms require only that the running sums of the data values, their squares, and a count of the number of data entries be stored. The final computation is performed by squaring the sum of the data values, then either dividing this large number by the total count of data entries and subtracting it from the sum of the squares of the data, another large number, or by subtracting it from the product of the sum of the squares of the data multiplied by the total count, an even larger number. The result is a (hopefully) small difference, which must then be divided by one less than the count of the data (in the first case) or by the product of one less than the count of the data and the count of the data (in the second case). Should we care? In an analog world or a world where humans carry out calculations using pencil and paper, the answer is no: any of the three formulas will work equally well. If you are an engineer designing a digital calculating device, you will probably choose either the second or third algorithm; these require only a limited number of storage registers, known in advance for any problem, to store the three running totals. The first algorithm needs a storage register for each datum entered by the user, as well as an additional register to store the sums of the data (to calculate the mean), and the sum of the squares of the differences (obtainable only after the myriad subtractions needed to calculate the individual differences have been completed, and their respective squares calculated). This requires many more operations, each of which takes time, and vastly larger storage capacity. While computer memory is now cheap, and central processing units are now extremely fast, nevertheless small, hand-held devices such as scientific calculators still have restricted memory capacity, and limited speed. And lazy computer programmers find the second and third algorithms attractively simple to implement. However, electronic calculators and computers use floating point numerical processors to actually carry out the calculations. These devices represent all numbers as integers having a fixed number of significant figures (e.g., 10^{-7}, 10^{-10}, 10^{-15}, etc.), multiplied by an integer power of ten (actually, most floating point processors use binary arithmetic, but the idea is the same). When you square a number, the processor keeps the most significant digits, and throws the rest away. When the numbers you square are large enough, you start throwing away the digits that contain the information about the variability between similar numbers. The result: using the second or third algorithm, instead of the first, will cause the computing device to give the wrong result when the number of significant digits required to perform the calculation exceeds the capacity of the floating point processor to represent the squares of the data accurately.

You can prove this easily for yourself. Consider the set of numbers {1,2,3}; this set has mean = 2, and sample standard deviation = 1. Now consider the set of numbers {11,12,13} and {101,102,103}; these have means 12, and 102 respectively but the sample standard deviation is still exactly 1. Indeed, the set {$10^n + 1$, $10^n + 2$, $10^n + 3$} has sample mean = $10^n + 2$, and standard deviation = 1, for any value of the exponent n. Using your favorite scientific calculator or computer software, calculate the sample standard deviation of the this set of numbers: {100001, 100002, 100003}. Now try this set: {1000000001, 1000000002, 1000000003}. And this set: {10000000000001, 10000000000002, 10000000000003}. Did you always get the number

"1" as the result? All digital computing devices will fail this test if you simply make the value of n large enough. What you need to know is how large a value of n makes *your* calculator or computer software fail. Then only work with numbers having no more than $(n - 1)$ significant digits when you want to calculate variances or standard deviations. A large number of test data sets designed to cause computational failures in computing machines are available from NIST (see bibliography).

10.6.4 Coefficient of Variation

The coefficient of variation is simply the standard deviation divided by the mean. From a statistical point of view, this is a difficult number to work with, since it is the ratio of two parameters, each of which has different statistical properties. If nobody ever rounded off the results of statistical calculations, one could always be confident of retrieving the value of the standard deviation from knowledge of both the coefficient of variation and the mean. Unfortunately, the only time one is likely to encounter this statistic is after somebody has finished rounding data for presentation, and such rounding may or may not have been properly performed. Using the sample data set, we find:

C.V. = 2.028153544% (rounded to 10 significant digits)

10.6.5 Multivariate Covariance and Correlation

When two or more types of measured values are considered jointly, they may be completely unrelated or it may be that a change in one type of measurement may be reflected, at least to some extent, as a change in another type of measurement. That is, the measurements are correlated. If they are correlated, then the dispersion of one set of measurements will affect the dispersion of the other set of measurements, and *vice versa*. The net effect is to constrain the overall allowable range of dispersion. The traditional measure of this joint dispersion is obtained from the covariance, which is the adjusted average of the products of the deviations of each of the individual measurements from their respected arithmetic means. Although no consensus symbolism for the covariance has been established, most often the symbols used to represent the variances of the measured values are used with subscripts indicating which pair of jointly measured values is being considered.

$$s_{13} = = \frac{\sum\limits_{i=1}^{i=n}(x_{1i} - \bar{x}_1)(x_{3i} - \bar{x}_3)}{n-1}$$

The product–moment correlation coefficient, usually symbolized by r, with subscripts if necessary to identify which pair of data sets out of a multivariate set of data are being considered, is simply the ratio of the covariance of these two data sets divided by the square root of product of their respective variances:

$$r_{13} = \frac{s_{13}}{\sqrt{s_1^2\, s_3^2}} = \frac{\sum\limits_{i=1}^{i=n}(x_{1i} - \bar{x}_1)(x_{3i} - \bar{x}_3)}{\sqrt{\left(\sum\limits_{i=1}^{i=n}(x_{1i} - \bar{x}_1)^2\right)\left(\sum\limits_{i=1}^{i=n}(x_{3i} - \bar{x}_3)^2\right)}}$$

Because the covariance can be either positive or negative (the variances, of course, are always positive), it is possible for r to be positive or negative. However, it can be shown that r can never be smaller than -1, nor larger than $+1$. Measures of correlation and covariance can be defined for any set of paired samples from any two populations.

10.6.6 Correlation and Causality

If the correlation between variables A and B is not zero, then there are four possibilities:

1. A causes B (which can only happen if A preceded B);
2. B causes A (which can only happen if B preceded A);
3. Something else causes both A and B (and therefore happened before either A or B were observed); or
4. An unlikely coincidence has occurred.

For example, for many years there was a strong positive correlation between the number of stork nests per hectare in the Netherlands, and the number of human babies born per hectare. This does not mean that storks bring babies, a common folktale told to children in Europe. More careful investigation revealed that unusually high numbers of stork nests (and unusually high numbers of babies born) were correlated with bountiful harvests during the previous growing season, which increased both the food supply available to the storks, and the prosperity of the farmers and other members of the community.

10.6.7 Error Propagation

A frequent problem encountered in scientific and engineering studies is that the final result we wish to obtain is actually a function of several experimental variables, each of which has a measured value and, of course, an associated dispersion, assuming that the measurements were made more than once. How should these individual measurements be combined to compute the best estimate of the final value? The naïve approach is to carry out one complete set of measurements, so that one obtains a single measurement for each of the individual components that are required to compute the overall result, then repeat the entire process again several times, calculating results for each replication each time, and then finally average the individual results, and compute an appropriate measure of dispersion for this average. If all of the individual component measurements were uncorrelated, this would work. However, in practice, some of the individual component measurements may be correlated with each other, and the resulting estimate of dispersion would then be incorrect.

In general, if the result is a continuous function of several variables:

$$y = f(x_1, x_2, \ldots, x_n)$$

then the variance of y can be approximated by taking only the linear terms of a Taylor expansion of f:

$$s_y^2 \cong \left(\frac{\partial f}{\partial x_1}\right)^2 s_1^2 + \left(\frac{\partial f}{\partial x_2}\right)^2 s_2^2 + \cdots + \left(\frac{\partial f}{\partial x_n}\right)^2 s_n^2$$
$$+ \left(\frac{\partial f}{\partial x_1}\frac{\partial f}{\partial x_2}\right) s_{12} + \left(\frac{\partial f}{\partial x_1}\frac{\partial f}{\partial x_3}\right) s_{13}$$
$$+ \cdots + \left(\frac{\partial f}{\partial x_{n-1}}\frac{\partial f}{\partial x_n}\right) s_{(n-1)n}$$

The variance and covariance terms comprise the elements of an $n \times n$ square matrix (the variance–covariance matrix), which we will see plays an important role in multivariate analysis. This relationship can be simplified for commonly encountered functions:

If: $y = ax_1 + bx_2$ then $\quad s_y^2 = a^2s_1^2 + b^2s_2^2 + 2abs_{12}$

If: $y = ax_1 - bx_2$ then $\quad s_y^2 = a^2s_1^2 + b^2s_2^2 - 2abs_{12}$

If: $y = ax_1 \pm b$ $\quad$ then $\quad s_y^2 = a^2s_1^2$

If: $y = \dfrac{a_ix_1 + a_2x_2 + \cdots + a_nx_n}{n}$ $\quad$ then
$$s_y^2 = \sum_i a_i^2 s_i^2 + 2 \sum_i \sum_{\substack{j \\ i \neq j}} a_i a_j s_{ij}$$

If: $y = \dfrac{a_ix_1 + a_2x_2 + \cdots + a_nx_n}{n}$ $\quad$ then

$$s_y^2 = \frac{\sum_i a_i^2 s_i^2}{n^2}$$ if the x_i are uncorrelated

If: $y = \ln(x)$ $\quad$ then $\quad s_y^2 = \dfrac{s_x^2}{\overline{x}^2}$

Products and ratios give rise to more complex results, but some simplified formulae can be obtained if the coefficients of variation of each of the variables $x_1, x_2, \ldots x_n$ are small, and all of the variables $x_1, x_2, \ldots x_n$ are uncorrelated:

If: $y = \dfrac{x_1x_2 \ldots x_m}{x_{m=1}x_{m+2} \Lambda x_n}$ $\quad$ then $\quad s_y^2 = y^2 \sum_i \dfrac{s_i^2}{x_i^2}$

These rules are independent of the actual function, so long as it is continuous, and its mean and variance are both defined. Remember that even a discrete population that contains at least one element has a mean and variance; what restricts propagation of error calculations according to the rules above is the assumption that the population has a continuous distribution. However, nothing has been said so far about the shape of any continuous distributions we may encounter.

Using the rules above, the variance

of a mean is: $s_{\overline{y}}^2 = \dfrac{s_y^2}{n}$

10.7 PROBABILITY

Thus far, we have developed some descriptive tools, but have not considered probability and risk assessment to any great extent. Probability theories arose out of the study of games of chance by European mathematicians in the 1600s and 1700s. From the outset, two different points of view on probability have coexisted. On the one hand, risk assessment from the individual gambler's perspective led to the development of rules for combining probability estimates to calculate the probability of a particular event based upon other contingent probabilities, beginning with the publication, in 1763, of Thomas Bayes' essay on probability as a tool for inductive reasoning. On the other hand, risk assessment from the casino operator's perspective grew out of the work of Laplace and Gauss. This work culminated in the development of tests of significance based on frequency of occurrence when subsets of data are obtained from potentially infinite populations by Karl Pearson and William Gosset (writing under the pen name "Student") in the first decade of the twentieth century. These different interpretations are known as the Bayesian and frequentist approaches to probability.

In the frequentist approach, the probability of an event is simply its relative frequency of occurrence. If you consider that the set of "true" values that you have actually measured can be just one of a number of samples drawn from some population, then mathematical models allow statements to be made about the frequency of obtaining the set of data you actually observed with respect to other samples that might have been obtained. Adherents of frequentist methods claim that this approach allows purely objective inferences about the "true" or ideal values (the parameters of the model) describing the population distribution, while overlooking the fact that users of this technique may need to make certain unsupportable assumptions about the nature of the frequency distribution from which they are supposedly sampling (for example, that it is "normal" or Gaussian).

Frequentist methods can be justified in principle when the set of measurements at hand is a subset of a finite population of potential or actual measurements. Such a data set can, in principle, be enumerated by actual census. Deming has called such investigations enumerative studies.[2] Enumerative studies are common in political, business, and social science applications of statistical methods. The probability distributions used in enumerative studies cover only a finite number of possible measurements, and the parameters describing these probability distributions are in principle measurable if sufficient time and resources can be made available. The probability of obtaining the particular subset of measurements at hand could then be deduced from these known parameters describing the entire population.

However, most investigations performed by scientists and engineers in the course of developing pharmaceutical products are not enumerative; rather, they are what Deming called analytic studies. The purpose of analytic studies is to make inferences about future measurements based upon measurements that have already been completed. The probability distributions used in analytic studies potentially cover an infinite number of possible measurements, and the parameters describing these probability distributions are in principle immeasurable, no matter how much time or how many resources could be devoted to the task. Whatever inferences are drawn from analytic studies by inductive reasoning must necessarily be based on assumptions about the probability distribution, typically the normal probability distribution, that are impossible to ever confirm by actual measurement.

In the Bayesian approach, probability represents one's subjective degree of belief that an event will occur. These subjective beliefs are combined with "true" objective data obtained by actual measurement using Bayes' theorem to make probability statements concerning the likelihood that future measurements will fall within certain boundaries or cluster around a certain value; these statements can be continuously refined as new measurements become available.

When a weather forecaster said yesterday that there is a 30% chance of rain today, and you look out the window, then either it is raining or it is not. It is not raining 30%. What does the 30% figure mean, then? The frequentist forecaster is saying that, based upon previous experience, when the cloud cover, barometric pressure, etc., were "essentially the same" as the weather conditions were yesterday, it rained on 30% of the following days. The Bayesian weather forecaster, adopting the point of view of a gambler, is saying that he (or she) was willing to give odds of 3:7 that it would rain today if you had placed your bet before midnight yesterday. The Bayesian forecaster is also saying that, based on previous experience, when the cloud cover, barometric pressure, etc., were "essentially the same" as the weather conditions were yesterday, he (or she) would have broken even betting at 3:7 odds that it would rain the following day. In either case, the forecaster assumes a persistence of structure in making this prediction—that is, whatever factors were operative on previous days will be operative today. There will be no comets crashing into the earth or volcanic eruptions or other unforeseen (and unforeseeable) events that might trigger a cloudburst. Unpredictable events such as these introduce uncertainty. Forecasting is based on risk, that is, an assessment of the probability of a future occurrence based upon past experience. Statistical methods may be applied to estimating risks, but there is no way to predict uncertainties.

Bayesians use factual data to augment interpretation of their prior beliefs; frequentists use unprovable assumptions about the hypothetical probability distributions characteristic of analytic studies to interpret factual data. Debating whether the frequentist or Bayesian approach is correct is akin to debating whether an electron is best described as a particle or a wave. The answer, in each case, is "yes." Scientists and engineers wishing to make optimal projections of future performance from limited process data must apply both concepts of probability as part of a continuous knowledge building process.

10.7.1 Chebyshev's Inequality

Mathematics provides a solution to this conundrum: the Russian mathematician P. L. Chebyshev was able to develop a mathematical proof that, for any probability distribution $f(x)$ with finite first and second moments (which correspond to the mean μ and variance σ^2), one can assign a probability to the interval:

$$P\left\{x: \mu - h\sigma < x \le \mu + h\sigma\right\} \ge 1 - \frac{1}{h^2}$$

So long as the probability distribution meets the very minimal requirements (having a finite first and second moment), it does not matter what its actual shape is. The probability of finding any particular value within ± 2 standard deviations from the mean is at least 75%; within ± 3 standard deviations it is 88.8%; within ± 6 standard deviations it is at least 97.2%. Now, of course, if you were somehow able to convince yourself (and others) that the data you are studying actually were sampled from an infinite set of data having a normal probability distribution, these probabilities become much greater: for ± 2 standard deviations, the probability increases to 95.4%, while for ± 3 standard deviations it increases to 99.7%, and for ± 6 standard deviations it increases to some number so close to 100% that the difference is too small to bother with. However, if the data were not sampled from a normal probability distribution, those probability values no longer apply. The values obtained from Chebyshev's inequality are still valid, however, as worst-case limits, so long as you exclude uncertain events, and restrict your attention only to risky events.

Empirically, one finds that Chebyshev's limits are ultraconservative. Even for some truly odd-shaped distributions (such as the uniform rectangular distribution and the right triangular distribution), the probabilities are much higher than Chebyshev's lower bound. It is reasonable to assume that at the probability of finding a value within ± 2 standard deviations from the mean is at least 90% for any realistic distribution that might be encountered in practice, with at least 98% of values within ± 3 standard deviations.[3] Thus, the machinery of statistical inference, based upon the assumption of normality, works pretty much as advertised, except that the probability values obtained from a model Gaussian distribution represent a somewhat liberal estimate of the true probability. The actual probability lies closer to the estimate obtained by assuming normality than to the bounding value computed from Chebyshev's inequality. As long as you do not quibble about overly precise probability values to make inferences, the numerical estimates of probability based on the assumption of normality should be adequate.

10.7.2 The Normal Probability Assumption

Many statisticians attempt to justify using a normal probability distribution by appealing to the central limit theorem of probability, which states that the distribution of sums of randomly variable measured values approaches a normal probability distribution as the number of terms in the sum increases. Although this is certainly provable mathematically, it is less easy to see how this theorem applies to real measurement data. Real measurement processes may include multiple unit operations, each of which has outputs subject to random variation that must be combined together, using the propagation of error rules discussed previously, to estimate the overall best measured value, and its associated dispersion. However, real measurement processes typically have just one or two sources of variation that dominate the process. It can be shown mathematically that when no single source of error dominates, and multiple sources of error must be incorporated in the final estimate of error (an unusual case, to be sure), the combined errors can appear as if they were normally distributed even when as few as five independently uncorrelated sources of error of comparable magnitude are combined together, no matter how bizarre the distribution of actual errors for each source might be. But the central limit theorem states that it is only asymptotically true that the resulting distribution of errors actually follows a normal probability distribution.

More commonly, the argument is stated in a different way: if any population is sampled, then the means of samples from that population tend to have a frequency distribution that is closer to the normal distribution than the population from which the samples were taken. And if the means themselves are sampled, then the means of the samples of means will tend to have a frequency distribution that even more closely resembles the normal distribution. This follows mathematically from the central limit theorem. So, by repeatedly taking means of means of means … of samples, we can get a set of numbers that have a frequency distribution that is arbitrarily close to the normal distribution. This is very true. But nobody who makes measurements that people actually use to guide decision-making ever does this. At best, we are only concerned about the distribution of means of samples, not the means of means of (many repetitions) of means of samples.

An assertion of normality for any particular sample of real measurements based on argument from the central limit theorem is just so much hand waving. It is true that real measured data often appears as if it had been obtained by sampling a process that can be adequately modeled using the normal probability distribution; after all, that is how Laplace and Gauss deduced the form of the so-called normal error law! But since the normal probability distribution is just a convenient mathematical abstraction that was initially selected because it fitted real data rather well, to claim that real data are normally distributed is a circular argument. There simply is no way that anybody can actually prove that a set of real experimental data was drawn from a population with a normal probability distribution, although it is possible to provide a probabilistic estimate that such a set was drawn from a distribution that was *not* the normal probability distribution.

An alternative to assuming normality is to propose the use of an empirically selected probability distribution instead. This seems attractive, but also has problems. To be useful in assigning probabilities to future events, the cumulative distribution function must be easily integrated, which limits the mathematical form of suitable functions. As additional data become available, the best fitting empirical model will change, rendering previous probability assignments obsolete. A better approach is to be skeptical of overly precise probability assignments, particularly if a slight change in probability would lead to choosing a different course of action.

10.8 INTERVAL ESTIMATION

With the foregoing points of view in mind, we now assume, for the purpose of the following discussion, that the set of measurements we have obtained are a sample from a potentially infinite number of measurements in a population; in most instances we will also assume that the frequency distribution of this population really can be described by a normal probability distribution with mean μ, and variance σ^2, even though we know we can never prove this assumption. These are the standard assumptions of frequentist statistical methods. We want to define rules that put boundaries on population parameters μ and σ^2, based on the statistics $\bar{x}$ and s^2 calculated from our set of measurement data. In the frequentist case, we assume that the population parameters are fixed values. The boundaries generated by the rule for constructing the interval are variables that will change from sample data set to sample data set. Probabilities are assigned to whether or not the rule so defined encompasses the fixed parameter estimate. Bayesians assign probabilities to the parameters or statistics instead of to the rules; interval estimates (called "credible" intervals) indicate the degree of belief that a parameter or statistic has a value within the stated interval. In the Bayesian interpretation, we assume that the population parameters are variables, and that the boundaries

generated for constructing the intervals are fixed by the data. Probabilities are assigned to whether or not the parameter estimates so defined are encompassed by the fixed rule. It is possible to construct interval estimates using either the frequentist or Bayesian approach that are identical in range with the same associated probability values; only the interpretation of what this probability means differs between the two approaches.

10.8.1 Confidence Intervals

Confidence intervals define boundaries enclosing a region in which we expect to find a population parameter with a specified probability. In most textbooks, the author uses α to represent the probability that the parameter *is not* in the interval, so the probability that the parameter *is* in the interval is simply $1 - \alpha$. Obviously, for any particular interval based on statistics computed from any particular set of measurement data, the population parameter of interest either is in the interval or it is not. If we adopted the frequentist viewpoint, and were somehow able to repeatedly make sets of measurements like the particular set of measurements we are considering right now then, in the long run, over many such replicate sets of measurements, we would find the population parameter within the boundaries constructed by the rule for obtaining the confidence interval estimate the percentage of time specified when we chose the rule. If we prefer the Bayesian approach, we would instead state that we were willing to lay odds of $(1 - \alpha)$:α that the population parameter will be found within the boundaries constructed by the rule for obtaining the credible interval estimate derived from our particular set of measurements. It turns out that if we are Bayesians with little prior knowledge of what value of the parameter to expect, and we are forced to rely only on the measurements at hand, we will find that we will identify exactly the same boundary points for our credible interval estimate that our frequentist colleagues chose. Furthermore, if we are frequentists, and have some prior knowledge about the reliability of our measurements so that we can assign appropriate weighting factors to them, then we will identify exactly the same boundary points for our confidence interval that our Bayesian colleagues, using the same prior information, would have selected for their credible interval estimate. The numbers do not change; only our interpretation of what probability means to us changes. Since the frequentist approach is more commonly used in introductory texts, it is the approach that will be used in the following discussion.

Mean

A two-sided $100(1 - \alpha)\%$ confidence interval for the population mean μ is (assuming normality, and giving equal weight to every measurement):

$$P\left\{\mu: \bar{x} - t_{(1-\alpha/2,n-1)}s\sqrt{\frac{1}{n}} < \mu \leq \bar{x} + t_{(1-\alpha/2,n-1)}s\sqrt{\frac{1}{n}}\right\}$$
$$= 1 - \alpha$$

where $t_{(1-(\alpha/2),n-1)}$ represents the $(1 - \alpha/2)$ percentile of Student's t distribution with $n - 1$ degrees of freedom. This distribution takes into account the fact that s is only an approximate estimate of the population standard deviation.

For the sample data set previously used to demonstrate computation of the mean, and setting $\alpha = 0.05$, we find:

$$n = 5$$
$$t_{0.975,4} = 2.7764509$$

so that the 95% two-sided confidence interval for the population mean is:

$9582.6590658 < \mu \leq 10077.7656650$ (rounded to the same number of significant digits used to calculate the mean).

We'll consider rounding later. However, it should be apparent that the sample mean could have been rounded at least to the nearest integer or even to the nearest ten units without appreciably affecting the width of this confidence interval. Also, the probability value (95%) is only valid if the real frequency distribution is actually the normal distribution, which of course can never be proven, but must be taken on faith.

To better visualize the effect of increasing the number of degrees of freedom used to estimate the sample mean and standard deviation, the upper and lower confidence limits for estimating the mean of a normally distributed population were plotted as a function of the number of degrees of freedom as shown in Figure 10.15.

Note that the width of the confidence interval estimate depends upon the size of the sample standard deviation, as well as upon the value of Student's t for the number of degrees of freedom. The sample must have at least six degrees of freedom (i.e., seven measured values) to obtain a confidence interval estimate for the population mean that is within ± 1 standard deviation of the sample mean with 95% confidence, assuming that the measurement data from which the sample was drawn are normally distributed with mean μ and variance σ^2. To be within ± 0.5 standard deviations, at least 17 degrees of freedom are needed.

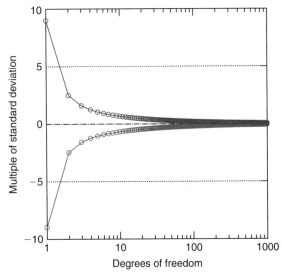

FIGURE 10.15   Effect of sample size on confidence limits for the sample mean

To be within ± 0.1 standard deviations, 386 degrees of freedom are required. No matter how many measurements are made, the interval will always have finite width.

Median

A two-sided $100(1 - \alpha)\%$ confidence interval for the population median can be constructed using the ranks of the observations in the set of measurements we have already obtained for certain values of α. The calculation of probability is based upon the binomial distribution. First, find, if possible:

$$P\left\{B_{u-1,n,0.5} - B_{l-1,n,0.5}\right\} \geq 1 - \alpha$$

for $0 < l < u \leq n$, where n is the number of measurements in the set of measurements we have. This may not always be possible if n is small; in that case, set $l = 1$ and $u = n$ and calculate the binomial probabilities $B_{1,n,0.5}$ and $B_{n,n,0.5}$.

For the sample data set previously used to demonstrate computation of the mean, and setting $\alpha = 0.05$, we find:

$$n = 5, B_{1,n,0.5} = 0.9687, B_{n,n,0.5} = 0.0313$$

so the interval [9568.279745, 10043.677788] (using the same number of significant digits initially reported) contains the population median with 93.74% probability, assuming only that the frequency distribution of the measurements is continuous (i.e., the data are analog, not digital). In order to obtain a 95% confidence interval bounded by the measurements that define the range of the data, at least six measurements are required. However, with nine measurements, the probability of finding the population median within the region bounded by the second smallest and second largest values in the set of measurements obtained is greater than 95%, assuming only that the data come from a population that has a continuous frequency distribution. Only a set of twelve measurements are required to define a confidence interval bounded by the third lowest and third highest values in the set of measurements with 95% probability. Thus, if the occurrence of "wild" values is anticipated, due to the frequency with which outright blunders might occur, simply increasing the number of measured values obtained from six to twelve will automatically exclude the two smallest and two largest values in the data set from the values required to construct an interval estimate of the median. Also note that we have made no assumption that the frequency distribution of deviations from the population median is normal, but only that it is continuous.

Standard Deviation

A two-sided $100(1 - \alpha)\%$ confidence interval for the population standard deviation σ is (assuming normality and giving equal weight to every measurement):

$$P\left\{\sigma: s\sqrt{\frac{n - 1}{\chi^2_{(\alpha/2, n-1)}}} < \sigma \leq s\sqrt{\frac{n - 1}{\chi^2_{(1-\alpha/2, n-1)}}}\right\} = 1 - \alpha$$

where χ^2 represents the appropriate percentile of the χ^2 distribution with $n - 1$ degrees of freedom. This distribution takes into account the fact that s is only an approximate estimate of the population standard deviation.

For the sample data set previously used to demonstrate computation of the mean, and setting $\alpha = 0.05$, we find:

$$n = 5$$

$$\chi^2_{0.025, 4} = 11.1432620, \quad \chi^2_{0.975, 4} = 0.4844190$$

so that the 95% two-sided confidence interval for the population standard deviation is:

$119.4503855 < \sigma \leq 572.9057096$ (rounded to the same number of significant digits used to calculate the standard deviation).

Again, we'll consider rounding later. Also, the probability value (95%) is only valid if the real frequency distribution is actually the normal distribution, which of course can never be proven, but must be taken on faith. In addition, note how imprecisely we can estimate the population standard deviation based on

this small sample. It should be apparent that the sample standard deviation could have been rounded at least to the nearest integer or even to the nearest ten units without appreciably affecting the width of this confidence interval.

To better visualize the effect of increasing the number of degrees of freedom used to estimate the sample standard deviation, the upper and lower confidence limits for estimating the standard deviation of a normally distributed population were plotted as a function of the number of degrees of freedom, as shown in Figure 10.16.

Note that logarithmic scales are used for both axes.

Suppose we wanted to estimate the population standard deviation with 95% confidence that the true value was bounded by an interval no more than ±10% of the true value, assuming that the population was characterized by a normal frequency distribution. How many measurements would we need to collect to estimate the standard deviation of the sample in order to achieve this goal? The answer may surprise you: at least 234 measurements. And to be within ±5% of the "true" value with 95% confidence, you would need to collect at least 849 measurements. In the ordinary course of events, research and development scientists and engineers will never gather sufficient data to ever estimate the population standard deviation of an assumed normal probability distribution with any degree of precision. If we are willing to tolerate an error in estimating the true value as large as ±50%, we still need at least at least 18 replicate measurements to obtain a confidence interval estimate that would include the standard deviation of a normally distributed population with "95%" confidence. This

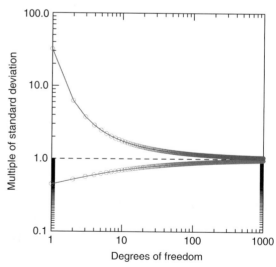

FIGURE 10.16   Effect of sample size on confidence limits for the sample standard deviation

experimentally estimated standard deviation is used to construct an interval estimate for the mean. So, it should be readily apparent that we have an estimated standard deviation, known very imprecisely, which we will use to construct an interval estimate for the mean based on a probability derived from an assumption of normality that can never be proven. We must not be persnickety about keeping too many significant digits in our final estimates of either the boundaries of our interval estimate or the probability we associate with it.

Median Absolute Deviation from the Median

A two-sided $100(1 - \alpha)\%$ confidence interval for the median absolute deviation from the population median can be constructed using the ranks of the absolute differences between the observations in the set of measurements we have already obtained, and the median of that set of observations for certain values of α using the same procedure described above for finding a confidence interval for the median itself. However, it is seldom useful to include the lowest-ranking deviation, which will always be zero for odd-numbered data sets or close to zero for even-numbered data sets.

For the sample data set previously used to demonstrate computation of the mean, and setting $\alpha = 0.05$, we find:

$$n = 5, B_{2,n,0.5} = 0.8125, B_{n,n,0.5} = 0.0313$$

so the interval [142.168995, 282.204964] (using the same number of significant digits initially reported) contains the median absolute deviation from the population median with 78.12% probability, assuming only that the frequency distribution of the measurements is continuous (i.e., the data are analog, not digital).

10.8.2 Prediction Intervals

We use prediction intervals when our interest lies in predicting future observations, the means of future sets of measurements or the standard deviations of future sets of measurements.

Individual New Value or Mean of a New Sample

A two-sided $100(1 - \alpha)\%$ prediction interval for the mean $\bar{x}_m$ of a future set of m measurements is:

$$P\left\{ \bar{x}_m : \bar{x} - t_{\left(1 - \alpha/2, n-1\right)} s\sqrt{\frac{1}{n} + \frac{1}{m}} < \bar{x}_m \right.$$
$$\left. \leq \bar{x} + t_{\left(1 - \alpha/2, n-1\right)} s\sqrt{\frac{1}{n} + \frac{1}{m}} \right\} = 1 - \alpha$$

where t represents the appropriate percentile of Student's t distribution with $n - 1$ degrees of freedom. This distribution takes into account the fact that s is only an approximate estimate of the population standard deviation. The samples are also assumed to be uncorrelated and, of course, drawn from the same normally distributed population. If the new sample is obtained under different circumstances, such that the mean and variance of the population being sampled are affected, then the probability statement is no longer correct.

Standard Deviation of a New Sample

A two-sided $100(1 - \alpha)\%$ prediction interval for the population standard deviation s_m of a future set of m measurements is:

$$P\left\{ s_m : s\sqrt{\frac{1}{F_{\left(1 - \alpha/2, n-1, m-1\right)}}} < s_m \right.$$
$$\left. \leq s\sqrt{F_{\left(1 - \alpha/2, n-1, m-1\right)}} \right\} = 1 - \alpha$$

where F represents the appropriate percentile of the F distribution with $n - 1$ and $m - 1$ degrees of freedom. This distribution takes into account the fact that s is only an approximate estimate of the population standard deviation.

To get a suitably small value of the F-statistic so that the error in estimating the standard deviation is less than $\pm 10\%$, both n and m must be large; if both are 426, for example, then you will have a sufficient number of replications if you are willing to assume that the random deviations in both sets of measurements come from a population with a normal probability distribution. With only 10 replicates in each sample, the error is ± 50.

Again, the samples are also assumed to be uncorrelated and, of course, drawn from the same population. If the new sample is obtained under different circumstances, such that the mean and variance of the population being sampled are affected, then the probability statement is no longer correct.

10.8.3 Tolerance Intervals

We use tolerance intervals when our interest lies in characterizing the entire population of potential measurements from which the current set of measurements was supposedly obtained as a random sample. Tolerance intervals are used to set boundaries that, with the stated probability, will enclose at least the stated percentage of possible measured values.

Tolerance intervals may be thought of as confidence intervals that set boundaries for a specified range of values, rather than a single parameter or statistic.

Tolerance Interval for a Central Proportion of a Normally Distributed Population

A two-sided $100(1 - \alpha)\%$ tolerance interval to contain at least $100p\%$ of measurements taken from the center of a normally distributed population is:

$$P \left\{ 100p\% \text{ of } x_i : \overline{x} - g_{(1-\alpha,p,n)}s \\ < 100p\% \text{ of } x_i \leq \overline{x} + g_{(1-\alpha,p,n)}s \right\}$$

where $g_{(1-\alpha,p,n-1)}$ is obtained using the non-central Student's t distribution.[4] This distribution takes into account the fact that s is only an approximate estimate of the population standard deviation.

For the sample data set previously used to demonstrate computation of the mean, and setting $\alpha = 0.05$ and $100p\% = 99\%$, we find:

$$n = 5$$

$$g_{0.95,0.99,5} = 6.598$$

so that the 95% two-sided tolerance interval bounding 99% of the population (centered on the mean) from which the set of measurements was a sample is:

$8514.7572261 < 99\%$ of measurements ≤ 11145.6675047 (rounded to the same number of significant digits used to calculate the mean).

Again, we'll consider rounding later. Also, the probability value (95%) is only valid if the real frequency distribution is actually the normal probability distribution, which of course can never be proven, but must be taken on faith.

Again, the samples are also assumed to be uncorrelated and, of course, drawn from the same population. If the new sample is obtained under different circumstances, such that the mean and variance of the population being sampled are affected, then the probability statement is no longer correct.

Tolerance Interval for a Central Proportion of a Population with a Continuous Frequency Distribution

A two-sided $100(1 - \alpha)\%$ tolerance interval encompassing $100p\%$ of measurements that are continuously distributed (i.e., analog, not digital) can be constructed without assuming that the real frequency distribution of the measurement data are the normal

distribution by using the ranks of the observations in the set of measurements we have already obtained for certain values of α. Unfortunately, rather large sets of data are required for this to have any practical utility. For example, if we use the extreme highest and lowest measurements in a set of data to define the tolerance limits, then to assure with 95% probability that at least 99% of the population was encompassed by these limits, we would need at least 130 measurements.[5]

10.8.4 Rounding

At last we have the tools to deal with the whole question of rounding. From the preceding section on propagation of error, it should be clear that failing to carry through a sufficient number of significant digits in calculations could give rise to serious bias in the results of chain calculations. If the minimum difference between two possible digital measurements d_- and d_+ is $w = d_+ - d_-$, and the "true" analog value can, with equal probability, lie anywhere within this interval, then the "true" value behaves as if it were a member of a class of measurements having a rectangular frequency distribution bounded by d_- and d_+ with mean $w/2$ and variance $w^2/12$. If the variance of the analog measurement is σ^2, then the variance of either of the two closest digital representations of the analog number is:[6]

$$\sigma^2_{d\pm} = \sigma^2 + \frac{w^2}{12}$$

So long as width w of the interval is less than 0.49σ, the value of σ is not altered by more than $\pm 1\%$. Similarly, so long as the maximum width of the interval is less than 0.155σ, the value of σ is not altered by more than $\pm 0.1\%$. We have seen that estimates of a normally distributed population standard deviation with an accuracy of $\pm 10\%$ with ~95% confidence require that there be more than 234 measurements in the set, so that any estimate of the population standard deviation reported with an accuracy of $\pm 1\%$ is clearly sufficient.

If we round the standard error of the mean $s/\sqrt{n}$ calculated from the set of actual measurements, so that it has only one significant digit if the leading digit is 2 through 9, or two significant digits if the leading digit is 1, then the resulting value will not differ from a value having a greater number of significant digits by more than ~0.5σ. All other values (e.g., the mean, median, probability interval boundaries, etc.) should be rounded to the same number of significant digits. This result holds for any continuous frequency distribution; the assumption of normality is not required.

For our sample data set, $s = 199.3718004$ and $n = 5$, so $s/\sqrt{n} = 89.1617797$. Applying the above rule, after rounding $s/\sqrt{n} = 9 \times 10^1 = 90$. So the data set mean $= 9830$, the data set median $= 9850$, the data set range $= 480$, the data set interquartile range $= 300$, the data set variance $= 40000$ and the coefficient of variation is 2%. In addition, if we assume that the measurements come from a population with a frequency distribution that is a normal distribution, then we can state with 95% confidence that the population mean is between 9580 and 10080 (note that we round down for a lower limit and up for an upper limit), the population standard deviation is between 110 and 580, and that 99% of the population measurements are between 8510 and 11150. Similarly, with 93% confidence, the median is between 9560 and 10050, and with 78% confidence the population median absolute deviation from the median is between 140 and 290.

Although rounding an estimated standard error to only one or two significant figures may seem a profligate waste of information, and the temptation to increase the number of significant figures to be retained may be strong (or required by institutional practices), there really is no usable information conveyed by extra digits unless the number of degrees of freedom used to estimate the standard error is large. A modified rule that provides extra assurance if the rounded numbers might possibly be used in further computations is to round the data set standard error of the mean to two significant digits if it has fewer than 14 degrees of freedom; if the degrees of freedom are between 15 and 49, retain three significant digits if the leading digit is a 1, and if the degrees of freedom are between 50 and 99, retain three significant digits if the leading digit is 1 or 2, retain three significant digits in other cases only if the degrees of freedom for estimating the standard error are 100 or more.[7]

For our sample data set, $s = 199.3718004$ and $n = 5$, so $s/\sqrt{n} = 89.1617797$. Applying the above rule, after rounding $s/\sqrt{n} = 89$. So the data set mean $= 9830$, the data set median $= 9850$, the data set range $= 475$, the data set interquartile range $= 297$, the data set variance $= 39601$, and the coefficient of variation is 2.0%. In addition, if we assume that the measurements come from a population with a frequency distribution that is a normal distribution, then we can state with 95% confidence that the population mean is between 9582 and 10078 (note that we round down for a lower limit and up for an upper limit), the population standard deviation is between 119 and 573, and that 99% of the population measurements are between 8514 and 11147. Similarly, with 93% confidence, the median is between 9568 and 10044, and with 78% confidence the population median absolute deviation from the median is between 140 and 290.

10.9 PROCESS MODELING AND EXPERIMENTAL DESIGN

Philosopher Karl Popper once said, "Science is the art of systematic oversimplification." Scientists and engineers systematically oversimplify complex processes by reducing them to mathematical models. Recall that George Box claimed, "All models are wrong, but some are useful." Among the useful models are stochastic models—models that explicitly contain a term (or terms) representing the (predictable based on past performance!) random variation inherent in all processes.

Consider an example: a pharmaceutical formulator manufactures a batch of tablets containing an active ingredient, coats them with a water-soluble enteric coating, and sends a sample of thirty tablets to be assayed for potency. The analyst selects ten tablets at random, and carefully weighs each tablet in the subsample, and then assays each individual tablet using a complex chromatographic method. The formulator wants to estimate the effect of weight variation on content uniformity of the tablets. What is the relationship between the amount of active ingredient per tablet, and the weight of each individual tablet? Can tablet weight be used to predict the amount of drug in a tablet?

Of course, the first step in answering these questions is to plot the data. Having done so, the formulator might theorize that the potency might be roughly proportional to the tablet weight, allowing, of course, for the added weight of the coating. If there were no random fluctuations to account for, all of the plotted data should lie on a straight line. They don't. Instead, they exhibit some scatter about a line drawn through the plotted points, as shown in Figure 10.17.

The line itself slopes slightly upwards. How could this be represented mathematically?

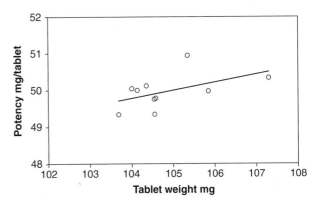

FIGURE 10.17   Potency versus tablet weight example

10.9.1 Models, Parameters, and Hypotheses

We recall from analytical geometry that the equation for a straight line can be written:

$$y = b_0 + b_1 x$$

where b_0 and b_1, the *parameters* of the model, represent the y-intercept and slope of the line, respectively. However, this model does not accurately predict the data actually observed, since it ignores the random fluctuations we see. It is too oversimplified. Upon reflection, we realize that there must be some random variation associated with the weighing process, as well as some variation associated with the chromatographic assay, which may include both systematic bias and random fluctuation. There may also be some random variation in the composition of the powder blend used to make each tablet. Also, the coating contains no drug, although the weight of the coating is included in the total weight of each tablet. Furthermore, the tablets may not be uniformly coated, so some provision must also be made to include this source of random variation. Thus, a more accurate model might be:

$$y_i = b_0 + b_1 \left[(x_i + e_{xi}) - (b_3 + e_{ci}) \right](1 + e_{ui}) + e_{ai}$$

where y_i is the measured potency of the ith tablet, b_0 is the average bias of the chromatography assay, e_{ai} is the variation for the ith tablet due to random variation in the chromatography process, x_i is the weight of the ith tablet, e_{xi} is the random variation in the tablet weighing process, b_3 is the average weight of the coating applied to each tablet, e_{ci} is the random variation in the weight of the coating applied to the ith tablet, and e_{ui} is the random variation in content uniformity of the powder blend used to make the ith tablet. Note that sources of bias (b_0 and b_3) have been represented as if they were parameters of the model, since they are presumed to be constant for all tablets, while the various random errors (e_{xi}, e_{ci}, e_{ui}, and e_{ai}) are subscripted to indicate that they each have unique values (which may be positive or negative) for each tablet. After some algebra, and assuming that the random fluctuations are sufficiently small so that the product of two random fluctuations can be ignored, we can rewrite the model as:

$$y_i = (b_0 - b_1 b_3) + b_1 x_i + b_1 (e_{(x+c)i} + (x_i - b_3)e_{ui}) + e_{ai}$$

This is still a challenging model to fit to the data using conventional approaches; in particular, there are errors associated with both the x and y variables.

Recognizing that the tablet weights vary over only a small range, the errors associated with an individual tablet can be pooled together without much loss

of accuracy, and the constant parameters can also be lumped together, leaving:

$$y_i \cong c + bx_i + e_i$$

This somewhat oversimplified model, which completely ignores any errors associated with the x variables, can easily be fitted to the data using standard techniques. It can be used to predict the approximate potency assay value from the tablet weight if another tablet from the same batch were to be assayed. However, it does confound all of the sources of variability, making it impossible to discern whether the variability that is observed arises primarily from the measurement process or the production process. Thus, this model is not very useful as a tool for process improvement.

Although we know the model is wrong, it may be useful at an early stage in development. The formulator may want to know if the variation in tablet weight is important in predicting potency. A confidence interval estimate for the parameter b in the simplified model might, for example, include both positive and negative estimates. For the data plotted, and assuming that the errors are normally distributed, a 95% confidence interval for b covers the interval $[-0.09, +0.53]$. For this example, clearly zero is not only a possible value for b, but also a probable value. And if b were zero, then the effect of tablet weight variation is too small to measure. We would say that b is not a statistically significant parameter, and therefore tablet weight was not a statistically significant predictor of potency. This is a risky conclusion.

10.9.2 Confidence Interval Estimation and Hypothesis Testing

The evaluation of the effect of random variation is the motivation for statistical hypothesis testing. The goal is to make an assertion (a hypothesis) about a model parameter, and to provide a probability estimate of the truth or falsehood of the assertion. Mathematically, the process of performing a statistical test of a hypothesis is identically equivalent to the process of constructing a confidence interval estimate for the parameter. The two approaches are one and the same when it comes to implementation. However, when viewed from the perspective of hypothesis testing, some additional insight can be obtained.

Any hypothesis is either true or false. The purpose of statistical hypothesis testing is to assign a probability that the hypothesis is true, and to assign a probability that the hypothesis is false. The two probabilities must sum to 100%. Whenever you ask a question that has two, and only two, possible answers (e.g., is this statement true or false?), then there are always exactly four possible outcomes:

1. You conclude the statement is true, when in fact it really is true.
2. You conclude the statement is false, when in fact it really is false.
3. You conclude the statement is true, when in fact it really is false (Type I mistake).
4. You conclude the statement is false, when in fact it really is true (Type II mistake).

(Note: Most statistics books use the vernacular term "error" instead of "mistake.")

The probability of making a Type I mistake is the probability associated with the confidence interval estimate of the parameter. The probability of making a Type II mistake is more difficult to determine. It involves posing alternate hypotheses, and systematically evaluating these, because the probability of making a Type II mistake is dependent entirely on which of the alternate hypotheses is actually "true" compared the hypothesis being tested.

In the section immediately above, we noted that the formulator found that a 95% confidence interval estimate for the model parameter b was wide enough to include zero. The formulator could conclude that there was not sufficient evidence that the effect of weight variation was different from zero, and tentatively conclude that the statement "the potency does not depend on the tablet weight" is true. A more useful way to perform a hypothesis test is equivalent to finding the probability associated with the shortest confidence interval that just excludes the target value (in this case, zero); for example, the formulator can assert, with 86% confidence, that if the random errors were normally distributed, then a confidence interval estimate for the parameter b would not include the value zero. Another way of putting this is that there is a 14% chance that b is different from zero. If the formulator would assert that "the potency does not depend on the tablet weight" based on this evidence, we might disagree. We might find the probability not sufficiently compelling, and conclude that the formulator had made a Type I mistake. A moment's reflection should be sufficient to convince any reader that the potency must depend upon the tablet weight; if the tablet weighed half as much (say, it broke in two before it was coated) or twice as much (two tablets stuck together during the coating process), the measured potency would be dramatically different. All the model tells you is that, based on the amount of random variation actually seen, the formulator doesn't have sufficient evidence to convincingly demonstrate

this from the measurements actually collected. A more carefully designed experiment (e.g., including tablets deliberately made with widely different target weights) or better control over the production process variation and analytical process variation, would reveal this by making the confidence interval estimate for b smaller and smaller, until it no longer included zero (or, conversely, until a confidence interval that just excluded zero had a larger and larger probability associated with it).

10.9.3 Are Two Processes Different or the Same?

Textbook examples of statistical hypothesis tests are always framed to test whether two sets of data are different. They do this by actually testing the opposite hypothesis, that is, the hypothesis that two sets of data are samples drawn from the same population. If the probability that the samples are the same is sufficiently small, we conclude that they are most likely different.

What if this is not the question you want to pose? What if you want to establish that two processes are the "same" instead? You would need to test a different hypothesis: that the two sets of data differed by more than some specified critical amount. If you do not have enough evidence to convincingly demonstrate that two processes are different by at least that amount, then it is fair to conclude that the difference between the two sets of data are small enough not to be of concern. This does not mean that the two sets of data are samples from the exactly the same population; all it means is that whatever populations the data sets are drawn from, the populations do not differ enough for the difference to have practical consequences. There is no amount of evidence that can ever demonstrate that two sets of data come from identically the same population. If you can show that the measured difference is smaller than the allowed difference, conclude that the two processes are interchangeable for practical purposes.

10.9.4 More Complex Models

Models of real processes are often complex; many factors, either those under the control of the process designer or those that are not, can influence the measured outcomes of a process. A model may contain simply additive terms or multiplicative terms. If the model contains only additive terms, representing the effects of single factors, then the factors act independently of each other. When the model contains more complex terms involving combinations of factors, then the factors are not independent, but interact with each other. The development of a new process may require the investigation of the effects of multiple factors; we apply the scientific method plan to a systematic investigation to discover potential factors, study the effect of changing them, draw conclusions, and modify the process. This proceeds iteratively until we are satisfied that the process can be operated consistently to produce the desired results. The application of statistical methods has led to the development of experimental designs that efficiently produce information (signals), with minimum confusion resulting from random variation (noise). The primary tools for analyzing data obtained from experiments designed in accordance with statistical principles are regression modeling, and the analysis of variance.

10.9.5 Regression Models and the Analysis of Variance

The concepts of designed experiments based on statistical considerations evolved out of agricultural research in the early part of the twentieth century, and were first elegantly described in Ronald Fisher's pioneering text published in 1935. For many years thereafter, the emphasis of most advances in this area were based on improving and extending the analysis of variance (ANOVA) method that Fisher had invented. ANOVA uses a specialized subset of linear statistical models that are the subject of a broader technique, known as regression analysis, developed several decades earlier by Francis Galton and Karl Pearson. The actual computations involved in performing either regression analysis or the more restricted models developed for the analysis of variance are most efficiently performed using linear algebra to manipulate a vector (or matrix) of measured responses $\mathbf{Y}$, and a matrix of design factors $\mathbf{X}$ to estimate a vector of model parameters β:

$$\mathbf{Y} = \mathbf{X}\beta + \varepsilon$$

The only real difference between a linear regression model and an ANOVA model is the design matrix. Regression models traditionally use continuous numerical design variables. ANOVA models often use categorical design variables (also called factors); appropriate integer values can be assigned using well-defined rules so that regression calculations can be performed. Computers don't know the difference; they just crunch the numbers. ANOVA models also have certain elements of symmetry that can lead to problems when traditional desk calculator methods for performing the calculations are used, and some

of the data required by the design is missing; these computational problems vanish when linear algebra methods developed to perform regression analysis are used to perform the computations. Purists may make much ado about missing data in ANOVA calculations, but as long as the design variables are properly coded, and the missing values are not critical to the design (e.g., one of several planned replicate measurements is missing), the necessary calculations can be made, model parameters can be estimated, and probability values needed for making inferences can be calculated.

10.9.6 One-way ANOVA with One Nominal Factor

The simplest type of ANOVA model can be written as either a "cell means" model:

$$y_{ij} = \mu_i + e_{ij}$$

where the mean responses to each of the i different levels of the nominal factor are computed separately, or as a "factor effects" model:

$$y_{ij} = \mu + \tau_i + e_{ij}$$

where an overall mean is first estimated, and then the differences from that mean due to each level of the nominal factor are estimated separately. In either case, i can be as low as 2, and the maximum value of j does not need to be the same for each level. If $i = 2$, then this design is identical to the use of Student's t-test to compare the means of two independent samples. You can use the cell means model with $i = 1$ to compare the differences between pairs of measurements subjected to two different levels of a categorical factor; this is equivalent to the use of Student's paired t-test to compare the differences between two samples.

10.9.7 Two-Way ANOVA with Two Nominal Factors

The two-way model has two nominal factors. The cell means model is the same as for a one-way model, but of course the interpretation of the resulting means is different. More useful is the factor effects model:

$$y_{ijk} = \mu + \alpha_i + \beta_j + (\alpha\beta)_{ij} + e_{ijk}$$

This model allows explicit estimation of the main effects of the factors A and B, as well as their interaction, AB. Frequently, a two-way ANOVA model is selected when the objective is to determine whether or not the interaction of the two factors is significant; if not, their effects on the experimental response are independent and additive.

10.9.8 Regression Analysis with One Continuous Factor

The simplest regression model is one we have already encountered as an example:

$$y_i = \beta_0 + \beta_1 x_i + e_i$$

This looks similar to the one-way model, except that now the experimentally-controlled factor is a continuous numerical variable, and a functional relation (in this case, a proportional relation) is presumed to exist between the controlled factor and the measured result. We have used the terms "factor," and "variable," interchangeably and colloquially to represent model elements that are controlled by the experimenter or designer. Some authors choose to use the word factor to denote nominal scale design elements (categorical variables), and variable to denote continuously variable design elements (numerical variables). To be certain that your audience understands your model, be certain to specify whether the design elements you are studying are nominal (categorical) or continuously variable.

10.9.9 Regression Analysis with Multiple Continuous Factors

It is possible to have two or more continuously variable factors, and quite complex models can be used:

$$y_i = \beta_0 + \beta_1 x_{i1} + \beta_2 x_{i2} + \beta_{11} x_{i1}^2 + \beta_{22} x_{i2}^2 + \beta_{12} x_{i1} x_{i2}$$

This is the full quadratic polynomial response model used in response–surface modeling, for example.

10.9.10 Regression with Nominal and Continuous Variables (ANCOVA)

Models can have both nominal and continuous variables, as in the analysis of covariance:

$$y_{ijkh} = \mu + \alpha_i + \beta_j + (\alpha\beta)_{ij} + \gamma x_{ijk} + e_{ijkh}$$

This is a typical model for a stability study, where the nominal factors might be container size and manufacturing plant, for example, and the continuous variable is the storage time.

10.9.11 Nonlinear Models

The models so far considered have all been linear in the parameters. That is, the models consist of additive terms, each containing a single model parameter, even though some of the terms may include two or more factors or variables multiplied together. All linear models can always be analyzed as cell means models. Often models of interest to scientists and engineers are more complex, and the individual model terms contain two or more parameters, such as the model for the potency of a substance undergoing pseudo-first-order degradation as a function of time:

$$y_{ij} = \beta_0 e^{-\beta_1 x_i} + e_{ij}$$

Nonlinear models require more advanced computational techniques. Briefly, one must somehow obtain initial estimates of the model parameters; once these are in hand, they can be refined by iterative calculations until better estimates are obtained. There is usually no way to obtain the final estimates of the parameters directly in one step, although sometimes close approximations can be achieved. For example, taking logarithms of both sides of the first-order kinetic model above converts the model into a linear form if the error term is ignored. Fitting this linear model to the data gives good initial estimates of the model parameters that can then be further refined using nonlinear modeling techniques.

10.9.12 Data Snooping (Data Mining)

Data snooping (or data mining) is the process of hunting for patterns in data as the basis for formulating a model. This is a critical activity that serves the useful purpose of suggesting further experiments that need to be performed. However, some researchers make the mistake of collecting data first without any specific plan or model in mind, hunting for some pattern in the results, selecting a model to be fitted based on the pattern observed, and then claiming that the model fits the data. Such an approach invalidates any probability statements the researcher may want to make, since any inference is circular: the model is most likely because the most likely model was fitted to the data. The correct way to proceed is to propose the model, but then design a completely new experiment to test the model, collect new data, and fit the proposed model to the new data. If the model fits the new data, then the pattern suggested by the original data set is confirmed. If you see a pattern in data, by all means explore the possibility that the pattern is real by conducting an experiment. Patterns found in old data not subjected to experimental confirmation could arise by chance, and are meaningless.

10.9.13 Outliers

When a designed experiment is performed, and one or more of the measurements is aberrant, then one of two possibilities must be considered:

1. The measurement is invalid, because the researcher made a mistake in obtaining the sample to be measured, in performing the measurement, in recording the results, in performing the calculations used in the model-fitting process or a meteor striking the earth caused tremors that disturbed the instruments used to make the measurements or some other unforeseeable event interfered with the execution of the measurement process; or
2. The model is wrong.

Many researchers cherish their models, and are very reluctant to accept the second possibility. Sometimes a large financial investment may hinge on the results; for example, an out-of-specification result in a stability experiment might trigger a product recall. Can't we just throw away the "bad" data? Isn't there some statistical procedure for determining whether or not anomalous data should be retained or discarded? The answers to these questions are "no" and "no."

The best defense is a good offense: design your experiments so that even if "mistakes" are made or "problems" occur, the results will still be salvageable. Statisticians have contrived so-called robust methods for summarizing data and making inferences from the data that are insensitive to an occasional wild value. We have already seen that the median is less sensitive to extreme values in a data set than the mean; if the procedure required to obtain a measured value is exceedingly complex and mistake-prone, then collecting larger data sets and using the median might be more fruitful than using a more conventional approach based on calculating sample means. So long as this is applied as the standard procedure for performing the measurement process, and everyone who uses the resulting measurements concurs, robust methods should be acceptable.

Sometimes a tiered strategy can be designed: use a certain sample size, and note the variability actually observed; if it exceeds a certain critical value, increase the sample size, and collect additional data. This approach is used for several pharmacopeial tests, such as content uniformity testing, and chromatography system repeatability testing.

An important strategy is to incorporate validity checks in the measurement process. These fall under the general heading of system suitability tests or controls. A control sample can be analyzed with every set of experimental samples; by keeping records of the results obtained for the control sample, you can establish whether or not the measurement process itself is under statistical control (that is, operating in a predictable and reliable manner). If the measurement process is out of control, then the measurement results may be rejected as invalid. But *all* of the results must be rejected once the process is found to be out of control, and *no* results can be accepted until the process is back in control, as demonstrated by achieving consistent and reproducible results for the control sample. Results that appear anomalous cannot be discarded if the system is in control, and results that appear valid must be discarded if the system appears to be out of control.

Making additional measurements of a different kind, such as weight, volume, color, temperature, time of sampling, logon name of computer user, etc., (so called "metadata," or data about the data) can be an extremely important tool for providing additional evidence that a sample collected for measurement was obtained and processed under proper, controlled conditions. Metadata are critically important for robotic systems, which often run unattended and unobserved. Such systems are prone to both catastrophic failure, as well as temporary glitches that invalidate any measurements obtained during the time period when the robot was malfunctioning. Determining just when such failures have occurred is important. Data collected when the robot was malfunctioning is, of course, invalid, and should be summarily rejected. Similarly, human operators should be instructed to stop immediately any sampling or measurement process during which they know that they have made a mistake, and to log the event.

There are many statistical outlier tests (see the bibliography). What is important is that these methods are tools for identifying outliers. They are not tools for rejecting outliers, no matter what they may be called. If one or more outliers are discovered, every effort should be made to determine the root cause of the outlying value, if possible. Of course, it may be that some unknown and unforeseeable event was the real cause; no amount of effort attempting to recreate the circumstances surrounding the suspect result ever yields anything remotely resembling the observed outlier. In addition, the impact of the outlier on any inferences made from the data should be checked by repeating the data analysis, both with and without inclusion of the outlier. If the inferences made are unaffected, fine; but if a different conclusion would be drawn if the outlier were excluded, additional investigation may be needed. Certainly, one is not justified by statistical hypothesis testing alone to exclude data that critically affect decisions. Indeed, such data may point the way to the discovery of new and improved methods for operating the process. If additional data are obtained, and the supposed outlying value can be reproduced (within the expected experimental error), then this is strong evidence that the model itself is wrong, leading to the development of an improved model. A reproducible outlier is not an outlier!

10.10 THE MEASUREMENT PROCESS

Scientists and engineers make measurements so that inferences can be made about the object being measured. These measurements will exhibit some natural variability if they are repeated. This natural variability arises from two sources: the inherent variability of the process or product being measured, and the inherent variability of the act of obtaining a measurement.

$$\sigma^2_{measurement} = \sigma^2_{production\ process} + \sigma^2_{measurement\ process}$$

The act of obtaining a measurement can be considered a separate process. Since our primary interest is usually in the variability of the production process, it is important that the variability of the measurement process be small enough to permit estimating the variability of the production process. But how small is small enough?

In industrial manufacturing, it is common to require that the measuring process be sufficiently accurate so that $\sigma_{measurement\ process} = 0.204\sigma_{production\ process}$. This is equivalent to requiring that the ratio of the variance of the production process to the variance of the measurement process be 24:1, or that the intraclass correlation coefficient (ICC), defined as the ratio of the variance of the production process to the total variance, equals 0.96. Only 4% of the total variance is due to measurement error if this is true. Manufacturing industries that produce hardware items typically rely upon measurement processes that are both well-defined and stable, such as measurements of mass, dimension or other physical properties that have highly accurate and precise reference standards, so achieving this level of measurement precision is feasible.

If we allow $\sigma_{measurement\ process} = 0.5\sigma_{production\ process}$, this is equivalent to requiring that the ratio of the variance of the production process to the variance of the measurement process be 4:1 or ICC = 0.8; in this case 20% of the total variance is due to measurement error; this level of measurement performance is frequently achievable in pharmaceutical processes. Some workers prefer to set a higher standard; a 9:1 variance ratio ($\sigma_{measurement\ process} = 0.333\sigma_{production\ process}$, ICC = 0.9, so that 10% of the total variance is due to measurement error) is commonly recommended,[8] but this distribution of errors between measurement and production can be difficult to achieve in pharmaceutical processes. Indeed, since it is utterly impractical to estimate a standard deviation during the development of a new process with an accuracy of ±10%, an even less stringent requirement may suffice. Empirically, a 5:6 variance ratio ($\sigma_{measurement\ process} = 1.09\sigma_{production\ process}$, ICC = 0.45, so that 55% of the total variance is due to measurement error) still can provide usable data;[9] this will assure there can be at least 5 or more digitally distinct readings within $\pm 3\sigma_{measurement}$. Since reducing the variation of the measurement process costs time, money, and manpower, it is important to choose a level of performance consistent with the end needs of the user of the data. It is also important to recognize that an overly generous allocation of the total error budget to the measurement process may make reduction of the product process variation extremely difficult to achieve. The measurements of most concern to the pharmaceutical product developer with respect to variability are those that involve chemical analysis.

10.10.1 Models and Assay Design in Analytical Chemistry

Since measurement is a process, like all processes it can be modeled mathematically. Most of the recent literature focuses on the calibration curve assay design as if it were the only model appropriate for use in making chemical measurements; other designs may be equally appropriate.

10.10.2 Direct Assays (Titrations)

The simplest type of chemical measurement is titration: a reagent of known activity is added to the test sample until an equivalence point is detected. The amount or volume of the added reagent is then used as a measure of the activity of the test material in the test sample. This same model applies to any measurement process that relies on application of an increasing stimulus to the test object until a sudden and catastrophic change in the state of the test object can be detected. The amount of applied stimulus then serves as a measure of the test object property. A one-way ANOVA model describes this process adequately.

10.10.3 Slope–Ratio Assays

The next most common type of measurement is the proportional response model. A standard preparation (or different dilutions of a standard preparation), and a test sample (or different dilutions of a test sample), are each measured. The ratio of the measured response to the test sample, and the measured response(s) to the standard preparation(s), is directly proportional to the ratio of the amount of test material in the test sample to the amount of test material in the standard preparation(s). The model for this assay design has been described in detail.[10,11]

10.10.4 Parallel Line and Ligand-binding Assays

Another type of assay design more commonly encountered in biotechnology is the ligand-binding assay:

$$y_i = \beta_0 + \frac{\beta_1 - \beta_0}{1 + 10^{\beta_4(\log_{10} x_i - \log_{10} \beta_3)}} + e_i$$

This is obviously nonlinear in the parameters; a simplified version (when $\beta_0 = 0$, and $\beta_4 = 1$) can be linearized to give the parallel line assay design. Logarithmic functions of the independent variable x_i (the dose of the ligand), and the parameter β_3 (the dose of the ligand required to achieve half-maximal response, sometimes called the ED$_{50}$), are used because it is conventional in pharmacology research to plot the measured response versus the logarithm of the dose to produce the familiar sigmoid log dose response curve. Parameter β_4 (the Hill parameter) is a measure of cooperativity of receptor binding sites; when $\beta_4 = 1$, there is no cooperativity. Another form of the equation, familiar to biochemists, is the linear ligand dose scale version:

$$y_i = \beta_0 + \frac{\beta_1 - \beta_0}{1 + \left(\dfrac{x_i}{\beta_3}\right)^{\beta_4}} + e_i$$

When there isn't any nonspecific binding ($\beta_0 = 0$), then this is the familiar Hill equation, and when $\beta_4 = 1$, this reduces to the rectangular hyperbola encountered in simple enzyme kinetics. Volumes have been written about optimal design when these simpler models can be used.

10.10.5 Calibration Lines and Curves

Most of the literature on the application of statistical experimental design and inference to analytical chemistry treats this model (the simple regression model described previously) in detail. What are sometimes omitted are details for constructing a prediction

interval estimate for the concentration of an unknown, given a linear calibration curve. If the calibration curve constructed after measuring the responses corresponding to n standards having different known concentrations x_{s_i} is modeled by:

$$y_{s_i} = \beta_0 + \beta_1 x_{s_i} + e_i,$$

then we predict the mean concentration of the kth of l unknown samples $\hat{x}_{u_k}$ from the mean of m_k measured responses $\hat{y}_{u_k}$ (where $m_k \geq 1$) to be:

$$\hat{x}_{u_k} \approx \frac{\hat{y}_{u_k} - \beta_0}{\beta_1} \pm \frac{t_{1-\alpha,n-2-l+\sum m_k} S_{pooled}}{\beta_1}$$
$$\times \sqrt{\frac{1}{n} + \frac{1}{m_k} + \frac{(\hat{y}_{u_k} - \hat{y}_s)^2}{\beta_1 \sum\limits_{i=1}^{i=n} x_{s_i}^2 - \dfrac{\left(\sum\limits_{i=1}^{i=n} x_{s_i}\right)^2}{n}}}$$

where the above prediction interval estimate (which is approximately correct for reasonably small values of s_{pooled}) is calculated using:

$$\hat{y}_{u_k} = \frac{\sum\limits_{j=1}^{j=m_k} y_{u_{jk}}}{m_k}, \text{ the mean of the set of measurements for the } k\text{th unknown sample,}$$

$$\hat{y}_s = \frac{\sum\limits_{i=1}^{i=n} y_{s_i}}{n}, \text{ the overall average of the measurements for the calibration standards,}$$

$$(n-2)s_Y^2 = \sum_{i=1}^{i=n} y_{s_i}^2 - \frac{\left(\sum\limits_{i=1}^{i=n} y_{s_i}\right)^2}{n}$$
$$- \frac{\left(\sum\limits_{i=1}^{i=n} x_{s_i} y_{s_i} - \dfrac{\left(\sum\limits_{i=1}^{i=n} x_{s_i}\right)\left(\sum\limits_{i=1}^{i=n} y_{s_i}\right)}{n}\right)^2}{\sum\limits_{i=1}^{i=n} x_{s_i}^2 - \dfrac{\left(\sum\limits_{i=1}^{i=n} x_{s_i}\right)^2}{n}}$$

$$(m_k - 1)s_{u_k}^2 = \sum_{j=1}^{j=m_k} y_{u_{ik}}^2 - \frac{\left(\sum\limits_{i=1}^{i=n} y_{u_{ik}}\right)^2}{m_k} \text{ for each unknown,}$$

$$\text{and } s^2_{pooled} = \frac{(n-2)s^2_Y + \sum_{k=1}^{k=l}(m_k-1)s^2_{u_k}}{n-2-l+\sum_{k=1}^{k=l}m_k},$$

the pooled variance.

From this rather complex equation, several facts become apparent after careful inspection: There must be at least two standards; any standards more than that minimum increase the number of degrees of freedom for estimating the pooled variance. There must be more than one measurement of an unknown for it to contribute to increasing the number of degrees of freedom for estimating the pooled variance. To reduce the overall variance, it is a good idea to spread the workload evenly between standards and samples; that is, set $m_k = n$, which also allows variation in the measured responses for the unknown samples to be combined with variation about the calibration line to provide a better estimate of the variance. It is also a good idea to select calibration standards to bracket the expected values of the unknown samples, so that the average response measured for all of the standards is as close as possible to the average response to a typical unknown sample; this will reduce the magnitude of the numerator in the fraction that appears under the radicand in the prediction interval equation. Finally, make the range of the standards as wide as possible, and increase the number of replicate standards at the lowest and highest concentrations at the expense of replicate closer to the middle of the range; this will increase the size of the term involving the concentrations of the standards that appears in the denominator of the fraction under the radicand in the prediction interval equation; however, these values must not be so far apart that the assumption of uniform variance over the entire range bracketed by the standards is compromised. Note also that a pooled estimate of the variance is used; many textbook formulae omit this, because the authors focus on generating a prediction interval for as yet unmeasured future samples, but in practice we will always measure the unknown samples along with the calibration standards. When you have additional data to estimate variation, use it. Our goal is to increase the number of degrees of freedom to as large a value as practical.

You will find more theoretically exact formulae for calculating the prediction interval above based on application of Fieller's theorem for calculating the variance of a ratio in some textbooks. A correction factor is introduced which is only important if the coefficient of variation of the slope of the calibration curve is greater than 10%. This is unlikely in practice, so that the effect of the correction factor is negligible.

The pooled estimated variance described above is, of course, a measure of the short-term repeatability of the calibration process exclusive of variation due to sample preparation, if samples and standards are not prepared identically. This may be the only estimate of precision available during the earliest stages of product development. Ideally, a better estimate of the overall precision of the measurement process (the long-term variance described below) should be used; although the long-term variance must be larger than the short-term variance, thus inflating the value of s used in the calculation, the number of degrees of freedom used to estimate it will be much larger, thus deflating the value of Student's t-statistic used in the calculation. Even more ideally, the interval estimate above should be considered as but one component of a more encompassing formal uncertainty analysis (also described below).

10.10.6 Accuracy, Precision, Bias, and Blunders

Accuracy is the degree of agreement between the set of measured values we actually obtain (the real "truth") and the unobservable value we expect to obtain (the theoretical "truth"). Generally, we consider measurements to be accurate if essentially the same result can be obtained using a completely different approach. As noted previously, there are only three sources of inaccuracy in the measurement process: ubiquitous and unpredictable random errors, so-called "common" causes of disagreement which form the basis for statistical estimation and inference, fixed systematic additive or multiplicative deviations, so-called "special" or "assignable" causes of disagreement that bias the results, and outright procedural mistakes or unforeseen events that may or may not produce detectable outliers.

10.10.7 Detecting and Eliminating Bias

Bias can creep into the measurement process in numerous ways, but by far the most common problem encountered in pharmaceutical product development is interference in the measurement process caused by components of the sample matrix other than the analyte of interest. Since these problems tend to be uniquely different for each measurement process, it is difficult to prescribe generic solutions. Often, making the preparation of samples and standards as similar as possible can minimize these problems. Schemes in which placebo formulations are cross-diluted with standard preparations and active formulations are cross-diluted with reagent blank preparations can compensate for formulation-related biases.

Another approach that often helps to identify possible sources of bias is to perform a cause-and-effect analysis of the measurement process itself; the Ishikawa "fishbone" diagrammatic approach is a graphical tool to facilitate this analysis.[12] Many measurement processes differ only in detail and the specific target analyte from similar measurement processes developed previously, so it is helpful to compile a checklist of previously observed sources of bias in these other similar processes as a guide to troubleshooting the current process.[13]

The single most useful technique with wide applicability is to create a standard reference material that can be used as a positive control sample to be assayed with each batch of unknown samples; by keeping accurate records of the measurements obtained for the control sample, measurement system performance failures are easier to detect; once detected, corrective and preventative actions can be proposed based on an investigation of the assignable causes of failure using the strategies and techniques that have been developed for quality control and quality assurance of other processes, such as manufacturing processes. This positive control can be used as a system-suitability check sample to verify continued adequate precision, thus serving two purposes.

It may not be possible to eliminate certain types of bias associated with the order in which events occur. Operator fatigue, uncontrollable instability of reagents, equipment wear-and-tear, and other factors that cause the performance of a system to degrade over time are all sources of bias. This type of bias can best be controlled by an experimental design trick called blocking; that is, larger groups of unknown samples can be broken down into smaller groups according to a special plan that allows the actual effects of changes in operational conditions to be measured as the contributions of separate experimental factors, such as day-to-day, operator-to-operator or system-to-system changes in average response. Blocking lets you obtain a direct measure of the effects of "special" causes of variation. If blocking is impractical, this type of bias can also be converted to random error through the simple expedient of processing the samples to be measured in random sequence. Although this inflates the variance due to "common" causes, it has the beneficial effect of converting unpredictable bias into predictable random variation. When all else fails, consider randomization of the order of presentation of samples for measurement as a potential "cure" to problems of bias due to temporal degradation in system performance. Usually,

a combination of planned blocking to eliminate the effects of bias from anticipated sources, and randomization to convert bias from unanticipated sources into predictable random error works best. Both of these techniques do introduce additional complexity into the experimental design. Complexity increases the likelihood that blunders will occur, so the application of both blocking and randomization should be approached judiciously. Procedural changes, such as the use of additional labeling or distinctive packaging, automated label reading devices, robotic sample handling equipment, and redundant metadata collection or measurement of additional covariates (including internal standards) may be needed to reduce the frequency of outright blunders to a tolerable level.

10.10.8 Precision

Consistent precision is the hallmark of a measurement process in statistical control. If a measurement process is in a state of statistical control, then the means of a large number of "identical" samples (such as samples of a standard reference material) assayed over a period of time tend to approach a limiting value. In addition, the fluctuation of the means of the individual data sets about this limiting value should be describable by a single frequency distribution indicative of a process with a stable variance (and therefore a constant standard deviation). If bias has indeed been conquered by imposition of suitable environmental and procedural controls, then, with the exception of rare outright blunders or other unforeseeable interferences, the only source of deviation of the measured values from their predicted values that remains is statistically predictable random fluctuation. Such data can be described and used to make inferences using statistical tools. Measurement systems that are subject to uncontrolled bias or so difficult to execute that they are plagued by numerous blunders are useless; such systems do not produce usable data.

10.10.9 Short-term Repeatability

Over short periods of time, many causes of random variation exert only small effects. When sets of measurements are performed within a short time frame, the variability within such sets of measurements is often seen to be less than the variability between sets of otherwise identical measurements performed over longer periods of time. Because this short-term variability provides information needed to calculate how many replicate measurements should be made at any one time to achieve a specified level of precision, it is called repeatability. One obvious way to improve the sensitivity of development experiments designed to estimate production process variation is to group all the samples together as a batch, and then have a single analyst prepare and analyze the samples in random order. This reduces the impact of any long-term variation in the measurement process. Repeatability is often measured by analyzing the successive differences in measurements obtained for replicate control samples.

10.10.10 Long-term Reproducibility

Some components of variation only exert effects over a longer term; different technicians may prepare samples with idiosyncratic variation in techniques, instrument components may be replaced (or entirely different equipment may be used), the environmental conditions (air temperature, humidity, light levels) under which the measurements are obtained may fluctuate, etc. These factors all come into play when different operators in different laboratories use different equipment to analyze samples from the same batch of material on different days. To some extent, it is a philosophical issue whether these contributors to variation should be considered fixed causes (correctable bias) or strictly random factors. After all, poorly performing technicians can be fired, and be replaced by more capable and competent employees, less reliable instrumentation can be replaced by more carefully designed and crafted models, environmental controls can be added to control room temperature, humidity, and light levels, etc. Nevertheless, technicians have "bad days," equipment components exhibit random fluctuations in performance that cannot be traced to any specific malfunction or design flaw, and even the best environmental controls can only maintain temperature, humidity, and light levels within (sometimes broad) design limits. Some sources of variation that we might think could be controllable bias are indeed random.

Because the long-term variability better reflects the consistency with which we expect to be able to obtain future measurements using the measurement process, and includes within it the short-term variability as a subcomponent, the long-term variability provides a better estimate of the overall precision of the measuring process. The establishment of reference standards, and the distribution of control samples that are included in every batch of samples to be measured, can used as tools with which to generate measurements that can be used to monitor long-term variability. The overall variability of the measurement process, which can also include estimates of unavoidable bias, is usually called the uncertainty of the measurement.

This is an unfortunate choice of terminology, since "uncertainty" really refers to unknowable and unforeseeable changes in measurement response caused by irreproducible outside interferences that afflict all human activities. It is perhaps more proper to call this overall variability, which includes both random fluctuations and fixed biases, the "reliability" of the measurement process, which is the term used in what follows; it is the same as the "uncertainty" used in some regulatory requirements.

10.10.11 Measurement Reliability Analysis Based on ANOVA with Random Factors

The classical statistical tool for evaluating overall measurement reliability (or "uncertainty") by estimating the magnitude of components of random variance is the analysis of variance using random factors. An experiment is designed to compare results obtained in a suitably large collection of laboratories where a suitably large number of different analysts use a suitably large number of different instruments to assay suitability large sets of samples taken from some suitably homogenous and stable batch of material over a suitably long period of time. In designing experiments to measure overall precision, the combined number of degrees of freedom assignable to random variation should also be suitably large. In practice, the question of "how large is suitably large?" is frequently not adequately addressed; practical constraints limit what can actually be achieved. The purpose of an experiment to estimate precision is to estimate a variance or standard deviation. As we have seen, large numbers of measurements are required to obtain even a crude estimate of a standard deviation with any accuracy. This is inherent in the properties of the χ^2 distribution, which is only appropriate to set interval bounds if the random deviations can be said to be drawn from a population with a normal probability distribution. The application of distribution-free statistical methods, to any but the simplest components of variance problems, is also problematic. Yet some knowledge is better than none; despite the practical difficulties of conducting large-scale components of variance experiments, they still should be an essential component of the evaluation of any new measurement process.

However, it is important to realize the limitations inherent in attempting to partition the overall variance into subcomponents when the degree of freedom for assessing the effect of a particular subcomponent is small. Since the estimates subcomponents are themselves random variables, it sometimes happens that a component may be estimated to have a negative value; this, of course, is nonsensical because variance components must always be greater than or at least equal to zero. A formal analysis of variance will reveal and quantify these difficulties to the extent that such quantification is possible given the limitations of the statistical methods currently available. Despite the flaws in this model, it is still useful. It is quintessentially a frequentist approach to the problem. This type of measurement reliability (or "uncertainty") estimation is described as the Type A method in the NIST SEMATECH on-line handbook (see bibliography).

10.10.12 Measurement Reliability Analysis Based on Prior Information and In-process Standards

A different approach to the problem of evaluating measurement reliability attempts instead to evaluate all components of the measurement process by breaking the process down into unit operations, each of which is separately evaluated. These individual estimates are then combined using the laws for propagation of error described previously, which hold true for any set of data having a unimodal frequency distribution. Ishikawa "fishbone" diagrams are frequently used as a diagrammatic approach to deconvolute contributions to the overall measurement reliability. Biases and random variability assignable to each unit operation are estimated based on prior history, manufacturing tolerances, vendor specifications, and other sources of information. This historical data, often well-defined, is combined with in-process measurements acquired in the course of operating the process under evaluation, such as repeatability of calibration or control sample measurements. Scientists and engineers more familiar with statistical methods based upon normal probability distributions may find this approach intellectually challenging, because rectangular and triangular frequency distributions are used to model the frequency distributions for some unit operations. Nevertheless, the practical utility of this approach has been demonstrated, and is being required by some regulatory authorities, especially in Europe. This approach can be useful to uncover additional sources of error (for example, difference in the way standards and samples are prepared).

Although this model also has some flaws, it is at least as useful as the random ANOVA components of variance model. However, this type of measurement reliability analysis relies extensively on historical precedent and data generated by similar, but different, processes. It is only as reliable as the extensions of inferences based on these other systems apply

to the system being evaluated. It is quintessentially a Bayesian approach to the problem. The CITAC/ EURACHEM references in the bibliography describe how to perform this type of measurement reliability (or "uncertainty") analysis; it is described as the Type B approach in the NIST SEMATECH online handbook.

10.10.13 Reporting Measurement Reliability

Whether or not a formal measurement reliability analysis has been performed, the use of any measurement data to make inferences relies upon an honest estimate of the overall bias and precision of the measurement process. Even now, although reviewers demand an assessment of variability, some measurements are reported as simple point estimates, with no indication at all of their precision or accuracy. Too frequently, data are reported with only an estimate of the short-term variability. When you are evaluating data generated by others, pay particular attention to how estimates of measurement reliability are reported. Data with no estimate of reliability are essentially useless. Data with an estimate of short-term repeatability may have limited value. Only data presented with an analysis of sources of bias and long-term reproducibility can be trusted for making inferences. When you report measurements you have made, you owe your clients a frank appraisal of the reliability of the numbers you provide.

10.10.14 Multivariate Methods

The discussion of the measurement process has so far focused on systems that generate individual numerical values. Modern analytical methods often generate complex data sets (entire spectra, for example) that quantitatively reflect some property of interest in the sample (such as the concentrations of particular analytes in a mixture). The basic principles outlined above still apply, but multivariate statistical methods must now be used. For processes that can be modeled using a model that is linear in its parameters, the vector of measured responses becomes a matrix of measured responses; the vector of parameter estimates becomes a matrix of parameter estimates, and the matrix of independent variables (or factors) remains a matrix of independent factors (or variables). The vector of random errors becomes a matrix of random errors having the same dimensions as the matrix of measured responses. Other than this increased complexity, the modeling process stays the same, and computations using linear algebra can still be used to solve the problem. That is, it would be possible to use ordinary linear algebra methods if there were no apparent colinearity caused by large partial correlations within the data. So, in many cases, the generalized Moore–Penrose inverse matrix must be used. Methods based on principal component analysis and latent-variable regression methods are used to simplify the models.

One wrinkle introduced by practitioners of multivariable analysis is so-called partial least-squares (PLS) regression analysis. This is a mathematical technique that employs a training set of standards to develop a calibration model, which is then used to infer properties of unknowns based on multiple measured responses obtained for those unknowns. Correlations between the measured responses with the controlled variables, as well as between the controlled variables with each other, are included in the modeling process. It is not unlike the traditional single covariate calibration curve approach if you follow the naïve approach of plotting the independent variable for the standards on the Y-axis (treating them as if the x values were what was being measured) versus the measured values for the standards on the X-axis (treating them as if the y values were what was known), and then use the resulting calibration line to infer the corresponding x values for the unknowns from their measured y values. Since multivariate analysis frequently relies on the use of measured values for controlled variables, as well as for the dependent variables, the PLS technique is a sensible approach and has proved valuable in practice.

10.11 THE PRODUCTION PROCESS

A process is a process is a process, and much of what has been said already about the measurement process also applies to the production process. The focus in this section will be on more complex experimental designs.

10.11.1 Controlled and Uncontrolled Factors

As noted above, some authors distinguish nominal variables or factors from continuous variables or factors by restricting the use of the name factor to describing nominal variables. Another viewpoint, perhaps more useful to the process designer, is whether variables (factors) are controlled or uncontrolled. The formulator can specify that a formulation contain 35% of an excipient, for example, this should be thought of as a controlled variable because the amount can be specified in advance and measured. If performing a wet granulation, the amount of fluid required may not be known in advance, but may be determined at the time that the granulation is manufactured by measuring some property of the granulation itself (e.g., its water content) or some operating parameter of the equipment used to make the granulation (e.g., the power consumed by the granulator motor); these are also controlled factors, since the formulator can specify moisture content or motor power, and also measure these. Other process variables, such as the relative humidity in the corridor connecting the room where weighing operations are performed with the room where mixing operations are performed, may not be controlled. The goal of the process designer is to identify all of the factors or variables that contribute to the success or failure of the process, determine acceptable ranges for each, control those that must be confined to their acceptable ranges artificially, and monitor those that do not require such confinement. For a complex process, many process variables might be discovered.

10.11.2 Response Surface Modeling: The Design Space

The design space for a process is simply the n-dimensional space defined by the n process variables that have been identified, along with the acceptable ranges for each of the variables. The design space for a pharmaceutical product can be quite complex; the rest of this book is devoted to exploring the subspaces within the design space for various unit operations that can be linked together to form a complete process. A goal of the process designer is to be able to predict measured properties of the product, based on knowing and understanding the effect of the process variables on these properties. The process designer constructs a statistical model to make these predictions. If there were only two process variables and one product property, for example, then a three-dimensional plot of the measured property of the product versus the selected values of the process variables would be a two-dimensional surface (the response surface), the goal of the process designer would be to determine the loci of points on this surface (the design surface, in this two-dimensional example) that met the desired quality characteristics for the property of the product, and from this plot the designer would determine the ranges of the process variables to ensure that the product property would remain within this boundary. If there are m product properties that must be controlled by n process variables, then the objective remains the same: to determine the region on the n-dimensional hyperspace in the $n + m$ dimensional hyperspace that meets quality expectations, and identify the appropriate ranges of the n process variables that will ensure that the m product properties will lie within acceptable ranges. The region in the n-dimensional hyperspace defined by these ranges is the design space.

10.11.3 Classical Factorial Designs

Classically, it was realized that the analysis of variance model with multiple factors could be used to model experiments in which two or more factors, each at two or more levels, were used to control the output of a process. Actually, this is a misstatement; classically, Ronald Fisher realized that an experiment comprising the study of the effects of multiple factors (such as amount or type of applied fertilizer, amount of tillage and type of seed), each at different levels, on the output of a process (such as crop yield), could be modeled using an analysis of variance model, which is why, of course, he invented it. The empirical ANOVA model usually used is linear in the model parameters. In actuality, a more complex nonlinear model might have greater physical meaning. The usefulness of any fitted model to predict future performance must always be evaluated.

10.11.4 Confounding Variables: Fractional Factorials

Once the mathematics of ANOVA were understood, experimenters realized that not all factor combinations were equally informative; some factor combinations generated more useful and interesting predictions of the process output than did others. In more complex designs with multiple factors, certain combinations were found that provided information primarily on the main effects of each factor acting independently; other combinations provided information on two-way interactions between pairs of factors, yet other combinations provided information on three-way or higher order interactions. Experimenters found that most of the useful information was derived from knowledge of the main effects and simple two-way interactions of the factors. The effects of higher-level interactions were often indistinguishable from noise (the inherent random variations in the measured process output). If so, then why waste time, money, and resources studying these worthless combinations that only gave information about higher level interactions? By simply deleting these combinations, only a fraction of the original planned experiment needed to be done; the fractional factorial experiment was born.

However, these systematic deletions do cause some problems. Mathematically, it was found that when some of the factor combinations were deleted, the effects that they did contribute to (the higher-order interactions) became manifest in the combinations that remained. For example, in a four-factor experiment with factors A, B, C, and D, it might be the case that if there was really a significant ABC interaction, it would no longer be possible to distinguish this from, say, the main effect of factor D. This masquerade is called confounding of variables. See the bibliography section on *Experimental Design* for further information.

10.11.5 Screening Designs

If fractional designs are stripped to the barest essentials, so that only main effects can be measured, the result is a so-called screening design. Of course, the problem of confounding is disastrous if it should occur in a screening experiment. Screening designs are mostly useful for eliminating certain factors from further study; if no main effect is observed, drop the factor.

10.11.6 Taguchi Designs

The Japanese quality expert Taguchi elaborated even more complex experimental designs to segregate the controlled variables from uncontrolled environmental factors. These designs may be useful in some aspects of product development.

10.11.7 Model Assumptions

Typically, designed experiments require certain assumptions to be made about the measurements:

1. The random deviations from the values predicted by the model can all be viewed as a sample from a larger population of potentially observable deviations that has a single, constant, frequency distribution with mean $\mu = 0$, and variance σ^2. (The variability is not a function of any of the design variables or the measured response.)
2. The random variations are independent, and uncorrelated with each other. (The outcome of the last measurement has no effect on the next measurement in a sequence of measurements.)
3. The model is correct. (All sources of bias have been included in the model.)
4. The design variables are all known, invariant, quantities (if numeric) or qualities (if nominal).
5. If probabilistic inferences are to be made, the probability distribution associated with the

random deviations from the model is the normal distribution with mean $\mu = 0$, and variance σ^2. (Of which, of course, we can never be sure.)

It is important to examine the results of modeling carefully to see if there is any evidence that any of the modeling assumptions are invalid. Finding such evidence is cause to reject the model, and try another. Failure to find such evidence really doesn't prove anything; excessive variation, choosing too limited a range for the independent variables or failure to account for timing issues may make it difficult or impossible to find convincing evidence that one or more model assumptions have been violated. You can never prove that a model is correct; however, you can discover convincing evidence that a model is inadequate, and thereby eliminate it from further consideration.

10.11.8 Choosing an Experimental Design

Follow Albert Einstein's advice and make everything as simple as possible, but not simpler. A study-everything-at-once design is difficult to plan, difficult to execute, and difficult to interpret. It also costs a lot of money, and takes a lot of time. On the other hand, a one-factor-at-a-time design misses important interactions between variables, and may lead to completely wrong conclusions.

One approach which considers all of the factors simultaneously, but varies only one factor at a time, is simplex optimization. Although potentially quite time-consuming, this process will eventually lead to an optimum outcome. It is an approach worth considering when the set of variables to be explored is small, and the time required to execute an experiment to produce a measured outcome is short. This approach requires making a series of consecutive decisions, each of which introduces the potential for error. A mis-step could lead to a false optimum.

Another approach with some merit is the grid search: every possible combination of every possible factor is studied, in parallel on a small scale, over a range of several possible levels for each variable. This type of design is sometimes used to make efficient use of robotic equipment. It is an approach worth considering when the process can be easily miniaturized and automated. This approach has been used with some success to screen potential liquid formulations for poorly soluble drugs, for example. However, it generates massive amounts of data, much of which may have little or no value.

Previous experience with development of analogous products should always serve as a guide. The amount of lubricant needed in a tablet formulation, for example, can be roughly estimated from the amounts used in previous successfully manufactured tablets.

Break down complex manufacturing operations into simpler unit operations. Develop models to predict the properties of the intermediate products obtained after each operation, based on variation of the input variables to each stage. Once you understand how each stage works, work backwards through the process to define ranges for each of the inputs to the last stage that yields acceptable product. Then define ranges for inputs to the next to the last stage that define an acceptable range of outputs that can serve as an input to the final stage, and so on.

10.11.9 Data Analysis and Model Simplification

If the model used to design the experiment was selected appropriately, some factors that have been included may turn out to have had little effect on the properties of the product that was produced, at least over the range that you explored. If this range provides an adequate working range for future work, choose the central value for further studies, and keep it constant in future experiments. You may need to go back and challenge the final process by again testing each of the extremes used in the initial experiment, but at least the intermediate workload will be reduced.

Since most experimental designs are based on models that are linear in their parameters, and since, as we have already seen, ANOVA models can be fitted to experimental data using mathematical methods developed for fitting regression models to data, one technique for model simplification that can be explored is stepwise regression analysis to eliminate model parameters with low explanatory power. Many textbooks on modeling describe how to use forward stepwise regression to sequentially add first the most important controlled variable, then the next most important controlled variable, and so on, until essentially all of the variations that can be explained by factors controlled by the experimenter have been explained. Another approach to simplification is so-called backward elimination. In this approach, a complete model, with all of the controlled variables and every combination and permutation of possible interactions included, is first fitted to the data. Then one by one, each variable is removed from the model, and the model is refitted. Whichever variable had the least effect when it was removed is eliminated from the model, and the process of testing each remaining variable for removal is repeated. Novices are frequently surprised to discover that each of these simplification processes can lead to wildly different final models. Furthermore, relying on algorithms built into statistical software to control the addition or selection process can lead to bizarre results. Problems occur with factorial models that have complex interactions; it is impossible to interpret factorial models that have higher order interactions unless all of the lower order interactions and main effects used to generate the higher order term are also included in the model:

Right: $y_{hijkl} = \alpha_i + \beta_j + \gamma_k + \delta_l + \alpha_i\beta_j + \gamma_k\delta_l + e_{hijkl}$

Right: $y_{hijkl} = \alpha_i + \beta_j + \gamma_k + \delta_l + \alpha_i\beta_j + \beta_j\gamma_k + \alpha_i\gamma_k + \alpha_i\beta_j\gamma_k + e_{hijkl}$

Wrong: $y_{hijkl} = \alpha_i + \gamma_k + \delta_l + \beta_j\gamma_k + \alpha_i\gamma_k + \alpha_i\beta_j\gamma_k + e_{hijkl}$

Remember: these are probabilistic models. It is entirely possible that through sheer bad luck, you just happened to get a set of measurements that suggests a particular model should be used, when in fact the measurements for only one or two experimental factor combinations support this. Various diagnostic tools can help to identify data points with exceptionally high influence; if these data points were simply somewhat more variable than usual values, and they were the only evidence supporting inclusion of a particular model term, particularly a higher order interaction term, then some additional confirmation should be sought. Doubtful models should be tested, and confirmed by additional experimentation. Be cautious.

10.11.10 Evolutionary Operation

Once the most important controlled variables have been identified, further optimization of the process can be achieved, in practice, by making minor adjustments in just a few of the controlling factors. Factorial experimental designs can be employed sequentially, for example. This is an ongoing strategy for process improvement that can be implemented once the basic process itself has been established, and is up and running. (For a discussion and example, see Box, Hunter & Hunter.)

10.11.11 Process Stability and Capability

A well-designed process will operate consistently and predictably, on target with minimum variation. Of course it is impossible for any process to produce two or more product units that are exactly alike in every detail. Some variability is inherent in every

process. A customer who demands perfection can never be satisfied. The traditional approach adopted with the advent of mass production processes for manufacturing durable goods, each of which could be individually inspected using non-destructive methods, was to establish sets of specifications that the product of the process was required to meet for the product to be acceptable to the customer. A successful process was one that was capable of turning out products that consistently met customer expectations, and was defined by specifications. That is, what you get must meet specifications. Anything that meets specifications is O.K., no matter how close or how far the measured properties of the products of the process are to the specified limits. Entire batches could be tested one item at a time, and inspectors could then sort the items in a batch into "good" and "bad" units. Individual items that failed to meet specifications would be rejected, and possibly reworked. However, this categorical approach to quality assurance and control leaves much to be desired. It is difficult to apply to pharmaceutical products, many of which must be subjected to destructive testing. If a sample from a batch fails to meet specifications, there is no choice but to scrap the entire batch.

The modern approach is to define process capability as the reproducibility that the process is actually able to achieve with respect to the extent of variability demonstrated by measured properties of the product. What you get is what you have. Specifications that impose narrower limits on variability than the process is naturally capable of achieving will result in continued process failures until, and if, process variability can be reduced. The natural process capability is often defined numerically as six standard deviations of the measured property of the process product, expressed in measurement units. The process capability ratio, a summary statistic that reveals the extent to which a process can generate product that will meet specifications, is computed by dividing the width of the interval, in measurement units, defined by the upper and lower specification limits, by the natural process capability:

$$C_p = \frac{USL - LSL}{6\sigma}$$

This begs the question: what is σ?

10.11.12 Statistical Process Control Revisited

The estimation of variability for the measurement process typically makes allowance for differences between short-term repeatability, and long-term reproducibility. Traditional quality assurance programs developed for manufacturers of "widgets" or other discrete hardware items produced as individual units, such as integrated circuits or automobiles, seldom distinguish between long-term and short-term variability; indeed, differences in variability between production lines or manufacturing sites are viewed as assignable causes to be eliminated. Pharmaceutical products are not "widgets;" rather, pharmaceutical products are more usefully viewed as processed materials akin to other bulk materials, such as sheet metal, photographic film or food products, produced either by continuous processes or batch processes with many batches per year of a given product type.[14] The measurement process itself is often a major component of the overall variation of the complete process. Pharmaceutical processes typically exhibit five sources of variation:

- lot-to-lot variation around the process average;
- package-to-package variation around the true lot average;
- within-package variation around the true unit package average;
- short-term measurement repeatability affecting samples tested at the same test time; and
- long-term measurement reproducibility encompassing all other sources of measurement error.

The major challenge to product development scientists and engineers is simply the paucity of lots produced during the development of a new product. This harkens back to the issue of obtaining a confidence interval estimate for the standard deviation. Unfortunately, frequentist statistical components of variance estimation using five-way ANOVA with random factors (lots, packages, dosage forms, analytical repeatability, and analytical reproducibility) is doomed to failure if the number of demonstration lots produced during the development cycle is too small. (One author suggests that a minimum of sixty degrees of freedom for each of the five sources of variation be used;[14] who makes sixty-one lots during product development?)

10.11.13 In-process Monitoring and Control Using Process Analytical Technology

One proposed solution is to increase the number of measurements made during operation of the process, and to use this data to estimate overall variability of the process. This can be viewed intellectually as simply an extension of the Bayesian approach to estimating uncertainty of the measurement process by combining uncertainties associated with unit operations using propagation-of-error calculations. No formal rules have yet been established to extend this concept to the overall pharmaceutical production process; it is an ongoing area of contemporary research. Publications describing multivariate statistical process control and process analytical technology should be consulted for the latest advances in this new field.

10.11.14 Process "Wellness"

The concept of process "wellness" has been developed to express the concept that the suitability for use of the end-product of a pharmaceutical process may depend on more than just end point testing to assure conformance to specifications.[15,16,17] Sometimes it may be possible to achieve the same measured quality-indicating properties on the final product by following different process paths, and certain path-dependent properties not measured as part of the end point tests may affect the usability of the product. The set of multiple quality-indicating measurements that collectively characterize the product of the process, and the process itself, must display on-target performance over time, with minimum variability for the process to be considered in statistical control.

10.12 SOFTWARE

A number of well-designed and tested statistical software packages are available commercially. Any software package you choose should be evaluated for accuracy using standard test data. The software vendor should also supply adequate documentation describing models and algorithms used to perform calculations. Nearly all statistical work performed in support of pharmaceutical product development requires that calculations be performed using double-precision arithmetic; some older software may have been designed to run in single precision mode to enhance computational speed, but rounding errors nearly always make the results too inaccurate to be useful.

10.13 SUMMARY

Any scientific or engineering endeavor that generates measurement data necessarily uses more or less appropriate statistical techniques, and methods of inference, to present and interpret the data. A number of different techniques are available that rely to different extents on the use of the normal probability frequency distribution; conservative probability statements can still be made without making this assumption using distribution-free methods. The accurate estimation of variability is challenging; much more data than is typically available is required by traditional frequentist probability assessments. Bayesian approaches offer a different path to the assessment of variability by combining probabilities estimated from detailed study of sub-processes. Developing a new pharmaceutical product requires the design and testing of manufacturing and measurement processes. The resulting process produces quality products when measurements indicative of product quality are on target with minimum variance.

Selected Bibliography

History of Statistics

The interested reader can learn more about the historical antecedents of modern statistics by reading:

Stigler, S.M. (1986). *The History of Statistics: The Measurement of Uncertainty Before 1900*. Belkap Press of Harvard University Press, Cambridge, MA, and London. [Korean translation by Jae Keun Jo. (2005). Hangilsa Publishing Co., Ltd.].

Stigler, S.M. (1999). *Statistics on the Table: The History of Statistical Concepts and Methods*. Harvard University Press, Cambridge, MA.

Hald, A. (1986). *A History of Probability and Statistics and their Applications Before 1750*. Wiley, New York.

Hald, A. (1998). *A History of Mathematical Statistics from 1750 to 1930*. Wiley, New York.

Reprints of some early seminal works can be found in:

Newman, J.A.R. (1956). *The World of Mathematics, Volume III*. Simon and Schuster, New York.

A useful website with links to historical materials is maintained by Peter M. Lee at the University of York:

Lee, P. M. Materials for the History of Statistics, http://www.york.ac.uk/depts/maths/histstat/welcome.htm

Basic Statistics for Scientists and Engineers

The following books provide coverage of basic statistics written from the perspective of the scientist or engineer:

Natrella, M. G. (1963). *Experimental Statistics*. National Bureau of Standards Handbook, 91. Washington, D.C., US Government Printing Office (out of print).

This book, originally written for the US Army, covers statistical concepts and fundamentals of data analysis using frequentist methods in language even an army sergeant can understand; highly recommended if you can find a copy. It has been supplanted by the greatly expanded *NIST/SEMATECH e-Handbook of Statistical Methods*, http://www.itl.nist.gov/div898/handbook/. This online statistics text covers every possible statistical method that can possibly be encountered in product development or at least attempts to do so. Free downloadable statistical software is available for use with this web site maintained by the US government. The online version is so exhaustive that it comes across as less user-friendly than Mary Natrella's pioneering work.

Berry, D.A. (1996). *Statistics: A Bayesian Perspective*. Wadsworth, Belmont, CA.

An introductory text requiring minimal mathematical preparation, which teaches statistical thinking using a Bayesian approach; a useful antidote to the myriad texts based on frequentist methods

to promote a different perspective on problem analysis, and data interpretation. The approach taken is somewhat more natural to the scientific method than the conventional frequentist approach. The author provides numerous examples dealing with substantive scientific issues, many related to healthcare. Read this along with Natrella's book, and you'll be able to communicate effectively with statistically more knowledgeable colleagues.

Bolton, S. (1997). *Pharmaceutical Statistics: Practical and Clinical Applications*, 3rd edn. Marcel Dekker, New York & Basel.

A basic statistics book, written from the perspective of industrial pharmacy, using frequentist methods. Read Natrella & Berry first, then use this book as your workday reference.

Caulcutt, R. & Boddy, R. (1983). *Statistics for Analytical Chemists*. Chapman and Hall, London.

Written from the perspective of an analytical chemist using frequentist methods.

Dudewicz, E.J. (1999). Basic Statistical Methods. In: *Juran's Quality Handbook*, J.M. Juran, & A.N. Godfrey, (eds). McGraw-Hill, New York.

Mandel, J. (1984). *The Statistical Analysis of Experimental Data*. Dover, New York.

Written from the perspective of an analytical chemist using frequentist methods.

Meier, P.C. & Zünd, R.E. (1993). *Statistical Methods in Analytical Chemistry*. John Wiley & Sons, New York.

Written from the perspective of an analytical chemist using frequentist methods.

Sokal, R.R. & Rohlf, F.J. (1995). *Biometry: The Principles and Practice of Statistics in Biological Research*, 3rd edn. W. H. Freeman, New York.

Written from the perspective of a biologist using frequentist methods.

Graphical Design

The following books are a useful introduction:

Kosslyn, S.M. (1993). *Elements of Graph Design*. W.H. Freeman, New York.

Cleveland, W.S. (1985). *The Elements of Graphing Data*. Wadsworth Advanced Books and Software, Monterey, CA.

A reprint is available from Hobart Press, Summit, NJ.

Cleveland, W.S. (1993). *Visualizing Data*. Hobart Press, Summit, NJ.

Anyone who wants to become proficient at communicating numerical data visually should read these books on graphic design by Professor Tufte.

Tufte, E.R. (2001). *The Visual Display of Quantitative Information*, 2nd edn. Graphics Press, Cheshire, CT.

Tufte, E.R. (1990). *Envisioning Information*. Graphics Press, Cheshire, CT.

Tufte, E.R. (1997). *Visual Explanations*. Graphics Press, Cheshire, CT.

Interval Estimation

Hahn, G.J. & Meeker, W.Q. (1991). *Statistical Intervals: A Guide for Practitioners*. John Wiley & Sons, New York.

A comprehensive monograph focusing on frequentist methods.

Statistical Inference

Miller, R.G., Jr. (1981). *Simultaneous Statistical Inference*, 2nd edn. Springer-Verlag, New York.

An advanced text that covers subjects found in introductory texts more thoroughly.

Experimental Design: Fundamentals

Box, G.E.P., Hunter, W.G. & Hunter, J.S. (2005). *Statistics for Experimenters: Design, Innovation, and Discovery*, 2nd edn. Wiley, New York.

Hunter, J.S. (1999). Design and Analysis of Experiments. In: *Juran's Quality Handbook*, J.M. Juran, & A.N. Godfrey, (eds). McGraw-Hill, New York.

Haaland, P.D. (1989). *Experimental Design in Biotechnology*. Marcel Dekker, New York.

Manly, B.F.J. (1992). *The Design and Analysis of Research Studies*. Cambridge University Press, Cambridge, UK.

Experimental Design: Advanced Topics

Chow, S.-C. & Liu, J.-P. (1995). *Statistical Design and Analysis in Pharmaceutical Science: Validation, Process Controls and Stability*. Marcel Dekker, New York.

Advanced topics in the application of statistical methods to industrial pharmacy.

Cornell, J.A. (1990). *Experiments with Mixtures: Designs, Models and the Analysis of Mixture Data*, 2nd edn.. John Wiley & Sons, New York.

All pharmaceutical formulations are mixtures; this monograph covers the design of experiments where the sum of all components must be 100%.

Finney, D.J. (1978). *Statistical Method in Biological Assay*, 3rd edn.. Charles Griffin, London.

The classic text on biological assays; out of print.

Nelson, W. (1990). *Accelerated Testing: Statistical Models, Test Plans and Data Analysis*. John Wiley & Sons, New York.

The book on stress testing and failure mode investigation.

Tranter, R.L. (2000). *Design and Analysis in Chemical Research*. CRC Press, Boca Raton, FL.

Covers a wide range of topics at a more advanced level, including multivariate methods.

Linear Models

Draper, N.R. & Smith, H. (1998). *Applied Regression Analysis*, 3rd edn. Wiley, New York.

A classic text with a good discussion on model building and how to select the best model.

Neter, J., Kutner, M.H., Nachtsheim, C.J. & Wasserman, W. (1996). *Applied Linear Statistical Models: Regression, Analysis of Variance and Experimental Designs*, 4th edn. Irwin, Chicago, IL.

A comprehensive textbook suitable for both beginning and advanced readers.

Milliken, G.A. & Johnson, D.E. (1992). *Analysis of Messy Data. Vol. I: Designed Experiments*. Chapman & Hall, London.

Worked examples of difficult problems.

Milliken, G.A. & Johnson, D.E. (1989). *Analysis of Messy Data. Vol II: Nonreplicated Experiments*. Chapman & Hall/CRC, Boca Raton, FL.

More worked examples of difficult problems.

Milliken, G.A. & Johnson, D.E. (2002). *Analysis of Messy Data. Vol. II: Analysis of Covariance*. Chapman & Hall/CRC, Boca Raton, FL.

Even more worked examples of difficult problems.

Nonlinear Models

Seber, G.A.F. & Wild, C.J. (1989). *Nonlinear Regression*. John Wiley & Sons, New York.

An advanced text.

Outliers

Barnett, V. & Lewis, T. (1994). *Outliers in Statistical Data*, 3rd edn.. John Wiley & Sons, Chichester, UK.

A comprehensive text focused on outlier detection.

Rousseeuw, P.J. & Leroy, A.M. (1987). *Robust Regression and Outlier Detection*. John Wiley & Sons, New York.

Although outlier detection is a major topic, this book offers suggestions for robust methods that are immune to interference from outliers.

Statistics Applied to Quality Assurance

CITAC/EURACHEM. (2000). *Quantifying Uncertainty in Analytical Measurement*. Available online at: http://www.measurementuncertainty.org/mu/EC_Trace_2003_print.pdf

CITAC/EURACHEM. (2002). *Guide to Quality in Analytical Chemistry*. Available online at: http://www.eurachem.ul.pt/guides/CITAC EURACHEM GUIDE.pdf

Funk, W., Dammann, V. & Donnevert, G. (1995). *Quality Assurance in Analytical Chemistry*. VCH, Weinheim.

Neidhart, B. & Wegscheider, W. (2001). *Quality in Chemical Measurements: Training Concepts and Teaching Materials*. Springer-Verlag, Berlin.

Searle, S.R., Casella, G. & McCulloch, C.E. (1992). *Variance Components*. John Wiley & Sons, New York.

Shewhart, W.A. (1986). *Statistical Method from the Viewpoint of Quality Control*. Dover, Mineola, NY.

A reprint of the original work with a new foreword by W. Edwards Deming.

Taylor, J.K. (1987). *Quality Assurance of Chemical Measurements*. Lewis, Chelsea, MI.

Wadsworth, H.M. (1999). Statistical Process Control. In: *Juran's Quality Handbook*, J.M. Juran, & A.N. Godfrey, (eds). McGraw-Hill, New York.

Wheeler, D.J. & Lyday, R.W. (1989). *Evaluating the Measurement Process*, 2nd edn. SPC Press, Knoxville, TN.

Wheeler, D.J. (1995). *Advanced Topics in Statistical Process Control: The Power of Shewhart's Charts*. SPC Press, Knoxville, TN.

See also the book edited by Tranter listed under *Experimental Design: Advanced Topics*.

Multivariate Analysis

For the statistically faint of heart, a lucid introduction to the concepts of multivariate statistics, especially factor analysis and principal component analysis, can be found in:

Gould, S.J. (1996). *The Mismeasure of Man*. Norton, New York & London.

See especially Chapter 6, entitled "The Real Error of Cyril Burt: Factor Analysis and the Reification of Intelligence."

A basic overview is:

Manley, B.F.J. (1994). *Multivariate Statistical Methods: A Primer*, 2nd edn. Chapman & Hall, London.

See also the book edited by Tranter listed under *Experimental Design: Advanced Topics*.

Other advanced books include:

Brown, P.J. (1993). *Measurement, Regression, and Calibration*. Clarendon Press, Oxford.

Statistical Software

Sample datasets useful for testing and evaluating statistical software are available from the US National Institute of Science and Technology: NIST Statistical Reference Datasets (StRD), http://www.itl.nist.gov/div898/strd/

NIST also has the downloadable free statistical software programs *Dataplot* and *Omnitab* (the predecessor to the commercially available *Minitab*) at: http://www.itl.nist.gov/div898/software.htm. The current release of the commercial product is available, for a fee, at: http://www.minitab.com/

The American Statistical Association (http://www.amstat.org) reviews statistical software frequently in its journals, particularly *The American Statistician*, and some of these reviews can be downloaded from their web site.

A number of statistical software packages are available commercially. Many of these offer extremely sophisticated data analysis tools to support skilled professionals, and require some computer programing skills to make full use of their capabilities. Even simple commercial spreadsheet programs, such as Microsoft *Excel*, have some statistical data evaluation functionality built-in. Since software versions change rapidly, and newer versions may have expanded capabilities, no recommendations will be made here; readers are encouraged to read published reviews in current journals. However, the use of the *SAS®* software, available commercially from the SAS Institute (http://www.sas.com/) has been popular with many pharmaceutical regulatory authorities.

Other References

1. Deming, W.E. (1986). Foreword. In: *Statistical Method from the Viewpoint of Quality Control*, W.A. Shewhart, (ed.). Dover, Mineola, NY.
2. Deming, W.E. (1975). On probability as a basis for action. The American Statistician 29, 146–152.
3. Wheeler, D.J. (1995). *Advanced Topics in Statistical Process Control: the Power of Shewhart's Charts*. SPC Press, Knoxville, TN. pp. 116–122.
4. Odeh, R.E. & Owen, D.B. (1980). *Tables for Normal Tolerance Limits, Sampling Plans and Screening, Table 3*. Marcel Dekker, New York.

Abbreviated versions of this table can be found in: Hahn, G. J. & Meeker, W. Q. (1991). *Statistical Intervals: A Guide for Practitioners*, Tables A.1a, A.1b and A.10. New York: John Wiley & Sons, also in: Juran, J. M. & Godfrey, A. B. (1999). *Juran's Quality Handbook*, 5th edn, Table V. McGraw-Hill, New York.

5. Juran, J.M. & Godfrey, A.B. (1999). *Juran's Quality Handbook*, 5th edn. Table V. McGraw-Hill, New York.
6. ASTM E29 Standard Practice for Using Significant Digits in Test Data to Determine Conformance with Specifications. ASTM, West Conshohocken, PA.
7. ASTM E29 Standard Practice for Using Significant Digits in Test Data to Determine Conformance with Specifications. ASTM, West Conshohocken, PA.
8. Gookins, E.F. (1999). Inspection and Test. In: *Juran's Quality Handbook*, J.M. Juran, & A.B. Godfrey, (eds), 5th edn. McGraw-Hill, New York.
9. Wheeler, D.J. & Lyday, R.W. (1989). *Evaluating the Measurement Process*, 2nd edn. SPC Press, Knoxville, TN.
10. Finney, D.J. (1978). *Statistical Method in Biological Assay*, 3rd edn. Charles Griffin, London.
11. Yeh, C. (1981). Uses of Bioassay in Drug Development: Dose-Response Relationships. In: *Statistics in the Pharmaceutical Industry*, C.R. Buncher, & J.Y. Tsay, (eds). Marcel Dekker, New York.
12. Ishikawa, K. (1976). *Guide to Quality Control*. Asian Production Organization, Tokyo.
13. Taylor, J.K. (1987). *Quality Assurance of Chemical Measurements*. Lewis, Chelsea, MI.
14. Marquardt, D.W. (1999). Process Industries. In: *Juran's Quality Handbook*, J.M. Juran, & A.B. Godfrey, (eds), 5th edn. McGraw-Hill, New York.
15. Kourti, T. (2004). Process analytical technology and multivariate statistical process control. Wellness index of process and product—Part 1. Journal of Process Analytical Technology 1(1), 13–19.
16. Kourti, T. (2005). Process analytical technology and multivariate statistical process control. Wellness index of process and product—Part 2. Journal of Process Analytical Technology 2(1), 24–28.
17. Kourti, T. (2005). Process analytical technology and multivariate statistical process control. Wellness index of process and product—Part 2. Journal of Process Analytical Technology 3(3), 18–24.

BIOPHARMACEUTICAL AND PHARMACOKINETIC EVALUATIONS OF DRUG MOLECULES AND DOSAGE FORMS

Oral Absorption Basics: Pathways, Physico-chemical and Biological Factors Affecting Absorption

Zhongqiu Liu, Stephen Wang and Ming Hu

11.1 BARRIERS TO ORAL DRUG DELIVERY

Barriers to oral drug delivery, the most popular and economical route of drug administration, are composed of poor solubility and dissolution, absorption barriers, presystemic metabolism, and excretion. For drugs whose targets are easily accessible, those that overcome all of these barriers, and reach systemic circulation, are considered bioavailable. Other drugs that have to reach target organs such as the central nervous system (CNS) and drug-resistant cancer cells that are difficult to access, must first be transported across additional physiological barriers (e.g., blood–brain barrier) to their targets. Such barriers may represent a further hurdle we have to overcome in order to deliver orally administered drugs to these targets.

Drugs need to be rapidly dissolved in the aqueous environment of the gastrointestinal tract so that they have a chance to be adequately absorbed. This seemingly simple process is actually a significant challenge to the development of new oral drug candidates, especially those that are derived from high throughput screening, which tends to favor selection of lipophilic molecules that bind well to receptors as drug candidates, but that have less than desirable biopharmaceutical properties.

The important issue to recognize is that the transit time for solid dosage forms or undissolved drug solids in the upper gastrointestinal tract (i.e., stomach and small intestine) typically ranges from 2–6 hours.[1] Therefore, dissolution rates must be sufficiently rapid to allow the solids to be dissolved within this time window for absorption to occur.

Once drug molecules are dissolved in gastric fluid, they must remain soluble throughout the GI tract. This is not trivial, since the pH of the gastrointestinal tract changes from highly acidic (pH ~1.5) in the stomach to slightly basic (pH ~8) in the lower small intestine and colon. This factor should be considered in designing solubility and dissolution experiments.

Dissolved drugs are absorbed via a variety of transcellular and paracellular pathways across the intestinal tract. The paracellular pathway is defined as drug transport through the junctions between the cells, whereas the transcellular pathway is defined as drug transport through both apical and basolateral cellular membranes, as well as through the internal aqueous environment of the cells themselves. Transcellular pathways also include both passive diffusion and carrier-mediated transport, whereas transport by the paracellular pathway is mainly passive. Drugs are absorbed primarily in the small intestine, where the absorption area is very large (100 m^2 or an area

Developing Solid Oral Dosage Forms: Pharmaceutical Theory and Practice
ISBN: 978-0-444-53242-8

equivalent to that of a tennis court). Absorption in the colon is generally limited, and can be highly variable because of the variability in undigested food, bacteria, and water content. Because of these factors, gastrointestinal transit plays a central role in the absorption of drugs.

After drugs are absorbed into the intestinal cells, they may be subjected to first-pass metabolism by a variety of intestinal enzymes. Escaping intestinal metabolism does not guarantee bioavailability, however, as drugs absorbed from the stomach and intestine (large and small), with exception of those absorbed from the terminal rectum, are subjected to additional first-pass metabolism by the liver. Metabolites formed in the intestinal cells can be excreted back to the intestinal lumen, directly or indirectly, after they are taken up by the liver cells, and are then excreted via the bile. Metabolites formed in the hepatocytes can also be excreted via the bile. Alternatively, all metabolites formed in the enterocytes or hepatocytes may also stay in the blood, where they are eliminated via the kidneys.

11.1.1 Intestinal Barrier

The intestinal tract is traditionally recognized as an organ for absorption. However, it is not an organ where absorption occurs without selection. Selection is based on several factors. First is the size of the molecules; large molecules are not absorbed unless the quantities are minute, as in the case of antigen delivery (e.g., polio vaccine). Instead, a variety of liver and intestinal enzymes degrade many macromolecules such as proteins, polypeptides, polysaccharides, and others, into much smaller molecules. These smaller molecules are often hydrophilic, and require the assistance of transporters to take them up into the cells. This size restriction is enabled by the mechanical barrier of the intestinal cells, which is comprised of the mucous-coated cell membranes and the tight junctions between cells.

For small molecules, many can diffuse into the system with ease via passive diffusion, but some cannot because of the presence of efflux transporters (e.g., p-glycoprotein) that reduce the overall entrance of certain lipophilic substances by actively excreting them back into the intestinal lumen. Small molecules that are taken up by the intestinal cells can be rapidly metabolized by both phase I and phase II enzymes in the enterocytes. Phase II enzymes appear to be the major metabolic enzymes that are capable of deactivating a large number of polyphenols and phenolics.[2] Excretion of phase I metabolites is usually straightforward, with the vast majority using the same pathway

as the parent compound. Excretion of many phase II metabolites, especially those that are highly hydrophilic, requires the action of efflux transporters.[2] These transporters are often coupled to the phase II enzymes to achieve optimal functionality.

Lastly, expression of enzymes and transporters is highly region-dependent within the intestinal tract. Duodenal expression of an enzyme or a transporter is usually, if not always, different from that in the terminal ileum and colon.[3,4] These region-dependent expressions of activity can often be used as an indicator that a transporter or enzyme is involved by using an experimental system (regional intestinal perfusion) that can deliver drugs to specific targeted regions within the gastrointestinal tract.

11.1.2 Hepatic Barrier

The hepatic barrier is quite different from the intestinal barrier, in that the liver barrier tends to be quite uniform. The primary barrier in the liver is the presence of vast amounts of metabolic enzymes, which tend to inactivate lipophilic substances absorbed from the intestine that have escaped intestinal metabolism. Both phase I and phase II enzymes are expressed in abundant quantities and varieties in the liver. The main phase I enzyme system in liver is the cytochrome P450 superfamily of mixed-function oxidases. These enzymes often produce metabolic products that can be further conjugated (via phase II enzymes) to hydrophilic moieties, so that the final metabolites are highly hydrophilic. Hydrophilic metabolites are often then excreted to the bile or plasma, where they will be carried to the kidneys and eliminated in urine.

Another important component of the liver barrier is the presence of various efflux transporters that line the bile canicular membrane.[5] These transporters are capable of excreting parent compounds, phase I metabolites, and phase II metabolites, out of the hepatocytes into the bile, which are then excreted back into the upper intestinal tract. Similar to what happens in the intestine, the functions of metabolic enzymes and efflux transporters can be interdependent, resulting in faster, and more extensive, metabolism than predicted. These coupling processes have been labeled as "double jeopardy" and "revolving door" processes (Sections 11.5.1 and 11.5.2)

11.2 PATHWAYS OF DRUG ABSORPTION

Absorption is the process of transferring chemical substances from the gastrointestinal tract through its wall into the bloodstream and lymphatic stream. In general, there are no specific differences in absorption between drugs and food, but there are different mechanisms of absorption, and also differences in absorption at different parts of the GI tract. Absorption of drugs depends on both physico-chemical factors, including formulation factors (e.g., rates of disintegration and rates of drug release from polymeric dosage forms) and drug factors (e.g., solubility and lipophilicity), as well as biological factors (e.g., stomach emptying rate and intestinal transit time).

There are two main mechanisms of drug transport across the gastrointestinal epithelium: transcellular (i.e., across the cells) and paracellular (i.e., between the cells). The transcellular pathway is further divided into simple passive diffusion, carrier-mediated transport (active transport and facilitated diffusion) and endocytosis. These pathways are illustrated in Figure 11.1. In general, transport across healthy intestinal epithelium by the paracellular route (pathway C) is minimal, due to the presence of tight junctions between the cells. Only small hydrophilic molecules are allowed to pass between the cells, unless a modulator of the tight junctions (pathway F) is present.[6,7] Transcellular transport of a molecule can take place by a passive mechanism (pathway A) or by a specific carrier (pathway B). For passive flux of a molecule to occur, it must have the correct physico-chemical properties (e.g., size, charge, lipophilicity, hydrogen bonding potential, and solution conformation) to cross both the apical and basolateral membranes, which are lipophilic, and diffuse through the cytoplasm, an aqueous environment separating the two membranes.[8] However, compounds that are absorbed by this route may be substrates for intracellular metabolism and apically polarized efflux mechanisms (pathway G), such as p-glycoprotein, which transport compounds from the cell inside back into the intestinal lumen.[8,9] Compounds may also be absorbed transcellularly by utilizing naturally-occurring carriers that will transport them from the lumen into the cell. Some drugs are absorbed via carrier-mediated pathways. For instance, L-dopa and oral cephalosporins are absorbed by amino acid and dipeptide transporters, respectively.[10,11] Endocytosis of compounds (pathway D) is minimal in the adult small intestine, and is not a probable mechanism for drug absorption in the intestine. Most orally administered drugs are absorbed by passive transport (pathway A).[8]

11.2.1 Paracellular Diffusion

The paracellular pathway involves transport of materials through the aqueous pores, between the cells rather than across them. This pathway differs from all the other absorption pathways described below. In the intestine, cells are joined together by means of closely fitting tight junctions on their apical side. The tightness of these junctions can vary considerably between different epithelia in the body. The intercellular spaces occupy only about 0.01% of the total surface area of the intestinal epithelium. Generally, absorptive epithelia, such as that of the small intestine, tend to be leakier than other epithelia. The paracellular pathway progressively decreases in importance down the length of the gastrointestinal tract, since the number and size of pores between the epithelial cells decrease.

The paracellular route of absorption is important for the transport of ions, such as calcium, and for the transport of sugars, amino acids and peptides at concentrations above the capacity of their carriers. Small hydrophilic and charged drugs, which do not distribute into cell membranes, can also cross the gastrointestinal epithelium via the paracellular pathway. The molecular weight cut-off for the paracellular route is usually considered to be 200 Daltons, although some larger drugs have been shown to be absorbed via this route. The paracellular pathway can be divided into a convective ("solvent drag") component and a diffusive component. The convective component is the rate at which the compound is carried across the epithelium via water flux. Paracellular diffusion is relatively unimportant as a mechanism for drug absorption.

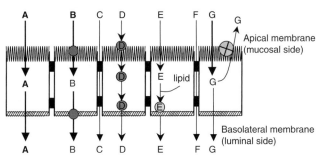

FIGURE 11.1 Potential modes of absorption of drug molecules across the intestinal epithelium: (A) transcellular passive diffusion; (B) carrier mediated transcellular diffusion; (C) paracellular diffusion; (D) transcellular diffusion by endocytosis; (E) transcellular diffusion and incorporation into lipid particles; (F) paracellular diffusion with a modulator of tight junctions; (G) transcellular diffusion modified by a polarized efflux

11.2.2 Passive Diffusion

Passive diffusion is the preferred route of absorption most likely to be used by low molecular weight lipophilic drugs. In this process, drug molecules pass through lipoidal membranes via passive diffusion from a region of high concentration in the intestinal lumen to a region of lower concentration in the blood. This lower concentration is maintained primarily by blood flow, which carries absorbed drug away from the intestinal tissues. The rate of transport is determined by physico-chemical properties of the drug, the nature of the intestinal membrane and the concentration gradient of the drug across the membrane. The process initially involves the partitioning of the drug between the aqueous fluids within the gastrointestinal tract and the lipoidal-like membrane of the epithelial cells. The drug in solution in the membrane diffuses through the epithelial cells within the gastrointestinal barrier into blood flowing in the capillary network within the lamina propria. Upon reaching the blood, the drug will be rapidly pumped away, so maintaining a much lower concentration than that at the absorption site. If the cell membranes and fluid regions making up the gastrointestinal–blood barrier can be considered as a single membrane, then the stages involved in gastrointestinal absorption could be represented by the model shown in Figure 11.2. The mechanism of the passive pathway follows Fick's law, whereby the absorption rate is proportional to the drug concentration and the surface area. Note that given the different lipid and protein compositions of the apical and basolateral membranes, the rate of passage across these two barriers could be different for the same molecule. It has also been assumed that the substance being absorbed exists solely as a single chemical species. Many drugs, however, are weak electrolytes that exist in aqueous solution as both unionized and ionized forms. Because the unionized form of a weak electrolyte drug exhibits greater lipid solubility compared to the corresponding ionized form, the gastrointestinal membrane is more permeable to the unionized species. Thus, the rate of passive absorption of a weak electrolyte drug is related to the fraction of total drug that exists in the unionized form in solution in the gastrointestinal fluids at the site of absorption. This fraction is determined by the dissociation constant of the drug (e.g., its pK_a) and by the pH of the aqueous environment. According to the pH-partition hypothesis, if the pH on one side of a cell membrane differs from the pH on the other side of the membrane, then first the drug (weak acid or base) will be ionized to different degrees on respective sides of the membrane; moreover, the total drug concentration (ionized plus nonionized drug) on either side of the membrane will be unequal. On the other hand, the compartment in which the drug is more highly ionized will contain the greater total drug concentration. For these reasons, a weak acid compound will be rapidly absorbed from the stomach (pH ~1.2), whereas a weak base will be poorly absorbed from the stomach.

11.2.3 Carrier-mediated Transport

Theoretically, a lipophilic drug may pass through the cell or go around it. If the drug has a low molecular weight and is lipophilic, the lipid cell membrane is not a barrier to drug diffusion and absorption. In the intestine, drugs and other molecules can go through the intestinal epithelial cells either by diffusion or by a carrier-mediated mechanism. Numerous specialized carrier-mediated transport systems are present in the body, especially in the intestine for the absorption of ions and nutrients required by the body. This mechanism of carrier-mediated transport involves specific interaction between the molecule and the transporter or carrier and is saturable; it is utilized by small hydrophilic molecules as shown in Figure 11.3. Two kinds of transport exist: active and passive carrier-mediated transports. The active carrier-mediated transport mechanism is either Na^+- or H^+-linked with bi-functional carriers. This process requires metabolic energy, and can act against a concentration gradient of the substrate. On the other hand, passive

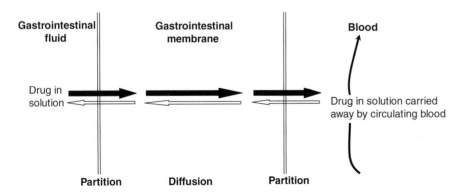

FIGURE 11.2 Diagrammatic representation of absorption via passive diffusion

carrier-mediated transport does not require metabolic energy, and so is driven by the concentration gradient of substrate. These carrier-mediated mechanisms are utilized by some drugs as routes for entering cells. The best-documented examples are β-lactam and cephalosporin antibiotics,[12] which are substrates for the proton-driven dipeptide transporter. The peptide mimetic ACE inhibitors, such as captopril, are also absorbed by carrier-mediated systems.[13]

11.2.4 Active Transport

In contrast to passive diffusion, active transport involves the participation by proteins located in the apical cell membrane of the columnar absorption cells that act as transporters. A carrier or membrane transporter is responsible for binding a drug, and transporting it across the membrane by a process as illustrated in Figure 11.3. Some substances may be absorbed by simultaneous carrier-mediated and passive transport processes. Generally, the contribution of carrier-mediated processes to the overall absorption rate decreases with concentration and at a sufficiently high concentration is negligible.

Active transport allows compounds to be transported against a concentration gradient across a cell membrane, i.e., transport can occur from a region of lower concentration to one of higher concentration. It is an energy-consuming process. The energy is obtained from the hydrolysis of ATP either by direct interaction with the transport carrier protein or indirectly from the transmembrane sodium gradient and/or transmembrane electrical potential difference maintained by normal cellular energy metabolism. Because cellular metabolic energy is required for active transport, the process is also temperature-dependent. There are many carrier-mediated active transport systems or membrane transporters in the small intestine, which can be present either on the apical or on the basolateral cell membrane. These include peptide transporters,

nucleoside transporters, sugar transporters, bile acid transporters, amino acid transporters, organic anion transporters, efflux transporters of multidrug resistant proteins (like MDR1 (multidrug resistant), MRPs (multidrug resistant proteins), BCRP (breast cancer resistant protein)) and vitamin transporters.

Unlike passive absorption, where the rate of absorption is directly proportional to the concentration of the absorbable species of the drug at the absorption site, active transport proceeds at a rate that is proportional to the drug concentration only at low concentrations. At higher concentrations the carrier mechanisms become saturated, and further increases in drug concentration will not increase the rate of absorption, i.e., the rate of absorption remains constant.

Another characteristic of carrier-mediated transport is competition occurring when two similar substrates vie for the same transfer mechanism resulting in inhibition of absorption of one compound by the other.

In summary, active transport mechanisms may be involved as follows:

1. transport requires the presence of one or more carrier proteins;
2. ATP energy is required for activation;
3. the process shows temperature-dependence; and
4. transport can be competitively inhibited by substrate analogs or specific inhibitors.

Active transport also takes place in the intestine, kidney, and liver.

Peptide Transporter

Most oral chemical drugs rely on passive diffusion to cross cell membranes. However, some orally administered peptidomimetic drugs are absorbed via the intestinal transepithelial peptide transport system as shown in Figure 11.4.[14,15] According to this model, the transmembrane proton gradient and resulting membrane potential difference provides the driving force for peptide uptake into intestinal epithelial cells via proton-dependent peptide transporters located in the apical membranes.[16] Peptides that are resistant to hydrolysis by intracellular peptidases are transported across the basolateral membrane via the basolateral peptide transporters.[17] The Na$^+$/H$^+$-exchanger generates and maintains the inward proton gradient on the luminal surface, while the Na$^+$/K$^+$-ATPase present in the basolateral membrane maintains a low intracellular sodium concentration. Because protons are cotransported with peptides across the epithelial membrane, this system is also referred to as the H$^+$-dependent peptide cotransport system.[16] Peptide transporters can accept di- and tri-peptides as physiological substrates, indicating that

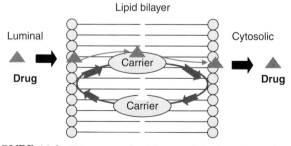

FIGURE 11.3 Diagrammatic representation of carrier-mediated transport of a drug across intestinal membrane

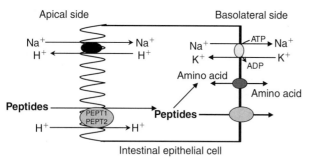

FIGURE 11.4   The accepted model for intestinal transepithelial peptide transport

they have much broader substrate specificity than other nutritional transporters. Consequently, foreign compounds structurally resembling small peptides, such as β-lactam antibiotics, are recognized by the peptide transporters. Thus, peptide transporters work not only as nutritional transporters, but also as drug transporters (Figure 11.4).

Currently, the peptide transporters are divided into two types: those localized at the brush border membranes of epithelial cells and those localized at the basolateral membranes of intestinal and renal epithelial cells. About a decade ago, two border-type peptide transporters were identified and designated PEPT1 and PEPT2. PEPT1 and PEPT2 are polytropic integral membrane proteins with 12 predicted membrane-spanning domains with both NH_2- and COOH-terminal ends facing the cytosol. The mammalian PEPT1 protein comprises 701–710 amino acids, depending on species and is highly glycosylated.[18–20] As shown by *in vitro* translation studies in the presence of microsomes, PEPT1 has a molecular mass of ~75 kDa, whereas digestion with endoglycosidase A shifted the mass to 63 kDa.[20] The PEPT2 protein is also glycosylated, with a molecular mass of the mature protein of ~107 kDa, and a nonglycosylated mass of 83 kDa.[21] Western blot analysis of protein preparations of intestine and kidney identified PEPT1 and PEPT2 immunoreactivity as glycosylated proteins with molecular masses of ~75 and 100 kDa, respectively.[22,23] The Pept2 gene encodes a 729-amino acid protein[23] with 48% amino acid identity to PEPT1 predominantly in transmembrane domains (TMD) with the least similarity in the large extracellular loop connecting TMD 9 and 10. The genomic organization of the peptide transporter genes has also been elucidated. The human Pept1 and Pept2 genes have been mapped to chromosomes 13q33-34 and 3q13.3-q21, respectively.[19,24]

Intestinal PEPT1 can transport L-valine ester prodrugs such as valacyclovir; this observation provided a major step forward toward the development of novel drug delivery systems. Additional peptide transporters, which have similar substrate specificity to PEPT1 and PEPT2 but possess other distinct functional properties, are localized at basolateral membranes of intestinal and renal epithelial cells.[25] The absorption of peptide-like drugs through the intestinal epithelia requires the crossing of two distinct membranes; i.e., uptake by epithelial cells from the lumen across the brush border membrane followed by transfer to the blood across the basolateral membranes. Although orally active β-lactam antibiotics are efficiently absorbed from the intestine they are difficult to move across the basolateral membranes by passive diffusion because of their physico-chemical properties. Based on those findings, it was reported that the peptide transporters are also expressed in the basolateral membranes of intestinal epithelial cells. Through the characterization of peptide-like drug transport via the basolateral membranes of Caco-2 cells grown on microporous membrane filters, it was demonstrated that a peptide transporter, distinct from PEPT1, is expressed in the basolateral membranes of intestinal epithelial cells.[26,27] On the other hand, the intestinal peptide transporters, especially PEPT1, have been a key target molecule for prodrug approaches.[28] According to this approach, prodrugs that are appropriately designed in the form of di- or tri-peptide analogs can be absorbed across the intestinal brush border membranes via PEPT1, and may be absorbed intact or hydrolyzed intracellularly by peptidases or esterases prior to exit from the cell. In addition to PEPT1, the intestinal basolateral transporter has been demonstrated to have the ability to transport nonpeptidic compounds such as δ-ALA, which is a precursor of porphyrins and heme, and plays an important role in the production of heme-containing proteins.[27] The transport of δ-ALA by PEPT1 and the basolateral peptide transporter can explain the good bioavailability of δ-ALA (approximately 60% in a human study).[27,29]

Amino Acid Transporter

The endothelial lining of blood vessels provides a barrier for the exchange of nutrients, and is itself actively involved in the local control of vascular homeostasis. Multiple transport systems mediate the influx of cationic, neutral, sulfonic, and anionic amino acids across the plasma membrane of mammalian cells. Molecular cloning approaches have led to the identification of Na^+-dependent and Na^+-independent amino acid transports. Table 11.1 summarizes the classical nomenclature used to designate these different amino acid transport systems. The ionic dependency and K_m values corresponding to the different transport systems were

TABLE 11.1 Mammalian amino acid transport systems and identified transporters (Giovanni et al., 2003)

Transporter system	Associated protein or cDNA	Amino acid selectivity	Ionic dependency	$K_{m,\ \mu}M$
CAT-associated transport				
y^+	CAT-1	Cationic	No	70–250
	CAT-2A or CAT-2/2α	Cationic	No	2150–5200
y^+	CAT-2B or CAT-2/2β	Cationic	No	38–380
$y^{+?}$	CAT-3	Cationic	No	40–120
	CAT-4	Cationic(Arg)	No	450–910
Heterodimeric glycoprotein (4F2hc, CD98)-associated transport				
y^+L	y^+LAT1	Neutral/cationic	Na$^+$(neutral)	340
y^+L	y^+LAT2	Neutral/cationic	Na$^+$(neutral)	6–10
L	LAT1/LAT2	Large neutral	No	30–300
x_c^-	xCT	Cystine/glutamate	No	40–92
Asc	Asc-1	Small neutral	No	9–23
rBAT-associated transport				
$B^{0,+}$	$b^{0,+}$, AT	Neutral/cationic cystine	No	88
Unknown heavy chain-associated transport				
Asc	Asc-2	Small neutral	No	2.9
Na$^+$ and/or Cl$^-$ or H$^+$-associated transport				
A	ATA1/2/3(SAT1/2/3 or SA 1/2/3)	Neutral/N–Me group	Na$^+$	>200
N	SN 1/2/3	Gln, Asn, His	Na$^+$/H$^+$	150–1600
ABS	ASCT 1/2*	Neutral	Na$^+$	9–464
$B^{0,+}$	ATB$^{0,+}$	Neutral/cationic	Na$^+$/Cl$^-$	23–140
Pro	PROT*	Praline	Na$^+$/Cl$^-$	6
Gly	GLYT ½*	Glycine	Na$^+$/Cl$^-$	17
Beta-like	mTAUT*	β-amino-acids	Na$^+$/Cl$^-$	3–13
	GAT-1-3	GABA and/or β-amino acid	Na$^+$/Cl$^-$	1–20
	BGT-1			
	EAAT1-5*	Glu and/or Asp	Na$^+$, OH$^-$/HCO$_3$	18–97
X^-_{AG}		Glu, Asp	Na$^+$	~200
X^-_{AG}		Glu	No	~230

compiled from the cited publications, and do not necessarily reflect transport properties of all cell types.[30]

The different carrier proteins mediating transport of cationic amino acids include the Na$^+$-independent systems y^+, y^+L, $b^{0,+}$, b^+, and Na$^+$-dependent system $B^{0,+}$. System b^+, originally described in mouse blastocysts, is highly specific for cationic amino acids, whereas the other systems can also transport neutral amino acids. System y^+ is the principal cationic amino acid transport system expressed in NO producing cells, and thus most likely plays a key role in regulating L-arginine supplies for NOS. Although there

is limited information on ASCT, PROT, GLYT, TAUT, and EAAT associated amino acid transport in vascular cells, recent evidence indicates that bovine aortic endothelial cells express a taurine transporter sharing a high degree of sequence homology with that of the mTAUT cDNA isolated from brain.[31]

There are similarities between the transport of cationic amino acids in renal proximal tubule and the small intestine. This became clear from the observation that, in patients with the renal abnormality cystinuria, the transport of lysine and ornithine was also defective in the intestinal tract. For this reason, and with considerable prescience, it was reported that the genetic defect underlying cystinuria was shared by the small intestine. This notion was compatible with early studies that indicated that in the *in vitro* hamster intestine there is net transport against a concentration gradient for the three basic amino acids, and that these amino acids share the same transport system as cystine.[32]

To date, both Na^+-dependent and Na^+-independent transport systems for cationic amino acids have been identified in the brush border of the small intestine. There is also evidence that efflux across the basolateral membrane constitutes that rate-limiting step of transepithelial cationic amino acid transport. Thus, during lysine transport across the intact epithelium, the intracellular amino acid concentration may exceed by fivefold that in the lumen, whereas for neutral amino acids, the accumulation of solute in the tissue is much less.[33,34]

The principles of transepithelial cationic amino acid transport exemplified in the intestine are also applicable to the kidney. In the kidney, there is controversy concerning both Na^+-dependence and electrogenicity of the brush border transport of cationic amino acids. Thus, in studies using membrane vesicles, it has been variously concluded that there is Na^+-dependent secondary active transport,[35] that there is electogenic but Na^+-independent transport,[36] and that there is electroneutral transport in the absence of Na^+.[37] A model for the reabsorption of cationic amino acids in the kidney was recently proposed, and is shown in Figure 11.5.

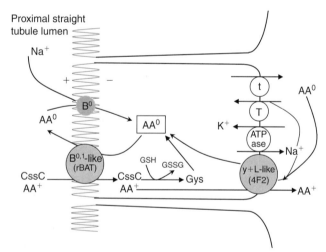

FIGURE 11.5 Model for renal reabsorption of cationic amino acids (AA^+) and cystine (CssC). Participation of various broad-scope systems ($b^{0,+}$, y^+L, and $B^{0,+}$) and interactions with neutral aminoacids (AA^0) are indicated. Note proposed role of rBAT ($b^{0,+}$) and 4F2 (y^+L) proteins in apical and basal membranes, respectively. GSH: glutathione; GSSG: oxidized glutathione (redrawn from Deves et al., 1998)

Organic Anion Transporting Peptide

Organic anion transporters (OATs) and organic cation transporters (OCTs) are two of the major transporter families responsible for absorption, distribution, and elimination of environmental xenobiotics, plant or animal toxins and drugs. Although both transport systems have distinct substrate preferences with OAT for those carrying negative changes and OCT for those carrying positive charges, they share several common features: similar predicted transmembrane topology, interaction with numerous structurally and pharmacologically diverse compounds, and expression in tissues as varied as kidney, liver, intestine, brain and placenta. Four members of the OAT family have been identified so far: OAT1, OAT2, OAT3 and OAT4. These OATs have primary structures of 526–568 amino acid residues and a predicted secondary structure of 12 transmembrane domains. These transporters are expressed in a variety of tissues, including kidney, liver, brain and placenta, and are multispecific with a wide range of substrate recognition. For the organic cation transporters, six members of the OCT family have been identified, i.e., OCT1, OCT2, OCT3, OCTN1, OCTN2 and OCTN3. Based on their primary structures, OCTs and OCTN3 are distinct subfamilies within the OCT group. Like OATs, common structural features of OCT family members include 12 transmembrane domains, a large hydrophilic loop between transmembrane domains 1 and 2 carrying several potential glycosylation sites and multiple potential phosphorylation sites localized on the large intracellular loop between transmembrane domains 6 and 7.[38]

OAT1 and OAT3 transporters belong to the classically described organic anion transporter in the kidney proximal tubules, which utilizes a tertiary transport process to move organic anions across the basolateral membrane into the proximal tubule cells for subsequent exit/elimination across the apical membrane into urine. This tertiary process in the basolateral membrane includes the following steps:

1. Na^+ K^+-ATPase pumps Na^+ out of the cells;
2. this Na^+ gradient then moves dicarboxylates into the cells through a Na/dicarboxylate cotransporter ($SDCT_2$), which process, in conjunction with ongoing cellular metabolic activity, sustains an outwardly directed dicarboxylate gradient; and
3. this dicarboxylate gradient then drives transfer of organic anions into the cells through OAT1 or OAT3, serving as organic anion/dicarboxylate exchangers.

Whether or not other members of the OAT family, such as OAT2 and OAT4, use a similar transport mechanism remains to be found. After being transported across the basolateral membrane into the proximal tubule cells, organic anions will exit across the apical membrane into the urine for elimination. However, the mechanism for this apical step is not completely understood.[39,40]

The characteristics of organic cation transport by OCT1, OCT2 and OCT3 are electrogenic activity, transport directional reversibility and independence from Na^+.[41] For OCTNs, the transport modes depend on the substrates tested. Transporters hOCTN1 and rOCTN1 mediate pH-dependent and Na^+-dependent transport of TEA.[42,43] However, mOCTN1 mediates carnitine transport in a Na^+-dependent manner.[44] OCTN2, which has significant affinities both for carnitine and TEA, transports carnitine in a Na^+-coupled manner, but transports other organic cations including TEA in a Na^+-independent manner.[45,46] OCTN2-mediated transport is also electrogenic as demonstrated recently with the two-electrode voltage clamp technique and pH-dependent.[47] In contrast to OCTN2, OCTN3-mediated transport of carnitine is Na^+-independent.[44]

Three synthetic opioid peptides, DPDPE, DADLE and deltorphin II have been shown to be transported by certain members of the OATP/Oatp family. This includes the rodent Otap1, Oatp2 and Oatp4,[48,49] and human OATP-A, OATP-C, and OATP-8.[49–52] Enkephalins may also be recognized by some of these transporters. The primary location of most of these transporters is the basolateral membrane of hepatocytes.[48,50,53–55] Therefore, these transporters play a critical role in the uptake of opioid peptides by the liver for subsequent elimination into bile. OATP-A is located in brain capillary endothelial cells in humans,[49,52] and hence is expected to be an important determinant of transfer of opioid peptides across the blood–brain barrier. There is evidence for marked changes in the ability of OATP-A to transport opioid peptides, due to genetic polymorphisms.[52]

11.2.5 Facilitated Transport

This carrier-mediated process differs from active transport, in that it cannot transport a substance against a concentration gradient of that same substance. Therefore, facilitated diffusion does not require an energy input, but it does require a concentration gradient for its driving force as does passive diffusion. When substances are transported by facilitated diffusion they are transported down the concentration gradient, but at a much faster rate than would be anticipated based on the molecular size and polarity of the molecule. The process, like active transport, is saturable and is subject to inhibition by competitive inhibitors. In terms of drug absorption, facilitated diffusion seems to play a very minor role, except in the case of nucleoside analogs.

Nucleosides are precursors of nucleic acid biosynthesis, which process is fundamental to the control of growth and metabolism in all living systems. Nucleosides are hydrophilic and diffuse slowly across cell membranes. To facilitate the salvage of these precursors for nucleotide biosyntheses, cells have evolved complex transport systems consisting of multiple carrier proteins known as the nucleoside transporters. The physiologic roles of these transporters include the salvaging of precursors for DNA and RNA synthesis and regulation of adenosine-mediated neuromodulation by controlling its concentrations at the receptor site. Many of the therapeutic nucleoside analogs rely on nucleoside transporters to enter or exit cells. Consequently, the expression and functional characteristics of these transporters in the absorptive/excretory organs and target/non-target cells have an important impact on the pharmacokinetics, efficacy and toxicity of nucleoside analogs.[56]

Two major classes of nucleoside transport systems, equilibrative and concentrative, have been identified. The equilibrative system is comprised of facilitated carrier proteins, whereas the concentrative system consists of Na^+-dependent secondary active transporters. Within each major class, multiple subtypes with distinct substrate specificity and inhibitor sensitivity exist. The cloned equilibrative nucleoside transporters share significant sequence homology, and belong to a so-called equilibrative nucleoside transporter gene family, whereas genes encoding Na^+-dependent nucleoside transporters belong to a concentrative nucleoside transporter family.

In polarized cells, such as renal and intestinal epithelia and hepatocytes, the equilibrative nucleoside transporters (ENTs) and the concentrative nucleoside transporters (CNTs) are thought to asymmetrically distribute between the apical and basolateral membranes to mediate vectorial transepithelial flux of nucleosides (Figure 11.6). The equilibrative nucleosides transporters (ENT) mediate facilitated diffusion of nucleosides across membranes and function bidirectionally in accordance with the substrate concentration gradient. Based on the sensitivity to nitrobenzylthioinosine (NBMPR), a tight-binding and highly specific inhibitor, the equilibrative nucleoside transporters have been classified into two subtypes, *es* (equilibrative sensitive) and *ei* (equilibrative insensitive). The *es* subtype binds NBMPR with high affinity as a result of a noncovalent interaction at a high affinity binding site on the transporter protein. In contrast, the *ei* subtype is not affected by NBMPR at nanomolar concentrations and only becomes inhibited at high NBMPR concentrations.[57] Both *es* and *ei* transporters exhibit broad substrate selectivity, and are widely distributed in different cell types and tissues. More recently, the two transporters were renamed as ENT1 and ENT2, since, according to their characteristics, they belonged to a large ENT gene family whose members are also found in yeast, protozoa, insects and plants.[58] Moreover, two new mammalian ENT members (ENT3 and ENT4) with unknown functions were identified from the public sequence database. In contrast to the equilibrative transporters, which mediate passive downhill flux of nucleosides, the concentrative nucleoside transporters (CNT) mediate active uphill transport of nucleosides. These transporters utilize the inwardly-directed Na^+ gradient established by the ubiquitous Na^+-K^+-ATPase to move substrates into cells against their concentration gradients. Unlike the ENTs, the Na^+-dependent nucleoside transporters exhibit distinct substrate selectivity for purine or pyrimidine nucleosides, which are powerful neuromodulators that regulate a variety of physiological processes, including neurotransmission and cardiovascular activity. Based on functional studies in cell and tissue preparations, five Na^+-dependent nucleoside transport subtypes (N1–N5) were identified. The N1 (or *cif*) subtype is mainly purine-selective, but also transports uridine. The N2 (or *cit*) subtype is pyrimidine-selective, but also transports adenosine. The N3 (or *cib*) subtype is broadly selective, transporting both purine and pyrimidine nucleosides. The N4 subtype transports pyrimidine and guanosine. N4 was characterized in brush border membrane vesicles isolated from human kidney. The N5 subtype, which is NBMPR sensitive, and transports formycin B and

cladribine, was described only in human leukemia cell lines. To date, genes encoding N1–N3 transporters have been cloned, and belong to a CNT gene family. Genes encoding N4 and N5 activities have not been identified.[56]

The clinical significance of nucleoside transporters can be summarized as follows:

1. A number of anti-cancer nucleoside analogs rely on nucleoside transporters to enter cells to reach their cellular targets. For these drugs, expression of nucleoside transporters on the cancer cells is a prerequisite for the cytotoxicity of nucleoside analogs, while loss of nucleoside transporters in tumor cells can lead to drug resistance.

2. If a drug is a substrate for nucleoside transporters, the distribution of these transporters in various tissues/organs, particularly the absorptive and excretory organs, may influence its pharmacokinetic and toxicological properties.

3. Nucleoside transporters themselves could serve as drug targets. In conclusion, nucleoside transporters are critical in determining intracellular bioavailability and systemic disposition of therapeutic nucleoside analogs. Knowledge of nucleoside transporters is important in the evaluation and prediction of the kinetics, targeting, efficacy, and toxicities of nucleoside-derived drugs.

11.3 PATHWAYS OF DRUG METABOLISM

Drug metabolism usually involves a variety of enzymes which, by definition (from a biochemical perspective), typically help to increase efficiency (by acting as catalysts) of biotransformation of a substrate to a product through a lowering of the required threshold energy for this reaction. Two categories of drug metabolism are well-recognized in the field today: phase I and phase II drug metabolic processes. In general, phase I metabolism acts as the first step in the drug metabolic process, in that its products often, but not always, become substrates for phase II metabolism. For lipophilic endo- and xenobiotics that enter cells by passive diffusion or uptake transporters, phase I enzymes often represent the first enzymatic reaction that acts to clear them from body. Phase II reactions are the true "detoxification" pathways, producing metabolites that are generally much more water-soluble and can be readily excreted in bile or urine, and hence readily eliminated from the body.

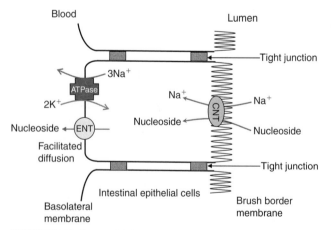

FIGURE 11.6 Model for transepithelial nucleoside flux mediated by Na^+-dependent nucleoside transporters (CNT) and equilibrative nucleoside transporters (ENT) in the lumen of the intestine

11.3.1 Phase I Metabolism

Phase I drug-metabolizing enzymes catalyze a wide array of chemical reactions that facilitate xenobiotics metabolism and elimination. A common theme apparent for all phase I enzyme reactions is that final products are usually modified to contain a functional group (e.g., hydroxyl, amino, sulfonic or carboxylic acid) that is chemically reactive.[59]

This gives support to the well-documented concept that phase II metabolic processes (e.g., glucuronidation, glycosidation, sulfation, methylation, acetylation, glutathione conjugation, amino acid conjugation, fatty acid conjugation, and condensation) are the "true" detoxification steps for xenobiotic elimination from the body (discussed in detail below). Because phase I reactions add functional groups onto a substrate so that phase II metabolism can occur, phase I metabolism can serve as a necessary prerequisite that allows the detoxification of xenobiotics.

Phase I metabolism also occurs during the process of nutrient digestion, which typically involves hydrolysis reactions. These reactions include the hydrolysis of proteins, polysaccharides, and polymeric nucleotides and nucleosides.[60,61] The end results of these hydrolysis reactions are typically to provide usable nutrients. Additional phase I reactions include hydrolysis of the ester bond, which is necessary for the processing of fatty acids and derivatives, again producing monoglycerides and fatty acids for absorption.[62] Some drugs may also undergo hydrolysis in the gastrointestinal tract and in the liver, but this is not common.

Hydrolysis

The necessity for hydrolysis for both absorption and metabolite conversion can be exemplified with the intestinal disposition pathways for compounds such as isoflavones. Natural isoflavones exist predominantly in the form of glycosides. In order for them to be absorbed, lactase phlorizing hydrolase that resides on the surface of the intestinal lumen must be utilized to cleave the sugar group off the isoflavone glycoside.[63,64] Only then can the isoflavone aglycone (no sugar group attached) be substantially absorbed from the intestine. Furthermore, hydrolysis by bacteria is also a necessary component in the enteric recycling of isoflavones, in the sense that phase II metabolites of isoflavones are hydrolyzed back to the isoflavone aglycone form in the intestine, which can then be reabsorbed.

Various substrates (not just isoflavones) are subjected to hydrolysis. Four main groups of compounds subjected to hydrolysis are amides, carbamates, hydrazides, and esters. The hydrolysis of esters usually takes place via both nonspecific and specific esterases. Amides can also be hydrolyzed slowly via nonspecific esterases in the plasma. However, amidases in the liver are more specific, and have shown higher hydrolytic capacity for amides. Hydrazide groups or carbamate groups are the least common functional groups that are subjected to hydrolysis.

Hydroxylation

Hydroxylation reactions are typically very common reactions for compounds that have at least one aromatic ring in their chemical structures. Therefore, hydroxy-derivatives are quite commonly seen in nature for both drugs and xenobiotics. Hydroxylation reactions are also observed for some aliphatic substrates. Of interest to cancer research is that unstable epoxide intermediates are formed in the course of some hydroxylation reactions; these intermediates have been shown, in some cases, to be carcinogenic.

The majority of research in the area of phase I metabolism has focused on cytochrome P450 (CYP450; 450 stands for the spectral absorption maximum of the enzyme at 450 nm after carbon monoxide binding). As a superfamily of enzyme proteins, CYP450 mixed-function oxidases play a very important role in the phase I oxidative metabolism of drugs, and are responsible for primary metabolism of a large variety of drugs *in vivo*.[66]

Because of their importance, great emphasis has been placed on the determination of the mechanistic details of CYP450 reactions. From a basic research perspective, the purpose for CYP450 in the elimination of xenobiotics is to prepare a substrate for phase II metabolism via the addition of reactive functional groups, typically hydroxyl groups. However, this is not to say that phase I metabolites cannot be excreted and eliminated from the body via both active and passive efflux. From a drug design point of view, a thorough understanding of CYP450 behavior in itself, as well as its activity with xenobiotics, will help to predict possible adverse reactions of drugs, as well as to provide solutions to improve drug efficacy and administration.[67] Regulatory agencies such as the US Food and Drug Administration (FDA) have also paid much attention to this subject. The FDA, in a recent draft guidance for industry concerning drug interaction studies, clearly emphasized that the metabolism of an investigational new drug should be defined during early drug development.

CYP450s with capacity for oxidation of various xenobiotics are located in the cellular endoplasmic reticulum. Because CYP450s have iron protoporphyrin IX as a prosthetic group, they are categorized as heme-containing enzymes. This heme iron is bonded to the rest of the enzyme by four pyrrole nitrogen atoms of protoporphyrin IX, and two ligands axial to the porphyrin plane. The two axial ligands (the fifth and sixth ligands) and their complex states of electronic configuration essentially allow CYP450s to oxidize a diverse variety of substrates. The overall main catalytic function of CYP450s is to split molecular oxygen. One oxygen atom is transferred to the substrate, typically inserted between a carbon atom and a hydrogen atom to form an alcohol or phenol or added across a double bond to form an epoxide, while the other oxygen atom is reduced to water by transfer of electrons from NADH via a specific CYP450 reductase enzyme.

Because of the enormous varieties of CYP450s that exist in nature, the classification of these enzymes has also been a rather complex issue, due to newly found isoforms that are constantly being published in the literature. Despite this confusion, Dr David R. Nelson has a very well-updated website that reports all of the known CYP450 genes across species. In addition, sequence alignments and information about known structures are also available at: http://drnelson.utmem.eud/CytochromeP450.html.

The nomenclature for CYP450 is based on gene sequence similarity. Through divergent evolution, many subclassifications of P450s have developed into gene families and subfamilies. In general, all CYP450s share ~40% in sequence identity with each other (e.g., CYP3A4 and CYP2D6). Therefore, all enzymes in the 3A and 2D subfamily share at least 40% in gene sequence. In addition, the nomenclature scheme dictates that a P450 isoform, such as CYP2D6, belongs to the 2D subfamily and is the sixth gene to have been completely sequenced in this subfamily. With respect to individual isoforms in a particular subfamily, for example CYP3A, the isoforms CYP3A4 and CYP3A5, while both in the same subfamily, share at least 70% of their respective gene sequences as they belong to the same subfamily.

Although the amino acid composition of CYP450s is very diverse, and enzyme mutations occur quite frequently in nature, the structures of CYPs are quite well conserved. Complicated pathologies resulting from mutated CYP450s, such as Antley–Bixler syndrome,[59] are seen in subjects with mutations in the genetic makeup of their CYPs. Another example in which genetic polymorphism can have great impact in patient reaction to drugs is seen in the case of warfarin (the S enantiomer has higher activity than the R form). CYP2C9 is the main isoform responsible for S-warfarin metabolism. Patients with polymorphisms primarily

Cyp2C9*2 and CYP2C9*3 (both hetero and homozygous) have major deficiencies in the metabolism of S-warfarin, and thus experience higher incidences of serious life-threatening bleeding resulting from bioaccumulation of S-warfarin.[68]

Oxidation reactions not related to CYP450 are also observed, and typically involve the metabolism of endogenous substrates. Oxidative metabolism has been called many names, and a list of common names for oxidative metabolism includes dehydrogenases (e.g., alcohol dehydrogenase), oxidases (e.g., amine oxidase), and aromatases (e.g., aromatase cytochrome P450 (P450arom)).[65]

Reductive Metabolism

Reductive metabolism in mammalian species is quite rare, and seldom occurs in the metabolism of drugs and xenobiotics. However, reductive metabolism, as well as ring fission, frequently occurs in the intestinal microflora.[69] The commonality that exists for reductive metabolic processes is that they require NADPH as a necessary component in the reaction mixture, but are generally inhibited by oxygen. This differs from mixed-function oxidase reactions, which require NADH, but where oxygen is required for reaction.

11.3.2 Phase II Enzymes

Phase II enzymes are conjugating enzymes in drug metabolic pathway classification. Although drugs can undergo phase I and phase II reactions simultaneously, one of the pathways typically dominates. For most prescription drugs, and drug candidates under development, the predominant pathway of metabolism is not phase II metabolism. Rather, phase II metabolism often occurs following phase I metabolism, which serves to eliminate drug molecules from the body.

There are some compounds whose main metabolic pathway is phase II conjugation. For example, this is the major metabolic pathway for polyphenols. Once absorbed, polyphenols are subjected to 3 types of conjugation: glucuronidation, sulfation, and methylation.[2,70–72] Glucuronidation and sulfation metabolize polyphenols into very hydrophilic conjugates, whereas methylation produces metabolites that have essentially the same if not slightly more lipophilic properties.[2] Regardless of whether methylation occurs, the methylated products are usually conjugated subsequently into glucuronides and sulfates, as long as there is a functional group available for conjugation into more hydrophilic metabolites. Therefore, conjugation enzymes that catalyze the formation of hydrophilic metabolites significantly impact the bioavailability of drugs or xenobiotics.

UDP-glucuronosyltransferases (UGTs)

Two superfamilies of phase II enzymes, UDP-glucuronosyltransferases (UGTs) and sulfotransferases (SULTs), catalyze the formation of hydrophilic phase II conjugates. UGTs are membrane-bound enzymes that are located in the endoplasmic reticulum of many tissues.[73] UGTs catalyze the transfer of a glucuronic acid moiety from UDP-glucuronic acid to their substrates, such as steroids, bile acids, polyphenols, dietary constituents, and xenobiotics. Mammalian UGTs belong to the UGT1A and UGT2B subfamilies.[73] Among the human UGT isoforms, UGT1A1, UGT1A6 and UGT1A9 appear to be broadly distributed, whereas UGT1A8 and UGT1A10 have more restrictive distribution. UGT2Bs appear to be less active (when measured *in vitro*) when compared to UGT1As, but are capable of metabolizing important pharmacological agents such as morphine and ezetimibe, generating metabolites that are more active than parent compounds.[74]

Sulfotransferases (SULTs)

SULTs are cytosolic enzymes that are soluble and highly active. They catalyze the transfer of a sulfate moiety from 3'-phosphoadenosine-5'-phosphosulfate to a hydroxyl group on various substrates.[75,76] Compared to UGT isoform-catalyzed metabolism, much less is known about how SULT isoforms metabolize their substrates and relevant structure-activity relationships. The latter may be due to the fact that sulfation is often the secondary metabolic pathway (to glucuronidation and other phase II reactions). Only a handful of UGT and SULT isoforms are commercially available, and commercially available SULTs are much more expensive than UGTs. Therefore, the isoforms that are specifically involved in the conjugation of polyphenols have not yet been clearly identified. However, sulfation still can account for a large percentage of the phase II metabolism at lower concentration, and may serve as the primary metabolic pathway for certain compounds such as resveratrol.[77]

Glutathione Transferases (GSTs)

Similar to UGTs and SULTs, glutathione transferases (GSTs) are also important for the detoxification process.[78,79] Their metabolic products are also highly polar, and need the assistance of efflux transporters to be removed from cells. Importantly, glutathione depletion can significantly affect the function of this enzyme. More so than UGTs and SULTs, GST appears to be superior in detoxifying carcinogenic and oxidizing agents. Xenobiotics and natural polyphenols are capable of inducing (in mammals) biosynthesis of GSTs that are critical to an organism's ability to fight oxidative stress and cancer.[78,79]

Methyltransferases and Other Conjugating Enzymes

Unlike UGTs and SULTs, methyltransferases such as catechol-O-methyltransferase catalyze the O-methylation of several catechol-containing polyphenols, forming metabolites that are just as polar or slightly less polar than the parent compound.[80] This O-methylation reaction is subjected to strong inhibitory regulation by S-adenosyl-L-homocysteine, which, e.g., is formed in large quantities during the O-methylation of tea polyphenols. Although methylation may not be a major metabolic pathway, its importance in the mechanisms of action of tea polyphenols cannot be underestimated, as methylated metabolites tend to have different activities, and some may resist inactivation via UGTs and SULTs.

Similar to methyltransferases, many other phase II enzymes, such as acetyltransferases, also produce less hydrophilic molecules, whereas glutamyltransferases and others will produce more hydrophilic metabolites that facilitate their elimination.

11.4 PATHWAYS OF DRUG ELIMINATION

Traditionally, research has focused on how to facilitate the absorptive transport of drugs. More recently, we have begun to pay more attention to active transport mechanisms by which molecules can undergo efflux out of the intestinal lumen. In addition to excreting or eliminating absorbed molecules, these transporters may also be responsible for the elimination of phase I and/or phase II metabolites of the drugs, as described in detail in the earlier sections of this chapter. Currently, several processes of active efflux have been identified. Active transport proteins, such as P-glycoprotein (P-gp), multidrug resistance-associated proteins (MRPs), and other organic anion transporters, play a major role in governing the intestinal absorption and metabolism of drugs. Together with the action of hepatic enzymes and efflux transporters, they determine the bioavailability of drugs and xenobiotics.

11.4.1 P-glycoprotein (P-gp)

The history of P-gp goes hand in hand with human cancer and chemotherapy. Upon discovery of cytotoxic drugs that can destroy cancer cells, researchers also discovered that drug resistance (for multiple drugs) can impede the effects of these drugs. P-gp was the first active transporter protein to be discovered at the time, a little over 30 years ago. Two research groups must be acknowledged as having made great contributions to the discovery of P-gp, and determining that this transporter is a major culprit responsible for multidrug resistance (MDR). In 1968, the Ling laboratory (University of Toronto) initially used somatic cell genetics to investigate colchicine resistance in Chinese hamster ovary cells, which linked P-gp to MDR.[81] In the meantime, Dr Gottesman's laboratory (National Cancer Institute) was able to clone amplified DNA sequences related to MDR phenotype in cell lines.[82] From both of these works we now know that the MDR gene and P-gp gene are the same. Today, we know that P-gp, and other more recently identified protein(s), act as efflux transporter pumps with a broad specificity for a variety of substrates.

P-gp is a member of a large diverse family (over 50 members) of ATP-binding cassette (ABC) transporters that facilitate efflux of xenobiotics and certain endogenous substances such as bile acids and bilirubin. Dependent on ATP, the P-gp structure shares extensive sequence homology and domain organization with other members of this superfamily. The most conserved region is the ATP-binding cassette domain, containing approximately 200–250 amino acids consisting of two nucleotide-binding domains (NBDs) located towards the cytoplasmic face of the membrane.[83] More specifically, P-gp contains 12 transmembrane regions split into two "halves," each containing an NBD.

P-gp, as well as other members of the multidrug resistance-type transporters, are organized and classified under the MDR/TAP (transporter associated with antigen processing) proteins subfamily. Within the ABC superfamily, MDR type transporters such as P-gp (also known as MDR1), MDR3, and BSEP (bile salt export pump, also known as a sister of P-gp) are grouped within the B subfamily, and thus designated as ABCB1, ABCB4, ABCB11, respectively.

Substrates for P-gp are typically lipophilic and cationic. As previously mentioned, a large number of compounds are substrates/inhibitors for P-gp, and include anticancer agents, antibiotics, antivirals, calcium channel blockers, immunosuppressive agents, and plant chemicals usually found in a normal diet.[84]

The role of P-gp is to limit the absorption of compounds by forceful efflux back into the lumen, the net effect of which limits bioavailability. Data from both *in vitro* and *in vivo* studies using human intestinal epithelial cell lines[85] and P-gp-knockout mice,[86] respectively, show that the disruption of P-gp activity can lead to some potentially hazardous problems with regard to

drug disposition, since elimination via excretion of a compound in the body will be substantially decreased (if the compound is predominantly eliminated by P-gp), thus leading to increased sensitivity to toxicity.

11.4.2 Multidrug-resistance Associated Proteins (MRPs)

Multidrug-resistance associated proteins (MRPs) were discovered much later than P-gps. For instance, MRP1 was first cloned in 1992 from a human small cell lung cancer cell line that did not express P-gp.[87] MRP2 was later cloned in 1996 from rat liver, designated as cMRP,[88] and from human liver, named canalicular multispecific organic anion transporter (cMOAT).[89] MRP3 was discovered later, and shown to be closest related to MRP1, sharing 58% amino acid identity.[90] Relatively little information exists currently with regards to both function and expression patterns of the more recently discovered MRPs (MRP7–9).

The core structure of P-gp, as well as MRPs, is comprised of 12 transmembrane regions split into two "halves" which each contain an NBD. MRPs structures are just a little bit more complex than P-gp. MRP1–3 and MRP6–7 have a total of 17 transmembrane regions, with an additional five transmembrane regions at the N-terminus. However, these additional five transmembrane regions do not have an additional NBD. More interestingly, MRP4 and MRP5 do not have these additional regions, and thus resemble P-gp with only 12 transmembrane regions.

The nomenclature for MRPs is consistently being updated via the discovery of more and more novel MRP transporters. The subfamily that incorporates MRPs is termed MRP/CFTR (cystic fibrosis transmembrane conductance regulator). This subfamily includes MRP1 to MRP9, CFTR, and SUR (sulfonylurea receptor) 1 and 2.

The substrates for MRPs are different with regard to each individual isoform and, of course, with regard to their localization. However, the overall mechanistic functions of MRPs are to eliminate compounds from the cell by way of efflux transport. For MRPs, studies have shown that these transporters can confer resistance to cytotoxic drugs, such as vincristine[91] and peptides,[92] heavy metal anions,[93] as well as endogenous metabolites, such as bilirubin glucuronides.[94] More specifically, MRP2 has been shown to be centrally involved in the detoxification process by means of its ability to secrete metabolites into bile. The importance of MRP2 is clearly evidenced in patients who suffer from Dubin–Johnson syndrome with defective MRP2, who have impaired ability to secrete glutathione conjugates, as well as bilirubin glucuronides.[95] MRP3 has shown affinity for bile salts with emphasis in mediating bile salt reabsorption. While it is clear that there are some major overlaps with regard to substrate specificity for these MRPs, they do seem to have some specific roles with regard to the disposition of xenobiotics, as well as endogenous compounds. In addition to this, much is yet to be discovered with regard to the substrate specificities, as well as their functions for the more recently discovered transporters (MRP7–9).

Disruption of MRP activity can differ greatly with regard to impact on the disposition process of xenobiotics or endogenous compounds. In general, various MRPs seem to overlap in substrate specificity, and thus a disruption of a specific MRP isoform, such as MRP3, will probably not result in major physiological dysfunction simply because MRP1 (if expressed and functional) can pick up the slack. However, this is not the case for all MRPs; certain isoforms (i.e., MRP2) seem to be more critically important to the body. As mentioned, the dysfunction of MRP2 in humans can lead to major consequences resulting in Dubin–Johnson syndrome.[95] Our laboratories have also found that MRP2 plays a vital role in the efflux of metabolite conjugates with respect to the enterohepatic recycling process for isoflavones and flavonoids.

11.4.3 Organic Anion Transporters

The discovery of organic anion transporters began almost 70 years ago. At that time, the anionic dye phenolsulphophthalein was observed to accumulate in very high concentrations in renal convoluted tubules, which suggested that a tubular secretion process might be operating.

Organic anion transporter 1 (OAT1) was first cloned in 1997 from rat kidney, and functionally identified as an organic anion transporter.[96,97] Organic anion and cation transporters share a predicted 12-transmembrane domain (TMD) structure with a large extracellular loop between transmembrane domain (TMD) 1 and 2, carrying potential N-glycosylation sites. Conserved amino acid motifs reveal a relationship to the sugar transporter family within the major transport facilitator superfamily.

Although type I and type II classifications for organic cation transporters are formally recognized, this is not the case with organic anion transporters. Currently, the most useful method is to recognize that OATs can be separated and classified with respect to molecular weight, net charge, and hydrophobicity. Type I OATs are relatively small (generally <400 KDa) and are associated with transport of monovalent compounds, such

as p-aminohippurate (PAH). Type II OATs are bulkier (generally >500 KDa), polyvalent in nature, and are associated with transport of compounds such as calcein.

Substrates for OATs typically include acids that have a net negative charge on carboxylate or sulfonate residues at physiological pH. Although OATs have the ability of endogenous transport via active secretion by the proximal tubule of compounds such as riboflavin, the principal function of OATs is to eliminate high levels of xenobiotic agents.[98] This includes many of the products of phase I and phase II hepatic biotransformation, as well as anionic drugs.[99]

The disruption or alteration of OATs activity due to either under-expression or over-expression of OATs is reflected in pathophysiological states. Essentially, the accumulation of uremic toxins (of which many are organic anions) in the kidney due to OATs dysfunction will reflect or lead to general renal disease.[100]

11.5 COUPLING OF ENZYMES AND EFFLUX TRANSPORTERS

Until recently, conjugating enzymes, such as UDP-glucuronosyltransferases (UGTs), and their ability to metabolize compounds (phase II metabolism) were believed to be the most important step in the disposition of a xenobiotic. The ability for UGTs to biotransform a lipophilic compound into a more hydrophilic metabolite (via the addition of a glucose sugar molecule) was initially believed to be the major biological barrier to the entry of xenobiotics/drugs into systemic circulation, and to represent one of the main pathways for their elimination.[2] However, this belief in the primacy of UGT activity does not comprehensively cover the overall disposition of xenobiotics and drugs. The fallacy lies in the fact that many conjugates are hydrophilic, and cannot permeate the cell membrane once they are biotransformed by UGTs. While UGT metabolism is a very necessary component for the disposition process of xenobiotics/drugs, more focus has recently been placed on the various transporters capable of transporting negatively-charged hydrophilic conjugates across the cellular membrane. In this section we will take a look at two theories that explain the mechanistic details and complexities of this coupling process.

11.5.1 Double Jeopardy Theorem

This theorem, in a slightly different form, was originally proposed to explain the mechanistic details that describe the coupling phenomenon between a phase I metabolic enzyme, such as CYP3A4, and an efflux transporter, such as P-gp (Figure 11.7). The theorem was originally proposed by Benet and coworkers to explain pharmacokinetic behavior of certain drugs that are substrates of both CYP3A and P-gp.[101,102]

Mechanistic Description of the Theorem

The mechanism of action for this coupling theory is a little less complex than the revolving door theory (Section 11.5.2). Essentially, the substrate is assumed to be absorbed (at the apical side of the membrane), and is met by the enzyme CYP450 (typically CYP3A4). This substrate is metabolized, and thus is termed as "prosecuted" for the first time by CYP3A4. After this, P-gp can take this one-time metabolized substrate, and transport it back into the intestinal lumen. However, it is important to note that some of this one-time metabolized substrate can pass through the other side (basolateral) of the membrane, and thus can reach the systemic circulation. But, if this one-time metabolized substrate is transported back into the intestinal lumen via P-gp, it can be absorbed one more time at the apical side of the membrane (further down the intestinal tract), and thus can be met again by the enzyme CYP450, and be subjected once again to metabolism. This repeat of the "prosecution" thus gives the term "Double Jeopardy" to this theory.

The consequences for the disruption of this, and any other coupling mechanisms, can vary depending on the substrate in question. Due to differences between substrate disposition profiles, the toxicity, and interactions with other drug disposition mechanisms, as well as compensatory mechanisms or effects by other enzymes or transporters in the system, will vary accordingly. With regard to the double jeopardy theory and thus more specifically with CYP450 and P-gp, the disruption of P-gp activity would result in less exposure time of the substrate in question at the apical membrane. This would lead to more substrate inside the intestine (i.e., increase in absorption), and thus could potentially increase the bioavailability of both the substrate and/or its metabolite in the systemic circulation. On the other hand, if CYP450 activity was disrupted, the amount of metabolite would decrease severely, thus perhaps allowing more substrate to reach the systemic circulation.

11.5.2 Revolving Door Theorem

The revolving door theory was proposed more recently, and hypothesizes that efficient coupling of the conjugating enzymes (UGTs) and efflux transporters enables both enterohepatic recycling and enteric recycling processes.[2] Therefore, unlike the previous theory, this "revolving door" theorem emphasizes the importance of efflux transporters, and their ability to enable the cellular excretion of hydrophilic metabolites (Figure 11.8). In addition, this theory also recognizes the transport of hydrophilic metabolites to both apical and basolateral sides of the membrane. This latter point adds complexity to this theory and its mechanism (Figure 11.8).

Mechanistic Description of the Theorem

The mechanism of the revolving door theory is best illustrated step-by-step for a model compound, such as the soy isoflavone genistein (aglycone). When genistein is absorbed into the intestinal lumen, it has two potential fates. One is that it will pass through the basolateral side of the membrane, and reach the systemic circulation. Research has found that this is mostly not the case, as the bioavailability for this compound upon ingestion is extremely low.[103] The more likely fate of genistein in the intestinal lumen is that it will be extensively metabolized by UGTs.[103,104] After biotransformation by UGTs, the genistein metabolites again have two more choices. One, the genistein metabolites, as organic anions, can be transported

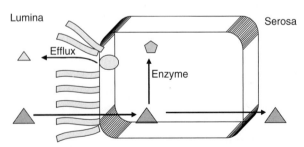

FIGURE 11.7 Schematic representation of the double jeopardy theory. Substrates are represented by triangles, whereas products of enzymes or metabolites are represented by pentagons

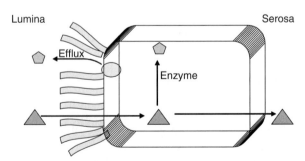

FIGURE 11.8 Schematic representation of the revolving door theory. Substrates are represented by triangles, whereas products of enzymes or metabolites are represented by pentagons

by efflux transporters (MRP1 and/or MRP3) located at the basolateral side of the lumen, and eventually reach the systemic circulation. The other choice is that both genistein and its metabolites will be transported back across the apical side of the intestinal lumen by efflux transporters such as MRP2 or perhaps BCRP. This efflux step, according to our research,[72] is most likely the rate-limiting step for this coupling process. In other words, the amount of metabolites made by UGTs does not significantly alter or influence the disposition of genistein or its metabolites, because disposition is ultimately dependent on the efflux step carried out by transporters. The revolving door theory places emphasis on the rate of the efflux step (i.e., the speed at which the revolving door is spinning) as the determining factor for the disposition of genistein and its metabolites.

Upon efflux into the intestinal lumen, genistein metabolites are converted back to the genistein aglycone through bacterial hydrolysis, and thus can re-enter the intestinal lumen; this whole process occurring at the intestinal level is known as enteric recycling. With regards to the liver, any genistein that gets past the UGTs in the intestine will be subjected to liver UGTs. These metabolites, as well as any metabolites that made it through the intestinal level, will be again secreted in bile into the intestinal lumen, and thus hydrolyzed and again ready for absorption. This process is known as enterohepatic recycling, and again the revolving door theory is very much involved in this scheme (Figure 11.9). This extensive metabolism at the enteric and hepatic level is also known as first-pass metabolism.

The consequences of disruption for this coupling theory are again dependent on the substrate and its metabolite(s) in question. The reason for this is because the body has an elaborate system of various metabolic enzymes (i.e., UGTs, SULTs), as well as efflux transporters (i.e., MRPs, BCRP, OATs) that have overlapping substrate specificities. Because of the fact that detoxification is an essential function for organism survival, organisms have developed a very complex system through evolution that has multiple enzymes and efflux transporters which can pick up the slack, should any one particular member become dysfunctional. Therefore, in order to severely disrupt coupling, a wide number and variety of enzymes (i.e., both UGTs and SULTs) will have to be made dysfunctional.

11.6 PHYSICO-CHEMICAL FACTORS AFFECTING DRUG ABSORPTION

We classify physico-chemical characteristics of a drug molecule or drug particle into those that are solely related to chemical structures, and those that are related to the physical shape (e.g., crystalline forms). Because of the biological constraints posed by the gastrointestinal barriers, we must consider the following physico-chemical properties: lipophilicity, size, charge, solubility, and dissolution.

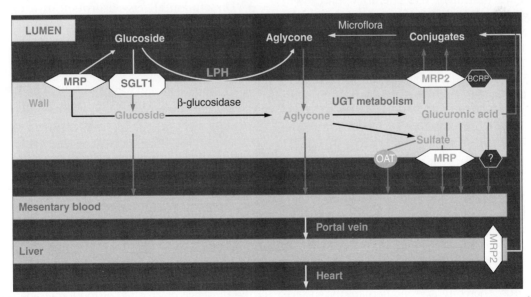

FIGURE 11.9   Schematic representations of both entero and enterohepatic recycling, using isoflavone aglycones as an example. Isoflavones are typically subjected to rapid hydrolysis with intestinal gut hydrolase. Absorption of aglycone is quite rapid, and is subjected to UGT metabolism with metabolites (typically efflux) at both the intestinal and hepatic level. Further hydrolysis from conjugates back to the aglycone form completes a cyclical recycling process where we see repeated absorption, followed by metabolism

11.6.1 Lipophilicity

Lipophilicity of drug candidate molecules is a major concern in the development of its dosage form, because drug molecules must penetrate the lipid bilayer of most cellular membranes, including that of the enterocytes. Therefore, it is generally believed that drug molecules must be lipophilic to have good absorption.

Lipophilicity of uncharged molecules can be estimated experimentally via a straightforward method of measuring the partition coefficient in a water/oil (e.g., water/octanol) biphasic system. For molecules that are weak acids or bases, one must consider the pH at which the majority of the species remain uncharged, versus that at which the majority of the species are charged. Based on the pH-partition theorem, absorption is favored when a molecule is uncharged, which works for drug molecules absorbed via passive diffusion.

This general trend that favors lipophilicity does not imply that the higher the lipophilicity, the better the absorption, as pH-partition theory suggests. Drug molecules, during transcellular absorption in the enterocytes, must first enter through the apical membrane, travel through the cytosolic domain, and then exit through the basolateral membrane. If a compound binds too tightly to the cell membrane, as the result of extremely high lipophilicity, it would be unable to enter the aqueous cytosolic domain, and so would be unable to exit from the lipophilic basolateral membrane into the aqueous lamina propria. Since mature enterocytes take about 10 days to develop, and function about 4 days after maturation, drugs stuck to the cell membranes (apical or basolateral) would eventually slough off when the mature cells perish as the result of their natural lifecycle. According to Lipinski's Rule of Five, this usually means the partition coefficient should be positive, but less than 100 000 to 1 (or $\log_{10}PC = 5$).[105,106] In another statistical study, the log PC was seen to be the best at $\log_{10}PC < 3$.[107]

11.6.2 Size

Passive absorption in the gastrointestinal tract is severely limited by the size of the penetrating drug molecule. This is probably due to the well-organized and packed structure of the cell membrane lipid bilayer. When a molecule is too large, the potential energy resulting from its concentration difference is not large enough to generate the high energy required to greatly disturb the bilayer, so a large molecule can insert into it, and then leave afterwards. Therefore, size and perhaps the surface area of a molecule are major factors that limit absorption via passive diffusion. According to Lipinski's Rule of Five, this means the optimal molecular weight is less

than 500.[105,106] In another similar paper, that molecular weight is extended to 550.[107] At any rate, very few drug molecules with large molecular weight are absorbed to any appreciable extent (>20%). Cyclosporin A is one of the exceptions, with good bioavailability, yet formulations with improved solubility were able to drive its absorption further.

11.6.3 Charge

Effects of charge on passive absorption of drugs are well-recognized. In general, charged molecules are not as permeable as the corresponding uncharged species when the compound is absorbed via passive diffusion. However, the effect of charge on the absorption of drugs via a carrier-mediated transport process is not simple. Some transporters favor neutral substrates, some positively charged, and others negatively charged.

11.6.4 Solubility

Solubility affects the absorption of drugs because it affects the driving force of drug absorption, the concentration of drug molecules at the site of absorption. This factor is discussed extensively elsewhere in this book. Solubility properties are discussed in greater detail in Chapter 1.

11.6.5 Dissolution

Dissolution affects absorption of drugs because it also affects the concentration of the drug that may be achieved. However, dissolution describes the process of solubilization, as represented by the dissolution rate. Drug molecules must have sufficient dissolution rates since drug particles are only in contact with the absorption area within the intestinal tract for a finite length of time. The dissolution process is discussed in more detail in Chapter 14.

11.7 BIOLOGICAL FACTORS AFFECTING DRUG ABSORPTION

The oral route of administration is the most common and popular route of drug dosing. The oral dosage form must be designed to account for extreme pH ranges, the presence or absence of food, degradative enzymes, varying drug permeability in the different regions of the intestine, and motility of the gastrointestinal tract. These are some of the barriers to absorption that a drug may encounter when it is released from its dosage form and has dissolved into the gastrointestinal fluids. The drug needs to remain in solution, and not become bound to food or other material within the gastrointestinal tract. It needs to be chemically stable in order to withstand the pH changes within the gastrointestinal tract, and it must be resistant to enzymatic degradation in the intestinal lumen.

For most drugs, the optimum site for drug absorption after oral administration is the duodenum region or upper portion of the small intestine. The unique anatomy of the small intestine and duodenum provides an immense surface area for the drug to diffuse passively. The large surface area of the intestine is due to the presence of valve-like folds in the mucous membrane on which are small projections known as "villi." These villi contain even smaller projections known as "microvilli," forming a brush border. Additionally, the duodenal region is highly perfused with a network of capillaries, which help to maintain a concentration gradient from the intestinal lumen and plasma circulation.

Gastric empting time, the presence or absence of food, the range of pH values within the gastrointestinal tract, and luminal enzymes are important factors affecting the plasma concentration profile of orally administered drugs. In addition, the intestinal transit rate also has a significant influence on drug absorption, since it determines the residence time of the drug at the absorption site. Consequently, the gastrointestinal (GI) absorption of orally administered drug is determined not only by the permeability of GI mucosa, but also by the transit rate in the GI tract.[108]

11.7.1 Transit Time

Once a drug is given orally, the exact location and environment of the drug product within the GI tract is difficult to discern. GI motility tends to move the drug through the alimentary canal, so that the drug does not stay at the absorption site for long. The transit time of the drug in the GI tract depends on the physio-chemical and pharmacologic properties of the drug, the type of dosage form, and various physiological factors.[109]

Intestinal propulsive movements will determine intestinal transit rate, and therefore the residence time of a drug in the intestine. Obviously, the greater the intestinal motility, the shorter the residence time, and the less time there is for the propulsive to process the drug. Peristaltic activity is increased after a meal as a result of the GI reflex initiated by distension of the stomach, and results in increased motility and secretion.

GI mixing movements are a result of contractions dividing a given region of the intestine into segments, producing an appearance similar to a chain of sausages. These mixing motions will tend to improve drug absorption, since mixing movement can increase dissolution rate, thereby influencing absorption, and the mixing process can increase the contact area between drug and membrane. Transit through the small intestine appears to be quite different, in a variety of ways, from movement through the stomach. Once emptied from the stomach, drug (such as pellets and tablets) will move along the small intestine and reach the ileocecal valve in about three hours. The transit time appears to be less dependent on the physical nature of the drug, such as liquid versus solid, and size of solids, compared to the response of the stomach. Furthermore, food appears not to influence intestinal transit as it does gastric emptying. There appear to be no gender-related differences in intestinal transit time, while vegetarians appear to have longer intestinal transit times compared to nonvegetarians.[110]

On the other hand, the colonic transit of pharmaceuticals is long and variable, and depends on the types of dosage form, diet, eating pattern, and disease. Contractile activity in the colon can be divided into two main types:

1. propulsive contractions or mass movements, which are associated with the aboral (away from mouth) movement of contents;
2. segmental or haustral contractions, which serve to mix the luminal contents, and result in only small aboral movements.

Segmental contractions are brought about by contraction of the circular muscle and predominate, whereas the propulsive contractions, which are due to contractions of the longitudinal muscle, only occur 3–4 times daily in normal individuals. Colonic transit is thus characterized by short bursts of activity, followed by long periods of stasis. Movement is mainly aboral, i.e., towards the anus. Colonic transit can vary from anything between 2 to 48 hours. In most individuals, mouth-to-anus transit times are longer than 24 hours.[108]

11.7.2 pH

The pH of GI fluids varies considerably along the length of the gastrointestinal tract. Gastric fluid is highly acidic, normally exhibiting a pH within the range 1–3.5 in healthy people in the fasted state. Following the ingestion of a meal, the gastric juice is buffered to a less acidic pH, which is dependent on meal composition. Typical gastric pH values following a meal are in the range 3–7. Depending on meal size, the gastric pH returns to the lower fasted-state values within 2–3 hours. Thus, only a dosage form ingested with or soon after a meal will encounter these higher pH values, which may affect the chemical stability of a drug, drug dissolution or absorption.[108]

The GI pH may influence the chemical stability of the drug in the lumen, its dissolution rate or its absorption, if the drug is a weak electrolyte. Chemical degradation due to pH-dependent hydrolysis can occur in the GI tract. The result of this instability is incomplete bioavailability, as only a fraction of the administered dose reaches the systemic circulation in the form of intact drug.[108]

11.7.3 Food

The presence of food in the GI tract can affect the bioavailability of the drug from an oral drug product. Digested foods contain amino acids, fatty acids, and many nutrients that may affect intestinal pH and solubility of drugs. Some effects of food on the bioavailability of a drug from a drug product include:

1. delay in gastric emptying;
2. stimulation of bile flow;
3. a change in the pH of the GI tract;
4. an increase in splanchnic blood flow;
5. a change in luminal metabolism of the drug substance; and
6. physical or chemical interaction of the meal with the drug product or drug substance.

One needs also to consider interactions between food and drugs other than binding, precipitation, absorption, chelation, changes in gastric and urinary pH, etc. For instance, grapefruit juice may considerably increase peroral bioavailability of many CYP3A4 substrates by reducing intestinal phase I metabolism by up to 3-fold, such as is found for felodipine, nifedipine, nisoldpine, and nitrendipine. Many drugs are transported back from the enterocyte into the gastrointestinal lumen by the P-gp efflux transporter system. However, components of grapefruit juice have higher affinity for P-gp than most drugs, so drug efflux may be inhibited, and bioavailability increases such as found for cyclosporine, vinca alkaloids, digoxin, fexofenadine, and others. Grapefruit juice components also have affinity for the organic anion transport polypeptide (OATP), where they inhibit the influx of drugs transported by this system from the enterocyte to plasma, thus decreasing a drug's bioavailability.[111]

The components of food may interact with drugs, resulting in substantial positive or negative therapeutic effects. This principle also applies to so-called dietary supplements, including botanicals, used for the treatment of numerous medical conditions.

11.7.4 Luminal Enzymes

The primary enzyme found in gastric juice is pepsin. Lipases, amylases, and proteases are secreted from the pancreas into the small intestine in response to ingestion of food. These enzymes are responsible for most nutrient digestion. Pepsins and the proteases are responsible for the degradation of protein and peptide drugs in the lumen. Other drugs that resemble nutrients, such as nucleotides and fatty acids, may also be susceptible to enzymatic degradation. The lipases may also affect the release of drugs from fat/oil-containing dosage forms. Drugs that are esters can also be susceptible to hydrolysis in the lumen. Bacteria, which are mainly localized within the colonic region of the GI tract, also secrete enzymes that have been utilized when designing drugs or dosage forms to target the colon.[108]

11.8 SUMMARY

This chapter presents a general description of all the barriers to oral bioavailability. Barriers to oral bioavailability have several components, including solubility and dissolution rate, absorption, metabolism, and excretion. We have not discussed transport of drugs to target organs, which may also serve as important barriers for drugs to become active in the CNS, tumor cells, and other difficult-to-access organs. Our understanding of the solubility and dissolution behaviors of solids has not changed very much in the last 20 years, in that we cannot predict solubility accurately. On the other hand, we have made great progress in the last 10 years in learning about the transport of drugs, but, unfortunately, more than 90% of human transporters have unknown functions and substrates. Therefore, we remain hopelessly inadequate in our ability to predict drug absorption accurately; the current state is reviewed in the following chapter. Finally, metabolism and excretion of drugs have received considerable attention from regulatory agencies due to drug interaction issues; prediction remains a challenge, especially *in vivo*, where enzymes and transporters may work together. We are hopeful that in the coming decade, we will make significant progress in this area by undertaking system biology, and other multidisciplinary approaches.

References

1. Hwang, S.J., Park, H. & Park, K. (1998). Gastric retentive drug-delivery systems. Critical Reviews in Therapeutic Drug Carrier Systems 15(3), 243–284.
2. Jeong, E.J., Liu, X., Jia, X., Chen, J. & Hu, M. (2005). Coupling of conjugating enzymes and efflux transporters: impact on

bioavailability and drug interactions. Current Drug Metabolism 6(5), 455–468.

3. Hu, M., Cheng, Z. & Zheng, L. (2003). Functional and molecular characterization of rat intestinal prolidase. Pediatric Research 53(6), 905–914.

4. Johnson, B.M., Zhang, P., Schuetz, J.D. & Brouwer, K.L. (2006). Characterization of transport protein expression in multidrug resistance-associated protein (Mrp) 2-deficient rats. Drug metabolism and disposition: The biological fate of chemicals 34(4), 556–562.

5. Klaassen, C.D. & Slitt, A.L. (2005). Regulation of hepatic transporters by xenobiotic receptors. Current Drug Metabolism 6(4), 309–328.

6. Fix, J.A., Engle, K., Porter, P.A., Leppert, P.S., Selk, S.J., Gardner, C.R. & Alexander, J. (1986). Acylcarnitines: drug absorption-enhancing agents in the gastrointestinal tract. The American Journal of Physiology 251(3 Pt 1), G332–340.

7. Nellans, H.N. (1991). (B) Mechanisms of peptide and protein absorption (1) Paracellular intestinal transport: Modulation of absorption. Advanced Drug Delivery Reviews 7(3), 339–364.

8. Lee, V.H.L. & Akira, Y. (1989). Penetration and enzymatic barriers to peptide and protein absorption. Advanced Drug Delivery Reviews 4(2), 171–207.

9. Collington, G.K., Hunter, J., Allen, C.N., Simmons, N.L. & Hirst, B.H. (1992). Polarized efflux of 2',7'-bis(2-carboxyethyl)-5(6)-carboxyfluorescein from cultured epithelial cell monolayers. Biochemical Pharmacology 44(3), 417–424.

10. Inui, K., Yamamoto, M. & Saito, H. (1992). Transepithelial transport of oral cephalosporins by monolayers of intestinal epithelial cell line Caco-2: specific transport systems in apical and basolateral membranes. The Journal of Pharmacology and Experimental Therapeutics 261(1), 195–201.

11. Hidalgo, I.J., Ryan, F.M., Marks, G.J. & Smith, P.L. (1993). pH-dependent transepithelial transport of cephalexin in rabbit intestinal mucosa. International Journal of Pharmacy 98, 83–92.

12. Caroline, H., Gochoco, F.M.R., Miller, J., Smith, P.L. & Hidalgo, I.J. (1994). Uptake and transepithelial transport of the orally absorbed cephalosporin cephalexin, in the human intestinal cell line, Caco-2. International Journal of Pharmaceutics 104(3), 187–202.

13. Hu, M. & Amidon, G.L. (1988). Passive and carrier-mediated intestinal absorption components of captopril. Journal of Pharmaceutical Sciences 77(12), 1007–1011.

14. Dantzig, A.H. & Bergin, L. (1988). Carrier-mediated uptake of cephalexin in human intestinal cells. Biochemical and Biophysical Research Communications 155(2), 1082–1087.

15. Dantzig, A.H., Duckworth, D.C. & Tabas, L.B. (1994). Transport mechanisms responsible for the absorption of loracarbef, cefixime, and cefuroxime axetil into human intestinal Caco-2 cells. Biochimica et Biophysica Acta 1191(1), 7–13.

16. Yang, C.Y., Dantzig, A.H. & Pidgeon, C. (1999). Intestinal peptide transport systems and oral drug availability. Pharmaceutical Research 16(9), 1331–1343.

17. Ganapathy, V. & Leibach, F.H. (1983). Role of pH gradient and membrane potential in dipeptide transport in intestinal and renal brush-border membrane vesicles from the rabbit. Studies with L-carnosine and glycyl-L-proline. The Journal of Biological Chemistry 258(23), 14189–14192.

18. Fei, Y.J., Sugawara, M., Liu, J.C., Li, H.W., Ganapathy, V., Ganapathy, M.E. & Leibach, F.H. (2000). cDNA structure, genomic organization, and promoter analysis of the mouse intestinal peptide transporter PEPT1. Biochimica et Biophysica Acta 1492(1), 145–154.

19. Liang, R., Fei, Y.J., Prasad, P.D., Ramamoorthy, S., Han, H., Yang-Feng, T.L., Hediger, M.A., Ganapathy, V. & Leibach, F.H. (1995). Human intestinal H+/peptide cotransporter. Cloning,

functional expression, and chromosomal localization. The Journal of Biological Chemistry 270(12), 6456–6463.

20. Saito, H., Okuda, M., Terada, T., Sasaki, S. & Inui, K. (1995). Cloning and characterization of a rat H+/peptide cotransporter mediating absorption of beta-lactam antibiotics in the intestine and kidney. The Journal of Pharmacology and Experimental Therapeutics 275(3), 1631–1637.

21. Boll, M., Herget, M., Wagener, M., Weber, W. M., Markovich, D., Biber, J., Clauss, W., Murer, H. & Daniel, H. (1996). Expression cloning and functional characterization of the kidney cortex high-affinity proton-coupled peptide transporter. Proceedings of the National Academy of Sciences of the United States of America, 93(1), 284–289.

22. Ogihara, H., Saito, H., Shin, B.C., Terado, T., Takenoshita, S., Nagamachi, Y., Inui, K. & Takata, K. (1996). Immuno-localization of H+/peptide cotransporter in rat digestive tract. Biochemical and Biophysical Research Communications 220(3), 848–852.

23. Rubio-Aliaga, I., Boll, M. & Daniel, H. (2000). Cloning and characterization of the gene encoding the mouse peptide transporter PEPT2. Biochemical and Biophysical Research Communications 276(2), 734–741.

24. Ramamoorthy, S., Liu, W., Ma, Y.Y., Yang-Feng, T.L., Ganapathy, V. & Leibach, F.H. (1995). Proton/peptide cotransporter (PEPT 2) from human kidney: functional characterization and chromosomal localization. Biochimica et Biophysica Acta 1240(1), 1–4.

25. Terada, T. & Inui, K. (2004). Peptide transporters: Structure, function, regulation and application for drug delivery. Current Drug Metabolism 5(1), 85–94.

26. Terada, T., Sawada, K., Ito, T., Saito, H., Hashimoto, Y. & Inui, K. (2000). Functional expression of novel peptide transporter in renal basolateral membranes. American Journal of Physiology. Renal physiology 279(5), F851–857.

27. Sawada, K., Terada, T., Saito, H. & Inui, K. (2001). Distinct transport characteristics of basolateral peptide transporters between MDCK and Caco-2 cells. Pflügers Archiv: European Journal of Physiology 443(1), 31–37.

28. Hu, M., Subramanian, P., Mosberg, H.I. & Amidon, G.L. (1989). Use of the peptide carrier system to improve the intestinal absorption of L-alpha-methyldopa: carrier kinetics, intestinal permeabilities, and in vitro hydrolysis of dipeptidyl derivatives of L-alpha-methyldopa. Pharmaceutical Research 6(1), 66–70.

29. Nakanishi, T., Tamai, I., Sai, Y., Sasaki, T. & Tsuji, A. (1997). Carrier-mediated transport of oligopeptides in the human fibrosarcoma cell line HT1080. Cancer Research 57(18), 4118–4122.

30. Mann, G.E., Yudilevich, D.L. & Sobrevia, L. (2003). Regulation of amino acid and glucose transporters in endothelial and smooth muscle cells. Physiological Reviews 83(1), 183–252.

31. Qian, X., Vinnakota, S., Edwards, C. & Sarkar, H.K. (2000). Molecular characterization of taurine transport in bovine aortic endothelial cells. Biochimica et Biophysica Acta 1509(1–2), 324–334.

32. Deves, R. & Boyd, C.A. (1998). Transporters for cationic amino acids in animal cells: discovery, structure, and function. Physiological Reviews 78(2), 487–545.

33. Cheeseman, C. (1992). Role of intestinal basolateral membrane in absorption of nutrients. The American Journal of Physiology 263(3 Pt 2), R482–488.

34. Cheeseman, C.I. (1983). Characteristics of lysine transport across the serosal pole of the anuran small intestine. Journal of Physiology 338, 87–97.

35. Hammerman, M.R. (1982). Na+-independent L-arginine transport in rabbit renal brush border membrane vesicles. Biochimica et Biophysica Acta 685(1), 71–77.

36. Hilden, S.A. & Sacktor, B. (1981). L-arginine uptake into renal brush border membrane vesicles. Archives of Biochemistry and Biophysics 210(1), 289–297.

37. Stieger, B., Stange, G., Biber, J. & Murer, H. (1983). Transport of L-lysine by rat renal brush border membrane vesicles. Pflügers Archiv: European Journal of Physiology 397(2), 106–113.

38. You, G. (2004). The role of organic ion transporters in drug disposition: an update. Current Drug Metabolism 5(1), 55–62.

39. Pritchard, J.B. & Miller, D.S. (1993). Mechanisms mediating renal secretion of organic anions and cations. Physiological Reviews 73(4), 765–796.

40. Sweet, D.H. & Pritchard, J.B. (1999). The molecular biology of renal organic anion and organic cation transporters. Cell Biochemistry and Biophysics 31(1), 89–118.

41. Koepsell, H., Gorboulev, V. & Arndt, P. (1999). Molecular pharmacology of organic cation transporters in kidney. The Journal of Membrane Biology 167(2), 103–117.

42. Tamai, I., Yabuuchi, H., Nezu, J., Sai, Y., Oku, A., Shimane, M. & Tsuji, A. (1997). Cloning and characterization of a novel human pH-dependent organic cation transporter, OCTN1. FEBS Letters 419(1), 107–111.

43. Wu, X., George, R.L., Huang, W., Wang, H., Conway, S.J., Leibach, F.H. & Ganapathy, V. (2000). Structural and functional characteristics and tissue distribution pattern of rat OCTN1, an organic cation transporter, cloned from placenta. Biochimica et Biophysica Acta 1466(1–2), 315–327.

44. Tamai, I., Ohashi, R., Nezu, J.I., Sai, Y., Kobayashi, D., Oku, A., Shimane, M. & Tsuji, A. (2000). Molecular and functional characterization of organic cation/carnitine transporter family in mice. The Journal of Biological Chemistry 275(51), 40064–40072.

45. Wu, X., Huang, W., Prasad, P.D., Seth, P., Rajan, D.P., Leibach, F.H., Chen, J., Conway, S.J. & Ganapathy, V. (1999). Functional characteristics and tissue distribution pattern of organic cation transporter 2 (OCTN2), an organic cation/carnitine transporter. The Journal of Pharmacology and Experimental Therapeutics 290(3), 1482–1492.

46. Wu, X., Prasad, P.D., Leibach, F.H. & Ganapathy, V. (1998). cDNA sequence, transport function, and genomic organization of human OCTN2, a new member of the organic cation transporter family. Biochemical and Biophysical Research Communications 246(3), 589–595.

47. Wagner, C.A., Lukewille, U., Kaltenbach, S., Moschen, I., Broer, A., Risler, T., Broer, S. & Lang, F. (2000). Functional and pharmacological characterization of human Na(+)-carnitine cotransporter hOCTN2. American Journal of Physiology. Renal Physiology, 279(3), F584–591.

48. Cattori, V., van Montfoort, J.E., Stieger, B., Landmann, L., Meijer, D.K., Winterhalter, K.H., Meier, P.J. & Hagenbuch, B. (2001). Localization of organic anion transporting polypeptide 4 (Oatp4) in rat liver and comparison of its substrate specificity with Oatp1, Oatp2 and Oatp3. Pflügers Archiv: European Journal of Physiology 443(2), 188–195.

49. Gao, B., Hagenbuch, B., Kullak-Ublick, G.A., Benke, D., Aguzzi, A. & Meier, P.J. (2000). Organic anion-transporting polypeptides mediate transport of opioid peptides across blood-brain barrier. The Journal of Pharmacology and Experimental Therapeutics 294(1), 73–79.

50. Kullak-Ublick, G.A., Ismair, M.G., Stieger, B., Landmann, L., Huber, R., Pizzagalli, F., Fattinger, K., Meier, P.J. & Hagenbuch, B. (2001). Organic anion-transporting polypeptide B (OATP-B) and its functional comparison with three other OATPs of human liver. Gastroenterology 120(2), 525–533.

51. Nozawa, T., Tamai, I., Sai, Y., Nezu, J. & Tsuji, A. (2003). Contribution of organic anion transporting polypeptide OATP-C to hepatic elimination of the opioid pentapeptide analogue [D-Ala2, D-Leu5]-enkephalin. The Journal of Pharmacy and Pharmacology 55(7), 1013–1020.

52. Lee, W., Glaeser, H., Smith, L.H., Roberts, R.L., Moeckel, G.W., Gervasini, G., Leake, B.F. & Kim, R.B. (2005). Polymorphisms in human organic anion-transporting polypeptide 1A2 (OATP1A2): Implications for altered drug disposition and central nervous system drug entry. The Journal of Biological Chemistry 280(10), 9610–9617.

53. Reichel, C., Gao, B., Van Montfoort, J., Cattori, V., Rahner, C., Hagenbuch, B., Stieger, B., Kamisako, T. & Meier, P.J. (1999). Localization and function of the organic anion-transporting polypeptide Oatp2 in rat liver. Gastroenterology 117(3), 688–695.

54. Konig, J., Cui, Y., Nies, A.T. & Keppler, D. (2000). Localization and genomic organization of a new hepatocellular organic anion transporting polypeptide. The Journal of Biological Chemistry 275(30), 23161–23168.

55. Konig, J., Cui, Y., Nies, A.T. & Keppler, D. (2000). A novel human organic anion transporting polypeptide localized to the basolateral hepatocyte membrane. American Journal of Physiology. Gastrointestinal and Liver Physiology 278(1), G156–164.

56. Kong, W., Engel, K. & Wang, J. (2004). Mammalian nucleoside transporters. Current Drug Metabolism 5(1), 63–84.

57. Griffith, D.A. & Jarvis, S.M. (1996). Nucleoside and nucleobase transport systems of mammalian cells. Biochimica et Biophysica Acta 1286(3), 153–181.

58. Cabrita, M.A., Baldwin, S.A., Young, J.D. & Cass, C.E. (2002). Molecular biology and regulation of nucleoside and nucleobase transporter proteins in eukaryotes and prokaryotes. Biochemistry and Cell Biology (Biochimie et Biologie Cellulaire) 80(5), 623–638.

59. Sue Masters, B. & Marohnic, C.C. (2006). Cytochromes P450—a family of proteins and scientists-understanding their relationships. Drug Metabolism Reviews 38(1–2), 209–225.

60. Jakoby, W.B. (1981). Detoxication and Drug Metabolism: Conjugation and Related Systems. Academic Press, New York. p. xxii.

61. Testa, B. & Jenner, P. (1976). Drug Metabolism: Chemical and Biochemical Aspects. Marcel Dekker, New York. p. xiii.

62. Numa, S.O. (1984). Fatty Acid Metabolism and its Regulation. Elsevier, Amsterdam New York. p. xi.

63. Liu, Y. & Hu, M. (2002). Absorption and metabolism of flavonoids in the caco-2 cell culture model and a perused rat intestinal model. Drug Metabolism and Disposition: The Biological Fate of Chemicals 30(4), 370–377.

64. Liu, Y., Liu, Y., Dai, Y., Xun, L. & Hu, M. (2003). Enteric disposition and recycling of flavonoids and ginkgo flavonoids. Journal of Alternative and Complementary Medicine 9(5), 631–640.

65. Conley, A. & Hinshelwood, M. (2001). Mammalian aromatases. Reproduction 121(5), 685–695.

66. Fisher, M.B., Campanale, K., Ackermann, B.L., VandenBranden, M. & Wrighton, S.A. (2000). In vitro glucuronidation using human liver microsomes and the pore-forming peptide alamethicin. Drug Metabolism and Disposition: The Biological Fate of Chemicals 28(5), 366–560.

67. Guengerich, F.P. (2006). Cytochrome P450s and other enzymes in drug metabolism and toxicity. The AAPS Journal 8(1), E101–111.

68. Dervieux, T., Meshkin, B. & Neri, B. (2005). Pharmacogenetic testing: Proofs of principle and pharmacoeconomic implications. Mutation Research 573(1–2), 180–194.

69. Bischoff, S.C. (2006). Food allergies. Current Gastroenterology Reports 8(5), 374–382.

70. Chen, J., Lin, H. & Hu, M. (2003). Metabolism of flavonoids via enteric recycling: Role of intestinal disposition. The Journal of Pharmacology and Experimental Therapeutics 304(3), 1228–1235.

71. Hu, M., Krausz, K., Chen, J., Ge, X., Li, J., Gelboin, H.L. & Gonzalez, F.J. (2003). Identification of CYP1A2 as the main isoform for the phase I hydroxylated metabolism of genistein and a prodrug converting enzyme of methylated isoflavones. Drug

Metabolism and Disposition: The Biological Fate of Chemicals 31(7), 924–931.

72. Wang, S.W., Chen, J., Jia, X., Tam, V.H. & Hu, M. (2006). Disposition of flavonoids via enteric recycling: Structural effects and lack of correlations between *in vitro* and *in situ* metabolic properties. Drug Metabolism and Disposition: The Biological Fate of Chemicals.

73. Mackenzie, P.I., Walter Bock, K., Burchell, B., Guillemette, C., Ikushiro, S., Iyanagi, T., Miners, J.O., Owens, I.S. & Nebert, D.W. (2005). Nomenclature update for the mammalian UDP glycosyltransferase (UGT) gene superfamily. Pharmacogenet Genomics 15(10), 677–685.

74. Burchell, B., Brierley, C.H. & Rance, D. (1995). Specificity of human UDP-glucuronosyltransferases and xenobiotic glucuronidation. Life Science 57(20), 1819–1831.

75. Gamage, N., Barnett, A., Hempel, N., Duggleby, R.G., Windmill, K. F., Martin, J.L. & McManus, M.E. (2006). Human sulfotransferases and their role in chemical metabolism. Toxicological Sciences: An Official Journal of The Society of Toxicology 90(1), 5–22.

76. Nimmagadda, D., Cherala, G. & Ghatta, S. (2006). Cytosolic sulfotransferases. Indian Journal of Experimental Biology 44(3), 171–182.

77. Walle, T., Hsieh, F., DeLegge, M.H., Oatis, J.E., Jr. & Walle, U.K. (2004). High absorption but very low bioavailability of oral resveratrol in humans. Drug Metabolism and Disposition: The Biological Fate of Chemicals 32(12), 1377–1382.

78. Coles, B.F. & Kadlubar, F.F. (2003). Detoxification of electrophilic compounds by glutathione S-transferase catalysis: Determinants of individual response to chemical carcinogens and chemotherapeutic drugs? Biofactors 17(1–4), 115–130.

79. Hayes, J.D., Flanagan, J.U. & Jowsey, I.R. (2005). Glutathione transferases. Annual Review of Pharmacology and Toxicology 45, 51–88.

80. Haga, S.B., Thummel, K.E. & Burke, W. (2006). Adding pharmacogenetics information to drug labels: Lessons learned. Pharmacogenet Genomics 16(12), 847–854.

81. Kessel, D., Botterill, V. & Wodinsky, I. (1968). Uptake and retention of daunomycin by mouse leukemic cells as factors in drug response. Cancer Research 28(5), 938–941.

82. Gottesman, M.M. & Ling, V. (2006). The molecular basis of multidrug resistance in cancer: the early years of P-glycoprotein research. FEBS Letters 580(4), 998–1009.

83. Hyde, S.C., Emsley, P., Hartshorn, M.J., Mimmack, M. M., Gileadi, U., Pearce, S.R., Gallagher, M.P., Gill, D.R., Hubbard, R.E. & Higgins, C.F. (1990). Structural model of ATP-binding proteins associated with cystic fibrosis, multidrug resistance and bacterial transport. Nature 346(6282), 362–365.

84. Evans, A.M. (2000). Influence of dietary components on the gastrointestinal metabolism and transport of drugs. Therapeutic Drug Monitoring 22(1), 131–136.

85. Hunter, J., Hirst, B.H. & Simmons, N.L. (1991). Epithelial secretion of vinblastine by human intestinal adenocarcinoma cell (HCT-8 and T84) layers expressing P-glycoprotein. British Journal of Cancer 64(3), 437–444.

86. Schinkel, A.H., Mayer, U., Wagenaar, E., Mol, C.A., van Deemter, L., Smit, J.J., van der Valk, M.A., Voordouw, A.C., Spits, H., van Tellingen, O., Zijlmans, J.M., Fibbe, W.E. & Borst, P. (1997). Normal viability and altered pharmacokinetics in mice lacking mdr1-type (drug-transporting) P-glycoproteins. Proceedings of the National Academy of Sciences of the United States of America 94(8), 4028–4033.

87. Cole, S.P., Bhardwaj, G., Gerlach, J.H., Mackie, J.E., Grant, C.E., Almquist, K.C., Stewart, A.J., Kurz, E.U., Duncan, A.M. & Deeley, R.G. (1992). Overexpression of a transporter gene in a multidrug-resistant human lung cancer cell line. Science 258(5088), 1650–1654.

88. Buchler, M., Konig, J., Brom, M., Kartenbeck, J., Spring, H., Horie, T. & Keppler, D. (1996). cDNA cloning of the hepatocyte canalicular isoform of the multidrug resistance protein, cMrp, reveals a novel conjugate export pump deficient in hyperbilirubinemic mutant rats. The Journal of Biological Chemistry 271(25), 15091–15098.

89. Paulusma, C.C., Bosma, P.J., Zaman, G.J., Bakker, C.T., Otter, M., Scheffer, G.L., Scheper, R.J., Borst, P. & Oude Elferink, R.P. (1996). Congenital jaundice in rats with a mutation in a multidrug resistance-associated protein gene. Science 271(5252), 1126–1128.

90. Belinsky, M.G. & Kruh, G.D. (1999). MOAT-E (ARA) is a full-length MRP/cMOAT subfamily transporter expressed in kidney and liver. British Journal of Cancer 80(9), 1342–1349.

91. Stride, B.D., Grant, C.E., Loe, D.W., Hipfner, D.R., Cole, S.P. & Deeley, R.G. (1997). Pharmacological characterization of the murine and human orthologs of multidrug-resistance protein in transfected human embryonic kidney cells. Molecular Pharmacology 52(3), 344–353.

92. de Jong, M.C., Slootstra, J.W., Scheffer, G.L., Schroeijers, A. B., Puijk, W.C., Dinkelberg, R., Kool, M., Broxterman, H.J., Meloen, R.H. & Scheper, R.J. (2001). Peptide transport by the multidrug resistance protein MRP1. Cancer Research 61(6), 2552–2557.

93. Cole, S.P., Sparks, K.E., Fraser, K., Loe, D.W., Grant, C.E., Wilson, G.M. & Deeley, R.G. (1994). Pharmacological characterization of multidrug resistant MRP-transfected human tumor cells. Cancer Research 54(22), 5902–5910.

94. Kawabe, T., Chen, Z.S., Wada, M., Uchiumi, T., Ono, M., Akiyama, S. & Kuwano, M. (1999). Enhanced transport of anticancer agents and leukotriene C4 by the human canalicular multispecific organic anion transporter (cMOAT/MRP2). FEBS Letters 456(2), 327–331.

95. Paulusma, C.C. & Oude Elferink, R.P. (1997). The canalicular multispecific organic anion transporter and conjugated hyperbilirubinemia in rat and man. Journal of Molecular Medicine 75(6), 420–428.

96. Sekine, T., Watanabe, N., Hosoyamada, M., Kanai, Y. & Endou, H. (1997). Expression cloning and characterization of a novel multispecific organic anion transporter. The Journal of Biological Chemistry 272(30), 18526–18529.

97. Sweet, D.H., Wolff, N.A. & Pritchard, J.B. (1997). Expression cloning and characterization of ROAT1. The basolateral organic anion transporter in rat kidney. The Journal of Biological Chemistry 272(48), 30088–30095.

98. Moller, J.V. & Sheikh, M.I. (1982). Renal organic anion transport system: pharmacological, physiological, and biochemical aspects. Pharmacological Reviews 34(4), 315–358.

99. Sweet, D.H., Bush, K.T. & Nigam, S.K. (2001). The organic anion transporter family: from physiology to ontogeny and the clinic. American Journal of Physiology. Renal Physiology 281(2), F197–205.

100. Deguchi, T., Kusuhara, H., Takadate, A., Endou, H., Otagiri, M. & Sugiyama, Y. (2004). Characterization of uremic toxin transport by organic anion transporters in the kidney. Kidney International 65(1), 162–174.

101. Benet, L.Z., Cummins, C.L. & Wu, C.Y. (2004). Unmasking the dynamic interplay between efflux transporters and metabolic enzymes. International Journal of Pharmaceutics 277(1–2), 3–9.

102. Cummins, C.L., Jacobsen, W. & Benet, L.Z. (2002). Unmasking the dynamic interplay between intestinal P-glycoprotein and CYP3A4. The Journal of Pharmacology and Experimental Therapeutics 300(3), 1036–1045.

103. Coldham, N.G., Zhang, A.Q., Key, P. & Sauer, M.J. (2002). Absolute bioavailability of [^{14}C] genistein in the rat; plasma

pharmacokinetics of parent compound, genistein glucuronide and total radioactivity. European Journal of Drug Metabolism and Pharmacokinetics 27(4), 249–258.

104. Setchell, K.D., Brown, N.M., Desai, P.B., Zimmer-Nechimias, L., Wolfe, B., Jakate, A.S., Creutzinger, V. & Heubi, J.E. (2003). Bioavailability, disposition, and dose-response effects of soy isoflavones when consumed by healthy women at physiologically typical dietary intakes. The Journal of Nutrition 133(4), 1027–1035.

105. Lipinski, C.A. (2003). Chris Lipinski discusses life and chemistry after the Rule of Five. Drug Discovery Today 8(1), 12–16.

106. Remko, M., Swart, M. & Bickelhaupt, F.M. (2006). Theoretical study of structure, pKa, lipophilicity, solubility, absorption, and polar surface area of some centrally acting antihypertensives. Bioorganic & Medicinal Chemistry 14(6), 1715–1728.

107. Wenlock, M.C., Austin, R.P., Barton, P., Davis, A.M. & Leeson, P.D. (2003). A comparison of physiochemical property profiles of development and marketed oral drugs. Journal of Medicinal Chemistry 46(7), 1250–1256.

108. Aulton, M.E. & Cooper, J.W. (1988). *Pharmaceutics: The Science of Dosage Form Design*, 1st edn. Churchill Livingstone, Edinburgh, New York. p. xv, p. 734.

109. Kimura, T. & Higaki, K. (2002). Gastrointestinal transit and drug absorption. Biological & Pharmaceutical Bulletin 25(2), 149–164.

110. Shargel, L., Wu-Pong, S. & Yu, A.B.C. (2005). *Applied Biopharmaceutics & Pharmacokinetics*, 5th edn. McGraw-Hill, Medical Pub., Division, New York. p. xx, p. 892.

111. Ritschel, W.A. & Kearns, G.L. (2004). American Pharmaceutical Association. In: *Handbook of Basic Pharmacokinetics—Including Clinical Applications*, 6th edn. American Pharmacists Association, Washington, DC. p. xii.

12

Oral Drug Absorption, Evaluation, and Prediction

Yongsheng Yang and Lawrence X. Yu

12.1 INTRODUCTION

A very important question during drug discovery and development is probably whether a drug will be bioavailable after its oral administration. Good oral bioavailability generally facilitates formulation design and development, reduces intra-subject variability, and enhances dosing flexibility. Oral bioavailability can be mathematically represented by the equation:

$$F = F_a \times F_g \times F_h$$

where:

F_a is the fraction of drug absorbed
F_g is the fraction that escapes metabolism in the gastrointestinal tract
F_h is the fraction that escapes the hepatic metabolism.

Therefore, oral drug absorption is one of the main factors governing the bioavailability of drugs. The absorption of drugs from the gastrointestinal tract is largely controlled by:

1. dissolution rate and solubility, which determine how fast a drug reaches a maximum concentration in the luminal intestinal fluid; and
2. intestinal permeability, which relates to the rate at which dissolved drug will cross the intestinal wall to reach the portal blood circulation.

The determination of the dissolution, solubility, and permeability properties of drugs can thus provide information about their absorption. This chapter will

focus on these properties. It begins with a discussion of the Biopharmaceutical Classification System (BCS). It then proceeds with the introduction of techniques available to evaluate intestinal permeability, and the mathematical models to predict oral drug absorption. It is concluded with a discussion of future trends in oral drug absorption evaluation and prediction.

12.2 BIOPHARMACEUTICS CLASSIFICATION SYSTEM (BCS)

The BCS is a scientific framework for classifying a drug substance based on its aqueous solubility and intestinal permeability.[1] According to this system, drug substances can be classified into four groups:

1. high solubility–high permeability;
2. low solubility–high permeability;
3. high solubility–low permeability; and
4. low solubility–low permeability (Table 12.1).

When combined with the *in vitro* dissolution characteristics of the drug product, the BCS considers three major factors: solubility, intestinal permeability, and dissolution rate, all of which govern the rate and extent of oral absorption from immediate-release (IR) solid oral dosage forms. Since the introduction

---

*The opinions expressed in this report by the authors do not necessarily reflect the views or policies of the Food and Drug Administration (FDA).

TABLE 12.1   Biopharmaceutics classification system

Biopharmaceutics class	Solubility	Permeability
I	High	High
II	Low	High
III	High	Low
IV	Low	Low

of the BCS, its validity and applicability have been the subject of extensive research and discussion.[2–5] The BCS framework has implications in the selection of candidate drugs for full development, prediction, and elucidation of food interaction, choice of formulation principle, including suitability for oral extended-release administration, and the possibility of *in vitro/in vivo* correlation in the dissolution testing of solid formulations.[3,6–7] The regulatory applications of BCS are demonstrated by an improved SUPAC-IR guidance,[8] a dissolution guidance,[9] and a Food and Drug Administration (FDA) guidance on waiver of *in vivo* bioequivalence studies for BCS class I drugs in rapid dissolution immediate-release solid oral dosage forms.[10]

12.2.1 FDA Guidance on Biowaivers

In August 2000 the FDA issued a guidance for industry on waivers of *in vivo* bioavailability (BA), and bioequivalence (BE) studies, for IR solid oral dosage forms based on the BCS.[10] This guidance provides recommendations for sponsors of investigational new drug applications (INDs), new drug applications (NDAs), abbreviated new drug applications (ANDAs), and supplements to these applications who may request biowaivers for highly soluble and highly permeable drug substances (class I) in IR solid oral dosage forms that exhibit rapid *in vitro* dissolution, provided the following conditions are met:

1. the drug must be stable in the gastrointestinal tract;
2. excipients used in the IR solid oral dosage forms have no significant effect on the rate and extent of oral drug absorption;
3. the drug must not have a narrow therapeutic index; and
4. the product is designed not to be absorbed in the oral cavity.

The guidance also outlines methods for determination of solubility, permeability, and dissolution.

Determination of Solubility Classification

According to the BCS approach, the equilibrium solubility of a drug substance under physiological pH conditions needs to be determined. The pH-solubility profile of the test drug substance should be established at $37 \pm 1°C$ in aqueous media with a pH in the range of 1–7.5. The number of pH conditions for a solubility determination can be based on the ionization characteristics of the test drug substance. For example, when the pKa of a drug is in the range of 3–5, solubility should be determined at pH = pKa, pH = pKa + 1, pH = pKa − 1, and at pH = 1, and 7.5. A minimum of three replicate determinations of solubility at each pH condition is recommended. Standard buffer solutions described in the United States Pharmacopeia (USP) can be used for solubility studies.[11] If these buffers are not suitable for physical or chemical reasons, other buffer solutions can be used. It is necessary to verify the solution pH after the equilibrium has been reached. Methods other than the traditional shake–flask method, such as acid or base titration methods, can also be used with justification to support the ability of such methods to predict equilibrium solubility of the test drug substance. A validated stability-indicating assay should be used to determine the concentration of the drug substance in selected buffers. A drug substance is considered highly soluble when the highest dose strength is soluble in 250 ml or less of aqueous media over the pH range of 1.0–7.5, otherwise, the drug substance is considered poorly soluble. The volume estimate of 250 ml is derived from typical BE study protocols that prescribe administration of a drug product to fasting human volunteers with a glass (about 8 ounces or 250 mL) of water.

Determination of Drug Substance Permeability

The permeability classification is based directly on measurements of the rate of mass transfer across human intestinal membrane, and indirectly on the extent of absorption (fraction of dose absorbed, not systemic BA) of a drug substance in humans. The FDA biowaiver guidance[10] cites the use of human pharmacokinetic studies, and intestinal permeability methods, as acceptable methods to determine permeability classification. In many cases, a single method may be sufficient. When a single method fails to conclusively demonstrate a permeability classification, two different methods may be advisable. In the absence of evidence suggesting instability in the gastrointestinal tract, a drug substance is considered to be highly permeable when the extent of absorption in humans is 90% or more, based on a mass balance determination or in comparison to an intravenous reference dose. Otherwise, the drug substance is considered to be poorly permeable.

Mass balance and absolute bioavailability studies

In mass balance studies, unlabeled, stable isotopes or a radiolabeled drug substance are used to determine the extent of absorption of a drug. A sufficient number of subjects should be enrolled to provide a reliable estimate of extent of absorption. Due to the highly variable outcomes for many drugs, this method is less preferable.

Oral BA determination using intravenous administration as a reference can be used. Depending on the variability of the studies, a sufficient number of subjects should be enrolled in a study to provide a reliable estimate of the extent of absorption. When the absolute BA of a drug is shown to be 90% or more, additional data to document drug stability in the gastrointestinal fluid is not necessary.

Intestinal permeability

The FDA biowaiver guidance[10] recommends that the following methods be considered appropriate to determine the permeability of a drug substance from the gastrointestinal tract for passively transported drugs:

1. *in vivo* human intestinal perfusion;
2. *in vivo* or *in situ* animal intestinal perfusion;
3. *in vitro* permeation studies using excised human or animal intestinal tissues; or
4. *in vitro* permeation studies across a monolayer of cultured epithelial cells.

An apparent passive transport mechanism can be assumed when one of the following conditions is satisfied:

1. a linear pharmacokinetic relationship between the relevant clinical dose range and the area under the concentration–time curve (AUC) of a drug is demonstrated in humans;
2. lack of dependence on initial drug concentration in the perfusion fluid for the *in vivo* or *in situ* permeability is demonstrated in an animal model; and
3. lack of dependence of the measured *in vitro* permeability on initial drug concentration is demonstrated in donor fluid and transport direction, using a suitable *in vitro* cell culture method.

To demonstrate suitability of a permeability method intended for application of the BCS, a rank-order relationship between test permeability values and the extent of drug absorption data in human subjects should be established using a sufficient number of model drugs. The model drugs should represent a range of low (e.g., <50%), moderate (e.g., 50–89%), and high (>90%) absorption, and should have available information on mechanism of absorption and reliable estimates of the extent of drug absorption in humans. For *in vivo* intestinal perfusion studies in humans, six model drugs are recommended. For *in vivo* or *in situ* intestinal perfusion studies in animals and for *in vitro* cell culture methods, twenty model drugs are recommended.

After demonstrating suitability of a method, and maintaining the same study protocol, it is not necessary to retest all selected model drugs for subsequent studies intended to classify a drug substance. Instead, a low and a high permeability model drug should be used as internal standards. These two internal standards, in addition to the fluid volume marker (or a zero permeability compound such as PEG 4000), should be included in permeability studies. The choice of internal standards should be based on compatibility with the test drug substance (i.e., they should not exhibit any significant physical, chemical or permeation interactions). The model drugs suggested for use in establishing suitability of a permeability method are listed in Table 12.2. When it is not feasible to follow this protocol, the permeability of internal standards should be determined in the same subjects, animals, tissues or monolayers, following evaluation of the test drug substance. The permeability values of the two internal standards should not differ significantly between different tests, including those conducted to demonstrate suitability of the method. At the end of an *in situ* or *in vitro* test, the amount of drug in the membrane should be determined.

Comparison of Dissolution Profile[12]

In the BCS guidance, an IR drug product is considered rapidly-dissolving when no less than 85% of the labeled amount of the drug substance dissolves within 30 minutes, using USP Apparatus I at 100 rpm (or Apparatus II at 50 rpm) in a volume of 900 ml or less in each of the following media:

1. 0.1 N HCl or simulated gastric fluid without enzymes;
2. a pH 4.5 buffer; and
3. a pH 6.8 buffer or simulated intestinal fluid without enzymes.

Otherwise, the drug product is considered to be a slow-dissolution product.

According to the scientific principles of the BCS, the *in vivo* differences in drug dissolution may be

TABLE 12.2 The model drugs suggested for use in establishing suitability of a permeability method. Potential internal standards (IS), and efflux pump substrates (ES) are identified

Drugs	Permeability class
Antipyrine	High (potential IS candidate)
Caffeine	High
Carbamazepine	High
Fluvastatin	High
Ketoprofen	High
Labetalol	High (potential IS candidate)
Metoprolol	High (potential IS candidate)
Naproxen	High
Theophylline	High
Verapamil	High (potential ES candidate)
Amoxicillin	Low
Atenolol	Low
Furosemide	Low
Hydrochlorthiazide	Low
Mannitol	Low (potential IS candidate)
α-Methyldopa	Low
Polyethylene glycol (400)	Low
Polyethylene glycol (1000)	Low
Polyethylene glycol (4000)	Low (zero permeability marker)
Ranitidine	Low

(Do) is characterized by the volume required for solubilizing the maximum dose strength of the drug:

$$\mathrm{Do} = \frac{M/Vo}{C_s} \qquad (12.1)$$

where:

C_s is the solubility
M is the dose
Vo is the volume of water taken with the dose, which is generally set to 250 mL.

Dissolution number (Dn) is characterized by the time required for drug dissolution, which is the ratio of the intestinal residence time (t_{res}), and the dissolution time (t_{diss}):

$$\mathrm{Dn} = \frac{t_{res}}{t_{diss}} = \frac{3DC_s}{r^2\rho} \times t_{res} \qquad (12.2)$$

where:

D is diffusivity
ρ is density
r is the initial particle radius.

Absorption number (An) is characterized by the time required for absorption of the dose administered, which is a ratio of residence time and absorptive time (t_{abs}):

$$\mathrm{An} = \frac{t_{res}}{t_{abs}} = \frac{P_{eff}}{R} \times t_{res} \qquad (12.3)$$

where:

P_{eff} is the permeability
R is the gut radius.

Drugs with complete absorption show Do <1, while Dn and An >1. This approach is used to set up a theoretical basis for correlating *in vitro* drug product dissolution with *in vivo* absorption.[1] To follow the movement of a dosage form through the GI tract, the entire process needs to be broken down into several component parts, in order to see it mechanistically. The fundamental starting point is to apply Fick's first law to the absorption across the intestinal membrane:

$$J_w = P_w \times C_w \qquad (12.4)$$

where:

J_w (x, y, z, t) is the drug flux (mass/area/time) through the intestinal wall at any position and time. P_w (x, y, z, t) is permeability of intestinal membrane and C_w (x, y, z, t) is the drug concentration at the intestinal membrane surface.

This equation is a local law pertaining to each point along the intestinal membrane. It is assumed that sink conditions (drug concentration equals zero) exist, and

translated into the *in vivo* differences in drug absorption. If the *in vivo* dissolution is rapid in relation to gastric emptying, oral drug absorption is likely to be independent of drug dissolution. Therefore, similar to oral solutions, demonstration of *in vivo* bioequivalence may not be necessary, as long as the inactive ingredients used in the dosage form do not significantly affect the absorption of drugs. Thus, for BCS class I (high solubility/high permeability) drug substances, demonstration of rapid *in vitro* dissolution using the recommended test methods would provide sufficient assurance of rapid *in vivo* dissolution, thereby assuring human *in vivo* bioequivalence.

12.2.2 Scientific Basis for BCS

The key parameters controlling drug absorption are three dimensionless numbers: dose number, dissolution number, and absorption number, representing the fundamental processes of membrane permeation, drug dissolution, and dose, respectively. Dose number

that P_w is an effective permeability. The plasma may be assumed to be the physiological sink, since concentrations in the plasma are generally several orders of magnitude lower than that in the intestinal lumen in humans.[13] The drug absorption rate, i.e., the rate of loss of drug from the intestinal lumen, assuming no luminal reactions, at any time is:

$$\text{Absorption rate} = \frac{dm}{dt} = \iint_A P_w C_w dA \qquad (12.5)$$

Where: the double integral is over the entire gastro-intestinal surface. The total mass, M, of drug absorbed at time t is:

$$M(t) = \int_0^t \iint_A P_w C_w dA dt \qquad (12.6)$$

These mass balance relations are very general, since the surface can be of arbitrary shape, and the concentration at the membrane wall, and permeability, can have any dependence on position and time. For full generality the permeability Pw must be considered to be position-dependent as well as time-dependent.

Based on Equations 12.5 and 12.6 above, the following principle for bioavailability may be stated that if two drug products, containing the same drug, have the same concentration time profile at the intestinal membrane surface then they will have the same rate and extent of absorption. This statement may further imply that if two drug products have the same *in vivo* dissolution profile under all luminal conditions, they will have the same rate and extent of drug absorption. These general principles assume that there are no other components in the formulation that affect the membrane permeability and/or intestinal transit. Accordingly, the fraction absorbed (F) of a solution follows an exponential function, and can be calculated by the following equation.[14]

$$F = 1 - e^{-2An} \qquad (12.7)$$

To establish *in vitro/in vivo* correlation (IVIVC), several factors have to be considered. These *in vitro* dissolution tests can only model the release and dissolution rates of the drug, and it is only when these processes are rate-limiting in the overall absorption that IVIVC can be established.[7] For class I drugs, the complete dose will be dissolved already in the stomach and, provided that the absorption in the stomach is negligible, the gastric emptying will be rate-limiting, and therefore IVIVC is not expected. Thus, *in vitro* dissolution testing can be expected to be "over-discriminating" for these drugs, since tablets showing different *in vitro* dissolution profiles will provide the same rate and extent of BA.[15] Class II drugs are expected to have a dissolution-limited absorption,

and an IVIVC can be established using a well-designed *in vitro* dissolution test. But the IVIVC will not be likely for class II drugs if absorption is limited by the saturation solubility in the gastrointestinal tract, rather than by the dissolution rate.[16] In this situation, the drug concentration in the gastrointestinal tract will be close to the saturation solubility, and changes in the dissolution rate will not affect the plasma concentration profile or the *in vivo* BA. The absorption of class III drugs is limited by their intestinal permeability, and no IVIVC should be expected. However, when the drug dissolution becomes slower than the gastric emptying, a reduction of the extent of BA will be found at slower dissolution rates, since the time during which the drug is available for transport across the small intestinal barrier will then be reduced. The class IV drugs present significant problems for effective oral delivery. Very limited or no IVIVC is expected.

12.3 INTESTINAL PERMEABILITY EVALUATION: CULTURED CELLS

Successful design of orally bioavailable molecules requires that the molecules:

1. be stable to chemical and enzymatic degradation (e.g., within the intestinal lumen, intestinal wall, liver, and circulation);
2. be able to traverse the intestinal epithelial barrier to the portal circulation; and
3. can pass through the liver, and enter the systemic circulation intact at a concentration sufficient to elicit the appropriate pharmacologic response.

Various methodologies can be used for evaluation of intestinal permeability and drug absorption; each has advantages and disadvantages. Therefore, it is the judicious use of these techniques that can help identify drug candidates that will be well-absorbed in humans.

Numerous *in vitro* methods have been used in the drug selection process for assessing the intestinal absorption potential of drug candidates. Compared to *in vivo* absorption studies, evaluation of intestinal permeability *in vitro*:

1. requires less compound;
2. is relatively easier and, in the case of segmental absorption studies, avoids complicated surgery and maintenance of surgically prepared animals;
3. is more rapid and has the potential to reduce animal usage since a number of variables can be examined in each experiment;
4. provides insights into the mechanisms (e.g., carrier-mediated versus passive) routes

(e.g., transcellular versus paracellular), and segmental differences (e.g., small versus large intestine) involved in transepithelial transport; and

5. is analytically more simple because compounds are being analyzed in an aqueous buffer solution as opposed to whole blood or plasma.

However, one universal issue with all the *in vitro* systems is that the effect of physiological factors, such as gastric emptying rate, gastrointestinal transit rate, gastrointestinal pH, etc., cannot be incorporated into the data interpretation.

Each *in vitro* method has its distinct advantages and drawbacks. Based on the specific goal, one or more of these methods can be used as a screening tool for selecting compounds during the drug discovery process. The successful application of *in vitro* models to predict drug absorption across the intestinal mucosa depends on how closely the *in vitro* model mimics the characteristics of the *in vivo* intestinal epithelium. Although it is very difficult to develop a single *in vitro* system that can simulate all the conditions existing in the human intestine, various *in vitro* systems are used routinely as decision-making tools in early drug discovery.

Various cell monolayer models that mimic *in vivo* intestinal epithelium in humans have been developed and widely used. The cell lines are now routinely cultivated as monolayers for studies of the transepethelial transport of drugs. The examples of some selected cell culture models are summarized in Table 12.3.

12.3.1 Caco-2 cells

The Caco-2 cell line was first isolated in the 1970s from a human colon adenocarcinoma.[17] During growth Caco-2 cells go through processes of proliferation, confluency, and differentiation.[18] When grown under standard conditions on semipermeable membranes, fully differentiated Caco-2 cells are very similar to normal enterocytes with regard to their morphological characteristics. Primarily, they have functional tight junctions, and they develop apical and basolateral domains and brush border cytoskeleton. Because the permeation characteristics of drugs across Caco-2 cell monolayers correlate with their human intestinal mucosa permeation characteristics,[18] it has been suggested that Caco-2 cells can be used to predict the oral absorption of drugs in humans. In the past decade, there has been a dramatic increase in the use of Caco-2 cells as a rapid *in vitro* screening tool in support of drug discovery within the pharmaceutical industry, as well as in the mechanistic studies.[18–22]

As reported,[19,23] the Caco-2 cells are usually grown in culture T-flasks (75 cm^2 or 175 cm^2), in a CO$_2$ incubator at 37°C, and 5% CO$_2$. The culture medium is Dulbecco's Modified Eagle Medium (DMEM), supplemented by 0.1 mM nonessential amino acids, 100 U/mL penicillin, 0.1 g/mL streptomycin, 10 mM sodium bicarbonate, and 10% fetal bovine serum (FBS). At a confluency of 70%–80% the cells are split at a ratio of 1:3 to 1:5. For use in the transport experiments, the cells are harvested with trypsin-EDTA, and seeded on polycarbonate filters (0.4 μm pore size, 1.13 cm^2 growth area) inside Transwell® cell culture chambers at a density of approximately 75 000 cells/cm^2 (Figure 12.1). The culture medium is refreshed every 24 to 48 hrs. Transport studies are usually done after 21 days in culture, when expression of transporters, e.g., P-glycoprotein (P-gp), reaches its maximum.[24]

To assure the integrity of the monolayer during the course of the experiment, quality control was done by measuring the transepithelial electrical resistance

TABLE 12.3   Cultured cells commonly used for permeability assessment

Cell type	Species or origin	Special characteristics
Caco-2	Human colon adenocarcinoma	Most well-established and frequently used cell model Differentiates and expresses some relevant efflux transporters Expression of influx transporters is variable (laboratory to laboratory)
MDCK	Madin-Darby canine kidney epithelial cells	Polarized cells with low intrinsic expression of ATP-binding cassette(ABC) transporters Ideal for transfections
LLC-PK1	Pig kidney epithelial cells	Polarized cells with low intrinsic transporter expression Ideal for transfections
2/4/A1	Rat fetal intestinal epithelia cell	Temperature-sensitive Ideal for paracellularly absorbed compounds (leakier pores)
TC-7	Caco-2 subclone	Similar to Caco-2
HT-29	Human colon	Contains mucus-producing goblet cells
IEC-18	Rat small intestine cell line	Provides a size-selective barrier for paracellularly transported compounds

(TEER) values, and the permeability of mannitol. Caco-2 cells with TEER value greater than $250\,\Omega \times cm^2$ (24 wells) were used in the study. Caco-2 permeability of ^{14}C- or ^3H-mannitol should have been lower than $0.5 \times 10^{-6}\,cm/s$. In each experiment, three markers (known intestinal absorption) should have been included. The apparent permeability (P_{app}) coefficient expressed in cm/sec was calculated from the following equation:

$$P_{app} = \frac{V_R}{A \times C_0} \times \frac{dC}{dt}$$

where:

V_R is the volume in the receiver chamber (mL)
A is the filter surface area (cm^2)
C_0 is the initial donor concentration of the drug ($\mu g/mL$)
dC/dt is the initial slope of the cumulative concentration ($\mu g/mL$) in the receiver chamber with time (s).

The use of Caco-2 cell culture model in the prediction of intestinal drug absorption has been extensively studied. The first study attempting to correlate passive drug permeability in Caco-2 monolayers with drug absorption in humans after oral administration suggested that the cell monolayers might be used to identify drugs with potential absorption problems.[18] Completely absorbed drugs were found to have high permeability coefficients ($P_{app} > 1 \times 10^{-6}\,cm/s$), whereas incompletely absorbed drugs had low permeability coefficients ($P_{app} < 1 \times 10^{-6}\,cm/s$) in Caco-2 cells. Several studies suggested that Caco-2 cells ranked the permeabilities of drugs in the same order as more complex absorption models, such as *in situ* perfusion models.[25–29] These correlation studies were mainly performed with passively transported drugs (Figure 12.2). The effective permeabilities of three

different classes of drugs were investigated in Caco-2 cells, and in human jejunum *in situ* using a double balloon technique and single pass perfusion.[30–31] The effective permeabilities of the rapidly and completely absorbed compounds (transported by the passive transcellular route) differed only 2- to 4-fold between the Caco-2 cell and human intestinal perfusion models, indicating that Caco-2 cells are an excellent model of the passive transcellular pathway, the most common drug permeation route in the intestine. However, the correlation of the permeabilities of the slowly and incompletely absorbed drugs in the Caco-2 cells, and human jejunum was qualitative rather than quantitative. These drugs were transported at a 30- to 80-fold slower rate in the Caco-2 cells than in the human jejunum. It is also very difficult to compare the absolute permeability coefficient value of individual compounds reported in the literature, particularly with compounds that primarily permeate via the paracellular route. The variability may be attributed to differences in culture conditions, and composition of cell subpopulation. Nevertheless, within each individual laboratory, completely absorbed drugs can be easily separated from poorly-absorbed compounds by this cell model.

12.3.2 Madin–Darby Canine Kidney Cells (MDCK)

The Madin–Darby canine kidney (MDCK) line, established in the 1950s, is another most-frequently used cell line for permeability assessment. MDCK cells are grown in culture medium modified eagle

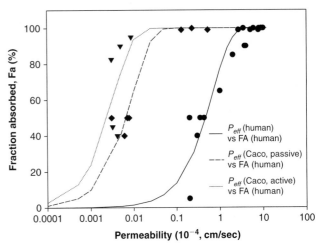

FIGURE 12.2 The relationship between human jejunal effective permeability, Caco-2 monolayer permeability and fraction dose absorbed in human[28]

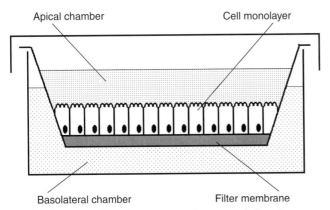

Apical chamber
Cell monolayer
Basolateral chamber
Filter membrane

FIGURE 12.1 Typical experimental set-up of Caco-2 system used to study the transport of molecules across a monolayer

medium (MEM), supplemented with 2% sodium bicarbonate, 1% glutamine, and 5% fetal bovine serum (FBS). Like Caco-2 cells, MDCK cells have been shown to differentiate into columnar epithelium, and to form tight junctions when cultured on semipermeable membranes.[32] The use of MDCK cell lines as a model to evaluate the intestinal permeation characteristics of compounds was first reported by Cho.[33] More recently, several other researchers investigated the use of MDCK cells as a tool for assessing the membrane-permeability properties of early drug discovery compounds.[32,34] Given the fact that Caco-2 cells are derived from human colon carcinoma cells, whereas MDCK cells are derived from dog kidney cells, the major differences between Caco-2 and MDCK cells are the absence or presence of active transporters and drug metabolizing enzymes.

With respect to permeability screening, differences can be expected between Caco-2 cells and MDCK cells, especially for actively transported compounds. The Caco-2 and MDCK cells were experimentally compared for their predictability of permeability of new compounds. For that purpose the permeability of a series of 12 compounds was measured in both cell types. None of them was a P-gp substrate. A very good correlation (r^2 value of 0.88) was observed in the permeability values over the tested range of low to high permeable compounds. The Spearman's rank correlation coefficient for MDCK to Caco-2 P_{app} was 0.87. Irvine[32] also concluded that, at least for passively absorbed compounds, MDCK cells can be used as an alternative for Caco-2 cells. Although a high rank correlation coefficient of 0.93 for MDCK to Caco-2 P_{app} was observed, the relationship between the permeability in cells, and the absorption in humans, was less strongly correlated in MDCK. Permeability values tended to be lower in MDCK cells than in Caco-2 cells. Species difference should also be considered before using MDCK cells as a primary screening tool for permeability in early drug discovery. One of the major advantages of MDCK cells over Caco-2 cells is the shorter cultivation period (three days versus three weeks). A shorter cell culture time becomes a significant advantage, considering reduced labor, and reduced downtime in case of cell contamination.

12.3.3 Other Cells

TC-7 is one of the subclones isolated from Caco-2 cells. A comparison in apparent drug permeability was made between TC-7 cell, and its parental Caco-2 cells.[35] The results showed that TC-7 clone had very similar cell morphology to Caco-2 cells. The permeability of mannitol and PEG-4000 was identical in both cell lines, but TC-7 had a significantly higher TEER value at 21 days in culture and beyond. Permeability values of passively absorbed drugs obtained in TC-7 clone correlated equally well as in parental Caco-2 cells, to the extent of absorption in humans. Thus, on the basis of morphological parameters, biochemical attributes, and drug permeability characteristics, the TC-7 subclone appears to be similar to Caco-2 cells, and presents a suitable alternative to parental cells for intestinal drug permeability studies.

Lewis lung carcinoma-porcine kidney 1 (LLC-PK1) cells have also been explored as an alternative to Caco-2 cells for assessing the permeability of test compounds.[36] Several investigators have reported the utility of porcine cell line for characterizing the passive absorption discovery compounds.[37]

A new cell model, 2/4/A1, which originates from fetal rat intestine, is found to be able to better mimic the permeability of the human small intestine, particularly with regard to passive transcellular and para-cellular permeability.[38–39] This immortalized cell line forms viable differentiated monolayers with tight junctions, and brush border membrane enzymes, as well as transporter proteins. The paracellular pore radius of 2/4/A1 cell was determined to be 9.0 ± 0.2Å, which is similar to the pores in the human small intestine, whereas the pore size in Caco-2 is much smaller ($\sim 3.7 \pm 0.1$Å). Since the tight junctions in Caco-2 cell lines appear unrealistically tighter than those in the epithelial cells in human intestine, the 2/4/1A cells were proposed as a better model to study passively transported compounds via paracellular routes. The transport rate of poorly-permeable compounds (e.g., mannitol and creatinine) in 2/4/1A monolayers was comparable with that in the human jejunum, and was up to 300 times faster than that in the Caco-2 monolayers, suggesting that the 2/4/1A cell line will be more predictive for compounds that are absorbed via the paracellular route.

12.3.4 Limitations of Cultured Cell Models

There are a few important factors that limit the use of cultured cell models. One of the limitations is that the carrier-mediated drug intestinal absorption is poorly predicted. Caco-2 cell model primarily measures passive drug transport (both transcellular and paracellular). Caco-2 cell can express some transporters (e.g., peptide transporters, organic cationic transporter, organic anion transporter), but they are quantitatively underexpressed when compared to that *in vivo*. For example, beta-lactam antibiotics, such as cephalexin and amoxicillin, known substrates of dipeptide transporters, were poorly permeable across the Caco-2 cell, despite the fact that they are completely absorbed *in vivo*.[40] The Caco-2 cell model is likely to generate false negatives with actively transported drug candidates. In addition to the lack of expression of various transporters, the variable expression of those transporters is another issue associated with the use of the Caco-2 cell model.

The lack of correlation for paracellularly transported compounds is another limitation. Low molecular weight hydrophilic compounds (e.g., ranitidine, atenolol, furosemide, hydrochlorothiazide, etc.) also displayed low permeability in this cell model, despite the fact that the extent of absorption in humans is greater than 50%. In other words, Caco-2 cell model can only serve as a one-way screen, such that compounds with high permeability in this model are typically well absorbed *in vivo*; however, compounds with low permeability cannot be ruled out as poorly absorbed compounds *in vivo*.

Also, there is the lack of metabolic enzymes in cell models. Cytochrome P450 (CYP) 3A4 is the most prominent oxidative enzyme present in the intestine, and plays a significant role in first-pass metabolism.[41] An ideal cell-based intestinal permeability tool would be one that simulates the human gastrointestinal enterocytes not only in lipid bilayer characteristics, but also in metabolic enzyme activity. Although Caco-2 cell models are known to express adequate amounts of hydrolase, esterase, and brush border enzymes, they fail to simulate the complete *in vivo* intestinal environment, because they do not express appreciable quantities of CYP3A4, the principle CYP present in human enterocytes.

Moreover, the use of an appreciable amount of organic co-solvent is limited. The integrity of tight junctions is easily compromised by commonly used organic solvents (e.g., methanol, ethanol, polyglycol, polyethelene glycol, etc.) even at a small concentration (more than 1–2% v/v). Therefore, a significant percentage of new drug candidates with poor aqueous solubility cannot be evaluated in this model. Furthermore, cultured cell systems cannot be used to adequately evaluate these compounds that can non-specifically bind to plastic devices.

In most cases, the preparation of fully functional cell monolayer generally requires a 3-week cell culture period, with 8–9 laborious cell feeding. However, the preparation time can be substantially reduced by modifying both the coating material and growth medial.[40] A shorter cell culturing period to generate functional monolayer not only increases the overall productivity, but also reduces the chance of bacterial/fungal

contamination so that it minimizes the downtime. Despite these limitations, cultured cell model still is the most widely used intestinal cell culture system at present, and it is providing valuable information to decision-making processes in early drug discovery.

12.4 INTESTINAL PERMEABILITY EVALUATION: *EX-IN VIVO*

12.4.1 The Everted Gut Sac Technique

The everted sac approach, introduced in 1954 by Wilson and Wiseman,[42] has been widely used to study intestinal drug transport. Everted sacs are prepared from rat intestine by quickly removing the intestine from the decapitated animal, flushing with a saline solution, everting it over a glass rod (diameter 3 mm), filling it with fresh oxygenated culture medium, and dividing it into sacs approximately 2–4 cm in length with silk suture (Figure 12.3). Sacs (mucosal side outside) are then submerged in culture medium containing the drug of interest, and accumulation in the inner compartment is measured. Under optimal conditions, sacs remain viable for up to 120 minutes. To check sac viability and integrity, glucose concentration can be monitored inside and outside the everted sac during the experiments. It can be considered as a two-compartment system: the epithelial cell, and the entire sac. The kinetics of uptake into the epithelial tissue can be calculated by assaying material in the cells, while the kinetics of transfer across the entire epithelial layer can be calculated by measuring material that is found inside the sac at the end of the incubation period. The system has been used to study the uptake of liposomes and proteins,[43–44] bioadhesive lectins, and synthetic non-degradable polymers.[45–46]

The improved everted sac technique is a useful tool to study the mechanisms of uptake of molecules. Test

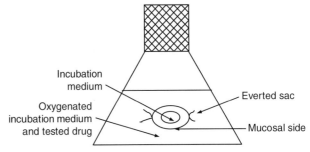

FIGURE 12.3 Everted sac: the sac is incubated with shaking in oxygenated tissue culture medium. Each sac is removed at the required time point and drug is analyzed in the serosal space and tissue

compounds are incubated with the sac at various concentrations, and for differing time periods, to obtain the kinetics of uptake. At the end of the incubation the compounds are analyzed in the tissue, and the serosal space, and as tissue protein is measured the uptake is expressed per unit protein for normalization. In the case of passive membrane diffusion, the compound is detected in both tissue and serosal space, and uptake will be linearly concentration-dependent. For carrier-mediated transports, uptake will be saturable, and subject to competition by other substances transported by the carriers. Test compounds should be detected in both tissue and serosal space. In the case of active mechanisms there will be inhibition by the metabolic inhibitors added to the system. Endocytosis is slow, and may or may not be saturable, depending on whether it is receptor mediated, and inhibited by both metabolic inhibitors and inhibitors of microtubule assembly like colchicine. Compound will be detected in the tissue, and very small amounts in the serosal space. If it is transported by paracellular route, there will be no test compound in the tissue, only in the serosal space, and translocation should be concentration-dependent. In addition, disruption of the tight junctions with Ca^{2+} chelators EDTA or EGTA should increase the uptake of molecules by the paracellular route.

Given the presence of P-gp activity along the rat intestine, the everted gut sac model can also be useful to study the action of intestinal P-gp on intestinal drug absorption. By comparing the transport kinetics of a substrate in the absence or the presence of potential P-gp inhibitors, the method can be used to evaluate the role of P-gp in the intestinal drug absorption, and to screen for putative P-gp inhibitors.[47] An understanding of the site specificity of absorption is most important in optimizing oral drug delivery, particularly in developing controlled-released formulations. The everted sac system affords a simple technique to investigate differences in drug absorption along the gastrointestinal tract. The everted sac system is also a useful tool for screening absorption enhancers. The transport mechanism that is modified by the enhancers can be verified by using specific model compounds to measure the absorption in the presence and absence of enhancers. For example, quinine or digoxin for membrane diffusion, amino acids or dipeptides for carrier transport, and mannitol for the paracellular route can be used for this purpose. The everted gut sac has potential for studying the metabolism of drugs by the intestinal mucosa. If drugs are metabolized by cell surface enzymes in the intestine, then the metabolic products will be detected in the medium following incubation. If the drug is absorbed into the cells, then

it may be susceptible to first-pass metabolism within the enterocytes. The products of this metabolism may themselves be transported, in which case they would be detected in the serosal space or they may be confined to the interior of the cells.

Thus, the everted gut sac system has a number of advantages. It is simple, quick, very reproducible, and inexpensive. The regional differences in drug absorption can be studied and differentiated with this system. It can provide information on the mechanism of drug absorption, and be used to test the effects of enhancers and formulations on absorption. The system also has some disadvantages. The major disadvantage is that it is an animal model, there exists variability between animals, and the absorption results obtained with this model may not always reflect the real absorption profile in humans. In addition, the test compounds have to cross all the layers (including muscle) of the small intestine, instead of just the intestinal mucosa. Furthermore, the sink condition cannot be established, due to the small volume inside the sac.

12.4.2 Ussing Chamber

The Ussing chamber technique to be described here resulted from the pioneering work of Ussing and coworkers, who in the late 1940s and early 1950s published a series of papers describing transepithelial ion fluxes.[48] This technique has subsequently been modified by Grass and Sweetana to study drug transport.[49] This technique utilizes small intestinal sheets which are mounted between two compartments. The mucosal and serosal compartments are usually supplied with Krebs–Ringer bicarbonate buffer (KRB) which is continuously gassed with a mixture of $O_2:CO_2$ (95:5). The test compound is added to either the mucosal or serosal side of the tissue to study transport in the absorptive or secretory direction, respectively. Apparent permeability coefficients (P_{app}) are calculated as for Caco-2 transport experiments from the appearance rate of the compound in the receiver compartment.

One application of the Ussing chamber technique is to study transepithelial drug transport in combination with intestinal metabolism.[50–51] Another wide application of the Ussing chamber system is to investigate the regional differences in intestinal absorption.[52–53] Advantages of the technique are that the amount of drug needed to perform a study is relatively small, and the collected samples are analytically clean. Unlike the *in vitro* cultured cell model, the presence of the apical mucus layer makes the system more relevant to *in vivo* conditions. The published results[52] from a rat Ussing chamber study with 19 drugs exhibiting a wide range of physico-chemical properties demonstrated that the Ussing chamber model was useful in classifying compounds with high or low permeability, according to the BCS system. In addition, as the model offers the possibility to study bidirectional drug transport, as well as concentration dependency of transport and the effect of specific transport inhibitors, Ussing chambers have been used to assess the role of drug transporter in intestinal absorption.[53] Furthermore, species differences with respect to intestinal absorption characteristics can be determined,[20] which can be useful during the selection of a suitable animal model for drug bioavailability studies. Finally, the Ussing chamber model has been used to demonstrate transport polarity of compounds that are substrates of P-gp or multidrug resistance associated protein.[54–55] It should be noted that during preparation of the Ussing chamber system, dissection of the epithelial tissue is rather difficult to perform, and the serosal muscle layers can be only partially removed, which may result in an underestimation of transport, which appears to be an issue, especially for lipophilic drugs.

12.4.3 *In Situ* Method

This method was first introduced in the late 1960s. Intestinal segments of the anesthetized animals are cannulated and perfused by a solution of the drug, and the amount of the drug which is taken up from the perfusate can be calculated (Figure 12.4). Input of the drug compound can be closely controlled in terms of concentration, pH, osmolarity, intestinal region, and flow rate. Among the various preclinical models that are used to study drug absorption, the *in situ* method is the nearest to the *in vivo* system. For instance, the barriers that a compound has to cross to reach the portal blood circulation are identical in the *in situ* and *in vivo* situations. The blood supply, innervation, and clearance capabilities of the animal remain intact. This method provides a unique possibility for studying the intestinal events under isolated status without the complication of biliary excretion and enterohepatic circulation. Similar to the Ussing chamber technique, the *in situ* method can also be used for regional absorption studies and observing the gross effects of enhancer.[56] Therefore, the method has been widely used for the selection of drug candidates, and to confirm the permeability results obtained from *in vitro* experiments (e.g., Caco-2). For example, the antiviral agent adefovir has low permeability, and poor oral absorption. When it is

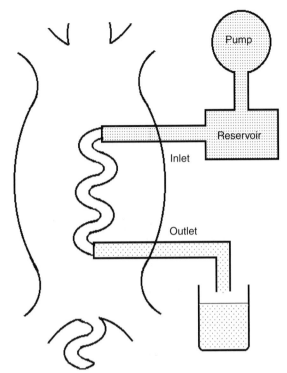

FIGURE 12.4 The *in situ* study of drug uptake by the single-pass perfusion technique. Rat is anesthetized and an intestinal segment is cannulated and perfused with the solution containing the compound of interest. The amount of the compound taken up from the solution can be calculated from the difference between the inlet and the outlet concentration of the compound

converted to a prodrug, adefovir dipivoxil, the oral absorption is significantly improved. This enhanced absorption was demonstrated by Caco-2 monolayer,[57] and further confirmed by *in situ* perfused rat ileum.[58] The prediction of the extent of absorption in humans from rat intestinal perfusion data was demonstrated for a series of compounds with variable absorption (5~100%) in humans.[59] A high correlation between effective permeability values determined in rat and human jejunum has been demonstrated.[60] Therefore, *in situ* perfusion of rat jejunum are considered to be a useful tool to classify compounds according to BCS, provided that appropriated reference compounds are included to account for inter-laboratory variations for passively and actively transported drugs.[61]

The basic experimental procedure for the single pass *in situ* method has been described by Fagerholm.[60] Rats are fasted for at least 12 hrs, anaesthetized, and then an intestinal segment (10–20 cm) is isolated and cannulated. This segment is rinsed with an isotonic solution, before being constantly perfused with the solution containing the compound of interest. The perfusate is then collected at determined intervals.

Complete recovery of PEG-4000 (a non-absorbable marker), stable water flux, and P_{eff} coefficient (effective permeability coefficient) with time for compounds transported both passively (antipyrine), and by a carrier-mediated mechanism (glucose), indicate that viability of the intestinal tissue is maintained during the experiment. P_{eff} of antipyrine can also be used as an indication of extensive change of the mesenteric blood flow. The effective permeability coefficient (P_{eff}) is calculated as follows:

$$P_{eff} = \frac{-Q_{in} \times \ln(C_{out}/C_{in})}{2\pi rL}$$

Where, C_{in} and C_{out} are the inlet and outlet concentration of the compound in the perfusate, Q_{in} is the flow rate of perfusion medium entering in the intestinal segment, and $2\pi rL$ is the mass transfer surface area within the intestinal segment that is assumed to be the area of a cylinder, with length L and radius r. The accessibility of the luminal compartment enables an estimation of intestinal metabolism. However, perfusion systems give no information about events at the cellular or membrane level. The measurement of the rate of disappearance of the drug concentration in the perfusate does not always represent the rate of absorption of the drug into the systemic circulation, in particular if presystemic or intracellular intestinal metabolism occurs. This problem can be overcome if this technique is applied in combination with measurements of the concentration of the drug in the portal vein. The method is also limited, since it requires a large number of animals to obtain statistically significant absorption data. Relatively high amounts of test compounds are also required to perform studies, which is not feasible in early drug discovery. It was also demonstrated that surgical manipulation of intestine, combined with anesthesia, caused a significant change in the blood flow to the intestine, and had a remarkable effect on absorption rate.[62-63] Furthermore, the method uses perfused intestinal flow rates higher than those *in vivo*, and, as a consequence, the *in situ* intestine is fully distended and the luminal hydrostatic pressure increases. This distension may affect the intestinal permeability or absorptive clearance.[64]

12.4.4 Intestinal Perfusion in Man

Intestinal perfusion techniques were first used in man with the aim of studying the absorption and secretion mechanisms or the role of gastric emptying in drug absorption. The basic principle of these techniques is to infuse a solution of the test compound, and a non-absorbable marker such as PEG-4000, into an intestinal segment and to collect perfusate samples after the perfusion has passed through the segment. The difference between the inlet and the outlet concentration of the compound in the solution is assumed to have been absorbed.

Three main single-pass perfusion approaches have been employed in the small intestine:

1. open system – a triple lumen tube including a mixing segment;
2. semi-open system – a multilumen tube with a proximal occluding balloon; and
3. closed system – a multilumen tube with two balloons occluding a 10 cm long intestinal segment.[65-70]

In the triple lumen tube method, entering perfusion solution and gastrointestinal fluids are mixed in a "mixing segment," and at the distal end of the mixing segment a sample is taken which is considered to be the inlet concentration of the test segment. The absorption is then calculated from a second outlet sample taken at the end of the test segment, which usually is 20–30 cm distal to the mixing segment.[68-69] A major disadvantage of this method is that the composition of the perfusate will alter along both mixing and test segments, which makes it difficulty to define the absorption conditions, and therefore to determine reference drug permeability at well-controlled luminal conditions. Perfusate can flow in either direction, and it is difficult to estimate the actual segment length in this open system.

The semi-open system introduced by Ewe and Summerskill[70] overcomes the problem of proximal contamination by using an occluding balloon proximal to the test segment. This method decreases proximal leakage, and therefore the luminal composition will be maintained at equilibrium, and drug permeability can be determined under well-controlled conditions. However, both of these methods generally use rather high perfusion flow rates, typically between 5 and 20 ml/min, which are significantly higher than physiological flow rates of 1–3 ml/min. The recovery of liquid was low and variable, and the length of the intestinal segment studied unknown.

Lennernäs et al.[13] developed a new intestinal perfusion instrument that consists of a multichannel sterile tube with two inflatable balloons, creating a 10 cm length segment, and allowing segmental intestinal perfusion (Figure 12.5). The multichannel tube contains six channels: the four wider channels in the center of the tube, of which two are for infusion, and two are for aspiration of perfusate, respectively. The two remaining peripheral smaller channels are used for the administration of the marker substance or for drainage. The tube is introduced orally after local anesthesia, and when the tube has been positioned the balloons are inflated, creating a closed intestinal segment. The segment is rinsed, perfused with a free drug perfusate, and then perfused with the perfusion solution containing the test compound. The absorption rate is calculated from the disappearance rate of the compound from the perfused segment. The absorption rate can be calculated in different ways, but the intestinal P_{eff} most likely provides the best description of the transport process across the intestinal barrier.[1,60–61] The effective permeability (P_{eff}) is calculated as follows:

$$P_{eff} = \frac{Q_{in} \times (C_{in} - C_{out})}{C_{out} \times 2\pi Rl}$$

where:

Q_{in} is the inlet perfusion rate
C_{in} and C_{out} are the inlet and outlet concentration of the compound in the perfusate
R is the radius
l is the length of the intestinal segment.

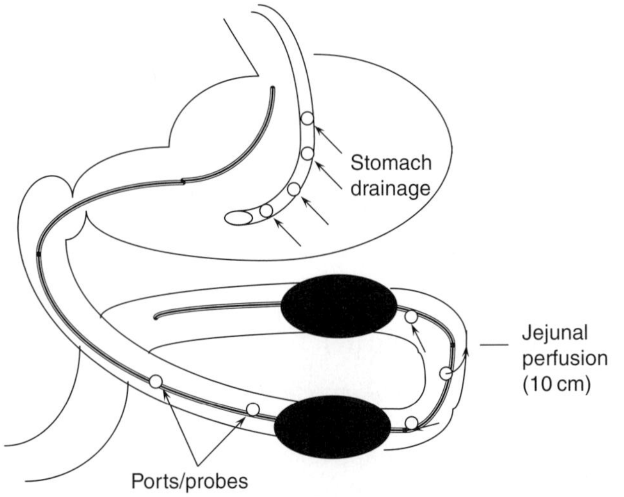

The viability of the mucosa is monitored by the transmucosal transport of D-glucose and L-leucine, and complete recovery of a non-absorbable marker, PEG-4000, in the perfusate leaving the jejunum segment.[13,60,66–67] This regional human jejunal perfusion technique has been validated, and there is a good correlation between the measured effective permeability values and the extent of absorption of drug in man determined by pharmacokinetics studies[61] (Figure 12.6). While the technique can give valuable pharmacokinetic data with human subjects, it is too complex to be used for mass or routine screening studies.

12.5 IN SILICO METHODS

Computational or virtual screening has received much attention in the last few years. *In silico* models that can accurately predict the membrane permeability of test drugs based on lipophilicity, H bonding capacity,

FIGURE 12.5 The multichannel tube system with double balloons enabling segmental perfusion in man. The difference between the inlet and the outlet concentration of the compound in the solution is assumed to have been absorbed

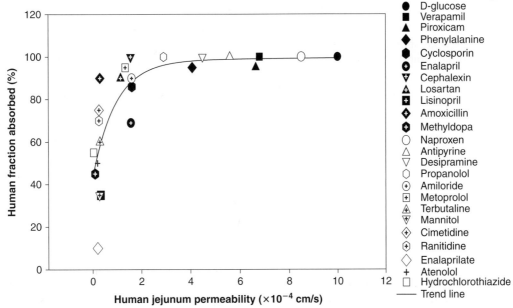

FIGURE 12.6 The relationship between human jejunal effective permeability and fraction dose absorbed[1]

molecular size, polar surface area (PSA), and quantum properties, have the potential to specifically direct chemical synthesis, and, therefore revolutionize drug discovery processes. Such an *in silico* predictive model would minimize extremely time-consuming steps of synthesis, as well as experimental studies of thousands of test compounds. Lipinski et al.[71] proposed an *in silico* computational method for qualitatively predicting the developability of compounds. The "Rules of Five" predicted lower developability for compounds with more than five H bond donors, ten H bond acceptors, molecular weight greater than 500 or clog *P* greater than 5. Using this empirical model, useful predictions were achieved for closely related analog series of compounds. Additionally, a number of *in silico* methods, including compartmental absorption and transit (CAT) model,[72] the quantitative structure–bioavailability relationship (QSBR) model,[73–74] and quantitative structure–property relationship (QSPR) model,[75–77] have been developed for predicting oral drug absorption and bioavailability in humans.

12.5.1 CAT Model

Based on the transit modes,[78–79] the CAT model was developed by considering gastric emptying, small intestinal transit, *in vivo* dissolution/precipitation, linear absorption, saturable absorption, drug metabolism, influx and efflux transporters, and hepatic metabolism. Along with the pharmacokinetic model, the CAT model describes how a drug gets into the blood, how much it gets into the blood, how fast it gets into the blood, and how long it stays there, (i.e., absorption, distribution, metabolism, and excretion (ADME)). It is a dynamic, mechanistic model that simulates and predicts the rate and extent of drug absorption from the human small intestinal tract. The transit flow in the human small intestine is described by seven compartments, where a drug transfers from one to the next one in a first-order fashion. The colon is considered only as a reservoir, the colonic transit flow is not considered in the model. The CAT model is developed based on the following assumptions:

1. absorption from the stomach and colon is insignificant compared with that from the small intestine;
2. transport across the small intestinal membrane is passive or active; and
3. a drug moving through the small intestine can be viewed as process-flowing through a series of segments.

Each segment is described by a single compartment with linear transfer kinetics from one to the next, and

all compartments may have different volumes and flow rates, but the same residence times. The CAT model can simulate the effect of gastric emptying on absorption, estimate the rate of drug absorption, and couple easily with compartmental pharmacokinetic models. This model has been modified and extended to be the advanced compartmental absorption and transit (ACAT) model, which laid foundations for the commercial software, GastroPLUS™. With this physiologically based simulation software program, the rate and extent of oral drug absorption can be predicted. Since the determination of human P_{eff} is complex and expensive, the *in situ* rat or dog intestinal permeability values are used instead. The human P_{eff} is estimated based on the measured permeability in rat or dog, using a built-in correlation. The data from epithelial cell culture models such as Caco-2 and MDCK can also be used for the purpose of prediction. The software has been licensed and used by numerous pharmaceutical companies around the world.

12.5.2 Quantitative Structure Bioavailability Relationships (QSBR)

The earlier QSBR model for the prediction of human oral bioavailability was built up by using the method of fuzzy adaptive least-squares, and a combination of continuous, discrete and indicator variables.[80] In the study, 188 noncongeneric diverse organic compounds were used. They were divided into three groups, nonaromatics, aromatics, and heteroaromatics groups. When models were produced for each of the chemical classes using $\log P$, $(\log P)^2$, and molecular weight, the statistical reliability of these models was poor. After discrete and indicator variables were added for the various structural fragments present in the compounds, new models were developed with improved statistical significance. Some interesting insights into the impact of various structural fragments on human oral bioavailability were yielded by using these models, but caution needs to be taken since these observations were based purely on the sign of the coefficient.

Recently, the quantitative structure–bioavailability relationship of 232 structurally diverse drugs was studied.[73] The oral bioavailability determined in human adults was assigned one of four ratings, and analyzed in relation to physico-chemical and structural factors by the ordered multi-catagorical classification method using the simplex technique (ORMUCS) method. A systematic examination of various physico-chemical parameters relating primarily to absorption was carried out to analyze their effects on the bioavailabilty classification of drugs in the data set. Lipophilicity, expressed as the distribution coefficient at pH 6.5, was found to be a significant factor influencing bioavailability. The observation that acids generally had better bioavailability characteristics than bases, with neutral compounds between, led to define a new parameter, $\Delta \log D(\log D_{6.5} - \log D_{7.4})$, which allows a better classification of compounds. An additional 15 structural descriptors relating primarily to well-known metabolic processes yielded a satisfactory equation that had a correct classification rate of 71%, and a Spearman rank correlation coefficient of 0.851, despite the diversity of structure and pharmacological activity in the compound set. In leave-one-out tests, an average of 67% of drugs was correctly classified with a correlation coefficient of 0.812. The relationship identified significant factors influencing bioavailability, and assigned them quantitative values expressing their contribution. The predictive power of the model was evaluated using a separate test set of 40 compounds, of which 60% were correctly classified. Potential uses are in drug design, prioritization of compounds for synthesis, and selection for detailed studies of early compound leads in drug discovery programs.

In another approach using oral bioavailability data of 591 compounds, a regression model was built employing 85 structural descriptors.[74] The final regression model had an $r^2 = 0.71$. An analysis of the available experimental bioavailability data demonstrated that the mean experimental error was 12%. Comparing this model with the predictive ability of the Lipinski rule of five, in general, it was found that the structure-based model performed better than the rule of five in terms of reducing the number of false positives. However, it should be borne in mind that the rule of five is not a method for predicting bioavailability, rather, it is a method of defining drug absorption properties. Thus, it is not surprising that it did not perform as well as the structure-based model, since there is no consideration of the chemical properties that govern clearance in the rule of five.

One advantage of the structure-based model is that it is able to identify the impact of certain functional groups on bioavailability. Those groups, like tetrazole and 4-aminopyridine, are highlighted as having a significant negative effect on bioavailability, while 1-methylcyclopentyl alcohol is a group with a significant positive effect on bioavailability. Although the model does not provide any mechanistic explanation for these findings, in terms of effect on absorption or clearance, this model can still be used to estimate the bioavailability of new compounds.

Genetic programming, a specific form of evolutionary computing, has recently been used for predicting oral bioavailability.[81] The results show a light improvement compared to the ORMUCS (ordered multi-catagorical classification method using the simplex technique) approach. These methods demonstrate that at least qualitative predictions of oral bioavailability seem possible directly from the structure.

12.5.3 Quantitative Structure Permeability Relationships (QSPR)

A number of QSPR models have been proposed for predicting $\log P_{app}$ and human intestinal absorption. The choice of proper descriptors is the key to a successful QSPR model. There are a great number of descriptors available for use in QSPR studies, ranging from simple molecular weight and molecular surface area, to the grid interaction of energies between a probe and target molecules. Most of the reported QSPR models utilize PSA as an indicator of intestinal permeability and absorption. For a diverse set of 17 compounds, it was shown that the $\log P_{app}$ measured from Caco-2 monolayers correlates well with the molecular weight and the PSA obtained for a single conformation.[82] In another study, twenty structurally diverse model drugs, ranging from 0.3 to 100% absorbed, were investigated.[83] These compounds also displayed diversity in physico-chemical properties such as lipophilicity, hydrogen bonding potential, and molecular size. The dynamic molecular surface properties of the compounds were calculated, taking into account their three-dimensional shape and flexibility. A sigmoidal relationship was established between the absorbed fraction after oral administration to humans and the dynamic PSA ($r^2 = 0.94$). Similarly, the Boltzmann-averaged dynamic solvent-accessible surface area obtained from molecular dynamics simulations was related to the intestinal absorption.[84]

Artursson and coworkers[85] extended the PSA model by including the dynamic nonpolar surface area (NPSA) component for prediction of the transmembrane permeability to the oligopeptide derivatives. Relationships between the dynamic molecular surface properties and intestinal epithelial permeability, as determined in Caco-2 cell monolayers, were used to develop a model for prediction of the transmembrane permeability to the oligopeptide derivatives. A theoretical model that takes both the polar and nonpolar part of the dynamic molecular surface area of the investigated molecule into consideration was derived. The model provided a strong relationship with transepithelial permeability for the oligopeptide derivatives. However, the PSA, NPSA, and H-bond atom count were not determined to be the critical elements responsible for the observed cellular permeability of the 21 peptide and peptidomimetic compounds tested by a different group.[86] This suggests that QSPR models based on log P, PSA or NPSA, while helpful for deriving meaningful correlations within a narrow structure class, may not extend universally. Recently, a quantitative model for predicting human intestinal absorption was proposed by combining a genetic algorithm and a neural network scoring function.[87] A data set of 86 drug and drug-like compounds with measured values of human intestinal absorption taken from the literature was used to develop and test a QSPR model. A nonlinear computational neural network model was developed by using the genetic algorithm with a neural network fitness evaluator. The calculated human intestinal absorption model performs well, with root-mean-square errors of 9.4 units for the training set, 19.7 units for the cross-validation (CV) set, and 16.0 units for the external prediction set. However, the major drawback rests in the compounds selection, since a single model was used to describe both passive and carrier-mediated absorption mechanisms. In addition, with 52/67 (52 out of 67) compounds exhibiting >75% intestinal absorption, the training set data primarily contains compounds with high absorption, and therefore may result in a biased model. Most recently, a genetic algorithm was applied to build up a set of QSPR models for human absolute oral bioavailability, using the counts of molecular fragments as descriptors. It was claimed that the correlation coefficient was improved significantly, and the standard errors reduced dramatically.[88] Kitchen and Subramanian[89] reported that QSPR models were developed for estimating both log P_{app}, and human intestinal absorption. QSPR models for computing log P_{app}, and human intestinal absorption, were derived independently by using evenly-distributed datasets. The results showed that the multivariate-statistics approach performs best for estimating the P_{app}, while a single variable such as PSA describes the human intestinal absorption process satisfactorily. The log P_{app} models derived in this study also demonstrate that intestinal permeability is governed by several parameters. Since the correlations and validations are better for P_{app}, and that it is a simple experiment, the authors claimed that the log P_{app} models are more likely to extend to new compounds.

12.6 FUTURE TRENDS

Recent advances in molecular biology and combinatorial chemistry have changed the way in which pharmaceutical companies conduct drug discovery research. The biggest challenge is to screen a large number of drug candidates, and find lead compounds in a very short period of time. The *in silico* techniques have been used to meet this challenge. The significant advance has been made in the prediction of intestinal permeability using *in silico* techniques over the last decade, but what is most needed now are more, and reliable, data to form the foundation of computational models that are capable of integrating the existing knowledge of intestinal permeability, and permitting us to see relationships implicated in the data. More, and high quality, data should also permit the application of non-linear models to better fit the observed curvilinear relationships between physico-chemical properties/descriptors and permeability.

However, effective use of cell culture techniques has dramatically improved the efficiency of permeability screening at the discovery phase. There have been substantial advances in the fields of miniaturization and automation with respect to cell culture techniques. Most biological screening assays are performed in the miniaturized models, such as 384- or 1536-well plates for ultra-high throughput screening.[90–91] In contrast to the successful use of miniaturization in biological activity screening, cell-based intestinal permeability screening has not made similar advances. Currently, permeability studies using cell monolayer are conducted in automation-friendly 12- or 24-well transwell plates. The implementation of Caco-2 cells in 96-well plate format for both permeability and P-gp interaction studies were reported.[92–94] The utilization of a 96-well Caco-2 cell system will significantly increase throughput, reduce cost, and decrease the amount of compound required for permeability assessment. However, further miniaturization using 384-well filter plate has been difficult because of very small cell monolayer surface area. Automation, on the other hand, has made significant progress. Cell-based permeability studies are now regularly conducted by robotic equipment with minimum human intervention. A fully automated Caco-2 cell system has a throughput in the order of 500 to 2000 compound studies per month, without a proportional increase in resources.[95] Robotic systems, coupled with miniaturization devices, can be extremely valuable because of the precision and high-speed handling of repetitive tasks, and will definitely lead the way to an era of high technology laboratories working smoothly with minimal human intervention. Furthermore, some of the technological innovations can be made to reduce the time for cell growth. The efforts towards improvements in culturing media, adjustments of seeding density, and use of modified transwell plates have already shortened cell growth time.[40,93] These shortened cell models function as well as the regular cell models. Further improvement in this area, with respect to cell culture techniques, will certainly be the focus of development efforts in the near future.

12.7 CONCLUSION

Optimizing bioavailability of orally administered drug is one of the most important aims for the pharmaceutical industry. In order to achieve this goal, however, high throughput, cost-effective, highly discriminating, and predictive models for the absorption of drug molecules in man will be required. The current *in silico* approaches seem to hold promise of fulfilling this need, although larger and more chemically diverse data sets will be needed, and much more optimization work remains to be done before these models will be reliable enough to accurately predict intestinal absorption. However, the conventional experimental methods for assessing absorption characteristics are not streamlined to keep pace with the large number of compounds synthesized by combinatorial chemistry. The available experimental models have various pros and cons, and their wise use can increase the likelihood of progressing drugs with favorable oral absorption characteristics. Therefore, permeability prediction methods that are rapid and require no usage of animal tissues (physico-chemical and *in silico* methods) can be used as primary screening models for evaluation of compounds in very early drug discovery. Such methods can afford a very fast and economical way of screening out libraries of compounds with minimum usage of resources. Once the primary screening has been performed, the secondary screening can be achieved using automated high throughput *in vitro* systems (cell culture-based or animal tissue-based) for selecting and optimizing the chemical leads to identify potential drug candidates. Finally, traditional approaches for the evaluation of drug absorption, such as *in situ* rat intestinal perfusion techniques, and *in vivo* animal studies, should also be utilized to further prevent "false positives" and "false negatives" from getting into the development process. Thus, it is the prudent use of the various permeability evaluation techniques at the right stage of drug discovery that can ensure that only drug candidates with a high developability potential are moved forward into the development pipeline.

References

1. Amidon, G.L., Lennernas, H., Shah, V.P. & Crison, J.R. (1995). A theoretical basis for a biopharmaceutic drug classification: The correlation of *in vitro* drug product dissolution and *in vivo* bioavailability. Pharmaceutical Research 12, 413–420.

2. Yu, L.X., Amidon, G.L., Polli, J.E., Zhao, H., Mehta, M.U., Conner, D.P., Shah, V.P., Lesko, L.J., Chen, M-L., Lee, V.H. & Hussain, A.S. (2002). Biopharmaceutics classification system: The scientific basis for biowaiver extensions. Pharmaceutical Research 19, 921–925.

3. Polli, J.E., Yu, L.X., Cook, J.A., Amidon, G.L., Borchardt, R.T., Burnside, B.A., Burton, P.S., Chen, M-L., Conner, D.P., Faustino, P.J., Hawi, A., Hussain, A.S., et al. (2004). Summary workshop report: Biopharmaceutics classification system-Implementation challenges and extension opportunities. Journal of Pharmaceutical Sciences 93, 1375–1381.

4. Cheng, C-L., Yu, L.X., Lee, H-L., Yang, C-Y., Lue, C-S. & Chou, C-H. (2004). Biowaiver extension potential to BCS class III high solubility-low permeability drugs: Bridging evidence for metformin immediate-release tablet. European Journal of Pharmaceutical Sciences 22, 297–304.

5. Wu, C.Y. & Benet, L.Z. (2005). Predicting drug disposition via application of BCS: transport/absorption/elimination interplay and development of a biopharmaceutics drug disposition classification system. Pharmaceutical Research 22, 11–23.

6. Fleisher, D., Li, C., Zhou, Y., Pao, L.H. & Karim, A. (1999). Drug, meal and formulation interactions influencing drug absorption after oral administration. Clinical implications. Clinical Pharmacokinetics 36, 233–254.

7. Lennernäs, H. & Abrahamsson, B. (2004). The use of biopharmaceutic classification of drugs in drug discovery and development: current status and future extension. The Journal of Pharmacy and Pharmacology 57, 273–285.

8. Guidance for Industry. (1995). Immediate Release Solid Oral Dosage Forms: Scale-Up and Post-Approval Changes. November, CDER/FDA.

9. Guidance for industry. (1997). Dissolution Testing of Immediate Release Solid Oral Dosage Forms. August, CDER/FDA.

10. Guidance for industry. (2000). Waiver of *In Vivo* Bioavailability and Bioequivalence Studies for Immediate Release Solid Oral Dosage Forms Based on a Biopharmaceutics Classification System. August, CDER/FDA.

11. Buffer solutions. (2006). USP-NF Online. United States Pharmacopeia 29/National Formulary 24. Accessed December 12, 2006.

12. Dissolution. (2006). USP-NF Online. United States Pharmacopeia 29/National Formulary 24. Accessed December 12, 2006.

13. Lennernäs, H., Ahrenstedt, O., Hällgren, R., Knutson, L., Ryde, M. & Paalzow, L.K. (1992). Regional jejunal perfusion, a new *in vivo* approach to study oral drug absorption in man. Pharmaceutical Research 9, 1243–1251.

14. Oh, D.M., Curl, R.L. & Amido, G.L. (1993). Estimating the fraction dose absorbed from suspensions of poorly soluble compounds in humans: A mathematical model. Pharmaceutical Research 10, 264–270.

15. Rekhi, G.S., Eddington, N.D., Fossler, M.J., Schwarts, P., Lesko, L.J. & Augsburger, L.L. (1997). Evaluation of *in vitro* release rate and *in vivo* absorption characteristics of four metoprolol tartrate immediate-release tablet formulations. Pharmaceutical Development and Technology 2, 11–24.

16. Yu, L.X. (1999). An integrated model for determining causes of poor oral drug absorption. Pharmaceutical Research 16, 1883–1887.

17. Delie, F. & Rubas, W. (1997). A human colonic cell line sharing similarities with enterocytes as a model to examine oral absorption of the Caco-2 model. Critical Reviews in Therapeutic Drug Carrier Systems 14, 221–286.

18. Hidalgo, I., Raub, T. & Borchardt, R. (1989). Characterization of human colon carcinoma cell line (Caco-2) as a model system for intestinal epithelial permeability. Gastroenterology 96, 739–749.

19. Artursson, P. & Karlsson, J. (1991). Correlation between oral drug absorption in humans and apparent drug permeability coefficients in human intestinal epithelial (Caco-2) cells. Biochemical and Biophysical Research Communications 175, 880–885.

20. Rubas, W., Jezyk, N. & Grass, G.M. (1993). Comparison of the permeability characteristics of a human colonic epithelial (Caco-2) cell line to colon of rabbit, monkey, and dog intestine and human drug absorption. Pharmaceutical Research 10, 113–118.

21. Borchardt, R. (1995). The application of cell culture systems in drug discovery and development. Journal of Drug Targeting 3, 179–182.

22. Autursson, P., Palm, K. & Luthman, K. (1996). Caco-2 mono-layers in experimental and theoretical predictions of drug transport. Advanced Drug Delivery Reviews 22, 67–84.

23. Volpe, D.A., Ciavarella, A.B., Asafu-Adjaye, E.B., Ellison, C.D., Faustino, P.J. & Yu, L.X. (2001). Method suitability of a Caco-2 cell model for drug permeability classification. AAPS PharmSci. 2001 AAPS Annual Meeting Supplement.

24. Anderle, P., Niederer, E., Rubas, W., Hilgendorf, C., Spahn-Langguth, H., Wunderli-Allenspach, H., Merkle, H.P. & Langguth, P. (1998). P-glycoprotein (P-gp) mediated efflux in Caco-2 cell monolayers: The influence of culturing conditions and drug exposure on P-gp expression levels. Journal of Pharmaceutical Sciences 87, 757–762.

25. Kim, D.C., Burton, P.S. & Borchardt, R.T. (1993). A correlation between the permeability characteristics of a series of peptides using an in vitro cell culture model (Caco-2) and those using an in situ perfused rat ileum model of the intestinal mucosa. Pharmaceutical Research 10, 1710–1714.

26. Conradi, R.A., Wilkinson, K.F., Rush, B.D., Hilgers, A.R., Ruwart, M.J. & Burton, P.S. (1993). In vitro/in vivo models for peptide oral absorption: Comparison of Caco-2 cell permeability with rat intestinal absorption of rennin inhibitory peptides. Pharmaceutical Research 10, 1790–1792.

27. Wils, P., Warnery, A., Phung-Ba, V. & Scherman, D. (1994). Differentiated intestinal epithelial cell lines as in vitro models for predicting the intestinal absorption of drugs. Cell Biology and Toxicology 10, 393–397.

28. Walter, E., Janich, S., Roessler, B.J., Hilfinger, J.M. & Amidon, G.L. (1996). HT29-MTX/Caco-2 cocultures as an in vitro model for the intestinal epithelium: in vitro-in vivo correlation with permeability data from rats and humans. Journal of Pharmaceutical Sciences 85, 1070–1076.

29. Yee, S. (1997). In vitro permeability across Caco-2 cells (colonic) can predict in vivo small intestine absorption in man—fact or myth. Pharmaceutical Research 14, 763–766.

30. Lennernäs, H., Ahrenstedt, Ö., Hallgren, R., Knutson, L., Ryde, M. & Paalzow, L.K. (1992). Regional jejunal perfusion, a new in vivo approach to study oral drug absorption in man. Pharmaceutical Research 9, 1243–1251.

31. Lennernäs, H., Palm, K., Fagerholm, U. & Artursson, P. (1996). Correlation between paracellular and transcellular drug permeability in the human jejunum and Caco-2 monolayers. International Journal of Pharmaceutics 127, 103–107.

32. Irvine, J.D., Takahashi, L., Lockhart, K., Cheong, J., Tolan, J.W., Selick, H.E. & Grove, J.R. (1999). MDCK (Madin-Darby canine kidney cells): a tool for membrane permeability screening. Journal of Pharmaceutical Sciences 88, 28–33.

33. Cho, M., Thompson, D., Cramer, C., Vidmar, T. & Scieszka, J. (1989). The Madin-Darby canine kidney (MDCK) epithelial cell monolayer as a model cellular transport barrier. Pharmaceutical Research 6, 71–79.

34. Putnam, W.S., Ramanathan, S., Pan, L., Takahashi, L.H. & Benet, L.Z. (2002). Functional characterization of monocarboxylic acid, large neutral amino acid, bile acid and peptide transporters, and P-glycoprotein in MDCK and Caco-2 cells. Journal of Pharmaceutical Sciences 91, 2622–2635.

35. Gres, M., Julian, B., Bourrie, M., Roques, C., Berger, M., Boulenc, X., Berger, Y. & Fabre, G. (1998). Correlation between oral drug absorption in humans, and apparent drug permeability in TC-7 cells, a human epithelial cell line: comparison with the parental Caco-2 cell line. Pharmaceutical Research 15, 726–733.

36. Li, H., Chung, S.J. & Shim, C.K. (2002). Characterization of the transport of uracil across Caco-2 and LLC-PK1 cell monolayers. Pharmaceutical Research 19, 1495–1501.

37. Adachi, Y., Suzuki, H. & Sugiyama, Y. (2003). Quantitative evaluation of the function of small intestinal P-glycoprotein: comparative studies between in situ and in vitro. Pharmaceutical Research 20, 1163–1169.

38. Tavelin, S., Taipalensuu, J., Hallbook, F., Vellonen, K.S., Moore, V. & Artursson, P. (2003). An improved cell culture model based on 2/4/A1 cell monolayers for studies of intestinal drug transport: Characterization of transport routes. Pharmaceutical Research 20, 373–381.

39. Tavelin, S., Taipalensuu, J., Soderberg, L., Moore, V., Chong, S. & Artursson, P. (2003). Prediction of the oral absorption of low-permeability drugs using small intestine-like 2/4/A1 cell monolayers. Pharmaceutical Research 20, 397–405.

40. Chong, S., Dando, S., Soucek, K. & Morrison, R. (1996). In vitro permeability through Caco-2 cells is not quantitatively predictive of in vivo absorption for peptide-like drugs absorbed via the dipeptide transporter system. Pharmaceutical Research 13, 120–123.

41. Artursson, P. & Borchardt, R.T. (1997). Intestinal drug absorption and metabolism in cell cultures: Caco-2 and beyond. Pharmaceutical Research 14, 1655–1658.

42. Wilson, T.H. & Wiseman, G. (1954). The use of sacs of everted small intestine for the study of the transference of substances from the mucosal to the serosal surface. The Journal of Physiology 123, 116–125.

43. Rowland, R.N. & Woodley, J.F. (1981). The uptake of disteary-phosphatidylcholine/cholesterol liposomes by rat intestinal sac in vitro. Biochimica et Biophysica Acta 673, 217–223.

44. Rowland, R.N. & Woodley, J.F. (1981). The uptake of free and liposome entrapped horse radish peroxidase by rat intestinal sacs in vitro. FEBS letters 123, 41–44.

45. Carreno-Gomez, B., Woodley, J.F. & Florence, A.T. (1999). Study on the uptake of nanoparticles in everted gut sacs. International Journal of Pharmaceutics 183, 7–11.

46. Pato, J., Mora, M., Naisbett, B., Woodley, J.F. & Duncan, R. (1994). Uptake and transport of poly(N-vinylpyrrolidone-co-maleic acid) by the adult rat small intestine cultured in vitro: effect of chemical structure. International Journal of Pharmaceutics 110, 227–237.

47. Barthe, L., Bessouet, M., Woodley, J.F. & Houin, G. (1998). An improved everted gut sac as a simple and accurate technique to measure paracellular transport across the small intestine. European Journal of Drug Metabolism and Pharmacokinetics 23, 313–323.

48. Ussing, H.H. & Zerahn, K. (1951). Active transport of sodium as the source of electric current in the short-circuited isolated frog skin. Acta Physiologica Scandinavica 23, 110–127.

49. Grass, G.M. & Sweetana, S.A. (1988). In vitro measurement of gastrointestinal tissue permeability using a new diffusion cell. Pharmaceutical Research 5, 372–376.

50. Smith, P., Mirabelli, C., Fondacaro, J., Ryan, F. & Dent, J. (1988). Intestinal 5-fluorouracil absorption: Use of Ussing chambers to assess transport and metabolism. Pharmaceutical Research 5, 598–603.

51. Annaert, P., Tukker, J.J., van Gelder, J., Naesens, L., de Clercq, E., van Den Mooter, G., Kinget, R. & Augustijins, P. (2000). *In vitro, ex vivo,* and *in situ* intestinal absorption characteristics of the antiviral ester prodrug adefovir dipivoxil. Journal of Pharmaceutical Sciences 89, 1054–1062.

52. Ungell, A.L., Nylander, S., Bergstrand, S., Sjöberg, Å. & Lennernäs, H. (1998). Membrane transport of drugs in different regions of the intestinal tract of the rat. Journal of Pharmaceutical Sciences 87, 360–366.

53. Biosset, M., Botham, R.P., Haegele, K.D., Lenfant, B. & Pachot, P.I. (2000). Absorption of angiotensin II antagonists in Ussing chambers, Caco-2, perfused jejunum loop and *in vivo*: Importance of drug ionization in the *in vitro* prediction of *in vivo* absorption. Eur.J.Pharm. 10, 215–224.

54. Naruhashi, K., Tamai, I., Inoue, N., Muraoka, H., Sai, Y., Suzuki, N. & Tsuji, A. (2001). Active intestinal secretion of new quinolone antimicrobials and the partial contribution of P-glycoprotein. The Journal of Pharmacy and Pharmacology 53, 699–709.

55. Gotoh, Y., Suzuki, H., Kinoshita, S., Hirohashi, T., Kato, Y. & Sugiyama, Y. (2000). Involvement of an organic anion transporter (Canalicular multispecific organic anion transporter/multidrug resistance-associated protein 2) in gastrointestinal secretion of glutathione conjugates in rats. The Journal of Pharmacology and Experimental Therapeutics 292, 433–439.

56. Hu, M., Roland, K., Ge, L., Chen, J., Li, Y., Tyle, P. & Roy, S. (1998). Determination of absorption characteristics of AG337, a novel thymiddylate synthase inhibitor, using a perfused rat intestinal model. Journal of Pharmaceutical Sciences 87, 886–890.

57. Annaert, P., Kinget, R., Naesens, L., de Clercq, E. & Augustijins, P. (1997). Transport, uptake, and metabolism of the bis(pivaloyloxymethyl)-ester prodrug of 9-(2-phosphonylmethoxyethyl)adenine in an *in vitro* cell culture system of the intestinal mucosa (Caco-2). Pharmaceutical Research 14, 492–496.

58. Okudaira, N., Tatebayashi, T., Speirs, G.C., Komiya, I. & Sugiyama, Y. (2000). A study of the intestinal absorption of an ester-type prodrug, ME3229, in rats: Active efflux transport as a cause of poor bioavailability of the active drug. The Journal of Pharmacology and Experimental Therapeutics 294, 580–587.

59. Stewart, B.H., Chan, O.H., Lu, R.H., Reyner, E.L., Schmid, H.L., Hamilton, H.W., Steinbaugh, B.A. & Taylor, M.D. (1995). Comparison of intestinal permeabilities determined in multiple *in vitro* and *in situ* models: Relationship to absorption in humans. Pharmaceutical Research 12, 693–699.

60. Fagerholm, U., Johansson, M. & Lennernäs, H. (1996). Comparison between permeability coefficients in rat and human jejunum. Pharmaceutical Research 13, 1336–1342.

61. Lennernäs, H. (1998). Human intestinal permeability. Journal of Pharmaceutical Sciences 87, 403–410.

62. Uhing, M.R. & Kimura, R.E. (1995). The effect of surgical bowl manipulation and anesthesia on intestinal glucose absorption in rats. The Journal of Clinical Investigation 95, 2790–2798.

63. Yuasa, H., Matsuda, K. & Watanabe, J. (1993). Influence of anesthetic regimens on intestinal absorption in rats. Pharmaceutical Research 10, 884–888.

64. Chiou, W. (1994). Determination of drug permeability in a flat or distended stirred intestine. International Journal of Clinical Pharmacology and Therapeutics 32, 474–482.

65. Knutson, L., Odlind, B. & Hällgren, R. (1989). A new technique for segmental jejunal perfusion in man. The American Journal of Gastroenterology 84, 1278–1284.

66. Lennernäs, H., Fagerholm, U., Raab, Y., Gerdin, B. & Hällgren, R. (1995). Regional rectal perfusion, a new *in vivo* approach to study rectal drug absorption in man. Pharmaceutical Research 12, 426–432.

67. Lennernäs, H., Lee, I.D., Fagerholm, U. & Amidon, G.L. (1997). A residence-time distribution analysis of the hydrodynamics within the intestine in man during a regional single-pass perfusion with Loc-I-Gut: *In-vivo* permeability estimation. The Journal of Pharmacy and Pharmacology 49, 682–686.

68. Gramatté, T., el Desoky, E. & Klotz, U. (1994). Site-dependent small intestinal absorption of ranitidine. European Journal of Pharmacology 46, 253–259.

69. Gramatté, T., Oertel, R., Terhaag, B. & Kirch, W. (1996). Direct demonstration of small intestinal secretion and site-dependent absorption of the beta-block tailinolol in humans. Clinical Pharmacology and Therapeutics 59, 541–549.

70. Ewe, K. & Summerskill, W.H. (1965). Transfer of ammonia in the human jejunum. The Journal of Laboratory and Clinical Medicine 65, 839–847.

71. Lipinski, T., Lombardo, F., Dominy, B. & Feeney, P. (1997). Experimental and computational approaches to estimate solubility and permeability in drug discovery and development settings. Advanced Drug Delivery Reviews 23, 3–25.

72. Yu, L.X. & Amidon, G.L. (1999). A compartmental absorption and transit model for estimating oral drug absorption. International Journal of Pharmaceutics 186, 119–125.

73. Yoshida, F. & Topliss, J.G. (2000). QSAR model for drug human oral bioavailability. Journal of Medicinal Chemistry 43, 2575–2585.

74. Andrews, W.C., Bennett, L. & Yu, L.X. (2000). Predicting human oral bioavailability of a compound: development of a novel quantitative structure-bioavailability relationship. Pharmaceutical Research 17, 639–644.

75. Sugawara, M., Takekuma, Y., Yamada, H., Kobayashi, M., Iseki, K. & Miyazaki, K. (1998). A general approach for the prediction of the intestinal absorption of drugs: regression analysis using the physicochemical properties and drug-membrane electrostatic interaction. Journal of Pharmaceutical Sciences 87, 960–966.

76. Winiwarter, S., Bonham, N.M., Ax, F., Hallberg, A., Lennernäs, H. & Karlen, A. (1998). A general approach for the prediction of the intestinal absorption of drugs: Regression analysis using the physicochemical properties and drug-membrane electrostatic interaction. Journal of Medicinal Chemistry 41, 4939–4949.

77. Bermejo, M., Merino, V., Garrigues, T.M., Pla-Delfina, J.M., Mulet, A., Vizet, P., Trouiller, G. & Mercier, C. (1999). Validation of a biophysical drug absorption model by the PATQSAR system. Journal of Pharmaceutical Sciences 88, 398–405.

78. Yu, L.X., Crison, J.R. & Amidon, G.L. (1996). Compartmental transit and dispersion model analysis of small intestinal transit flow in humans. International Journal of Pharmaceutics 140, 111–118.

79. Yu, L.X. & Amidon, G.L. (1998). Characterization of small intestinal transit time distribution in humans. International Journal of Pharmaceutics 171, 157–163.

80. Hirono, S., Nakagome, I., Hirano, H., Matsushita, Y., Yoshii, F. & Moriguchi, I. (1994). Non-congeneric structure-pharmacokinetic property correlation studies using fuzzy adaptive least-squares: Oral bioavailability. Biological & Pharmaceutical Bulletin 17, 306–309.

81. Bains, W., Gilbert, R., Sviridenko, L., Gascon, J.M., Scoffin, R., Birchall, K., Harvey, I. & Caldwell, J. (2002). Evolutionary computational methods to predict oral bioavailability QSPRs. Current Opinion in Drug Discovery & Development 5, 44–51.

82. van de Waterbeemd, H. (2002). High-throughput and *in silico* techniques in drug metabolism and pharmacokinetics. Current Opinion in Drug Discovery & Development 5, 33–43.

83. Palm, K., Stenberg, P., Luthman, K. & Artursson, P. (1997). Polar molecular surface properties predict the intestinal absorption of drugs in humans. Pharmaceutical Research 14, 568–571.

84. Krarup, L.H., Christensen, I.T., Hovgaard, L. & Frokjaer, S. (1998). Predicting drug absorption from molecular surface properties based on molecular dynamics simulations. Pharmaceutical Research 15, 972–978.

85. Stenberg, P., Luthman, K. & Artursson, P. (1999). Prediction of membrane permeability to peptides from calculated dynamic molecular surface properties. Pharmaceutical Research 16, 205–212.

86. Goodwin, J.T., Mao, B., Vidmar, T.J., Conradi, R.A. & Burton, P.S. (1999). Strategies toward predicting peptide cellular permeability from computed molecular descriptors. Journal of Peptide Research 53, 355–369.

87. Wessel, M.D., Jurs, P.C., Tolan, J.W. & Muskal, S.M. (1998). Prediction of human intestinal absorption of drug compounds from molecular structure. Journal of Chemical Information and Computer Sciences 38, 726–735.

88. Wang, J., Krudy, G., Xie, X.Q., Wu, C. & Holland, G. (2006). Genetic algorithm-optimized QSRP models for bioavailability, protein binding, and urinary excretion. Journal of Chemical Information and Modeling 46, 2674–2683.

89. Kitchen, D.B. & Subramanian, G. (2006). Computational approaches for modeling human intestinal absorption and permeability. Journal of Molecular Modeling 12, 577–589.

90. Kariv, I., Cao, H., Marvil, P.D., Bobkova, E.V., Bukhtiyarov, Y.E., Yan, Y.P., Patel, U., Coudurier, L., Chung, T.D. & Oldenburg, K.R. (2001). Identification of inhibitors of bacterial transcription/translation machinery utilizing a miniaturized 1536-well format screen. Journal of Biomolecular Screening 6, 233–243.

91. Lahoz, A., Gombau, L., Donato, M.T., Castell, J.V. & Gomez-Lechon, M.J. (2006). In vitro ADME medium/high-throughput screening in drug preclinical development. Mini Reviews in Medicinal Chemistry 6, 1053–1062.

92. Van de Waterbeemd, H. (2005). From in vivo to in vitro/in silico ADME: Progress and challenges. Expert Opinion on Drug Metabolism & Toxicology 1, 1–4.

93. Alsenz, J. & Haenel, E. (2003). Development of a 7-day, 96-well Caco-2 permeability assay with high-throughput direct UV compound analysis. Pharmaceutical Research 20, 1961–1969.

94. Balimane, P.V., Patel, K., Marino, A. & Chong, S. (2005). Utility of 96-well Caco-2 system for increased throughput of P-gp screening in drug discovery. European Journal of Pharmaceutics and Biopharmaceutics 58, 99–105.

95. Fung, E.N., Chu, I., Li, C., Liu, T., Soares, A., Morrison, R. & Nomeir, A.A. (2003). Higher-throughput screening for Caco-2 permeability utilizing a multiple sprayer liquid chromatography/tandem mass spectrometry system. Rapid Communications in Mass Spectrometry 17, 2147–2152.

13

Fundamentals of Dissolution

Jianzhuo Wang and Douglas R. Flanagan

13.1 INTRODUCTION

Orally administered solid dosage forms generally undergo disintegration, dissolution, and absorption to enter the blood stream and reach the site of action. For drugs with low solubility, dissolution is often the rate-limiting step, and directly affects the rate and extent of drug absorption. Various dissolution tests have been developed that have become tools for predicting *in vivo* performance, and monitoring product quality. The basic theoretical aspects of solid dissolution are discussed in this chapter, which is focused on dissolution of small drug molecules in aqueous media.

13.2 MECHANISM AND THEORIES OF SOLID DISSOLUTION

A prerequisite for drug molecules to be transported into the bulk solution is that they detach from the solid surface, and form solvated molecules. This process is called "solvation," which is a physico-chemical reaction. Solvated molecules then need to transfer from the solid–liquid interface to the bulk solution, which is a mass transport process. This mass transport process generally controls dissolution rates. Diffusion usually plays a key role in this transport process, while convection also is important in cases of agitated media.

13.2.1 Thermodynamic Considerations

No matter whether a solid is crystalline or amorphous, neighboring molecules are closely associated with each other through intermolecular forces. Dissolution involves the breaking of these existing intermolecular interactions, and the formation of new interactions with solvent—usually water. The solid dissolution process generally involves two sequential steps: the first step is the interaction between solid and solvent molecules to form solvated molecules (solvation), which takes place at the solid–liquid interface. The second step is the mass transport of solvated molecules from the solid–liquid interface to the bulk solution. These two steps govern the rate and extent of solid dissolution. Solubility, a basic property for solids, controls the first step. Transport, on the other hand, usually controls the second step, which is generally slower than the first step. Overall, dissolution is governed by solubility and transport processes.

We can view the first step of dissolution as a physico-chemical reaction, which is governed by the same principles as regular chemical reactions. The solvation process is reversible, and solubility is reached when the reaction reaches equilibrium. This process can be described by its Gibbs free energy (ΔG):

$$\text{Drug} + \text{Solvent} \rightleftharpoons \text{Solvated Drug} \qquad (13.1)$$

$$\Delta G = \Delta H - T\Delta S \qquad (13.2)$$

This reaction involves both the breakage of existing intermolecular interactions (drug–drug, solvent–solvent), and the formation of new intermolecular interactions (drug–solvent). The net entropy (ΔS) change for this reaction is generally positive (dissolution causes an increase in disorder) which is favorable for dissolution. Therefore, the extent of dissolution is often determined by the net enthalpy change (ΔH).

If the net enthalpy change is negative or close to zero, the reaction will continue until all available solid is dissolved. The empirical rule, "like dissolves like," therefore has its thermodynamic basis. On the other hand, if the net enthalpy change (ΔH) is positive, the reaction will progress until equilibrium is reached ($\Delta G = 0$). A saturated solution is obtained.

The reaction rate V is described kinetically by:

$$V = k_1[\text{Drug}][\text{Solvent}]$$

$$k_1 = Ae^{-E_a/RT} \qquad (13.3)$$

The overall rate of dissolution is controlled by the slower step of the two-step dissolution process. Thermodynamically, the activation energy E_a for the formation of solvated drug should be less than the energy to break water–water or drug–drug intermolecular interactions. Since hydrogen bonding is among the strongest intermolecular interactions, the activation energy for reaction (13.1) in many cases should be less than the energy of water–water hydrogen bond, which is approximately 19 kJ/mol. In liquid water, hydrogen bonds are constantly being broken and reformed, because thermal energy is sufficient to cause cleavage of these interactions. Therefore, at room temperature, the rate of solvation is generally so fast that equilibrium is almost instantaneous. Compared to the rate of solvation, mass transport from the solid–liquid interface to bulk solution involves molecules moving a large distance compared to molecular dimensions, which is usually much slower and becomes the rate-limiting step.

13.2.2 Dissolution by Pure Diffusion

For solid dissolution processes, convection generally accompanies diffusion in transporting dissolved molecules. Dissolution through pure diffusion without any contribution from some form of convection is rare. Even without mixing, density gradients caused by concentration differences or thermal effects due to the heat of solvation can lead to natural convection. However, we can consider a hypothetical situation in which dissolution is purely diffusional.

Assume a small drug particle is placed at the bottom of a large beaker full of water. The water is kept unstirred so that there is no convection. The drug particle may dissolve by diffusion, which is equivalent to having a diffusion layer of growing thickness. In this case, dissolution becomes a pure diffusional phenomenon.

When a particle dissolves by pure diffusion, the concentration at every point away from the solid–liquid interface increases, but the concentration gradient at any distance from the particle decreases with time. The overall dissolution rate of the particle keeps decreasing. Depending on the solubility and solvent volume, there can be two possible results. If the amount needed to saturate the solvent is equal to or more than the particle weight, the particle will eventually completely dissolve; if the amount needed to saturate the solvent is less than the particle weight, a saturated solution will eventually form which coexists with a smaller particle.

No matter what the final result is, we will not be able to see the formation of a pseudo-steady state in this dissolution process. A pseudo-steady state can be reached if, during some finite time in the dissolution process, the concentration gradient becomes relatively constant with time. The existence of a pseudo-steady state would make the dissolution rate expression simpler mathematically. However, in this case, the concentration gradient may be constantly changing, and we may not be able to apply the pseudo-steady state treatment. Later we will see cases where pseudo-steady state is applicable.

13.2.3 Diffusion Layer Model

Noyes and Whitney first proposed the basic transport-controlled model for solid dissolution.[1] They suggested that when surface area is constant, the dissolution rate is proportional to the difference between solubility and the bulk solution concentration:

$$\frac{dQ}{dt} = k(C_s - C_b) \qquad (13.4)$$

where:
dQ/dt is the dissolution rate
k is a constant (mass transfer coefficient)
C_S is solubility
C_b is bulk solution concentration.

Nernst[2] and Brunner[3] then suggested that rapid equilibrium (i.e., saturation) is achieved at the solid–liquid interface during dissolution, and then diffusion occurs across a thin layer of stagnant solution, called the diffusion layer, into the bulk solution. Diffusion across this diffusion layer is rate-controlling in most cases, which effectively converts the heterogeneous dissolution process into a homogeneous process of liquid-phase diffusion. This model, as shown in Figure 13.1, is also called the film model. Dissolution rate can be expressed as:

$$\frac{dQ}{dt} = DA\frac{(C_s - C_b)}{h} \qquad (13.5)$$

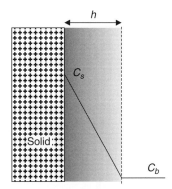

FIGURE 13.1 Diffusion layer model for a planar surface dissolution (C_S is solubility, C_b is bulk solution concentration, h is diffusion layer thickness)

where:

D is diffusion coefficient

A is solid surface area

h is diffusion layer thickness.

Nernst and Brunner's concept of a diffusion layer being a stagnant or unstirred layer of liquid adhering to the solid surface is hydrodynamically unrealistic, but allows the complex dissolution processes to be analyzed in a tractable fashion. The diffusion layer model is widely used, due to its simplicity and applicability to a wide range of dissolution phenomena. However, the notion of a stagnant liquid layer near the solid surface is not supported by fluid dynamics. Liquid motion was observed at distances from solid surfaces much closer than a typical diffusion layer thickness. So, the diffusion layer is actually a boundary layer, with a concentration gradient as well as a velocity gradient. Another limitation of the diffusion layer model is that it does not give a means to calculate independently a diffusion layer thickness based on hydrodynamics. Thus, it does not allow computation of the diffusional flux, *a priori*. Diffusion layer thicknesses can be obtained only by fitting equations to experimental data.

13.2.4 Convective Diffusion Model

The limitations of the diffusion layer model call for further examination of dissolution processes in order to develop an improved model. There are two mechanisms for the transport of solute molecules from a solid in a moving liquid. First, there is molecular diffusion as a result of a concentration gradient; secondly, solute molecules are carried along by the moving solvent (i.e., convection). Dissolution is usually a combination of these two mechanisms, which is called convective diffusion. In convective diffusion models,

the contribution of both convection and molecular diffusion are taken into account. The general equation for convective diffusion in three dimensions is given below:

$$\frac{\partial C}{\partial t} = D \left(\frac{\partial^2 C}{\partial x^2} + \frac{\partial^2 C}{\partial y^2} + \frac{\partial^2 C}{\partial z^2} \right) - v_x \frac{\partial C}{\partial x} - v_y \frac{\partial C}{\partial y} - v_z \frac{\partial C}{\partial z} \tag{13.6}$$

v_x, v_y and v_z are liquid velocities in the x, y and z directions in Cartesian coordinates.

This equation is an extension of Fick's second law of diffusion, with the addition of convection terms. It is a second-order partial differential equation with variable coefficients. To determine the net concentration change at a particular point at any time we also need to know the liquid flow pattern, and the boundary and initial conditions. This equation can be solved exactly for only a very limited number of special cases. Some of these cases will be discussed later.

In the convective diffusion model, solvent stream movement depends on its distance from the solid surface. At distances far from the solid surface, convection dominates over diffusion for transport of solute molecules. At distances very close to the solid surface, the solvent stream movement is slow, while the concentration gradient is large. In such regions, the contribution of diffusion to the solute molecule movement is comparable to or larger than convection. This region is also called the diffusion layer, but it is different from Nernst's concept. Levich pointed out the differences between Nernst's layer and the convective diffusion-based diffusion layer:[4]

1. Solvent in Nernst's layer is considered stagnant while it has a velocity gradient in the convective diffusion model.
2. In Nernst's model, mass transport in the direction parallel to solid surface is disregarded. In convective diffusion theory, convection and diffusion both across and along the diffusion layer are taken into account.
3. Nernst's layer is considered to have constant thickness everywhere, while the thickness of the diffusion layer based on convective diffusion theory varies substantially along the solid surface depending on position and solvent motion. In fact, the diffusion layer has no clear-cut boundary; it is simply a region where the concentration gradient is at a maximum.

Unlike Nernst's diffusion layer model, the convective diffusion model is more hydrodynamically realistic, and it does allow us to predict solid dissolution rates. However, it is usually complicated to apply convective diffusion to derive accurate expressions for solid dissolution because of the need to describe the fluid dynamics accurately.

13.3 PLANAR SURFACE DISSOLUTION

Modeling planar surface dissolution is easier than modeling particulate dissolution because the mathematics is simpler. The simplest expression describing planar surface dissolution is the empirical Noyes–Whitney equation. The diffusion layer model is almost as simple. Measuring dissolution rate from a well-defined surface has been a popular way of characterizing pharmaceutical solids. Determination of intrinsic dissolution rate is one example. Though the Noyes–Whitney equation is capable of describing such a process, planar surface dissolution can be more accurately described with convective diffusion models based on different hydrodynamic conditions.

13.3.1 Intrinsic Dissolution Rate

When other parameters, such as agitation intensity and surface area, are fixed, dissolution rate can be viewed as a property of the solid. This loosely defined property is called the "intrinsic" dissolution rate. Due to the close relationship between the intrinsic dissolution rate and solubility, measuring the intrinsic dissolution rate becomes an alternative method for solubility estimation when equilibrium solubility cannot easily be obtained experimentally. For example, measurement of intrinsic dissolution rates is a powerful tool for the evaluation of solubility differences between polymorphs or solvates. The equilibrium solubility of an anhydrous crystal form may not be determined if it converts to a hydrate when in contact with water. The solubility difference of an anhydrous versus a hydrate crystal form can be estimated by studying the difference in initial intrinsic dissolution rates as the conversion occurs.

Since dissolution rate is always affected by agitation intensity, surface area, and container configuration, determination of intrinsic dissolution rates requires a method with good reproducibility. The rotating disk method, which is schematically demonstrated in Figure 13.2, is often the method of choice. The disk is compressed from pure material, and has a planar surface. The compressed disk is put into the holder so that only one flat surface is in contact with the solvent. The disk is then rotated at a constant (or varying) speed, and the dissolution rate is measured. When a diffusion

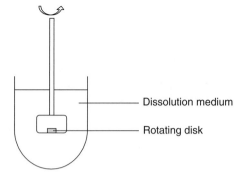

FIGURE 13.2 Rotating disk apparatus for measuring intrinsic dissolution rate

layer model is applied, a diffusion layer thickness can easily be determined from the dissolution rate data.

The hydrodynamics for a rotating disk system presents a good case of applying a convective diffusion model. According to Levich, using a convective diffusion model, the solvent flow pattern can be depicted as shown in Figure 13.3.[5,6] Far from the disk, the fluid moves axially toward the disk. In a thin layer near the disk surface, the liquid acquires a rotating motion, and moves radially away from the center of the disk. This system is one of the few cases that can be solved exactly with convective diffusion theory. The dissolution rate (dQ/dt) is given by:

$$\frac{dQ}{dt} = 1.95 D^{2/3} C_s u^{-1/6} \omega^{1/2} R^2 \qquad (13.7)$$

where:

D is the diffusion coefficient
C_S is the solubility
u is the kinematic viscosity
ω is the rotational speed
R is the disk radius.

The convective diffusion model for dissolution of a rotating disk also provides a means to estimate the diffusion layer thickness, as shown below:

$$h = 1.61 D^{1/3} u^{1/6} \omega^{-1/2} \qquad (13.8)$$

An interesting study using the rotating disk is by McNamara and Amidon, who applied convective diffusion models to reactive dissolution.[7,8]

13.3.2 Convective Diffusion Model for Flow Past a Planar Surface

In addition to dissolution from a rotating disk, the case of planar surface dissolution can be modeled with relative ease. When the solvent flows parallel to a flat surface of a solid, there is a velocity gradient, as

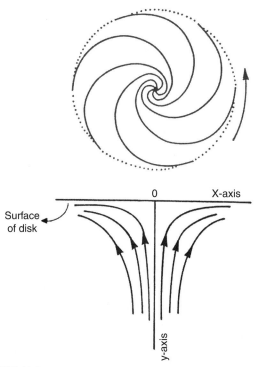

FIGURE 13.3   Liquid flow pattern around a rotating disk apparatus

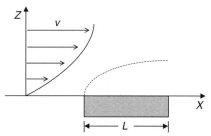

FIGURE 13.4   Convective–diffusion model for dissolution of a planar surface with liquid flow parallel to the surface. The dashed curve indicates the boundary layer region. X and Z are coordinate axes, L is the solid surface length, v is the bulk fluid velocity

If the tablet is circular with a radius of r, the equation becomes:

$$\frac{dQ}{dt} = 2.157\, D^{2/3} C_s \alpha^{1/3} r^{5/3}   \quad (13.11)$$

The results obtained by Nelson and Shah were confirmed by Neervannan et al. using numerical methods to solve the convective diffusion equations.[14]

13.4 PARTICULATE DISSOLUTION

Modeling planar surface dissolution is important for understanding dissolution mechanisms. However, dissolution of solid dosage forms usually involves solid particles. Most rapid release oral dosage forms first disintegrate into small particles, which then dissolve for the drug to be bioavailable. The same dissolution theories that apply to planar surface dissolution are also applicable to particle dissolution. However, the dissolution of solid particles is more complicated, because total surface area changes during dissolution. Also, particles have various shapes and size distributions that make modeling their dissolution process even more complicated.

13.4.1 Diffusion Layer-based Dissolution Models

Three diffusion-controlled models have been reported (as presented in Chapter 7) for monosized spherical particle dissolution under sink conditions, as shown below:

shown in Figure 13.4. Both molecular diffusion normal to the surface, and the forced convection parallel to the surface, contribute to the dissolution of the solid. For such a flat surface, the diffusion boundary layer is well characterized, and can be used to calculate the dissolution rate. An equation derived by Levich can be applied to dissolution of a rectangular tablet of length L (in the direction of flow) and width b:[9]

$$\frac{dQ}{dt} = 0.68 D^{2/3} C_s u^{-1/6} v^{1/2} b L^{1/2}   \quad (13.9)$$

where:

D is the diffusion coefficient
C_S is the solubility
u is the kinematic viscosity
v is the bulk fluid velocity.

Nelson and Shah also developed a convective diffusion model for planar surface dissolution under parallel flow.[10–13] For rectangular tablets with length L (in the direction of flow), and width b, the dissolution rate is:

$$\frac{dQ}{dt} = 0.808 D^{2/3} C_s \alpha^{1/3} b L^{2/3}   \quad (13.10)$$

where:

α is the rate of shear in the boundary layer
b is the tablet width (normal to flow)
L is the tablet length (parallel to flow).

$$W^{1/3} = W_0^{1/3} - K_{1/3} t \qquad K_{1/3} = \left(\frac{4\pi \rho N}{3}\right)^{1/3} \frac{DC_s}{\rho h}$$

$$(13.12)$$

$$W^{1/2} = W_0^{1/2} - K_{1/2}t \qquad K_{1/2} = \left(\frac{3\pi\rho N}{2}\right)^{1/2}\frac{DC_s}{k'\rho}$$

$$(13.13)$$

$$W^{2/3} = W_0^{2/3} - k_{2/3}t \qquad K_{2/3} = \left(\frac{4\pi\rho N}{3}\right)^{2/3}\frac{2DC_s}{\rho}$$

$$(13.14)$$

where:

W is the particle weight at time t

W_0 is the initial particle weight

$K_{1/3}$, $K_{1/2}$, and $K_{2/3}$ are composite rate constants

ρ is the density of the particle

N is the number of particles

D is the diffusion coefficient

C_S is the solubility

h is the diffusion layer thickness

k' is a constant.

Equation 13.12 was reported by Hixson and Crowell, and is known as the cube-root law.[15,16] It was derived originally based on the assumption that dissolution rate is proportional to the surface area of spherical particles. It can also be derived using a simple diffusion layer model. Equation 13.13 is a semi-empirical expression reported by Niebergall et al., and has a square-root dependency on weight.[17] Equation 13.14 has a two-thirds-root dependency on weight, and was derived by Higuchi and Hiestand for dissolution of very small particles.[18,19]

Each of the above three particle dissolution models gives satisfactory fits to certain experimental dissolution data.[16,17,19] However, the choice of the model to fit experimental data is somewhat arbitrary. Though they appear different in form, the three equations are often difficult to distinguish when applied to experimental data. Veng Pedersen and Brown evaluated these three models experimentally by studying dissolution of tolbutamide powder.[20] By taking into account the particle size distribution in their computer model, they found that the cube-root model worked best with the smallest mean squared deviation for the fitted curve. However, the fitting results of the cube-root and the square-root models were almost equally good.

By accounting for the curvature of the concentration gradient in the diffusion layer around a spherical particle, Wang and Flanagan derived a general solution for diffusion-controlled single particle dissolution (Equations 13.15 and 13.16)[21]. Their analysis shows that the concentration gradient inside a diffusion layer is not linear (Figure 13.5). Mathematical analysis shows that the three classical particle dissolution rate expressions are approximate solutions to the general solution.

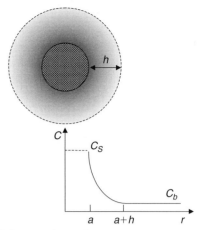

FIGURE 13.5　Pseudo-steady state concentration gradient around a spherical particle

The cube-root law is most appropriate when particle size is much larger than the diffusion layer thickness; the two-thirds-root expression applies when the particle size is much smaller than the diffusion layer thickness. The square-root expression is intermediate between these two models.

$$\frac{DC_S}{\rho h}t = a_0 - a - h\ln\frac{h+a_0}{h+a} \qquad (13.15)$$

$$\frac{DC_S}{\rho h}t = \left(\frac{3w_0}{4\pi\rho}\right)^{\frac{1}{3}} - \left(\frac{3w}{4\pi\rho}\right)^{\frac{1}{3}} - h\cdot\ln\frac{h+\left(\frac{3w_0}{4\pi\rho}\right)^{\frac{1}{3}}}{h+\left(\frac{3w}{4\pi\rho}\right)^{\frac{1}{3}}} \qquad (13.16)$$

In deriving the general solution for diffusion-controlled particle dissolution, pseudo-steady state is an important assumption. For example, dissolution from a planar surface under sink conditions reaches steady state when the dissolution rate becomes constant; hence the concentration gradient in the diffusion layer becomes time-invariant. In any short time interval, the number of molecules moving into the diffusion layer from one side equals the number of molecules moving out of the diffusion layer from the other side.

For particle dissolution, a similar state can often be reached in which the number of molecules moving into the diffusion layer from one side approximately equals to the number of molecules moving out of the diffusion layer from the other side. This assumption requires that, within the time for an average molecule to cross the diffusion layer, the change of particle surface area is negligible.

An interesting result derived from the general particle dissolution model is given by Equation 13.17, which demonstrates that the dissolution rate per unit surface area (surface-specific dissolution rates) depends upon particle size, with smaller particles having higher surface-specific dissolution rates. Bisrat et al.[22] and Anderberg et al.[23,24] reported a dependence of surface-specific dissolution rates upon particle size. Their results showed the same trend as predicted here. The surface-specific dissolution rate increased (after correcting for solubility dependence on particle size) with decreasing particle size. This increase was especially pronounced for particle sizes below ~5 μm.

$$J = DC_S \left(\frac{1}{h} + \frac{1}{a} \right) \qquad (13.17)$$

13.4.2 Convective Diffusion-based Particulate Dissolution Model

The convective diffusion model has the advantage of being more hydrodynamically realistic. Applying convective diffusion to spherical particle dissolution has the potential of being able to predict dissolution rate more accurately.

Levich derived an equation for convective diffusion from a sphere. Assuming liquid flow around a particle is in creeping motion while the boundary layer is small compared to particle size, Levich derived an expression for mass transport to a free-falling sphere based on convective diffusion.[4] This expression is applicable when the Reynolds number is much less than 1, while the Peclet number is much larger than 1 (see Chapter 29). When this expression is applied to spherical particle dissolution, it can be written as:

$$\frac{dQ}{dt} = 7.98 \cdot C_s D^{2/3} v^{1/3} a^{4/3} \qquad (13.18)$$

where:
Q is the amount dissolved
t is time
C_S is solubility
D is the diffusion coefficient
"v" is the bulk solvent velocity
"a" is the particle radius.

The dissolution rate per unit area (J) is obtained by normalizing the total dissolution rate (Equation 13.18) by particle surface area ($4\pi a^2$), which leads to:

$$J = 0.635 \cdot C_S D^{2/3} v^{1/3} a^{-2/3} \qquad (13.19)$$

The significance of Equation 13.19 is that the dissolution rate per unit area depends on surface curvature. For the same total surface area, smaller particles have higher dissolution rates. Though the expressions are different, this conclusion qualitatively agrees well with the previous general diffusion layer model for spherical particle dissolution (Equation 13.17). Applying the above equation for diffusional flux under such flow conditions leads to the following equation for particle weight undissolved (w) with time:

$$w^{5/9} = w_0^{5/9} - 2.35 \cdot C_S D^{2/3} v^{1/3} \rho^{-4/9} t \qquad (13.20)$$

For dissolution of N monosized spherical particles, the equation becomes:

$$W^{5/9} = W_0^{5/9} - K_{5/9} t$$

$$K_{5/9} = 2.35 \cdot C_S D^{2/3} v^{1/3} \rho^{-4/9} N^{5/9} \qquad (13.21)$$

For dissolution of a polydisperse particle system, the overall dissolution profile can be obtained by summing the contributions from each particle:

$$W_t = \sum_{i=1}^{N} w_{ti} \qquad (13.22)$$

where:
W_t is total particle weight remaining at time t
w_{ti} is weight remaining of particle i at time t
N is number of particles.

Since all the parameters in Equation 13.21 can be determined independently, it is possible to calculate particle dissolution profiles *a priori* without resorting to parameters that must be calculated from the dissolution data (i.e., diffusion layer thickness).

The derivation of Equation 13.21 based on Levich's expression is a novel approach in modeling particle dissolution. Independently of this study, Abdou[25] and Shah et al.[26] also presented equations similar to Equation 13.21. Their equations were slightly different from Equation 13.21, possibly due to editorial errors.

13.4.3 Dissolution Under Non-sink Conditions

For solid dissolution, a changing bulk solution concentration complicates the modeling of this process. The assumption of sink conditions makes the mathematical derivation easier. The particle dissolution models summarized above are such examples. However, many dissolution processes take place under non-sink conditions, particularly for sparingly soluble compounds.

If the change of solvent volume (V) during dissolution is minimal, the concentration in the bulk solution can be expressed as:

$$C_b = \frac{Q}{V} \qquad (13.23)$$

where:

Q is the amount dissolved

V is the solvent volume.

For spherical particle dissolution, concentration in the bulk solution is expressed as:

$$C_b = \frac{\frac{4}{3}\pi\rho(a_0^3 - a^3)}{V} \qquad (13.24)$$

By introducing Equations 13.23 and 13.24 to the aforementioned particle dissolution models, the particle dissolution models discussed above can be extended to non-sink conditions. Hixson and Crowell actually derived equations for particle dissolution under non-sink conditions. They also discussed a special situation in which the initial total particle weight is equal to the saturation capacity of the solvent. However, their equations were presented in a way that was inconvenient to apply.[15] These equations were later derived and discussed by Short et al.,[27] and also by Pothisiri and Carstensen.[28] Patel and Carstensen found that these non-sink condition models held up to 80–90% dissolved for dissolution of p-hydroxybenzoic acid and sodium chloride.[29]

13.4.4 Effects of Particle Shape

All of the three classical particle dissolution models were developed for spherical particles. Obviously, real pharmaceutical powders usually have irregular shapes. It is desirable to know how much deviation irregular particle shapes can contribute to the dissolution profile. Veng Pedersen and Brown investigated this problem theoretically.[30] Assuming exact isotropic dissolution, they derived the equations governing the dissolution profile for ten common crystal shapes. They found the dissolution of each crystal shape can usually be approximated by a hypothetical spherical particle dissolution. Deviation became large after a large portion of the particle had dissolved.

Dali and Carstensen studied the effect of particle shape on dissolution behavior using single potassium dichromate crystals.[31] They incorporated a semi-empirical shape factor to fit the dissolution profile of a crystal to that of a spherical particle of equivalent volume. Assuming that deviations from the cube-root law were completely due to the shape factor, they found that the shape factor is not constant, but changes as a particle dissolves.

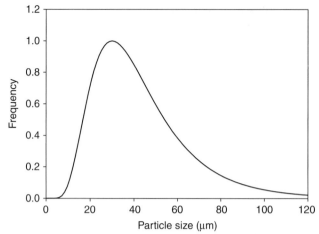

FIGURE 13.6   Typical log-normal particle size distribution for pharmaceutical powders

13.4.5 Polydispersity Effects

Classical particle dissolution models, like the cube-root law, are intended only for single or monodisperse particle dissolution. However, pharmaceutical powders are composed of particles of various sizes. Sieve cuts from powders have often been used in dissolution experiments. Based on theoretical calculations, Brooke pointed out that, when treated as monosized powders, the error can be as much as 3% for the narrowest sieve cuts depending on particle size distribution across the cut. For wider sieve cuts, errors of 6–10% are possible.[32] Therefore, a theoretical treatment for polydispersity effects is necessary even for fairly narrowly-distributed powders. Most pharmaceutical powders are produced by milling and, as a result, tend to give skewed particle size distributions as shown in Figure 13.6. Such a distribution can be converted to a Gaussian distribution by plotting the x-axis on a logarithmic scale. Such a distribution is log-normal. Most theoretical investigations for poly-dispersed particle dissolution assume the particle size distribution to be log-normal.

Higuchi et al. studied dissolution of a polydispersed methylprednisolone powder by approximating a log-normal distribution with a simpler function.[19] By convoluting the approximate particle size distribution function with the two-thirds-root particle dissolution model, the total particle dissolution profile was calculated. Reasonably good agreement between experimental results and theory was obtained in the study of methylprednisolone powder dissolution.

Brooke derived an exact equation for dissolution of a log-normal distributed powder, based on the cube-root single particle dissolution model.[33] Though the calculations are tedious, they can be performed with a calculator, and a normal distribution table. Brooke's expression is:

$$
\begin{aligned}
W_\tau = {} & r e^{3(\mu + 3\sigma^2/2)} \left(1 - F\left[\frac{\ln(\tau) - (\mu + 3\sigma^2)}{\sigma} \right] \right) \\
& - 3r\tau e^{2(\mu + \sigma^2)} \left(1 - F\left[\frac{\ln(\tau) - (\mu + 2\sigma^2)}{\sigma} \right] \right) \\
& + 3r\tau^2 e^{(\mu + \sigma^2/2)} \left(1 - F\left[\frac{\ln(\tau) - (\mu + \sigma^2)}{\sigma} \right] \right) \\
& - r\tau^3 \left(1 - F\left[\frac{\ln(\tau) - \mu}{\sigma} \right] \right)
\end{aligned}
$$

(13.25)

where $\displaystyle F(x) = \frac{\sqrt{2}}{2\pi} \int_{-\infty}^{x} e^{-x^2/2}\, dx$

and $\displaystyle \tau = \frac{2kC_S}{\rho t}$

where:

W_τ is the weight undissolved
μ is the mean particle diameter
σ is its standard deviation
$r = \pi\rho N / 6$
C_S is the particle solubility
ρ is the particle density
k is a constant.

Brooke also pointed out that many actual powders follow truncated distributions. Therefore, it is possible that applying an untruncated distribution or ideal lognormal distribution would lead to errors. If the exact equation is used to represent a distribution that is truncated, the result is erroneously adding some larger or smaller particles than actually exist. However, the error due to the addition of smaller particles is minimal, while the error due to the addition of larger particles can be significant. This arises because, for the same number of particles, the total weight of the larger particles is much higher than that for smaller particles. Brooke then presented an equation for dissolution of truncated lognormal distributed powders which is applicable before the critical time (i.e., before the smallest particles disappear).[34] Veng Pedersen and Brown presented complex expressions for polydispersed powder dissolution under sink or non-sink conditions, based on the three classical single particle dissolution models.[35–37]

With faster computational tools, it is less important to have a single equation convolving a size distribution function with a particular basic particle dissolution model to predict a dissolution profile. As long as the size distribution is available, the total dissolution profile can be calculated by treating each narrow size fraction separately, and adding the contributions of each fraction together. The added advantage for this approach is that particle size does not need to follow any specific distribution. Several powder dissolution studies have been conducted using this method, and satisfactory results were obtained.[38–40]

In all of the above methods dealing with polydispersed particles, it is assumed that each particle dissolves independently. This may not be true under certain experimental conditions. A commonly encountered problem in particle dissolution is aggregation. In such cases, the dissolution of one particle is affected by the existence of other particles. The above multi-particle dissolution expressions do not apply to such situations.

References

1. Noyes, A.A. & Whitney, W.R. (1897). The rate of solution of solid substances in their own solutions. Journal of the American Chemical Society 19, 930–934.
2. Nernst, W. (1904). Theorie der reaktionsgeschwindigkeit in heterogenen systemen. Zeitschrift für Physikalische Chemie 47, 52–55.
3. Bruner, E. (1904). Reaktionsgeschwindigkeit in heterogenen systemen. Zeitschrift für Physikalische Chemie 47, 56–102.
4. Levich, V.G. (1962). Physicochemical Hydrodynamics, 2 edn. Prentice-Hall, Englewood Cliffs, New Jersey. pp. 57–60.
5. Levich, V.G. (1962). Physicochemical Hydrodynamics, 2 edn. Prentice-Hall, Englewood Cliffs, New Jersey. pp. 61–72.
6. Grant, D.J.W. & Brittain, H.G. (1995). Solubility of pharmaceutical solids. In: Physical Characterization of Pharmaceutical Solids, H.G. Brittain. (ed.) Marcel Dekker, Inc, New York, NY. p. 359.
7. McNamara, D.P. & Amidon, G.L. (1986). Dissolution of acidic and basic compounds from the rotating disk: Influence of convective diffusion and reaction. Journal of Pharmaceutical Sciences 75, 858–868.
8. McNamara, D.P. & Amidon, G.L. (1988). Reaction plane approach for estimating the effects of buffers on the dissolution rate of acidic drugs. Journal of Pharmaceutical Sciences 77, 511–517.
9. Levich, V.G. (1962). Physicochemical Hydrodynamics, 2 edn. Prentice-Hall, Inc. Englewood Cliffs, New Jersey. pp. 87–91.
10. Nelson, K.G. & Shah, A.C. (1975). Convective diffusion model for a transport-controlled dissolution rate process. Journal of Pharmaceutical Sciences 64, 610–614.
11. Shah, A.C. & Nelson, K.G. (1975). Evaluation of a convective diffusion drug dissolution rate model. Journal of Pharmaceutical Sciences 64, 1518–1520.
12. Nelson, K.G. & Shah, A.C. (1987). Mass transport in dissolution kinetics I: Convective diffusion to assess the role of fluid viscosity under forced flow conditions. Journal of Pharmaceutical Sciences 76, 799–802.
13. Shah, A.C. & Nelson, K.G. (1987). Mass transport in dissolution kinetics II: Convective diffusion to assess role of viscosity under conditions of gravitational flow. Journal of Pharmaceutical Sciences 76, 910–913.
14. Neervannan, S. et al. (1993). A numerical convective-diffusion model for dissolution of neutral compounds under laminar flow conditions. International Journal of Pharmaceutics 96, 167–174.
15. Hixson, A.W. & Crowell, J.H. (1931). Dependence of reaction velocity upon surface and agitation I: Theoretical consideration. Industrial and Engineering Chemistry 23, 923–931.

16. Hixson, A.W. & Crowell, J.H. (1931). Dependence of reaction velocity upon surface and agitation II: Experimental procedure in study of surface. Industrial and Engineering Chemistry 23, 1002–1009.

17. Niebergall, P.J., Milosovich, G. & Goyan, J.E. (1963). Dissolution rate studies II: Dissolution of particles under conditions of agitation. Journal of Pharmaceutical Sciences 52, 236–241.

18. Higuchi, W.I. & Hiestand, E.N. (1963). Dissolution rates of finely devided drug powders I: Effect of a distribution of particle sizes in a diffusion-controlled process. Journal of Pharmaceutical Sciences 52, 67–71.

19. Higuchi, W.I., Rowe, E.L. & Hiestand, E.N. (1963). Dissolution rates of finely divided drug powders II: Micronized methylprednisolone. Journal of Pharmaceutical Sciences 52, 162–164.

20. Pedersen, P.V. & Brown, K.F. (1976). Experimental evaluation of three single-particle dissolution models. Journal of Pharmaceutical Sciences 65, 1442–1447.

21. Wang, J. & Flanagan, D.R. (1999). General solution for diffusion-controlled dissolution of spherical particles. I. Theory. Journal of Pharmaceutical Sciences 88, 731–738.

22. Bisrat, M. & Nystrom, C. (1988). Physicochemical aspects of drug release VIII: The relation between particle size and surface specific dissolution rate in agitated suspensions. International Journal of Pharmaceutics 47, 223–231.

23. Anderberg, E.K., Bisrat, M. & Nystrom, C. (1988). Physicochemical aspects of drug release VII: The effect of surfactant concentration and drug particle size on solubility and dissolution rate of felodipine, a sparingly soluble drug. International Journal of Pharmaceutics 47, 67–77.

24. Anderberg, E.K. & Nystrom, C. (1990). Physicochemical aspects of drug release X: Investigation of the applicability of the cube root law for characterization of the dissolution rate of fine particulate materials. International Journal of Pharmaceutics 62, 143–151.

25. Abdou, H.M. (1989). Theory of dissolution. In: *Dissolution, Bioavailability and Bioequivalence*. Mack Publishing Company, Easton, PA. pp. 11–36.

26. Shah, A.C., Nelson, K.G. & Britten, N.J. (1991). Dissolution kinetics of spherical tablet in stirred media: 2. Functional dependency of solubility and diffusivity. Pharmaceutical Research 8, S–182.

27. Short, M.P., Sharkey, P. & Rhodes, C.T. (1972). Dissolution of hydrocortisone. Journal of Pharmaceutical Sciences 61, 1732–1735.

28. Pothisiri, P. & Carstensen, J.T. (1973). Nonsink dissolution rate equation. Journal of Pharmaceutical Sciences 62, 1468–1470.

29. Patel, M. & Carstensen, J.T. (1975). Nonsink dissolution rate equations. Journal of Pharmaceutical Sciences 64, 1651–1656.

30. Pedersen, P.V. & Brown, K.F. (1976). Theoretical isotropic dissolution of nonspherical particles. Journal of Pharmaceutical Sciences 65, 1142–1437.

31. Dali, M.V. & Carstensen, J.T. (1996). Effect of change in shape factor of a single crystal on its dissolution behavior. Pharmaceutical Research 13, 155–162.

32. Brooke, D. (1975). Sieve cuts as monodisperse powders in dissolution studies. Journal of Pharmaceutical Sciences 64, 1409–1412.

33. Brooke, D. (1973). Dissolution profile of log-normal powders: Exact expression. Journal of Pharmaceutical Sciences 62, 795–798.

34. Brooke, D. (1974). Dissolution profile of log-normal powders II: Dissolution before critical time. Journal of Pharmaceutical Sciences 63, 344–346.

35. Pedersen, P.V. & Brown, K.F. (1975). Dissolution profile in relation to initial particle distribution. Journal of Pharmaceutical Sciences 64, 1192–1195.

36. Pedersen, P.V. (1977). New method for characterizing dissolution properties of drug powders. Journal of Pharmaceutical Sciences 66, 761–766.

37. Pedersen, P.V. & Brown, K.F. (1977). General class of multiparticulate dissolution models. Journal of Pharmaceutical Sciences 66, 1435–1438.

38. Mauger, J.W., Howard, S.A. & Amin, K. (1983). Dissolution profiles for finely divided drug suspensions. Journal of Pharmaceutical Sciences 72, 190–193.

39. Lu, A.T.K., Frisella, M.E. & Johnson, K.V. (1993). Dissolution modeling: Factors affecting the dissolution rates of polydisperse powders. Pharmaceutical Research 10, 1308–1314.

40. Almeida, L.P.D. et al. (1997). Modeling dissolution of sparingly soluble multisized powders. Journal of Pharmaceutical Sciences 86, 726–732.

14

Dissolution Testing of Solid Products

Michelle Long and Yisheng Chen

14.1 INTRODUCTION

The dissolution test is a key test of solid oral dosage form performance that can be a rich source of information for quality control, formulation, and process development and, most importantly, for evaluation of performance *in vivo*. In fact, a dissolution test with demonstrated predictability for *in vivo* performance can be used to request a waiver of bioequivalency studies from regulatory authorities, thus significantly reducing development time and costs by avoiding lengthy and expensive clinical trials. In its simplest definition, the dissolution test provides a measure of the extent and rate of drug release from a dosage form into an aqueous medium under a set of specified test conditions. The drug release profile is a result of a combination of the properties of the active pharmaceutical ingredient (API), formulation design, manufacturing process, and the chemical and mechanical environment of the test method selected to monitor drug release. The contributions and influence of these factors must be carefully evaluated in order to develop meaningful dissolution test methods.

The connection between the dissolution test and *in vivo* performance is based on the fact that before an active pharmaceutical agent can be absorbed, it must first be dissolved in the aqueous contents of the gastrointestinal (GI) tract. Dokoumetzidis and Macheras,[1] in their review of the history of dissolution testing, credit Edwards[2] with publishing the first studies describing the relationship between rates of dissolution and absorption. Over the subsequent 50 years to the present day, the interest in developing *in vitro* tools to describe, and ultimately predict, *in vivo* performance has been a central focus of biopharmaceutical research. Amidon and his coworkers have developed comprehensive models to describe the transit of drug suspensions through the gastrointestinal tract using chemical engineering concepts coupling mass transfer and fluid dynamics.[3-4] These models established the basic relationships among drug solubility, dissolution rate, and GI membrane permeability. New dimensionless parameters were introduced including the dose number, which relates the dose applied to the ability to solubilize the ingested dose, and the absorption number, which relates the drug permeability to the residence time. These models were the basis for establishment of the Biopharmaceutical Classification System (BCS),[5] which has provided a solid framework for interpretation of dissolution studies in the regulatory approval process.[6] With the advent of modified-release dosage forms, where the amount of drug available is controlled deliberately by the formulation, traditional dissolution testing apparatuses have been adopted, and new ones developed, for monitoring drug release. Extended-release dosage forms have the potential to provide direct correlations between the *in vitro* measured drug release and *in vivo* absorption, and regulatory flexibility for certain formulation and process changes is allowed when such a correlation exists.[7-8]

Because there is no other *in vitro* performance test with such a close link to *in vivo* performance, dissolution and drug release studies are a regulatory requirement for the development, and ultimate

Developing Solid Oral Dosage Forms: Pharmaceutical Theory and Practice
ISBN: 978-0-444-53242-8

approval, of all solid oral drug products.[9] Multiple approaches and instrumentation are available for characterizing drug release, reflecting the multitude of dosage form designs and their distinctive properties. Recognition that the design and operation of the apparatus, and the selection of medium, could influence the drug release profile, coupled with an appreciation of the relationship between a properly correlated drug release profile and oral absorption led to the standardization of practices and equipment through the US Pharmacopeia. The USP <711> describes the various apparatuses used in dissolution studies, and has been recently harmonized with the European Pharmacopoeia and the Japanese Pharmacopoeia. Additional guidance for the development and application of dissolution testing is provided in various FIP position papers[10–11] and regulatory guidances.[8,9,12]

This chapter will begin with a general discussion of the major components to consider in designing a dissolution test method, including a description of the available apparatuses, and a discussion of test media. Subsequent sections focus on applications for testing both immediate release and modified-release products. These will include examples demonstrating the correlation of dissolution test results to *in vivo* performance, and for selecting and monitoring critical quality and process control attributes. A final section will discuss method validation, selection of specifications, and *in vitro–in vivo* correlations.

For the ensuing discussion, the USP, FDA, and ICH guidances are referenced extensively. The authors acknowledge that differences in requirements and definitions do exist in, for example, the EMEA guidances and Japanese Pharmacopoeia. Therefore the reader is encouraged to ensure that the appropriate regulatory expectations are met, based on the intended use and market for the products tested. The objective of this chapter is to explain the scientific basis for design and interpretation of dissolution tests, and the references cited aid in that effort.

14.2 COMPONENTS OF DISSOLUTION TEST METHOD DEVELOPMENT

Development of any analytical test for a drug product must begin with a review of the existing information on the drug substance and the drug product. The intent of the test must also be determined. The complexity of a dissolution test for quality control purposes, for example, may be different from one developed to produce an *in vitro–in vivo* correlation (IVIVC). Similarly, the choice of test con-

ditions for an eroding matrix tablet may be different from those for a disintegrating tablet, even when the same drug is used to prepare both formulations. The major considerations for dissolution test method development are the medium composition, including its pH, and the apparatus type employed, along with its associated operating parameters. The process of selecting the conditions can be iterative or can use formal designed experiments. In order to explain the influence of each component they are described separately below.

14.2.1 Dissolution Apparatuses

There are seven apparatuses defined in the USP general Chapter <711>. This chapter was recently harmonized with the EP and JP to create common definitions and operating parameters for all drug release monitoring. Of the seven apparatuses, Apparatus V (paddle over disk) and Apparatus VI (rotating cylinder) are not used for oral drug products and will not be discussed.

The main apparatuses used for dissolution testing of solid oral dosage forms are Apparatus I and Apparatus II (Figure 14.1). Both of these apparatuses employ a single hemispherical bottom vessel containing the dissolution medium with a centered spindle. The temperature of the vessel is controlled within narrow limits by immersion in a constant temperature water bath or by other suitable technology. For Apparatus I, the dosage form is placed in a basket affixed to the end of the spindle. Agitation is achieved by rotating the basket; a rotational speed of 100 rpm is most commonly used. Experimental and theoretical flow visualization techniques employed by D'Arcy et al.[13] demonstrated that the medium enters the bottom of the basket in the axial direction, flows upward and then exits through the sides.

Apparatus II uses a paddle to induce agitation, with typical rotation speeds of 50–75 rpm. For Apparatus II, the dosage form is dropped directly into the vessel. In cases where the dosage form may float (e.g., capsule formulations), Apparatus I may be more appropriate. Alternatively, when using Apparatus II, the dosage form, either tablet or capsule, may be placed in a sinker designed to enclose the dosage form. There are various sinker designs (Figure 14.2), and the most common sinker, as described by the USP <711> and <1092>, consists of "a few turns of a wire helix." Soltero et al.[14] demonstrated that the sinker design could affect dissolution results by entrapping material or altering the hydrodynamics and slowing dissolution. In addition to inhibiting flotation, the

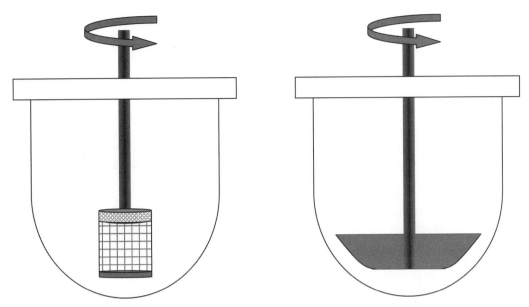

FIGURE 14.1 Schematic illustration of Dissolution Apparatus I (Basket) and II (Paddle)

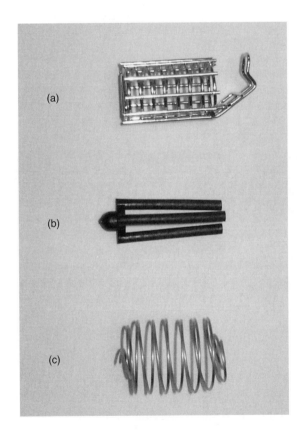

FIGURE 14.2 Example sinker designs. (a) Basket sinker; (b) three pronged sinker; (c) spiral sinker

sinker may be useful for assuring consistent placement of the dosage form in the bottom of the vessel. The hydrodynamic environment in the Apparatus II vessel is highly heterogeneous[15–16] and it has been demonstrated that position of the dosage form (e.g., side versus center of the vessel or height of the dosage form) can alter the rate of dissolution.[17–18]

For both Apparatuses I and II, the typical medium volume is 500–1000 mL with 900 mL most frequently used. Smaller and larger vessels are available to accommodate either low-dose or poorly-soluble compounds respectively. The rotational speed is selected as part of the method development process to whatever rotational speed can be justified as providing an appropriate measure of product performance.

Sampling from Apparatuses I and II can be conducted either manually or automatically, with filtration to eliminate undissolved particles. The sampling time is recorded as the point of initiation of sampling. Manual sampling is conducted using syringes equipped with cannulas of a prescribed length, to ensure sampling within the USP sampling zone (defined vertically as midway between the medium surface and the top of the paddle blade or basket, and radially as not less than 1 cm from the vessel wall). Dissolution vessels are typically fitted with covers containing sampling ports to facilitate reproducible sampling. These covers also minimize evaporation of the test medium during extended trials.[19] Automatic sampling devices employ sampling manifolds that either deliver the sample to a fraction collector or pass the aliquot through an online detector. Filtration can occur at the sampling port or inline. Whether manual or automatic methods are used, sampling can be conducted with or without replacement of the withdrawn media. With online detectors, the sampled aliquot can be returned to the vessel. In other cases, an equivalent volume of prewarmed media is delivered carefully to the vessel to prevent unacceptable alteration of the vessel hydrodynamics. Calculation of the amount of drug released versus time must be corrected for the volume changes that occur when the medium is not replaced.

The results obtained when using either the Apparatus I or II are sensitive to the configuration of the various components such as depth, centering, and verticality of the shaft, leveling of the bath, and imperfections in the vessels.[20,21] Vibration is another source of error in dissolution testing.[22] In order to ensure consistent performance across equipment and laboratories, the USP provides calibrator tablets of prednisone and salicylic acid, to be used to demonstrate that the bath configuration and operator practices meet specified standards. Bath performance verification is typically monitored on a semiannual basis or after major repairs, equipment or location changes. The prednisone tablet is a rapidly disintegrating tablet, and the salicylic acid tablet is a non-disintegrating tablet. The tests are conducted for both dosage forms with a single 30-minute sampling point. The acceptance criteria are established for each lot of tablets through collaborative studies with various laboratories around the world.[23] Each laboratory measures the release under a defined protocol, and the results are compiled to provide the average ranges used as the future acceptance criteria. The operating conditions and acceptance criteria are supplied in the package inserts with the calibrator tablets. The prednisone calibrator tablets have some stability issues, and the acceptance criteria for a given lot may be revised during their specified shelf life. The sensitivity and usefulness of the salicylic acid calibrator tablets has been questioned.[24] Recently, ASTM[25] has provided a test method for mechanical calibration of the Apparatus I and II, and the debate regarding the relative merits of mechanical calibration versus use of calibrator tablets continues.[26]

Less commonly used equipment for measuring drug release from solid oral products includes Apparatuses III, VII, and IV. Apparatus III uses a reciprocating cylinder to induce agitation, and to transport the dosage form through a series of vessels. This design allows for monitoring release through a series of media at different pH to simulate the pH gradient of the GI tract. The reciprocating action may also be a better model of the pulsatile hydrodynamics of the GI tract than the hydrodynamic environments of Apparatus I or II.[27] Apparatus VII is a similar design, with a smaller vessel volume (approximately 10 mL versus 250 mL for the Apparatus III), and a shorter stroke length. It is used for extended-release products

where the amount of drug released is low, and the smaller vessel volume improves the ability to quantify reliably the amount of drug released. Apparatus IV is a more recent addition. It is a flow-through system designed to have improved control over the hydrodynamics of the medium. The flow has a pulsatile motion to mimic intestinal flow. This design also allows for continuous changes in the medium, such as inducing a pH gradient.

In addition to the dissolution apparatuses, the original tablet performance test, disintegration, should not be discounted. The disintegration apparatus is defined in USP <701>. The test is straightforward, with individual tablets held in tubes capped with mesh screens that are agitated by reciprocation in the selected medium, typically water. The disintegration test provides a measure of the amount of time necessary for the dosage form to disintegrate into smaller pieces. It does not involve quantitative measurement of drug concentration. For a given product, disintegration test results can be sensitive to materials and process parameters such as levels of binder, disintegrant, lubricant, and compression force, or gelatin capsule cross-linking. This test was the primary performance test for tablets before the introduction of dissolution tests. It remains a useful performance test, especially for immediate release products with very rapid release across the physiological pH range, where it may be impractical to develop a meaningful dissolution test. The ICH Q6A guidance provides a decision tree using dissolution test data for justifying the use of disintegration in place of dissolution.[28]

14.2.2 Analytical Assay

For any selected apparatus, the amount of drug released must be monitored by a suitable analytical method, often referred to as the analytical finish. The concentration of each sample is then converted to the amount of drug released using an algorithm taking into account the sampling method and whether replacement of media occurred (Table 14.1). Although any analytical technique that is sensitive to the concentration of drug in solution can be used, the most common test methods use either UV/visible spectrophotometry or HPLC with UV detection. Each of the techniques has its benefits. Monitoring absorbance at UV or visible wavelengths requires minimal to no sample preparation. The rapid measurement is conducive to automation or providing measurements at closely spaced time points. With fiber optic sensors,

TABLE 14.1 Example calculations for %label claim (%LC) released at the nth time point based on medium replacement strategy and apparatus

Apparatus		Calculation
I and II	Without replacement of medium volume V_{pull}	$\%LC_n = \dfrac{1}{LC}\left\{ V_{pull}\sum_{i=1}^{n-1} c_i + c_n\left[V_{medium} - (n-1)V_{pull} \right] \right\} \times 100\%$
I and II	With replacement of fresh medium volume V_{pull}	$\%LC_n = \dfrac{1}{LC}\left[V_{pull}\sum_{i=1}^{n-1} c_i + c_n V_{medium} \right] \times 100\%$
I, II and IV	With recycling of analyzed sample	$\%LC_n = \dfrac{c_n V_{medium}}{LC} \times 100\%$
III and VII	Single sample from each cell containing medium volume V_{medium}	$\%LC_n = \dfrac{V_{medium}}{nLC}\sum_{i=1}^{n} c_i \times 100\%$

TABLE 14.2 Environmental pH and residence time in the gastrointestinal tract (fasted state)

	pH	Residence time
Stomach	1.5–2	0–3 hours
Duodenum	4.9–6.4	
Jejunum	4.4–6.4	3–4 hours
Ileum	6.5–7.4	
Colon	7.4	Up to 18 hours

the need for sampling can be eliminated by measurement of absorbance with *in situ* probes.[29] These probes provide the advantage of capturing a large number of data points over a short period of time, which is especially useful with fast-dissolving dosage forms that release within five minutes. A drawback of using spectrophotometry is the possibility of assay interference by excipients that absorb in the same wavelength region or by undissolved excipients that may scatter light and affect the results. Approaches to eliminate these interferences include baseline normalization, and the use of second derivatives of the absorbance profile.[30] HPLC avoids such interference with improved specificity resulting from the chromatographic separation. The current thrust for ever-faster chromatography[31] improves the potential for application of HPLC to automation, even with multiple time points. However, the expense and environmental consequences of the large amount of organic waste from the mobile phase used for HPLC should be acknowledged.

14.2.3 Medium Selection

General Considerations for Medium Selection

Evaluation of the appropriate testing medium begins by considering the *in vivo* transit of an oral dosage form. The journey through the GI tract involves changes of pH in the medium from approximately pH 1 or 2 in the stomach to pH 7.4 in the colon. The approximate pH and residence time along the GI tract in the fasted state is given in Table 14.2.[32] This information must be considered in evaluating the conditions under which a particular dosage form will be tested. For example, an immediate-release product is designed to release drug rapidly, typically in less than an hour. Therefore, one might choose a lower pH medium to simulate the conditions in the stomach. However, the choice of medium may also be influenced by the solubility and stability of the active pharmaceutical ingredient. Excipients in the formulation may also react differently based on the medium composition.[33–34] This is especially true when polymers are used as rate-controlling agents. Their swelling and release can be altered by medium pH, ionic strength, surfactants, and even counterion composition. For some formulations, an evaluation of the effect of coadministered food is important. Food will extend the residence time, and elevate gastric pH,[35] therefore alternative testing methods may be needed to compare effects with and without food.

The driving force for dissolution of drug into the aqueous medium is the concentration gradient, defined by the difference between the concentration of drug in solution I and the drug solubility (C_S). This relationship was originally described by Noyes and Whitney[36] with an empirical rate constant, k. Nernst and Brunner demonstrated that the rate constant was related to the exposed surface area and the rate of diffusion across a hydrodynamic boundary layer at the surface.[37] This led to the Nernst–Brunner equation:

$$\frac{dC}{dt} = \frac{DS}{Vh}(C_S - C) \qquad (14.1)$$

where D is the diffusion coefficient, which is a function of temperature and viscosity of the medium; S is the exposed surface area, usually related to particle size in disintegrating dosage forms or tablet size in eroding dosage forms; V is the volume of medium; and h is the thickness of the hydrodynamic boundary layer which is dependent on the fluid velocity. For modified-release formulations, the drug release rate is often driven by mechanisms other than dissolution, and is discussed separately.

In order to ensure that the dissolution test is measuring the properties of drug release without limitation by the experimental conditions, the medium is selected to ensure that the concentration gradient remains large, e.g., a sink condition, for the duration of the test. When the saturated solution concentration (i.e., solubility limit) is much greater than the concentration in solution, then the gradient can be considered constant. Thus, knowledge of the pH-solubility profile of the compound at 37°C (or the intrinsic solubility and the ionization constants which can be used to construct the pH-solubility profile) is required before selecting the dissolution medium. Sink conditions are achieved when the capacity for the selected medium to solubilize the dose is at least three times the amount necessary (USP <1088>). This capacity is the product of the solubility in the medium and the selected volume therefore, either can be adjusted as needed. For ionizable drugs the first choice for adjusting the medium to achieve sink conditions is to adjust the pH. The typical pH range for dissolution testing is from pH 1 (representing gastric pH) to pH 7.5 (representing intestinal pH). Table 14.3 provides

the most common media used in dissolution studies. Simulated gastric and intestinal fluids with enzyme are useful for digesting cross-linked gelatin. Simulated gastric fluid contains pepsin derived from porcine stomach mucosa, and the simulated intestinal fluid contains pancreatin.

Although purified water is acceptable, it is not the most preferred medium, because water has no buffering capacity. Buffered media should be considered where the dissolution of either the drug or excipients is pH-sensitive. In unbuffered media, dissolution of ionizable species may create a pH-microclimate where the pH at the surface of the particles or dosage form is different from the bulk solution pH. Also, for an ionizable drug with a significant loading in the dosage form, the dissolution of the drug may cause the pH of the bulk medium to change over the duration of the test. In either case, these changes in pH add an uncontrolled variable to the events occurring during dissolution, and may complicate the interpretation of results. When selecting buffered media, the pH of the medium after the dissolution test should be compared to the starting pH to ensure no changes have occurred, and that the appropriate buffering strength has been selected.

For poorly soluble compounds, the solubility in physiologically relevant buffer solutions may be insufficient to allow for the use of a practical volume of medium, therefore surfactants are commonly added to the medium to increase the solubility.[38] A detailed discussion of surfactant behavior in solution is beyond the intention of this chapter, and the reader is referred to other references.[39-40] In brief, surfactants are amphiphilic agents where the molecule has a distinct hydrophilic portion (which may be anionic, cationic, zwitterionic or nonionic) and a distinct hydrophobic portion, typically an aliphatic chain. This dichotomy causes the molecules to align at air–water or water–oil interfaces. When present above a certain concentration, called the critical micelle concentration (CMC), these molecules will self-associate to form micelles shielding the hydrophobic portions from contact with water. These lipophilic cores have the capacity to solubilize lipophilic molecules to increase their solubility in aqueous solution. The critical micelle concentration varies with the surfactant structure, temperature, and the concentration and type of added salt. Above the CMC, the solubility of a compound will generally increase linearly with surfactant concentration, which allows adjustments to meet sink conditions. Surfactants may also enhance dissolution rate by improving wetting of hydrophobic drugs or excipients. Table 14.4 lists surfactants commonly used in dissolution testing.

TABLE 14.3   Common media used in dissolution studies

pH	Medium	Comments
–	Purified water	
1–3	Hydrochloric acid	Between 0.1 and 0.001 N
1.2	Simulated gastric fluid, TS	With or without enzyme
4.1–5.5	Acetate buffer	50 mM
5.8–8.0	Phosphate buffer	50 mM, potassium or sodium
6.8	Simulated intestinal fluid, TS	With or without pancreatin

TABLE 14.4 Commonly-used surfactants in dissolution testing

Surfactant	Common names	Type
Sodium dodecyl sulfate	SDS, SLS, sodium lauryl sulfate	Anionic
Cetyl trimethyl ammonium bromide	CTAB, cetrimmonium bromide, hexadecyltrimethyl ammonium bromide	Cationic
Tween® family	Polysorbate 20, polyoxyethylene (20) laurate	Nonionic
	Polysorbate 80 polyoxyethylene (20) oleate	
Lauryl dimethylamine oxide	LDAO	Nonionic

TABLE 14.5 FaSSIF and FeSSIF media for simulating intestinal fasted and fed states[42]

Components	Fasted state (FaSSIF)	Fed state (FeSSIF)
Buffering agent	0.029 M KH_2PO_4	0.144 M acetic acid
NaOH	q.s. to pH 6.8	q.s. to pH 5
NaTaurocholate	5 mM	15 mM
Lecithin	1.5 mM	4 mM
KCl	0.22 M	0.19 M
Distilled water	q.s. to 1 L	q.s. to 1 L

The use of surfactants is not as great a deviation from physiological conditions as it may seem, given that bile salts and lecithin are surfactants present in intestinal fluids and bile, which are responsible for solubilizing poorly soluble foodstuffs in preparation for absorption.[41] Typically, natural surfactants are often too expensive for use in routine testing, so synthetic surfactants are used for test methods designed for quality control purposes. For studies where bile salts and lecithin are desired, Dressman and coworkers have proposed a set of dissolution media simulating the intestinal state under fed and fasted conditions (Table 14.5).[42] These media are useful during early formulation development to improve estimation of food effects or for correlation with *in vivo* studies.[43] Precautions should be taken in making comparisons of drug release measured using separate media preparations, as results may vary due to changes in composition based on the source of the reagents. For example, Wei and Löbenberg[44] compared dissolution using media prepared with bile salts and lecithin of different purity (high purity and crude), and found that dissolution profiles obtained with the lower quality preparation better simulated the *in vivo* absorption profile.

Medium selection is also influenced by the stability of the drug substance. In order to develop a practical test method, the compound should have demonstrated stability in the medium at 37°C to allow sufficient time for sampling and quantitation of the amount of drug in the medium. The pH-stability profile at 37°C should be available during the medium selection process. Susceptibility to light or oxidation should also be evaluated for additional precautions. Usually, such instability is an issue in formulation development, and leads to design controls to limit the

exposure of the compound to adverse environments *in vivo* or on the pharmacy shelf. For example, drug products containing acid labile drugs may be enteric coated so that release occurs in the higher pH regions of the small intestine to avoid exposure to the acidic environment of the stomach. The design of dissolution tests for these particular products is covered below in the review of modified-release dosage forms.

One additional procedure that should be evaluated once the medium composition is selected is deaeration. Deaeration can be achieved in several ways including heating, vacuum degassing, sparging with an inert gas such as helium, sonication, and combinations thereof. Entrapped gases in the dissolution medium can nucleate on the surfaces of Apparatus I baskets, on the dosage form or particles, creating a barrier between the dosage form and the medium. This reduces the dissolution rate, and can also be a major cause for variability in the results. The resulting bubbles may also affect the hydrodynamics in the vessel, and could increase the extent of release or variability of results. In one study reviewing the performance of calibrator tablets, deaeration was cited as a major contributor to failure of the calibrator tablets.[45] Gao et al. evaluated nine deaeration methods for eliminating total dissolved gases, and found that the USP method, an in-house method of equilibrating media at a pressure of 140–150 mm Hg (DPA method), and a spray-vacuum method were equivalent.[46] Further, they determined that the heating step currently prescribed by USP is not necessary when sufficient vacuum is used. Their results confirmed earlier reports that transfer of deaerated medium to the dissolution vessels is a primary source of reaeration.[47] The authors' recommendation was to limit the total dissolved gases to less than 60% saturation at room temperature, providing an adequate working range so that reaearation during media transfers or on heating to 37°C would not reach above 100% saturation.

Medium Selection for Encapsulated Products

Encapsulated products, whether solid or liquid filled, are another form of solid oral dosage form. The dissolution of the capsule shell adds an additional step to the release of drug, and usually results in a lag time for drug release. Capsules may be soft elastic capsules prepared by simultaneously filling and forming the capsule, or hard shell capsules composed of two halves that nest together. Hard shell capsules can be sealed by banding or through the use of solvents to allow encapsulation of liquids.

Capsule shells have historically been made of gelatin. Gelatin is prepared by hydrolyzing collagen sourced from bovine or porcine bone or skin. The process can be conducted under either acidic (Type A gelatin) or basic (Type B gelatin) conditions, resulting in differences in the isoelectric point (approximately 5 for Type A gelatin and 7 for type B), thus influencing the gelatin solubility.[48] Gelatin is a reactive material and will cross-link upon exposure to aldehydes, dyes, high humidity, and light exposure.[49] This reduces the solubility of the gelatin capsule, and may prevent or significantly delay opening, which, in severe cases, will result in reduced drug release and absorption.[50–51] When investigating incidents of cross-linking, it is important to realize that there are various sources of aldehydes, including impurities in excipients, by-products of excipient degradation such as occurs with oxidation of fatty acids, or even packaging materials.[52–53]

In the dissolution bath, cross-linked gelatin will appear as a swollen rubbery sac, known as a pellicle, in which material is entrapped. The presence of enzymes and the acidic environment of the stomach are usually able to digest cross-linked gelatin, so gelatin cross-linking poses more of a concern for *in vitro* testing rather than *in vivo* performance.[49,50,53] The Gelatin Capsule Working Group, a joint committee including representatives from the pharmaceutical industry, capsule manufacturers, academia, and the FDA Center for Drug Evaluation and Research, conducted a thorough study of the effects of cross-linking on both *in vitro* and *in vivo* performance.[50] They recommended a two-tier testing protocol for gelatin encapsulated products. This recommendation was adopted by the USP, and included in Chapter <711> in 1999. The Tier 2 method uses the same medium as prescribed in the first line dissolution test, but with the addition of proteolytic enzymes. For acidic media below pH 6.8, pepsin is used at a level of 7.5×10^5 units of activity/L. At higher pH, ≥ 6.8, pancreatin is used with an activity no more than 1750 units/L.

Because the expectation is that the presence of enzyme is the only difference between the Tier 1 medium and the Tier 2 medium, the first tier medium must be carefully selected to ensure proper evaluation of dosage form performance and suitability for the enzymes. The optimal pH for pepsin activity has been reported to be approximately 2,[54–55] and demonstrated to decrease at or above pH 6. Gallery et al.[55] demonstrated that pancreatin was less efficient than pepsin at the USP recommended levels even between pH 6 and 8, and called for increasing the level three-fold. For optimal use of enzymes, dissolution media at intermediate pH are not recommended. Surfactant selection also requires careful attention. Surfactants are known to denature enzymes or reduce their activity. Sodium dodecyl sulfate (SDS), in particular, should be avoided in the development of dissolution test methods for gelatin products. In addition to denaturing the enzymes, SDS has also been reported to interact with gelatin itself, and to reduce the dissolution rate in acid media forming a precipitate containing both gelatin and surfactant.[56]

With the concerns about bovine spongiform encephalopathy (BSE), the chemical reactivity of gelatin, and patient diets that eliminate animal products, alternative materials for capsule manufacture are being introduced. One of the more popular of these new materials is hydroxypropylmethylcellulose (HPMC). HPMC capsules include the natural polymer carageenan as a gelling agent. The strength of the carageenan gel is modified by the composition of dissolution media, especially cations and specifically potassium ions. This results in extended disintegration and dissolution times. Missaghi and Fassihi showed that in the presence of 50 mM potassium phosphate buffer at pH 6.8, the mean disintegration time of HPMC capsules was 270 seconds, versus 53 seconds for gelatin capsules.[57] Similarly, the dissolution of ibuprofen-filled capsules (App II, 50 rpm, 900 mL) demonstrated a lag time of 15 minutes before drug release occurred.[58] In non-potassium containing media, a lag before disintegration or drug release persists, but is not as pronounced. Also, a delay in capsule rupture has been demonstrated *in vivo*, but without statistically significant impact on pharmacokinetic parameters of ibuprofen.[58] Therefore, dissolution media for HPMC encapsulated products should avoid potassium salts, and use sodium salts where buffers are necessary.

14.3 DISSOLUTION TESTS FOR IMMEDIATE-RELEASE PRODUCTS

Immediate-release (IR) dosage forms are designed to allow drugs to dissolve freely in the GI contents, with no intention of delaying or prolonging the dissolution/absorption of the drugs upon administration. IR products could be rapidly-dissolving or slowly-dissolving, depending on the intrinsic dissolution rate of drug substances. For a rapidly-dissolving product, more than 85% of the API is expected to dissolve within 30 minutes using USP Apparatus I or II in $\leq 900\,ml$ of aqueous medium. If a drug is poorly soluble, a slower dissolution rate, and hence a longer dissolution time may be normal, although dissolution rate can be artificially accelerated using aggressive medium and testing conditions.

14.3.1 Dissolution Tests for Tablets or Solid-Filled Capsule Products

Most immediate-release products are tablets or capsules consisting of the drug, with additional excipients that act as fillers, disintegrants, and processing aids. Tablets will disintegrate on exposure to an aqueous environment, and then drug dissolution occurs from the resulting solid particles. Alternatively, the tablet may remain intact while erosion of the surface occurs to release the drug. For capsule formulations, the dissolution of the capsule shell is an added step in the process of drug release, and can result in a lag time before drug is detected in solution. Formulations of poorly soluble compounds may be more complex, employing different formulation techniques, e.g., the drug may be embedded in melt-extruded polymer matrices or semisolid formulations, such that drug release occurs through erosion of the matrix or formation of emulsions.[59] If dissolution of an IR product containing a highly soluble drug is demonstrated to be rapid with respect to gastric emptying time, then dissolution testing may provide a surrogate to *in vivo* bioequivalence studies.[6] Alternatively, very rapid dissolution may permit the use of disintegration testing in place of a dissolution test for release of drug product as per ICH guidelines.[28] For less soluble compounds where dissolution is the rate-limiting step to absorption, development of an IVIVC may be possible.

Initial studies for dissolution method development should focus on testing dosage forms in biorelevant and moderate hydrodynamic conditions. This will include testing in low pH media to mimic the stomach, usually monitoring release up to an hour.

An additional stage of dissolution testing in a pH 6.8 medium may be added to simulate transport to the intestinal tract. In Apparatus I or II this is achieved by adding a concentrated buffer to the existing acidic medium. Apparatus III, where the dosage form is transported through a series of separate vessels, can be used to develop a more gradual pH gradient. However, the design of the mesh basket that transports the dosage form may limit the utility to non-disintegrating dosage forms. More facile transitions in pH can be achieved using Apparatus IV.[60] Dissolution under intestinal conditions can be important for basic drugs that dissolve rapidly in gastric conditions, but then precipitate at higher pH, or alternatively for acidic compounds where dissolution will not begin until the intestinal tract is reached. When compounds are insufficiently soluble or when the dosage strength is high, the addition of surfactants or use of the FaSSIF and FeSSIF media can be considered.[38,43]

In the early stages of formulation development, the dissolution test should be viewed as a supportive tool in developing an understanding of the drug release mechanism and identifying the important parameters for formulation performance. During these studies, evaluation and analysis of drug release should not rely solely on the quantitative values obtained from HPLC or spectrophotometry. Visual observations of the performance of dosage forms are critical to help identify the major factors controlling drug release, and to provide insight into unanticipated effects such as floating dosage forms, changes in disintegration or coning. Visual observation is also important to include when using formally designed experiments to test formulation modifications or processing changes.

Interpretation and design of dissolution studies are considered with an assessment of the formulation properties that control drug release. For traditional tablets, the parameters affecting dissolution rate are the disintegration time, which in turn can be related to tablet hardness, disintegrant level, solubility, and intrinsic dissolution rate of the drug in the selected medium, and the drug and/or granule particle size.[61] The mechanism for dissolution enhancement from solid dispersion systems is less well understood.[59] Two general mechanistic classifications can be made for systems using water-soluble polymers. In the first class, release of solubilized drug is controlled by release or erosion of the matrix. In the second category, solid drug particles are released when the matrix rapidly erodes.

Table 14.6 provides a summary of the major drug and formulation factors capable of controlling drug release, and the dissolution method adjustments that can be made. Except for drug solubility and intrinsic dissolution rate, the other properties mentioned are linked to the processing parameters, e.g., milling, granulation processes, drying, and tableting. Careful attention must be paid to changes that occur during process modifications or scale-up that can alter properties driving dissolution behavior.[62] For example, granulation can be achieved by either wet or dry processes. If a drug has multiple solid forms, especially when it forms hydrates, it may convert to another form during wet granulation which will affect the intrinsic dissolution rate of the drug. Another example of processing effects occurs with magnesium stearate, used as a lubricant. Magnesium stearate is insoluble, and under the right processing conditions (high shear or temperature) can coat particles and inhibit or slow dissolution.[62]

During this method and formulation development stage, modeling of the dissolution profile can help identify dissolution rate-limiting factors and optimal operating conditions. There are many papers in the literature focused on unformulated drug, relating the solubility, dissolution rate, and permeability to ultimate bioavailability.[3,4,63] This has led to the development of physiologically-based pharmacokinetic software programs such as Gastroplus™ (Simulations Plus, Lancaster, CA), that also incorporate metabolic processes to provide a complete assessment of

TABLE 14.6 *In vitro* factors influencing drug dissolution

	Factor	Dissolution method variable
Drug properties	Aqueous solubility	Medium composition, pH, volume
	Intrinsic dissolution rate (function of solid form)	Hydrodynamics, pH
	Lipophilicity/ hydrophobicity	Surfactants for wetting or solubility
	Stability	pH adjustment, other additives, timing
Formulation properties	Disintegration/ deaggregation	Hydrodynamics
	Particle size	Hydrodynamics
	Particle density	Hydrodynamics
	Wettability	Deaeration, hydrodynamics, surfactants
	Insoluble fillers (coning)	Hydrodynamics

TABLE 14.7 Mathematical expressions for modeling dissolution profiles for immediate release products

Model name	Expression	Parameters
Nernst–Brunner	$\dfrac{dM}{dt} = \dfrac{DS}{h}(C_S - C)$	M: mass released at time t
Hixson–Crowell	$M_0^{1/3} - M^{1/3} = kt$	D: molecular diffusion coefficient
	$k = \left(\dfrac{\pi}{6\rho^2}\right)^{1/3} \dfrac{2DC_s}{h}$	C_S: solubility
	d_0: initial particle size	S: particle surface area
	ρ: particle density	h: hydrodynamic boundary layer thickness
Weibull	$M = M_0\left[1 - \exp\left(-\dfrac{t^b}{a}\right)\right]$	M_0: initial mass API
	a: scale constant	t: time
	b: shape constant	

bioavailability.[64] For developing quantitative models useful to interpretation of dissolution testing, these models may be difficult to apply. For example, particle size is often assumed to be homogeneous and fluid flow constant. In actual practice, the particle size may be highly heterogeneous, and the hydrodynamics in Apparatus I and II vessels result in regions with vastly different fluid flow regimes. This leads necessarily to the use of empirical models.

Various models used for interpreting dissolution rates of immediate-release products are listed in Table 14.7. The most commonly cited model is the Nernst–Brunner (N–B) equation that relates the dissolution rate (dM/dt) to the concentration gradient from the surface of a particle, the exposed surface area (S), and the diffusivity across a hydrodynamic boundary layer of thickness h. Hixson and Crowell expanded on the concept by incorporating the change in surface area as the particle dissolved.[65] These models are best applied to the early time points in a dissolution profile to ensure the assumptions of constant surface area (for the N–B equation), and sink conditions (for the Hixson and Crowell expression), are valid. Application of the Weibull equation[66] is a less phenomenological approach to modeling dissolution profiles. This stretched exponential provides an empirical model that incorporates the many different dissolution rates occurring in a real system due to factors such as particle size distributions. A lag time, either due to disintegration, capsule opening or finite time for wetting, can be incorporated into this model by substituting $t - t_{lag}$ for t in the expression.

Selection of the most appropriate model may not be apparent *a priori*. For example, Nicolaides et al. evaluated fits to *in vitro* dissolution data using a first order kinetic model, the Weibull distribution, and a theoretical model based on the Noyes–Whitney relationship, in an attempt to predict *in vivo* plasma profiles.[67] The authors used the difference factor, f_1, to compare the measured and simulated plasma profiles. They found that no model consistently provided the best fit. Nevertheless, with the Noyes–Whitney-based model, they were able to successfully describe the *in vivo* performance of seven of eleven formulations.

Formal experimental designs or multivariate analysis can be applied to evaluate the effect of processing parameters or physical characteristics both on the formulation, and for refining the dissolution test. The evaluation of effects can be analyzed by choosing release at a particular time point, area under the curve to a particular time point or parameters selected based on modeling the profile.[68]

14.3.2 Dissolution Tests for Liquid-filled Capsule Products

Liquid-filled capsule products have been the subject of debate with respect to the required application of dissolution testing for these solid oral dosage forms. In this type of dosage form the drug is completely solubilized, therefore, dissolution will only occur if the drug precipitates from solution after capsule opening. This may occur, for example, when acidic drugs are solubilized in a water-miscible solvent such as PEG 400, and the test medium is acidic. Alternatively, if the fill material is water-immiscible and maintains the drug in a solubilized state, the "dissolution" test is then sensitive to the rate of dispersion of the formulation or extraction of the drug from the carrier solvent.

Lipid-based drug delivery systems encompass a broad array of formulations designed to present a poorly aqueous soluble drug in a solubilized form to eliminate dissolution as the rate-limiting step to absorption. These formulations are based on blends of acylglycerides, fatty acids, fatty acid derivatives, and emulsifiers.[69,70,71] What happens on ingestion of the formulation depends on the components selected. Pouton has proposed a classification system[71] of lipid-based drug delivery formulations based on the balance between reliance on biological processing for emulsification versus intrinsic design of the formulation. Regardless of the lipid-based formulation classification, the overriding concept is that the active ingredient is solubilized, and dissolution of solid drug is not a factor controlling bioavailability.

Most lipid-based formulations are encapsulated in a gelatin capsule, which must rupture to release its contents. What happens next in a dissolution vessel depends on the composition of the formulation, the medium, and the apparatus settings. Often, lipid-based formulations are less dense than the aqueous medium, so release from the capsule is buoyancy driven. If the formulation has been designed to be self-emulsifying, the formulation will efficiently disperse into most aqueous media. Formulations such as those consisting simply of a triglyceride, with no additional cosolvent or emulsifier, will rapidly cream to the top of the vessel. In this case, dispersion of the formulation is strongly affected by apparatus parameters such as paddle speed. Because lipid-based formulations are generally used for poorly aqueous soluble compounds, most dissolution media for these formulations will include additional surfactant to maintain sink conditions for the active ingredient. Given that dissolution testing results in the formation of emulsions or microemulsions, the type of surfactant and concentration can influence the release profile, due to the ability to solubilize the formulation, minimize interfacial tension affecting emulsion droplet size or drive extraction of the active from the emulsion droplets. If a dissolution test method is to be developed for these formulations, the medium selected for dissolution testing should provide sink conditions for the drug, should not interfere with the activity of enzymes used to overcome cross-linking of gelatin in Tier 2 methods, and should avoid negatively interacting with the formulation.

Various alternative test methods have been proposed to measure drug release from lipid-based drug delivery systems. Pillay and Fassihi reported on drug release measurements for a self-emulsifying formulation using a two-phase system with an octanol receiver phase in an Apparatus II system.[72,73] One significant disadvantage to this method would be in the case of formulations that do not disperse well, and would immediately cream to the octanol phase. Additional methods have been proposed, such as the use of USP Apparatus IV, and use of lipases to mimic digestion.[74] These approaches are still in the exploratory stage, and have not undergone sufficient study to merit use as routine release tests for drug product, though they may be useful for early formulation development.

One can argue that for formulations where the drug remains solubilized in the dissolution medium or more importantly *in vivo*, the critical process related to *in vivo* exposure is capsule opening. Han and Gallery applied the ICH Q6A decision tree to demonstrate that disintegration provided an equivalent measure of drug release to dissolution for two separate encapsulated products.[75]

14.3.3 Method Development for Quality Control of Immediate-release Products

Once the basic formulation design has been selected, the dissolution test will usually be simplified to a point that demonstrates its sensitivity to the relevant rate-controlling properties. The acceptance of the Biopharmaceutics Classification System[5] has greatly clarified the development and justification of dissolution test methods for immediate-release dosage forms of highly soluble compounds (BCS class I and III). The BCS class I compounds are those that have high permeability and demonstrated high solubility, defined as requiring 250 mL or less to dissolve the highest dose across the range of pH 1 to pH 7.5. The class III compounds have high solubility, but low permeability. For these highly soluble compounds, the pH of the medium selected for testing the product is not driven by the compound's solubility. Instead stability or excipient sensitivity to pH may dictate medium pH.

Developing a sensitive test method will likely focus on the hydrodynamics of the apparatus, comparing results from Apparatus I and Apparatus II at the lower limits of the typical spindle rotational speed (100 rpm and 50 rpm respectively).[76] The use of alternative apparatuses are rarely justified. More aggressive hydrodynamic conditions may be needed for low dose compounds where the tablets contain a substantial amount of insoluble excipients used as diluents (e.g., calcium phosphate dibasic or microcrystalline cellulose). At low agitation speeds, these may form a mound or a cone in the center of the vessel where there is a hydrodynamic dead zone (e.g., directly under the Apparatus II paddle). This mound will entrap drug substance, and reduce the overall dissolution rate. Agitation speed can be increased to overcome this. Alternatively, PEAK™ vessels, which have a raised dimple in the center of the vessel, can be used to direct material to more favorable hydrodynamic regions while maintaining the use of lower agitation rates.[77] These vessels are non-standard, and justification for their use must be made.

BCS class II compounds are those that are highly permeable, but do not meet the criteria for solubility across the physiological pH range. In fact, many of these compounds are either acids or bases, with high solubility in part of the pH range from 1 to 7.5. Therefore, there is the opportunity to tune the rate of dissolution by adjusting the pH. Care must be taken to ensure that any discrimination provided by increasing the sensitivity of dissolution (e.g., by reducing the medium pH to a region of lower solubility) is meaningful to the *in vivo* performance of the product. If adequate solubility cannot be achieved by adjusting the pH, the use of surfactants may be justified.

As a tool for quality control of pharmaceutical products, a dissolution method should be capable of discriminating products made with different materials and/or processes. It is not uncommon for the grade and/or amount of excipients, such as polymers with different viscosities or the amount of disintegrant or lubricant, to affect the product dissolution rate. For a given formulation manufactured with the correct materials, processing methods such as direct compression versus wet granulation, and perhaps the processing endpoint, such as extent of wet granulation or lubrication, can affect product dissolution rate. Thus, the effects of materials and manufacturing process parameters on dissolution should be carefully evaluated during the method development stage. However, these aspects should be balanced with a perspective on the human physiological conditions to which the drug product is exposed, and the practical range of the manufacturing process, to avoid use of overly-sensitive test method conditions designed to emphasize the discrimination power of the method. While meaningful discriminatory power is desired for a quality control method, over-discrimination can lead to unnecessary limitations on manufacturing process ranges, and rejection of products that would otherwise perform well *in vivo*.

14.4 DRUG RELEASE TEST METHODS FOR MODIFIED-RELEASE PRODUCTS

The category of modified-release products encompasses a broad range of oral dosage form designs. These include enteric-coated tablets (including immediate-release), and extended-release products where drug release is controlled by the dosage form to occur over a period of hours. With these dosage forms, polymers often play a key role in modulating the release, and the medium composition will typically play a larger role than the hydrodynamics in influencing drug release. Polymer entanglement, swelling, and dissolution may be sensitive to pH, ionic strength, and in some cases the type of counterion in the medium. The general mechanisms controlling release include dissolution of a coating, matrix erosion, diffusion through a coating or matrix gel, drug dissolution, and osmotic pressure imbalances.

14.4.1 Drug Release Test Methods for Enteric Coated Products

Enteric coating is a special case of a mechanism using erosion or dissolution of a coating to control release. An enteric coating resists dissolution under acidic conditions, but is freely soluble at the more basic conditions of the intestinal tract. Enteric coating may be used to protect acid-labile drugs or to avoid gastric distress induced by high concentrations of some drugs, such as aspirin. When a dosage form design includes an enteric coat, the dissolution test will include two stages: an acid stage of pH 1 to demonstrate the integrity of the enteric coat, and a drug release phase at a higher pH (USP <711>). The amount released in the acid stage is commonly limited to 10% or less of the labeled content. The release in the buffer stage will be determined by the design of the dosage form, with typical release criteria for an IR or extended-release as appropriate. The dual stage testing can be conducted using two vessels, one at acidic conditions, and the other basic. In this case, the dosage form will be transferred between the two vessels. This can be impractical for multiparticulate dosage forms (for which Apparatus III may be more appropriate), and adds a time-consuming step that is not conducive to the workflow of a quality control laboratory. When a single vessel is used, the acid stage can be conducted, for example, in 500 mL of medium, and then the initiation of the buffer stage begins with the addition of a prewarmed buffer concentrate that will result in the final desired pH.

14.4.2 Drug Release Test Methods for Extended-release Products

Extended-release products are designed to provide a therapeutically effective amount of drug over a long period of time to improve patient compliance. They do so either by reducing the number of doses required per course of treatment or by increasing safety as a result of providing a consistent delivery of drug without excessively high initial plasma concentrations. Various mechanisms are available for controlling drug release. The use of semipermeable coatings or swelling matrices to control diffusion of the drug out of the dosage form is one such method. The use of poorly soluble matrices to control erosion of the surface of the dosage form with drug release concomitant with matrix dissolution is another. Control can also be achieved by utilizing the intrinsic dissolution rate limitations of poorly soluble drugs. Finally, osmotic pressure-driven release mechanisms can be incorporated into specially engineered dosage forms. Product design may utilize one or a combination of these mechanisms to achieve the desired *in vivo* release profile.

Mathematical models for different release mechanisms can be useful in the identification of formulation design variables and dissolution method parameters with significant influence on drug release. Examples of some common kinetic models are presented in Table 14.8. Most models cannot simulate the entire release profile, and usually are used to interpret the initial and intermediate-release regions. Selection of the appropriate model requires an understanding of the dosage form design, and many are specific to particular shapes. The major designs are discussed below with examples. The reader is referred to other resources for more comprehensive reviews.[78]

Reservoir systems are the most straightforward examples of diffusion-controlled dosage forms. These consist of a drug-containing core surrounded by a non-degrading membrane. The membrane may either swell slightly or contain soluble polymers to allow permeation of drug. The release of drug is controlled by the rate of diffusion through the membrane. Table 14.8 provides one model for the steady state release from a spherical system of outer radius R and inner radius R_i, thus the membrane thickness is $(R - R_i)$.[78] Drug release measurements can be used to demonstrate the effect of adjusting membrane thickness.

Swellable polymers can be used to create monolithic matrix systems for controlled-release. One of the most extensively used polymers for achieving this type of controlled-release is HPMC (hydroxypropylmethylcellulose). Swellable matrix systems are often described as diffusion controlled, but in fact are not so simply defined. In these systems, several rates are balanced against each other: the rate of polymer swelling, rate of drug dissolution and diffusion, and rate of erosion of polymer. The polymer swells on exposure to aqueous media. Drug entrapped in the matrix must dissolve, and then diffuse through the matrix before being released. Depending on the particular design of the dosage form (e.g., molecular weight of polymer or concentration of polymer), drug release may also occur due to erosion of the disentangled polymer chains. Peppas published a series of papers describing mass release as a power law relationship with time.[79,80,81] Interpretation of the exponent obtained by fitting the drug release profile (within the first 60% of the release) requires consideration of the shape of the dosage form to indicate the balance of contributions from Fickian diffusion, erosion or other non-Fickian mechanisms of release. More sophisticated models have been reported that more exactly model the various competitions between drug, water, and polymer

TABLE 14.8 Kinetic models for controlled release products

Model		
Rigter and Peppas[79,80]	$\dfrac{M}{M_0} = kt^n$	n: exponent dependent on shape and mechanism For a slab: • $n < 0.5$, diffusion controlled release • $n > 1$, erosion controlled release • $0.5 < n < 1$, mixed mechanism
Osmotic controlled release	$\dfrac{dM}{dt} = \dfrac{Ak}{h}\left(\Delta\pi - \Delta P\right)C_i$	A, h: membrane area and thickness $\Delta\pi$: osmotic pressure difference ΔP: hydrostatic pressure difference C_i: concentration of drug inside dosage form
Reservoir system	$M = 4\pi\dfrac{RR_i}{\left(R - R_i\right)}DC_i$	C_i: concentration of drug inside dosage form R: spherical particle outer radius R_i: spherical core radius

in the swelling process,[82] however, these are usually computationally intensive.

The simplicity of the power law relationship, and its accessibility for interpretation (once the applicable assumptions have been carefully considered), make it a powerful tool in developing drug release methods for controlled-release dosage forms. The change in the exponent can be particularly useful as a guide when developing a dissolution method to match the absorption profile obtained from deconvolution of *in vivo* data. Method variables, such as paddle speed or medium ionic strength, can affect the rate of polymer erosion and swelling, thus altering the mechanism of drug release. Colombo et al.[83] examined the effects of pH and ionic strength on drug release rates, they also used visual observations of diffusion and erosion fronts to demonstrate that ionic strength changes affected polymer erosion, and that although release rate was affected by pH, this was due to the pH-solubility

dependence of the drug, not to any particular effect on the polymer gel. Missaghi and Fassihi[27] presented the contributions of varying hydrodynamics to release from an eroding/swelling matrix through apparatus selection (I, II and III), and operating conditions. These authors concluded that *in vivo* studies are ultimately needed to support the significance of the *in vitro* test conditions selected.

Osmotic drug delivery systems typically consist of a non-erodable semipermeable membrane surrounding a swellable tablet core. The osmotic pressure difference across the semipermeable membrane, between the medium and the tablet core, controls the rate of water ingression into the tablet. The tablet will swell and push the drug suspension or solution out of the dosage form through ports formed during dosage form preparation or *in situ*. For highly soluble drugs, these dosage forms can be insensitive to drug release method parameters, such as rotational speeds or medium pH. This insensitivity can be an advantage in developing an IVIVC.

14.5 STATISTICAL COMPARISON OF DISSOLUTION PROFILES

As a measure of product performance, the results of dissolution testing are used to ensure consistency in manufacture. This includes demonstrating equivalency of release after manufacturing process, site changes or excipient changes. Executing experiments to demonstrate similarity or differences in product requires careful attention to potential sources of variation when testing is conducted. Variability between laboratories or analysts could result from the use of testing apparatus made by different manufacturers, differences in methods of deaeration or execution of mechanical checks, and the quality of analyst training.

Quantitative comparison of dissolution profiles is required to demonstrate sameness. Model-dependent and model-independent methods can be used.[84,85,86] The model-dependent methods rely on selecting the proper mathematical model (examples are provided in Table 14.7 and Table 14.8), and comparing the goodness of fit and change in fitted parameters. In many cases, these models represent an ideal case for dissolution of particles or diffusion from matrices of a defined geometry, and do not adequately capture the shape of the measured dissolution profile. For those cases where the models fit well, the comparison is made both on the extent and shape of the profile, ensuring consistency in potential exposure and the mechanism of release. Determining the correct model will require methods to compare fits such as minimization of χ^2, the f_1 and f_2 fit factors described below or alternative approaches.[87] For example, Polli used the Akaike Information Criterion to obtain a single numeric value against which to evaluate the appropriateness of a particular model for describing the dissolution profiles of metoprolol tartrate tablets.[88]

During comparison of profiles using quantitative models, incorporation of the normal variation of the fitted parameters, although potentially complex, is necessary in order properly to assess similarity.[84] Common statistical tools, such as t-tests or use of ANOVA, can be used to demonstrate sameness of the fitted parameters.

Model-independent approaches provide direct comparison of a test profile against a reference profile, without transformation to another mathematical expression. Calculations that can be made include the area under the curve of the percent released versus time profile or the amount released at a particular time point or time points.[86,89] Although these quantities may demonstrate that the amount of drug released is the same, they will not necessarily indicate whether the shape of the profile is similar. Yuksel et al.[86] described the use of ANOVA-based methodology whereby a multivariate ANOVA was used to demonstrate whether the test and reference profiles were parallel. This was then followed by use of ANOVA to identify differences between amount released at individual time points, and t-tests for significance.

The most commonly used model-independent approach that provides such information was introduced by Moore and Flanner[84] through the use of fit factors: the difference factor, f_1, and similarity factor, f_2. The difference factor provides the mean percent difference between two curves and is calculated as:

$$f_1 = \left\{ \left[\sum_{t=1}^{n} (R_t - T_t) \right] \bigg/ \sum_{t=1}^{n} R_t \right\} \cdot 100\% \qquad (14.2)$$

where:

n is the number of time points in the profile

R_t is the mean release of the reference product at time t

T_t is the mean release from the test product at time t.

Identical profiles will have an f_1 of zero. A value less than 15% is commonly taken to indicate sameness of profiles.

The similarity factor, f_2, is more commonly reported than the difference factor. The f_2 is a logarithmic transformation of the average sum squared error. The f_2 is given by:

$$f_2 = 50 \cdot \log \left\{ \left[1 + \frac{1}{n} \sum_{t=1}^{n} (R_t - T_t)^2 \right]^{-0.5} \cdot 100 \right\} \qquad (14.3)$$

When two profiles are identical, f_2 is 100. A 10% difference between profiles results in an f_2 of 50.[90] Therefore, an f_2 of greater than 50 is used to demonstrate similarity of profiles. The squaring of the difference ensures that positive and negative deviations from the reference profile do not cancel each other out. Because the f_2 calculation is a comparison of mean values, without implicitly including variability, the coefficient of variation is limited to less than 20% at early time points, and less than 10% at later time points. Also, to avoid overweighting the comparison, the calculation is limited to only one time point exhibiting greater than 85% release.[90]

14.6 SPECIFICATIONS

The dissolution specification for product release or shelf life stability of a drug product consists of both the validated test method and the acceptance criteria for the test itself. The expected acceptance criteria vary with the type of dosage form, and must be justified in terms of their relationship to *in vivo* performance, processing parameters, and the results of long-term stability studies. The purpose is to ensure consistent performance from lot-to-lot over the lifetime of the product, and may be useful to demonstrating product equivalency during scale-up or justification of certain post-approval changes. The acceptance criteria are determined from a comprehensive review of the dissolution data generated during development, including data from stability studies, with an emphasis on testing of products used in clinical studies.

14.6.1 Method Validation

Validation of a dissolution test method includes evaluation of the operating parameters of the test, and the acceptability of the analytical finish. The objective is to demonstrate the ability of the method to detect changes in the test product large enough to affect *in vivo* performance. The extent of validation may vary with phase of development; additional elements or more stringent criteria may be applied when the product is closer to commercialization.[91] The validation elements and criteria for acceptance that are expected for new drug applications are described in USP <1092> and guidances published by the International Conference on Harmonisation (ICH).[92,93] Characteristics evaluated during method validation include specificity, linearity, range, accuracy, repeatability, intermediate precision, robustness, and standard and sample solution stability. Specificity demonstrates that the analytical method is not affected by the presence of excipients or the medium. According to the USP, such interference should be less than 2% of the sample response. Linearity and range are established for samples and standards, bracketing the range of concentrations expected to be measured during the drug release test. Accuracy is determined in the presence of the excipients in one dosage unit, and may be evaluated at several concentrations of API (e.g., 20–120% of dosage form strength). Typical recovery criteria are 95–105% of the amount added. This evaluation can be combined with linearity and range studies. Repeatability is assessed for analysis of samples or standards, and is determined by replicate measurements of the sample and determining the acceptability of the resultant RSD. This evaluation can also be conducted simultaneously with accuracy, linearity, and range experiments. Intermediate precision is used to demonstrate that the method can be executed successfully under varying conditions, such as changes in instruments used, laboratories, test date, etc. Special attention must be given to ensuring that the variability of the test product is understood to assist in setting the acceptance criteria for intermediate precision of the method. Method robustness will demonstrate the acceptable range of deliberate variations to the method parameters, such as assay conditions (mobile phase ratios, wavelength, etc.), and dissolution parameters (e.g., agitation rate, medium composition, deaeration, etc.). Solution stability (both standards and samples) should also be determined under environmental conditions and of a duration expected during testing (e.g., room temperature, 37°C, refrigerated, light-exposed.). Recovery of 98–102% is a typical expectation. Additional validation elements may demonstrate the suitability of filter selections, and the use of autosamplers.

14.6.2 Acceptance Criteria

Immediate-release Products

The acceptance criterion for immediate-release products is typically described by a minimum amount of drug released (Q) at a single time point (usually less than or equal to 60 minutes). For rapidly releasing dosage forms, specification times of 15 or 30 minutes are not unusual. Products that release more slowly may require a second time point, for example, an initial time point of 15 minutes and a second at a later time to ensure complete release.[12] Testing of the product is conducted using a staged approach defined

TABLE 14.9 Stage testing for immediate-release dosage forms

Stage	Number of units tested	Passing criteria
1	6	No dosage unit releases less than +5%
2	6	Average release of 12 units $\geq Q$, and no single unit releases less than $Q - 15\%$
3	12	Average release of 24 units $\geq Q$, and not more than two units release less than $Q - 15\%$, and no unit releases less than $Q - 25\%$

by the USP (Table 14.9), and based on a combination of the results from individual tablets and the mean release values for up to 24 units tested (USP <711>). Hofer and Gray demonstrated how to estimate the amount of Stage 2 testing expected by including the variability of historical dissolution test results.[94] It is rarely acceptable to set acceptance criteria that will not result in some level of Stage 2 testing.

The acceptance criteria chosen must demonstrate discrimination against non-bioequivalent batches and/or expose the limits of acceptable process parameters. This can be shown by using profiles of various formulations generated during development, and those from testing during process range studies. A deliberate mapping study, where formulations with dissolution characteristics bracketing the target profile and created by alterations in processing are tested in clinical studies, provides a robust method for establishing dissolution specifications. The final specification time points and acceptance criteria will be determined through evaluation of the historical development data, and discussions with the various regulatory agencies. Although single point specifications are acceptable for quality control purposes, a full dissolution profile with an adequate number of points to describe the time-course for drug release should be established for scale-up or post-approval changes that require demonstration of equivalency or for bioequivalence study waivers.[6, 95]

Modified-release Products

Specifications for modified-release products are developed to ensure that the desired controlled-release attributes are achieved. Acceptance criteria will be established for multiple time points. Typically the first time point ensures against dose dumping, the final time point demonstrates complete release (>80% or lower if a plateau has been reached), and the intermediate time points prove control of the release. The acceptance criteria are defined relative to the mean dissolution profile of clinical study lots. The starting range

TABLE 14.10　Level testing for modified-release products

Level	Number tested	Criteria
A	6	• No individual value lies outside of stated ranges • No individual value is less than the stated amount at the final test time
B	6	• Average value of 12 units lies within each stated range • Average value of 12 units is not less than the stated amount at the final test time • No value is more than 10% outside of each range or below the amount at final test time
C	12	• Average value of 24 units lies within each stated range • Average value of 12 units is not less than the stated amount at the final test time • Not more than 2 units are more than 10% outside of each range or below the amount at final test time • No unit is more than 20% outside of each range or below the amount specified at final test time

of acceptable release at any time point is ±10% from the mean dissolution profile. Wider ranges may be accepted, though it may be necessary to demonstrate that clinical lots with the same range of variability were bioequivalent. Additionally, an IVIVC may be used to justify wider acceptance ranges (see Section 14.7).

Similar to the staged testing for immediate-release products, modified-release products are tested according to levels described in USP <711> (Table 14.10). Care must be taken to ensure that specified ranges for Level A testing are sufficiently stringent to ensure that non-bioequivalent lots do not pass when Level B and C criteria are applied.

14.7 IN VITRO–IN VIVO CORRELATION (IVIVC)

An established *in vitro–in vivo* correlation can be used to guide formulation development and will strengthen the justification for drug release specifications. It can also be used to avoid bioequivalency studies that are normally required for certain scale-up and post-approval changes. The utility of the correlation between *in vitro* release and the selected pharmacokinetic parameter (e.g., C_{max}, AUC) or drug plasma concentration is defined by its robustness. The regulatory guidances such as USP <1088> or the FDA Guidance for Industry on development of IVIVC[8] describe three types of correlations: Level A, B and C.

A Level A IVIVC is a point-to-point correlation between the *in vitro* release, and the amount absorbed *in vivo*. The amount absorbed is not measured directly, but obtained through deconvolution of, for example, the plasma concentration–time profile. The reader is referred to other sources for discussion of the techniques used to obtain the absorption profile.[96,97] Level A correlation is the most direct relationship to the plasma concentration profile, and provides the greatest regulatory advantage. It is typically attempted for extended-release dosage forms. A validated Level A IVIVC can be used to predict drug absorption, set dissolution specifications, obtain waivers of bioequivalence studies, and form the basis for justifying scale-up and post-approval manufacturing changes.

A Level B correlation is a correlation between the mean *in vitro* dissolution and mean *in vivo* dissolution or residence time, each obtained by application of statistical moment analysis to the full release profile. Because it is based on an aggregate quantity that is not uniquely reflective of the plasma concentration, a Level B IVIVC is not very meaningful, and hence is rarely used.

The final category is a Level C correlation for which a particular element of the dissolution profile (e.g., extent or rate of release) is related to a single pharmacokinetic parameter (e.g., C_{max} or AUC). This correlation, like Level B, also suffers from being less descriptive of the plasma concentration profile than a Level A correlation, but the utility of a Level C correlation can be strengthened by using information from multiple time points, and creating a multiple Level C correlation. This type of correlation may be most appropriate for immediate-release products where the time course for absorption is of short duration, and obtaining a sufficient number of data points in the *in vivo* profile for a Level A IVIVC is more difficult. A Level C correlation could be used to guide formulation development, and as supportive justification for setting dissolution specifications.

14.7.1 Developing an IVIVC

The development of an IVIVC requires a critical evaluation of the knowledge gained during formulation and dissolution method development regarding the mechanism of drug release and the parameters that most affect the kinetics of drug release from the dosage form. The following discussion is focused on development of a Level A IVIVC where it is more likely that the *in vitro* test conditions will be altered to develop a correlation. For a Level C correlation the AUC or C_{max} are obtained from several formulations, and correlations between amount released *in vitro* at one or more time points versus the selected pharmacokinetic parameters are developed, typically through linear regression analysis. Balan et al.[98] developed a highly predictive Level C IVIVC for metformin modified-release dosage forms, and suggested that Level C IVIVCs were useful for indicating the potential of developing a Level A IVIVC. The simplistic nature of the comparison in a Level C IVIVC is such that adjustments to the method will focus on separating or collapsing release values at individual time points. A Level A correlation uses the entire plasma concentration-time and *in vitro* release profiles, and is thus sensitive to the mechanism for drug release, which may be altered significantly by the design of the *in vitro* test conditions.

To develop a Level A IVIVC, evaluation begins with a plot of the fraction absorbed *in vivo* versus fraction released *in vitro*. This can be done with data from one or more formulations of different composition or drug products with different manufacturing histories (e.g., different scale, different manufacturing site.). Ideally, the relationship would be linear. If the *in vitro* kinetics are not a linear function of the *in vivo* data, a decision must be made whether this non-linearity will be addressed through scaling of the *in vitro* data (e.g., introduction of a lag time or transformation using a non-linear model) or through modifications of the dissolution test method. Unless a simple lag time is sufficient, in most cases, the dissolution method will be modified. The shape of the *in vivo* profile can then be used as a target for the *in vitro* data to match. Modifications to the dissolution method can include adjusting the agitation rate, the medium composition (e.g., pH, ionic strength or through additions of solubilizers) or even the apparatus used. The effects of these parameters on the release profiles of immediate-release and modified-release products were discussed in Sections 14.3 and 14.4. All of the same variables available during initial method development can be revisited for the purposes of developing an IVIVC. Statistically designed experiments, and the tools for profile comparisons described in Section 14.5, will facilitate efficient development. Qiu et al.[99,100,101] developed a Level A IVIVC for HPMC-based controlled-release formulations of divalproex sodium. Formulations used in the study included one with the target profile that had existing human clinical data, two that were designed to release drug at rates bracketing the reference formulation, and one additional formulation with a higher drug loading. Studies in dogs indicated that the *in vitro* method was not sufficiently discriminating, and a human clinical study was designed to obtain the *in vivo* data that would be used to guide modification of the *in vitro* method, and develop the IVIVC. Comparison of the *in vitro* results with the *in vivo* absorption profile illustrated that the

formulations released via a different kinetic mechanism *in vitro* versus *in vivo*. To refine the *in vitro* method, a Plackett–Burman design was used in two experiments to screen the drug release test method parameters including apparatus (I versus II), rotational speed, medium pH, presence of surfactant, ionic strength, and drug loading in the formulation. The results of these studies were interpreted in conjunction with an evaluation of the potential mechanisms of release from the dosage form, including the ability of HPMC matrices to release by both diffusion and erosion, and the effect of pH on the solubility of the drug. The final drug release conditions were determined by extrapolation of the results of a full factorial design beyond the range of surfactant concentration and pH studied. Although it is often tempting to take results of statistically designed experiments at their face value, the importance of thoughtful interpretation of results cannot be overemphasized. Such reflection may identify variables that had previously been missed, and avoid adding in variables that would be difficult to rationalize based on an understanding of the design of the formulation.

Once the initial correlation is established, the next step is to validate the IVIVC. Internal validation demonstrates that the pharmacokinetic parameters (such as AUC and C_{max}) are accurately estimated (prediction error <20%) when the *in vitro* data for the formulations used to develop the model are inputs. The robustness of the IVIVC is further demonstrated through external validation. For external validation, the *in vitro* release of a formulation manufactured independently of the formulations used to develop the IVIVC is used to predict the pharmacokinetic parameters. These are tested *in vivo*, and used for final development and internal validation of the IVIVC, whereby the *in vitro* dissolution profiles of each of the three formulations are used to predict the *in vivo* plasma concentration profile. If this validation is successful, the predictability of the model for additional formulations is evaluated, and used as external validation.

14.7.2 Setting Specifications Using an IVIVC

An established IVIVC can be used to develop acceptance criteria for release of drug products by using the predictive powers to demonstrate the range of *in vitro* release that will result in bioequivalent *in vivo* results. As with developing the IVIVCs, there are several methods proposed for developing the release criteria, from brute force calculations of *in vivo* parameters within varying *in vitro* release profiles, to more sophisticated probability models. A few examples of these methods are described below.

The simplicity of the correlation provided by a Level C IVIVC allows the most direct determination of an acceptable release range. Lake et al.[102] provide a nice example in developing a Level C IVIVC for immediate-release tablets of carbamazepine. In their study, they evaluated the potential for IVIVC with two different dissolution methods: one that used a medium containing the surfactant sodium dodecyl sulfate, and a second that used a hydrochloric acid medium. Although acceptable rank order of the formulations was achieved using both methods, the surfactant medium was chosen as it provided sink conditions for the dosage forms. The IVIVC was then explored for each time point in the profile with the best predictive capability for C_{max} demonstrated at the 20-minute time point. Then, using the C_{max} bioequivalence requirements of a point estimate in the range 0.75 to 1.35, the acceptance criteria at 20 minutes were 34–99%. This is clearly a much wider range than might have otherwise been accepted using the typical Q value of 80%.

The evaluation is less straightforward with a Level A IVIVC, where exploration of the *in vitro* space involves convolution of the entire profile to obtain the predicted pharmacokinetic parameters. A basic approach is described by Modi et al.,[103] who developed a linear IVIVC for an OROS® formulation system. The OROS® system design is based on controlled-release via an osmotic driving force, and typically results in a zero-order release profile both *in vitro* and *in vivo*. The IVIVC was validated both internally and externally, with mean prediction errors for AUC and C_{max} less than 15%. The authors applied the IVIVC to identify the limits of acceptable *in vitro* release by conducting "what-if" predictions of the AUC_{∞} and C_{max} after varying the width of the *in vitro* release specification. In their case, they demonstrated that a range of ±10% predicted a bioequivalent product, but ±12.5% failed the criteria for C_{max}. In this case, the IVIVC did not necessarily provide advantages in broadening the specifications beyond typical regulatory guidelines, but will still prove useful to waive bioequivalence studies for future site changes.

Additional examples of increasing sophistication for the development of specifications are described by Elkoshi[104] and Hayes et al.[105] Elkoshi[104] presented a generalized approach where a linear IVIVC exists, and the release rate is either zero or first-order. Two types of acceptance criteria were defined: a "minimum" range, and an "ideal" range. The "minimum" range is defined by the necessary linear relationship between the *in vivo* absorption rate constant and the *in vitro* release rate constant. Thus where ±20% C_{max} is acceptable for bioequivalence, the acceptable change in release rate k is ±20% of the release rate, k_r,

of the reference product. The "ideal" acceptance criteria are more complicated relationships derived from series expansions of the absorption and elimination processes defining C_{max}, and are best evaluated for their suitability by review of the paper. Hayes et al.[105] describe the use of simulations to optimize specifications when an IVIVC is in place to ensure optimal probability that products that pass the acceptance criteria for the *in vitro* method will be bioequivalent. In their example, the resultant acceptance criteria were narrower than ±10%, but the authors note that their example results are model- and parameter-specific, and not directly translatable to other products.

These examples illustrate that the greatest utility of an IVIVC may not be for gaining flexibility in specifications. However, a properly validated IVIVC is a useful tool for evaluating the acceptability of manufacturing and design changes.

14.8 SUMMARY AND FUTURE STATE

In vitro dissolution methods are developed to evaluate the potential *in vivo* performance of a solid oral dosage form, and as quality control tests demonstrating the appropriate performance of drug products. In recent years the convergence of the increased understanding of the physiological environment and processes of absorption, critical deconstruction of the mechanisms of release from formulations, and improved computational tools has led to a more sophisticated discussion of the role of dissolution testing in drug product design and control. It is clear that meaningful results and interpretation of dissolution data can be achieved only when the biopharmaceutical and physical properties of the drug products are well-understood, and that test methods are properly established through thorough studies during formulation and manufacturing process design and clinical development. For quality control of products, effects of formulation and process parameters on the dissolution of the resulting products must be characterized, so that discriminating methods can be developed to relate the dissolution behavior to changes in either formulation or process. These should then be checked for relevance to bioavailability to avoid over-discriminating methods that may lead to unnecessarily failing products. For evaluation of product *in vivo* performance, dissolution methods and specifications should be developed based on human data obtained from clinical studies, and ideally, lead to creation of a validated IVIVC.

The increased emphasis by regulatory bodies on demonstrating understanding and knowledge of dosage form performance provides exciting opportunities for dissolution and drug release research and development. The Biopharmaceutical Classification System, and especially the resultant regulatory guidances for BCS class I compounds, has provided a clear description of key concepts for drug release, i.e., the balance of solubility and permeability. The current evaluation of biorelevant media and solubilization of poorly soluble compounds will continue, and likely include increased use of alternative dissolution apparatuses, with Apparatus IV looking especially promising. The role of compound permeability, although not directly measured in a dissolution test, will also greatly influence design and interpretation of dissolution data. This will be especially true as the influence of drug transporters is better understood, which will likely lead to conversations about the transit times and absorption windows within which drug release must occur. Although not discussed extensively here, simulations and modeling not just of the physiological processes, but of fluid transport and mass transfer within the current apparatuses, will provide additional insight into the properties and phenomena occurring as dosage forms release drug. These understandings will then be used to design alternative tests or excipient controls that clearly demonstrate our understanding of the attributes critical to the dosage form performance.

References

1. Dokoumetzidis, A. & Macheras, P. (2006). A century of dissolution research: From Noyes and Whitney to the Biopharmaceutics Classification System. International Journal of Pharmaceutics 321, 1–11.
2. Edwards, L.J. (1951). The dissolution and diffusion of aspirin in aqueous media. Transactions of the Faraday Society 47, 1191–1210.
3. Sinko, P.J., Leesman, G.D. & Amidon, G.L. (1991). Predicting fraction dose absorbed in humans using a macroscopic mass balance approach. Pharmaceutical Research 8, 979–988.
4. Oh, D.M., Curl, R.L. & Amidon, G.L. (1993). Estimating the fraction dose absorbed from suspensions of poorly soluble compounds in humans: A mathematical model. Pharmaceutical Research 10, 264–270.
5. Amidon, G.L., Lennernas, H., Shah, V.P. & Crison, J.R. (1995). A theoretical basis for a biopharmaceutic drug classification—the correlation of in-vitro drug product dissolution and in-vivo bioavailability. Pharmaceutical Research 12, 413–420.
6. FDA Guidance for Industry. (2000). Waiver of In Vivo Bioavailability and Bioequivalence Studies for Immediate-Release Solid Oral Dosage Forms Based on a Biopharmaceutics Classification System.
7. FDA Guidance for Industry. (1997). SUPAC-MR: Modified Release Solid Oral Dosage Forms. Scale-Up and Postapproval Changes: Chemistry, Manufacturing, and Controls; In Vitro Dissolution Testing and In Vivo Bioequivalence Documentation.
8. FDA Guidance for Industry. (1997). Extended Release Oral Dosage Forms: Development, Evaluation, and Application of In Vitro/In Vivo Correlations.
9. US Pharmacopeial Convention. (2007). The United States Pharmacopeia 30/National Formulary 25. Rockville, MD.
10. Federation International Pharmaceutique (1981). FIP guidelines for dissolution testing of solid oral products. Die Pharmazeutische Industrie 42, 334–343.
11. Federation International Pharmaceutique (1996). FIP guidelines for dissolution testing of solid oral products, Final draft, 1995. Drug Information Journal 30, 1071–1084.
12. FDA Guidance for Industry. (1997). Dissolution Testing Of Immediate Release Solid Oral Dosage Forms.
13. D'Arcy, D.M., Corrigan, O.I. & Healy, A.M. (2006). Evaluation of hydrodynamics in the basket dissolution apparatus using computational fluid dynamics—Dissolution rate implications. European Journal of Pharmaceutical Sciences 27(2–3), 259–267.
14. Soltero, R.A., Hoover, J.M., Jones, T.F. & Standish, M. (1989). Effects of sinker shapes on dissolution profiles. Journal of Pharmaceutical Sciences 78(1), 35–38.
15. Kukura, J., Arratia, P.C., Szalai, E.S., Bittorf, K.J. & Muzzio, F.J. (2002). Understanding pharmaceutical flows. Pharmaceutical Technology October, 48–72.
16. Kukura, J., Arratia, P.E., Szalai, E.S. & Muzzio, F.J. (2003). Engineering tools for understanding the hydrodynamics of dissolution tests. Drug Development and Industrial Pharmacy 29(2), 231–239.
17. Gao, Z., Moore, T.W., Smith, A.P., Doub, W.H. & Westenberger, B.J. (2007). Studies of variability in dissolution testing with USP Apparatus 2. Journal of Pharmaceutical Sciences 96(7), 1794–1801.
18. Healy, A.M., McCarthy, L.G., Gallagher, K.M. & Corrigan, O.I. (2002). Sensitivity of dissolution rate to location in the paddle dissolution apparatus. The Journal of Pharmacy and Pharmacology 54, 441–444.
19. Tang, L.-J. & Schwartz, J.B. (1998). Introduction of dissolution error as a result of different openings in vessel covers. Pharmaceutical Development and Technology 3(2), 261–267.
20. Moore, T. W. et al. (1996). Pharmacopeial Forum, 22, 2423–2428.
21. Liddell, M.R., Deng, G., Hauck, W.W., Brown, W.E., Wahab, S.Z. & Manning, R.G. (2007). Evaluation of glass dissolution vessel dimensions and irregularities. Dissolution Technologies 14(1), 28–33.
22. Gao, Z., Moore, T. & Doub, W.H. (2007). Vibration effects on dissolution tests with USP Apparatuses 1 and 2. Journal of Pharmaceutical Sciences. online November 13.
23. Pharmaceutical Research and Manufacturers of America. (1997). The USP dissolution calibrator tablet collaborative study—an overview of the 1996 process. Pharmacopeial Forum 23(3), 4198–4237.
24. Oates, M., Brune, S., Gray, V., Hippeli, K., Kentrup, A., et al. (2000). Dissolution calibration: Recommendations for reduced chemical testing and enhanced mechanical calibration. Pharmacopeial Forum 26(4), 1149–1151.
25. ASTM International. (2007). Standard practice for qualification of basket and paddle dissolution apparatus. E2503-07.
26. Foster, T. & Brown, W. (2005). USP dissolution calibrators: Re-examination and appraisal. Dissolution Technologies 12(1), 6–8.
27. Missaghi, S. & Fassihi, R. (2005). Release characterization of dimenhydrinate from an eroding and swelling matrix: Selection of appropriate dissolution apparatus. International Journal of Pharmaceutics 293, 35–42.
28. International Conference on Harmonization of Technical Requirements for Registration of Pharmaceuticals for Human Use. (1999). ICH Harmonised Tripartite Guideline "Specifications: Test Procedures and Acceptance Criteria for New Drug Substances and New Drug Products: Chemical Substances Q6A."
29. Lu, X., Lozano, R. & Shah, P. (2003). In-situ dissolution testing using different UV fiber optic probes and instruments. Dissolution Technologies 10(4), 6–15.
30. Perkampus, H.H. (1992). UV-Vis Spectroscopy and Its Applications. Chapter 5, translated by H. C. Grinter & T. L. Threlfall. Springer-Verlag, Berlin.

31. Mazzeo, J.R., Neue, U.D., Kele, M. & Plumb, R.S. (2005). Advancing LC performance with smaller particles and higher pressure. Analytical Chemistry 77(23), 460A–467A.

32. Fleisher, D., Li, C., Zhou, Y., Pao, L.-H. & Karim, A. (1999). Drug, meal and formulation interactions influencing drug absorption after oral administration: Clinical implications. Clinical Pharmacokinetics 36(3), 233–254.

33. Koparkar, A.D., Augsburger, L.L. & Shangraw, R.F. (1990). Intrinsic dissolution rates of tablet filler-binders and their influence on the dissolution of drugs from tablet formulations. Pharmaceutical Research 7(1), 80–86.

34. Samyn, J.C. & Jung, W.Y. (1970). In vitro dissolution from several experimental capsule formulations. Journal of Pharmaceutical Sciences 59(2), 169–175.

35. Wilson, C.G. & Kilian, K. (2005). Gastrointestinal Transit and Drug Absorption. In: Pharmaceutical Dissolution Testing, J. Dressman, & J. Krämer, (eds). Taylor and Francis, Boca Raton, FL, pp. 97–125.

36. Noyes, A.A. & Whitney, W.R. (1871). The rate of solution of solid substances in their own solutions. Journal of the American Chemical Society 19, 930–934.

37. Nernst, W. (1904). Theorie der Reaktionsgeschwindigkeit in heterogenen Systemen. Zeitschrift für Physikalische Chemie. 47, 52–55.

38. Shah, V.P., Konecny, J.J., Everett, R.L., McCullough, B., Noorizadeh, A.C. & Skelly, J.P. (1989). In vitro dissolution profile of water-insoluble drug dosage forms in the presence of surfactants. Pharmaceutical Research 6(7), 612–618.

39. Rosen, M. (1989). Surfactants and Interfacial Phenomena. John Wiley & Sons, New York.

40. Attwood, D. & Florence, A.T. (2005). Surfactant Systems. Chapman and Hall, New York.

41. Hörter, D. & Dressman, J.B. (1997). Influence of physicochemical properties on dissolution of drugs in the gastrointestinal tract. Advanced Drug Delivery Reviews 25, 3–14.

42. Dressman, J.B., Amidon, G.L., Reppas, C. & Shah, V.P. (1998). Dissolution testing as a prognostic tool for oral drug absorption: immediate release dosage forms. Pharmaceutical Research 15(1), 11–22.

43. Galia, E., Nicolaides, E., Hörter, D., Löbenberg, R., Reppas, C. & Dressman, J.B. (1998). Evaluation of various dissolution media for predicting in vivo performance of class I and II drugs. Pharmaceutical Research 15(5), 698–705.

44. Wei, H. & Löbenberg, R. (2006). Biorelevant dissolution media as a predictive tool for glyburide a class II drug. European Journal of Pharmaceutical Sciences 29, 45–52.

45. Qureshi, S.A. & McGilveray, I.J. (1995). A critical assessment of the USP dissolution apparatus suitability test criteria. Drug Development and Industrial Pharmacy 21(8), 905–924.

46. Gao, Z., Moore, T.W., Doub, W.H., Westenberger, B.J. & Buhse, L.F. (2006). Effects of deaeration methods on dissolution testing in aqueous media: a study using a total dissolved gas pressure meter. Journal of Pharmaceutical Sciences 95(7), 1606–1613.

47. Degenhardt, O.S., Waters, B., Rebelo-Cameirao, A., Meyer, A., Brunner, H. & Toltl, N.P. (2004). Comparison of the effectiveness of various deaeration techniques. Dissolution Technologies 11(1), 6–11.

48. Hom, F.S., Veresh, S.A. & Miskel, J.J. (1973). Soft gelatin capsules I: Factors affecting capsule shell dissolution rate. Journal of Pharmaceutical Sciences 62(6), 1001–1006.

49. Digenis, G.A., Gold, T.B. & Shah, V.P. (1994). Cross-linking of gelatin capsules and its relevance to their in vitro-in vivo performance. Journal of Pharmaceutical Sciences 83(7), 915–921.

50. Gelatin Capsule Working Group (1998). Collaborative development of two-tier dissolution testing for gelatin capsules and gelatin-coated tablets using enzyme-containing media. Pharmacopeial Forum 24(5), 7045–7050.

51. Meyer, M.C., Straughn, A.B., Mhatre, R.M., Hussain, A., Shah, V.P., Bottom, C.B., Cole, E.T., Lesko, L.L., Mallinowski, H. & Williams, R.L. (2000). The effect of gelatin cross-linking on the bioequivalence of hard and soft gelatin acetaminophen capsules. Pharmaceutical Research 17(8), 962–966.

52. Chafetz, L., Hong, W-H., Tsilifonis, D.C., Taylor, A.K. & Philip, J. (1984). Decrease in the rate of capsule dissolution due to formaldehyde from Polysorbate 80 autooxidation. Journal of Pharmaceutical Sciences 73(8), 1186–1187.

53. Singh, S., Rao, K.V.R., Venugopal, K. & Manikandan, R. (2002). Alteration in dissolution characteristics of gelatin-containing formulations: A review of the problem, test methods, and solutions. Pharmaceutical Technology April, 36–58.

54. Piper, D.W. & Fenton, B.H. (1965). pH stability and activity curves of pepsin with special reference to their clinical importance. Gut 6, 506–508.

55. Gallery, J., Han, J.-H. & Abraham, C. (2004). Pepsin and pancreatin performance in the dissolution of crosslinked gelatin capsules from pH 1 to 8. Pharmacopeial Forum 30(3), 1084–1089.

56. Zhao, F., Malayev, V., Rao, V. & Hussain, M. (2004). Effect of sodium lauryl sulfate in dissolution media on dissolution of hard gelatin capsule shells. Pharmaceutical Research 21(1), 144–148.

57. Missaghi, S. & Fassihi, R. (2006). Evaluation and comparison of physicomechanical characteristics of gelatin and hypromellose capsules. Drug Development and Industrial Pharmacy 32, 829–838.

58. Cole, E.T., Scott, R.A., Cade, D., Connor, A.L. & Wilding, I. (2004). In vitro and in vivo pharmacoscintigraphic evaluation of ibuprofen hypromellose and gelatin capsules. Pharmaceutical Research 21(5), 793–798.

59. Craig, D.Q.M. (2002). The mechanisms of drug release from solid dispersions in water-soluble polymers. International Journal of Pharmaceutics 231, 131–144.

60. Perng, C.-Y., Kearney, A.S., Palepu, N.R., Smith, B.R. & Azzarano, L.M. (2003). Assessment of oral bioavailability enhancing approaches for SB-247083 using flow-through cell dissolution testing as one of the screens. International Journal of Pharmaceutics 250, 147–156.

61. Rogers, T.L., Gillespie, I.B., Hitt, J.E., Fransen, K.L., Crowl, C.A., Tucker, C.J., Kupperblatt, G.B., Becker, J.N., Wilson, D.L., Todd, C., Broomall, C.F., Evans, J.C. & Elder, E.J. (2004). Development and characterization of a scalable controlled precipitation process to enhance the dissolution of poorly water-soluble drugs. Pharmaceutical Research 21, 2048–2057.

62. Lukas, G. (1996). Critical manufacturing parameters influencing dissolution. Drug Information Journal 30, 1091–1104.

63. Kostewicz, E.S., Wunderlich, M., Brauns, U., Becker, R., Bock, T. & Dressman, J.B. (2004). Predicting the precipitation of poorly soluble weak bases upon entry in the small intestine. The Journal of Pharmacy and Pharmacology 56, 43–51.

64. Parrott, N. & Lavé, T. (2002). Prediction of intestinal absorption: comparative assessment of GASTROPLUS™ and IDEA™. European Journal of Pharmaceutical Sciences 17, 51–61.

65. Hixson, A.W. & Crowell, J.H. (1931). Dependence of reaction velocity upon surface and agitation: I Theoretical consideration. Industrial & Engineering Chemistry Research 23, 923–931.

66. Langenbucher, L. (1976). Parametric representation of dissolution-rate curves by the RRSBW distribution. Die Pharmazeutische Industie 38, 472–477.

67. Nicolaides, E., Symillides, M., Dressman, J.B. & Reppas, C. (2001). Biorelevant dissolution testing to predict the plasma profile of lipophilic drugs after oral administration. Pharmaceutical Research 18(3), 380–388.

68. Polli, J.E., Rekhi, G.S. & Shah, V.P. (1996). Methods to compare dissolution profiles. Drug Information Journal 30, 1113–1120.

69. Charman, W.N. (2000). Lipids, lipophilic drugs, and oral drug delivery—some emerging concepts. Journal of Pharmaceutical Sciences 89, 967–978.

70. Humberstone, A.J. & Charman, W.N. (1997). Lipid-based vehicles for the oral delivery of poorly water soluble drugs. Advanced Drug Delivery Reviews 25, 103–128.

71. Pouton, C.W. (2000). Lipid formulations for oral administration of drugs: non-emulsifying, self-emulsifying and self-microemulsifying drug delivery systems. European Journal of Pharmaceutical Sciences 2, 11 Suppl. S93–S98.

72. Pillay, V. & Fassihi, R. (1999). A new method for dissolution studies of lipid-filled capsules employing nifedipine as a model drug. Pharmaceutical Research 16, 333–337.

73. Pillay, V. & Fassihi, R. (1999). Unconventional dissolution methodologies. Journal of Pharmaceutical Sciences 88(9), 843–851.

74. Porter, C.J.H. & Charman, W.N. (2001). In vitro assessment of oral lipid based formulations. Advanced Drug Delivery Reviews, S127–S147.

75. Han, J.-H. & Gallery, J. (2006). A risk based approach to in vitro performance testing: a case study on the use of dissolution vs. disintegration for liquid filled soft gelatin capsules. American Pharmaceutical Reviews September/October.

76. Shah, V.P., Gurbarg, M., Noory, A., Dighe, S. & Skelly, J.P. (1992). Influence of higher rates of agitation on release patterns of immediate-release drug products. Journal of Pharmaceutical Sciences 81(6), 500–503.

77. Mirza, T., Joshi, Y., Liu, Q. & Vivilecchia, R. (2005). Evaluation of dissolution hydrodynamics in the USP, Peak™ and flat-bottom vessels using different solubility drugs. Dissolution Technologies 12(1), 11–16.

78. Arifin, D.Y., Lee, L.Y. & Wang, C.-H. (2006). Mathematical modeling and simulation of drug release from microspheres: Implications to drug delivery systems. Advanced Drug Delivery Reviews 58, 1274–1325.

79. Ritger, P.L. & Peppas, N.A. (1987). A simple equation for description of solute Fickian and non-Fickian release from non-swellable devices in the form of slabs, spheres, cylinders or discs. Journal of Controlled Release 5, 23–36.

80. Ritger, P.L. & Peppas, N.A. (1987). A simple equation for description of solute release II. Fickian and anomalous release from swellable devices. Journal of Controlled Release 5, 37–42.

81. Peppas, N.A. & Sahlin, J.J. (1989). A simple equation for the description of solute release. III Coupling of diffusion and relaxation. International of Journal of Pharmaceutics 57, 169–172.

82. Borgquist, P., Körner, A., Piculell, L., Larsson, A. & Axelsson, A. (2006). A model for the drug release from a polymer matrix tablet—effects of swelling and dissolution. Journal of Controlled Release 113, 216–225.

83. Colombo, P., Bettini, R., Massimo, G., Catellani, P.L., Santi, P. & Peppas, N.A. (1995). Drug diffusion front movement is important in drug release control from swellable matrix tablets. Journal of Pharmaceutical Sciences 84(8), 991–997.

84. Sathe, P.M., Tsong, Y. & Shah, V.P. (1996). In-vitro dissolution profile comparison: Statistics and analysis, model dependent approach. Pharmaceutical Research 13(12), 1799–1803.

85. Moore, J.W. & Flanner, H.H. (1996). Mathematical comparison of dissolution profiles. Pharmaceutical Technologies. June, 64–74.

86. Yuksel, N., Kanik, A.E. & Baykara, T. (2000). Comparison of in vitro dissolution profiles by ANOVA-based, model-dependent and -independent methods. International of Journal of Pharmaceutics 209, 57–67.

87. Ju, H.L. & Liaw, S.-J. (1997). On the assessment of similarity of drug dissolution profiles—a simulation study. Drug Information Journal 31, 1273–1289.

88. Polli, J.E. (1999). Dependence of in vitro-in vivo correlation analysis acceptability on model selections. Pharmaceutical Development and Technology 4(1), 89–96.

89. Tsong, Yi., Hammerstrom, T., Sathe, P. & Shah, V.P. (1996). Statistical assessment of mean differences between two dissolution data sets. Drug Information Journal 30, 1105–1112.

90. Shah, V.P., Tsong, Y., Sathe, P. & Liu, J.-P. (1998). In vitro dissolution profile comparison—statistics and analysis of the similarity factor, f_2. Pharmaceutical Research 15(6), 889–896.

91. Boudreau, S.P., McElvain, J.S., Martin, L.D., Dowling, T. & Fields, S. M. (2004). Method validation by phase of development: An acceptable analytical practice. Pharmaceutical Technology 28(11), 54–66.

92. ICH Q2A. (1995). International Conference on Harmonization: Guideline for Industry: Text on the Validation of Analytical Procedures, Availability. Federal Register 60(40), 11260–11262.

93. ICH Q2B. (1997). International Conference on Harmonization: Guidance for Industry Q2B Validation of Analytical Procedures: Methodology, Availability. Federal Register 62(96), 27464–27467.

94. Hofer, J.D. & Gray, V.A. (2003). Examination of selection of immediate-release dissolution acceptance criteria. Pharmacopeial Forum 29(1), 335–340.

95. FDA Guidance for Industry. (2003). Bioavailability and bioequivalence studies for orally administered drug products—general considerations.

96. O'Hara, T., Hayes, S., Davis, J., Devane, J., Smart, T. & Dunne, A. (2001). In vivo–in vitro correlation (IVIVC) modeling incorporating a convolution step. Journal of Pharmacokinetics and Pharmacodynamics 28(3), 2001.

97. Dunne, A., O'Hara, T. & Devane, J. (1997). Level A in vivo in vitro correlation: nonlinear models and statistical methodology. Journal of Pharmaceutical Sciences 86(11), 1245–1249.

98. Balan, G., Timmins, P., Greene, D.S. & Marathe, P.H. (2001). In vitro-in vivo correlation (IVIVC) models for metformin after administration of modified-release (MR) oral dosage forms to healthy human volunteers. Journal of Pharmaceutical Sciences 90(8), 1176–1185.

99. Qiu, Y., Cheskin, H.S., Engh, K.R. & Poska, R.P. (2003). Once-a-day controlled-release dosage form of Divalproex Sodium I: Formulation design and in vitro/in vivo investigations. Journal of Pharmaceutical Sciences 92(6), 1166–1173.

100. Qiu, Y., Garren, J., Samara, E., Cao, G., Abraham, C., Cheskin, H.S. & Engh, K.R. (2003). Once-a-day controlled-release dosage form of Divalproex Sodium II: Development of a predictive in vitro drug release method. Journal of Pharmaceutical Sciences 92(11), 2317–2325.

101. Dutta, S., Qiu, Y., Samar, E., Cao, G. & Granneman, G.R. (2005). Once-a-day controlled-release dosage form of Divalproex Sodium III: Development and validation of a Level A in vitro-in vivo correlation (IVIVC). Journal of Pharmaceutical Sciences 94(9), 1949–1956.

102. Lake, O.A., Olling, M. & Barends, D.M. (1999). In vitro/in vivo correlations of dissolution data of carbamazepine immediate release tablets with pharmacokinetic data obtained in healthy volunteers. European Journal of Pharmaceutics and Biopharmaceutics 48, 13–19.

103. Modi, N.B., Lam, A., Lindemulder, E., Wang, B. & Gupta, S.K. (2000). Application of in vitro-in vivo correlations (IVIVC) in setting formulation release specifications. Biopharmaceutics & Drug Disposition 21, 321–326.

104. Elkoshi, Z. (1999). Dissolution specifications based on release rates. Journal of Pharmaceutical Sciences 88(4), 434–444.

105. Hayes, S., Dunne, A., Smart, T. & Davis, J. (2004). Interpretation and optimization of the dissolution specifications for a modified release product with an in vivo-in vitro correlation (IVIVC). Journal of Pharmaceutical Sciences 93(3), 571–581.

Bioavailability and Bioequivalence

Hao Zhu, Honghui Zhou and Kathleen Seitz

15.1 GENERAL BACKGROUND

Substituting one oral dosage formulation for another has been a common practice for many years in the drug development industry, as well as in the clinic. During drug development, for example, industry scientists frequently evaluate different versions of investigational drug products or dosage formulations, and thereby often need to conduct bioequivalence studies. In turn, prescribing clinicians use the bioavailability and bioequivalence data provided on the product label to select an optimal treatment regimen for their patients. Consequently, the overall therapeutic success of any drug substitution in the clinic will ultimately depend on multiple factors. These factors include the pharmacokinetics of the comparator and reference drugs, as well as the appropriateness of the study design and statistical criteria that were used to initially demonstrate bioequivalence.

Bioequivalence has evolved as a specific regulatory requirement over the last 40 years. In the early 1960s, researchers noticed that the bioavailability of a therapeutic drug product could vary depending on its oral dosage formulation.[1] Almost 15 years later, in 1977, the US Food and Drug Administration (FDA) initially published their recommended procedures for sponsors to use in studies of bioequivalence.[1] Since then, the FDA has continued to refine and revise its guidance on bioequivalence, other international regulatory agencies have published their own guidelines, and pharmaceutical industry professionals worldwide have contributed their statistical expertise and

scientific opinions. Nevertheless, several major controversies have yet to be resolved. Issues pertaining to the selection of the most appropriate statistical criteria to use to sufficiently demonstrate bioequivalence are still frequently debated. Other topics of discussion include a determination of exactly when (or under what specific circumstances) should formal tests of bioequivalence be required from a regulatory standpoint, and for which type or class of drug.

Under the Food, Drug and Cosmetic (FD&C) Act of 1938 and the 1962 Kefauver–Harris Amendment, sponsors were required to provide safety and efficacy data to support all claims for the active ingredients in a new drug product before it could be approved for sale. Scientific standards later set by the FDA, however, have since allowed sponsors to lawfully make appropriate drug substitutions without necessarily having to conduct additional time-consuming, and expensive, clinical safety and efficacy studies. That is, in the absence of additional clinical studies (and under specific circumstances), an appropriate set of biopharmaceutical, pharmacokinetic, and statistical evaluations may now be used to establish that a test drug formulation is bioequivalent (and thereby therapeutically interchangeable) with a reference drug formulation.

The information included in this chapter will provide the reader with an overview of the clinical, pharmacokinetic, and statistical issues associated with bioavailability and bioequivalence studies of oral dosage formulations. The current international regulatory perspectives will also be presented, along with a detailed comparison of the various criteria presently being used in the pharmaceutical industry to demonstrate bioequivalence.

15.2 DEFINITIONS AND KEY CONCEPTS

Bioavailability essentially describes the overall rate and extent of drug absorption. Data from bioavailability studies are routinely used to identify a drug product's pharmacokinetics, optimize a therapeutic dose regimen, and support product labeling requirements. Bioequivalence, on the other hand, generally describes the extent to which the bioavailability of one particular drug product (i.e., the test product) compares with that of another known drug product (i.e., the reference product). Data from bioequivalence studies are often used to establish a link between different investigational drug formulations (e.g., an early phase 1 formulation versus a later phase 3 formulation). Bioequivalence studies may also be required during the post-approval period in certain situations, such as whenever a major change occurs in a manufacturing method for an approved drug product. Bioequivalence studies are also generally required to compare generic versions of a drug product with the corresponding reference-listed drug.

Regulatory requirements for bioavailability and bioequivalence data submitted with new drug applications (NDAs) and supplemental applications are specifically addressed in the US Code of Federal Regulations,[2] and a corresponding FDA guidance document has been published.[3] The following sections will provide an overview of the key concepts, and general underlying principles, of bioavailability and bioequivalence.

15.2.1 Bioavailability

When a drug is administered orally (or by any other extravascular route), a sufficient amount of the administered dose must be absorbed over a certain time period before the intended pharmacologic effect can manifest. Thus, the bioavailability of an orally administered drug clearly depends on a combination of factors, including the physiochemical characteristics of the drug formulation, and the physiological state of the gastrointestinal (GI) system.

Bioavailability of an oral dosage form is defined[3] as:

"the rate and extent to which the active ingredient or active moiety is absorbed from a drug product and becomes available at the site of action."

From a pharmacokinetic perspective, two specific types of bioavailability can be considered: absolute bioavailability, and relative bioavailability. Absolute bioavailability is a special case in which the systemic exposure of an extravascular dosage form is determined relative to that of its intravenous (IV) dosage form. Relative bioavailability, in contrast, compares the rate and extent of absorption of one dosage formulation (e.g., oral solution) to another dosage formulation (e.g., oral capsule). Relative bioavailability can also sometimes compare the rate and extent of absorption for one drug product with two different administration routes (e.g., intramuscular and subcutaneous).

For the most part, absolute bioavailability is generally determined by comparing the extent of drug absorption after an extravascular versus an intravenous (e.g., infusion or bolus) administration. Thus, valid extravascular and IV data are both typically required for the calculation of absolute bioavailability. In operational terms, this means two series of pharmacokinetic samples must be collected—one extravascular series, and one IV series—using a suitable biological matrix (e.g., blood, plasma or serum), and appropriate sampling schedules. In addition, drug concentrations from each series must be analyzed using a validated drug assay.

Measured concentration data from each series are then plotted, and the area under the drug concentration–time curves (AUC) estimated (e.g., by applying a numerical integration formula such as the trapezoidal rule). Assuming clearance remains constant AUC is directly proportional to the amount of drug absorbed. Thus absolute oral bioavailability (F) can be calculated:

$$F = \frac{D_{iv}}{D_{po}} \cdot \frac{AUC_{po}}{AUC_{iv}}$$

where:

D_{iv} and D_{po} are the intravenous and oral doses administered, respectively

AUC_{iv} and AUC_{po} are the AUC estimates for the intravenous and oral routes, respectively.

In contrast to absolute bioavailability, relative bioavailability essentially compares the rate and extent of absorption of one dosage formulation (e.g., oral solution) to that of another (e.g., oral capsule). Over the course of a typical drug development cycle, several relative bioavailability studies could potentially be required (e.g., to compare the *in vivo* performance of an earlier stage formulation versus the later stage formulation). Depending on the overall pace of drug development, new dosage formulations are often still being prepared while a new molecular entity progresses from the nonclinical stage into the early clinical stage. In cases where the final product is intended as a solid oral dosage form, for example, oral solutions or suspensions might be the only formulations ready for use. Solid prototype formulations, such as capsules, might also be ready for use in early phase 1; however these prototypes are often far from the final marketable form. Under these types of circumstances, therefore, an estimate of the drug's relative bioavailability is needed.

Relative bioavailability (F_{rel}) can be calculated:

$$F_{rel} = \frac{D_A}{D_B} \cdot \frac{AUC_B}{AUC_A}$$

where:

D_A and D_B are the doses administered for drug formulation A and B, respectively

AUC_A and AUC_B are the AUC estimates for the A and B formulations, respectively.

15.2.2 Bioequivalence

Bioequivalence is defined[3] as:

"the absence of a significant difference in the rate and extent to which the active ingredient or active moiety in pharmaceutical equivalents or pharmaceutical alternatives becomes available at the site of drug action when administered at the same molar dose under similar conditions in an appropriately designed study."

From a regulatory perspective, and for various strategic reasons, bioequivalence studies may need to be conducted before a product is approved for use in the clinic or during the post-approval period. Depending on the particular research objective, for example, a pre-approval bioequivalence study might be required in an NDA submission to demonstrate the therapeutic link between the early phase dosage formulation and the to-be-marketed formulation. Bioequivalence studies are also typically required in abbreviated NDAs for generic versions of brand name drugs.

Two oral drug products can generally be considered to be bioequivalent if their respective concentration–time profiles are so similar that it would be unlikely that they would produce clinically significant differences in the pharmacological response. In other words, bioequivalent drug products with essentially the same systemic bioavailability should thus be able to produce similar, and predictable, therapeutic effects. Pharmacokinetic assessments in bioequivalence studies of solid oral drug products, therefore, typically include statistical comparisons of AUC and maximum concentration (C_{max}). Different measures are sometimes needed to describe drug exposure. For example, partial AUC truncated to the median T_{max} of the reference product can be used to describe

early drug exposure. C_{max} is used to describe peak exposure. For a single dose study, both $AUC_{0-\tau}$ and $AUC_{0-\infty}$ are used to measure the total exposure. If a multiple dose study is appropriate, the $AUC_{0-\tau}$ at steady state (where τ is the dosing interval) is used to describe total exposure.

Pharmacodynamic assessments may also sometimes be performed. For instance, if the systemic exposure of the drug is too low to be reliably detected or if an appropriate bioanalytical methodology cannot be developed to support a pharmacokinetic assessment, an appropriate pharmacodynamic assessment (i.e., a reliable and predictable surrogate marker) may suffice. Pharmacodynamic measurements are usually not recommended if pharmacokinetic measurements are available.

Pharmacokinetic bioequivalence methods can be quite challenging for drugs with minimal systemic bioavailability. Drug classes that typically show minimal systemic bioavailability are ophthalmic, dermal, intranasal, and inhalation drugs. Nevertheless, pharmacodynamic assessments are not routinely used to show bioequivalence, for several reasons. First, very few validated, predictable surrogate biomarkers are available that are also considered acceptable surrogates by the regulatory authorities. Secondly, pharmacodynamic studies generally require prohibitively large sample sizes since intra- and inter-subject variability levels tend to be relatively high. Some examples of biological markers that have been successfully used for bioequivalence testing are skin blanching[4] with corticosteroids, and stomach acid neutralization with antacids.[5]

15.2.3 Pharmaceutical Equivalence and Therapeutic Equivalence

Drug products are considered to be pharmaceutical equivalents if they contain the same active ingredient, in the same amount, with identical dosage forms, and identical routes of administration. Furthermore, drug products are considered to be therapeutically equivalent only if they are pharmaceutical equivalents (as described above) that are expected to produce the same clinical effects, and have similar safety profiles when they are administered to patients under the same conditions as specified in the product labeling information.

Therapeutic equivalence is thus an ultimate measure of the interchangeability of two distinct drug products or formulations. Therapeutic equivalence may be reasonably inferred from results of appropriately designed *in vivo* pharmacokinetic bioequivalence studies.

15.3 STATISTICAL CONCEPTS IN BIOEQUIVALENCE STUDIES

A test (T) drug product and a reference (R) drug product can only be considered bioequivalent if equivalence of the rate and extent of drug absorption are demonstrated. This leads to three key questions:

1. What are the pharmacokinetic measures that can be used to best characterize the rate and extent of drug absorption?
2. What are the most appropriate statistical criteria to use to adequately demonstrate bioequivalence?
3. How should a study be designed to sufficiently, and appropriately, capture the information necessary to show bioequivalence?

Each of these major topics will be thoroughly discussed in the next several sections.

15.3.1 Selection and Transformation of Pharmacokinetic Measures

In general, the pharmacokinetic measures that are typically used to describe the rate and extent of drug absorption include C_{max}, time to reach C_{max} (T_{max}), and AUC. Whether this particular set of measures best reflects the actual rate and extent of drug absorption, however, continues to be debated and discussed among many members of the industry and the regulatory agencies.[6,7]

The two most commonly used pharmacokinetic variables in bioequivalence studies are AUC, and C_{max}. While C_{max}, and T_{max}, are both commonly used in standard *in vivo* pharmacokinetic studies to reflect absorption rate, C_{max} is specifically used in bioequivalence studies, whereas T_{max} is not used as often because of the high interindividual variability typically seen with this parameter. In addition to C_{max}, AUC is also routinely used in bioequivalence studies. Assuming the *in vivo* clearance of a drug is constant for a given individual, AUC is directly proportional to the amount of drug being absorbed, and thus ideally describes the extent of drug absorption.

To demonstrate equivalence, the mean AUC (or C_{max}) values for two different products are directly compared. Mathematically, the easiest way is to do this is to calculate the difference between the two mean values. As an extension, the difference between the two log-transformed means can likewise be calculated. Logarithmic transformation of AUC (or C_{max}) provides several important advantages. A ratio comparing log-transformed means can easily be converted back to a ratio of means in the normal scale, which can then be readily communicated to regulatory reviewers and prescribing clinicians. From a general clinical perspective the ratio of the mean AUC (or C_{max}), for the test versus the reference drugs, provides the most clinically relevant information. This is generally accepted in the industry, and has been recommended by the FDA Generic Drug Advisory Committee in 1991.[8,9,10]

From a pharmacokinetic perspective, pharmacokinetic measures in bioequivalence studies can be expressed in a multiplicative fashion. AUC, for example, can be expressed as:

$$AUC_{0-\infty} = \frac{F \cdot D}{CL}$$

where:
  D is the dose given to a subject
  CL represents the clearance
  F is the bioavailability which is the fraction of the dose being absorbed ($0 \leq F \leq 1$).

This equation clearly shows that each subject's AUC value is inversely proportional to a specific CL value. This multiplicative term (CL) can thus be regarded as a function of subject. However, in the statistical analysis of bioequivalence, all factors (e.g., treatment, subjects, and sequence) that contribute to the variation in pharmacokinetic measurements are considered to be additive effects. Westlake[11] contends that the subject effect is not additive, if data are analyzed on the original scale. Logarithmic transformation of AUC yields an additive equation:

$$\log AUC_{0-\infty} = \log D + \log F - \log CL$$

which is therefore preferable in bioequivalence analyses. Similar arguments can also be applied to C_{max}.

Finally, from a statistical perspective, AUC (or C_{max}) values in bioequivalence studies are often positively skewed, and the variances between the test and reference groups may differ. This generates an inconsistency in the two major assumptions (i.e., normality, and homoscedasticity of the variance) of the statistical analysis of bioequivalence. Log-transformation of AUC (or C_{max}) values, however, makes the distribution appear more symmetric, closer to the normal distribution, and achieves a relatively homogeneous variance. Thus, major international regulatory agencies generally recommend using log-transformations of pharmacokinetic measurements like AUC or C_{max} in bioequivalence analyses. However, one main drawback to using log-transformation is that, although the mean log AUC (or log C_{max}) values are compared between the test and reference groups, log-transformation essentially compares the median AUC (or C_{max}) values instead of the means from each group.[12]

15.3.2 Variability in Pharmacokinetic Measures of Bioavailability

The variability in pharmacokinetic measurements (e.g., log AUC or log C_{max} values) of bioavailability can be represented in two hierarchical layers.[13,14] That is, bioavailability measurements can vary at the individual subject level, and at overall population level. Whenever oral bioavailability measurements are repeated over time, for example, an individual subject's values may vary from time to time, even if the same drug product is administered each time. This series of measures can then collectively form a distribution where the mean value represents the inherent bioavailability, and the variance reflects the within-subject variability. Of note, in addition to the changes in subject-level information over time, any intra- or inter-lot variability arising from the manufacture of the drug product over time will also be reflected in the within-subject variability.

The second hierarchical layer of variability represents the overall population level variance. In the overall study population, individual subjects may have variations in their own inherent bioavailability. In all, these variations collectively form a distribution where the mean represents the population average of the bioavailability, and the variance reflects the between-subject variability. For example, in a non-replicated parallel bioequivalence study, patients are divided into two groups and given either a test (T) or reference I product. The jth subject in the trial would have a bioavailability measurement (e.g., log AUC or log C_{max}) of Y_{ij}, where i represents the product being given (i = T or R). Then Y_{ij} follows a distribution with mean μ_{ij}, and variance σ_{wi}^2 representing the within-subject variability for a given product. The individual means μ_{ij} (j = T or R) are jointly distributed with mean μ_j, and variance σ_{Bi}^2 (where σ_{Bi}^2 is the between subject variability).

The total variance for each formulation is then derived as the sum of the within- and between-subject variability $\sigma_{Tj}^2 = \sigma_{Bj}^2 + \sigma_{Wj}^2$.

This model allows the correlation (ρ), between μ_{iT} and μ_{iB}. Then the subject-by-formulation interaction variance component is defined as:

$$\sigma_D^2 = variance(\mu_{iT} - \mu_{iR})$$
$$= (\sigma_{BT} - \sigma_{BR})^2 + 2 \cdot (1 - \rho) \cdot \sigma_{BT} \cdot \sigma_{BR}$$

In general, a linear mixed-effect model is used to evaluate bioequivalence. For crossover designs or repeated measurements, the means are given additional structure by including period and sequence effects.

15.3.3 Statistical Criteria for Evaluating Bioequivalence

The statistical tools (i.e., criteria) available for use in bioequivalence analyses have evolved remarkably over the past few decades. This has mostly occurred through a joint effort by interested stakeholders (i.e., professionals in academia, industry, and regulatory agencies) to select the most appropriate tools to address research questions related specifically to bioequivalence. In the early 1970s, bioequivalence was evaluated with a basic comparison of the mean AUC and C_{max} values for the test versus reference drug products. That is, if the mean AUC and C_{max} values for the test product were within 20% of the mean values from the reference product, bioequivalence was concluded. Other relatively basic criteria (e.g., the 75/75 or 75/75–125 rules) have also been used to demonstrate bioequivalence. According to these criteria, if the ratio of the AUC and C_{max} of the test product versus those of the reference product was within 75% to 125% for at least 75% of the subjects, bioequivalence could be claimed.[15,16,17]

In accordance with the conclusions from a 1986 FDA Bioequivalence Task Force, the FDA began to recommend a more standard approach for *in vivo* bioequivalence studies in the early 1990s.[18] This approach is known as average bioequivalence, in which the statistical analysis of pharmacokinetic measurements (e.g., AUC and C_{max}) is based on the two one-sided test (TOST) procedures to determine if the average values from the test product are comparable to those of the reference product. Using this procedure, a 90% confidence interval for the difference of the pharmacokinetic measurements is calculated on a log scale. Bioequivalence is demonstrated if this calculated confidence interval falls within the predefined bioequivalence limits (i.e., ±0.22 with a log scale or 0.8 to 1.25 with a regular scale).

In the late 1990s, the FDA subsequently recommended two different approaches.[19] These new approaches are known as population bioequivalence, and individual bioequivalence, and each can be compared and contrasted to the standard approach (i.e., average bioequivalence). From a statistical point of view, for example, average bioequivalence focuses on comparing the population average values of the pharmacokinetic measurements from two product groups. By contrast, population bioequivalence and individual bioequivalence focus on comparing the average values, and their variances as well. These variance terms are included in the population and individual bioequivalence approaches to reflect the possibility that the test and reference drug products could differ in some ways other than in their average bioavailabilities.

Population bioequivalence assumes an equal distribution of the test and reference formulation bioavailabilities across all subjects in the population, and is intended to address the issue of drug prescribability. Drug prescribability refers to the clinician's choice for prescribing a particular drug product versus another product to a new patient. For example, a clinician can choose to prescribe either the brand name drug or any number of generic versions that have been shown to be bioequivalent. The underlying assumption of drug prescribability is that the brand name drug product and its generic versions may be used interchangeably in terms of general efficacy and safety.

Individual bioequivalence, however, focuses on drug switchability, and the assumption of equivariance of the distributions of the test and reference product bioavailabilities for each individual subject. Drug switchability describes the situation when a clinician prescribes an alternative drug product (e.g., a generic company's version) to a patient who has already been titrated to a steady, therapeutic level of a previously-prescribed drug product (e.g., an innovator company's drug product). Drug switchability is considered more critical, and also more clinically relevant, than drug prescribability, particularly for patients with chronic diseases requiring long-term drug therapy. Drug prescribability and drug switchability can be assessed by population bioequivalence and individual bioequivalence tests, respectively.[20,21] The population bioequivalence approach is not applicable to evaluations of drug switchability, however, because of a possible subject-by-formulation interaction.[22]

Average Bioequivalence

Average bioequivalence indicates that two products may be considered equivalent if the difference in their population average value is relatively small, and contained within a predefined acceptable range. Under current regulatory guidance, the lower and upper limits (δ_L and δ_U, respectively) of an acceptable range are defined as ± 0.22 in the log scale or from 0.8 to 1.25 in the original scale. The selection of the lower and upper limits for equivalence is somewhat arbitrary, and is usually attributed to the general clinical observation that for most drugs, a 20% change in dose does not significantly change the clinical outcome.

In average bioequivalence, the hypotheses to be tested include:

$$\text{Ho:} \mu_T - \mu_R \leq \delta_L \text{ or } \mu_T - \mu_R \geq \delta_l$$
$$\text{Ha:} \delta_L < (\mu_T - \mu_R) < \delta_U$$

where μ_T and μ_R are the population averages of the pharmacokinetic measurement (e.g., log AUC or log C_{max}) for the test and reference products, respectively, and δ_L and δ_U are the prespecified lower and upper limits, respectively.

Average bioequivalence is systematically evaluated through the following set of procedures. First, a non-replicated or replicated bioequivalence study is conducted, and intensive blood samples are obtained from subjects who received either the test or reference product. Next, a non-compartmental analysis is performed to obtain the pharmacokinetic measurements (e.g., AUC or C_{max}) and these results are log-transformed. A linear mixed-effect model is then fitted to the log AUC (or log C_{max}), in which subject and period effects are eliminated so that the product (or formulation) effect, $\mu_T - \mu_R$, can -be estimated. The standard error of the estimated product (or formulation) effect is estimated. The 90% confidence interval is then set by applying the standard error, and comparing it with the predetermined limits. If the 90% confidence interval falls within the predetermined upper and lower limits (i.e., δ_L and δ_U) bioequivalence can be concluded.

For bioequivalence analyses, the confidence interval approach is considered more plausible than the conventional hypothesis test approach. Conventional hypothesis tests (e.g., t test or F test), generally test the null hypothesis that $\mu_T - \mu_R = 0$. Once the null hypothesis is rejected under a certain preset alpha level (e.g., $\alpha = 0.05$), the type I error is under control, and the probability of falsely declaring inequivalence is also thereby controlled. However, controlling instead for the error of falsely declaring equivalence would actually be more meaningful in tests of bioequivalence. This relates to the power function in a conventional hypothesis test. Power functions cannot be directly tested. However, a confidence interval can be linked to the power function that is defined as the probability that the confidence interval would not include an alternative value. Bioequivalence can then be concluded at a risk no greater than 10%, once the 90% confidence interval has no common points with the equivalence limits or the 90% confidence interval falls within the equivalence limits.

Westlake[23] initially suggested that a confidence interval approach could be applied in bioequivalence studies and, when it was first introduced, he proposed using a confidence interval centered on the point of exact equivalence (i.e., $\mu_T - \mu_R = 0$). Kirkwood,[24] on the other hand, suggested using a conventional confidence interval, which is instead centered on the point estimate ($\hat{\mu}_T - \hat{\mu}_R$). Thus, with Westlake's approach, equivalence is accepted if the probability of equivalence is at least 90%. With Kirkwood's conventional confidence interval approach, however, equivalence is accepted if the limits are within the "shortest" 90% region. Kirkwood's approach has currently gained acceptance internationally, and is considered more stringent than Westlake's approach.

Other statistical approaches have also been used to assess average bioequivalence. Of these, Schuirmann's two one-sided test (TOST) approach[25] is considered important. With t–he TOST method, the question of equivalence is essentially transformed into two separate and independent questions:

1. is the difference of the average mean values of the pharmacokinetic measurements for the test and reference products larger than the value of the prespecified upper limit? Or,
2. is the difference of the average mean values smaller than the value of the prespecified lower limit?

Statistically, the null and alternative hypotheses for the first question are:

$$H_{0A}: \mu_T - \mu_R \leq \delta_L \text{ and } H_{1A}: \mu_T - \mu_R > \delta_L.$$

Likewise, the null and alternative hypotheses for the second question are:

$$H_{0B}: \mu_T - \mu_R \geq \delta_U \text{ and } H_{1B}: \mu_T - \mu_R < \delta_U.$$

Under conditions that both null hypotheses have been rejected, this leads to acceptance of both alternative hypotheses and their intersection, $\delta_L < (\mu_T - \mu_R) < \delta_U$. When the two independent tests are carried out at an alpha level equal to 0.05, this is equivalent to using the conventional 90% confidence interval approach. Thus, the confidence interval approach is also sometimes called the TOST approach.

Population Bioequivalence

Population bioequivalence is intended to ensure drug prescribability by assessing the total variances of the bioavailabilities of the test and reference products, in addition to their mean difference. The assumption for population bioequivalence is that there is an equal distribution within the test or reference formulation bioavailability across the entire subject population. Between the two formulations, however, the distributions might be different.

Population bioequivalence considers the scenario that the test and reference products are given to different (i.e., independent) subjects. Assuming the jth and j'th subjects are two independent subjects coming from the same study population and they both receive reference product ®, the expected squared difference for these two subjects can be expressed as:

$$E(R_j - R_{j'})^2 = [E(R_j - R_{j'})]^2 + Var(R_j - R_{j'})$$
$$= 0 + \sigma_{TR}^2 + \sigma_{TR}^2 = 2 \cdot \sigma_{TR}^2$$

where:

$E(R_j - R_{j'})^2$ is the expected squared difference

$[E(R_j - R_{j'})]$ is the expected value for the difference between the two subjects taking R.

Since the distribution equality assumption holds for any subject taking the same formulation, then $E(R_j - R_{j'}) = E(R_j) - E(R_{j'}) = 0$. And $Var(R_j - R_{j'})$ represents the variability for the jth and j'th subjects taking R. Since the subjects are considered to be independent and identically distributed, then:

$$Var(R_j - R_{j'}) = 2 \cdot \sigma_{TR}^2$$

Likewise, if the jth subject is given test product (T) and the j'th subject is given the reference product ®, the expected squared difference between T and R given to two different subjects can be expressed as:

$$E(T_j - R_{j'})^2 = [E(T_j - R_{j'})]^2 + Var(T_j - R_{j'})$$
$$= (\mu_T - \mu_R)^2 + \sigma_{TT}^2 + \sigma_{TR}^2$$

where $E(T_j - R_{j'})^2$ is the expected squared difference between T and R given to two different subjects. $Var(T_j - R_{j'})$ and $E(T_j - R_{j'})$ are the variance term and expected value, respectively, for the two subjects taking the two formulations. Then $E(T_j - R_{j'}) = (\mu_T - \mu_R)$ and the variance term can be simplified as: $Var(T_j - R_{j'}) = \sigma_{TT}^2 + \sigma_{TR}^2$, when the two distributions related to the two products are independent.

To ensure drug prescribability, an equation is needed to show the expected squared difference between T and R, given to two different subjects from the same patient population, compared with the expected squared difference for the reference product given to the two subjects. This formula can be shown as:

$$\frac{E(T_j - R_{j'})^2}{E(R_j - R_{j'})^2} = \frac{(\mu_T - \mu_R)^2 + (\sigma_{TR}^2 + \sigma_{TR}^2)}{2 \cdot \sigma_{TR}^2}$$

The square root of this ratio is known as the population difference ratio (PDR). The relationship between the PDR and the test formula of the population bioequivalence can be expressed as:

$$PDR = \left(\frac{\Theta_p}{2} + 1\right)^{0.5}$$

where:

$\Theta_p = \dfrac{(\mu_T - \mu_R)^2 + (\sigma_{TT}^2 - \sigma_{TR}^2)}{\sigma_{TR}^2}$ represents the test formula for population bioequivalence.

In an ideal situation, the PDR ratio should be equal to 1. In reality, however, if the PDR ratio is not substantially greater than 1, the two drug products can be considered to be populationally bioequivalent. The decision for population bioequivalence under current FDA guidance is illustrated using a mixed-scaling criteria. If $\sigma_{TR}^2 < \sigma_{TO}^2$, then the criteria is reference-scaled:

$$\Theta_p = \frac{(\mu_T - \mu_R)^2 + (\sigma_{TR}^2 - \sigma_{TR}^2)}{\sigma_{TR}^2} \leq \theta_P$$

where:

θ_P is the population bioequivalence criteria.

On the other hand, if $\sigma_{TR}^2 > \sigma_{TO}^2$, the criteria should be changed from reference-scaled to constant-scaled:

$$\Theta_p = \frac{(\mu_T - \mu_R)^2 + (\sigma_{TT}^2 - \sigma_{TR}^2)}{\sigma_{TO}^2} \leq \theta_P$$

where:

σ_{TO}^2 is a constant variance that represents the standard between-subject variability.

The FDA recommends[26] that the population bioequivalence criteria should satisfy:

$$\theta_P = \frac{(1.25)^2 + \varepsilon_P}{\sigma_{TO}^2}$$

where:

the value 1.25 comes from the average bioequivalence criteria

ε_P is the allowable variance

σ_{TO}^2 is the standard variance.

Recommended values for these parameters in the population bioequivalence approach are not as clear as they are for the individual bioequivalence approach; thus, some researchers use empirical or simulation methods to identify these values. Furthermore, if a confidence interval for Θ_p cannot be obtained directly, a bootstrap method may be used to calculate the bootstrap interval and this interval would then be compared using the predefined criteria.[27]

Individual Bioequivalence

Individual bioequivalence is designed to guarantee drug switchability. Switchability means that an individual who is currently taking one drug product can subsequently switch to an equivalent product without experiencing a major change in safety or efficacy. The main assumption here is that the within-subject distribution of the bioavailability for both products is equal.

Individual bioequivalence considers situations where either the same subject takes a reference product on two different occasions or the same subject takes the reference ® and test (T) products on different occasions. Assuming the reference product ® is given to the jth subject on different occasions, the expected squared difference between T and R can be expressed as:

$$E(R_j - R'_j)^2 = [E(R_j - R'_j)]^2 + Var(R_j - R'_j)$$
$$= 0 + \sigma_{WR}^2 + \sigma_{WR}^2 = 2 \cdot \sigma_{WR}^2$$

where $E(R_j - R'_j)^2$ represents the expected squared difference and $E(R_j - R'_j)^2$ is the expected value for the difference of the jth subject taking R on different occasions. The value should be zero, since it follows the same distribution. $Var(R_j - R'_j)$ is the variance term for the same subject taking R on different occasions. Following a similar argument as with population bioequivalence, this term is equivalent to $2 \cdot \sigma_{WR}^2$.

Assuming T and R are given to the same (i.e., jth) subject on different occasions, the expected squared difference between T and R can be expressed as:

$$E(T_j - R_j)^2 = [E(T_j - R_j)]^2 + Var(T_j - R_j)$$
$$= (\mu_T - \mu_R)^2 + \sigma_D^2 + \sigma_{WT}^2 + \sigma_{WR}^2$$

where $E(T_j - R_j)^2$ is the expected square difference, and $Var(T_j - R_j)$ represents the variance term for the same subject taking T and R. Following a similar argument as with population bioequivalence, the relationship can be simplified as the population average and variance terms, where σ_D^2 is known as the subject-by-formulation term.

To ensure drug switchability from T to R, an equation is constructed to examine whether the expected squared difference between T and R is comparable to the expected squared difference in R itself on different occasions. The formula is:

$$IDR = \left[\frac{E(T_j - R_j)^2}{E(R_j - R'_j)^2}\right]^{0.5}$$
$$= \left[\frac{(\mu_T - \mu_R)^2 + \sigma_D^2 + (\sigma_{WT}^2 + \sigma_{WR}^2)}{2 \cdot \sigma_{WR}^2}\right]^{0.5}$$

where IDR is the known individual difference ratio. The relationship between IDR and the test metric for individual bioequivalence can be derived:

$$IDR = \left(\frac{\Theta_I}{2} + 1\right)^{0.5}$$

Where $\Theta_I = \dfrac{(\mu_T - \mu_R)^2 + \sigma_D^2 + (\sigma_{WT}^2 - \sigma_{WR}^2)}{\sigma_{WR}^2}$ is the test equation for individual bioequivalence.

FDA guidance[26] suggests using a combination of scaled and unscaled criteria to determine the acceptance criteria. As with the population bioequivalence, the reference scale is used when $\sigma_{WR}^2 < \sigma_{WO}^2$. Here, individual bioequivalence can be concluded if:

$$\Theta_I = \frac{(\mu_T - \mu_R)^2 + \sigma_D^2 + (\sigma_{WT}^2 - \sigma_{WR}^2)}{\sigma_{WR}^2} \leq \theta_I$$

where:

θ_I is the individual bioequivalence limit.

On the other hand, the constant scale is applied when $\sigma_{WR}^2 > \sigma_{WO}^2$. Here, individual bioequivalence can be concluded if:

$$\Theta_I = \frac{(\mu_T - \mu_R)^2 + \sigma_D^2 + (\sigma_{WT}^2 - \sigma_{WR}^2)}{\sigma_{WO}^2} \leq \theta_I$$

where:

σ_{WO}^2 is a constant variance term representing a standard for the within-subject variance.

Proper selection of the values for σ_{WO}^2 and θ_I is important. The FDA guidance [26] proposes using the following equation and standard for determining the criteria.

$$\theta_I = \frac{(1.25)^2 + \varepsilon_I}{\sigma_{WO}^2}$$

The value 1.25 comes from the average bioequivalence criteria. ε_I is the variance allowance and σ_{WO}^2 is the standard variance term. In general, ε_I is a combined variance from the subject-by-formulation variance (σ_D^2) and the difference between the within-subject variability ($\sigma_{WT}^2 - \sigma_{WR}^2$). The value for ε_I is recommended as 0.05 and the value for σ_{WO}^2 is generally recommended as 0.2. Nevertheless, there is no known distribution related to θ_I. As with the population bioequivalence approach, using a bootstrap method to obtain the confidence interval is recommended in the preliminary FDA guidance.[19] To relieve the computational burden, efforts have also been made to derive a non-bootstrap method.

Differences between the Various Bioequivalence Criteria

The statistical criteria for average bioequivalence versus population and individual bioequivalence are thus very different. In average bioequivalence, the lower and upper limits (i.e., 0.8 and 1.25, respectively) are fixed preset values. This approach appears reasonable, since most oral drug products that have been shown to be bioequivalent using the average bioequivalence criteria have not generally demonstrated clinical failure. However, several important issues associated with using a fixed set of upper and lower limits have been identified, especially for bioequivalence tests of drugs with a narrow therapeutic window, and a highly variable bioavailability.[28,29,30,31,32]

For drugs with a narrow therapeutic window, for instance, even just a slight change in bioavailability could cause a significant change in drug concentration (i.e., either above or below the therapeutic window) that may lead to clinically important changes in safety or efficacy. The powerful immunosuppressant drug cyclosporine is a good example. Cyclosporine is primarily used to treat patients with organ transplants. This drug has a very narrow therapeutic window such that patients with subtherapeutic drug concentrations have an increased risk of graft rejection or loss, and patients with supratherapeutic concentrations are more likely to experience severe toxicities (e.g., irreversible renal damage). After successfully passing an average bioequivalence test, a generic version of cyclosporine became available. In 2001, however, a panel of transplant specialists and pharmacokineticists proposed that switching from the brand name cyclosporine to the generic version at the same dose level might not be appropriate.[33] Results of large multicenter studies conducted in renal, hepatic, and heart transplant recipients showed a 10% to 15% dose reduction would be appropriate for the generic version of cyclosporine. Nonetheless, this issue may not have surfaced at all if stricter bioequivalence criteria had been applied in the original bioequivalence study.[34,35]

On the other hand, for highly variable drugs with a wide therapeutic window, it may be more appropriate to consider less stringent bioequivalence criteria. Using the current guidance, for example, this type of drug product can sometimes fail a bioequivalence test because the high variability in bioavailability inherently produces a large confidence interval, suggesting a lack of statistical power. Thus, depending on the level of variability, the total number of subjects needed to obtain sufficient statistical power could reach several hundreds.[36,37]

In contrast to the average bioequivalence approach, the population and individual bioequivalence approaches allow for adjustment of the bioequivalence limits by scaling. Using an individual bioequivalence approach, for instance, reference scaling can be achieved through the within-subject variability of the reference product. Then, when a highly variable formulation is tested, the large within-subject variability compensates for this by elevating the limits by $\sigma_{WR}^2 \cdot \theta_I$. This approach would then allow a sponsor to examine a highly variable test product without recruiting a large number of subjects in the clinical trial. Drugs with a narrow therapeutic window may also benefit from this feature. Most drugs with a narrow therapeutic window have a low within-subject variability therefore, the bioequivalence limits can be reset to a much lower level.

The average bioequivalence approach inherently considers the population average values for the test or reference products. Population and individual bioequivalence approaches, on the other hand, include both the population averages, as well as the different bioavailability variance components, into one equation (i.e., aggregate criterion). While including the variance terms in the statistical test provides additional values, this may also raise some concerns. One big advantage to considering the bioavailability variance terms is known as a "reward of less variability." With a large enough sample size, a highly variable generic drug product could technically meet the requirements of a study using the average bioequivalence criteria. Nevertheless, patients may not actually benefit from this generic product. For example, although the bioequivalence study may have shown enough similarity in the population averages, the generic product's higher variability in bioavailability suggests lower quality.

In contrast, population and individual bioequivalence criteria both offer incentives for a company to manufacture a less variable (i.e., higher quality) product.[38,39,40,41,42] For instance, using the individual bioequivalence criteria, comparing $(\mu_T - \mu_R)^2 + \sigma_D^2 + (\sigma_{WT}^2 - \sigma_{WR}^2)$ with the scaled criteria. Assuming $(\mu_T - \mu_R)^2$ is small enough, making the $(\sigma_{WT}^2 - \sigma_{WR}^2)$ term small would be beneficial, and the product could pass the equivalence test. In other words, lowering the within-subject variability, the between-subject variability or both yields a smaller numerator value in constructing the test statistic for population or individual bioequivalence. Thus, the product has a better chance of passing the equivalence limits.

One disadvantage to including the variance term in the population and individual equivalence criteria, however, is also evident. Considering two formulations with remarkable differences in the population average values, reducing the within-subject or between-subject variability also helps to reduce the numerator value. With individual bioequivalence, for example, if σ_{WT}^2 is small enough, $(\sigma_{WT}^2 - \sigma_{WR}^2)$ can be negative, and the product can pass the equivalence test despite the large difference in the population averages $(\mu_T - \mu_R)^2$. A test product that may be substantially different from the reference product would still pass the individual or population bioequivalence criteria, and subsequently be approved for marketing.

These substantial differences for variance terms related to different formulations or drug products are quite likely, because the variances themselves tend to be variable. Further examination indicates that scaling can offset the trade-off in total variance. This introduces new concerns regarding the use of aggregate criteria where the variance terms are included.

Average, population, and individual bioequivalence metrics can be viewed as:

$$D_A = (\mu_T - \mu_R)^2$$

$$D_P = (\mu_T - \mu_R)^2 + (\sigma_{TT}^2 - \sigma_{TR}^2)$$

$$D_I = (\mu_T - \mu_R)^2 + (\sigma_{WT}^2 - \sigma_{WR}^2 + \sigma_D^2)$$

respectively. As such, average bioequivalence only accounts for the population average, whereas population bioequivalence and individual bioequivalence each consider the population average, as well as the variance components. Under specific conditions, however, these three bioequivalence tests can be interchangeable. For example, assuming the total variances on the test and reference products are the same (i.e., $\sigma_{TT}^2 = \sigma_{WR}^2$), then $D_A = D_P$. In other words, population bioequivalence can be viewed as average bioequivalence in this case. Likewise, individual bioequivalence is reduced to average bioequivalence when the between-subject variability is equal (i.e., $\sigma_{WT}^2 = \sigma_{WR}^2$), and the subject-by-formulation interaction variability equals 0. This relationship, however, does not guarantee a hierarchical structure among the three bioequivalence tests. Consequently, a test drug product that successfully passes the individual bioequivalence test does not automatically meet the criteria for population bioequivalence or average bioequivalence. This has been proven theoretically, and also demonstrated practically.[43] Zariffa et al.[44] conducted a retrospective study to evaluate approximately 22 datasets based on average, population, and individual bioequivalence methods. Their results showed that, based on the AUC values, 19 of the 22 datasets passed on average bioequivalence, all 22 passed on population bioequivalence, and 20 passed on individual bioequivalence. Interestingly, the three datasets that failed on average bioequivalence actually passed on population bioequivalence, and one of these three also passed on individual bioequivalence. The same overall pattern was seen when bioavailability was measured using C_{max}. Of the 16 datasets that passed on average bioequivalence, one dataset failed on both population bioequivalence and individual bioequivalence. Clearly, this lack of hierarchy among the three different bioequivalence approaches raises concern from industry and academia on the use of alternative approaches in bioequivalence studies.

The introduction of population and individual bioequivalence criteria reflects the ongoing effort in the search for a better statistical tool for bioequivalence analyses. Nevertheless, public debate has increased among the interested parties from regulatory, academia, and industry on various issues, including the theoretical basis, potential application, unresolved issues, and the strengths and limitations associated with each method. The current consensus is that average bioequivalence remains as the primary criterion for new products to gain access to the market. In the meantime, the FDA suggests that sponsors are free to explore the possibility of applying alternative approaches (e.g., population bioequivalence and individual bioequivalence)—after first consulting with the agency.

15.3.4 Bioequivalence Study Designs and Other Statistical Considerations

Bioequivalence studies require multidisciplinary perspectives, and major input from regulatory, pharmacokinetic, and statistical subject matter experts. Collaborative efforts from research scientists and biostatisticians are especially needed to ensure a successful bioequivalence study design.[45]

In a typical bioequivalence study, two products, T (test product), and R (reference product), are each administered. Standard bioequivalence study designs, therefore, include parallel and crossover designs. In a parallel study, subjects are randomly assigned to one of two treatment groups (i.e., T or R), and both treatment groups are followed in parallel. Consequently, each individual subject in a parallel study receives only one of the two drugs (i.e., either T or R) for the entire study. In a crossover study, each subject receives both drugs (i.e., T and R); one in one portion of the study and the other in a second portion (i.e., in succession). Essentially, subjects in a crossover study are randomly assigned to one of two sequence groups. Subjects in sequence group 1 (i.e., TR) receive the test

drug first, followed by the reference drug. Subjects in sequence group 2 (i.e., RT) receive the reference drug first, followed by the test drug.

Standard bioequivalence studies generally use a crossover design. Because drug clearance typically shows large between-subject variabilities, analyzing pharmacokinetic results for two products within the same subject is usually more powerful. One major concern with a crossover design, however, is the possibility of introducing a carryover effect where the drug administered in study period 1 could remarkably affect the product given in period 2. As such, a washout time is generally incorporated between the two periods to ensure that subjects return to baseline—both pharmacokinetically and pharmacodynamically—before the comparator drug is administered. Since a washout interval is inherently necessary for a crossover study design, but may not always be feasible (e.g., for drugs with a relatively long half life), a parallel study design may be appropriately used to test bioequivalence instead.

Bioequivalence studies can be conducted in a non-replicated or replicated fashion. The standard two-period, two-formulation, two-sequence crossover study uses a non-replicated design. In terms of statistical analysis criteria, therefore, an average bioequivalence approach is generally sufficient. A population bioequivalence approach may also be used in a non-replicated study, since the test and reference products are given to different subjects. The individual bioequivalence approach, on the other hand, requires that the same product should be given to the same subject more than once. This is done so that the within-subject variability can be assessed. Thus, only a replicated design should be considered when the individual bioequivalence approach is proposed.

For bioequivalence studies of immediate-release and modified-release formulations, the FDA generally recommends using a single-dose study design, rather than a multiple-dose design, because the single-dose study is considered to be more sensitive.

In bioequivalence studies, the study design also determines the appropriate statistical model for data analysis. In a simple parallel study design, the statistical analysis should be conducted including the between-subject variability to calculate the 90% confidence interval of the treatment mean difference. In a non-replicated crossover design, factors such as sequence, subjects nested in sequence, period, and treatment are usually included in the model as sources of variation. Then a generalized linear model should be applied in data analysis in order to obtain the 90% confidence interval.

15.4 OTHER GENERAL COMPONENTS OF BIOEQUIVALENCE STUDIES

15.4.1 Study Populations

Subjects that may be suitable for enrollment in a standard bioequivalence study would include healthy adult volunteers of at least 18 years of age who are capable of giving informed consent. Healthy volunteers are usually preferred over patients for bioequivalence studies for a number of important reasons. Practical advantages associated with enrolling healthy subjects include simpler inclusion and exclusion criteria, easier recruitment, homogenous population characteristics, and less use of concomitant medications. In addition, healthy volunteers are also generally more amenable to intensive pharmacokinetic sampling schedules. A major statistical argument in favor of using healthy subjects in bioequivalence testing is that the effects of formulation factors can be readily evaluated rather than the effects of inter- or intra-subject factors (e.g., age, race, sex, diet, and disease state) that are known to affect drug absorption, disposition or both.

In some cases, however, patient populations may be preferred over healthy volunteers for bioequivalence studies. For example, pharmacokinetic characteristics obtained in a patient population could be much different than those in healthy subjects, and therefore results from a bioequivalence study in patients would be more clinically meaningful. Likewise, patients would also sometimes be more appropriate than healthy volunteers for various ethical reasons. For example, bioequivalence studies of oncology drugs are generally conducted with cancer patients. Whether healthy volunteers or patients are enrolled, however, most regulatory agencies recommend a total sample size of at least 12 subjects.

15.4.2 Biofluid Matrices

Peripheral blood (e.g., plasma, serum or whole blood) is the most commonly used biofluid matrix for determining the systemic availability of a drug, and is thereby most often used in studies of bioavailability and bioequivalence. Venous blood samples are relatively easy to collect, even when pharmacokinetic sampling times are strict and assessment schedules are intensive. Urine is also sometimes used as a matrix in bioequivalence studies, although much less so than peripheral blood. However, urine can only be used if: 1) the main mechanism of drug elimination is urinary excretion of unchanged drug; and 2) the rate and

amount of excretion can be measured as accurately as possible (i.e., with urine samples collected at short enough intervals). Without an adequate sampling schedule, urine data may not be useful because of the inevitable variability in urinary pharmacokinetic parameter estimation. Other biofluid matrices such as saliva, cerebral spinal fluid, and lymphatic fluid are less frequently used for studies of bioavailability and bioequivalence.

15.4.3 Bioanalytical Methods

Bioanalytical methods used in bioavailability and bioequivalence studies should be accurate, precise, selective, sensitive, and reproducible.[3] Accuracy describes the closeness of the observed mean test results obtained with the bioanalytical method to the true (i.e., actual) concentration of the analyte. The accuracy of a particular method can be determined with replicate analysis of samples containing known amounts of the analyte. In addition, a minimum of five determinations per concentration should be measured.

Precision describes the closeness of the observed individual measures of an analyte when the method is applied repeatedly to multiple aliquots of single homogeneous determinations per concentration. At each concentration level above the lower limit of quantification, the determined precision should not exceed 15% of the coefficient of variation (CV). At the lower limit of quantification, precision should not exceed 20% of the CV. Precision can be further subdivided into the within-run intra-batch precision or repeatability.

Selectivity is defined as the ability of an analytical method to differentiate and quantify an analyte in the presence of other components in the sample. Substances in the biological matrix that may potentially interfere with the results include endogenous substances, metabolites, and degradation products. Sensitivity refers to the ability of the bioanalytical method to measure and differentiate an analyte in the presence of components that may be expected to be present. For example, these components may include metabolites, degradants, and impurities. Reproducibility compares the precision of the analytical method between two different laboratories. Reproducibility can also represent the precision of the method obtained under the same operating conditions over a short period of time.

In 2001, the FDA issued a separate guidance[46] on bioanalytical method validation primarily for use in clinical pharmacology, bioavailability, and bioequivalence studies requiring pharmacokinetic evaluation. Typical method development and validation of a bioanalytical method such as a chemical assay includes determinations of:

1. selectivity;
2. accuracy, precision, recovery;
3. calibration curve; and
4. stability of an analyte in spiked samples.

15.4.4 Drug Moieties

Biological fluid samples collected in bioavailability and bioequivalence studies are used to measure either the active drug ingredient or its active moiety in the administered dosage form (i.e., parent drug) and, when appropriate, its active metabolites.[3] For bioavailability studies, the FDA recommends that both the parent drug and its major active metabolites should be measured, if analytically feasible. For bioequivalence studies, on the other hand, the FDA does not recommend measuring the metabolites, since the parent drug concentration–time profile would better reflect changes in formulation performance. Nonetheless, the FDA also notes certain exceptions to this general approach:

- If parent drug levels are too low for reliable measurements in biological fluids over an appropriate time period, then measurement of a metabolite may be preferred.
- If presystemic metabolism results in the formation of a metabolite that contributes meaningfully to the product's safety and efficacy profile, then the metabolite and the parent drug should both be measured.

The FDA also suggests that measurement of individual enantiomers may be important for bioavailability studies, and that measurement of the racemate (i.e., using an achiral assay) is recommended for bioequivalence studies. Whether a generic company would be required to provide bioequivalence information on an enantiomer of a racemate is determined on a case-by-case basis.[47] In bioequivalence studies, the FDA only recommends measurement of individual enantiomers when all of the following conditions are met:

1. the enantiomers exhibit different pharmacodynamic characteristics;
2. the enantiomers exhibit different pharmacokinetic characteristics;
3. primary efficacy and safety activity resides with the minor enantiomer; and
4. nonlinear absorption is present for at least one of the enantiomers.

For drugs that exhibit nonlinear pharmacokinetics, results of bioequivalence studies that are based on the total drug may differ from those based on the individual enantiomers. Similar discrepancies have also been shown for a racemic drug with linear pharmacokinetics whose enantiomers substantially differ from each other in their pharmacokinetic characteristics.[48] Sponsors of generic drug applications of racemate drugs that exhibit nonlinear or otherwise unusual pharmacokinetics should therefore discuss the requirements with the appropriate regulatory agency before performing formal bioequivalence studies.

15.5 INTERNATIONAL REGULATORY PERSPECTIVES

Of the major worldwide regulatory agencies, most share similar ideas on the general concepts of bioavailability and bioequivalence. In most countries, for example, bioavailability and bioequivalence studies are critical to many regulatory decisions, including novel therapeutic drug approvals, generic drug product approvals, and various post-approval formulation changes. Consequently, many international regulatory authorities have published multiple guidance documents to suggest their recommendations for the design and conduct of bioavailability and bioequivalence studies.

15.5.1 US Food and Drug Administration

To date, the FDA has published a total of 18 bioequivalence-related guidances, 14 final, and 4 draft guidance documents. The titles and publication dates for the final and draft publications are listed in Table 15.1 and 15.2, respectively. Collectively, these FDA guidance documents cover a wide variety of issues that are particularly relevant to the design and conduct of bioavailability and bioequivalence studies.

The FDA generally indicates three main circumstances under which sponsors are expected to submit bioavailability and bioequivalence data. First, these data are expected as part of an investigational new drug (IND) application or NDA submission for most novel therapeutic drug products and formulations. Secondly, bioavailability and bioequivalence data are also routinely submitted along with an abbreviated NDA (ANDA) for generic versions of reference listed drugs. Finally, during the post-approval period, bioequivalence data is expected whenever a major change occurs (e.g., in the manufacturing process) of an already-approved drug.

TABLE 15.1   Final FDA guidance related to bioequivalence studies

No.	Issue date	Title
1	3/19/2003	Bioavailability and Bioequivalence Studies for Orally Administered Drug Products—General Considerations (Revised)
2	1/31/2003	Food-Effect Bioavailability and Fed Bioequivalence Studies
3	8/31/2000	Waiver of *In Vivo* Bioavailability and Bioequivalence Studies for Immediate Release Solid Oral Dosage Forms Based on a Biopharmaceutics Classification System
4	2/2/2001	Statistical Approaches to Establishing Bioequivalence
5	8/25/1997	Dissolution Testing of Immediate Release Solid Oral Dosage Forms
6	9/26/1997	Extended Release Oral Dosage Forms: Development, Evaluation, and Application of *In Vitro/In Vivo* Correlations
7	2/1/1987	Format and Content of the Human Pharmacokinetics and Bioavailability Section of an Application
8	8/21/2002	Liposome Drug Products: Chemistry, Manufacturing, and Controls; Human Pharmacokinetics and Bioavailability; and Labeling Documentation
9	6/2/1995	Topical Dermatologic Corticosteriods: *In Vivo* Bioequivalence
10	7/15/1993	Cholestyramine Powder: *In Vitro* Bioequivalence
11	11/15/1996	Clozapine Tablets: *In Vivo* Bioequivalence and *In Vitro* Dissolution Testing
12	3/4/1994	Phenytoin/Phenytion Sodium (capsules, tablets, suspension): *In Vivo* Bioequivalence and *In Vitro* Dissolution Testing
13	3/8/2001	Levothyroxine Sodium Tablets: *In Vivo* Pharmacokinetic and Bioavailability Studies and *In Vitro* Dissolution Testing
14	6/6/1994	Potassium Chloride Modified-Release Tablets and Capsules: *In Vivo* Bioequivalence and *In Vitro* Dissolution Testing

TABLE 15.2   Draft FDA guidance related to bioequivalence studies

No.	Issue date	Title
1	4/3/2003	Bioavailability and Bioequivalence Studies for Nasal Aerosols and Nasal Sprays for Local Action—2nd Draft
2	12/30/2003	Clozapine Tablets: *In Vivo* Bioequivalence and *In Vitro* Dissolution Testing, Revision
3	12/30/1997	*In Vivo* Bioequivalence Studies Based on Population and Individual Bioequivalence Studies
4	8/7/2002	Potassium Chloride Modified-Release Tablets and Capsules: *In Vivo* Bioequivalence and *In Vitro* Dissolution Testing (Revised)

Overall, the FDA presents its current thinking on various issues related to bioequivalence of different dosage formulations including oral formulations, liposomal delivery systems, topical and dermatologic products, nasal sprays, and local action products. Two guidance documents are specifically devoted to statistical analysis methods, one document provides guidance on data formatting, and another presents recommendations on evaluating food effects in bioequivalence studies. Food can directly or indirectly affect drug absorption, and different types of food (e.g., high fat meals) can directly interact with certain drug products. The existence of food can alter the pH value in the GI tract, change gastric emptying time, and increase bile secretion. Each of these effects can potentially change the bioavailability of a drug. As such, the FDA generally recommends a study of food effects on bioavailability for almost all new investigational drugs. The FDA also recommends that, for food

effect bioequivalence studies, the highest formulation strength that will be marketed should be tested.

For an ANDA application, a bioequivalence study under fasting and fed conditions is needed for all modified-release oral formulations. For fast-release oral formulations, a similar food effect bioequivalence study is also generally needed, except in the following situations:

1. when the compound is in class I of the Biopharmaceutical Classification System (BCS) where a food effect is generally not expected;
2. when the label indicates the product should be taken on an empty stomach; or
3. when no statements about food effects are noted in the label.

The FDA also mentions other important topics in these guidances, including the special topic of biowaivers. A biowaiver means that a bioequivalence claim will be accepted without the need for supporting data from a clinical study. The FDA indicates that a biowaiver can be granted if the test drug product meets several key requirements. Usually, orally soluble formulations such as elixirs, solutions, and syrups can be exempted from a bioequivalence study, because the drug is already dissolved and the excipients are assumed to have no effect on absorption of the active ingredients. For immediate-release oral formulations, a biowaiver may also be granted if the drug has a large therapeutic window, and can also be classified as a BCS class I compound. Nevertheless, the FDA clearly states that BCS-based biowaivers are not appropriate for drugs with a narrow therapeutic window.

The similarity of the *in vitro* dissolution profile between test product and reference product is generally sufficient to demonstrate bioequivalence. To quantify the difference in the dissolution profile between a test and reference product, the FDA mainly considers the similarity factor (f_2), which can be expressed as:

$$f_2 = 50 \cdot \log \left[100 \cdot \frac{1}{\sqrt[2]{1 + (1/n) \cdot \sum_{t=1}^{n} (R_t - T_t)^2}} \right]$$

where R_t and T_t are the cumulative percentage dissolved at the each of the selected time points from reference product and test product. Two dissolution curves are considered as similar when the f_2 value is greater than or equal to 50.

For most other drugs and formulations, the waiver of *in vivo* bioequivalence may be accepted at one or more lower-formulation strengths, based on a dissolution profile comparison with one *in vivo* bioequivalence proven at the highest strength. Additional factors, such as the drug's safety profile, the linearity of the pharmacokinetics in the dosing range, and a proportional similarity in formulation between the higher and lower strengths, are needed for consideration of a biowaiver. For food effect studies, if fed bioequivalence is demonstrated using the highest strength, *in vivo* bioequivalence studies may be waived at the lower strengths based on *in vitro* dissolution studies.

For extended-release formulations, *in vitro/in vivo* correlation (IVIVC) is an important tool to estimate *in vivo* bioavailability characteristics, and provides an alternative approach for considering a biowaiver. In addition, IVIVC can be applied to validate the dissolution method.[49]

The FDA defines three major categories for IVIVC. Level A IVIVC represents a point-to-point comparison between the *in vitro* dissolution and *in vivo* input rate across the dissolution (or absorption) time course. The input rate can usually be generated using the Wagner–Nelson[50] or Loo–Riegelman[51] methods and numerical deconvolution. A pharmacokinetic measurement, such as the fraction of drug absorbed, is generally compared to the fraction of drug dissolved. Usually, a linear correlation is established between the *in vitro* dissolution and *in vivo* input. Once such a relationship is found, the *in vitro* dissolution and *in vivo* input rate function are superimposable. Use of a timescaling factor is sometimes necessary (e.g., when differences are noted between the *in vitro* and *in vivo* conditions).

Level B IVIVC is based on statistical moment theory. In this case the comparison is between the mean *in vitro* dissolution time, and the mean residence time or mean *in vivo* dissolution time. Even though Level B IVIVC considers a summary message from the *in vitro* and *in vivo* profile, information regarding the shape of the profile is ignored.

Level C IVIVC is a single time point comparison for a dissolution parameter (e.g., $t_{50\%}$) to a pharmacokinetic parameter (e.g., AUC, C_{max}, or T_{max}). Multiple Level C IVIVC, however, is designed to compare one or several pharmacokinetic measurements (e.g., AUC and C_{max}) to the drug dissolution profile at multiple time points. Thus, Multiple Level C IVIVC may contain detailed information regarding the shape of the profile, although perhaps not as detailed as Level A IVIVC. From a regulatory perspective, then, Level A IVIVC is the most informative, followed by Multiple Level C IVIVC, and Level C IVIVC. Level B IVIVC appears to contain the least information. Finally, Level D IVIVC compares the rank of the profile, and is generally not considered as useful for regulatory purposes.

Typical IVIVC studies use test formulations with different release rates that should ideally cover slow, medium, and fast release ranges. Both *in vitro* dissolution and *in vivo* concentration–time profiles are needed. In general, sponsors can use Level A IVIVC, and sometimes Multiple Level C IVIVC, when applying for a biowaiver. The FDA will accept an IVIVC-based biowaiver when a lower strength formulation is developed, release-controlling excipients are changed or a manufacturing process has been altered.

The FDAs current guidance on bioavailability and bioequivalence also suggests that "sponsors consider additional testing and/or controls to ensure the quality of drug products." Nevertheless, clear recommendations for this type of study are not specified. For drug products containing complex mixtures of active ingredients or others that are derived from multiple synthetic stages or natural products, the FDA does not require quantitative assays for all of these components in order to demonstrate bioequivalence. Instead, the agency requires a characterization of the bioavailability measurements from several markers in the product.

15.5.2 European Agency for the Evaluation of Medicinal Products

Two major bioequivalence-related documents have been introduced recently by the European Agency for the Evaluation of Medicinal Products (EMEA).[52,53] One document is entitled, "Note for Guidance on Investigation of Bioavailability and Bioequivalence" and the other one is "Questions and Answers on the Bioavailability and Bioequivalence Guideline." Within these two publications, the EMEA offers its requirements and recommendations on the design and conduct of bioavailability and bioequivalence studies.

According to the EMEA, for example, the nature of the drug formulation under study should govern the selection of either a single- or multiple-dose study design. By convention, a single-dose study is typically recommended for standard bioequivalence studies. Nevertheless, a multiple-dose study is generally required for drugs with dose-dependent (i.e., nonlinear) kinetics, drugs with time-dependent kinetics (involving transporter induction and inhibition), and modified-release formulations. From a statistical standpoint, a multiple dose study may also be necessary to reduce intra-subject variability.

The EMEA recommends that appropriate subjects should be properly selected to minimize variability in bioequivalence studies. In general, the study population should comprise healthy volunteers, unless the drug's pharmacological and safety profile would put healthy volunteers at increased risk. Subjects who are between 18 and 55 years of age, with normal body weight and body mass index, should be recruited and standard laboratory tests and medical exams are needed to ensure normal health status. The EMEA guidance also emphasizes that sponsors should consider study populations with different genotypes and phenotypes.

For bioanalytical measurements, the EMEA specifies that the parent drug ingredient should be analyzed. Metabolites can also be measured. Peripheral blood samples are preferred. Urine samples can also be used for bioanalysis.

Proper dose selection is critical for drugs with nonlinear pharmacokinetics. The EMEA requires sponsors to test both the lowest and highest doses. If only one dose level is selected, the highest dose should be used for drugs with a greater than proportional increase

in AUC or C_{max}, while the lowest dose should be used for drugs with a less than proportional increase in AUC or C_{max}. However, the highest and lowest strengths are both required if dissolution is the reason for nonlinearity.

The EMEA specifically recommends the average bioequivalence approach using a 90% confidence interval of the log-transformed pharmacokinetic measurements (i.e., AUC and C_{max}). The agency does not recommend alternative approaches, such as population bioequivalence and individual bioequivalence, citing lack of sufficient evidence. In general, the agency specifies the lower and upper boundaries of the confidence interval should be set at 0.8 and 1.25 in the original scale, respectively. The guidance also permits some degree of flexibility in certain situations. For drugs with a narrow therapeutic window, for example, the bioequivalence acceptance range may be tightened, although alternative values are not specified. In addition, for highly variable drugs with a wide therapeutic window, the boundaries for the acceptance range may be expanded, as long as they are prespecified and scientifically justifiable.

The agency permits some innovative (e.g., pharmacokinetic/pharmacodynamic) approaches to evaluate the alternative acceptance range. In addition, if the pharmacokinetic/pharmacodynamic analysis is not available or insufficient, clinical safety and efficacy data can be applied, instead, to determine the appropriate range. T_{max} can also be included in the analysis, along with AUC and C_{max}, if the evidence suggests that T_{max} is related in some way to safety or efficacy. The EMEA suggests using a nonparametric approach to assess differences in T_{max}. Other pharmacokinetic measurements, such as minimum concentration (C_{min}), fluctuation, and half life, can also be included in the analysis.

Like the FDA, the EMEA also does not generally require sponsors to conduct bioequivalence studies for oral solutions. Bioequivalence studies of immediate-release oral formulations of BCS class I (i.e., highly soluble and highly permeable) drugs, for example, may not be necessary, based on additional information regarding the active ingredient and the dosage formulation. Briefly, the active moiety should have a relatively wide therapeutic window, with linear pharmacokinetics, and evidence of complete absorption for complete permeation. High solubility should be demonstrated at 37°C over a pH range of 1 to 8 in 250 mL of an aqueous solution. Although this pH range seems to be wider compared to that in the FDA guidance, the EMEA- and FDA-recommended pH levels (e.g., 1.0, 4.6, and 6.8) for buffers are very similar. The EMEA also notes that any excipients present in the formulation should not interact with the active moiety. Rapid and similar dissolution profiles should be demonstrated between the test and reference products over the pH range of 1 to 8 (here again, the suggested buffer solutions are very similar to those recommended by the FDA).

Manufacturing factors should also be considered to avoid potential effects on drug release. When different formulation strengths are manufactured, the EMEA may accept a single bioequivalence study (i.e., using only one of the formulation strengths) if the components and manufacturing processes are similar.

15.5.3 Health Canada

The Canadian health authority, Health Canada, has published a series of documents to explain their study requirements and general understanding of bioequivalence and bioavailability. These publications are presented as guidances, draft guidances, notices to industry, and advisory committee reports. Table 15.3 presents a selection of the major bioequivalence-related guidance from Health Canada.

In general, Health Canada's guidance for bioequivalence studies is divided into three main categories based on the pharmacological and pharmacokinetic properties of a drug and its dosage form. These categories include:

1. uncomplicated drugs in immediate-release formulation;
2. uncomplicated drugs in modified-release formulation; and
3. complicated drugs in immediate-release formulation.

Uncomplicated Drugs in Immediate-release Formulations

Many drugs are represented by the first category (i.e., uncomplicated drugs in immediate-release formulation), and these drugs are usually manufactured in common formulations such as tablets and capsules. Bioequivalence and bioavailability studies of these drugs are generally very standard. In most cases, Health Canada suggests a single dose bioequivalence study in normal healthy subjects. The Canadian agency's standard of bioequivalence is defined a little differently than that of the US. Health Canada's bioequivalence criteria include:

1. the 90% confidence interval of the relative mean AUC of the test to the reference product should be within the range of 80% to 125%;
2. the relative mean measured C_{max} of the test to reference product should be between 80% and 125%.

TABLE 15.3   Health Canada's guidance on bioequivalence

No.	Issue date	Title	Type
1	5/31/2006	Bioequivalence Requirements: Critical Dose Drugs	Guidance
2	7/21/2005	Bioequivalence Requirements: Comparative Bioavailability Studies Conducted in the Fed State	Guidance
3	10/8/1997	Conduct and Analysis of Bioavailability and Bioequivalence Studies—Part A: Oral Dosage Formulations Used for Systemic Effects	Guidance
4	11/10/1996	Conduct and Analysis of Bioavailability and Bioequivalence Studies—Part B: Oral Modified Release Formulations	Guidance
5	5/28/2004	Use of Metabolite Data in Comparative Bioavailability Studies	Draft Guidance
6	5/18/2004	Preparation of Comparative Bioavailability Information for Drug Submissions in the CTD Format	Draft Guidance
7	5/12/2004	Preparation of Comparative Bioavailability Information for Drug Submissions in the CTD Format	Draft Guidance
8	10/9/2001	Clinical Trial Applications for Comparative Bioavailability Studies for Pharmaceuticals	Draft Guidance
9	6/22/2005	Bioequivalence Requirements for Drugs for Which an Early Time of Onset or Rapid Rate of Absorption is Important (rapid onset drugs)	Notice
10	6/22/2005	Bioequivalence Requirements for Long Half-life Drugs	Notice
11	6/3/2004	Bioequivalence Requirements for Combination Drug Products	Notice
12	9/24/2003	Removal of Requirement for 15% Random Replicate Samples	Notice
13	12/15/1992	Expert Advisory Committee On Bioavailability: Report On Bioavailability of Oral Dosage Formulations of Drugs Used For Systemic Effects. Report C: Report On Bioavailability of Oral Dosage Formulations, Not In Modified Release Form, Of Drugs Used For Systemic Effects, Having Complicated or Variable Pharmacokinetics	Report

The Canadian authorities also suggest using log-transformed pharmacokinetic measurement, and that the data should be analyzed using an analysis of variance (ANOVA) method (i.e., similar to the average bioequivalence approach published in the FDA guidance).

Uncomplicated Drugs in Modified-release Formulations

For uncomplicated drugs in the secondary category, the modified-release formulation has an active drug release rate that differs in some ways from that of the conventional formulation. For Health Canada, formulations in this category can be further subdivided into three groups. Group I is a new compound that is developed using a modified-release formulation. Generally, development of a Group I formulation should follow standard pharmacokinetic study requirements, and efficacy and safety data need to be collected in different phases of clinical trials.

Group II mainly contains the first modified-release formulation developed from a conventional formulation. Group II formulations generally require a bioavailability comparison, since the absorption rate is expected differ between a conventional and a modified-release formulation. However, the extent of absorption still needs to be similar. For a Group II formulation study, sponsors must demonstrate that the bioavailabilities between the two formulations are comparable (i.e., the relative mean of $AUC_{0-\tau}$ is within 80% and 125% and the relative mean of C_{max} is not larger than 125% versus that of a conventional formulation at steady state).

Group III contains any subsequent modified-release formulations that are developed based on previously marketed modified-release formulations. For a bioequivalence study of a Group III formulation, the acceptance ranges are defined as: 1) 90% confidence interval of the relative mean steady state AUC should be within the limits of 80% and 125%; 2) the relative mean of C_{max} at steady state is within the range of 80% and 125%; and 3) the relative C_{min} at steady state of the test versus reference product should not be less than 80%.

According to the Health Canada guidance, the bioequivalence criteria focus on the relative means of AUC and C_{max}, not the confidence intervals. In addition, since prolonged-release formulations are more likely to increase intersubject variability, patients are preferred over healthy subjects for studies of bioavailability and bioequivalence, according to the Canadian authorities. For modified-release formulations, the guidance also recommends that studies should be conducted with subjects receiving the drug under both fasted and fed conditions. In addition, for formulations in Groups II and III, if accumulation is likely to occur, additional data are needed to evaluate the performance of different formulations at steady state.

Complicated Drugs in Immediate-release Formulations

Complicated drugs have special pharmacological or pharmacokinetic properties. For example, combination drug products, drugs with a long half life, or drugs with nonlinear pharmacokinetics can all be classified as complicated drugs.

Critical dose drugs are also represented in this category. Canadian regulators have specifically published a guidance to discuss bioequivalence issues related to critical dose drugs.[54] According to this guidance, critical dose drugs are defined as "those drugs where comparatively small differences in dose or concentration lead to dose- and concentration-dependent, serious therapeutic failures, and/or serious adverse drug reactions which may be persistent, irreversible, slowly reversible, or life threatening, which could result in inpatient hospitalization or prolongation of existing hospitalization, persistent or significant disability or incapacity, or death."

Drugs in this category generally have a narrow therapeutic window or are highly toxic. Drugs such as cyclosporine, digoxin, flecainide, lithium, phenytoin, and theophylline belong to this category. In these cases, a stronger assurance of similarity between the test and reference product is required by the Canadian regulatory agency. This is reflected in both the study design and bioequivalence criteria. As far as the study design, the test and reference products should be evaluated under both fasting and fed conditions, regardless of whether the label stipulates the drug may be taken with or without food. For safety reasons, the study should be conducted in a patient population rather than a healthy population. For drugs (e.g., cyclosporine) intended to be administered on a long-term basis, the agency suggests that samples should be taken at steady state, and at least five half lives later after switching from a reference to a test product.

The Canadian agency also requires tighter bioequivalence limits. For example, a 90% confidence interval for the geometric mean of AUC should be within 90% and 112%; the limits for C_{max} reflect the standard 80% to 125% criteria. If a steady state study is required, the relative mean C_{min} also needs to satisfy the 80% to 125% criteria.

TABLE 15.4 Health Canada's bioequivalence requirements for other complicated drugs with immediate-release dosage forms

Drug and dosage form	Types	Study design considerations	Additional parameters	Criteria
Drugs with nonlinear kinetics	Greater than proportional increases in AUC	Using at least the highest dose strength	None	None
	Less than proportional increases in AUC	Using at least the lowest dose strength	None	None
Combined drug products	Type I (active ingredients acting independently)	None	AUC for each component C_{max} for each component	90% CI for each component falls into BE criteria. Relative mean C_{max} for each component must be between BE criteria.
	Type II (Active ingredients acting synergistically)	None	C1/C2 (at t_{max1} and t_{max2}) C1(t last)/C2 (t last) AUC(t last)/AUC (t last)	Provide additional information
Drugs with early time of onset or rapid rate of absorption	None	None	CmaxAUC(ref t_{max})	90% CI fall into BE criteria. Relative mean falls into BE criteria.
Drugs with a long effective half life	None	Consider parallel, steady-state study, stable isotope	Truncated AUC, e.g., AUC(0–72)	None

Health Canada's bioequivalence requirements for other complicated drugs with immediate-release dosage forms are summarized in Table 15.4.

15.5.4 Japanese Ministry of Health, Labour and Welfare

Regulatory authorities from Japan's Ministry of Health, Labour and Welfare require both *in vitro* and *in vivo* studies to support a claim of bioequivalence.[55,56,57] These regulators also believe that, since an oral drug product needs to go through different pH environments within the GI tract, an *in vitro* dissolution test must be conducted under various conditions. These include dissolution tests in water, and in three different physiological pH media (pH values from 1.2 to 7.5), at a rotation speed of 50 rounds per minute (rpm) with a paddle method, and 100 rpm at a discriminative pH in order to mimic the pH changes inside the body.

For the Japanese Health Authority, the *in vitro* dissolution test also has an additional purpose. Data from this test helps to design an appropriate *in vivo* bioequivalence study. As per the Japanese guidance, if a significant difference is observed in the dissolution profile at a neutral pH, the *in vivo* bioequivalence study should consider using achlorhydric subjects whose stomach pH is higher than that of normal subjects. In addition, if the drug is intended for a special patient population (e.g., pediatric patients), and if the test and reference products differ significantly in one of the dissolution test conditions, the study population for the *in vivo* bioequivalence study should comprise patients rather than healthy volunteers. On the other hand, if the *in vitro* outcomes show that the test and reference products performed similarly in the dissolution test, the *in vivo* bioequivalence study can be conducted in healthy volunteers.

Similar to the FDA guidance, the Japanese guidance recommends using AUC and C_{max} as the measurements of bioavailability. The Japanese authorities also require the average bioequivalence criteria in which the 90% confidence interval is studied and compared with the predefined range of 80% to 125% in the original scale. Nevertheless, if the confidence interval does not fall within this range, the Japanese agency suggests that the products can still be considered as bioequivalent if three additional requirements are met. First, the dissolution profiles for the two products must be equivalent under all test conditions. Secondly, the ratio of the mean AUC (or C_{max}) for the test versus reference product must be within the range of 90% and 111%. Thirdly, the *in vivo* study must have used a sample size of at least 20 subjects.

Another major difference in the Japanese guidance on bioequivalence is that decisions on biowaivers are not made on the basis of the BCS.

15.6 WAIVERS BASED ON THE BIOPHARMACEUTICAL CLASSIFICATION SYSTEM

Bioequivalence can generally be claimed if the *in vivo* rate and extent of absorption (i.e., bioavailability) of the test drug does not significantly differ from that of the reference product. In specific cases, however, regulatory agencies waive the requirement for a formal *in vivo* bioequivalence study for certain drugs that have certain physiochemical and kinetic properties. For example, both the US and European regulators consider study waivers for immediate-release dosage forms of highly soluble, highly permeable, drug substances.[58]

Drugs can generally be classified for regulatory purposes using the BCS into four basic classes. Each class represents a specific combination of drug solubility and permeability characteristics. Table 15.5 lists the combinations of solubility and permeability that distinguish the four BCS classes.[59,60,61,62,63]

To date, waivers are considered only for BCS class I drugs (i.e., highly soluble, highly permeable drugs). Biowaivers for drugs in the other three BCS classes are under discussion.

According to the BCS definitions, a drug substance is considered highly soluble if its highest formulation strength can dissolve into, at most, 250 mL of aqueous media over a pH range from 1 to 7.5. The 250 mL amount is used since subjects in most bioequivalence studies are generally asked to drink this much water (i.e., a cup of water) together with the study drug. Likewise, the pH range is selected to reflect the various changes that occur in the pH levels throughout the GI tract. For example, the pH environment in the stomach is strongly acidic (i.e., pH of approximately 1 to 2), but more neutral in the ileum (i.e., pH of approximately 6.5 to 7.4).

Drug permeability, on the other hand, is determined by measuring the extent of intestinal drug absorption. That is, if at least 90% of a drug permeates through the intestinal membrane, the drug is classified as highly permeable. Drug permeation tests can be conducted in clinical or nonclinical studies such as animal studies or with *in vitro* models (e.g., Caco-2 cell culture).

Dissolution rate is another important factor that must be considered once the compound is formulated into a drug product. Per the FDA, a drug formulation can be classified as an immediate-release formulation if at least 85% of the drug dissolves within 30 minutes, in each of three different pH aqueous media (i.e., ranging from pH of 1.0 to 6.8), using US Pharmacopeia (USP) Apparatus I (i.e., the basket method) at 100 rpm or Apparatus II (i.e., the paddle method) at 50 rpm. The immediate-release formulation of a BCS class I drug thus has some favorable features. When a class I drug is taken with a cup of water, for example, the drug is immediately immersed in about 250 mL of water in the stomach. By definition, BCS class I drugs can be completely dissolved. Since gastric emptying time averages about 30 minutes, it is very likely that most ($\geq$ 85%) of the drug is released from the formulation into the GI fluid within this period of time. Assuming the ingredient has no significant impact on the extent and rate of drug absorption, the fast release nature of a BCS class I formulation and its high permeability make it unlikely that drug bioavailability would be absorption-site dependent. Transporter effects would also be negligible, because of the high permeability. High permeability also ensures a sink condition in the GI tract.

Consequently, for a very rapid release formulation, absorption rate is possibly controlled by gastric emptying time, and IVIVC is generally not expected. Theoretically, the *in vitro* dissolution test is only needed to ensure that the release of drug from the formulation is sufficiently rapid. However, the similarity of the *in vitro* dissolution profile provides more quality control over both the test and reference drug products. In general, a model-dependent or model-independent method (e.g., linear regression of the percentage of drug dissolved at different time points), a statistical comparison of the parameters derived from the Weibull function or the similarity factor (general f_2) can be calculated for comparison.

In the EMEA guidance, the "similarity of dissolution profile may be accepted as demonstrated" if at least 85% of the drug dissolves within 15 minutes. Thus, *in vivo* bioequivalence studies might not be needed if similarity in the dissolution profiles between the test and reference products can be demonstrated under different pH environments.

TABLE 15.5 Biopharmaceutical Classification System

BCS class	Solubility	Permeability
I	High	High
II	Low	High
III	High	Low
IV	Low	High

A BCS class III drug has high solubility and low permeability.[64,65] Under certain conditions, then, a biowaiver might also be considered for drugs in this category since the rate-limiting step for drug absorption is permeability, not dissolution. Similar to class I drugs, a class III drug is almost in solution by the time it reaches the small intestine. Ordinarily, *in vivo* bioequivalence studies are not required. Nevertheless, class III drugs may have a more complicated absorption process, and since permeability is low, the sink condition in the GI tract might not occur. In addition, for a class III drug, availability at the absorption site is much less sensitive compared to its permeation, which is usually quite variable. Physiological and formulation factors (e.g., GI transit time, variation in absorption at different sites along the GI tract, and the existence of fatty acid or surfactant in the formulation) can greatly affect the rate and extent of drug absorption. Therefore, more stringent criteria might be needed before biowaivers may apply to BCS class III drugs. Some researchers suggest, for example, that a more rapid dissolution rate criterion (i.e., ≥85% of drug dissolved within 15 minutes) might be necessary for consideration of a biowaiver for a class III drug.

BCS class II drugs are highly permeable with low solubility.[66] This drug class is also being considered for a biowaiver under more stringent conditions. For example, drug absorption for this group is likely to be governed by *in vivo* dissolution. Given that *in vitro* dissolution reflects *in vivo* dissolution, *in vivo* drug absorption and bioequivalence studies might not be needed for class II drugs. However, mimicking *in vivo* solubility at the absorption site in the small intestine can be challenging. The microenvironment at these regions may be highly variable, and very complicated. Factors such as pH levels, and the coexistence of bile salts or other surfactants, can largely change drug solubility, and thereby affect the rate and extent of absorption. Because of their characteristically low solubility, excipients may be added to a class II drug formulation to increase solubility. This may impact drug dissolution and permeation. Thus, more research is needed to establish reasonable criteria for class II drugs before a biowaiver could be considered.

From a regulatory point of view, the BCS categories can also be used to better understand the effect of food on the bioavailability and bioequivalence of different drugs and formulations.[67,68] In general, food effects are least likely for BCS class I drugs, since absorption is generally independent of pH and GI absorption site. For bioavailability studies, however, interactions such as complexations between the drug and food or food-related changes in the GI environment are still possible. In bioequivalence studies of class I drugs, food effects are not generally expected. However, for drugs in classes II through IV, and for all modified-release formulations, interactions between the drug and food are more likely, and might therefore need to be studied.

The BCS approach is an evolving concept. Establishing the most appropriate criteria for biowaivers based on BCS drug class is still under discussion. Yazdanian et al.[69] conducted a study to assess the *in vitro* dissolution properties, and *in vivo* absorption characteristics, of various nonsteroidal anti-inflammatory drugs (NSAIDs). Their results demonstrated that, while each of the drugs tested were known to be highly permeable, 15 of the 18 acidic drugs tested did not dissolve in 250 mL of solution at a low pH, because of low acidic dissociation constants (pKa). Using the current system, all 15 of these drugs are in BCS class II. Based on their *in vivo* dissolution and absorption behaviors, however, these drugs were more similar to drugs in class I. These results seem to call into question whether the current BCS definition for class I compounds might be too stringent for acidic drugs.

Interest has recently increased to link BCS with modified-release formulations by applying IVIVC. In general, class I and class II drugs are likely to demonstrate IVIVC, since *in vivo* sink conditions can be obtained and dissolution is the rate-limiting step. With an adequate IVIVC, the BCS approach would be an important tool for regulating modified-release formulations. The application may be limited, however, by the complexity of the drug absorption process, especially regarding site-dependent absorption and different transit times. Additional study is therefore needed to fully implement the BCS approach to IVIVC of modified-release formulations.

15.7 SUMMARY

Bioavailability and bioequivalence studies of solid oral drug forms are routinely performed throughout all stages of drug development, and for a variety of reasons. Bioavailability studies are often conducted during development, for example, to document the rate and extent of absorption for new drug products. Likewise, bioequivalence studies are usually conducted to demonstrate the similarity between the pharmacokinetics of a test versus a reference drug product. Data from bioavailability and bioequivalence studies are typically analyzed and submitted to various international regulatory authorities in support of INDs, NDAs, ANDAs, and other marketing submissions. Each of the major regulatory agencies has published multiple guidance documents for sponsors to use in designing and conducting bioavailability and bioequivalence studies. In turn, industry scientists and biostatisticians have also contributed their knowledge and expertise to the task of identifying the most appropriate criteria and research methods that should be used to demonstrate bioequivalence sufficiently. Relevant regulatory requirements continue to evolve, while several major controversies have yet to be resolved. Topics worthy of particular debate presently include the selection of the most appropriate statistical approach, and the potential for expansion of BCS-based decisions for biowaivers.[70]

References

1. Barrett, J.S., Batra, V., Chow, A., Cook, J., Gould, A.L., Heller, A.H., Lo, M.W., Patterson, S.D., Smith, B.P., Stritar, J.A., Vega, J.M. & Zariffa, N. (2000). PhRMA perspective on population and individual bioequivalence. Journal of Clinical Pharmacology 40, 561–570.
2. US Code of Federal Regulations. (2000). *Bioavailability and bioequivalence requirements*. US Government Printing Office, Washington, DC, Vol. 21, Part 320.
3. Food and Drug Administration. (2003). *Guidance for industry: bioavailability and bioequivalence studies for orally administered drug products—general considerations*. US Department of Health and Human Services, Rockville, MD.
4. Food and Drug Administration. (1995). *Guidance for industry: topical dermatologic corticosteroids: In vivo bioequivalence*. US Department of Health and Human Services, Rockville, MD.
5. Tandon, V. (2002). Bioavailability and bioequivalence. In: *Pharmacokinetics in Drug Discovery and Development*, R.D. Schoenwald (ed.). CRC Press, Boca Raton, FL, pp. 97–112.
6. Gibaldi, M. (1990). *Biopharmaceutics and Clinical Pharmacokinetics*, 4th edn. Lea & Febiger, Malvern, PA. pp. 151–153.
7. McGilveray, I. (1991). Consensus report on issues in evaluation of bioavailability. Pharmaceutical Research 8, 136–138.
8. Rani, S. & Pargal, A. (2004). Bioequivalence: An overview of statistical concepts. Indian Journal of Pharmacology 36, 209–216.
9. Midha, K.K., Ormsby, E.D., Hubbard, J.W., McKay, G., Hawes, E.M., Gavalas, L. & McGilveray, I.J. (1993). Logarithmic transformation in bioequivalence: Application with two formulations of perphenazine. Journal of Pharmaceutical Sciences 82, 1300.
10. Pabst, G. & Jaeger, H. (1990). Review of methods and criteria for the evaluation of bioequivalence study. European Journal of Clinical Pharmacology 38, 5–10.
11. Westlake, W.J. (1981). Response to Kirkwood TBL: Bioequivalence testing—a need to rethink. Biometrics 37, 589–594.
12. Chow, S.C., Peace, K.E. & Shao, J. (1991). Assessment of bioequivalence using a multiplicative model. Journal of Biopharmaceutical Statistics 1, 193–203.
13. Food and Drug Administration. (1999). *Draft guidance: average, population and individual approaches to establishing bioequivalence*. US Department of Health and Human Services, Rockville, MD.
14. Food and Drug Administration. (1999). Center for Drug Evaluation and Research (CDER). Statistical Information from the June 1999 Draft Guidance and Statistical Information for *In Vitro* Bioequivalence Data, Posted on August 18, 1999. US Department of Health and Human Services, Rockville, MD. Available at: http://www.fda.gov/cder/guidance/5383stats.pdf Accessed January 31, 2007.
15. Chereson, R. (1996). Bioavailability, bioequivalence, and drug selection. In: *Basic Pharmacokinetics*, M.C. Makoid (ed.). Available at: http://pharmacyonline.creighton.edu/pha443/pdf/pkin08.pdf Accessed January 31, 2007.
16. Williams, R.L., Adams, W., Chen, M.L., Hare, D., Hussian, A., Lesko, L., Patnaik, R. & Shah, V. (1976). Where are we now and where do we go next in terms of the scientific basis for regulation on bioavailability and bioequivalence? FDA Biopharmaceutics Coordinating Committee. European Journal of Drug Metabolism & Pharmacokinetics 25, 7–12.
17. Office of Technology Assessment. (1974). Drug bioequivalence. Recommendations from the Drug Bioequivalence Study Panel to the Office of Technology Assessment, Congress of the United States. Journal Pharmacokinetics & Biopharmaceutics 2, 433–466.
18. Food and Drug Administration. (1992). *Guidance for industry: statistical procedures for bioequivalence studies using a standard two-treatment crossover design*. US Department of Health and Human Services, Rockville, MD.
19. Food and Drug Administration. (1997). *Guidance for industry: in vivo bioequivalence studies based on population and individual bioequivalence approaches*. US Department of Health and Human Services, Rockville, MD.
20. Anderson, S. & Hauck, W.W. (1990). Consideration of individual bioequivalence. Journal of Pharmacokinetics and Biopharmaceutics 18, 259–273.
21. Hauck, W.W. & Anderson, S. (1994). Measuring switchability and prescribability: When is average bioequivalence sufficient? Journal of Pharmacokinetics and Biopharmaceutics 22, 551–564.
22. Ekbohm, G. & Melander, H. (1989). The subject-by-formulation interaction as a criterion of interchangeability of drugs. Biometrics 45, 1249–1254.
23. Westlake, W.J. (1976). Symmetrical confidence intervals for bioequivalence trials. Biometrics 32, 741–744.
24. Kirkwood, T.B.L. (1981). Bioequivalence testing—a need to rethink. Biometrics 7, 589–591.
25. Schuirmann, D.J. (1987). A comparison of the two one-sided tests procedure and the power approach for assessing the equivalence of average bioavailability. Journal of Pharmacokinetics and Biopharmaceutics 15, 657–680.
26. Food and Drug Administration. (2001). *Guidance for industry: statistical approaches to establishing bioequivalence*. US Department of Health and Human Services, Rockville, MD.
27. Quiroz, J., Ting, N., Wei, G.C. & Burdick, R.K. (2000). A modified large sample approach in the assessment of population bioequivalence. Journal of Biopharmaceutical Statistics 10, 527–544.
28. Chen, M.L., Patnaik, R., Hauck, W.W., Schuirmann, D.J., Hyslop, T. & Williams, R. (2000). An individual bioequivalence criterion: regulatory consideration. Statistics in Medicine 19, 2821–2842.
29. Schall, R. & Luus, H.G. (1993). On population and individual bioequivalence. Statistics in Medicine 12, 1109–1124.
30. Chen, M.L. & Lesko, J.L. (2001). Individual bioequivalence revisited. Clinical Pharmacokinetics 40, 701–706.
31. Hauck, W.W., Hyslop, T., Chen, M.L., Patnaik, R. & Williams, R.L. (2000). Subject-by-formulation interaction in bioequivalence: conceptual and statistical issues. FDA Population/Individual Bioequivalence Working Group. Food and Drug Administration. Pharmaceutical Research, 17, 375–380.

32. Zintzaras, E. & Bouka, P. (1999). Bioequivalence studies: biometrical concepts of alternative designs and pooled analysis. European Journal of Drug Metabolism & Pharmacokinetics 24, 225–232.

33. Pollard, S., Nashan, B., Johnston, A., Hoyer, P., Belitsky, P., Keown, P. & Helderman, H. (2003). A pharmacokinetic and clinical review of the potential clinical impact of using different formulations of cyclosporin A. Clinical Therapeutics 25, 1654–1669.

34. Cattaneo, D., Perico, N. & Remuzzi, G. (2005). Generic cyclosporine: more open questions than answers. Transplant International 18, 371–378.

35. Kahan, B.D. (2004). Therapeutic drug monitoring of cyclosporine: 20 years of progress. Trans. Proc. 36, 278S–291S.

36. Midha, K.K., Rawson, M.J. & Hubbard, J.W. (1999). Prescribability and switchability of highly variable drugs and drug products. Journal of Controlled Release 62, 33–40.

37. Tothfalusi, L. & Enderyi, L. (2001). Evaluation of some properties of individual bioequivalence (IBE) from replicated design studies. International Journal of Clinical Pharmacology and Therapeutics 39, 162–166.

38. Hsuan, F.C. (2000). Some statistical considerations on the FDA draft guidance for individual bioequivalence. Statistics in Medicine 19, 2879–2884.

39. Endrenyi, L. & Tothfalusi, L. (1999). Subject-by-formulation interaction in determination of individual bioequivalence: Bias and prevalence. Pharmaceutical Research 16, 186–190.

40. Wijnand, H.P. (2003). Assessment of average, population and individual bioequivalence in two- and four- period crossover design. Computer Methods and Programs in Biomedicine 70, 21–35.

41. Nankai, K., Fujita, M. & Tomita, M. (2002). Comparison of average and population bioequivalence approach. International Journal of Clinical Pharmacology and Therapeutics 40, 431–438.

42. Midha, K.K., Rawson, M.J. & Hubbard, J.W. (2005). The bioequivalence of highly variable drugs and drug products. International Journal of Clinical Pharmacology and Therapeutics 43, 485–498.

43. Vuorinen, J. & Turunen, J. (1996). A three-step procedure for assessing bioequivalence in general mixed model framework. Statistics in Medicine 15, 2635–2655.

44. Zariffa, N.M. & Patterson, S.D. (2001). Population and individual bioequivalence: Lessons from real data and simulation studies. Journal of Clinical Pharmacology 41, 811–822.

45. Willavize, S.A. & Morgenthien, E.A. (2006). Comparisons of models for average bioequivalence in replicated crossover designs. Pharmaceutical statistics 5, 201–211.

46. Food and Drug Administration. (2001). Guidance for industry: Bioanalytical method validation. US Department of Health and Human Services, Rockville, MD.

47. Nerurkar, S.G., Dighe, S.V. & Williams, R.L. (1992). Bioequivalence of racemic drugs. Journal of Clinical Pharmacology 32, 935–943.

48. Mehvar, R. & Jamali, F. (1997). Bioequivalence of chiral drugs. Clinical Pharmacokinetics 33, 122–141.

49. Emami, J. (2006). In vitro-in vivo correlation: From theory to applications. Journal of Pharmacy & Pharmaceutical Sciences 9, 169–189.

50. Wagner, J.G. & Nelson, E. (1963). Percent absorbed time plots derived from blood level and/or urinary excretion data. Journal of Pharmaceutical Sciences 52, 610–611.

51. Loo, J. & Riegelman, S. (1968). New method for calculating the intrinsic absorption rate of drugs. Journal of Pharmaceutical Sciences 57, 918–928.

52. Committee for Proprietary Medicinal Products (CPMP). (2001). Note for guidance on the investigation of bioavailability and bioequivalence (CPMP/EWP/QWP/1401/98). The European Agency for the Evaluation of Medicinal Products, London.

53. Committee for Medicinal Products for Human Use (CHMP). (2006). Efficacy Working Party Therapeutic Subgroup on Pharmacokinetics: questions & answers on the bioavailability and bioequivalence guideline (EMEA/CHMP/EWP/40326/2006). The European Agency for the Evaluation of Medicinal Products, London.

54. Health Products and Food Branch (2006). Guidance for industry: Bioequivalence requirements: Critical dose drugs. Health Canada, Ottawa, Ontario.

55. Drugs Division. (2000). Guideline for bioequivalence studies for formulation changes of oral solid dosage forms. The National Institute of Health Sciences (NIHS), Japan.

56. Drugs Division. (2000). Guideline for bioequivalence studies for different strengths of oral solid dosage forms. The National Institute of Health Sciences (NIHS), Japan.

57. Drugs Division. (1997). Guideline for bioequivalence studies of generic products. The National Institute of Health Sciences (NIHS), Japan.

58. Food and Drug Administration. (2000). Guidance for industry: waiver of in vivo bioavailability and bioequivalence studies for immediate-release solid oral dosage forms based on a biopharmaceutics classification system. US Department of Health and Human Services, Rockville, MD.

59. Yu, L.X., Amidon, G.L., Polli, J.E., Zhao, H., Metha, M.U., Conner, D.P., Shah, V.P., Lesko, L.J., Chen, M.L., Lee, V.H. & Hussain, A.S. (2002). Biopharmaceutics classification system: the scientific basis for biowaiver extensions. Pharmaceutical Research 19, 921–925.

60. Lindenberg, M., Kopp, S. & Dressman, J.B. (2004). Classification of orally administered drugs on world health organization model list of essential medicines according to the biopharmaceutics classification system. European Journal of Pharmaceutics and Biopharmaceutics 58, 265–278.

61. Lennernas, H. & Abrahamsson, B. (2005). The use of biopharmaceutic classification of drugs in drug discovery and development: Current status and future extension. The Journal of Pharmacy and Pharmacology 57, 273–285.

62. Rinaki, E., Valsami, G. & Macheras, P. (2003). Quantitative biopharmaceutics classification system: The central role of dose/solubility ratio. Pharmaceutical Research 20, 1917–1925.

63. Loberbeng, R. & Amidon, G.L. (2000). Modern bioavailability, bioequivalence and biopharmaceutics classification system. New scientific approaches to international regulatory standards. European Journal of Pharmaceutics and Biopharmaceutics 50, 3–12.

64. Cheng, C.L., Yu, L.X., Lee, H.L., Yang, C.Y., Lue, C.S. & Chou, C.H. (2004). Biowaiver extension potential to BCS class III high solubility low permeability drugs: Bridging evidence for metformin immediate release tablet. Journal of Pharmaceutical Sciences 22, 297–304.

65. Jantratid, E., Prakongpan, S., Amidon, G.L. & Dressman, J.B. (2006). Feasibility of biowaiver extension to Biopharmaceutics Classification System class III drug products, cimetidine. Clinical Pharmacokinetics 45, 385–399.

66. Rinaki, E., Dokoumetzidis, A., Valsami, G. & Macheras, P. (2004). Identification of biowaivers among class II drugs: Theoretical justification and practical examples. Pharmaceutical Research 21, 1567–1572.

67. Yu, L.X., Straughn, A.B., Faustino, P.J., Yang, Y., Parekh, A., Ciavarella, A.B., Asafu-Adjaye, E., Mehta, M.U., Conner, D.P., Lesko, L.J. & Hussain, A.S. (2004). The effect of food on

relative bioavailability of rapid dissolving immediate-release solid oral products containing highly soluble drugs. Molecular Pharmaceutics 1, 357–362.

68. Fleisher, D., Li, C., Zhou, Y., Pao, L. & Karim, A. (1999). Drug, meal and formulation interactions influencing drug absorption after oral administration. Clinical Pharmacokinetics 36, 233–254.

69. Yazdanian, M., Briggs, K., Jankovsky, C. & Hawi, A. (2004). The "high solubility" definition of the current FDA Guidance on Biopharmaceutical Classification System may be too strict for acidic drugs. Pharmaceutical Research 21, 293–299.

70. Meredith, P. (2003). Bioequivalence and other unresolved issues in generic drug substitution. Clinical Therapeutics 25, 2875–2890.

In Vivo Evaluation of Oral Dosage Form Performance

Honghui Zhou and Kathleen Seitz

16.1 INTRODUCTION

The oral route of administration is essentially the most common drug administration route, and perhaps one of the most convenient. This convenience often only comes, however, after many years of diligent research effort and progressive development programs. New solid oral dosage formulations, for example, must be strategically designed to successfully withstand the physiological milieu of the gastrointestinal (GI) tract, and then subsequently allow for adequate absorption of the drug into the systemic circulation. In addition, this complex sequence of events must be precisely orchestrated to occur within a clinically relevant time period so that the intended therapeutic response can be produced. The ultimate goal is to develop an efficacious, cost-effective, and convenient drug product that can be administered safely and reliably to patients.

Solid oral dosage formulations must, therefore, be designed to produce predictable and consistent systemic drug exposure in the human body. As such, the in vivo performance of any new oral formulation must be thoroughly evaluated during drug development. A systematic set of prospectively planned, and appropriately designed, in vivo pharmacokinetic studies should provide the data needed to achieve this task.

Information presented in this chapter is intended as a synoptic overview of the in vivo evaluation of solid oral dosage form performance. Readers should expect to gain a general understanding of some commonly used development approaches, as well as a focused perspective on the basic underlying pharmacokinetic principles.

16.2 GENERAL PURPOSE OF IN VIVO PERFORMANCE EVALUATIONS

Over the development cycle of a solid oral dosage form, a series of multiple in vivo performance evaluations—including clinical and nonclinical pharmacokinetic assessments—are usually conducted once a prototype formulation with acceptable in vitro characteristics has been identified. Data from in vivo animal studies can provide useful preliminary information about drug absorption rates and GI absorption sites, for example. Animal data can also offer early insights into potential mechanisms of drug distribution, metabolism, and elimination. Data from in vivo human studies, on the other hand, can provide clinically useful information about oral bioavailability, bioequivalence, and the effects of food or other factors (e.g., gastric pH) on the pharmacokinetic behavior of the final oral dosage form in human subjects. Human pharmacokinetic data can also provide relevant knowledge about the relationship between drug exposure and clinical response (e.g., safety and efficacy).

Successful development of a new solid oral dosage form ultimately depends on the absorption characteristics, and overall capacity of the drug product to modulate the magnitude and duration of an

Developing Solid Oral Dosage Forms: Pharmaceutical Theory and Practice
ISBN: 978-0-444-53242-8

anticipated pharmacological response. For most drugs with extravascular (e.g., oral, subcutaneous) routes of administration, absorption is usually a complex, multi-step process comprising many interrelated physico-chemical and physiological factors. After a solid dosage formulation is orally administered, for example, two basic processes must occur before the active drug substance can be absorbed into the systemic circulation: disintegration and dissolution. Disintegration generally involves the breakdown of the drug product into smaller particles. Dissolution denotes the process by which these smaller particles subsequently dissolve in a solvent. Factors that could potentially affect disintegration and dissolution of a solid oral dosage form include the physico-chemical properties (e.g., stability, solubility, and particle size) of the drug substance, the inherent characteristics of any added excipients (e.g., stabilizing or binding agents), and other condition-related factors (e.g., pH of the dissolution medium).

Key initial research objectives of *in vivo* performance evaluations of a new solid oral dosage form therefore typically include the following:

1. determine the product's ability to release the active drug substance from the dosage form;
2. identify residence times of both the dosage form and the released drug at the absorption site;
3. locate the GI regional site of drug absorption;
4. describe the capacity of the GI mucosal tract to absorb the drug; and
5. evaluate other physiological factors (e.g., gastric emptying rates and intestinal motility patterns) that may potentially affect the overall drug absorption process.

16.3 ANIMAL PHARMACOKINETIC EVALUATIONS

As the development phase of an investigational drug product progresses, *in vivo* animal studies are typically conducted before any human studies are initially performed. Animal models can effectively be used to screen prototypes of a solid oral dosage formulation, for example, and to obtain early pharmacokinetic knowledge of a pilot product's *in vivo* absorption characteristics. Fundamental animal data can also be used to identify the main absorption site within the GI tract, and document preliminary absorption mechanisms for the novel drug formulation. Consequently, animal data from *in vivo* pharmacokinetic evaluations are often used to support selection of an optimal formulation, and guide the overall design of the final product's dosage form.

Researchers generally need to consider two main issues when planning *in vivo* pharmacokinetic studies in animals. First, the appropriate animal species that will yield optimal results must be selected. Secondly, a reliable method of extrapolating the animal data must be identified that can adequately predict the drug's pharmacokinetic behavior in humans.

16.3.1 Animal Species Selection

Preclinical evaluation of a new drug's pharmacokinetics should be conducted in an animal species with anatomical and physiological characteristics that are relevant to the research objectives. Because of the inherent differences in the GI tract between many animal species and humans, for example, selecting an optimal animal model for an oral drug absorption study can be challenging. Preclinical studies of a new solid oral dosage form such as a tablet or capsule, for instance, would require an animal species that can accommodate the drug without any untoward physiological responses, such as mucosal trauma from ingesting the human-scale dosage form. Other important factors to consider when selecting one species over another include the anatomical arrangement of the animal's blood and lymph supply to the gut, as well as any characteristic secretory levels of gastric and pancreatic juices and normative interdigestive motility patterns.

Animal models that are routinely used to study the *in vivo* performance of human-scale oral dosage forms include primates, dogs, pigs, and rabbits. Smaller animals such as rats, mice, and other small rodents, on the other hand, are seldom used for these types of studies, because of the obvious physical limitations of their diminutive GI tracts. Nonhuman primates are relatively large animals, however, and may initially appear most suitable for standard *in vivo* pharmacokinetic studies of solid oral dosage forms. Primates such as macaque monkeys, for example, have adequate gut dimensions, and their GI morphology is also generally similar to that of humans. Nevertheless, several practical issues relating to higher resource costs, and restricted supply availability, often preclude the widespread use of nonhuman primates in oral drug absorption studies.

Rabbits are more readily available, and less costly than other animal models such as monkeys, pigs or dogs. Nevertheless, several important physiological and anatomical differences between rabbits and humans limit their use as an appropriate model in an oral drug absorption study. Several researchers have had some success in modifying the gastric-emptying characteristics of rabbits to be more aligned with that of humans.[1] In general, though, bioavailability of even immediate-release (IR) oral formulations cannot be sufficiently correlated between rabbits and humans. Pigs have also occasionally been used for oral bioavailability studies, but with limited overall success.[2,3,4]

Dogs, however, have been used more extensively than any of these other animal models for *in vivo* evaluations of oral drug absorption. Dogs essentially have suitable anatomy and physiology of the stomach. Typical gastric dimensions for mongrel dogs weighing 15–25 kg are particularly similar to those of humans, for example. In addition, dogs have GI motility cycles, gastric emptying patterns, physiological responses to feeding, and bile secretion profiles, that are also generally similar to those of humans.[5] Nonetheless, several important anatomical and physiological GI differences between dogs and humans must also be considered whenever pharmacokinetic studies of oral dosage forms are either being designed or reported.

The typical canine gastric emptying rate in a fed state is slower than that of humans, for example, and canine gastric pH is essentially higher than that of humans. Intestinal dimensions and GI transit times also vary from dogs to humans. For example, the length of a dog's small intestine is only about half the length of a human's, and a dog's colon is also generally shorter than a human colon. These anatomical differences may explain the overall faster transit time noted in dogs versus humans. In a fasted state, for example, transit time for dogs is approximately half the time for humans, and this generally holds true for different oral dosage forms including granules, pellets, and tablets. To account for this relatively accelerated transit time, *in vivo* dog models have occasionally been pretreated with drugs that can delay GI motility, and subsequently prolong intestinal residence time of the investigational oral dosage form.[6,7] In general, however, incomplete systemic availability is usually observed in dogs, particularly in studies of controlled-release (*CR*) dosage forms (e.g., where drug release times may exceed the GI transit time in dogs), and other dosage forms that are not otherwise well-absorbed in the colon.

Even though the dog has some characteristics that are similar to those of the human and may allow for reasonable extrapolation, other physiologic features unique to the dog can affect pharmacokinetics, making extrapolations between canines and humans unreliable. Some key differences are shown as following:[8]

- basal acid secretion in dogs (0.1–0.4 mEq/hour) is lower than that of humans (2–5 Eq/hour);[8]
- larger inter-individual variability in gastric pH in dogs than in humans;

- fasted dogs have a slightly higher (1–2 pH units) small intestinal pH than humans;[9]
- transit time in fasted dogs is approximately 2-fold shorter than in humans (111 versus 238 minutes);[9]
- dogs secrete bile salts at a higher rate (49–90 mmol/L) in comparison with humans (3–45 mmol/L);[10]
- some cytochromes P450 (CYP450) isozymes are unique to the dogs have been identified (e.g., 2B11, 2C21, 2D15, 3A12, 3A26).

Thus, the pharmacokinetic/absorption results obtained from the dogs should be interpreted with caution. Chiou et al. found that the absorption data in dogs, based on 43 compounds including bases, acids, zwitterions, and neutral compounds, did not predict the human absorption very well ($r^2 = 0.51$).[11] Moreover, it is also worth noting that the small number of animals along with the substantially large inherent inter-animal variability in physiologic characteristics may further complicate the human absorption projection.

Regardless of which species is used, animal data obtained from these types of early stage *in vivo* studies can clearly offer considerable insight, and early knowledge of a new oral dosage form's general pharmacokinetics. In addition, when these animal data are carefully used with an appropriate interspecies scaling method, the pharmacokinetic behavior in humans may also be better predicted.

16.3.2 Animal Data Extrapolation

Interspecies data extrapolation (i.e., scaling) is a routine practice in the biopharmaceutical industry, and often represents a necessary activity in the ethical development of novel therapeutic drugs and biologics. While *in vivo* animal studies of a new dosage form are typically required by international regulatory authorities, institutional review boards, and ethics committees before research studies may be performed with human subjects, the obvious challenge involves the appropriate interpretation of the animal data, and an accurate prediction of the human pharmacokinetic response.

Interspecies scaling is essentially based on the assumption that several anatomical, physiological, and biochemical similarities exist among animals of different species.[12,13] Pharmacokineticists and other researchers in the industry may use one of two basic scaling approaches: mechanistic (i.e., physiology-based) or mathematical (i.e., allometry-based) methods. The physiology-based methods that involve determinations of organ weights, tissue perfusion, and metabolic reaction rates, for example, are inherently more complicated, costly, and thus generally not as popular. In contrast, the simpler allometric methods that basically incorporate applied mathematical equations are seen more routinely in drug development programs, and may be particularly helpful in the selection of first-in-human dosage forms.[14,15]

The simple allometric method is based on a power function:

$$Y = aW^b$$

where:

Y is the pharmacokinetic parameter of interest (e.g., clearance)
W is body weight
a and b represent the equation coefficient and exponent, respectively.

Using the log transformation:

$$\log Y = \log a + b \log W$$

the parameter values are simply plotted against the body weight data on a log-log scale with a y-intercept equal to log a and a slope equal to b.

Practical limitations of using this simple method to predict human pharmacokinetic parameters have been documented, however, and revised methods have been proposed.[16] For example, one revised method includes brain weight in the equation, whereas another revision uses the animal's maximum life-span potential.[15]

The simple allometric method is based on a fundamental assumption that a pharmacokinetic parameter of interest is related to the body weight, no matter what the species of the animal is. Apparently this method ignores the interspecies differences in enzymatic metabolism, renal elimination capacity, absorption characteristics, gastric pH and emptying rate, and intestinal residence time, etc.

Regardless of which allometric method is ultimately selected, researchers must exercise a standard caution whenever animal pharmacokinetic data is extrapolated and used to predict estimates of human pharmacokinetic parameters. That is, predictive values for allometric interspecies scaling methods vary considerably, and are significantly influenced by a number of experimental factors including the selected study design, animal model, and drug product.[15] Nonetheless, several helpful journal publications and relevant literature reviews are available that presently offer practical advice to industry researchers who wish to apply interspecies scaling methods in pharmacokinetic studies of therapeutic drugs and biologics.[14–18]

16.4 HUMAN PHARMACOKINETIC EVALUATIONS

Successful clinical development of a safe and effective solid oral drug product is often preceded by multiple *in vivo* evaluations and iterative refinements in the investigational dosage formulation. An optimal dosage regimen must ultimately be identified that can maintain therapeutic drug concentrations and avoid toxicities. Human pharmacokinetic studies are, therefore, routinely performed to determine the bioavailability of a solid oral dosage form. Clinical pharmacokinetic studies are also conducted in humans to determine the potential effects of food, and other factors, on the pharmacokinetics of the drug. A sound understanding of the drug's absorption, distribution, metabolism, and elimination is essential to the development and approval of any solid oral drug product.

16.4.1 Bioavailability and Bioequivalence

Bioavailability and bioequivalence studies are often critical components of any new drug application. Bioavailability essentially describes the overall rate and extent of drug absorption for a given dosage formulation. Data from bioavailability studies are routinely used during drug development to identify the product's pharmacokinetics, optimize therapeutic dose regimens, and support product labeling requirements.

Bioequivalence, on the other hand, generally describes the extent to which the bioavailability of a particular drug product (i.e., the test product) compares with that of another known drug product (i.e., the reference product). Data from bioequivalence studies are often used to establish a link between different test formulations (e.g., an early phase 1 formulation versus a later phase 3 or to-be-marketed formulation). Post-approval bioequivalence studies may also be required, for example, when a major change occurs in a manufacturing method. Bioequivalence studies are also generally used to compare a generic version of a drug product with the corresponding reference-listed drug.

In general, oral bioavailability can simply be considered as the proportion of an orally administered dose that ultimately becomes available to the systemic circulation. When a drug is administered orally (or by any other extravascular route), for example, a sufficient amount of the administered dose must be absorbed during a certain time period before the intended pharmacologic effect can manifest. Thus, the bioavailability of an orally administered drug clearly depends on a combination of factors, including the physico-chemical characteristics of the drug formulation, and the physiological state of the GI system. Pharmacokineticists must therefore consider each of these factors when designing and conducting oral bioavailability and bioequivalence studies.

Two different types of oral bioavailability will be discussed in this chapter: absolute and relative bioavailability. Absolute oral bioavailability is a special case in which the systemic exposure of an oral dosage form is determined relative to that of its intravenous (IV) dose form. In contrast, relative oral bioavailability compares the rate and extent of absorption of one dosage formulation (e.g., oral solution) to another dosage formulation (e.g., oral capsule). Relative bioavailability can also sometimes compare the rate and extent of absorption for one drug with two different administration routes (e.g., intramuscular and subcutaneous).

Absolute Bioavailability

For the most part, absolute bioavailability is generally determined by comparing the extent of absorption achieved after extravascular drug administration to that obtained after IV drug administration. Thus, valid extravascular and IV data are both typically required for the calculation of absolute bioavailability. In operational terms, this means two series of pharmacokinetic samples must be collected—one extravascular series, and one IV series—using a suitable biological matrix (e.g., blood, plasma or serum), and appropriate sampling schedules. In addition, drug concentrations from each series must be analyzed using a validated drug assay. Measured concentration data from each series are then plotted and the area under the drug concentration–time curves (AUC) are estimated (e.g., by applying a numerical integration formula such as the trapezoidal rule).

Assuming clearance remains constant, AUC is directly proportional to the amount of drug absorbed. Thus absolute oral bioavailability (F) can be calculated:

$$F = \frac{D_{iv}}{D_{po}} \cdot \frac{AUC_{po}}{AUC_{iv}}$$

where:

D_{iv} and D_{po} are the IV and oral doses administered, respectively
AUC_{iv} and AUC_{po} are the AUC estimates for the IV and oral routes, respectively.

The amount of drug that ultimately reaches the systemic circulation after extravascular administration is almost always less than the administered dose (i.e., $F < 1$). How much less actually depends on many different factors, including drug solubility, permeability, lipophylicity, particle size, and dissolution rate. Physiological factors such as GI motility rates, gastric pH, and hepatic function are also influential. Absolute bioavailability can evidently vary among different dosage forms and different formulations of the same drug. An accurate determination of a new drug's absolute bioavailability is thus essential to the development of an effective therapeutic regimen.

An important review of absolute bioavailability data from over 400 drugs indicates that drugs with relatively low absolute bioavailability are often associated with relatively high interindividual variability in the pharmacological response produced.[19] Early detection of low absolute bioavailability in a new oral dosage form is crucial, particularly for a drug with a narrow therapeutic window. A drug with a narrow therapeutic window that also has a low absolute bioavailability often has a higher potential for drug-related adverse reactions. If the absolute bioavailability of a new dosage form is found to be lower than a preset criterion (e.g., 5% or 10%), strategic recommendations could be made to either terminate the development program altogether or cautiously continue with additional steps to further optimize the dosage formulation.

Absolute bioavailability may first be evaluated in a phase 1 clinical trial. First-in-human study designs, for example, often include several dose-escalating treatment groups where some treatment groups may receive oral formulations while others receive IV formulations. This type of design is inherently suited for evaluating absolute bioavailability, and will likely provide relevant data—as long as the total number of subjects will support the necessary statistical analysis.

One way to reduce the total number of subjects, and yet still ensure a sound statistical interpretation, is to use a two-period crossover study design where each subject receives both oral and IV formulations (e.g., the oral formulation in study period 1 and the IV formulation in period 2). Study periods 1 and 2 are separated by an adequate washout period of approximately 5 to 7 times the drug's half life. The duration of the washout period should be long enough to prevent carryover of an appreciable amount of drug from the first treatment period into the next. This study design is therefore most suitable for drugs with relatively short half lives, but may not be practical for drugs with relatively long half lives (e.g., several days instead of hours).

Relative Bioavailability

In contrast to absolute bioavailability, where the comparison basically involves an oral drug versus its IV formulation, relative bioavailability essentially compares the rate and extent of absorption of one dosage formulation (e.g., oral solution) to that of another (e.g., oral capsule). Over the course of a typical drug development cycle, several relative bioavailability studies could potentially be required (e.g., to compare the *in vivo* performance of an earlier stage formulation versus a later stage formulation). Depending on the overall rate of drug development, new dosage formulations are often still being prepared while a new molecular entity progresses from the nonclinical stage into the early clinical stage. In cases where the final product is intended as a solid oral dosage form, for example, oral solutions or suspensions might be the only formulations ready for use. Solid prototype formulations such as capsules might also be ready for use in early phase 1, however, these prototypes are often far from the final marketable form.

Relative bioavailability (F_{rel}) can be calculated:

$$F_{rel} = \frac{D_A}{D_B} \cdot \frac{AUC_B}{AUC_A}$$

where:

D_A and D_B are the doses administered for drug formulation A and B, respectively
and AUC_A and AUC_B are the AUC estimates for the A and B formulations, respectively.

A two-period crossover design is usually used to assess relative bioavailability for a drug with a relatively short elimination half life. Other crossover designs such as a three-period or higher-order design can also be used to efficiently compare the relative bioavailability among three or more different dosage formulations. Crossover designs may not be feasible, however, for drugs with long elimination half lives (e.g., greater than 10 days).

Additional information on the design and conduct of bioavailability studies, including statistical approaches to consider in the overall evaluation of absolute and relative bioavailability, are reviewed in greater detail in an FDA guidance document,[20] and also in Chapter 15 (Bioavailability and Bioequivalence) of this book.

Bioequivalence

From a regulatory perspective, and for various reasons, bioequivalence studies may need to be conducted before a product is approved for use in the clinic or during the post-approval period. Depending on the research objective, for example, a pre-approval study might be required in a new drug application (NDA) submission to demonstrate bioequivalence between the early and late phase dosage formulation or between the phase 3 and to-be-marketed formulation. In addition, bioequivalence studies are routinely required in abbreviated NDAs for generic versions of brand name drugs.

Two oral drug products can generally be considered to be bioequivalent if their respective concentration–time profiles are so similar that it would be unlikely they would produce clinically significant differences in the pharmacological response. In other words, bioequivalent drug products with essentially the same systemic bioavailability should thus be able to produce similar, and predictable, therapeutic effects. Pharmacokinetic assessments in bioequivalence studies of solid oral drug products therefore typically include statistical comparisons of AUC and C_{max}.

Chapter 15 (Bioavailability and Bioequivalence) provides additional information on bioequivalence studies, along with a thorough discussion of the related research objectives, study designs, statistical principles, and regulatory requirements.

16.4.2 Effects of Food and Other Substances on Oral Drug Absorption

The presence of food in the GI tract can significantly affect the oral bioavailability of a drug. Changes in gastric pH following ingestion of a meal, for instance, can alter drug absorption due to incomplete dissolution or disintegration of the drug product. Likewise, the nutritional and caloric content of a meal can influence drug absorption, because of subsequent effects on gastric emptying times, tissue perfusion rates or nutrient–drug interactions. Substantial, unpredictable, and potentially unmanageable food effects could ultimately lead to discontinuation of a clinical development program. Thus, *in vivo* evaluations of potential food effects on the extent of absorption (i.e., bioavailability) are routinely performed for most solid oral dosage forms.

Although food-effect studies are usually conducted in animal models (e.g., dogs) first, animal results may not sufficiently predict what could happen in humans. Therefore, *in vivo* food-effect studies with human subjects should be planned as early as possible, especially for drugs with low oral bioavailability or limited aqueous solubility. As early as phase 1 (e.g., a first-in-human study), the potential effects of food on oral bioavailability could be investigated simply by adding a food-effect treatment group. Subjects assigned to this group receive the drug first while in a fasted state (i.e., period 1), and then again while in a fed state (i.e., period 2). As with all crossover study designs, an adequate washout period must separate the two treatment periods.

It has been well-documented that food can influence the oral bioavailability of a drug by affecting one or more of the factors (e.g., bile flow, splanchnic blood flow, gastrointestinal pH, gastric emptying, physical/chemical interactions with the drug).[21,22] Custodio and colleagues wrote an excellent review paper about food-effect prediction based on the Biopharmaceutics Drug Disposition Classification System (BDDCS).[23] They predicted that high fat meals are not expected to have a significant effect on total systemic exposure for class I drugs, because of the high gut permeability and high intestinal fluid solubility possessed by this class of drugs; for class II compounds, which are highly metabolized and therefore are often dual substrates of enzymes and transporters, an increase in bioavailability is predicted; for class III compounds, which are poorly metabolized and poorly permeable and therefore are often reliant on uptake transporters, a decrease in bioavailability is predicted.

If a drug development team ultimately plans to include data from a food-effect study in the product label, the study design should comply with the current regulatory guidance on food-effect studies. According to the FDAs guidance,[24] for example, key recommendations for food-effect bioavailability and fed bioequivalence studies basically comprise the following:

- randomized, balanced, single-dose, two-treatment (i.e., fasting and fed), two-period, two-sequence crossover design;
- adequate washout period between treatment periods;
- either healthy volunteers from the general population or subjects from the patient population (if more appropriate);
- a high-fat, high-calorie meal (i.e., 50% of total calories from fat; 800 to 1000 calories).

The FDA also stipulates that an adequate sample size must be used to support the appropriate statistical analysis. For instance, the FDA suggests planning for enough subjects so that a minimum of 12 complete the study.[24] However, a larger sample size might be required if previous pharmacokinetic studies indicate high levels of inter- or intra-subject variability. An equivalence approach is particularly recommended for the statistical analysis of data from food-effect studies. A detailed discussion of this statistical approach, and its practical application in the analysis of bioavailability and bioequivalence data, is presented in the previous chapter.

In general, food effects on bioavailability are least likely to occur with a highly soluble, highly permeable, *IR* drug product, such as a Biopharmaceutic Drug Classification System (BCS) class I drug. As such, food-effect studies for many BCS class I drugs are not

ordinarily conducted. On the other hand, regulatory agencies do recommend food-effect studies for all other IR drugs (i.e., BCS Class II, III, and IV), as well as all MR drugs, and any drug with a narrow therapeutic window regardless of BCS classification.

If a substantial and potentially clinically important food effect is identified, additional studies may be needed to determine whether the effect can be managed in the clinic. For example, one additional study could evaluate the potential effects of different meal types (e.g., high-fat, high-carbohydrate or high-fiber meals) on drug absorption. Another study could likewise investigate the effect of staggered meal times. Results from either of these studies could help clarify the underlying mechanism, and provide the data needed to support a development team's decision to proceed or discontinue. The following example describes one such instance.

A food-effect treatment group was incorporated into the design of a first-in-human, single-ascending-dose study to evaluate the effect of food on the oral bioavailability of Compound A. Results from this study in a small number of subjects showed an approximate 5- to 8-fold increase in oral bioavailability when Compound A was ingested with a high-fat meal. To further investigate this apparently substantial effect, a formal food-effect study was planned with two different meal types: a high-fat meal (i.e., approximately 50% fat content) typically recommended by the FDA, and a low-fat meal (i.e., approximately 15% fat content). A conventional crossover study design was used (i.e., since the half life of Compound A was relatively short), and pharmacokinetic samples were collected in each of three study periods: 1) fasted; 2) fed with the low-fat meal; and 3) fed with the high-fat meal.

The study results indicated that the highest mean plasma concentration profile of Compound A was produced with the high-fat meal. In addition, Figure 16.1

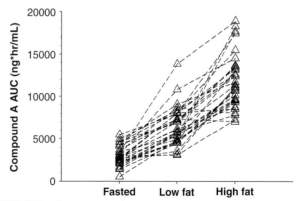

FIGURE 16.1 Area under the concentration-time curve (AUC) of Compound A by food-effect treatment group

shows that when compared to the bioavailability in the fasted condition, bioavailability of Compound A was approximately 5-fold higher with the high-fat meal, and approximately 2- to 3-fold higher with the low fat meal.

These findings confirmed the results from the earlier food-effect study. The researchers concluded that the oral bioavailability of Compound A was substantially altered by food, and that the effect was directly related to the fat content of the meal. The clinical implications were clear. Unlike phase 1 settings, where meal conditions can be strictly controlled, meal conditions in late phase clinical settings cannot be as restrictive, for obvious practical reasons. As such, the food-effect on Compound A could potentially become unmanageable in the clinic, and most likely increase the risk of adverse events.

Other food-effect studies can be conducted during the clinical phases of oral drug development. Food effects on drug pharmacokinetics can be further assessed in a meal-timing study, for example, where meal times are staggered around the oral drug administration time. With this type of study, the drug pharmacokinetics can be evaluated under conditions that reflect actual situations in which patients self-administer drugs at varying time intervals around the actual prescribed times (e.g., 1 minute before as opposed to 30 minutes before a meal).

Researchers used a meal-timing study to investigate the pharmacokinetics of tegaserod, a selective 5-HT4 receptor partial agonist drug.[25] In previous clinical studies, oral bioavailability was reduced when tegaserod was administered during a meal.[26] Another study was therefore proposed to further investigate the pharmacokinetics of tegaserod using five different dose administration time intervals. The study[25] was a randomized, open-label, two-phase, five-period crossover study design. In the first phase, healthy subjects received a single oral dose of tegaserod at 30 and 15 minutes before the start of the meal. In the second phase, the same subjects received a single oral dose 1 minute before the start of the meal, 2.5 hours after the start of meal or with a continued 4-hour postdose fast. Each subject received all five treatments in a randomized manner, and a standard 600-calorie, high-fat meal was provided.

Results showed that systemic exposure to tegaserod (i.e., AUC) was significantly lower under each of the four fed conditions, versus that of the fasted condition.[25] That is, regardless of whether tegaserod was administered before or after a meal, oral bioavailability was reduced. The researchers therefore concluded that, although meal timing did not apparently affect tegaserod pharmacokinetics, the administration of food reduced AUC by approximately 50%.[25]

Ingested substances other than solid food can also significantly affect the bioavailability of certain oral drugs. Clinically relevant drug interaction effects are well-documented for substances such as grapefruit juice, antacids, and various herbal supplements. Grapefruit juice, for example, increases the oral bioavailability of drugs that are substrates of the cytochrome P450 enzyme 3A (CYP3A). This effect is attributed to certain ingredients in grapefruit juice that can inhibit the intestinal activity of CYP3A, even when the juice is consumed in ordinary dietary quantities. Grapefruit juice may also inhibit the drug transporter, P-glycoprotein. In general, drug interaction studies with grapefruit juice are recommended if the investigational drug is a CYP3A substrate. A typical randomized, open-label, two-period crossover design can be used with grapefruit juice (or water) given at the time of drug administration, and then 30 and 90 minutes later. To maximize potential effects, double-strength grapefruit juice is sometimes used.

Concomitant use of antacids with other oral medications is quite common, and can be linked to specific drug–drug interactions. Certain drug classes, such as quinolone antibiotics, nonsteroidal anti-inflammatory drugs (NSAIDs), and cephalosporins, have shown interactions with coingested antacids. Tetracycline has been shown to form insoluble complex molecules with antacids (i.e., via metal ion chelation) that may sharply reduce tetracycline absorption.[27] Other notable drug–drug interactions have been reported when an antacid was coadministered with quinidine, ketoconazole, and oral glucocorticoids.[28]

The typical interaction effect associated with most antacids presents as either reduced or delayed absorption of the coadministered drug. Other antacids (e.g., magnesium hydroxide and sodium bicarbonate) can paradoxically increase the rate of absorption, and sometimes the extent of absorption, for certain drugs including NSAIDs (e.g., ibuprofen), and sulphonylurea antidiabetic agents (e.g., glipizide).[29] Weakly acidic drugs such as ibuprofen and glipizide ordinarily have low water solubility, and become nonionized at normal gastric pH. Administration of antacids such as magnesium hydroxide and sodium bicarbonate that elevate gastric pH, however, can increase the solubility and absorption of these sparingly water soluble drugs (e.g., NSAIDs).

Drug–drug interaction studies of oral drugs with antacids may be readily performed during the clinical phase of drug development. A typical antacid study uses a two-period crossover design: one period with the test drug administered alone, and another period with the test drug administered along with the antacid. Interaction studies with antacids are also usually conducted with healthy subjects.

16.4.3 Effects of Gastric pH on Oral Drug Absorption

Gastric acidity can significantly affect the oral bioavailability of some drugs. Gastric pH under fasting conditions may range from 2 to 6. After a meal, the rate of parietal cell hydrochloric acid secretion is typically increased, and gastric pH can drop below 2. Changes in gastric pH can affect the disintegration and dissolution of many oral dosage formulations, and thus alter the drug's pharmacokinetics. Depending on the drug's physiochemical properties, and the intended pharmacological response, an increase or decrease in system exposure may result.

Unlike the gastric pH, the small intestine pH at first decreases in response to a meal with the arrival of acidic chime from the stomach, but later the fasted state pH is re-established as a result of pancreatic bicarbonate output.[30]

Pretreatment with a histamine 2 receptor blocker (e.g., ranitidine) can increase gastric pH, and subsequently reduce the systemic exposure of certain drugs. The oral bioavailability of enoxacin, for example, decreased by 26% when subjects were pretreated with ranitidine.[31] Lange and his coauthors[32] found that coadministration of itraconazole with an acidic solution (e.g., a cola beverage) could counteract the decrease in systemic exposure that occurs with ranitidine pretreatment. These findings suggest that coadministration of an acidic beverage may be an effective way to enhance the oral bioavailability of itraconazole in patients who are hypochlorhydric or who may be using gastric acid suppressants.

Various physico-chemical and physiological factors, such as crystalline form, aqueous solubility and lipophilicity of a drug, pKa of a drug, and the gastrointestinal pH profile, can influence the saturation solubility of a drug in the gastrointestinal tract. The interplay between the pKa of a drug and the pH gradient along the gastrointestinal tract may determine the degree of ionization of a drug, and eventually the extent of its absorption into systemic circulation.[30]

Some drugs and their active metabolites may also exhibit pH-dependent pharmacokinetics. An *in vivo* pharmacokinetic study of tegaserod (the aforementioned selective 5-HT4 receptor partial agonist) provides one such example. Tegaserod exhibits extensive first-pass metabolism through two main pathways. After oral administration, tegaserod initially undergoes presystemic, pH-dependent hydrolysis in the stomach, followed by a subsequent oxidation, and glucuronidation into its major metabolite, 5-methoxy-indole-3-carbonic acid glucuronide.[33] To assess the effect of gastric pH on the systemic exposure of tegaserod and this metabolite, a randomized, open-label, single-dose, three-period crossover study was performed.[34]

After an overnight fast, subjects were randomly assigned to one of three treatment groups:

1. a single oral dose of omeprazole on the evening before and morning of tegaserod dose administration, followed by a sodium bicarbonate buffer (pH 4.5) to attain a gastric pH above 3.5, then a single oral dose of tegaserod;
2. a single subcutaneous dose of pentagastrin to attain a gastric pH below 2, followed by a single oral dose of tegaserod; and
3. oral tegaserod without any pretreatment.

The pharmacokinetic data showed that, while plasma tegaserod concentrations significantly decreased at pH <2.0, concentrations of the active metabolite significantly increased at pH <2.0. In addition, plasma concentrations of the metabolite subsequently decreased at pH >3.5. These results confirmed the data from the earlier investigation that indicated tegaserod undergoes pH dependent hydrolysis in the human stomach.[34]

16.4.4 Regional Absorption Site Assessments and Imaging Studies

The amount of time that a drug actually spends at or near a GI absorption site (i.e., residence time) is determined by several factors, such as gastric emptying rates and intestinal transit times, as well as various drug product characteristics. MR (e.g., CR) oral dosage forms, for example, are designed to release drug over a specific or extended length of time compared to that of IR oral dosage forms. This modification typically requires development of a drug product that can remain in the GI tract long enough for absorption to occur sufficiently before the rest of the capsule or tablet is eliminated. *In vivo* performance evaluations of MR oral dosage forms should, therefore, include regional absorption studies along with the standard set of pharmacokinetic assessments.

A series of *in vitro* dissolution profiles and their corresponding pharmacokinetic profiles for MR formulations with different release profiles and an IR formulation can be obtained experimentally. Methods of convolution/deconvolution can be used to extract the *in vivo* absorption profiles from both dissolution and pharmacokinetic data. If necessary, an ideal pharmacokinetic profile can be postulated and simulated first, along with a known absorption profile, an *in vivo* release profile for an MR formulation can be predicted and a prototype can be prepared accordingly. A pharmacokinetics-guided approach can effectively support the selection and optimization of MR formulations.

Several sophisticated procedures and imaging techniques have been used to evaluate regional absorption and pharmacokinetics of IR and MR oral drugs.[35] Gamma scintigraphy, for example, is a noninvasive imaging technique that uses a gamma camera to visualize and localize radiolabeled substances in various organs of the body. This technique has specifically been applied in the drug development industry to evaluate the *in vivo* human performance of a variety of oral drugs, including an IR formulation of a dual angiotensin-converting enzyme and neutral endopeptidase inhibitor,[36] as well as a sustained-release formulation of 5 aminosalicylic acid (5-ASA).[37] These two case studies will be presented to further illustrate the practical utility of a gamma scintigraphic approach to the *in vivo* evaluation of solid oral dosage form performance.

In the first study,[36] 13 healthy subjects were enrolled in a randomized, open-label, single-dose, five-period crossover study of M100240, a dual angiotensin-converting enzyme and neutral endopeptidase inhibitor. The purpose of the study was to obtain an assessment of the absolute bioavailability of an IR formulation of M100240, along with an assessment of the regional absorption of M100240 in various segments of the GI tract, including the proximal and distal small bowel and colon.

A remotely triggered, specially designed, radiolabeled capsule was used in combination with a gamma camera to localize capsule positions, and thereby provide controlled, targeted drug delivery. These Enterion™ capsules (Phaeton Research, Nottingham, UK) were first filled with M100240, and then sealed. The capsules were also radiolabeled with 1 MBq of ^{111}In and administered with 180 mL of tap water, to which 4 MBq of ^{99m}Tc-diethylenetriaminepentaacetic acid (DTPA) had been added. Scintigraphic images were obtained at 10-minute intervals, both before capsule activation (i.e., targeted drug release), and up to 4 hours postactivation, and then at 20-minute intervals from 4 to 8 hours postactivation. Pharmacokinetic blood samples were also collected and analyzed.

The absolute bioavailability of M100240 was estimated as 49%, and the relative bioavailability estimates (i.e., relative to the oral IR tablet form) were 94%, 97%, and 41% in the proximal small bowel, distal small bowel, and ascending colon, respectively.[36] Thus, the proximal and distal small bowel apparently represented the primary absorption site, while modest absorption also occurred in the colon. Overall, the researchers noted that the data from this regional

imaging study were particularly important for the development and optimization of prototype MR formulations of M100240.[36]

In the next example, drug absorption of a sustained-release oral formulation of 5-ASA was evaluated throughout multiple regions of the GI tract, using a combination of pharmacokinetic and gamma scintigraphic assessment methods.[37] Nine healthy volunteers participated in the study. Each subject received a single dose of radiolabeled (0.8 MBq of ^{153}SM) 5-ASA on two occasions (i.e., once in a fasted condition and once in a fed condition). Anterior and posterior images were obtained using a gamma camera at 20-minute intervals during the first 4 hours postdose, then at 30-minute intervals through 10 hours postdose, and finally at 12 and 24 hours postdose. Serial pharmacokinetic samples were obtained and analyzed.

Overall results of the study[37] showed that, for this sustained-release oral formulation of 5-ASA, drug release was generally detectable within 30 to 60 minutes postdose, and began in the stomach or proximal small intestine. Scintigraphic images also confirmed that peak plasma concentrations of 5-ASA generally occurred when the drug was in the small intestine or ascending colon, and that drug release also generally occurred throughout the rest of the GI tract. In addition, the pharmacokinetic behavior of this sustained-release formulation of 5-ASA was not significantly affected by the presence of food. The authors concluded that the regional absorption patterns for this sustained-release 5-ASA oral formulation were clinically relevant, since this formulation is intended for use in the treatment of inflammatory bowel disease, such as Crohn's disease.[37]

The incorporation of gamma scintigraphy and safer radiolabeling methods into the *in vivo* evaluations of oral drug formulations has provided many advantages to researchers in the drug development industry. For example, conventional phase 1 studies of oral MR formulations may typically require several years to complete.[38] Now, however, human GI site-specific pharmacokinetic data can be readily obtained from a gamma scintigraphic absorption study. Timely and quantitative results from these studies can then be communicated to strategic development teams, so that faster business decisions can be made. Furthermore, additional studies may be planned, depending on the outcome, to further optimize the lead product if needed or develop a back-up compound instead. Finally, from a regulatory perspective, validated gamma scintigraphic methods may also provide surrogate means to demonstrate therapeutic bioequivalence for locally-acting GI drug products.[39]

16.5 *IN VIVO* PHARMACOKINETIC METRICS

Complete characterization of the *in vivo* time course of drug absorption is crucial for the design and optimization of a therapeutic drug product. Information about *in vivo* drug release, *in vitro–in vivo* correlation, and absorption kinetics, for example, are all needed to support a successful drug development program. Once a product's entire *in vivo* time course (i.e., drug concentration–time profile) is identified, some additional *in vivo* metrics are commonly derived that may be used to further describe the drug's overall *in vivo* performance. Selected examples of these metrics will now be defined, and general practical descriptions will be provided. Metrics of particular importance in the evaluation of *CR* oral drug formulations are included.

- AUC: area under the drug concentration–time curve. AUC is generally used to represent the extent of drug absorption.
- C_{max} and T_{max}: maximal drug concentration and time to reach maximal drug concentration, respectively. C_{max} and T_{max} are generally used to represent the rate of absorption. C_{max} is also used along with AUC to collectively represent the extent of absorption.
- C_{min}: minimal drug concentration.
- C_{avg}: the ratio of $AUC_{0-\tau}$ to τ. $AUC_{0-\tau}$ is AUC during one dosing interval at steady state after multiple dose administration, and τ is a dosing interval.
- Degree of fluctuation (DOF): also known as peak–trough fluctuation ratio. DOF can be used to assess the steady state performance of a CR dosage form:

$$DOF = \frac{C_{max} - C_{min}}{C_{avg}}$$

- Retard quotient (R_Δ): is defined by the following equation:

$$R_\Delta = \frac{HVD_{CR}}{HVD_{IR}}$$

where *HVD* (i.e., half-value duration) is defined as the time span in which the plasma concentration exceeds $\frac{1}{2} C_{max}$. R_Δ quantifies the factor by which *HVD* is prolonged for a CR product (i.e., relative to that of the IR product), and is independent of the dose administered. However, this parameter R_Δ does not provide

information regarding the duration within the therapeutic range. When the minimum effective concentration of a given drug is not known, the trough concentration of an IR product at steady state may be used instead.

- Controlled-release effectiveness (CRE): is defined by the following equation:

$$CRE = \frac{AUC_{\Delta C}^{CR}}{AUC_{\Delta C}^{IR}}$$

where $AUC_{\Delta C}^{CR}$ is the AUC within the C_{max} and C_{min} limits over a dosing interval for the *CR* product, and $AUC_{\Delta C}^{IR}$ is the AUC within the C_{max} and C_{min} limits over a dosing interval for the *IR* product. This approach is based on the assumption that a CR product should yield plasma concentration levels that lie within the minimum and maximum levels produced by sequential dose administrations of the IR product. Treatment equivalence can generally be demonstrated by a CRE ratio near unity.

16.6 *IN VIVO* ABSORPTION PATTERN DIAGNOSTICS

Simply put, pharmacokinetics describes the processes and time courses of drug absorption, distribution, metabolism, and elimination. In addition, pharmacokinetics allows for these processes to be explained in terms of how they relate to the intensity and time course of a pharmacologic response (e.g., therapeutic effect or toxicity). Absorption is a particularly complex, yet essential, process that allows a released drug substance to enter the systemic circulation. Drug concentration–time profiles are generally used to describe and evaluate the overall absorption process. These profiles are typically created from drug concentration data (i.e., blood, plasma or serum samples) collected over the time course of an *in vivo* pharmacokinetic study.

Concentration–time profiles for oral drug formulations can generally be separated into two basic categories: typical or atypical. A typical oral drug absorption profile represents a process that follows simple first- or zero-order kinetics. In contrast, an atypical absorption profile may represent one of several possible irregular absorption processes. Practical evaluation of all oral drug absorption profiles, therefore, requires a combination of a thorough understanding of the drug's physiochemical properties, expert pattern diagnostics, and advanced knowledge of the drug's disposition kinetics (i.e., from a previous evaluation using the IV formulation).

Oral drug absorption processes are generally assumed to follow first-order kinetics (i.e., the amount of drug in the system decreases logarithmically over time). As such, the first-order absorption rate constant is readily obtained using a simple compartmental pharmacokinetic modeling approach. This assumption of first-order absorption kinetics is not always true, however, and a cursory visual inspection of a drug concentration–time profile can sometimes be misleading. Concentration–time profiles for a drug exhibiting biexponential disposition, for example, could appear to potentially reflect a one-compartment model. In reality, however, the absorption part of the profile may actually be masking the distribution portion.[40]

Typical oral drug absorption may also sometimes follow zero-order kinetics (i.e., the amount of drug in the system essentially decreases at a constant rate). Typical absorption profiles for drugs with zero-order absorption initially rise to a sharp peak, and then quickly decline without an intermediate plateau. Examples of drugs that exhibit zero-order absorption kinetics include griseofulvin,[41] hydroflumethiazide,[42] and erythromycin.[43] Nevertheless, for conventional *in vivo* evaluations of IR oral drug performance, most pharmacokinetic models generally assume first-order absorption, unless an assumption of zero-order absorption has been previously documented.

The oral absorption process can also sometimes be characterized by absorption kinetics other than first- or zero-order. For example, atypical absorption kinetics may include parallel first-order absorption, mixed zero- and first-order absorption, Weibull-type absorption, and an absorption window with or without Michaelis–Menten absorption.[40] An extensive discussion of atypical drug absorption profiles, and helpful information on pharmacokinetic strategies to identify them, can be found in a recently published review in the Journal of Clinical Pharmacology.[40]

16.7 GENERIC ALTERNATIVE: OPPORTUNITY OR THREAT?

Paracelsus wrote, "A drug can be an insert substance, a poison, or a therapeutic agent dependent upon how it is used, and the dosage in which it is given." This quote is also appropriate to switching from some branded drugs to their generic alternatives to treat certain diseases. In most cases, the availability of generic drugs is widely applauded as an opportunity to reduce expenditure on drug costs, and deploy limited resources more wisely and effectively. The current streamlined approval process of regulatory agencies for generic products, based on both pharmaceutical equivalence and pharmacokinetic bioequivalence, facilitates timely availability of many high-quality yet low-cost generic drugs to more patients. Nevertheless, the rigor of the scientific rationale behind the pharmacokinetic bioequivalence is short of perfect, and has undergone heated debate since the very concept has been introduced. Although switching a patient from a branded drug to a generic alternative may save the difference in the cost of acquisition of the two products, in certain cases, this must be done with extreme care, and consistent monitoring.[44] These inequivalence concerns become more imperative when we deal with drugs qualifying for the following criteria (so called "critical-dose drug"): narrow therapeutic range, requirement for blood level monitoring, administration based on body weight or other highly individualized dosing requirements, serious clinical consequences if overdosing or underdosing occurs, and manifestation of steep dose response relationships for efficacy, toxicity, or both.[45] Some examples include (but are not limited to) neurological, immunosuppressive, anticoagulant, and antiarrhythmic drugs.[46]

The current FDA-recommended pharmacokinetic bioequivalence testing serves well for most of the drugs in immediate-release formulations, and generally should enable clinicians to routinely substitute generic for innovator products. The traditional exposure matrices in bioequivalence tests, C_{max} and AUC, can do a fairly good job in claiming the equivalence of two pharmacokinetic profiles arising from immediate-release formulations. It has become known that C_{max} is a relatively poor and insensitive parameter in characterizing the pharmacokinetic profile from products with multiple peaks, commonly seen in modified-release formulations. The overall absorption pattern of a product, a reflection of multiple peaks, troughs, peak sizes, and ascending sections created by the immediate- and extended-release fractions of the total dose and release technology, is best characterized with an early exposure metric, AUC_{pR}. AUC_{pR} (or area under the curve to the population median t_{max} of the reference formulation), may be used as a supplemental essential metric, in addition to AUC and C_{max}.

Two recent examples may well underscore these concerns. One example is Wellbutrin XL 300 versus Budeprion XL 300. Long-acting antidepressant Wellbutrin XL 300, a branded product from GlaxoSmithKline, uses a membrane-based drug-delivery technology that is currently patent-protected. A generic form of this product is Budeprion XL 300.

A different drug-release technology, i.e., erodable tablet technology, is used instead in the generic version. Both drugs contained the same amount of active ingredient (bupropion). Apparently the generic product had passed the proof of "bioequivalence" to the brand name product in humans, and subsequently gained FDA approval. Since the launch of Budeprion XL 300 mg, multiple incidences of increased side-effects and decreased efficacy of the generic version have been reported. When both products were subjected to the *in vitro* dissolution testing described in the FDAs approval letters, the release rates for both were actually quite different. Whereas Wellbutrin XL 300 had released 8% of its bupropion HCL after two hours, Budeprion XL 300 had released four times as much. Similar disparity was also observed after four hours. It is interesting to note that after eight hours the dissolution results for both products became comparable. The higher release rate in the first several hours observed in the generic version of Wellbutrin XL 300 may imply that more active drug would enter into the systemic circulation faster than the originator product, and it could explain why a higher incidence of side-effects (such as nausea and anxiety) typical of too much buproprion were reported when the generic product was administered. Another example is the citizen petition (DOCKET 2005-0420/CP1) from Shire to the FDA on January 19, 2006. Shire was able to demonstrate that the standard bioequivalence criteria are not sufficiently rigorous when assessing the potential impact of changes to extended-release formulations in which the pharmacokinetic profile is expected to have a meaningful impact on therapeutic effect. Study results of a completed pharmacokinetic study were submitted. This study evaluated the relative bioavailability of ADDERALL XR® capsules and ADDERALL® tablets versus an oral solution of mixed amphetamine salts in healthy subjects. All three formulations are equal-strength, but contain distinct formulations of mixed amphetamine salts. Though these three formulations exhibited different pharmacokinetic profiles, especially between ADDERALL XR® capsules and ADDERALL® tablets versus an oral solution, bioequivalence testing based on C_{max} and AUC of these three formulations failed to distinguish them. This study further underscores the lack of adequate scientific rigor, and the insensitivity of the currently employed standard bioequivalence criteria.

Caution should be exercised when the pharmacokinetic profiles of two modified-release formulations (e.g., generic versus innovator products) are not essentially superimposable, additional parameters should be considered for switchability evaluation besides C_{max}, AUC, and food effect. These considerations should include (but not be limited to) t_{max}, degree of fluctuation, trough level, partial AUC, active metabolites, etc. A better-defined regulatory guidance may be warranted to test the *in vivo* pharmacokinetic equivalence for modified-release products.

16.8 SUMMARY

The *in vivo* performance of any new solid oral dosage form can be thoroughly evaluated with a strategic set of prospectively planned, and appropriately designed, pharmacokinetic studies. Data from *in vivo* pharmacokinetic studies provide essential information about drug absorption characteristics, GI absorption sites, bioavailability, and the effects of food and other related factors on the behavior of the drug product. Data from *in vivo* animal studies can specifically offer early knowledge of an investigational drug's general pharmacokinetics, and can potentially be used to predict pharmacokinetic behavior in humans. Most importantly, however, data from *in vivo* human pharmacokinetic studies can offer clinically relevant insight into the relationship between systemic drug exposure and the pharmacologic response.

Solid oral dosage formulations must be strategically designed to produce predictable, and consistent, systemic drug exposure in the human body. The ultimate goal is to develop an efficacious, cost-effective, and convenient drug product that can be administered safely and reliably to patients.

References

1. Maeda, T., Takenaka, H., Yamahira, Y. & Noguchi, T. (1979). Use of rabbits for GI drug absorption studies: Physiological study of stomach-emptying controlled rabbits. Chemical & Pharmaceutical Bulletin 27, 3066–3072.
2. Hussain, M., Abramowitz, W., Watrous, B.J., Szpunar, G.J. & Ayres, J.W. (1990). Gastrointestinal transit of nondisintegrating, nonerodible oral dosage forms in pigs. Pharmaceutical Research 7, 1163–1166.
3. Hildebrand, H., McDonald, F.M. & Windt-Hanke, F. (1991). Characterization of oral sustained release preparations of iloprost in a pig model by plasma level monitoring. Prostaglandins 41, 473–486.
4. Kostewicz, E., Sansom, L., Fishlock, R., Morella, A. & Kuchel, T. (1996). Examination of two sustained release nifedipine preparations in humans and in pigs. European Journal of Pharmaceutical Sciences 4, 351–357.
5. Dressman, J.B. & Yamada, K. (1991). Animal models for oral drug absorption. In: *Pharmaceutical Bioequivalence*, P.G. Welling, F.L. Tse, & S. Dighe, (eds). Marcel Dekker, New York. pp. 235–266.
6. Yamakita, H., Maejima, T. & Osawa, T. (1995). Preparation of controlled release tablets of TA-5707F with wax matrix type and their *in vivo* evaluation in beagle dogs. Biological & Pharmaceutical Bulletin 18, 984–989.

7. Yamakita, H., Maejima, T. & Osawa, T. (1995). *In vitro/in vivo* evaluation of two series of TA-5707F controlled release matrix tablets prepared with hydroxypropyl methyl cellulose derivatives with entero-soluble or gel formation properties. Biological & Pharmaceutical Bulletin 18, 1409–1416.

8. Tibbitts, J. (2003). Issues related to the use of canines in toxicologic pathology—issues with pharmacokinetics and metabolism. Toxicologic Pathology 31(Suppl.), 17–24.

9. Dressman, J.B. (1986). Comparison of canine and human gastrointestinal physiology. Pharm Res 3, 123–131.

10. Kararli, T.T. (1995). Comparison of the gastrointestinal anatomy, physiology, and biochemistry of humans and commonly used laboratory animals. Biopharm Drug Dispos 16, 351–380.

11. Chiou, W.L., Jeong, H.Y., Chung, S.M. & Wu, T.C. (2000). Evaluation of using dog as an animal model to study the fraction of oral dose absorbed of 43 drugs in humans. Pharm Res 17(2), 135–140.

12. Mordenti, J. (1986). Man versus beast. Journal of Pharmaceutical Sciences 75, 1028–1040.

13. Dedrick, R.L. (1973). Animal scale-up. Journal of Pharmacokinetics and Biopharmaceutics 1, 435–461.

14. Boxenbaum, H. & Dilea, C. (1995). First-time-in-human dose selection: Allometric thoughts and perspectives. Journal of Clinical Pharmacology 35, 957–966.

15. Mahmood, I. & Balian, J.D. (1999). The pharmacokinetic principles behind scaling from preclinical results to phase 1 protocols. Clinical Pharmacokinetics 36, 1–11.

16. Mahmood, I. (1999). Allometric issues in drug development. Journal of Pharmaceutical Sciences 88, 1101–1106.

17. Mahmood, I. (2002). Interspecies scaling: Predicting oral clearance in humans. American Journal of Therapeutics 9, 35–42.

18. Mahmood, I. (2003). Interspecies scaling of protein drugs: Prediction of clearance from animals to humans. Journal of Pharmaceutical Sciences 93, 177–185.

19. Sietsema, W.K. (1989). The absolute oral bioavailability of selected drugs. International Journal of Clinical Pharmacology, Therapy, and Toxicology 27, 178–211.

20. Food and Drug Administration (2003). *Guidance for industry: Bioavailability and bioequivalence studies for orally administered drug products—general considerations.* US Department of Health and Human Services, Rockville, MD.

21. Food and Drug Administration (2002). *Guidance for Industry: Food-Effect Bioavailability and Fed Bioequivalence Studies.* Food and Drug Administration, Rockville, MD.

22. Schmidt, L.E. & Dalhoff, K. (2002). Food–drug interactions. Drugs 62, 1481–1502.

23. Custodio, J.M., Wu, C.Y. & Benet, L.Z. (2008). Predicting drug disposition, absorption/elimination/transporter interplay and the role of food on drug absorption. Advanced Drug Delivery Reviews 60(6), 717–733.

24. Food and Drug Administration (2002). *Guidance for industry: Food-effect bioavailability and fed bioequivalence studies.* US Department of Health and Human Services, Rockville, MD.

25. Zhou, H., Khalilieh, S., Lau, H., Guerret, M., Osborne, S., Alladina, L., Laurent, A. & McLeod, J. (1999). Effect of meal timing not critical for the pharmacokinetics of tegaserod (HTF 919). Journal of Clinical Pharmacology 39, 911–919.

26. Appel-Dingemanse, S., Lemarechal, M-O., Kumle, A., Hubert, M. & Legangneux, E. (1999). Integrated modeling of the clinical pharmacokinetics of SDZ HTF 919, a novel selective 5-HT4 receptor agonist, following oral and intravenous administration. British Journal of Clinical Pharmacology 5, 483–492.

27. Gugler, R. & Allgayer, H. (1990). Effects of antacids on the clinical pharmacokinetics of drugs. An update. Clinical Pharmacokinetics 18, 210–219.

28. Sadowski, D.C. (1994). Drug interactions with antacids. Mechanisms and clinical significance. Drug Safety 11, 395–407.

29. Neuvonen, P.J. & Kivisto, K.T. (1994). Enhancement of drug absorption by antacids. An unrecognized drug interaction. Clinical Pharmacokinetics 27, 120–128.

30. Horter, D. & Dressman, J.B. (2001). Influence of physicochemical properties on dissolution of drugs in the gastrointestinal tract. Advanced Drug Delivery Reviews 46, 75–87.

31. Lebsack, M.E., Nix, D., Ryerson, B., Toothaker, R.D., Welage, L., Norman, A.M., Schentag, J.J. & Sedman, A.J. (1992). Effect of gastric acidity on enoxacin absorption. Clinical Pharmacology and Therapeutics 52, 252–256.

32. Lange, D., Pavao, J.H., Wu, J. & Klausner, M. (1997). Effect of a cola beverage on the bioavailability of itraconazole in the presence of H2 blockers. Journal of Clinical Pharmacology 37, 535–540.

33. Appel, S., Kumle, A., Hubert, M. & Duvauchelle, T. (1997). First pharmacokinetic-pharmacodynamic study in humans with a selective 5-hydroxytryptamine4 receptor agonist. Journal of Clinical Pharmacology 37, 229–237.

34. Zhou, H., Khalilieh, S., Campestrini, J., Appel-Dingemanse, S., Lachman, L. & McLeod, J.F. (2000). Effect of gastric pH on plasma concentration of tegaserod (HTF 919) and its major metabolite in healthy subjects. Gastroenterol 118, A1206.

35. Perkins, A.C. & Frier, M. (2004). Radionuclide imaging in drug development. Current Pharmaceutical Design 10, 2907–2921.

36. Martin, N.E., Collison, K.R., Martin, L.L., Tardif, S., Wilding, I., Wray, H. & Barrett, J.S. (2003). Pharmacoscintigraphic assessment of the regional drug absorption of the dual angiotensin-converting enzyme/neutral endopeptidase inhibitor, M100240, in healthy volunteers. Journal of Clinical Pharmacology 43, 529–538.

37. Hardy, J.G., Harvey, W.J., Sparrow, R.A., Marshall, G.B., Steed, K.P., Macarios, M. & Wilding, I.R. (1993). Localization of drug release sites from an oral sustained-release formulation of 5-ASA (Pentasa) in the gastrointestinal tract using gamma scintigraphy. Journal of Clinical Pharmacology 33, 712–718.

38. Wilding, I.R. & Heald, D.L. (1999). Visualization of product performance in the gut: what role in the drug development/regulatory paradigm. Journal of Clinical Pharmacology 39, 6S–9S.

39. Wilding, I. (2002). Bioequivalence testing for locally acting gastrointestinal products: What role for gamma scintigraphy? Journal of Clinical Pharmacology 42, 1200–1210.

40. Zhou, H. (2003). Pharmacokinetic strategies in deciphering atypical drug absorption profiles. Journal of Clinical Pharmacology 43, 211–227.

41. Bates, T.R. & Carrigan, P.J. (1975). Apparent absorption kinetics of micronized griseofulvin after its oral administration on single- and multiple-dose regimens to rats as a corn oil-in-water emulsion and aqueous suspension. Journal of Pharmaceutical Sciences 64, 1475–1481.

42. McNamara, P.J., Colburn, W.A. & Gibaldi, M. (1978). Absorption kinetics of hydroflumethiazide. Journal of Clinical Pharmacology 18, 191–193.

43. Colburn, W.A., Di Santo, A.R. & Gibaldi, M. (1977). Pharmacokinetics of erythromycin on repetitive dosing. Journal of Clinical Pharmacology 17, 592–600.

44. Nuss, P., Taylor, D., De Hert, M. & Hummer, M. (2004). The generic alternative in schizophrenia—opportunity or threat? CNG Drugs 18(12), 769–775.

45. Sabatini, S., Ferguson, R.M., Helderman, J.H., et al. (1999). Drug substitution in transplantation: a National Kidney Foundation white paper. American Journal of Kidney Diseases 33, 389–397.

46. Reiffel, J.A. (2001). Issues in the use of generic antiarrhythmic drugs. Current Opinion in Cardiology 16(1), 23–29.

In Vitro–In Vivo Correlations: Fundamentals, Development Considerations, and Applications

Yihong Qiu

17.1 INTRODUCTION

For decades, developing *in vitro* tests and models to assess or predict *in vivo* performance of pharmaceutical products has been sought after as a means of screening, optimizing, and monitoring dosage forms. With solid oral dosage forms, it most frequently starts with an attempt to link the results of an *in vitro* release test and *in vivo* pharmacokinetic studies. Through exploring the association or relationship between *in vitro* dissolution/release and *in vivo* absorption data, an *in vitro–in vivo* relationship (IVIVR) may be identified with a drug product. Such a relationship is often qualitative or semi-quantitative in nature (e.g., rank order). When a predictive relationship or model is established, and validated between differences in the *in vitro* dissolution rate, and known differences in *in vivo* absorption, it is designated as *in vitro–in vivo* correlation (IVIVC).

In vitro–in vivo correlations (IVIVC) of oral solid products have received considerable attention from the industry, regulatory agencies, and academia over the past decade, particularly since the publication of the FDA Guidance of dissolution testing of immediate-release (IR), and IVIVC of extended-release (ER) dosage forms in 1997,[1,2] and subsequent note for guidance issued by the European regulatory authorities, EMEA.[3,4] As a result, there has been increased confidence and success in using *in vitro* tests to evaluate or predict *in vivo* performance of solid drug product, especially ER dosage forms, based on

IVIVC.[5,6,7,8,9,10,11,12] With an established IVIVC, the dissolution data can be used not only as a quality control tool, but also for guiding and optimizing product development, setting meaningful specifications, and serving as a surrogate for bioavailability studies. This chapter will discuss basic principles, methodology, and evaluation utilized in establishing IVIVC models, as well as applications of IVIVC in developing solid dosage forms with a primary focus on ER products. Additional topics addressed include the importance of understanding drug, dosage form, and their *in vitro* and *in vivo* behaviors, as related to the strategy and approach of exploring and developing an IVIVC.

17.1.1 *In Vitro–In Vivo* Correlation (IVIVC)

In vitro–in vivo correlation (IVIVC) is defined by the USP and FDA respectively as follows:[1,13]

USP: The establishment of a relationship between a biological property or a parameter derived from a biological property produced by a dosage form, and a physicochemical characteristic of the same dosage form.

FDA: A predictive mathematical model describing the relationship between an *in vitro* property (usually the extent or rate of drug release), and a relevant *in vivo* response (e.g., plasma concentration or amount of drug absorbed).

Evaluation of *in vitro–in vivo* correlations by different levels was first proposed for oral dosage forms in the

Developing Solid Oral Dosage Forms: Pharmaceutical Theory and Practice
ISBN: 978-0-444-53242-8

USPs Information Chapter <1088>,[14] and was later adopted globally. Presently, IVIVC is categorized by the FDA into levels A, B, C, and Multiple C, depending upon the type of data used to establish the relationship, and the ability of the correlation to predict the complete plasma profile of a dosage form.[2]

- **Level A**: a predictive mathematical model for the relationship between the entire *in vitro* release time course, and the entire *in vivo* response time course, e.g., the time course of plasma drug concentration or amount of drug absorbed.
- **Level B**: a predictive mathematical model for the relationship between summary parameters that characterize the *in vitro* and *in vivo* time courses, e.g., models that relate the mean *in vitro* dissolution time to the mean *in vivo* dissolution time or to mean residence time *in vivo*.
- **Level C**: a predictive mathematical model for the relationship between the amount dissolved *in vitro* at a particular time (e.g., Q_{60}) or the time required for dissolution of a fixed amount (e.g., $t_{50\%}$), and a summary parameter that characterizes the *in vivo* time course (e.g., C_{max} or AUC).
- **Multiple Level C**: predictive mathematical models for the relationships between the amount dissolved at several time points of the product, and one or several pharmacokinetic parameters of interest.

Level A is the most informative, and most useful from a regulatory perspective, in that it represents a point-to-point relationship between *in vitro* release and *in vivo* release/absorption from the dosage form. It can be used to predict the entire *in vivo* time course from the *in vitro* data. Multiple Level C is also useful, as it provides the *in vitro* release profile of a dosage form with biological meaning. Level C can be useful in the early stages of product development or setting meaningful specification, although it does not reflect the complete shape of the plasma concentration–time curve. Level B utilizes the principles of statistical moment analysis. However, it is least useful for regulatory applications, because different *in vitro* or *in vivo* profiles may produce similar mean time values.

17.1.2 IVIVC and Product Development

The value of IVIVC in product development has been recognized since the early 1960s. Exploring *in vitro–in vivo* associations or correlations is very useful in guiding formulation and process development. A validated IVIVC can facilitate formulation changes, process scale-up, setting meaningful dissolution specifications, and support the use of dissolution as a surrogate for *in vivo*

studies, since IVIVC provides a biological meaning to the results of the *in vitro* test.[2] Thus, availability of a well-defined, predictive IVIVC of high quality can result in a significant positive impact on product quality, and reduced regulatory burden.

The approaches and challenges of developing IVIVC have undergone extensive discussions and debates since the 1980s.[15,16,17,18,19,20] In general, there is increased uncertainty associated with developing an IVIVC for IR oral dosage forms, because the *in vivo* apparent drug absorption is often a function of a multitude of variables, many of which are difficult to isolate or mimic *in vitro*. For example, an IVIVC for IR dosage forms of highly water-soluble drugs (BCS classes I and III) may not be possible,[2] because gastric emptying or membrane permeation is usually the rate-limiting step. Compared to IR products, an IVIVC is more amenable to ER dosage forms where drug release is rate-limiting in the absorption process. With ER products a patient is often exposed to specific plasma levels over an extended period of time (e.g., up to 24 hours); bio-relevant *in vitro* methods are desired to assure consistent *in vivo* performance. Hence, the FDA has recommended investigation of the possibility of an IVIVC in the development of ER dosage forms.[2]

17.2 DEVELOPMENT AND ASSESSMENT OF AN IVIVC

The FDA guidance on IVIVC of ER oral dosage forms issued in 1997[2] provides a comprehensive scientific framework and regulatory guideline to IVIVC model development, evaluation, and applications. In general, establishing an IVIVC involves:

1. study design;
2. model building; and
3. model validation based on appropriate statistical assessment.

17.2.1 Study Design and General Considerations

Development of an IVIVC requires *in vitro* and *in vivo* data for formulations with varying *in vitro* release rates, and corresponding *in vivo* differences. These data may come from studies at early or late stages of product development, such as bioavailability studies conducted in the formulation screening stage or an *in vivo* study specifically designed to explore IVIVC.[21,11,22] The *in vitro* release rates, as measured by percent dissolved for each formulation studied, should differ adequately (e.g., by 10%).[2]

To obtain useful data for establishing an IVIVC, a discriminating dissolution methodology is essential. Based on the FDA guidance,[2] in vitro data are preferably generated in an aqueous medium using USP Apparatus I (basket) or II (paddle), operating within an appropriate range of rotation speeds (e.g., 50–100 rpm). In other cases, USP Apparatus III (reciprocating cylinder) or IV (flow through cell) may also be used. Generally, any in vitro test method may be used to obtain the dissolution characteristics of the dosage forms, as long as it is shown to be predictive of in vivo performance. The dissolution profiles of at least 12 individual dosage units should be determined for IVIVC purposes. The coefficient of variation (CV) for the mean dissolution profiles of a single batch should be less than 10%.

According to the FDA guidance,[2] bioavailability studies for IVIVC development should be performed in humans with enough subjects to adequately characterize the absorption profiles of the drug products. Although crossover studies are preferred, parallel studies or cross-study analyses are also acceptable. The latter may involve normalization with a common reference treatment. The reference product in developing an IVIVC may be an intravenous solution, an aqueous oral solution or an immediate-release product of the drug. In addition, IVIVCs are usually developed in the fasted state. When a drug is not tolerated in the fasted state, studies may be conducted in the fed state.

17.2.2 IVIVC Modeling

The principles and methodologies of IVIVC modeling and assessment have been extensively addressed and reviewed in the literature.[23,24,25] Developing an IVIVC model begins with understanding the following mathematical principles for characterizing in vivo drug release/absorption profiles or parameters associated with different types of IVIVC models.

Convolution and Deconvolution Techniques Used in Level A Correlation

Convolution and deconvolution methods are essential tools for establishing a Level A IVIVC. Convolution is a model-independent technique used in linear system analysis. Based on the superposition principle in a linear time-invariant system, a response, $C(t)$, to an arbitrary input, $f(t)$, of the system can be obtained using the following convolution integral:[26]

$$C(t) = f(t) * C_\delta(t) = \int_0^\infty C_\delta(t - \tau)f(\tau)d\tau \quad (17.1)$$

$C_\delta(t)$ is the unit impulse response that defines the characteristic of the system. It is the response of the system to an instantaneous unit input, usually attainable from an IV bolus or oral solution. By the same principle, $f(t)$ can be obtained by deconvolution, the inverse operation of convolution. Their applications in IVIVC are illustrated in Figure 17.1, and representative systems are provided in Table 17.1. The definition of a system is flexible, and is determined by the nature of the time functions involved.[27] Depending on the specific $C_\delta(t)$, and input responses used to define a system, $f(t)$ obtained by deconvolution in IVIVC may represent the dissolution process, absorption process or the two processes combined.

In exploring IVIVC models, Level A correlation is usually estimated by a two-stage procedure, i.e., deconvolution followed by correlating the fraction dissolved in vitro with the fraction released or absorbed in vivo. It may also be evaluated via a single-stage procedure, i.e., convolution followed by comparison of the observed with predicted plasma profiles. According to Equation 17.1, the in vitro drug release and the in vivo input (release/absorption) estimated by deconvolution of the unit impulse response with the observed plasma data are either directly superimposable or may be made to be superimposable by the use of a scaling factor when a 1:1 IVIVC exists. Similarly, the plasma concentration profile observed following oral administration should be in good agreement with that obtained by convolution of the unit impulse response with in vitro release data if there is a Level A IVIVC.

General solution

The exact solution of convolution or deconvolution can be obtained by operation of Laplace transforms if each functional form is defined:

$$L\{C(t)\} = L\{(C_\delta * f)(t)\} = L\{C_\delta(t)\}L\{f(t)\} \quad (17.2)$$

$$f(t) = L^{-1}\{\bar{f}(s)\} = L^{-1}\left\{\frac{\bar{c}(s)}{\bar{c}_\delta(s)}\right\} \quad (17.3)$$

L and L^{-1} denote the Laplace transform, and inverse Laplace transform, respectively. Deconvolution methods include explicit (e.g., numerical point-area and midpoint methods, least squares curve fitting using polyexponential, polynomial, and spline functions), and implicit methods (e.g., prescribed function or deconvolution via convolution).[28,29,30,31,32,33,34,35,36,37,38,39]

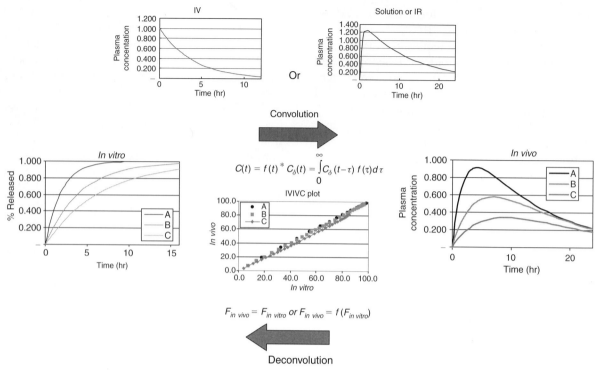

FIGURE 17.1   Illustration of convolution and deconvolution in IVIVC development

TABLE 17.1   Illustration of system definitions for oral administration

Case	Unit impulse response $C_\delta(t)$	Input response $C(t)$	Input function $f(t)$
I	Plasma levels from iv bolus	Plasma levels from oral solution	Absorption in GI
II	Plasma levels from iv bolus	Plasma levels from oral solid dosage form	Dissolution and absorption in GI
III	Plasma levels from oral solution (or IR dosage form as an approximation)	Plasma levels from oral solid dosage form	Dissolution in GI

Since the disposition of most drugs can be described by polyexponentials:

$$C_\delta(t) = \sum_{i=1}^{n} A_i e^{-\alpha_i t} \qquad (17.4)$$

The *in vivo* input function $f(t)$ can be obtained using Equation 17.3. For example, in the case of single-exponential disposition ($n = 1$), $C_\delta(t) = A_1 e^{-\alpha_1 t}$, and hence, $f(t)$, the input rate, is given by:[39]

$$f(t) = \frac{[C'(t) + \alpha_1 C(t)]}{A_1} \qquad (17.5)$$

The amount of drug absorbed from time 0 to t, $X_a(t)$, is then obtained by integration:

$$X_a(t) = \int_0^t f(t) dt = \frac{[C(t) + \alpha_1 \int_0^t C(t) dt]}{A_1} \qquad (17.6)$$

In cases where $C(t)$ or $f(t)$ cannot be fitted to an explicit function, numerical methods are used to deal with the raw data. In actual applications, nonlinear regression software can be used, e.g., WinNonlin by Pharsight Corporation. Recently, the company released an add-on IVIVC toolkit which expands on WinNonlin's deconvolution capabilities by adding convolution and IVIVC specific analysis. PDx-IVIVC is another software web application hosted by GloboMax. Users can access the application via the Internet. MS Excel has also been shown to be a useful tool for IVIVC applications.[40]

Model-dependent deconvolution

Two commonly used deconvolution methods for estimating the apparent *in vivo* drug absorption profiles following oral administration of a dosage form are Wagner–Nelson, and Loo–Riegelman methods.[41] These are model-dependent approaches based on mass balance. The Wagner–Nelson equation is derived from a one-compartment model and the mass balance, $X_a = X_t + X_e$, where X_a, X_t, and X_e are amounts of drug absorbed, in the "body," and eliminated at time t, respectively. By derivation, the amount of drug absorbed up to time T, $(X_a)_T$, is given by: $(X_a)_T = VC_T + kV \int_0^T C t dt$, where V is the volume of the central compartment, C_T is concentration of drug in the central compartment at time T, and k is the first-order elimination rate constant. In the study of IVIVC, this is often expressed in terms of fraction (F) of the dose (D) absorbed for comparison with fraction released *in vitro*:

$$F_a(T) = \frac{(X_a)_T}{(X_a)\infty} = \frac{C + k \int_0^T C t dt}{k \int_0^\infty C t dt} \quad (17.7)$$

$F_a(T)$ or FD is the fraction of the bioavailable drug absorbed at time T. It should be noted that Equation 17.7 is the same as Equation 16.6. Therefore, the Wagner–Nelson method represents a special case of deconvolution with single-exponential disposition. Because Equation 17.7 may be applied to extravascular data without intravenous data, it is frequently used in IVIVC modeling. In the absence of intravenous data, the apparent *in vivo* fractional absorption profile can be estimated by using the terminal phase elimination rate constant, k, and partial areas under the plasma concentration curve according to Equation 17.7. However, it should be pointed out that:

1. the k value should be derived from the true elimination phase, which may be difficult for drugs with prolonged absorption phase and/or long half life; and
2. only apparent absorption is estimated using this method.

The approximate equation used in absorption analysis for the two-compartment model was first published by Loo and Riegelman in 1968.[42] Wagner published an Exact Loo–Riegelman method for a multi-compartment model in 1983.[43] It is a general equation for absorption analysis of one- to three-compartment models, and requires IV data for the calculation of absorption profiles. For biexponential disposition, mass balance leads to: $(X_a)_T = X_c + X_p + X_e$, where X_c and X_p are amounts of drug in the central and peripheral compartments at time T, respectively. By derivation,[43] $(X_a)_T$ can be determined:

$$\frac{(X_a)_T}{Vc} = C_T + k_{10} \int_0^T C_t dt + k_{12} e^{-k_{21}T} \int_0^T C_t e^{k_{21}t} dt \quad (17.8)$$

Here k_{12}, k_{21}, and k_{10} are the microconstants that define the rates of transport between compartments. On the basis of mass balance, $(X_a)_T = X_c + X_{p1} + X_{p2} + X_e$, a similar equation can be derived for triexponential disposition. The corresponding Exact Loo–Riegelman equations are given as:

$$\frac{(X_a)_T}{Vc} = C_T + k_{10} \int_0^T C_t dt + k_{12} e^{-k_{21}T}$$
$$\int_0^T C_t e^{k_{21}t} dt + k_{13} e^{-k_{31}T} \int_0^T C_t e^{k_{31}t} dt \quad (17.9)$$

Equations 17.8 and 17.9 require prior intravenous data for application. It can be shown that the Loo–Riegelman method is also a special case of deconvolution, where *in vivo* disposition is described by two or three exponentials.[39] The theoretical and practical aspects of absorption analysis using model-dependent approaches have been thoroughly discussed by Wagner.[41]

Mean Time Parameters Used in Level B Correlation

Level B correlation is based on correlating mean time parameters that characterize the *in vitro* and *in vivo* time courses, e.g., the *in vitro* or *in vivo* mean dissolution time (MDT), and *in vivo* mean residence time (*MRT*). Mean time parameters have commonly been utilized in pharmacokinetic studies, and used to describe *in vitro* release. They are useful in studying specific models, as well as less differentiated, more general system models. Many important concepts, definitions, and computations on this subject have been thoroughly discussed by Veng-Pedersen[44] and Podczeck.[45]

In vivo *parameters*

By definition, *MRT* is the average total time the drug molecule spends in the introduced kinetic space. It depends on the site of input, and the site of elimination. When the elimination of the molecule follows first-order kinetics, its *MRT* can be expressed by:[44]

$$MRT = \frac{\int_0^\infty t C(t) dt}{\int_0^\infty C(t) dt} = \frac{AUMC}{AUC} \quad (17.10)$$

AUMC is the area under the moment curve. Estimates for *MRT* can be calculated by fitting $C(t)$ to a polyexponential equation followed by integration or by using trapezoidal rules.

For non-instantaneous input into a kinetic space, such as oral absorption, the *MRT* estimated from extravascular data includes a contribution of the mean transit time for input, known as mean absorption time (MAT, mean arrival time or mean input time).[44] The MAT of drug molecules represents the average time taken to arrive in that space, and it can be estimated as:

$$MAT = \frac{\int_0^\infty t f_{in}(t) dt}{\int_0^\infty f_{in}(t) dt} = \frac{AUMC}{AUC} \qquad (17.11)$$

Here $f_{in}(t)$ denotes an arbitrary rate of input into the kinetic space. For oral delivery, the MAT can be determined according to the equation:

$$MAT = MRT_{po} - MRT_{iv} \qquad (17.12)$$

The MAT term thus obtained represents the mean transit time involved in an apparent absorption process in the GI tract. When the formulation contains solid drug, the MAT includes in vivo dissolution, as well as absorption. If data of the same drug given in solution state are available, the in vivo mean dissolution time (MDT) can be estimated by:

$$MDT_{solid} = MAT_{solid} - MAT_{soln} = MRT_{solid} - MRT_{soln} \qquad (17.13)$$

In vitro parameters

The measured amount of drug substance in a cumulative release profile can be considered as a probability that describes the time of residence of the drug substance in the dosage form. Therefore, a dissolution profile may be regarded as a distribution function of the residence times of each drug molecule in the formulation.[45] By definition, the mean dissolution time (MDT) is the arithmetic mean value of any dissolution profile. If the amount of the drug remaining in the formulation is plotted as a function of time, the arithmetic mean value of the residence profile is the mean residence time (MRT) of the drug molecules in the dosage form.

The techniques that are used to calculate MDT or MRT can be divided into model-independent (e.g., pragmatic plane geometry and prospective area), and model-dependent methods (e.g., polyexponential, Weibull, and overlapping parabolic integration).[45] In general, model-independent approaches are used when release kinetics are unknown. These methods are based on area calculations from the amount released at various times. The following simple method is often used to determine the MDT and MRT using trapezoidal rules:[45]

$$MDT = \frac{\int_0^\infty (M_{max} - M(t)) dt}{M_{max}} = \frac{ABC}{M_{max}} \qquad (17.14)$$

$$MRT = \frac{\int_0^\infty t A(t) dt}{\int_0^\infty A(t) dt} \qquad (17.15)$$

ABC is the area between the drug dissolution curve and its asymptote. $A(t)$ is the amount of drug remaining in the dosage form at time t. $M(t)$ and M_{max} are the amount of drug released at time t, and the maximal amount released, respectively. The model-dependent methods are based on the derived parameters of functions that describe the release profiles. It should be noted that one important source of errors in calculations comes from the often incomplete release. The calculation of the moments in such cases is based on the maximum drug release. For systems that have a complete drug release, the size of errors depends on the number of data points, and the curve shape.[45]

Summary Parameters Used in Level C Correlation

The extent and rate of drug release from a dosage form are often characterized by one or more of the single measurements (e.g., Q_{60}, $t_{50\%}$, or $t_{85\%}$), particularly when there are not enough data points available to define the time functions of the profiles or there are simply no suitable models that describe the dissolution curves. These parameters are most often obtained either directly from the dissolution measurements or by interpolation. Although they do not adequately characterize the whole dissolution process, they are utilized both in quality control in vitro, and are commonly used in Level C correlation studies. The in vivo parameters used to correlate with the in vitro parameters are bioavailability parameters reflecting the rate and extent of absorption (e.g., AUC, T_{max}, and C_{max}).

Establishment of a Level A IVIVC Model

Establishing an IVIVC model requires in vitro data from formulations with different release rates (e.g., fast, medium, and slow) and a discriminating in vitro test methodology. The corresponding in vivo response can be plasma concentrations or the amount of drug released and/or absorbed in vivo. The latter is obtained from the observed plasma concentration–time curve by deconvolution. There are advantages and disadvantages for either type of response variable. When plasma concentration is used as a response variable (single-stage approach), the link between the *in vitro* release profile with the *in vivo* plasma concentration profile has clear clinical relevance, because many pharmacokinetic parameters, such as C_{max}, T_{max}, and AUC, are directly derived from the plasma concentration–time profile. Using the amount of drug released/absorbed as a response variable (two-stage approach) is intuitively straightforward, because the *in vitro* and *in vivo* parameters are directly compared.

Two-stage approach

A deconvolution-based IVIVC model is established using a two-stage approach that involves estimation of the *in vivo* release/absorption profile from plasma concentration–time data using an appropriate deconvolution technique (e.g., Wagner–Nelson, numerical deconvolution) for each formulation. Subsequently, the calculated *in vivo* percentage absorbed or released is correlated with the percentage released *in vitro*, as illustrated in Figure 17.2 using a basic linear model with intercept (a) and slope (b):

$$(\% \text{ absorbed})_{in\ vivo} = a + b\ (\% \text{ released})_{in\ vitro} \quad (17.16)$$

A slope closer to 1 indicates a 1:1 correlation, and a negative intercept implies that the *in vivo* process lags behind the *in vitro* dissolution. A positive intercept has

no clear physiological meaning. It can be a result of relatively high variability or curvature at the early time points. When the *in vitro* data are not in the same time scale as the *in vivo* absorption, it is usually necessary to incorporate a scaling factor, such as time-shifting and time-scaling parameters, within the model. Nonlinear models, while uncommon, may also be appropriate.[46] The two-stage approach is the most frequently used in building IVIVC models.

Single-stage approach

An alternative modeling approach based on convolution can be utilized to directly predict the time course of plasma concentrations using Equation 17.1 in a single step.[47] Based on the assumption of equal or similar release rates between *in vitro* and *in vivo*, the input rate, *f(t)*, is modeled as a function of the *in vitro* release data, with or without time scaling to predict the *in vivo* plasma profiles by convolution with the dose-normalized plasma data from an IV or IR reference dose. The IVIVC is assessed and validated by statistically comparing the predicted with the observed plasma levels. This convolution-based modeling approach focuses on the ability to predict measured quantities, rather than the indirectly estimated "*in vivo*" fraction absorbed and/or released. Thus, the results are more readily evaluated in terms of the effect of *in vitro* release on *in vivo* performances, e.g., AUC, C_{max}, and duration above minimum effective concentrations (*MEC*). For instance, in using this approach

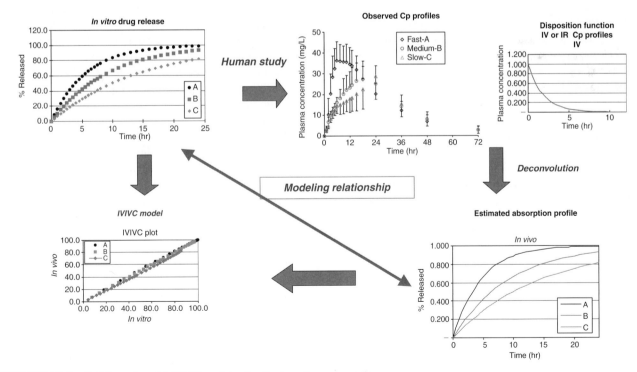

FIGURE 17.2 Building a Level A IVIVC model using the two-stage approach

to estimate the plasma concentrations from the *in vitro* data, a polyexponential unit impulse response with lag time could be used in the model as follows:

$$C_\delta(t) = \sum_{i=1}^{nex} A_i * e^{-a_{(i)}(t-t_{lag})} \qquad (17.17)$$

Here, "*nex*" is the number of exponential terms in the model, t_{lag} is the absorption lag time, and C_t is the plasma concentration at time t. The input rate may be modeled as a function of the *in vitro* cumulative amount dissolved. For example, Veng-Pedersen et al. reported a scaled convolution-based IVIVC approach by which the dissolution rate curve was first obtained via differentiation of a monotonic quadratic spline fitted to the dissolution data. Using time and magnitude scaling, the dissolution curve was then mapped into a drug concentration curve via a convolution by a single exponential, and the estimated unit impulse response function. The model was tested by cross-validation, and demonstrated to be predictive of the systemic drug concentration profiles from the *in vitro* release data using four different tablet formulations of carbamazepine.[48]

It should be noted that the single-stage approach is based on the assumption of a linear, time-invariant relationship between input (drug release) and plasma concentrations. Multiple formulations with different release rates are usually used in establishing an IVIVC. If a significant fraction of the dose of the slow releasing formulations is released beyond the site(s) of drug absorption (i.e., truncated absorption), overestimation of plasma concentrations can occur, because Equation 17.1 predicts the same dose-normalized AUC as the reference dose used to estimate $C_\delta(t)$.[47] To address the potential discrepancies between *in vitro* and *in vivo* release/absorption, Gillespie proposed an extended convolution-based IVIVC model using a function relating cumulative amounts released or release rate *in vitro* (x_{vitro}) to that *in vivo*, (x_{vivo}), $x_{vivo} = f(x_{vitro})$. Thus, plasma concentrations of multiple ER formulations can be more accurately predicted by substituting $f(t)$ with x_{vivo} in Equation 17.1 if there is an IVIVC. Selection of a specific functional form of x_{vivo} can be based on a mechanistic understanding of the *in vitro–in vivo* relationship or semi-empirically based on the goodness of model fitting. Certain plausible relationships include linear, nonlinear or time-variant functions, linear or nonlinear timescaling for taking into account the effects of lag time, truncated absorption or saturable presystemic metabolism.[47,49] For ER systems, the apparent absorption *in vivo* is limited by drug release from the dosage form of which the kinetics are determined by the system design. In many cases, the release kinetics can be described by one of the following models, zero-order,

first-order, square-root of time or one of Peppas's exponent models.[50] Therefore, the parametric function, $C(t)$, describing the plasma concentrations of an ER dosage form can be defined via convolution of $C_\delta(t)$ with the input, $f(t)$, prescribed from the *in vitro* model according to Equation 17.1. For instance, the functional form of $C(t)$ can first be obtained by convolution of a prescribed function of input (e.g., first-order) with a known unit impulse response. The unknown parameters remaining in the $C(t)$ equation are those from the prescribed input function, $f(t)$, which can then be solved by fitting the $C(t)$ equation to the observed plasma concentrations. The resulting $f(t)$ is compared with the observed *in vitro* data to evaluate the IVIVC. This approach is also known as deconvolution through convolution.

In predicting $C(t)$ by convolution, data from an IV or oral solution is desirable because it provides an estimate of $C_\delta(t)$ independent of the ER data. However, such a reference dose is not always available, particularly for compounds having low aqueous solubility. Nevertheless, estimation of $C(t)$ by convolution for evaluation of IVIVC is still possible using only data from ER formulations.[49] In such cases, the prescribed parametric functional forms of both $C_\delta(t)$ and $f(t)$ can be mechanistically or empirically selected, and substituted into Equation 17.1. The parameters of $C_\delta(t)$ are then estimated by fitting the overall convolution model to the plasma concentrations of ER formulations. Predictive performance of the IVIVC is evaluated by comparing the predicted and observed results. It should be pointed out that the ability of the model to predict changes of the *in vivo* plasma concentrations with varying release rates should be validated by separately or simultaneously fitting the data from multiple formulations. By doing so, a $C_\delta(t)$ function can be reliably defined. Thus, one of the most critical requirements of this approach is to use at least two ER formulations with different release rates in the assessment of IVIVC.[49]

While the use of the two-stage procedure is more widespread, the convolution approach has gained increased interest. O'Hara et al. compared odds and identity models that include a convolution step using data sets of two different products, and a nonlinear mixed-effects model fitting software to circumvent the unstable deconvolution problem of the two-stage approach.[51] Gaynor et al. used a simulation study to show that the convolution modeling approach produces more accurate results in predicting the observed plasma concentration–time profile.[52]

Establishment of a Level C IVIVC Model

Building a Level C IVIVC model is rather straightforward. It involves correlating the amount dissolved at various time points with C_{max}, AUC or other suitable bioavailability parameters. Data from at least three formulations of different dissolution rates are required for establishing a linear or nonlinear relationship between *in vitro* and *in vivo* parameters, because each data point of the correlation plot corresponds to only one formulation. A single point Level C correlation may facilitate formulation development or allow a dissolution specification to be set at the specified time point. The information is generally insufficient for justifying a biowaiver. A multiple point Level C correlation may be useful to support a biowaiver if the correlation has been established over the entire dissolution profile with one or more bioavailability parameters of interest. A relationship should be demonstrated at each time point with the same parameter, such that the effect on the *in vivo* performance of any change in dissolution can be assessed. When such a multiple Level C correlation is achievable, the development of a Level A correlation is often likely. A multiple Level C correlation should be based on at least three dissolution time points covering the early, middle, and late stages of the dissolution profile.[2]

17.2.3 Evaluation of a Correlation

To ensure a useful and reliable Level A IVIVC, the FDA guidance requires that the model should be demonstrated consistently with two or more formulations with different release rates. Therefore, the first important step in evaluating the appropriateness of the model is to test whether a single correlation fits all tested formulations. One of the statistical assessment approaches is to compare the fit of a reduced model, where all tested formulations are fitted to a single correlation line with that of a full model where each formulation is fitted to a different correlation line.[24] If both models fit well, the IVIVC is considered validated. If the full model fits well, but the reduced model does not, or if the full model is statistically different from the reduced model at a significance level of 0.05, the IVIVC becomes formulation dependent, and therefore is invalid. It is noted that the time scaling factor, if used, should also be the same for all formulations. Different time scales for each formulation indicate absence of an IVIVC.[2]

Following the establishment of a Level A IVIVC model, it is necessary to demonstrate that prediction of *in vivo* performance from the *in vitro* dissolution characteristics is accurate and consistent. The FDA guidance suggests evaluating the goodness of fit by measuring the prediction error (PE), i.e., differences between observed and predicted values over a range of *in vitro* release rates. As illustrated in Figure 17.3, determination of PE involves calculation of the *in vivo* absorption (input) profiles from the *in vitro* data using the established IVIVC model, followed by

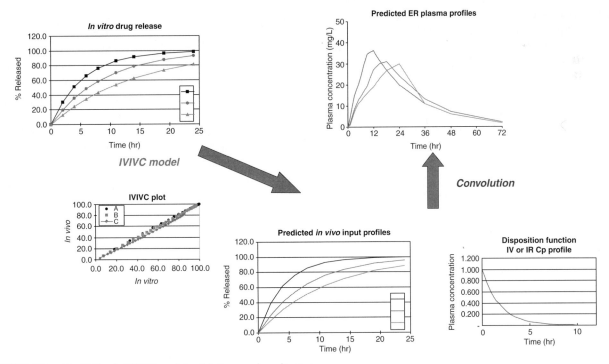

FIGURE 17.3   Prediction in IVIVC model validations and applications

prediction of the corresponding plasma concentration profiles via convolution. The guidance further elaborates approaches to validate the model internally and externally. The internal validation can be accomplished through measuring PE using data from the same study used to develop the IVIVC. The internal PE evaluates how well the model describes the data used to develop the IVIVC. It could be adopted for cases where the IVIVC was derived using two or more formulations with different release rates, provided the drug is not considered a narrow therapeutic index drug. The external validation approach requires data set that was not used in the development of the IVIVC, such as formulations with different release rates, formulations with minor manufacturing process changes or formulations from a different manufacturing batch obtained from a different study. External validation is desirable and affords greater "confidence" in the model.

The criteria used in the FDA guidance on IVIVC are as follows: for predicted C_{max} and AUC, the mean absolute percent prediction error (% PE) should not exceed 10%, and the PE for individual formulations should not exceed 15%. A PE of 10% to 20% indicates inconclusive predictability, and illustrates the need for further study using additional data sets. For drugs with narrow therapeutic index, external validation is required despite acceptable internal validation, whereas internal validation is usually sufficient with non-narrow therapeutic index drugs. In general, the less data available for initial IVIVC development and evaluation of predictability, the more additional data may be needed to define completely the IVIVCs predictability. Some combination of three or more formulations with different release rates is considered optimal.[2]

For Level C correlations, assessment of the predictability will depend on the type of application for which the correlation is to be used. These methods and criteria are the same as those for a Level A correlation.

17.3 CONSIDERATIONS IN IVIVC DEVELOPMENT

Defining a quantitative and reliable relationship between *in vitro* drug release and *in vivo* absorption is highly desired for rational development, optimization, and evaluation of solid dosage forms and manufacturing process. A validated IVIVC can significantly: (1) increase the development efficiency by reducing the time and resources required for formulation and process development, scale-up, and optimization; (2) ensure product quality by setting meaningful specifications; and (3) reduce regulatory burdens by using an *in vitro* test as a surrogate for an *in vivo* bioavailability study required for certain post-approval changes. Therefore, exploring and developing an IVIVC where possible should be an important part of solid oral product development.

Since the early 1990s, extensive colloquiums and research publications have primarily focused on development methodology, modeling, evaluation, and applications of IVIVC, most of which are based on the premise of availability of *in vitro* and *in vivo* information appropriate for establishing an IVIVC. However, it should be emphasized that obtaining suitable *in vitro* and *in vivo* data is not a given, and IVIVC development is more than modeling and statistical assessments. To achieve an IVIVC, at least two formulations that differ in *in vivo* and *in vitro* performance should be available. In fact, many failed attempts in achieving an IVIVC for solid products can usually be attributed to a lack of a predictive *in vitro* test or an *in vivo* difference among test formulations. Thus, it is crucial to understand the importance of the drug's physico-chemical and biological properties, delivery technology, formulation design, *in vitro* test methodology, and their interrelationship with the gastrointestinal tract (GIT) in developing an IVIVC and associated strategy.

17.3.1 *In Vivo* Absorption Versus *In Vitro* Test Considerations

In developing an IVIVC, the *in vitro* parameters commonly utilized are the amounts of drug released that can be determined with precision under controlled conditions. These are a function of both drug and dosage form characteristics, and the test methodologies. The *in vivo* response is usually dissolution and absorption estimated from availability of the drug in systemic circulation that typically has high variability. It is a function of a multitude of physico-chemical, biological, physiological variables, formulation, and their interactions. For test formulations that exhibit varying apparent *in vivo* absorption characteristics, the most critical element in establishing an IVIVC is the ability of *in vitro* tests to correlate quantitatively with *in vivo* performance. To assess the challenges and opportunities of developing a biorelevant or meaningful *in vitro* test, it is imperative to first understand the absorption characteristics and complexity of the drug substance and dosage forms of interest in the GI tract.

Apparent Drug Absorption from the GI Tract

The *in vivo* drug release and subsequent absorption from a solid product, particularly a modified-release dosage form, takes place in one of the most complex environments where the interplay of the GI tract with the dosage form, as well as with intra-lumenally released drug, is highly dynamic. The process is known to be influenced by: (1) drug properties (solubility, ionization, stability, solid phase, lipophilicity, permeability, surface area, wetting property, etc.); (2) dosage form design (dose, release mechanism, composition, type and size of dose unit, sensitivity to shear force, drug release location or duration, etc.); and (3) GI physiology and biology (motility, residence time, food, lumen contents, fluid volume, transport pathways and mechanism, enterohepatic recycling, permeability, surface area, metabolism, transporters, microflora, etc.). This type of information is highly valuable in anticipating and evaluating *in vitro* and *in vivo* behavior of the drug molecule and dosage form as related to IVIVC. Detailed information on drug absorption can be found in Chapters 11–12.

In Vitro Test Method

Among various *in vitro* physico-chemical tests, dissolution testing is one of the most important tools for product quality assessment, process control, and for assuring sameness after making formulation/process changes. While different dissolution tests have been applied to determine drug release, including the commonly used compendial methods (e.g., basket, paddle or reciprocating cylinder), the dissolution rate of a specific dosage form is, in many cases, an arbitrary parameter that often varies with the test methodology, and offers little relevance to *in vivo* performance.[24,55] Part of the reason is that none of the existing *in vitro* methods represents or mimics the dynamic and complex *in vivo* conditions and the wide range of variables involved in the drug absorption from solid dosage forms in the GI tract.

Over the years, the exploration and development of various tests have been carried out in an attempt to match *in vivo* data and/or to simulate specific aspects of the GI condition. These studies can be divided into three broad categories, listed in Table 17.2. The common approach used in these studies is to match *in vivo* data by adjusting the *in vitro* differentiation and release rate of different test formulations through altering hydrodynamics, mixing, creating shear force, etc.[6] It should be noted that most tests are static, and only capable of imitating one or two aspects of

physiological conditions. For example, some test methods are focused on test medium and/or apparatus variables. Other models based on multiple compartments or vessels are designed to simulate successive dynamic processes occurring in the GI tract. The most complicated *in vitro* model is a multicompartment dynamic computer-controlled system designed to simulate the human stomach and small intestine (TIM-1), and large intestine (TIM-2), respectively.[53,54] The system is intended for gathering information about the effects of various gastrointestinal conditions on the biopharmaceutical behavior of drug and delivery systems. However, setting up experiments and generating data are time-consuming and extremely labor intensive. It is unsuitable for routine product quality control. In addition, its utility and application in IVIVC development remain to be proven.

In summary, the state-of-the-art has yet to allow development of a universal predictive model independent of drug molecule and dosage form characteristics, because no *in vitro* test system can reproduce the complex dynamic processes, as well as physiological and biological conditions, *in vivo*.[6,55] Nevertheless, it remains possible to develop a predictive test when *in vivo* drug release is the dominant controlling factor in the rate of appearance of the drug in the blood. Furthermore, continued pursuit of such a test not only will potentially bring considerable benefit to product development and control, but also will help improve scientific understanding of *in vitro* and *in vivo* drug release. Therefore, an IVIVC should be developed on a case-by-case basis.

17.3.2 Drug and Formulation Considerations

The essential conditions for developing an IVIVC include: (1) the apparent *in vivo* absorption is dissolution rate limited; (2) *in vitro* dissolution and/or erosion is the critical dosage form attribute; (3) test formulations exhibit different *in vivo* performance; and (4) the *in vitro* test is discriminating (IVIVR) and/or predictive (IVIVC). When these conditions are met, IVIVC is deemed feasible. Through integrating knowledge of drug properties, delivery technology, formulation, and biopharmaceutics, it is possible to design proper studies for exploring IVIVC, to analyze expected or unexpected results, and to refine experiments when necessary.

Immediate-release (IR) Dosage Forms

An IVIVC is more difficult to achieve for IR dosage forms. With rapid drug release, apparent drug absorption of the dosage form usually occurs in the upper

TABLE 17.2   Types of *in vitro* drug release tests for IVIVC development

Type	Examples	Test variables	Reference
Standard pharmacopoeial methods	USP I, II, III or IV	Hydrodynamics; agitation; pH; ionic strength; surfactant; enzyme; use of fat, milk; etc.	56, 57, 58, 59, 60, 61, 62
Modified standard methods	USP II + polystyrene beads USP II + stationary basket USP II + two-phase Milk/fat as test medium FeSSIF/FaSSIF as test medium *Ex-vivo* gastrointestinal fluid	Hydrodynamics; shear stress; mechanical attrition; mixing; pH; test medium; release vs. dissolution; etc.	62, 63, 64, 65, 66, 67, 68, 69, 70, 71, 72, 73, 74
New models	Rotating dialysis cell Flow-through cell drop method TNO (Dynamic *in vitro* GI models) Dynamic multi-compartment	pH; food; mixing; motility; transit; secretion; microflora; etc.	75, 76, 77, 78, 79, 80, 81, 82

[56]Humbert, et al. (1994). *In vitro–in vivo* correlation of a modified-release oral form of ketotifen: *In vitro* dissolution rate specification. J. Pharm. Sci. 83(2), 131–136.

[57]Qiu, Y., Cheskin, H., Briskin, J. & Engh, K. (1997). Sustained-release hydrophilic matrix tablets of zileuton: Formulation and *in vitro/in vivo* studies. J. Controlled Release, 45, 249–256.

[58]Ku, M. et al. (1998). Optimization of sustained-release diltiazem formulations in man by use of an *in vitro/in vivo* correlation. J. Pharm. Pharmacol. 50, 845–850.

[59]Mu, X. et al. (2003). Development and evaluation of bio-dissolution systems capable of detecting the food effect on a polysaccaride-based matrix system. J. Controlled Release, 93, 309–318.

[60]Katori, N. et al. (1995). Estimation of agitation intensity in the GI tract in humans and dogs based on *in vitro/in vivo* correlation. Pharm. Res. 12(2), 237–243.

[61]Shameem, M. et al. (1995). Oral solid controlled release dosage forms: role of GI-mechanical destructive forces and colonic release in drug absorption under fasted and fed conditions in humans. Pharm. Res. 12(7), 1049–1053.

[62]Aoki, et al. (1992). Evaluation of the correlation between *in vivo* and *in vitro* release of phenylpropanolamine HCl from controlled release tablets. Int. J. Pharm. 85, 65–73.

[63]Macheras, P. et al. (1989). An *in vitro* model for exploring CR theophylline sustained or controlled release systems: *In vitro* drug release profiles. Int. J. Pharm. 54, 123–130.

[64]Wingstrand, et al. (1990). Bioavailability from felodipine extended release tablets with different dissolution properties. Int. J. Pharm. 60, 151–156.

[65]Grundy, J.S. et al. (1997). Studies on dissolution testing of the nifedipine gastrointestinal therapeutic system. I. Description of a two-phase *in vitro* dissolution test. J. Controlled Release 48, 1–8.

[66]Pillay, V. & Fassihi, R. (1999). Unconventioal dissolution methodologies. J. Pharm. Sci. 88, 843–851.

[67]Parojčić, J., Vasiljević, D., Ibrić, S. & Djurić, D. (2008). Tablet disintegration and drug dissolution in viscous media: Paracetamol IR tablets. Inter. J. Pharm. 355(1–2), 93–99.

[68]Nicolaides, E., Symillides, M., Dressman, J.B. & Reppas, C. (2001). Biorelevant dissolution testing to predict the plasma profile of lipophilic drugs after oral administration. Pharm. Res. 18(3), 380–388.

[69]Vertzoni, M., Fotaki, N., Kostewicz, E., Stippler, E., Vertzoni M., Leuner, C., Nicolaides, E. & Dressman, C. (2004). Dissolution media simulating the intralumenal composition of the small intestine: physiological issues and practical aspects. J. Pharm. Pharmacol. 56(4), 453–462.

[70]Al-Behaisi, S., Antalb, I., Morovjána, G., Szúnyoga, J., Drabanta, S., Martonb, S. & Klebovich, I. (2002). *In vitro* simulation of food effect on dissolution of deramciclane film-coated tablets and correlation with *in vivo* data in healthy volunteers. Eur J. Pharm. Sci. 15(2), 157–162.

[71]Müllertz, A. (2007). Biorelevant Dissolution Media. In: *Solvent Systems and their Selection in Pharmaceutics and Biopharmaceutics*, P. Augustijns & M.E. Brewster (eds). Springer, New York, pp. 151–177.

[72]Jones, H.M., Parrott, N., Ohlenbusch, G. & Lave, T. (2006). Predicting pharmacokinetic food effects using biorelevant solubility media and physiologically based modelling. Clinical Pharmacokinetics 45(12), 1213–1226.

[73]Pedersen, B.L., Brøndsted, H., Lennernäs, H., Christensen, F.N., Müllertz, A. & Kristensen, H.G. (2000). Dissolution of hydrocortisone in human and simulated intestinal fluids. Pharm Res. 17, s.183.

[74]Dressman, J.B. & Reppas, C. (2000). *In vitro–in vivo* correlations for lipophilic, poorly water-soluble drugs. Eur J. Pharm. Sci. 11(S2), S73–S80.

[75]El-Arini, et al. (1990). Theophylline controlled release preparations and fatty food: An *in vitro* study using the rotating dialysis cell method. Pharm. Res. 7, 1134–1140.

[76]Morita, R. et al. (2003). Development of a new dissolution test method for an oral controlled release preparation, the PVA swelling controlled release system (SCRS). J. Controlled Release, 90(1), 109–117.

[77]Minekus, M. & Havenaar, R. (1996). *In vitro* model of an *in vivo* digestive tract. US patent 5 525 305.

small intestine, where many potentially confounding variables that affect apparent absorption often exist. The short absorption phase, in most cases, is difficult to characterize, making Level A IVIVC modeling less likely than Level C or Multiple Level C modeling. Thus, the feasibility of an IVIVC is often drug dependent. In the case of BCS class II drugs, when dissolution is rate-limiting for drug absorption, and an IVIVC may be possible. For example, Level C IVIVC or IVIVR have been reported for carbamazepine and phenytoin.[56,57] For soluble BCS class I drugs, IVIVC is less likely unless drug dissolution is significantly slowed due to formulation or the compound has borderline solubility classification. For instance, Gordon and Chowhan investigated four different ketorolac IR tablet formulations in healthy subjects, and established a Level C IVIVC between dissolution and the rate of *in vivo* absorption, though the extent of absorption remained essentially unchanged.[58] IVIVC is rare for BCS class III drugs for which gastric emptying and/or permeability is usually the rate-controlling step in drug absorption. However, depending on the drug property and product design, IVIVR or IVIVC may sometimes be found. For example, in a study comparing 7 generic IR formulations of tetracycline with the innovator product, poor dissolution was correlated with low bioavailability.[84] Opportunity for an IVIVR or IVIVC may sometimes exist for BCS class IV drugs, for which both dissolution and permeability may limit the rate of *in vivo* absorption depending on the relative rate of the two, and whether the low permeability classification is borderline or due to metabolism.[59] Various physico-chemical, biopharmaceutical, and physiological factors that need to be considered in developing an IVIVC of IR oral dosage forms were recently reviewed by Li et al.[60] It should be noted that most of the so-called "IVIVCs" reported in the literature for IR dosage forms technically cannot be considered IVIVC, because many were not subject to the rigorous validation process discussed in the previous section.

Extended-release (ER) Dosage Forms

Compared to IR products, an IVIVC is, in general, more desirable and readily defined for ER solid dosage forms. In fact, it is often expected that an *in vitro* release test is predictive or has *in vivo* relevance, because drug input from the GI tract is, by design, controlled by drug release from the dosage form. With an ER dosage form, the apparent absorption takes place in the small intestine, ascending colon and/or throughout the large intestine, depending on the product design.[61] A longer absorption phase over an extended period of time means that it is possible to develop Level A, B, C or Multiple Level C IVIVC models. However, the feasibility of an IVIVC remains dependent on drug molecule, delivery technology, and formulation design of the dosage forms.

In the case of BCS class I compounds, the *in vivo* apparent absorption is primarily limited by drug release from either a diffusion or an osmotically controlled ER system with fewer significant confounding factors. Thus, an IVIVC is more likely. With BCS class II drugs, solubility-to-dose ratio, drug release mechanism, as well as release duration, can significantly influence the *in vitro* and *in vivo* relationship. In addition, drug particle dissolution following its release (metering) from the dosage form may also play a significant role depending on the dose and physico-chemical characteristics of the drug substance. Detailed discussion is provided in an example in the Case Study section of this chapter. IVIVC for a typical BCS class III or IV drug is more difficult to obtain, because of the various factors often involved in its apparent absorption from the GI tract, including low and variable membrane permeability, competing absorption pathways and their regional dependency, etc. In fact, many of the drugs in BCS class III or IV are either not feasible for ER development or exhibit very limited absorption windows, such as ranitidine, atenolol, furosemide, erythromycin, cefazolin, amoxicillin, hydrochlorothiazide, methotrexate, acyclovir, neomycin, etc.

[78]Blanquet, S., Zeijdner, E., Beyssac, E., Meunier, J., Denis, S., Havenaar, R. & Alric, M. (2004). A dynamic artificial gastrointestinal system for studying the behavior of orally administered drug dosage forms under various physiological conditions. Pharm. Res. 21, 37–49.

[79]Hu, Z., Kimura, G., Murakami, M., Yoshikawa, H., Takada, K. & Yoshikawa, A. (1999). Dissolution test for a pressure-controlled colon delivery capsule: Rotating beads method. J Pharm Pharmacol. 51(9), 979–89.

[80]Gu, C.H., Rao, D., Gandhi, R.B., Hilden, J. & Raghavan, K. (2005). Using a novel multicompartment dissolution system to predict the effect of gastric pH on the oral absorption of weak bases with poor intrinsic solubility. J. Pharm. Sci. 94(1), 199–208.

[81]He, X., Kadomura, S., Takekuma, Y., Sugawara, M. & Miyazaki, K. (2003). An *in vitro* system for prediction of oral absorption of relatively water-soluble drugs and ester prodrugs. Int. J. Pharm. 263, 35–44.

[82]Souliman, S., Blanquet, S., Beyssac, E. & Cardot, J. (2006). A level A *in vitro/in vivo* correlation in fasted and fed states using different methods: Applied to solid immediate release oral dosage form. Eur J. Pharm. Sci. 27(1), 72–79.

TABLE 17.3   Example of extended-release systems and food effect on bioavailability parameters

Product	Dosage form	C_{max}	AUC	T_{max}
Theophylline	IR tablet	Decrease (30–50%)	No change	Increase
Theo-Dur	Coated beads	Decrease (60%)	Decrease (50%)	Increase
Theo-24	Coated beads	Increase (120%)	Increase (60%)	No change
Theo-Dur	Matrix tablet	No change	No change	No change
Uniphyl	Matrix tablet	Increase (70%)	Increase (70%)	Increase
Verapamil	IR tablet	Decrease (15%)	No change	Increase
Isoptin SR	Matrix tablet	Decrease (50%)	Decrease (50%)	Increase
Verelan PM	Coated beads	No change	No change	No change
Test Formulation 1*	Coated tablet	No change	No change	Increase
Test Formulation 2*	Coated beads	No change	No change	Increase
Covera HS	OROS tablet	No change	No change	No change

*Clin Pharmacol Ther., July, 77–83, 1985.

Dosage form behavior as related to IVIVC development depends on drug properties, delivery technology, and formulation design. During drug release from ER systems across different segments of the GI tract, both drug and dosage form are subject to a wide range of environment and conditions, such as varying surface area, absorption pathways, permeability, metabolism, mixing, secretion, lumen content, and amount of fluid, etc. As a result, the *in vivo* absorption from an ER system may significantly vary with regions, making its estimation for IVIVC modeling unreliable. This is because of the significant deviation from the basic assumption of Case III in Table 17.1, as the unit impulse input always takes place in the upper GI tract. In addition, *in vitro* and *in vivo* mechanisms may differ or change, depending on the drug and formulation design. Increased variability of the apparent absorption often observed with ER products may also be exacerbated by improper or less robust formulation designs. A review of the literature indicates a wide range of *in vivo* performance and/or relationships with *in vitro* drug release for many drugs formulated using different or similar types of delivery technologies. For example, part of the *in vivo* behavior of a solid product can be inferred from the effect of food on its PK characteristics (i.e., food effects). Food intake is known to directly and indirectly induce changes in the GI environment and conditions, including gastric emptying and intestinal motility, mixing, mechanical and shear stress, lumen content, pH, viscosity, ionic strength, osmolality, secretions (bile salts, digestive enzymes, etc.), metabolic enzymes, and transporters. There is no general *in vitro* or animal model that is predictive of the effect of such changes on drug absorption. However, the potential impact of these changes on *in vivo* performance may be used as an indirect gauge for evaluation of the robustness of an ER solid product in IVIVC development. A survey of food effects on AUC and C_{max} of 47 selected marketed ER products[62] shows that out of 32 soluble APIs, 7 exhibit food effects on AUC, 8 on C_{max}, while among 15 insoluble APIs, 6 exhibit food effects on AUC, and 14 on C_{max}. Four out of seven osmotic pump products displayed food effects on AUC or C_{max}. Table 17.3 shows ER products of two well-known drugs and their food effects.[63] It is evident that both ER technology and formulation play a significant role in how a product performs in the GI tract. Therefore, opportunity and success of developing an IVIVC for an ER dosage form depends on the individual active compound, as well as on delivery system and formulation design. Table 17.4 is a comparison of three broad types of ER drug delivery systems discussed in Chapters 20 and 21, with respect to the characteristics related to IVIVC. Among the three types of ER technologies, it is well-known that the drug release from an osmotic system is generally insensitive to *in vitro* test conditions, thus offering a higher chance of matching *in vivo* drug release. However, once the *in vitro* test fails to predict, it is much more difficult to achieve IVIVC via altering the *in vitro* drug release of an osmotic system. On the other hand, drug release from the other two types of systems (reservoir and matrix) is most often dependent on drug properties, *in vitro* test methodology and conditions, thus providing greater flexibility and opportunity of adjusting test variables to match *in vitro* data with *in vivo* profiles. It should be pointed out that, for matrix systems, drug release rate and mechanism are also affected by the system strength and integrity that often vary with formulation design.

TABLE 17.4 Common extended-release systems and IVIVC

ER system	Characteristics
Matrix	• *In vitro* release is sensitive to *in vitro* test conditions • *In vivo* results depend on individual drugs and formulation design • Hydrophilic matrix: Gel strength and system integrity also affect rate and mechanism of drug release *in vivo* • Possible to alter *in vitro* test condition for obtaining IVIVC
Reservoir	• *In vitro* release is usually sensitive to *in vitro* test conditions • *In vivo* results depend on individual drugs and formulation design • Possible to adjust test condition for obtaining IVIVC
Osmotic pump	• *In vitro* release is generally insensitive to test conditions • *In vivo* results depend on individual drugs • Higher probability of obtaining IVIVC • Lack of flexibility to adjust test condition to match *in vivo* performance

As a result, different formulations of the same drug molecule may exhibit different sensitivity to the test variables, which in turn can influence their respective *in vitro–in vivo* relationships. Therefore, it is important to evaluate key formulation attributes and variables that influence the behavior of a specific dosage form.

17.4 IVIVC DEVELOPMENT STRATEGIES AND APPROACH

Among the many challenges encountered in the development of solid dosage forms is the scientific and regulatory need to explore an IVIVR and establish an IVIVC when feasible. Thus, it is important to create an IVIVC strategy, define an appropriate approach and integrate it into the entire product development lifecycle in the project planning stage, prior to initiating any development activities.

17.4.1 Strategy and General Approach

Exploration of IVIVC may start in the early, mid or late stage of product development depending on the objective and resources of a development program. For example, an IVIVC can be investigated through review and evaluation of the historical *in vitro* and *in vivo* data or initiation of an IVIVC study at a later stage of development. This type of retrospective development strategy is usually either driven by regulatory requirements, or due to a lack of understanding of IVIVC and its importance in rational development of solid product. To fully realize its potential, IVIVC development should begin at an early stage, and continue throughout the formulation development cycle if necessary. A prospective or concurrent development strategy requires integrated evaluation of drug substance, ER technology, and IVIVC feasibility, followed by incorporating an IVIVC investigation in formulation screening and development studies. When the IVIVC is explored as a part of the first *in vivo* formulation screening studies or subsequent development studies, it can be used to aid the development of a project timeline, planning of formulation/process studies, and scale-up activities. If an IVIVC exists, it is advantageous to establish and validate the model at an early stage to facilitate and accelerate subsequent product development, thereby saving time and resources associated with certain necessary bioequivalence studies. It also helps set development and regulatory strategy. If an IVIVC is unlikely, a different product development strategy will have to be defined, for example, by including bioequivalence studies required to support process scale-up and/or certain formulation changes in the development of an ER dosage form.

In the first stage of developing ER product, two or more prototype formulations with different *in vitro* release rates are usually tested in humans, in order to identify a formulation with a predefined PK performance. With properly designed formulations and *in vitro* tests, the study can also serve to explore and develop an IVIVC concurrently. For example, to enhance the chance of success or gain insight into IVIVR, it is helpful to build similar robustness in the prototype formulations to ensure consistent release control mechanism *in vivo*. This can be achieved via formulation design and additional testing prior to the *in vivo* test in humans. The former can be accomplished by considering key formulation variables in designing the prototypes that are likely to affect *in vivo* performance, such as type and level of the rate-controlling materials, properties and loading of the drug and fillers, operating principle, size and shape of the delivery system, etc. The latter may involve challenging the prototypes through testing *in vitro* behaviors (integrity, rank order of drug release, etc.) under different conditions (apparatus, medium, type and intensity of mixing, physico-chemical and mechanical stress) or studying in an appropriate animal model. To fully exploit information and potential of such *in vivo* studies for IVIVC, it is also beneficial to select and remain focused on one type of delivery technology in dosage form development. As discussed in Chapter 20, when testing prototype formulations with drug release profiles that bracket the theoretical target absorption profile *in vivo*, different outcomes may be obtained depending on the drug, formulation design and *in vitro* test methodology. Figure 17.4 illustrates four examples of possible *in vitro–in vivo* relationships of such a study. Unless a quantitative IVIVC is obtained in the first study (Example I), further investigation is required to pursue an IVIVC depending on the outcome. Generally, if little difference is found in the *in vivo* performance, the *in vitro* test is considered over-discriminating (Example IV). It would still be beneficial to modify test conditions to achieve the similar *in vitro* performance for guiding formulation modification in subsequent *in vivo* studies. If formulations show *in vivo* differences (rank order or under-discriminating), *in vitro* test conditions can be modified to correspond with *in vivo* data. Adopting such an IVIVC strategy, and making it a part of dosage form development often involves the following sequential steps:

1. Evaluate *in vivo* behaviors based on the understanding of drug's properties, dosage form, and their interplays with the GI tract.
2. Identify and investigate the mechanism/variables that influence or control both *in vitro* and apparent *in vivo* drug release.
3. Study test variables to identify conditions that:
   (a) Differentiate between formulations with different *in vivo* behaviors, and

(b) Decipher the dosage form behavior and its relationship with the release controlling variables (e.g., critical formulation, processing parameters).
4. Design an *in vitro* test that matches *in vivo* performance (if feasible).
5. Establish, evaluate, and validate the IVIVC.

It is evident that for formulations with varying PK profiles, developing an IVIVC relies heavily on the successful design of a discriminating *in vitro* test method.

17.4.2 Design of a Predictive *In Vitro* Test

The first step in developing a predictive *in vitro* test is to ensure IVIVC feasibility, i.e., that drug release from dosage form controls drug inputs in the GI tract. While the *in vitro* data generated for IVIVC are typically drug release data, the estimated "*in vivo* release" or apparent absorption is drug availability *in vivo*. As discussed previously, the latter is often a function of many other variables, in addition to drug release. Thus, the possibility of using an *in vitro* release test to predict *in vivo* performance is drug and formulation dependent, and should be explored on a case-by-case basis.

In the case of IR dosage form, where dissolution is limiting the rate of absorption (e.g., certain BCS class II drugs), it is sometimes possible to develop a biorelevant dissolution test for predicting differences in bioavailability among different formulations and dosing conditions. To achieve an *a priori* correlation, common approaches include altering test apparatus or

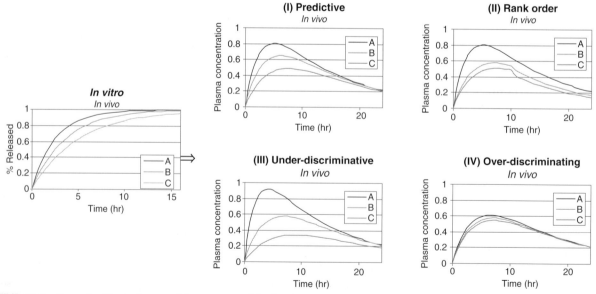

FIGURE 17.4   Examples illustrating possible outcomes of the first bioavailability study of prototype ER formulations with varying *in vitro* release rates

conditions, via simulating the volume of the contents and hydrodynamics in the gastrointestinal lumen or using model compositions of the gastric and intestinal contents, before and after meal intake, as the dissolution media. For example, to simulate the composition, volume, and hydrodynamics of the contents in the gastrointestinal lumen, one uses model compositions of the gastric and intestinal contents, before and after meal intake, as the dissolution media.[68] However, success as measured by meeting the rigorous IVIVC criteria for IR has been scarce, primarily because of the many confounding variables involved in apparent absorption *in vivo*.

In comparing *in vivo* with *in vitro* data of ER dosage forms, it is important to take into consideration the drug's properties, stability, and absorption pathways in relation to the effect of pH, transit time, region of drug release, food, ER technology utilized, and release control mechanisms.[6] This type of integrated knowledge is essential in anticipating and evaluating possible interplays of drug-GIT, formulation-GIT, and drug-formulation interactions, and their impact on the relationship between *in vivo* and *in vitro* data. While the results of an *in vivo* study are invariant, analysis of the drug, delivery system, and formulation design can provide greater insight into the *in vivo* absorption behavior to help assess the IVIVC opportunity and develop a prognostic method.

In general, the observed deviation of *in vivo* apparent absorption or release mechanism from that *in vitro* may be attributed to a lack of robustness of the delivery system, a particular composition in its operating environment or due to physico-chemical and biological properties, such as low solubility, enterohepatic recycling, pre-systemic saturable metabolism and its dose dependency, truncated absorption, effect of the absorbed drug or metabolite on the motility and transporter, etc. These types of confounding factors, if not corrected, often make an IR reference inappropriate as the unit impulse response to estimate *in vivo* absorption.[24] For example, the *in vivo* absorption of oxybutynin osmotic pump was found to be not only higher than that of the IR reference, but also significantly longer (>24 hours) than the *in vitro* drug release (15 hours) and the average GI residence time of solid dosage forms as well, resulting in a lack of IVIVC.[64] The former could be attributed to reduced gut metabolism in the lower bowel. However, the latter observation was not understood because oxybutynin has neither known pharmacological effects on GI motility like opioid analgesics,[65] nor does it undergo enterohepatic recycling. Wang et al. reported an IVIVC for a pulsatile release dosage form of methylphenidate (Ritalin® LA), although the double peaks observed in

plasma concentration–time profile resulted from two separate immediate-releases that were 4 hours apart.[66] This is likely a result of the favorable absorption properties of methylphenidate and decreased dissolution rate of the second IR due to its changing release environment in the lower bowel.

Sako et al.[67] investigated the effect of composition of a hydrophilic matrix on *in vivo* release of acetaminophen. Three formulations containing different fillers showed similar *in vitro* dissolution profiles using different agitation intensity, but had considerably different *in vivo* performance (Figure 17.5). The observed discrepancy was believed to result from the varying gel strength of the matrix systems. In developing an *in vitro* test that differentiates the formulation behaviors, the test method was modified by subjecting the tablets to mechanical stress after 1 hour of dissolution (shaking with glass beads for 10 min), which resulted in drug release profiles similar to the *in vivo* performance. It should be mentioned that, in addition to creating artificial shear and attrition,[60,94] other techniques that are useful to characterize gel microstructure, formation, and strength of a hydrophilic matrix system include magnetic resonance imaging (MRI) microscopy, confocal microscopy, rheometry, texture analyzer, dynamic mechanical analyzer (DMA), and increasing ionic strength in the dissolution medium.[68,69,70,71,72,73,74]

For high dose-to-solubility ratio drug substances that undergo drug dissolution upon delivery (metering) from the ER device, varying regional dissolution and absorption environments (e.g., surface area, amount of water, motility, enzymes, transporters, etc.) may become significant factors affecting the apparent *in vivo* absorption, and thus the IVIVC. For example, a discrepancy between the *in vitro* and *in vivo* data for a nifedipine osmotic pump was believed to be a result of the inability of conventional *in vitro* tests to separate release (metering) from dissolution, due to the large volume of test medium used throughout testing.[75] Generally, the *in vitro* test can become over- or under-discriminative of the *in vivo* results when particle dissolution upon release from an ER system plays a role in absorption, especially if a significant portion of the dose is delivered in the lower bowel. An additional challenge in exploring a predictive *in vitro* test for an insoluble compound like nifedipine is that its extent of absorption also depends on the particle size (or dissolution rate) of the drug upon its release from the ER system,[76] which is difficult to reflect using a conventional test method. Furthermore, the potential influence of the solid phase of an insoluble drug substance on *in vitro* dissolution and *in vivo* absorption may also complicate the *in vitro* and *in vivo*

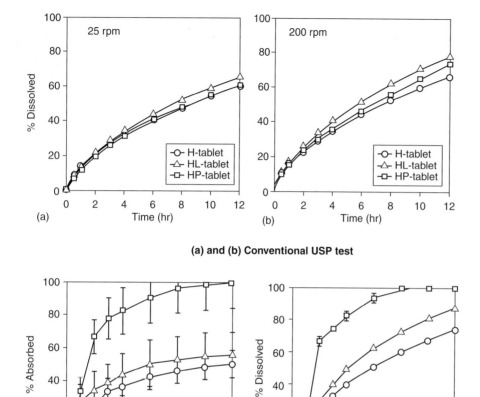

(a) and (b) Conventional USP test

FIGURE 17.5 *In vitro* drug release and *in vivo* absorption profiles of three hydrophilic matrix formulations of acetaminophen. Reprinted with permission: J. Controlled Release 81(1–2), 165–172, 2002

relationship. For example, a solid phase transition that occurs *in situ* or results from precipitation during drug release[77,78] may impact *in vitro* and *in vivo* drug release in a different manner. It should be noted that these types of differences again may affect the validity of using IR reference as the unit impulse response to estimate *in vivo* absorption.[24]

In investigating IVIVC for dosage forms with more complex release profiles or containing more than one drug substances (e.g., pulsatile release and fixed dose combinations), it is essential to take into consideration properties of both individual actives, and their release characteristics. Depending on the release design feature, separate test methods may sometimes be required to match the *in vivo* absorption of the individual drugs or one part of the profiles. It is also possible that a predictive test can only be developed for one of the actives or a portion of the dose and release profiles. For example, for a bimodal release profile consisting of an IR followed by an ER or an ER followed by an IR delivery (Figure 17.6), it

may be feasible to develop an IVIVC for only one (ER) or both portions of the curve. For products containing more than one drug with synchronized or divergent release profiles, various IVIVC outcomes are possible depending on each drug's BCS class, biological properties, dose, and IR-to-ER ratio. In any case, a predictive test method will always be useful whether it is for one or both drugs, a portion of or the entire absorption profiles, in setting dissolution specification, and guiding or justifying changes to part of the formulation and process of interest.

In the method development process, the challenge frequently encountered is that the *in vitro* release not only differs from *in vivo* release/absorption in rate and extent, but may also exhibit a different release mechanism when a routine pharmacopeial method is used (e.g., USP II, 75 rpm, SIF). A general approach to developing an *in vitro* test for IVIVC, requires identification of the mechanism that controls *in vivo* drug release.[6,79] For delivery systems that are sensitive to release environment, the effects of test variables on release kinetics

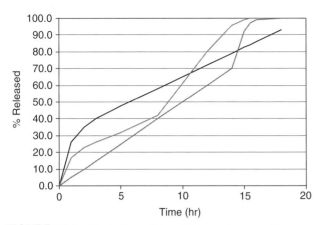

FIGURE 17.6 Illustration of bimodal drug release profiles

needs to be investigated in order to understand how formulation variables and dosage form behaviors respond to environmental changes. In certain cases, formulations can be subject to more stressed conditions (e.g., shear stress, high osmolarity, ionic strength or agitation intensity, multiple apparatuses, etc.) to test robustness or to show differences. Subsequently, a qualitative or quantitative relationship between drug release and key test variables may be established to guide the selection of a test condition that allows *in vitro* data to match both the mechanism and rates of *in vivo* release. A well-executed experimental design is of great value in defining this type of relationship.

Once an *in vitro* method that correlates with *in vivo* absorption is established, its value as a quality control tool of a drug product is significantly enhanced. It serves as a tool to distinguish between acceptable and unacceptable drug products with respect to *in vivo* performance. It should be emphasized that a newly developed method cannot be considered reliable and acceptable unless it has been validated, and demonstrated to be predictive of different formulations with varying *in vivo* performance.

17.5 APPLICATIONS AND LIMITATIONS

The most important aspect of developing an IVIVC is to identify an *in vitro* test that can serve as an indicator of how well a product will perform *in vivo*. According to the FDA Guidance on IVIVC for extended-release solid dosage forms,[2] a validated IVIVC can be used: (1) for setting meaningful dissolution specifications to ensure product quality; and (2) for requesting a biowaiver so that the regulatory burdens, cost, and time associated with product

development or post-approval changes can be significantly reduced.

17.5.1 Setting Dissolution Specifications

In vitro dissolution specifications are established to ensure batch-to-batch consistency, and to differentiate between acceptable and unacceptable drug products, thus minimizing the possibility of releasing lots that might not have the desired *in vivo* performance. In general, dissolution behaviors of the clinical bioavailability batches are used to define the amount released at each time point.[1,2] Dissolution specification setting for IR products should be based on consideration of BCS classification, and is discussed in detail in the regulatory guidance.[1] The difficulty arises in determining the acceptable variation around each time point for ER dosage forms. For NDAs or ANDAs, the specifications are based on the biobatch of a drug product. In the absence of an IVIVC, the range at any dissolution time point specification has to be within ±10% of the mean profile obtained from the biobatch. Deviations greater than 20% would be acceptable, provided that the batches at the specification limits are bioequivalent.[1,2] For ER products, a minimum of three time points covering early, middle, and late stages of the profile are required with a dissolution of at least 80% at the final time point.

A validated Level A IVIVC allows for the setting of dissolution specifications, such that all lots within the limits of the specifications are bioequivalent. In general, the convolution approach, as illustrated in Figure 17.3, is often used and the specifications should be set on mean data using at least 12 dosage units. In determining the release limits, the dissolution curves defined by the upper and lower extremes established from the biobatch are convoluted to project the corresponding *in vivo* plasma concentration profiles. A maximum difference of 20% in the predicted C_{max} and AUC is allowed between lots with the fastest and slowest release rates.[2] Alternatively, an acceptable set of plasma profiles, representing formulations with faster and slower release rates relative to the biobatch, can be used to set dissolution specifications by deconvolution based on the principles illustrated in Figure 17.2. These curves, selected based on extremes of 20% difference in C_{max}, and AUC, are deconvoluted and the resulting input curves are used to establish the upper and lower dissolution specification ranges at each time point via the IVIVC model.

In the case of Level C and multiple Level C IVIVC models, specification ranges should be set at the correlation time point, such that there is a maximum of 20% difference in the predicted AUC or C_{max}.[2] If the correlation involves more than one parameter, the one resulting in tighter limits should be used. In addition, drug release at the last time point should be at least 80%. Lake et al. reported an example of applying Level C IVIVC to set biorelevant dissolution specifications using four carbamazepine IR tablets.[80]

Although the general procedure and criteria for the establishment of dissolution specifications that ensure bioequivalence based on IVIVC has been proposed,[2,81,82] few discussions have centered on detailed processes and practical considerations in setting meaningful and realistic specification limits in product development. Elkoshi[83] described a procedure based on release rates that confines C_{max}, and AUC, values within any desired range to set the "minimum range" specifications for both zero-order and first-order release products. In reviewing the methods for setting dissolution specifications, Hayes et al.[84] evaluated the most commonly adopted "deterministic interpretation" approach, that is, those batches passing the *in vitro* specifications would be bioequivalent, and those failing the specifications would not be bioequivalent if tested *in vivo*. According to the authors, the deterministic interpretation may not be appropriate, and conditional probability needs to be considered due to random variation. Through a computer simulation based on an IVIVC model, the conditional probabilities are shown to depend on the choice of dissolution specifications. The authors further described a method for optimizing the dissolution specifications that takes production into consideration. A practical procedure of using IVIVC to establish a dissolution specification based on scientific, regulatory, and manufacturing considerations is provided in the Case Study section of this chapter.

17.5.2 Supporting Waiver of *In Vivo* Bioavailability Studies

In addition to serving as a quality control test, comparative dissolution tests have been used to waive bioequivalence or bioavailability studies required for both IR and MR solid dosage forms under certain circumstances. Comprehensive regulation, scientific rationales, considerations, approaches, and evaluation criteria associated with these biowaivers have been clearly laid out in various regulatory guidelines. According to the FDA guidance,[1,85] the biowaiver request for INDs, NDAs, ANDAs, and post-approval changes of IR solid dosage forms should be based on the consideration of the drug's BCS class,[86] therapeutic index, and potential effect of excipients on bioavailability. The global regulations with respect to biowaivers for IR solid oral products in the USA, the EU, Japan,

and from the World Health Organization (WHO), were reviewed recently.[5] Biowaiver monographs of a series of BCS class I and III compounds proposed by the BCS Working Group of the International Pharmaceutical Federation (FIP) have also been published in the Journal of Pharmaceutical Sciences to stimulate new biowaiver discussion and methods,[87] although many of them (e.g., BCS class III) have not been accepted by regulatory agencies. These drug substances include acetaminophen, acetazolamide, aciclovir, atenolol, amitriptyline hydrochloride, cimetidine, chloroquine phosphate, chloroquine sulfate, chloroquine hydrochloride, ethambutol dihydrochloride, ibuprofen, isoniazid, metoclopramide hcl, prednisolone, prednisone, propranolol hydrochloride, pyrazinamide, ranitidine hydrochloride, and verapamil hydrochloride.

For modified-release products, a dissolution test based on a validated IVIVC can also be used for obtaining a waiver of demonstrating *in vivo* bioavailability, often required for NDAs, ANDAs, scale-up, and post-approval changes.[2,88] The criteria for granting biowaivers using IVIVC are: (a) the difference in predicted means of C_{max} and AUC is no more than 20% from that of the reference product; and (b) dissolution meets specifications. According to the FDA guidance, the categories of biowaivers are also based on the therapeutic index of the drug, the extent of the validation performed on the developed IVIVC, and dissolution characteristics of the formulation. For instance, for non-narrow therapeutic index drugs, an IVIVC developed with two formulations can be used for biowaivers in Level 3 manufacturing site changes and Level 3 non-release controlling excipient changes defined in the SUPAC Guidance for MR Solid Dosage Forms.[115] If an IVIVC is developed using three formulations or two formulations with external validation, biowaivers may include: (1) Level 3 process changes; (2) complete removal or replacement of non-release controlling excipients without affecting release mechanism; (3) Level 3 changes in the release controlling excipients; and (4) change of strength (lower than the highest strength).

17.5.3 Limitations and Additional Considerations

Limitations to the IVIVC methodology reside in the physico-chemical, biological, and pharmacokinetic properties of the drug substance, the formulation design, as well as the methodology used to model, evaluate, and validate the IVIVC.

In the development of an IVIVC, the basic assumption of linear system analysis is that the drug candidate exhibits linear pharmacokinetic disposition. Thus, saturable absorption, absorption windows, rate-dependent absorption or rate-dependent pre-systemic metabolism, enterohepatic recycling, etc., are important factors to consider when modeling and validating an IVIVC, because they directly or indirectly result in deviation from the assumption of linearity.[12,89,90,91,92] In addition, an IVIVC should not be developed using plasma concentrations of racemate when there are stereoselective dissolution or absorption differences between the two enantiomers.[93] More importantly, the dissolution process should be the rate-limiting step in the absorption process, as discussed previously. In most cases, IVIVC models are being established using average *in vivo* response, thus ignoring the inter- and intra-subject variability. For drugs that have relatively high inter-subject variability, it is important to take into account the inter- and intra-subject variability in constructing and evaluating an IVIVC model.[24,94,95] Lastly, the *in vivo* studies used for developing an IVIVC are conducted in healthy volunteers under a well-controlled environment. Factors that might affect the performance of the dosage form or physiology should also be considered,[96,97] such as food effects, disease state, age (pediatric and geriatric), and drug–drug or drug–GIT interactions might affect the GI motility and/or the GI transit time.

The state-of-the-art is such that an IVIVC is typically only valid for one particular type of dosage form containing certain rate-controlling excipients with the same release mechanism. Even with the same type of solid dosage form, such as tablet, different release mechanisms (e.g., diffusion versus osmosis) often necessitate development of separate IVIVCs for the same drug molecule. In IVIVC modeling, the absorption parameters obtained with the most widely used Wagner–Nelson method reflect only the rate, and not the extent of absorption. Problems can arise from a correlation established using formulations that have different systemic bioavailability. For example, decreased or truncated absorption in the lower GI tract may occur with slow releasing formulations, due to less liquid available for dissolution, lower surface area, presence of bacterial metabolism or short residence time. As a result, the IVIVC will be apparently formulation-dependent if not corrected. This is illustrated using a simulated example. Two formulations (I and II) were originally designed to release a drug over approximately 8 and 14 hours (Figure 17.7a). Following oral administration, decreased bioavailability of formulation II was observed because the "window" of absorption was found to be 8 hours (Figure 17.7b). The apparent *in vivo* absorption profiles of the two formulations obtained by the Wagner–Nelson method are also shown in Figure 17.7a. A comparison between the *in vitro* release and *in vivo* absorption indicates a good 1:1 relationship for formulation I, and a significant deviation from the relationship for formulation II as a result of overestimation of the *in vivo* absorption. Therefore, in developing an IVIVC, the reduced AUC needs to be accounted for, for instance, by using a time-dependent function: $X_{in\ vivo} = g(t)\ X_{in\ vitro}$, where $g(t)$ is a step function for truncated or site-dependent absorption.

17.6 CASES STUDIES

17.6.1 Effect of Solubility on IVIVC

Nifedipine is practically insoluble. Its *in vivo* apparent absorption from osmotic pump or matrix systems consists of sequential steps of release or metering of drug particles followed by particle dissolution, and permeation across the intestinal membrane. This is indirectly supported by the known dependency of bioavailability on drug particle size discussed previously. Conventional USP tests using a large volume of test medium containing solubilizer to create

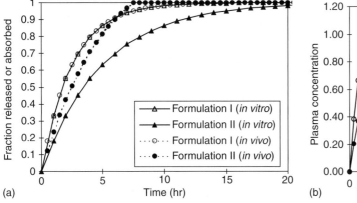

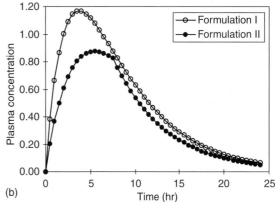

FIGURE 17.7 *In vitro* release versus *in vivo* absorption profiles obtained by Wagner–Nelson method (a) based on simulated plasma concentration profiles of two ER formulations with different release rates (b)

sink condition are incapable of separating particle dissolution from drug release. In investigating the IVIVC of a Push-Pull™ osmotic pump formulation of nifedipine, Grundy[65] et al. designed a two-phase test to measure the rate of drug "transfer" from an aqueous phase into an organic phase, i.e., the processes of release of suspension from the device, particle dissolution, and subsequent partitioning into the organic phase (Figure 17.8a).

The authors demonstrated that a zero-order rate of drug transfer (0.96 mg/h) obtained from such test system closely matched the estimated *in vivo* absorption rate of 1.03 mg/h (30 mg strength), as compared to a rate of 1.7 mg/h based on conventional test. As a result, an improved 1:1 Level A IVIVC was obtained for all strengths ($R^2 > 0.99$).

Similarly, the impact of drug solubility on IVIVR was also evaluated in a study comparing an ER hydrophilic matrix formulation containing crystalline and amorphous phases of a compound with high dose-to-solubility ratio.[98] Tablets with different *in vitro* release rates were prepared, primarily by varying the level of the rate-controlling polymer. It was found that a conventional USP method using 900 ml of test medium significantly overestimated the minor *in vivo* difference of formulations containing crystalline drug. The same method provided a rank order IVIVR for formulations that contained the more soluble amorphous drug and exhibited substantially different *in vivo* plasma profiles.

17.6.2 Developing a Predictive *In Vitro* Test

Depakote® ER tablet is a hydrophilic-matrix based extended-release system with high drug loading.[99,10,11] It provides nearly 24 hours of apparent zero-order *in vivo* absorption (Figure 17.9). The active ingredient, divalproex sodium, is a stable and permeable compound with pH-dependent solubility. During early formulation development, the *in vitro* drug release of three different formulations were all found to be slower, and showed inadequate separation compared to *in vivo* absorption (under-discriminating), when a

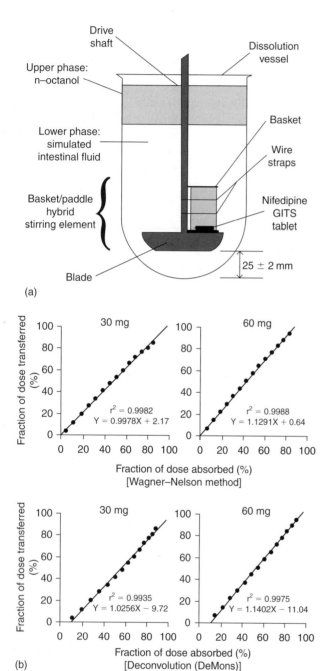

FIGURE 17.8 A two-phase *in vitro* test system (a) designed for improving IVIVC of ER dosage form of an insoluble drug, nifedipine (b). Reprinted with permission: J. Controlled Release, 48(1–8), 9–17, 1997.

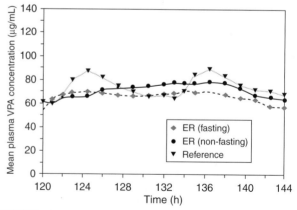

FIGURE 17.9 Mean steady-state plasma concentration profiles of once-daily Depakote® ER tablet dosed under fasting and non-fasting conditions with twice-daily enteric Depakote® tablet as reference

conventional test was used (Figure 17.10a). In addition, the mechanism of *in vitro* release was diffusion-controlled, whereas the apparent absorption profile obtained by deconvolution showed zero-order absorption, suggesting a predominantly erosion-controlled *in vivo* release (also supported by steady state plasma concentration curves in Figure 17.9).

In order to develop a new *in vitro* method that predicts *in vivo* absorption, statistically designed studies were carried out to investigate the effects of various *in vitro* testing variables on drug release. The variables investigated included agitation intensity, apparatus, surfactant, pH, and ionic strength of the dissolution medium. Based on these factorial studies and statistical analysis, a new set of testing conditions was determined and demonstrated to correlate with *in vivo* drug absorption for various ER formulations, using both two-stage and single-stage approaches (Figure 17.10b).[24] Statistical evaluation of the *in vitro* method based on a hypothesis test indicated that the same IVIVC equation holds for three different formulations (Figure 17.11a). A mixed effects model was used for data analysis, in which the dependence among observations from the same subject in the human pharmacokinetic study was taken into account. Figure 17.11b shows the agreement between observed and predicted plasma profiles of the tablets. The IVIVC has since been successfully validated internally and externally on multiple occasions over a period of eight years. More importantly, it has been applied for control of product quality, setting of meaningful drug release specifications, and for timely identification and correction of undesired dissolution trending of commercial

batches that could not have been detected had the conventional dissolution test been used as a QC tool.[100]

This study illustrates a useful approach in identifying a predictive method for the development of IVIVC, i.e., adjusting dissolution test conditions to correlate *in vitro* data with *in vivo* behaviors of the formulations.

17.6.3 Illustration of Setting an Optimal Dissolution Specification

The choice of dissolution specifications has profound implications for the routine production of the solid products. If the specification range is unnecessarily narrow, the probability of failing a batch is increased, due to inherent variability of both the product and its manufacturing process. If a wide range is set for passing batches or the range is solely based on individual product and process capability, *in vivo* performance may not always be ensured, especially in the absence of an IVIVC. One of the most significant advantages of establishing dissolution acceptance criteria using IVIVC is that it offers a greater flexibility for identifying a specification that maximizes the probabilities of assured product *in vivo* performance and successful commercial production. More specifically, it allows searching an optimal range in a multidimensional space defined by the needs of bioequivalence, quality control, manufacturing, and regulation. One of the challenges in arriving at such an optimal specification prior to regulatory submission is a lack of precise measures of product and process capability at production scale due to an

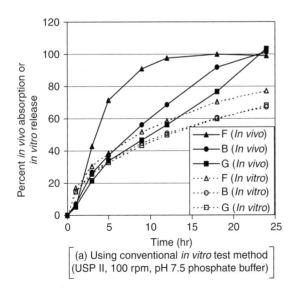

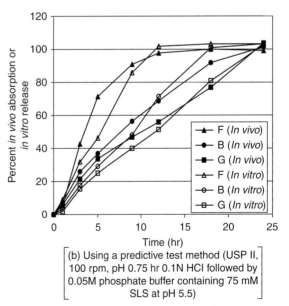

FIGURE 17.10   Mean *in vivo* absorption versus *in vitro* release profiles of three formulations

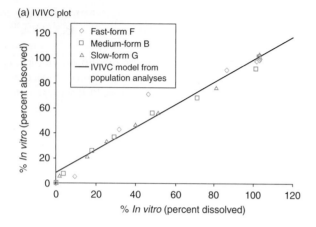

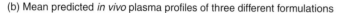

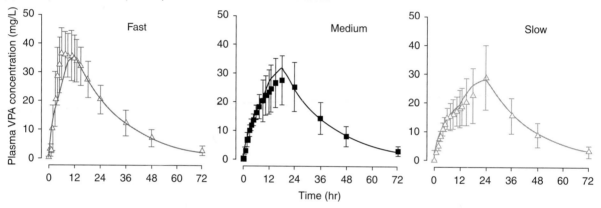

FIGURE 17.11   Results of *in vivo–in vitro* correlation studies of extended release Divalproex sodium tablets

TABLE 17.5   Illustration of assessment of multiple sets of dissolution specification based on IVIVC and manufacturing considerations

Specification set confined by IVIVC	Q (2 hr)*	Q (8 hr)	Q (12 hr)	L3 failure rate (%)	L1 pass rate (%)	L2 pass rate (%)	L3 pass rate (%)
I	UL(1)	LL–UL(1)	LL–(1)	0.0	89.3	10.2	0.5
II	UL(2)	LL–UL(2)	LL–(2)	0.0	78.2	12.3	0.5
III	UL(3)	LL–UL(3)	LL–(3)	0.1	75.4	24.4	0.1
IV	UL(4)	LL–UL(4)	LL–(4)	0.2	72.9	26.1	0.8

*Note: LL = Lower limit; UL = Upper limit

inadequate database. Nevertheless, for an ER dosage form, the following steps can be taken by utilizing available information, and a validated IVIVC, to best estimate meaningful dissolution limits that control product quality while maximizing the probability of production success:[125]

- Generate multiple sets of acceptable ranges for the specification based on the pivotal biobatch and a validated IVIVC model (Table 17.5). These ranges may be obtained by varying limits at individual time points, and should be confined by the predicted C_{max} and AUC (i.e., ≤ 20%).
- Review and combine all existing dissolution data of hundreds or thousands of individual tablets including pilot batches, scale-up and stability batches and perform statistical analysis to estimate the inherent variability.
- Perform simulation experiments by repeated random sampling using Monte Carlo methods based on estimated variability, e.g., simulating 5000 production lots by randomly sampling 5000 groups of 6 tablets.

- Test the simulation results against different sets of limits to estimate the probability of passing stages 1–3 (L1, L2, and L3), and assess the probability of batch failures (Table 17.5).

The usefulness and effectiveness of this approach can be subsequently confirmed in commercial production post product approval.

17.7 SUMMARY

The general concepts, theory, modeling methodology, assessment, and applications of *in vitro–in vivo* correlation have been established and extensively investigated, although differences of scientific opinions remain in the details of model development and evaluation. The state-of-the-art is such that there is no universal *in vitro* model that can mimic or reproduce the highly complex and dynamic GI environment or predict *in vivo* performance of solid oral dosage forms. Therefore, development of an IVIVC needs to be carried out on a case-by-case basis.

Compared with an IR product, an IVIVC is generally more likely for ER dosage forms where drug absorption is normally limited by drug release. To increase the chance of success, it is crucial to evaluate IVIVC feasibility, *in vitro*, and *in vivo* results, by applying integrated knowledge of physico-chemical and biological characteristics of drug substance, dosage form design, and their interplay with the GI tract. It is also important to make an IVIVC strategy an essential part of the dosage form development program.

Once an IVIVC is developed and validated, the predictive *in vitro* test can be used as a reliable tool for quality control, a surrogate for *in vivo* studies, and a guide for setting meaningful *in vitro* specifications. It is highly desirable that an IVIVC-based *in vitro* method is suitable for implementation in QC laboratories, such that any potential or unexpected changes of *in vivo* performance of a product during production can be detected to ensure safety and efficacy of every commercial batch.

References

1. Guidance for Industry. (1997). *Dissolution Testing of Immediate Release Solid Oral Dosage Forms.* US Department of Health, Food and Drug Administration, Center for Drug Evaluation and Research (CDER), August.
2. Guidance for Industry. (1997). *Extended Release Oral Dosage Forms: Development, Evaluation, and Application of In vitro/In vivo Correlations.* US Department of Health, Food and Drug Administration, Center for Drug Evaluation and Research (CDER), September.
3. Note for Guidance on Development Pharmaceutics. (1998). European Agency for the Evaluation of Medicinal Products, Human Medicines Evaluation Unit, Committee for Proprietary Medicinal Products, CPMP/QWP/155/96. London, UK, January.
4. Note for Guidance on Modified Release Oral and Transdermal Dosage Forms. (1999). Section II (Pharmacokinetic and Clinical Evaluation); European Agency for the Evaluation of Medicinal Products, Human Medicines Evaluation Unit, Committee for Proprietary Medicinal Products, CPMP/EWP/280/96. London, UK, July.
5. Guptaa, E., Barendsb, D.M., Yamashitaa, E., Lentzc, K.A., Harmszed, A.M., Shahe, V.P., Dressman, J.B. & Lipper, R.A. (2006). Review of global regulations concerning biowaivers for immediate release solid oral dosage forms. E. J. Pharm. Sci. 29(3–4), 315–324.
6. Qiu, Y. (2006). Design and applications of predictive *in vitro* tests for *in vitro–in vivo* correlations of oral extended-release dosage forms. Am. Pharm. Review 9(1), 94–99.
7. Souliman, S., Blanquet, S., Beyssac, E. & Cardot, J-M. (2006). A level A *in vitro/in vivo* correlation in fasted and fed states using different methods: Applied to solid immediate release oral dosage form. Eur. J. Pharm. Sci. 27(1), 72–79.
8. Rossia, R.C., Diasa, C.L., Donatoa, E.M., Martinsa, L.A., Bergolda, A.M. & Fröehlich, P.E. (2007). Development and validation of dissolution test for ritonavir soft gelatin capsules based on *in vivo* data. Inter. J Pharm. 338(1–2), 119–124.
9. Morita, R., Honda, R. & Takahashi, Y. (2003). Development of a new dissolution test method for an oral controlled release preparation, the PVA swelling controlled release system (SCRS). J. Controlled Release 90(1), 109–117.
10. Qiu, Y., Garren, J., Samara, E., Abraham, C., Cheskin, H.S. & Engh, K.R. (2003). Once-a-day controlled-release dosage form of Divalproex Sodium II: development of a predictive *in vitro* release method. J. Pharm. Sci. 92(11), 2317–2325.
11. Dutta, S., Qiu, Y., Samara, E., Cao, G. & Granneman, G.R. (2005). Once-a-day controlled-release dosage form of Divalproex Sodium III: Development and validation of a level a *in vitro–in vivo* correlation (IVIVC). J. Pharm. Sci. 94, 1949–1956.
12. Sirisuth, N., Augsburger, L.L. & Eddington, N.D. (2002). Development and validation of a non-linear IVIVC model for a diltiazem extended release formulation. Biopharm. & Drug Disposition 23(1), 1–8.
13. Tabusso, G. (1992). Regulatory Aspects of Development Pharmaceutics (2). Regulatory Affairs J. (12), 909–912.
14. Pharmacopeial Forum. (1993). *In vitro* and *in vivo* evaluation of dosage forms. 19, 5366–5379.
15. Skelly, J.P., et al. (1987). Report of the workshop on controlled release dosage forms: Issues and controversies. Pharm. Res. 4, 75–78.
16. Pharmacopeial Forum Stimuli Article. (1988). *In vitro–in vivo* correlation for extended release oral dosage forms. 4160–4161.
17. Skelly, J.P. & Shiu, G.F. (1993). *In vitro/in vivo* correlations in biopharmaceutics: Scientific and regulatory implications. Eur. J. Drug Metab. Pharmacokin. 18, 121–129.
18. Siewert, W. (1993). Perspectives of *in vitro* dissolution tests in establishing *in vitro/in vivo* correlations. Eur. J. Drug Metab. Pharmacokin. 18, 7–18.
19. Skelly, J.P., et al. (1990). *In vitro* and *in vivo* testing and correlation for oral controlled/modified-release dosage forms. Pharm. Res. 7(9), 975–982.
20. Khan, M. Z. (1996). Dissolution testing for sustained or controlled release oral dosage forms and correlation with *in vivo* data: Challenges and opportunities. 140, 131–143.
21. Mojaverian, P., et al. (1997). *In vivo–in vitro* correlation of four extended release formulations of pseudophedrine sulfate. J. Pharm. Biomed. Analysis 15, 439–445.

22. Mojaverian, P., et al. (1992). Correlation of *in vitro* release rate and *in vivo* absorption characteristics of four chlorpheniramine maleate extended release formulations. Pharm. Res. 9, 450–456.

23. Young, D., DeVane, J. & Butler, J. (eds). (1997). *In vitro–In vivo Correlations*. Plenum Press, New York, NY.

24. Qiu, Y., Samara, E. & Cao, G. (2000). *In vitro/In vivo* Correlations in the Development of Solid Controlled Release Dosage Forms. In: *Handbook of Pharmaceutical Controlled Release Technology*, D.L. Wise, A.M. Klibanov, R. Langer, A.G. Mikos, N.A. Peppas, D.J. Trantolo, G.E. Wnek, & M.J. Yaszeski, (eds). Marcel Dekker, Inc., New York, NY. pp. 527–549.

25. Murthy, D.C., Sunkara, G. & Young, D. (eds). (2007). *Pharmaceutical Product Development: In vitro-In vivo Correlation*. Informa Healthcare USA Inc, New York.

26. Cutler, D.J. (1978). Linear system analysis in pharmacokinetics. J. Pharmacokin. Biopharm. 6, 265–282.

27. Moller, H. (1989). Deconvolution Techniques and their use in Biopharmaceutics. In: *Drug Delivery to the Gastrointestinal Tract*, J.G. Hardy, S.S. Davis, & C.G. Wilson, (eds). Ellis Horwood Ltd., Chichester. pp. 179–194.

28. Cutler, D.J. (1978). Numerical deconvolution by least squares: Use of polynormils to represent the input functions. J. Pharmacokin. Biopharm. 6, 243–263.

29. Langenbucher, F. (1982). Numerical convolution/deconvolution as a tool for correlating *in vitro* with *in vivo* drug bioavailability. Pharm. Ins. 4, 1166–1172.

30. Gillespie, W.R. & Veng-Pedersen, P. (1985). A ployexponential deconvolution method. Evaluation of the "gastrointestinal bioavailability" and mean *in vitro* dissolution time of some ibuprofen dosage forms. J. Pharmacokin. Biopharm. 13, 289–307.

31. Vajda, S., Godfrey, K.R. & Valko, P. (1988). Numerical deconvolution using system identification methods. J. Pharmacokin. Biopharm. 16, 85–107.

32. Verotta, D. (1993). Two constrained deconvolution methods using spline functions. J. Pharmacokin. Biopharm. 21, 609–636.

33. Vaubhan, D.P. & Dennis, M. (1978). Mathematical basis of the point area deconvolution method for determining *in vivo* input functions. J. Pharm. Sci. 67, 663–665.

34. Veng-Pedersen, P. (1980). Model independent method of analyzing input in linear pharmacokinetic systems having polyexponential impulse response. 1: Theoretical analysis. J. Pharm. Sci. 69, 298–304.

35. Veng-Pedersen, P. (1980). Model independent method of analyzing input in linear pharmacokinetic systems having polyexponential impulse response. 2: Numerical evaluation. J. Pharm. Sci. 69, 305–312.

36. Veng-Pedersen, P. (1980). Novel deconvolution method for linear pharmacokinetic systems with polyexponential impulse response. 1: Theoretical analysis. J. Pharm. Sci. 69, 312–318.

37. Veng-Pedersen, P. (1980). Novel approach to bioavailability testing: Statistical method for comparing drug input calculated by a least squares deconvolution technique. J. Pharm. Sci. 69, 319–324.

38. Madden, F.N., Godfrey, K.R., Chappell, M.J., Hovorka, R. & Bates, R.A. (1996). A comparison of six deconvolution techniques. J. Pharmacokin. Biopharm. 24, 283–299.

39. Veng-Pedersen, P. Personal Communications.

40. Langenbucher, F. (2003). Handling of computational *in vitro/in vivo* correlation problems by Microsoft Excel: III. Convolution and deconvolution. Eur. J. Pharm. and Biopharm. 56(3), 429–437.

41. Wagner, J.G. (1993). Absorption Analysis and Bioavailability. In: *Pharmacokinetics for the Pharmaceutical Scientist*. Technomic Pub. Co. Inc., Lancaster, PA. pp. 159–206.

42. Loo, J. & Riegelman, S. (1968). New method for calculating the intrinsic absorption rate of drugs. J. Pharm. Sci. 57, 918–928.

43. Wagner, J.G. (1983). Pharmacokinetic absorption plots from oral data alone or oral/intravenous data and an exact Loo–Riegelman equation. J. Pharm. Sci. 72, 838–842.

44. Veng-Pedersen, P. (1989). Mean time parameters in pharmacokinetics. Definition, computation and clinical implications (Part I). Clin. Pharmacokin. 17, 345–366.

45. Podczeck, F. (1993). Comparison of *in vitro* dissolution profiles by calculating mean dissolution time (MDT) or mean residence time (MRT). Int. J. Pharm. 97, 93–100.

46. Sirisuth, N., Augsburger, L.L. & Eddington, N.D. (2002). Development and validation of a non-linear IVIVC model for a diltiazem extended release formulation. Biopharm. & Drug Disposition 23(1), 1–8.

47. Gillespie, W.R. (1997). Convolution-based approaches for *in vivo-in vitro* correlation modeling. Adv. Exp. Med. Biol. 423, 53–65.

48. Veng-Pedersen, P., Gobburu, J.V.S., Meyer, M.C. & Straughn, A.B. (2000). Carbamazepine level-A *in vivo-in vitro* correlation (IVIVC): A scaled convolution based predictive approach. Biopharm. Drug Disposition 21(1), 1–6.

49. Gillespie, W.R. (1997). *In vivo* modeling strategies for IVIVC for modified release dosage forms. AAPS/CRS/FDA Workshop on Scientific Foundation and Applications for the Biopharmaceutics Classification System and *In vitro–In vivo* Correlations, Arlington, VA. April.

50. Ritger, P.L. & Peppas, N.A. (1987). A simple equation for description of solute release I. Fickian and non-Fickian release from non-swellable devices in the form of slabs, spheres, cylinders or disks. J. Controlled Release 5, 23–26.

51. O'Hara, T., Hayes, S., Davis, J., Devane, J., Smart, T. & Dunne, A. (2001). Journal of Pharmacokinetics and Pharmacodynamics 28(3), 277–298.

52. Gaynor, C., Dunne, A. & Davis, J. (2007). A comparison of the prediction accuracy of two IVIVC modeling techniques. J. Pharm. Sci. Early View, 7 November.

53. Blanquest, S., et al. (2004). A dynamic artificial gastrointestinal system for studying the behavior of orally administered drug dosage forms under various physiological conditions. Pharm. Res. 21(4), 585–589.

54. Minekus, M., et al. (1999). A computer-controlled system to simulate conditions of the large intestine with peristaltic mixing, water absorption and absorption of fermentation products. Appl. Microbiol. Biotechnol. 53, 108–114.

55. Zahirula, M. & Khan, I. (1996). Dissolution testing for sustained or controlled release oral dosage forms and correlation with *in vivo* data: Challenges and opportunities. Int. J. Pharm. 140(2), 131–143.

56. Humbert., et al. (1994). *In vitro–in vivo* correlation of a modified-release oral form of ketotifen: *In vitro* dissolution rate specification. J. Pharm. Sci. 83(2), 131–136.

57. Qiu, Y., Cheskin, H., Briskin, J. & Engh, K. (1997). Sustained-release hydrophilic matrix tablets of zileuton: Formulation and *in vitro/in vivo* studies. J. Controlled Release 45, 249–256.

58. Ku, M., et al. (1998). Optimization of sustained-release diltiazem formulations in man by use of an *in vitro/in vivo* correlation. J. Pharm. Pharmacol. 50, 845–850.

59. Mu, X., et al. (2003). Development and evaluation of biodissolution systems capable of detecting the food effect on a polysaccharide-based matrix system. J. Controlled Release 93, 309–318.

60. Katori, N., et al. (1995). Estimation of agitation intensity in the GI tract in humans and dogs based on *in vitro/in vivo* correlation. Pharm. Res. 12(2), 237–243.

61. Shameem, M., et al. (1995). Oral solid controlled release dosage forms: Role of GI-mechanical destructive forces and colonic release in drug absorption under fasted and fed conditions in humans. Pharm. Res. 12(7), 1049–1053.

62. Aoki., et al. (1992). Evaluation of the correlation between *in vivo* and *in vitro* release of Phenylpropanolamine HCl from controlled release tablets. Int. J. Pharm. 85, 65–73.

63. Macheras, P., et al. (1989). An *in vitro* model for exploring CR theophylline sustained or controlled release systems: *In vitro* drug release profiles. Int. J. Pharm. 54, 123–130.

64. Wingstrand., et al. (1990). Bioavailability from felodipine extended release tablets with different dissolution properties. Int. J. Pharm. 60, 151–156.

65. Grundy, J.S., et al. (1997). Studies on dissolution testing of the nifedipine gastrointestinal therapeutic system. I. Description of a two-phase *in vitro* dissolution test. J. Controlled Release 48, 1–8.

66. Pillay, V. & Fassihi, R. (1999). Unconventional dissolution methodologies. J. Pharm. Sci. 88, 843–851.

67. Parojčić, J., Vasiljević, D., Ibrić, S. & Djurič, Z. (2008). Tablet disintegration and drug dissolution in viscous media: Paracetamol IR tablets. Inter. J. Pharm. 355(1–2), 93–99.

68. Nicolaides, E., Symillides, M., Dressman, J.B. & Reppas, C. (2001). Biorelevant dissolution testing to predict the plasma profile of lipophilic drugs after oral administration. Pharm. Res. 18(3), 380–388.

69. Vertzoni, M., Fotaki, N., Kostewicz, E., Stippler, C., Leuner, E., Nicolaides, J. & Dressman, C. (2004). Dissolution media simulating the intralumenal composition of the small intestine: physiological issues and practical aspects. J. Pharm. Pharmacol. 56(4), 453–462.

70. Al-Behaisi, S., Antalb, I., Morovjána, G., Szúnyoga, J., Drabanta, S., Martonb, S. & Klebovich, I. (2002). *In vitro* simulation of food effect on dissolution of deramciclane film-coated tablets and correlation with *in vivo* data in healthy volunteers. Eur J. Pharm. Sci. 15(2), 157–162.

71. Müllertz, A. (2007). Biorelevant Dissolution Media. In: *Solvent Systems and Their Selection in Pharmaceutics and Biopharmaceutics*, P. Augustijns, & M.E. Brewster, (eds). Springer, New York. pp. 151–177.

72. Jones, H.M., Parrott, N., Ohlenbusch, G. & Lave, T. (2006). Predicting pharmacokinetic food effects using biorelevant solubility media and physiologically based modelling. Clinical Pharmacokinetics 45(12), 1213–1226.

73. Pedersen, B.L., Brøndsted, H., Lennernäs, H., Christensen, F.N., Müllertz, A. & Kristensen, H.G. (2000). Dissolution of hydrocortisone in human and simulated intestinal fluids. Pharm. Res. 17, s183.

74. Dressman, J.B. & Reppas, C. (2000). *In vitro–in vivo* correlations for lipophilic, poorly water-soluble drugs. Eur J. Pharm. Sci. 11(S2), S73–S80.

75. El-Arini., et al. (1990). Theophylline controlled release preparations and fatty food: An *in vitro* study using the rotating dialysis cell method. Pharm. Res. 7, 1134–1140.

76. Morita, R., et al. (2003). Development of a new dissolution test method for an oral controlled release preparation, the PVA swelling controlled release system (SCRS). J. Controlled Release 90(1), 109–117.

77. Minekus, M. & Havenaar, R. (1996). *In vitro* model of an *in vivo* digestive tract. US patent 5(525), 305.

78. Blanquet, S., Zeijdner, E., Beyssac, E., Meunier, J., Denis, S., Havenaar, R. & Alric, M. (2004). A dynamic artificial gastrointestinal system for studying the behavior of orally administered drug dosage forms under various physiological conditions. Pharm. Res. 21, 37–49.

79. Hu, Z., Kimra, G., Murakami, M., Yoshikawa, Y., Takada, K. & Yoshikawa, K. (1999). A dissolution test for a pressure-controlled colon delivery capsule: Rotating beads method. J. Pharm. Pharmacol. 51(9), 979–989.

80. Gu, C.H., Rao, D., Gandhi, R.B., Hilden, J. & Raghavan, K. (2005). Using a novel multicompartment dissolution system to predict the effect of gastric pH on the oral absorption of weak bases with poor intrinsic solubility. J. Pharm. Sci. 94(1), 199–208.

81. He, X., Kadomura, S., Takekuma, Y., Sugawara, M. & Miyazaki, K. (2003). An *in vitro* system for prediction of oral absorption of relatively water-soluble drugs and ester prodrugs. Int. J. Pharm. 263, 35–44.

82. Souliman, S., Blanquet, S., Beyssac, E. & Cardot, J. (2006). A level A *in vitro/in vivo* correlation in fasted and fed states using different methods: Applied to solid immediate release oral dosage form. Eur J. Pharm. Sci. 27(1), 72–79.

83. Lake, O.A., Olling, M. & Barends, D.M. (1999). *In vitro/in vivo* correlations of dissolution data of carbamazepine immediate release tablets with pharmacokinetic data obtained in healthy volunteers. Eur. J. Pharm. Biopharm. 48(1), 13–19.

84. Shah, V.F. & Williams, R.L. (1994). *In Vitro* and *In Vivo* Correlations: Scientific and Regulatory Perspectives. In: *Generics and Bioequivalence*, A.J. Jackson, (ed.). CRC Press, Inc., Boca Raton, FL. pp. 101–111.

85. Gordon, M.S. & Chowhan, Z. (1996). *In vivo/in vitro* correlations for four differently dissolving ketorolac tablets. Biopharm. Drug Dispos. 17(6), 481–492.

86. Law, D., Schmitt, E.A., Marsh, K., Everitt, E.A., Wang, W., Fort, J.J., Krill, S.L. & Qiu, Y. (2004). Ritonavir-PEG 8000 amorphous solid dispersions: *in vitro* and *in vivo* evaluation. J. Pharm. Sci. 93, 563–570.

87. Li, S., He, H., Lakshman, J., Parthiban, I., Yin, H. & Serajuddin, A.T.M. (2006). IV-IVC considerations in the development of immediate-release oral dosage form. J. Pharm. S. 94(7), 1396–1417.

88. Qiu, Y. & Zhang, G. (2000). Research and Development Aspects of Oral Controlled Release Systems. In: *Handbook of Pharmaceutical Controlled Release Technology*, D.L. Wise, A.M. Klibanov, R. Langer, A.G. Mikos, N.A. Peppas, D.J. Trantolo, G.E. Wnek, & M.J. Yaszeski, (eds). Marcel Dekker, Inc., New York, NY. pp. 465–503.

89. Physicians Desk Reference. (2005). 59th edition. Thomson Healthcare, Stamford, CT.

90. Ju, T.R. (2003). *AAPS Short Course "Developing IVIVC for Oral MR Products: Drug Property, Formulation Design and Dissolution Considerations."* Salt lake City, UT.

91. Pitsiu, M., Sathyan, G., Gupta, S. & Verotta, D. (2001). A semi-parametric deconvolution model to establish *in vivo–in vitro* correlation applied to OROS oxybutynin. J. Pharm. Sci. 90(6), 702–712.

92. Drover, D.R., Angst, M.S. & Valle, M. (2002). Input characteristics and bioavailability after administration of immediate and a new extended-release formulation of hydromorphone in healthy volunteers. Anesthesiology 97, 827–836.

93. Wang, Y., Lee, L., Somma, R., Thompson, G., Bakhtiar, R., Lee, J., Rekhi, G.S., Lau, H., Sedek, G. & Hossain, M. (2004). *In vitro* dissolution and *in vivo* oral absorption of methylphenidate from a bimodal release formulation in healthy volunteers. Biopharm. Drug. Dispos. 25(2), 91–98.

94. Sako, K., Sawadaa, T., Nakashimaa, H., Yokohama, S. & Sonobe, T. (2002). Influence of water soluble fillers in hydroxypropyl-methylcellulose matrices on *in vitro* and *in vivo* drug release. J. Controlled Release 81(1–2), 165–172.

95. Verbekena, D., Neirinckb, N., Van Der Meerenb, P. & Dewettinck, K. (2005). Influence of κ-carrageenan on the thermal gelation of salt-soluble meat proteins. Meat Science 70(1), 161–166.

96. Melia, C.D., Rajabi-Siahboomic, A.R. & Bowtell, R.W. (1998). Magnetic resonance imaging of controlled release pharmaceutical dosage forms. Pharmaceutical Science & Technology Today 1(1), 32–39.

97. Richardson, J.C., Bowtellb, R.W., Mäderc, K. & Melia, C.D. (2005). Pharmaceutical applications of magnetic resonance imaging (MRI). Advanced Drug Delivery Reviews 57(8), 1191–1209.

98. Roshdy, M., Schnaare, R.L., Sugita, E.T. & Schwartz, J.B. (2002). The effect of controlled release tablet performance and hydrogel strength on *in vitro/in vivo* correlation. Pharm. Dev. Technol. 7(2), 155–168.

99. Bajwa, G.S., Hoebler, K., Sammon, C., Timmins, P. & Melia, C.D. (2006). Microstructural imaging of early gel layer formation in HPMC matrices. J. Pharm. Sci. 95(10), 2145–2157.

100. Yang, L., Johnson, B. & Fassihi, R. (1998). Determination of continuous changes in the gel layer thickness of poly(ethylene oxide) and HPMC tablets undergoing hydration: A texture analysis study. Pharm. Res. 15(12), 1902–1906.

101. Meyvisa, T.K.L., Stubbea, B.G., Van Steenbergenb, M.J., Henninkb, W.E., De Smedt, S.C. & Demeestera, J. (2002). A comparison between the use of dynamic mechanical analysis and oscillatory shear rheometry for the characterisation of hydrogels. Inter. J. Pharm. 244(1–2), 163–168.

102. Grundy, J.S., Anderson, K.E., Rogers, J.A. & Foster, R.T. (1997). Studies on dissolution testing of the nifedipine gastrointestinal therapeutic system. II. Improved *in vitro-in vivo* correlation using a two-phase dissolution test. J. Controlled Release 48(1), 9–17.

103. Hegasy, A. & Ramsch, K. Solid medicament formulations containing nifedipine, and processes for their preparation. United States Patent 5 264 446.

104. Katzhendler, I., Azoury, R. & Friedman, M. (1998). Crystalline properties of carbamazepine in sustained release hydrophilic matrix tablets based on hydroxypropyl methylcellulose. Journal of Controlled Release 54(1), 69–85.

105. Li, X., Zhi, F. & Hu, Y. (2007). Investigation of excipient and processing on solid phase transformation and dissolution of ciprofloxacin. Int. J. of Pharm. 328(2), 177–182.

106. Rohrs, B.R. (2003). Dissolution assay development for *in vitro–in vivo* correlations. Am. Pharm. Rev. 6(1), 8–12.

107. Lake, O.A., Olling, M. & Barends, D.M. (1999). *In vitro/in vivo* correlations of dissolution data of carbamazepine immediate release tablets with pharmacokinetic data obtained in healthy volunteers. European Journal of Pharmaceutics and Biopharmaceutics 48(1), 13–19.

108. Piscitelli, D.A. & Young, D. (1997). Setting dissolution specifications for modified-release dosage forms. Adv. Exp. Med. Biol. 423, 159–166.

109. Uppoor, V.R.S. (2001). Regulatory perspectives on *in vitro* (dissolution)/*in vivo* (bioavailability) correlations. J. Controlled Release 72(1–3), 127–132.

110. Elkoshi, Z. (1999). Dissolution specifications based on release rates. J. Pharm. Sci. 88(4), 434–444.

111. Hayes, S., Dunne, A., Smart, T. & Davis, J. (2004). Interpretation and optimization of the dissolution specifications for a modified release product with an *in vivo-in vitro* correlation (IVIVC). J. Pharm. Sci. 93(3), 571–581.

112. Guidance for Industry (2000). *Waiver of In vivo Bioavailability and Bioequivalence Studies for Immediate-Release Solid Oral Dosage Forms Based on a Biopharmaceutics Classification System.* US Department of Health, Food and Drug Administration, Center for Drug Evaluation and Research (CDER), August.

113. Biopharmaceutics Classification System (BCS) Guidance. US Department of Health, Food and Drug Administration, Center for Drug Evaluation and Research (CDER), Office of Pharmaceutical Sciences. (http://www.fda.gov/cder/OPS/BCS_guidance.htm).

114. International Pharmaceutical Federation (FIP), Board of Pharmaceutical Sciences, Working Group on Biopharmaceutics Classification System (BCS). [http://www.fip.org/www2/sciences/index.php?page=pharmacy_sciences&pharmacy_sciences=ps_sig_bcs]

115. Guidance for Industry. (1997). *SUPAC-MR: Modified Release Solid Oral Dosage Forms Scale-Up and Postapproval Changes: Chemistry, Manufacturing, and Controls; In vitro Dissolution Testing and In vivo Bioequivalence Documentation.* US Department of Health, Food and Drug Administration, Center for Drug Evaluation and Research (CDER), September.

116. Siewert, M. (1993). Perspectives of *in vitro* dissolution test in establishing *in vivo/in vitro* correlations. Eur. J. Drug Metab. Pharmacokinet. 18(1), 7–18.

117. Cardot, J.M. & Beyssac, E. (1993). *In vitro/in vivo* correlations: Scientific implications and standardisation. Eur. J. Drug Metab. Pharmacokinet. 18(1), 113–120.

118. Sirisuth, N. & Eddington, N.D. (2002). The influence of first pass metabolism on the development and validation of an IVIVC for metoprolol extended release tablets. Eur. J. Pharm. Biopharm. 53(3), 301–309.

119. Mistry, B., Leslie, J.L. & Eddington, N.D. (2002). Influence of input rate on the stereospecific and nonstereospecific first pass metabolism and pharmacokinetics of metoprolol extended release formulations. Chirality 14(4), 297–304.

120. Qiu, Y., Law, D. & Krill, S. (1995). Use of total plasma concentration of a drug given as racemate in absorption analysis is not valid for drug exhibiting stereoselective disposition and/or absorption. Proc. 22nd Int. Sym. on Controlled Release of Bioactive Materials 280.

121. Cao, G.L. & Locke, C. (1997). Assessing whether controlled release products with differing *in vitro* dissolution rates have the same *in vivo–in vitro* relationship. In: *In Vitro–In Vivo Correlations*, D. Young, J. Devane, & J. Butler, (eds). Plenum Press, New York. pp. 173–180.

122. Kortejärvi, H., Malkki, J., Marvola, M., Urtti, A., Yliperttula, M. & Pajunen, P. (2007). Level A *in vitro-in vivo* correlation (IVIVC) model with Bayesian approach to formulation series. J. Pharm. Sci. 95(7), 1595–1605.

123. Grundy, J.S. & Foster, R.T. (1996). The nifedipine gastrointestinal therapeutic system (GITS). Evaluation of pharmaceutical, pharmacokinetic and pharmacological properties. Clin. Pharmacokinet. 30(1), 28–51.

124. Schug, B.S., Brendel, E., Chantraine, E., Wolf, D., Martin, W., Schall, R. & Blume, H.H. (2002). The effect of food on the pharmacokinetics of nifedipine in two slow release formulations: pronounced lag-time after a high fat breakfast. Br. J. Clin. Pharmacol. 53(6), 582–588.

125. Qiu, Y. (2005). Strategy and approach in developing *in vitro-in vivo* correlations. Proc. 3rd CPA/AAPS Joint Symposium on: Modern Theory and Practice of Pharmaceutical Sciences in Research and Development of Oral Dosage Form. Shanghai. pp. 261–270.

126. Qiu, Y., Cheskin, H., Engh, K. & Poska, R. (2003). Once-a-day controlled-release dosage form of Divalproex Sodium I: Formulation design and *in vitro/in vivo* investigations. J. Pharm. Sci. 92(6), 1166–1173.

127. Qiu, Y. (2005). *In vitro–in vivo* correlations of oral solid dosage forms: Basics, development methodology, modeling, evaluation and applications. Proc. 3rd CPA/AAPS Joint Symposium on: Modern Theory and Practice of Pharmaceutical Sciences in Research and Development of Oral Dosage Form. Shanghai. pp. 250–260.

## PART III

DESIGN, DEVELOPMENT, AND SCALE-UP OF FORMULATION AND PROCESS

Integration of Physical, Chemical, Mechanical, and Biopharmaceutical Properties in Solid Oral Dosage Form Development

Xiaorong He

18.1 INTRODUCTION

In today's drug development world, combinatorial chemistry, high-throughput screening, and genomics have provided a technologic platform that produces hundreds of thousands of new chemical entities with therapeutic potential each year. It has been estimated that for every successful drug compound, 5000 to 10 000 compounds must be introduced into the drug-discovery pipeline. On average, it takes $800 million, and 10 to 15 years, to develop a successful drug. The reasons for failure are many. One thing is always true though—a marketable dosage form with the desired drug delivery properties must be developed to commercialize a product. Drug development requires a concerted effort among experts in the fields of pharmacology, chemistry, toxicology, metabolism, clinical research, and formulation development to ensure that a dosage form is safe, efficacious, robust, and manufacturable.

In order to initiate formulation development of a marketable product, important physico-chemical properties of a new chemical entity need to be determined early in the discovery process. This information is helpful in selecting the most promising lead molecules for further development. Once a lead candidate is selected for clinical testing, it is important to understand biopharmaceutical properties of the drug candidate with respect to its absorption and disposition *in vivo*. This is helpful in making appropriate

formulation choices to maximize the drug's bioavailability, which is believed to result in optimum therapeutic efficacy. Once the formulation is selected, and ready to enter phase 2 clinical trials, it is important to characterize mechanical properties of the formulation to ensure that it can be manufactured at a large scale in a reproducible and effective manner. This chapter will discuss the impact of physico-chemical properties, mechanical properties, and biopharmaceutical properties on various aspects of dosage form development. It will become apparent that a sound understanding of the interplay of this multitude of factors is a prerequisite to make science-based decisions for development of a bioavailable, stable and robust marketable product.

18.2 PHYSICAL AND CHEMICAL PROPERTIES

Physico-chemical properties of drug candidates may have a significant impact on manufacturing, storage, and performance of drug products. Key physical chemical properties, such as solubility and permeability, may also have significant ramifications on oral absorption of a drug *in vivo*. Therefore, measurement of physico-chemical properties not only helps to guide dosage form selection, but also provides insights into how drug products should be processed and stored to ensure quality. This section discusses the potential impact of key physico-chemical properties on various aspects of oral dosage form development. Relevant physico-chemical properties include aqueous solubility, dissolution rate, partition coefficient, biological membrane permeability, ionization constant, polymorphism, crystallinity, particle size/particle morphology, surface area, density, porosity, melting point, hygroscopicity, and solution stability and solid-state stability. It should be kept in mind that many of these properties are dependent on the solid form, and complete characterization of each of the most relevant solid forms is needed to provide a complete physico-chemical picture.

18.2.1 Aqueous Solubility

The solubility of a solid substance is defined as the concentration at which the solution phase is in equilibrium with a given solid phase at a stated temperature and pressure. It can be described by the van't Hoff equation as follows:[1]

$$-\log X = \frac{\Delta H_f}{2.303R}\left(\frac{T_0 - T}{TT_0}\right) + \log \gamma \qquad (18.1)$$

where:

X = solubility of a solute in mole fraction
ΔH_f = heat of fusion, that is, the heat absorbed when a solid melts
T_0 = melting point of the solid solute in absolute degrees
T = absolute temperature of the solution
γ = activity coefficient.

γ is determined by the intermolecular forces of attraction that must be overcome in removing a solute molecule from the solid phase and depositing it in the solvent. The stronger the solute–solute interaction, the higher the value of γ. In an ideal solution, the interactions between the solute and solvent molecules are identical to the solute–solute and solvent–solvent molecule interactions; under this condition the activity coefficient equals unity.

The aqueous solubility of a drug molecule is one of the key factors that influence the extent of drug absorption after oral administration. A prerequisite for a drug to exert its pharmacological effect is that the drug molecule has to be absorbed. In order for absorption to take place, the drug needs to be in solution at the site(s) of absorption. The following equation describes the flux of drug molecules across the intestinal membrane for an orally administered drug:

$$\text{Flux} = P_m \times (C_i - C_b) \qquad (18.2)$$

where:

P_m = intestinal membrane permeability
C_i = aqueous drug concentration (unionized) in the intestine
C_b = portal blood concentration.

Following oral administration, a solid dosage form enters the gastrointestinal tract where it disintegrates and dissolves to release drug. The small intestine, given its enormous surface area, is the primary site for absorption of the majority of marketed drug products. Most marketed drugs are absorbed through a passive diffusion process, where the concentration gradient, $(C_i - C_b)$, provides the driving force for molecules to diffuse across the intestinal wall to enter the systemic circulation. Generally, ionizable species are too polar to diffuse across the lipid-rich membranes of intestinal cells. Therefore, the concentration of the unionized form should be considered in Equation 18.2. The drug concentration in the lumen of the intestinal tract may approach or equal its aqueous solubility if dissolution and release of drug from the dosage form is sufficiently rapid. From Equation 18.2 then, it is apparent that the flux of drug across the intestine is directly proportional to its aqueous solubility. For drugs that have high intestinal membrane permeability, the membrane diffusion process is relatively fast. In this case, aqueous solubility may limit the rate and extent of drug absorption.

Generally, solubility is determined by adding excess drug to well-defined aqueous media, and agitating until equilibrium is achieved. It is important to control temperature, drug purity, and to allow sufficient time for equilibrium to be established, in order to assure high quality solubility data. In particular, it is important to evaluate the suspended solid form present at equilibrium, as conversion to another solid form (e.g., polymorph, pseudopolymorph, hydrate, salt) may occur during equilibration. If a form change occurs, the measured solubility is more likely representative of the solubility of the final form present, rather than the starting material. Given the importance of solubility on drug absorption, solubility determination has become a routine test in preformulation development. High-throughput screening methods are often used to measure or classify solubility of a large number of drug candidates rapidly in a variety of solvents. Despite its shortcomings as being a dynamic measure (i.e., not at equilibrium), and increased variability due to higher throughput, high-throughput solubility screening does offer valuable information to guide selection of an appropriate formulation strategy, especially for poorly soluble compounds. The impact of solubility on formulation selection will be discussed later in Section 18.4 (the Biopharmaceutical Properties section) of this chapter.

18.2.2 Dissolution Rate

The dissolution rate of a solute from a solid can be described by the Noyes–Whitney equation as follows:[2]

$$\frac{dC}{dt} = \frac{A \times D}{h}(S - C) \qquad (18.3)$$

where:

dC/dt = dissolution rate of drug
A = the surface area of solid
D = aqueous diffusion coefficient
h = aqueous diffusion layer thickness
S = aqueous drug solubility at the surface of the dissolving solid
C = concentration of drug in the bulk aqueous phase.

From the Noyes–Whitney equation, the dissolution rate is seen to be directly proportional to the aqueous solubility, S, as well as the surface area, A, of drug exposed to the dissolution medium. It is a common practice, when developing an immediate release dosage form of poorly soluble drug, to increase drug dissolution rate by increasing the surface area of a drug through particle size reduction.

Since drug dissolution has to occur before a drug can exert its pharmacological effect, the dissolution rate of an oral dosage form may be manipulated to time the pharmacological response. For certain therapeutic classes, such as antihypertension, pain relief, and antiseizure, it may be desirable to develop a fast-dissolving dosage form to achieve rapid relief of symptoms. For chronic therapy, it may be desirable to have a sustained-release dosage form to achieve once daily dosing to improve patient compliance. In some cases, it may be desirable to have a pulsated release where some immediate release provides rapid relief of symptoms, followed by sustained drug release to maintain the drug above its therapeutic concentration over a long period of time.

Given the diversity of drug release profiles, and their potential impact on therapeutic performance, dissolution tests have become an integral part of drug product development as a quality control tool. They are particularly important for drugs that have a high-risk potential for bioequivalence and bioavailability problems. A dissolution profile of percentage drug released in the dissolution medium as a function of time can be generated using one of the four types of dissolution apparatus approved by the United States Pharmacopeia.[3] In vitro dissolution profiles may not be predictive of in vivo results, because it is difficult to simulate the complex make-up of gastrointestinal fluid

and the agitation dynamics of the human GI tract. However, when an *in vivo–in vitro* correlation can be established, the *in vitro* dissolution test may then be used to justify drug product changes post-regulatory approval, without conducting a bioequivalence study in humans.[4]

18.2.3 Partition Coefficient

The partition coefficient is defined as the concentration ratio of unionized drug distributed between two phases at equilibrium:

$$P = \frac{[A]_o}{[A]_w} \qquad (18.4)$$

The logarithm (base 10) of the partition coefficient ($\log_{10}P$) is often used in the pharmaceutical and medicinal chemistry literature; environmental and toxicological sciences have more traditionally used the term K or K_{ow}.

For ionizable drugs where the ionized species does not partition into the organic phase, the apparent partition coefficient, D, can be calculated from the following:

Acids: $\log_{10}D = \log_{10}P - \log_{10}(1 + 10^{(pH-pKa)})$ (18.5)

Bases: $\log_{10}D = \log_{10}P - \log_{10}(1 + 10^{(pKa-pH)})$ (18.6)

The octanol–water partition coefficient, ($\log_{10}P_{ow}$), has been widely used as a measurement for defining the relative lipophilicity of a drug. The octanol–water system was selected in part because octanol is flexible, and contains a polar head and a nonpolar tail, which resembles biological membrane components. Hence, the tendency of a drug molecule to leave the aqueous phase and partition into octanol is viewed as a measure of how efficiently the drug will partition into, and diffuse across, biological barriers such as the intestinal membrane.

The application of partition coefficient data to drug delivery and quantitative structure activity relationships (QSARs) grew rapidly in the 1960s and 1970s to become a routinely studied physico-chemical parameter in medicinal chemistry and pharmaceutics.[5] Partition coefficients are relatively simple to measure, but the measurement is often time-consuming and challenging.[6] This, in part, stimulated the development of computational methods to estimate partition coefficient to meet the demand of rapid through-put development. Several recent reviews have cited programs and methods that are commercially available.[7–9] In general, the greatest success in predicting partition coefficient is likely to be achieved with the development of specific relationships within a defined chemical space. What this means for medicinal chemists is that measurement of representative compounds within a therapeutic class may very likely allow more accurate prediction of the properties of the entire class.

18.2.4 Permeability

There are essentially four mechanisms by which a drug molecule may cross the intestinal membrane to be absorbed. These are passive diffusion, carrier mediated transport, endocytosis, and paracellular transport. Among these, the most prevalent mechanism of drug transport is passive diffusion, which can be described by Fick's law, which has been simplified by Riggs:[10]

$$\left(\frac{dQ_b}{dt}\right)_{g \to b} = D_m \cdot A_m \cdot R_{m/aq} \cdot \left(\frac{C_g - C_b}{\Delta X_m}\right) \quad (18.7)$$

where:

$(dQ_b/dt)_{g \to b}$ = rate of appearance of drug in the blood when the drug diffuses from the gut fluids (g)
D_m = diffusion coefficient of the drug through the membrane
A_m = surface area of the absorbing membrane available for drug diffusion
$R_{m/aq}$ = partition coefficient of the drug between the membrane and the aqueous gut fluids
$C_g - C_b$ = concentration gradient across the membrane, representing the difference in the free drug concentration in the gut fluids (C_g) and the drug concentration in the blood (C_b) at the site of absorption
ΔX_m = thickness of the membrane.

Permeability determines the ability of a drug molecule to penetrate biological membrane in a passive diffusion process. It largely depends on three interdependent physico-chemical parameters: lipophilicity; polarity; and molecular size.[11,12] Drug lipophilicity is an important indicator of permeability, because partitioning of a drug into lipophilic epithelial cells is a necessary step for passive diffusion. A common measure of lipophilicity is the octanol-water partition coefficient (log P), which was discussed in greater detail in Section 18.2.3. In principle, a lipophilic drug with high log P tends to have higher membrane permeability as it can partition more easily into the lipid bilayer. However, drugs with excessively high lipophilicity may become sequestered in the cell, with little improvement in permeability across the membrane. In a recent study by Lipinski and coworkers,[13] only about 10% of the compounds that entered late stage clinical testing (phase 2) had a log P greater than 5.

Additional factors that appear to influence permeability are polarity and molecular weight. Membrane permeability is determined by the balance between the drug–water and drug–membrane intermolecular forces. Polar compounds with an excessive number of hydrogen bond donors and hydrogen bond acceptors form strong interactions with water, which has been correlated to poor permeability. Compounds with very high molecular weight (greater than 500 Daltons) also have poor permeability. Based on a review of physicochemical properties of marketed drugs,[14] Lipinski and others have proposed an empirical "Rule of Five," which states that a drug candidate is likely to have poor oral absorption or poor permeability if a molecule exceeds two or more of the following "limits:"

- There are more than 5 hydrogen bond donors (number of NH + number of OH);
- There are more than 10 hydrogen bond acceptors (number of nitrogens + number of oxygens);
- The molecular weight is greater than 500;
- Log P is greater than 5.

This "Rule of Five" only applies to compounds that undergo passive diffusion transport. The "Rule of Five" has been proven quite useful in selection of new drug candidates with optimum absorption characteristics in the early stages of drug design.

18.2.5 Ionization Constant

Ionization properties of acidic or basic drugs have important ramifications on a wide range of issues including dissolution, membrane partition, complexation, chemical stability, and drug absorption. The Henderson–Hasselbalch equation provides an estimate of the ionized and unionized drug concentration at a function of pH, shown by the following equations:

For acidic drugs:
$$pKa = -\log_{10}(Ka) = pH + \log_{10}([HA]/[A^-]) \quad (18.8)$$

For basic drugs:
$$pKa = pH + \log_{10}([HB^+]/[B]) \quad (18.9)$$

where:

K_a = ionization constant
$[HA]$ = concentration of the unionized acid
$[A^-]$ = concentration of the ionized acid
$[HB^+]$ = concentration of the unionized base
$[B]$ = concentration of the ionized base.

Determination of pK_a is of particular interest to development scientists because solubility, and consequently absorption, is a function of pK_a and pH. The total aqueous solubility is the sum of the concentrations of ionized and unionized species, shown as the following:

For acidic drugs:

$$\log_{10}(S_T) = \log_{10}(S_a)(1 + 10^{(\text{pH}-\text{p}Ka)}) \qquad (18.10)$$

For basic drugs:

$$\log_{10}(S_T) = \log_{10}(S_b)(1 + 10^{(\text{p}Ka-\text{pH})}) \qquad (18.11)$$

where:

S_T = total aqueous solubility
S_a = intrinsic solubility of the free acid
S_b = intrinsic solubility of the free base.

As shown by a typical solubility profile in Figure 18.1,[15] the solubility of acidic or basic drugs can be altered by orders of magnitude with changing pH. Taking a free base, for example, at a pH higher than the $\text{p}K_a$ of the ionizing group, the predominant form present in solution is the unionized form; hence the total solubility is essentially equal to the intrinsic solubility of the free base. At a pH equal to its $\text{p}K_a$, the drug is 50% ionized and the total solubility is equal to twice the intrinsic solubility. As the pH decreases significantly below the $\text{p}K_a$, the total solubility rapidly increases as the percentage ionized is dramatically increasing. In fact, for each unit decrease in pH, the total aqueous solubility will increase 10-fold, until it reaches the limit of the solubility of the ionized form. The reverse trend will be observed for weak acids. The total solubility of a weak acid and its corresponding conjugate form increases with increasing pH, as long as the ionized form continues to be soluble. Such dramatic increase in solubility underlies the rationale of selecting a soluble salt for development. Although ionization helps rapid dissolution of the drug, ionized species cannot passively diffuse across lipid membranes or pass through the tight junctions that link adjacent intestinal absorptive cells. Another concern of using a soluble salt is that it tends to precipitate *in vivo* with changing pH. For example, a soluble salt of weak base could rapidly dissolve at the low pH in the stomach, but as the drug enters the intestine where the pH approaches neutral, precipitation of the free base could occur. Such changes have been proposed as an explanation for the poor bioavailability of highly soluble salts of weak bases. Lastly, it is important to recognize that oral absorption cannot be accurately predicted by pH alone. It is influenced by a host of factors such as the rate of dissolution, lipid solubility, common ion effects, and metabolism in the GI tract.

A $\text{p}K_a$ value can be determined by a variety of analytical methods, including titrametric and spectroscopic methods, as well as measurements of aqueous solubility

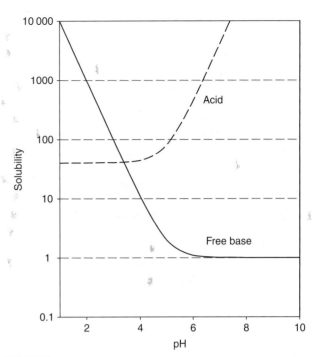

FIGURE 18.1 pH-solubility profile for a free base and its corresponding acid (copied from Figure 3 in reference 15)

as a function of pH. The $\text{p}K_a$ may also be reasonably estimated by predictive tools, based on a variety of approaches. These include the application of linear free energy relationships based on group contributions, chemical reactivity, and calculated atomic charges.

18.2.6 Polymorphism

Polymorphs differ in molecular packing (crystal structure), but share the same chemical composition.[16] Hydrates or solvates are often called "pesudopolymorphs" because, in addition to containing the same given drug molecule, hydrates or solvates also contain molecules of solvents that are incorporated into the crystal lattice. It is very common that drug substances can crystallize into different polymorphs and pesudopolymorphs. Polymorphism has a profound implication on formulation development, because polymorphs may exhibit significantly different solubility, dissolution rate, compactibility, hygroscopicity, physical stability, and chemical stability.[16] Succinylsulfathiazole is an excellent example to illustrate the complexity of the polymorphic issue. It crystallizes into at least six anhydrate polymorphs (forms I, II, III, IV, V, and VI), and three monohydrate crystal forms (H_I, H_{II}, and H_{III}), as well as an acetone solvate and an *n*-butanol solvate.[17] The solubility differences among the anhydrate polymorphs are as large as a factor of 4, and those between the anhydrate and hydrate crystal forms are as large as a factor of 12. Higher solubility and faster dissolution rates may lead to significantly better oral bioavailability, such as is the case with chloramphenicol palmitate.[18] Although use of a faster dissolving polymorph may have clinical benefit, it is important to keep in mind that a polymorph with a higher solubility or faster dissolution rate is also metastable (i.e., a higher energy form) and tends to convert to a thermodynamically more stable form over time. The conversion between solid forms is affected by multiple factors, such as solvent used, relative humidity, temperature, mechanical agitation, etc. Conversion from a metastable form to a stable form could lower a drug's oral bioavailability, and lead to inconsistent product quality. Therefore, companies prefer to select the thermodynamically most stable polymorph for development. It is important to keep in mind that polymorphic form conversion may still occur, even when a stable crystal form is chosen for development. In a recent review article, Zhang et al. reviewed how polymorphic conversion may occur in common pharmaceutical processes, such as milling, wet granulation, drying, and compression.[19]

18.2.7 Crystallinity

One definition of a crystalline material is that the component molecules are arranged or "packed" in a highly ordered fashion. In contrast, an amorphous material lacks the long-range order of crystals, but it probably possesses some short-range order (over a few Ångstroms). All crystals contain some disordered or amorphous regions. The degree of crystallinity refers to the ratio of crystalline to amorphous contents in a sample. Samples with low crystallinity or high amorphous content usually exhibit higher solubility, and a faster dissolution rate than pure crystalline samples. An amorphous form may be formulated to enhance the oral bioavailability of a poorly soluble drug. For example, a solid dispersion of amorphous ritonavir in polyethylene glycol (PEG) dissolved much faster than did a physical mixture containing crystalline ritonavir and PEG.[20] This dissolution enhancement was translated into a marked improvement in both AUC, and C_{max} in beagle dogs.[21] However, physical and chemical instability of amorphous material has prevented widespread applications of using an amorphous form for bioavailability enhancement. An amorphous form is thermodynamically less stable than a crystalline form. Thus, it will eventually crystallize to a slower dissolving form, if given enough time. Batch variation in amorphous content makes it difficult to reproduce drug dissolution profiles, and possibly oral

absorption, from batch to batch. The rate of crystallization may depend on many factors, such as temperature, relative humidity, processing history, excipients, etc. In particular, water can markedly accelerate the crystallization rate of an amorphous form by lowering its glass transition temperature (Tg), one of the most important parameters characterizing an amorphous form. Below the Tg, "the molecules are configurationally frozen in the glassy state," whereas above the Tg, an amorphous solid is said to be in the "rubbery" state, where its molecules have substantial configurational mobility.[16] Thus, it is important to keep amorphous forms stored below their Tg to reduce the rate of crystallization. In addition to physical instability, there is a large body of evidence to show that an amorphous form is less stable than the crystalline form chemically. For example, Pikal showed that cephalothin sodium samples with the highest level of amorphous content were the least stable.[22] Given the above issues, amorphous forms are rarely chosen for development of an oral solid dosage form.

18.2.8 Particle Size, Particle Morphology, and Surface Area

The micromeritic properties of solids, such as surface area, particle size, and particle shape have far-reaching impact on the bioavailability, processability, physical stability, and chemical stability of solid oral dosage forms. First of all, the rate at which a solid dissolves is directly proportional to its surface area exposed to the dissolution medium. Therefore, particle size reduction which leads to increased surface area has long been used to enhance the dissolution rate and bioavailability of a poorly soluble drug. Particle size, particle shape, and surface area also have a significant impact on the processability and product quality of pharmaceutical dosage forms. For a low dose direct compression formulation, where drug content uniformity is of particular concern, the particle size of the drug substance has to be small enough to meet the US Pharmacopeia requirement on content uniformity.[23] For example, Zhang and Johnson showed low dose blends containing a larger drug particle size (18.5 μm) failed to meet the USP requirement, whereas a blend containing smaller particle sizes (6.5 μm) passed.[24] Yalkoswky translated the requirements of the USP content uniformity test into physical and mathematical parameters. Assuming spherical particle sizes with a log-normal distribution, the mean particle size and particle size distribution required to ensure a high probability of passing the content uniformity test can be calculated.[25]

Particle size and shape of a solid may also affect powder flow properties. Many pharmaceutical active ingredients crystallize in needle-shaped crystals that are difficult to filter, and exhibit poor flow properties. Milling of long needle crystals can enhance flow properties, and improve content uniformity of dosage forms. However, excessively small particles tend to be cohesive, and exacerbate flow problems. The flow of small particles (less than $10\,\mu m$) through an orifice is restricted, because the cohesive forces between the particles are of the same magnitude as gravitational forces. A formulation with poor powder flow properties tends to create large tablet weight variation during compression. In addition to flow properties, compactibility of pharmaceutical powders may also be impacted by micromeritics of a solid. Nyström proposed that the primary factors impacting compactibility are how compact bonds are formed, and the surface area over which these bonds are active.[26] Since these two factors are difficult to evaluate experimentally, more indirect secondary factors such as particle size, shape, and surface texture are often used instead for correlation with tablet strength. For example, Alderborn and Nyström studied the effect of particle size on the mechanical strength of tablets for a series of materials with particle size ranging from 90–1000 μm.[27] Three types of relationship between particle size and tensile strength were found. For lactose and sodium citrate, tablet tensile strength increases as the particle size of the starting material decreases. For plastically deforming materials, such as cubic sodium chloride, tablet strength increases with increasing particle size. For aggregated calcium phosphate, tablet tensile strength is relatively independent of input material's particle size. It is important to keep in mind that micromeritic properties of starting materials can be significantly modified after processing. Therefore, it is important to characterize the micromeritic properties of the input materials, as well as the formulated product, to get a complete picture on how micromeritic properties may affect content uniformity, dissolution and manufacturability.

18.2.9 Derived Properties: Density and Porosity

Density and porosity are two important pharmaceutical properties that can be derived from the information on particle size distribution, particle shape, and surface area. Since pharmaceutical particles often contain microscopic cracks, internal pores, and capillary spaces, density can be defined in more than one way. There are three types of density defined for pharmaceutical powders:

1. True density is defined as the density of the material itself, exclusive of the voids or inter-particle pores larger than molecular or atomic dimensions in the crystal lattice. The true density can be predicted from the crystal lattice, and is often determined experimentally using a helium pycnometer.

2. Bulk density, which takes into account macroscopic inter-particle space, is defined as powder mass divided by its bulk volume without any tapping. Powder bulk density depends primarily on particle size distribution, particle shape, and the tendency of particles to adhere to each other. Some particles may pack loosely, leading to fluffy and light powder, while others may contain smaller particles that sift between larger particles to fill the void, leading to dense and heavy powder. Bulk density is often used to calculate the batch size for blender and granulator.

3. Tapped density is measured after a powder sample is subjected to mechanically tapping. The measurement procedure for bulk density and tapped density can be found in the US Pharmacopeia.[28] Bulk density and tapped density can be used to calculate compressibility index and Hausner ratio, which are measures of the propensity of a powder to flow and be compressed:

$$\text{Compressibility index} = \frac{(\text{Tap density} - \text{Bulk density})}{\text{Tap density} \times 100\%} \quad (18.12)$$

$$\text{Hausner ratio} = \frac{\text{Tap density}}{\text{Bulk density}} \quad (18.13)$$

A free-flowing powder should have a low compressibility index, because the inter-particle forces are not as significant as in a poorly-flowing powder, which implies the value of bulk density is close to that of the tapped density. As a general rule of thumb, a compressibility index of higher than 30% indicates poor powder flow.

Porosity can be derived from powder density, and is an important granule characteristic. Granule porosity is typically determined by mercury porosimetry, where mercury can fill inter- and intra-particle voids under pressure, but fails to penetrate the internal pores of the particles. It is generally believed that porous granules dissolve faster than dense granules, since pores allow water to penetrate granules more readily. Fluid bed granulation is known to produce smaller and more porous granules than high shear wet granulation. Therefore, fluid bed granulation may be a more appealing choice to process poorly soluble compounds when slow dissolution is of primary concern.

18.2.10 Melting Point

Melting point is defined as the temperature at which the solid phase exists in equilibrium with its liquid phase. Therefore melting point is a measure of the "energy" required to overcome attractive forces that hold a crystal together. Crystal lattices having greater molecular symmetry or the presence of hydrogen donor groups both significantly increase intermolecular interactions in the solid-state, and increase melting point. Melting point can be determined by any of several commonly used methods, including visual observation of the melting of material packed in a capillary tube (Thiele arrangement), by hot-stage microscopy or other thermal analysis methods, such as differential scanning calorimetry (DSC). It provides useful information for an investigator to assess and quantify the presence of impurities, as well as the presence or interconversion of polymorphs and pseudopolymorphs. Melting points and the energetic of desolvation can also be evaluated, as can the enthalpies of fusion for different solid forms. A comparison of melting points of polymorphs also provides a perspective on the relative stability of polymorphic forms.[29] For monotropic polymorphs, the highest melting polymorph is the most stable form at all temperatures. As for enantiotropic polymorphs, the highest melting polymorph is only the most stable form above the transition temperature.

From a manufacturing perspective, low melting materials tend to be more difficult to handle in conventional solid dosage forms. As a general rule of thumb, melting points below about 60°C are considered to be problematic. Temperatures in conventional manufacturing equipment, such as fluid bed dryers and tablet presses, can exceed 50°C. During the milling process, hot spots in the milling chamber may have much higher temperatures. While amorphous solids do not have a distinct melting point, they undergo softening as temperatures approach their glass transition temperatures. Alternative dosage forms (e.g., liquid type) may be required for liquid or low melting materials.

18.2.11 Hygroscopicity

Moisture uptake is a significant concern for pharmaceutical powders. Many drug substances and pharmaceutical excipients, particularly water-soluble salts, can sorb atmospheric moisture. Moisture has been shown to have a significant impact on the physical stability, chemical stability, flowability, and compactibility of drugs, excipients, and formulations. For example, moisture facilitates conversion between anhydrous forms and crystal hydrates, thus impacting the physical stability of a solid. To form a crystal hydrate, water molecule(s) must occupy a specific crystallographic site, which can be determined by X-ray unequivocally. For deliquescent compounds, materials can adsorb sufficient water to completely dissolve once a critical atmospheric humidity (RH_0) is exceeded. As for chemical stability, there is a large body of evidence to show that water can facilitate solid-state reactions by enhancing the molecular mobility of the reactants or by participating in hydrolysis as a reacting species.[16] For moisture-sensitive compounds like aspirin, hydrolysis can occur during the process of applying an aqueous film coating to aspirin tablets.[30] Therefore, it is important to control film coating process parameters, such as the inlet air relative humidity and spray rate, to minimize the amount of water adsorbed during processing. On the other hand, moisture may improve powder flow and uniformity of the bulk density as water helps dissipate a powder's triboelectrostatic charge. Appropriate amounts of moisture may also act as a binder to facilitate compaction. Given the above, a sound understanding of the hygroscopic properties of a formulation provides valuable guidance on making decisions related to processing, packaging, storage, and handling.

Water sorption and equilibrium moisture content can depend upon the atmospheric humidity, temperature, surface area, and exposure, as well as the mechanism for moisture uptake. In general, water adsorption to the surface of crystalline materials will result in very limited moisture uptake. Zografi suggested that surface water does not amount to more than 1 to 3 molecular layers.[31-32] A 0.1% water uptake would be predicted for monolayer coverage of a crystalline material with an average particle size of $1\,\mu m$.[32] Pharmaceutical powders are typically in the range of $1-200\,\mu m$ in diameter, and tend to adsorb water at a level that is orders of magnitude higher than 0.1%. It has been hypothesized that water must be taken into the solid by disordered or high-energy regions, such as defects and amorphous sites. Moisture sorption has, in fact, been used to quantitate the amorphous content of predominantly crystalline materials.

18.2.12 Chemical Stability

The importance of solution and solid-state stability is well-recognized in the pharmaceutical industry.

A marketable drug must be stable under a wide range of conditions of temperature and relative humidity to ensure a satisfactory shelf life. For oral solid dosage forms, it is generally considered that 2-year storage at room temperature is the minimum acceptable shelf life. This allows sufficient time for manufacture of drug substance and drug product, shipping, storage, and finally sale to and use by consumers. Loss of potency and impurity growth are important considerations in determining the shelf life. While perhaps 5% loss of drug may be considered acceptable by regulatory agencies, the shelf life of a product is often limited by formation of a much lower level of degradation products. The International Conference on Harmonization (ICH) Q3B (R2)[33] specifies the reporting, identification, and qualification thresholds for impurities in new drug products. Depending on the maximum daily dose, a level of 0.1% to 1% of degradation products will likely require identification or qualification.[33]

Solution Stability

For oral solid products, it is important to test solution stability, because a drug has to dissolve in the gastric or intestinal fluids prior to absorption. The stomach is generally quite acidic for a majority of people, and the residence time in the stomach varies between 15 minutes and a few hours depending on food intake. Therefore, it is important to conduct stability testing under acid conditions over a period of a couple of hours at 37°C, to ensure no significant appearance of degradation products of unknown toxicity. Residence time in the small intestine is approximately 3 hours, while residence time in the large intestine ranges up to 24 hours. The intestinal pH may range from 5 to 7. If a drug molecule is stable in solution with the pH ranging from 5 to 7 at 37°C for up to 24 hours, significant decomposition in the intestine will not be likely to occur. For a majority of drug candidates, solution stability is tested in buffered aqueous solution at pH of 1.2 to 2, and in the range of pH 5 to 7. However, for a compound with known stability problems, a complete pH-degradation rate profile can provide valuable information regarding the degradation mechanism and degradation products.

Solid-state Stability

Solid-state decomposition may occur through several pathways, i.e., hydrolysis, oxidation–reduction, racemization, decarboxylation, ring cleavage, and photolysis.[16] Among these, hydrolysis and oxidation–reduction are most frequently encountered.

Most solid-state degradation of pharmaceuticals has been analyzed with either zero-order or first-order kinetics.[34] Occasionally the Prout–Tompkins equation has been used.[35]

To speed up stability testing, accelerated stability studies are often carried out on drug substance and drug product at higher temperatures, such as 40°, 50° or even 70°C, under dry or humid conditions. It is a rule of thumb that the shelf life determined at 40°C/75% RH is about one-fourth of that at room temperature. Extrapolation of shelf life is based on the assumption that a solid-state reaction follows Arrhenius kinetics, and that an activation energy determined at higher temperatures can be used to calculate the rate and shelf life at room temperature. The assumption is valid if the reaction occurring at higher temperatures also occurs at room temperature, and follows the same degradation pathway. However, it is not uncommon that degradation products produced at temperatures such as 60°C and 70°C may never occur at room temperature. Generally though, according to the guidance document Q1A(R2), the FDA allows the projection of shelf life for New Drug Applications based on studies under accelerated conditions, but data at the recommended storage temperature is generally required to support the actual shelf life of marketed products.

18.3 MECHANICAL PROPERTIES

Oral pharmaceutical dosage forms are usually composed of multiple components, including an active ingredient that exerts pharmacological action, and inactive ingredients (or excipients) that enable processing of the active ingredient into a drug product, and facilitate disintegration and dissolution of the drug product upon ingestion. This multi-component system is quite complicated, because the drug and excipients may have widely differing density, shape, surface charge, particle size distribution, and crystal hardness, which significantly influence how well the material can be processed. Thus, it is important to understand how mechanical properties of a formulation and its individual components can influence common pharmaceutical unit operations, such as granulation, compression, milling, and mixing. This section will focus solely on oral solid dosage forms, which constitute the majority of marketed drug products.

18.3.1 Compression and Compaction

The processes of tableting, roller compaction, and extrusion all involve application of mechanical forces to induce compression and compaction of solid particles to form a compact dosage form with sufficient strength. When external forces are applied to a powder mass, the powder bed initially undergoes volume reduction by rearranging solid particles to achieve minimum packing volume. Further compression induces volume reduction through particle deformation. Three common types of deformations are elastic deformation, plastic deformation, and brittle fracture. Elastic deformation is reversible, and typically undesirable, because a compact formed by elastic deformation tends to expand to its original volume during decompression, leading the compact to laminate. Plastic deformation, which is irreversible by nature, may occur when the applied forces reach beyond the elastic limit or yield point. During plastic deformation, materials undergo further volume reduction, and particles are brought to close contact for bonding to occur. Plastic deformation predominates in materials that are soft and pliable, such as microcrystalline cellulose and clays. Conversely, for hard and brittle materials, such as dicalcium phosphate and lactose, the materials may fragment into smaller pieces when the shear strength exceeds the tensile or breaking strength of the materials, a phenomenon known as brittle fracture. Extensive fragmentation creates large clean surfaces, which provide opportunities for bonding between particles to occur. Both plastic deformation and brittle fracture produce strong compacts by forming a large number of contact points where intermolecular attractive forces can develop. In principle, the following material properties favor formation of a strong compact:[36]

1. materials with limited elastic deformation;
2. materials that are highly fragmenting or very plastically deforming;
3. fine particulate materials that have large surface area;
4. starting materials possessing high surface roughness which is capable of forming a large number of weak attractive forces.

18.3.2 Mechanical Property Characterization

Tensile Strength

Compactibility reflects a material's ability to produce compact strength (tensile strength) as a function of solid fraction. Here, solid fraction is calculated by subtracting porosity from unity. Pharmaceutical powder compacts tend to be brittle. For this reason, a simple tensile test by stretching the specimen is rarely used. The most commonly used technique to test breaking or tensile strength of pharmaceutical compacts is a diametral compression test, more commonly known as hardness testing. Taking the Schleuniger hardness tester as an example, a tablet is placed between two opposing platens. A platen driven by an electric motor presses the tablet at a constant load rate against a stationary platen until the tablet breaks. The instrument reports the tablet "hardness value" in both kilopound and Strong Cobb units. Tablet hardness is not a very precise terminology since hardness has a specific meaning in material science, associated with indentation, which will be discussed in this section. Nonetheless, tablet hardness can be converted to tensile strength, which is independent of tablet shape and dimension. For a round tablet, tensile strength can be calculated as the following:

$$\sigma = \frac{2P}{\pi Dt} \qquad (18.14)$$

where:

σ = tablet tensile strength
P = fracture load or tablet hardness
D = tablet diameter
t = tablet thickness.

Indentation Hardness

Unlike tensile strength, which describes the global strength of a specimen, indentation hardness describes the "local" plasticity of a material. Hardness may be defined as the resistance of a material to plastic deformation. To measure a material's hardness, either a pendulum is allowed to strike it from a known distance or an indenter is allowed to fall under gravity onto the surface of the specimen, leaving an indentation. The resistance of the material to indentation or the dynamic indentation hardness can be calculated by dividing the energy of impact to indentation volume. Under the same impact energy, soft materials tend to have a larger indentation, and thereby lower hardness than hard materials. Rowe and Roberts have collected data from the literature on indentation hardness of a variety of common drugs and excipients measured on compacts and crystals.[37]

Young's Modulus

Tensile strength and dynamic hardness alone are not sufficient to describe a material's mechanical properties. For this reason, Young's modulus was introduced to describe the stiffness and toughness of a material. For elastic deformation:

$$E = \frac{\sigma_d}{\varepsilon} \qquad (18.15)$$

where:

E = Young's modulus of elasticity
σ_d = deformation stress
ε = deformation strain.

Young's modulus of elasticity can be determined by several tests, including flexure testing using both four- and three-point beam bending, compression testing, and indentation testing on both crystals and compacts. Rowe and Roberts collected data from the literature on Young's modulus of elasticity of a variety of common drugs and excipients measured by flexure testing.[37] In general, the values of Young's modulus can vary over two orders of magnitude, ranging from high moduli for hard rigid materials (e.g., calcium phosphate) to low moduli for soft elastic materials (e.g., polymers).

Yield Stress from Heckel Plots

Compressibility reflects the ability of a material to undergo volume reduction under pressure. One of the most commonly used models to depict force–volume relationships is the Heckel equation:[38]

$$-\log E = K_y P + K_r \qquad (18.16)$$

where:

E = porosity of the tablet
K_y = a material-dependent constant inversely proportional to its yield strength S ($K_y = 1/3S$) or mean yield pressure P ($K_y = 1/P$)
K_r = porosity of the powder bed where the pressure is zero. This relates to the initial packing stage.

The compression pressure, P, can be calculated by dividing the compression force with tablet surface area. For a flat round tablet:

$$P = \frac{4F}{\pi D^2} \qquad (18.17)$$

where:

F = compression force
D = tablet diameter.

E can be calculated for any stage during compression. For a round tablet, E is calculated using the following equation:

$$E = 100 \times \left[1 - \frac{4w}{\rho_t \times \pi \times D^2 \times H} \right] \qquad (18.18)$$

where:

w = tablet weight
ρ_t = true density of the tableting mass
H = thickness at the point of compression. It can be obtained from relative punch displacement measurement.

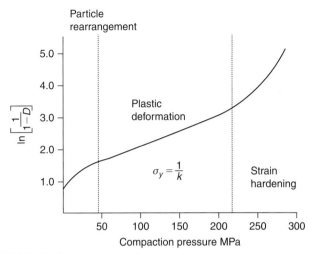

FIGURE 18.2 Schematic diagram of the Heckel plot (copied from Figure 5 in reference 38)

A unique feature of the Heckel plot resides in its ability to differentiate plastic deformation from brittle fracture. Materials that readily undergo plastic deformation have a relatively higher slope than those that undergo brittle fracture, implying the former has a lower yield pressure. Another advantage of the Heckel plot is that it depicts the physical significance of a compression event, shown in Figure 18.2.[38] Three events may occur—particle rearrangement at low pressure, plastic deformation (or fragmentation) occurs at medium to high pressure, and strain hardening at very high pressure.

Tableting Indices

A few decades ago, Hiestand developed a unique set of tableting indices that integrated some of the tests discussed earlier to characterize the mechanical properties of materials under careful experimental control.[39] Hiestand believed that a prerequisite to precise mechanical measurement was to produce compacts without internal fracture. Unfortunately, compacts made from the conventional uniaxial press tend to develop fracture lines, due to large die wall pressures developed during decompression. To solve this problem, he designed a triaxial press with a diagonally-split die to compress materials into square compacts. Unlike the conventional press, which can only relieve pressure vertically, the triaxial press can expand both horizontally and vertically, at a controlled rate, during decompression. Hiestand argued that if the mean die wall pressure and the mean punch pressures were held equal, the internal shear stresses should be less than the strength of the compact, in which case no fracture lines would be developed.

The three indices that Hiestand used to characterize the mechanical properties of materials are the bonding indices (BI), brittle fracture index (BFI), and strain index (SI). BI is calculated as the following:

$$BI_b = \frac{\sigma_T}{H_0} \tag{18.19}$$

$$BI_w = \frac{\sigma_T}{H_{30}} \tag{18.20}$$

where:

BI_b = best case bonding index
σ_T = tensile strength of the compact
H_0 = instantaneous indentation hardness where the indentation volume was obtained when the steel ball strikes the compact and immediately rebounds
BI_w = worst case bonding index
H_{30} = indentation hardness with a dwell time of 30 minutes. The indentation volume was obtained when the steel ball was held in contact with the compact for 30 minutes.

Hiestand believed that BI is a better indicator for a compact's bond strength than the conventionally used tensile strength, because tablets with excellent tensile strength may still have problems of capping and lamination. By incorporating the term of dynamic hardness, it is believed that BI more accurately reflects the actual bond strength of the compact. The higher the BI, the stronger is the bond strength of the compact. The value of dynamic hardness H depends on the dwell time over which an indentation is made. When the dwell time is really long, such as 30 minutes, the dynamic hardness H_{30} is lower than the instantaneous dynamic hardness H_0, and more so for viscoelastic materials. In theory, viscoelastic materials tend to produce stronger bonds than non-viscoelastic materials.[40] Therefore, both the magnitude of bonding indices, and the differences between BI_b and BW_b, should be considered. A large difference indicates the tablet strength can be dramatically improved by slowing down the machine speed.

The brittleness of a material may be measured by its brittle fracture index, calculated as:

$$BFI = 0.5 \times \left(\frac{\sigma_f}{\sigma_{f0}} - 1 \right) \tag{18.21}$$

where:

BFI = brittle fracture index
σ_f = tensile strength of a compact without a hole
σ_{f0} = tensile strength of a compact with a hole.

Two sets of square compacts were prepared using the triaxial press. One set contains a circular hole, whereas the other does not. The tensile strength of the compact with the hole (σ_f), is compared to that without (σ_{f0}). If the material is completely brittle, elastic theory predicts that the ratio of σ_f to σ_{f0} is close to 3. Most pharmaceutical materials are not completely brittle, and they are capable of relieving highly localized stress around the hole through plastic deformation. Therefore, the lower the BFI, the more plastic a material is. When BFI is less than 0.2, experiences teaches that there will not be a problem with tablet fracture on a rotary press unless the bonding (BI) is really weak.

The strain index, SI, may be used to reflect a relative value of the elastic strain following plastic deformation. It shows to what extent fracture of a compact is contributed to elastic recovery. SI is calculated as the following:

$$SI = \frac{H_0}{E'} \tag{18.22}$$

$$1/E' = \frac{\Sigma(1 - v^2)}{E} \tag{18.23}$$

where:

SI = strain index
E = Young's modulus
v = Poisson's ratio.

E' can be determined from the same indentation experiment used to measure the dynamic hardness, H_0. Hiestand measured tableting indicies of several common excipients, shown in Table 18.1.[39]

18.3.3 Practical Implications of Mechanical Property Characterization

Mechanical properties of drug substances and drug products can have a significant impact on

TABLE 18.1   Examples of values observed for tableting indices (modified from Table 3 in reference 39)

Material ($\rho_r = 0.9$)	$BI_W \times 10^2$	$BI_b \times 10^2$	BFI	$SI \times 10^2$
Avicel[a]	3.4	13.5	0.03	2.3
Sorbitol	0.46	13.7	0.03	0.94
Lactose, spray dried	0.36	1.1	0.12	1.8
Sucrose	0.40	2.3	0.68	1.5
Ibuprofen[b]	0.76	4.1	0.06	0.6
Aspirin	2.1	5.1	0.19	0.7
Caffeine	1.4	4.5	0.47	1.3
Phenacetin	0.88[c]	1.4	0.43	1.0
$CaSO_4 \cdot 2H_2O$	0.79	1.3	0.08	1.2

[a]PH-101, microcrystalline cellulose
[b]Lot-to-lot variation regularly observed
[c]Compression pressure slightly $>H_0$

manufacturability in multiple unit operations, such as compression, milling, and granulation. For example, during compression, a compression blend needs to have adequate flow from the hopper to the feed frame, and from the feed frame into the die. Otherwise, it is difficult to obtain consistent tablet weight. In addition, the compression blend needs to have reasonable compactibility, so that it can form a strong compact on a high-speed rotary press. Characterization of mechanical properties of the drug substance will help select appropriate formulation excipients and manufacturing processes for development of a robust product. This is especially important for high drug load formulations, where the mechanical properties of a drug may significantly impact final properties of the drug product. In a high drug load formulation containing drug with poor flow and/or compaction properties, one may choose to wet granulate or roller compact the formulation to improve flow and compaction properties of drug product. Granulation technology may also be selected for low dose formulation (e.g., the drug loading is <1% w/w) to improve content uniformity. For a drug substance that has reasonable mechanical properties, the drug can be blended with appropriate excipients, and the resulting blend can then be directly compressed on the tablet press. Direct compression is the simplest and most cost-effective way to manufacture a tablet dosage form. Of course, selection of a manufacturing process also strongly depends on the type of dosage form to be manufactured. For compounds that require specialty formulation to enhance oral bioavailability, additional manufacturing steps may be needed prior to compression or encapsulation of a formulation into a final dosage form. For example, milling may be required to reduce the particle size of drug substance to facilitate drug dissolution. How the drug substance fractures under impact, cutting or shear action may determine the fracture energy required, and the extent of particle size reduction. Therefore, understanding the impact of mechanical properties of a drug and formulation on each unit operation at a relevant scale is a recipe for successful scale-up of a robust product.

18.4 BIOPHARMACEUTICAL PROPERTIES

18.4.1 The Biopharmaceutical Classification System (BCS)

It is often believed that the magnitude of the therapeutic response increases as the drug concentration in the body increases. A more rapid and complete absorption tends to produce more rapid and uniform pharmacological responses. Based on this premise, one of the key objectives in designing an oral dosage form is to facilitate rapid and complete oral absorption, which is influenced by a multitude of factors, including physico-chemical properties of the drug and dosage form components, and physiological aspects of the human digestion system. To simplify this complicated picture, Amidon proposed a Biopharmaceutics Classification System (BCS), which categorized drugs according to two key physico-chemical parameters—solubility, and permeability.[41] These two factors were selected because most orally administered drugs are absorbed via a passive diffusion process through the small intestine, where the extent of oral absorption is largely influenced by a drug's membrane permeability and solubility, as is evident from the following equation:[42]

$$M = A \cdot t_{res} \cdot P_{eff} \cdot C_{app} \qquad (18.24)$$

The amount of drug absorbed (M) is proportional to the surface area available for absorption (A), the residence time (t_{res}) during which the drug stays within the site(s) of absorption, the effective membrane permeability (P_{eff}), and the apparent luminal drug concentration (C_{app}). As shown in Table 18.2, the BCS categorized drugs into four classes. Class I compounds have high solubility and high permeability; class II compounds have low solubility and high permeability; class III compounds have high solubility and low permeability; and class IV compounds have both low solubility and low permeability.

The Food and Drug Administration (FDA) has issued guidelines to define what is considered high solubility and high permeability.[43] According to this guideline, a high solubility drug is defined as one that, in the largest dose strength, fully dissolves in 250 mL of aqueous medium with the pH ranging from 1 to 7.5 at 37°C. Otherwise, drugs are considered poorly soluble. In other words, the highest therapeutic dose must dissolve in 250 mL of water at any physiological pH.

TABLE 18.2 The biopharmaceutics classification system[41]

Categories		Permeability	
		High	Low
Solubility	High	Class I	Class III
	Low	Class IIa (solubility limited)	Class V
		Class IIb (dissolution rate limited)	

In the same guidance as mentioned above, a drug is considered highly permeable if the extent of oral absorption is greater than 90%, based on mass-balance or in comparison to an intravenous reference dose.[43] Since oral absorption data is not easy to generate, researchers have been using *in vitro* permeability in predictor models such as Caco-2 or *in situ* perfusions to generate *in vitro* permeability data. A list of compounds has been compiled to allow researchers to establish a correlation between *in vitro* permeability measurements, and *in vivo* absorption. Generally speaking, a drug with a human permeability greater than $2–4 \times 10^{-4}$ cm/sec would be expected to have greater than 95% absorption.[42] Another rule of thumb is that compounds with permeability greater than metoprolol are considered highly permeable.

At the time the BCS was proposed, its primary objective was to guide decisions with respect to *in vivo* and *in vitro* correlations and the need for bioequivalence studies. It turns out that the BCS can also provide a useful framework to identify appropriate dosage form designs that are aimed at overcoming absorption barriers posed by solubility and permeability related challenges. For example, a variety of solubilization technologies are available to formulate BCS class II compounds whose absorption is limited by poor solubility and/or slow dissolution rate. It is within the BCS context that dosage form development strategies will be discussed in the following sections. Table 18.3 summarizes dosage form options for each of the biopharmaceutical classes.[15]

18.4.2 BCS Class I: High Solubility and High Permeability

BCS class I compounds are highly soluble and highly permeable. Table 18.4[44] lists class I compounds that are on the World Health Organization (WHO) list of essential medicines, and have been classified based on known solubility and permeability data in the literature. Compounds belonging to this class are normally expected to dissolve quickly in gastric and intestinal fluids, and readily cross the intestinal wall through passive diffusion. If the intent is to achieve fast and complete oral absorption, a conventional immediate release dosage form should be fit for purpose. Lieberman et al. have written a series of excellent books on formulation and process development of immediately released tablet and capsule formulations.[45] Although class I compounds are expected to have excellent oral absorption, given their high solubility and high permeability, additional absorption barriers may exist beyond the scope of the BCS.

TABLE 18.3 Dosage form options based on biopharmaceutics classification system (modified from Table 5 in reference 15)

Class I: High solubility high permeability	Class II: Low solubility high permeability
• No major challenges for immediate release dosage forms	Formulations designed to overcome solubility or dissolution rate problems: • Salt formation • Particle size reduction • Metastable forms • Solid dispersion • Complexation • Lipid based formulations • Precipitation inhibitors
Class III: High solubility low permeability	**Class IV: Low solubility low permeability**
Approaches to improve permeability: • Prodrugs • Permeation enhancers	• Formulation would have to use a combination of approaches identified in class II and class III to overcome dissolution and permeability problems • Strategies for oral administration are not really viable. Often use alternative delivery methods, such as intravenous administration

Other absorption barriers: metabolically or chemically unstable compounds*

Approaches to avoid luminal degradation:
• Enteric coating (for acid labile compounds)
• Lipid vehicles (micelles or emulsions/microemulsions)
• Prodrugs

Approaches to minimize pre-systemic metabolism:
• Coadministration of a drug with an enzyme inhibitor
• Lymphatic delivery (to avoid first pass metabolism) e.g., lipid prodrugs
• Explore effect of excipients on enzymatic inhibition

Approaches to minimize efflux mechanism:
• Coadministration with a P-gp efflux pump inhibitor
• Provide enough luminal concentration to saturate the efflux transporter
• Design prodrugs to evade efflux transporter
• Use of excipients that may inhibit efflux mechanism

Approaches to utilize carrier-mediated transport:
• Design prodrugs that are substrates for transporters

*Compounds in this class may have acceptable solubility and permeability, but can still pose significant absorption challenge if they undergo luminal degradation, pre-systemic elimination or are effluxed by p-glycoproteins.

For example, luminal complexation and degradation can significantly limit the amount of drug available for absorption. Even after the drug crosses the intestinal membrane, it may be metabolized within the

TABLE 18.4 Examples of BCS class I compounds (modified from Table 1 in reference 44)

Drug	Indication	Dose (mg)
Amiloride	Diuretic	5 (hydrochloride)
Chloroquine	Antimalarial agent	100 (phosphate), 150 (sulfate)
Cyclophosphamide	Antineoplastic	25
Diazepam	Antidepressant	2, 5
Digoxin[a]	Cardiac glycoside	0.625, 0.25
Doxycycline	Antibiotic	100 (hydrochloride)
Fluconazole	Antifungal	50
Levodopa[b] + (Carbidopa)	Parkinson's disease	100 + 10, 250 + 25
Levonorgestrel	Hormone	0.15 (+0.03 ethinylestradiol); 0.25 (+0.05 ethinyl-estradiol); 0.75 (pack of two) + D43
Metronidazole	Antibiotic	200–500
Phenobarbital	Sedative and anticonvulsant agent	15–100
Phenoxy-methyl penicilline	Antibiotic	250 (potassium)
Prednisolone	Glucocorticoid	5
Primaquine	Antimalarial	7.5, 15 (diphosphate)
Propranolol[b]	β-blocker	20, 40 (hydrochloride)
Pyrazinamide	Tuberculosis	400
Riboflavin[a]	Vitamin	5
Salbutmaol[b]	β-sympatho mimetic	4 (sulfate)
Stavudine	Antiviral	15, 20, 30, 40
Theophylline	Antiasthmatic	100, 200, 300
Zidovudine[b]	Antiviral	300 (tablet), 100, 250 (capsule)

[a]Substrates for active transport
[b]First pass effect

enterocytes/hepatocytes and/or pumped out of the cells due to efflux mechanisms. Potential formulation approaches to overcome these additional absorption barriers will be discussed in Section 18.4.6.

18.4.3 BCS Class II: Low Solubility and High Permeability

BCS class II compounds have high permeability but low aqueous solubility. Table 18.5 lists BCS class II compounds that are on the WHO list of essential medicines, and have been classified based on known

TABLE 18.5 Examples of BCS class II compounds (modified from Table 1 in reference 44)

Drug	Indication	Dose
Carbamazepine	Antiepileptic	100, 200
Dapsone	Antirheumatic/leprosy	25, 50, 100
Griseofulvin	Antifungal	125, 250
Ibuprofen	Pain relief	200, 400
Nifedipine[a]	Ca-channel blocker	10
Nitrofurantoin	Antibacterial	100
Phenytoin	Antiepileptic	25, 50, 100
Sulfamethoxazole	Antibiotic	100, 400
Trimethoprim	Antibiotic	100, 200
Valproic acid	Antiepileptic	200, 500 (sodium salt)

[a]First pass effect

solubility and permeability data in the literature.[44] This list is shorter than that for the class I compounds listed in Table 18.4. The list does not reflect the trend that an increasing number of class II compounds are emerging through the development pipeline due to recent advances in combinatory chemistry and high throughput screening.

By definition, poor solubility and/or slow dissolution are the rate-limiting steps for oral absorption of BCS class II compounds. For compounds with a very large dose-to-solubility ratio, poor solubility is likely to be the rate-limiting step for absorption. In other words, the compounds may dissolve quickly enough to reach their equilibrium solubility, but the solubility is too low to establish a wide enough concentration gradient to drive passive diffusion. Formulation technologies, such as use of a more soluble salt, use of a metastable form, amorphous solid dispersions, complexation and lipid formulations, can at least transiently significantly solubilize a drug at the site of absorption, thereby leading to faster and more complete oral absorption. In contrast to solubility-limited compounds, some compounds have decent solubility with respect to their dose, but dissolve too slowly to achieve an adequate concentration gradient across the intestinal wall. For these types of compounds, solubilization technologies cited above should also work, because dissolution rate increases proportionally with solubility enhancement. In addition to these solubilization technologies, simple technologies such as particle size reduction serve as an effective tool to significantly increase the dissolution rate. In principle, a 10-fold reduction in particle size increases the surface area, as well as the dissolution rate, by 100-fold, assuming primary particles do not agglomerate. The following section discusses the advantages and limitations of major formulation technologies for class II compounds.

Salt Formation

Use of a soluble salt is one of the most common approaches to deal with class II compounds, since the solubility and dissolution rate of a salt can be many-fold higher than that of the free acid or free base. As shown in Figure 18.1, a free acid continues to dissolve as pH increases until it reaches the solubility limit of the salt. Salt screening is an indispensable step in pre-formulation characterization. In addition to solubility and dissolution rate, one has to fully evaluate other properties of a salt, such as physical and chemical stability, hygroscopicity, crystallinity, polymorphism, ease of synthesis, and toxicity, before selecting an appropriate salt for product development. Salt selection largely depends on the pK_a of the salt. It is generally accepted that a minimum difference of 3 units between the pK_a value of the salt-forming moiety of the drug and that of the salt counterion is required to form stable salts.[46] As listed in Table 18.6, a wide variety of counterions have been successfully used in pharmaceuticals, among which sodium and potassium salts are often first considered for weakly acidic drugs, whereas hydrochloride salts are often first considered for weakly basic drugs.

However, salt formulation does not always work. First of all, it is not feasible to form salts of neutral compounds, and it may be difficult to form salts of very weak bases or acids. Even if a stable salt can be formed, conversion from a salt to a poorly soluble free acid or free base can occur both *in vitro* and *in vivo*. For example, a hydrochloride salt of a free base may initially dissolve at the low pH in the stomach. But, as it enters the intestine where pH increases, the drug concentration becomes supersaturated with respect to its equilibrium total solubility of ionized and unionized species at that pH; the free base may precipitate, resulting in less complete absorption. In such cases, precipitation inhibitors may be used to prevent conversion from a salt to its free base, thereby significantly improving the bioavailability of rapidly dissolving salts.

Particle Size Reduction

Particle size reduction is an effective tool to enhance the dissolution rate of poorly soluble drugs. It is well accepted that particle size reduction can enhance

TABLE 18.6 Selected counterions suitable for salt formation[47]

	Anions	Cations
Preferred	Citrate*	Calcium*
Universally accepted by regulatory agencies with no significant limit on quantities	Hydrochloride*	Potassium*
	Phosphate*	Sodium*
Generally accepted	Acetate*	Choline
Generally accepted but with some limitation on quantities and/or route of administration	Besylate	Ethylenediamine
	Gluconate	Tromethamine
	Lactate	
	Malate	
	Mesylate*	
	Nitrate*	
	Succinate	
	Sulfate*	
	Tartrate*	
	Tannate	
	Tosylate	
Suitable for use	Adipate	Arginine
More limited approval with some limitation on quantities which are acceptable in safety studies or human use and/or route of administration	Benzoate	Glycine
	Cholate	Lycine
	Edisylate	Magnesium
	Hydrobromide	Meglumine
	Fumarate	
	Maleate*	
	Napsylate	
	Pamoate	
	Stearate	

*Commonly used

in vivo absorption and bioavailability of poorly soluble drugs. As shown in Table 18.7,[48] size reduction can significantly enhance dissolution, but has little impact on solubility unless the particle size is reduced to less than 100 nm.

Most often, pharmaceutical compounds are milled to improve content uniformity, ease of processing, and/or dissolution rate. For dry powder milling, the most commonly used mills in pharmaceutical manufacturing are cutter, hammer, roller, and fluid energy mills, which can reduce the particle size of a drug substance to 1–100 μm.[49] Smaller particle sizes in the range of 200 nm to 1 μm may be achieved using a wet ball mill, with its milling chamber filled with grinding media and drug suspension. There are several

TABLE 18.7 Effect of particle size on solubility and dissolution rate

Particle size	S/S_{∞}[a]	$A_r/A_{10\mu m}$[b]	Theoretical impact on dissolution rate[c]
10 μm	1.00	1	No impact
1 μm	1.01	10	10-fold increase
100 nm	1.13	100	113-fold increase
10 nm	3.32	1000	3320-fold increase

[a]$Ln(S/S_{\infty}) = 2\gamma M/(\rho RTr)$,[48] where γ stands for surface tension of the solids, M stands for molecular weight, ρ stands for density of the solids, R is the gas constant, T is the absolute temperature, r is the particle size of a solid. Assuming $\gamma = 300$ dyne, $M = 300$ Dalton, $\rho = 1$ g/cm^3, $T = 25°C$, one could calculate the ratio of solubility of the solid with particle size r to that of the solid with infinitely large solubility (S/S_{∞});

[b]$A_r/A_{10\mu m}$ stands for the surface area ratio of the solid with particle size r to that of the solid with particle size of 10 μm, assuming spherical shape;

[c]Impact of particle size reduction on dissolution rate can be calculated from the Noyes–Whiteny equation, where dissolution rate at the sink condition is proportional to surface area and solubility. The dissolution rate of a 10 μm particle is used as the reference for calculation.

disadvantages associated with milling. First of all, heat and mechanical impact generated during the milling process can cause both physical and chemical instability. In addition, small particles tend to agglomerate due to cohesive forces. Agglomeration reduces the effective surface area of a drug, thereby somewhat negating the benefit of size reduction on dissolution enhancement. Excipients such as surfactants, sugars, polymers or other excipients may be added to a formulation to minimize aggregation and improve wetting.

Metastable Forms

An active pharmaceutical ingredient (API) may exhibit diverse polymorphism or may be amorphous. As discussed in Sections 18.2.6 and 18.2.7, solid-state form differences may significantly impact physicochemical, mechanical, and biopharmaceutical properties of solids. By definition, metastable forms have higher Gibbs free energies than the stable form. The higher energy translates into higher solubility, and faster intrinsic dissolution rate, as dictated by the equation below:

$$\Delta G_{A-B} = RT \ln(\text{Solubility}_A/\text{Solubility}_B) \quad (18.25)$$

ΔG_{A-B} is the Gibbs free energy difference between two polymorphs, A and B. Thus, it is not surprising

that metastable forms may exhibit higher bioavailability than their stable crystalline counterpart. As early as 1960, Aguiar and his coworkers demonstrated that the bioavailability of chloramphenicol depended on the polymorphic composition of its prodrug chloramphenicol palmitate,[18] which must be hydrolyzed by pancreatin prior to intestinal absorption. The *in vitro* ester hydrolysis of the metastable polymorph B of chloramphenicol palmitate was much more significant than that of the stable form A. As a result, peak chloramphenicol blood concentration increased proportionally to the percentage of form B in the A/B polymorphic mixture. Augiar and Zelmer further showed that the metastable form B had a much higher solubility, and dissolved faster than the stable form A.[50] It was hypothesized that the solubility differences led to polymorphic-dependent ester hydrolysis, and ultimately explained the differences in oral absorption. However, use of a faster-dissolving solid form does not always result in an improved pharmacokinetic profile. For example, Kahela et al. reported that the anhydrous and dehydrate forms of carbamazepine had very similar bioavailability in humans, despite the fact that the anhydrous form dissolved much more slowly than the dehydrate in 0.1 N HCl *in vitro*.[51] Compared to metastable crystalline forms, amorphous solids have even higher solubility and faster dissolution rates than any crystalline modification. Hancock and Parks predicted the metastable solubility value of the amorphous drugs to be 16 to 1000 times higher than that of the stable crystalline form.[52] However, the measured solubility of amorphous compounds was much less, due to rapid recrystallization of amorphous materials upon contact with water.

Despite the potential benefits of faster dissolution and higher solubility associated with metastable forms, they are seldom the candidates of choice for formulation development. Most often, innovator companies spend significant resources early in the development process to search for the thermodynamically most stable polymorph for development. The perceived physical and chemical instability of a metastable form has limited its application as a standard drug delivery technology. The concern is real, as illustrated by the catastrophic event occurring at Abbott Laboratories when a metastable form of Ritonavir was developed unintentionally. When a stable form was later discovered, Abbott failed to produce the metastable form consistently, and this led to lot-to-lot variation in capsule product dissolution, and withdrawal of the capsule product from the market. Abbott had to reformulate ritonavir capsules using the stable form, which resulted in the loss of millions of dollars in sales while the capsule product was off the market. Despite the physical and chemical instability associated with metastable forms, there are ways to stabilize a metastable form with appropriate choices of excipients and formulation design. Excellent review articles in the field of theory and practice of polymorphism are available. Relevant topics include the impact of polymorphism on developability,[53] physico-chemical properties, mechanical properties and bioavailabilities,[54] practical perspectives of phase transformations occurring in manufacturing process,[19] employment of process analytical technology (PAT) to monitor polymorphic conversion,[55] practice,[56] and regulatory considerations of polymorphism in generic drug approvals.[57]

Solid Dispersions

About five decades ago, Sekiguchi and Obi made the first solid dispersion by melting sulfathiazole and urea, followed by cooling in an ice bath.[58] The resultant eutectic mixture exhibited faster dissolution and better bioavailability than conventional formulations. Since then, solid dispersions have become one of the most studied drug delivery technologies to solubilize and enhance dissolution rates of class II compounds. The term "solid dispersion" is often used to encompass a diverse group of solid mixtures. Shown in Figure 18.3, solid dispersions can be categorized into simple eutectic mixtures, solid solutions, and physical mixtures of the microcrystalline drug dispersed in carriers.[59] Solid solutions can be further classified based on their miscibility into continuous versus discontinuous solid solutions. Alternatively, solid solutions may be classified according to the way in which solute molecules (such as the drug) are distributed in the solvent (such as carriers).[60] As depicted in Figure 18.3, the solute molecules may be dispersed in the solvent in three fashions, namely substitutional crystalline, interstitial crystalline, and amorphous solid solutions. The mechanism of drug release from solid dispersions in water-soluble polymers has been reviewed recently.[59] It is generally believed that a solid dispersion can enhance the dissolution rate of a poorly soluble drug through one or a combination of the following factors:

1. Increased surface area: a drug exists either as very fine crystalline particles or molecular dispersion in a solid dispersion. Therefore, the surface area of the drug is significantly increased as compared to the conventional formulation.
2. Surface modification through intimate contact with hydrophilic carriers: in the case where a physical mixture or eutectic mixture is formed, the surface properties of drug particles are modified through

intimate contact with a hydrophilic polymer, such that the drug wets more easily.

3. Increased solubility through formation of a solid solution: in the case of a solid solution, a drug forms a molecular dispersion in the hydrophilic carrier. Since the drug is already present in the molecular state as a "solid solution," the step of drug dissolution is bypassed.

The dissolution rate of the dosage form is determined by the characteristic of the carrier. The great variety of pharmaceutically approved carriers that can be used to formulate solid dispersions have been reviewed in several articles.[60,61] Such carrier systems include polyethylene glycol (PEG), polyvinylpyrrolidone (PVP) and its copolymers, cellulose derivatives, acrylate polymers, sugar and its derivatives, emulsifiers, organic acids and its derivatives.

Although solid dispersions offer great potential for enhancing the bioavailability of BCS class II compounds, decades of research have only resulted in a few marketed drug products. These include griseofulvin-PEG-dispersion (marketed by Wander as Gris-PEG®), Nabilone-PVP dispersion (marketed by Lilly as Cesamet), as well as a troglitazone formulation (marketed by Parke-Davis as Rezulin®). Rezulin had to be withdrawn from the market due to drug-related toxicity. As Serajuddin pointed out in his review article,[62] what has limited widespread application of solid

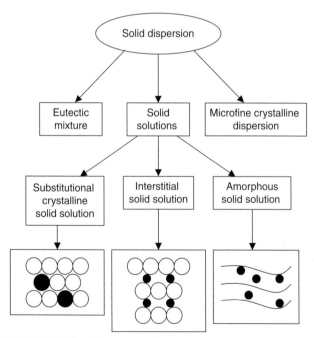

FIGURE 18.3   Classification of solid dispersions

dispersions as a drug delivery technology are technical challenges related to method of preparation, material processability, and dosage form variability. In terms of method of preparation, solid dispersions are typically prepared by either hot-melt or co-solvent techniques. The hot-melt method involves melting a drug with its carrier, followed with subsequent cooling, and this may not be suitable for thermolabile compounds. The co-solvent technique involves dissolving the drug and carrier in a common solvent, followed by solvent evaporation. Since solid dispersions often use hydrophilic carriers with hydrophobic drugs, it is difficult to find a common solvent to dissolve both components. Regardless of processing method, solid dispersion materials are often soft, waxy, and possess poor compressibility and flowability, which may pose challenges to material handling and compression. Physical instability and lack of reproducibility also limit the commercial application of solid dispersions. It is not uncommon to produce wholly or partially amorphous drug during processing, which will eventually transform to a more stable crystalline form over time. The rate of transformation may be greatly influenced by storage conditions and formulation composition, as well as processing methods. Recently, interest has grown in utilizing hot-melt extrusion to manufacture solid dispersion dosage forms. Hot-melt extrusion can produce granules or pellets of solid dispersion with uniform size, shape and density, which can be manufactured and scaled-up with relative ease. A recent success achieved through hot-melt extrusion is highlighted by the development of Kaletra® tablets (Abbott).[63] Kaletra® was initially marketed as a softgel capsule (SGC) formulation, because the two active ingredients, lopinavir and ritonavir, were poorly soluble and could not achieve adequate bioavailability when formulated in a conventional tablet. Kaletra® SGC requires refrigerated storage, and has to be taken either as 6 capsules once daily or 3 capsules twice a day. Kaletra® tablets, which are a solid dispersion prepared through hot-melt extrusion, have much better patient compliance, as they can be stored at room temperature and the required dose is only 4 tablets once a day.

Complexation

Interest in complexation technologies has grown considerably due to increased applications of cyclodextrins (CDs), which are cyclic oligosaccharides obtained from enzymatic conversion of starch. The parent or natural CDs that are of pharmaceutical relevance are α-, β-, and γ-CDs, which contain 6, 7, or 8 glucopyranose units joined through 1–4 bonds, respectively. The 3-D structure of the CD shows a hydrophobic cavity, into which a drug molecule can enter to form an inclusion complex. The hydrophilic exterior of the CD allows the complex to interact favorably with aqueous environments. In order for the drug to be absorbed into systemic circulation, it has to be dissociated from the drug–CD complex first. The kinetics of inclusion complex formation and dissociation between a CD and drug molecule is very fast, with a half life of much less than one second.[64] Dilution and competitive displacement are two major mechanisms that contribute to complex formation and the dissociation process. Many drugs interact most favorably with β-CD because the 6.0–6.5Å opening of β-CD is optimal for many biomedically relevant molecules.[65] Unfortunately, β-CD has the lowest solubility (1.8% in water at 25°C) among the three CDs, thereby limiting its solubilization capacity. To enhance solubility of the β-CD, as well as to improve its safety, derivatives of β-CD have been developed. Among them, hydroxypropyl-β-cyclodextrin (HP-β-CDs), and sulfobutylether-β-cyclodextrins (SBE-β-CDs, mainly as SBE7-β-CD, while 7 refers to the average degree of substitution), have captured interest in formulating poorly soluble drugs in immediate-released dosage forms.

Many papers have reviewed the versatile applications of CDs in the field of oral, parenteral, ophthalmic, nasal, and topical drug delivery.[66–68] This discussion will focus on the oral application of CDs only. CDs can be used to solubilize, stabilize, taste mask, and ameliorate the irritancy and toxicity of drug molecules in solid oral dosage forms. It is well demonstrated in the literature that complexation with CD can significantly enhance oral bioavailability of poorly soluble compounds, such as cinnarizine,[69] carbamazepine,[70] itraconazole,[71] and insulin[72] in animals. The effect of CDs on bioavailability enhancement was also demonstrated in human studies with compounds such as ursodeoxycholic acid (UDCA),[73] estradiol,[74] and dipyridamole.[75] The enhanced bioavailability is in part attributed to increased rate of drug dissolution from the drug–CD complex, and in part may be attributed to the effect of CD as a potential penetration enhancer. Studies showed that CD might complex with membrane components, such as cholesterol, thereby modifying the transport properties of the membrane and facilitating drug absorption.[76]

CD and its derivatives may decrease local tissue irritation through a decreased free drug concentration resulting from formation of the inclusion complex. For example, studies showed that piroxicam,[77] and naproxen,[78] caused fewer gastric lesions when dosed with a β-CD formulation. In addition, modified CDs, such as carboxymethyl derivatives (e.g., CME-β-CD), exhibit pH-dependent solubility, and therefore can be used to protect acid-labile compounds in enteric formulations. CME-β-CD complexes have been used with diltiazem,[79] and molsidomine,[80] to investigate their acid protection potential.

The safety of the parent CDs and their derivatives has been reviewed by Thompson.[67] Alpha- and beta-CDs are known to cause renal toxicity after intravenous injection,[81] but it is generally considered safe to administer CDs orally due to their poor oral absorption from the GI tract. For example, the oral bioavailability of β-CD was reported to be less than 4%.[82,83] Although oral administration of CDs may cause minimal concerns related to systemic toxicity, CDs may cause local tissue irritation. As discussed earlier, CDs may destabilize membranes through their ability to extract membrane components, such as cholesterol and phospholipids. To address the safety concerns associated with parent CDs, especially to minimize renal toxicity observed with the parenteral formulations, various derivatives of the parent CDs were developed. Two of the most promising derivatized CDs are HP-β-CD and (SBE)$_{7M}$-β-CD. Both CDs were found to be safe when administered parenterally in humans and animals. In addition, (SBE)$_{7M}$-β-CD was found less likely to disrupt lipid membranes, due to electronic repulsion between it and the lipid components.[67] Other disadvantages of CDs and their derivates are relatively high cost, and the need to be used in a large quantity. For example, for a drug with a molecular weight similar to that of the CD and a dose of 400 mg, at least 400 mg of CD is required to form a 1:1 inclusion complex. This has limited the use of CDs to only low dose formulations.

Lipid-based Formulations

Lipid-based formulations represent a unique solution to delivery of poorly soluble compounds. Their mechanism of absorption enhancement is multi-faceted. First, a drug is often already dissolved in a lipid dosage form, thereby bypassing the often-slow dissolution step. Secondly, a good lipid formulation may form a fine colloidal dispersion through lipid digestion or self-emulsification. This will help keep the drug in solution, and facilitate rapid drug absorption. Thirdly, certain lipids and surfactants may increase intestinal permeability,[84,85] mitigate intestinal efflux,[86,87] and reduce first-pass metabolism by promoting lymphatic transport[88] to further improve oral bioavailability. Several excellent papers have reviewed lipid formulation strategies and efforts to understand their mechanisms of action.[89–91]

A lipid dosage form typically consists of one or more drugs dissolved in a blend of lipophilic excipients such as triglycerides, partial glycerides, surfactants or co-surfactants.[91] Common types of lipid formulations include lipid suspensions and solutions, micelles, microemulsions, macroemulsions (or emulsions), self-emulsifying lipid formulations, and liposomes (Table 18.8).[92] The simplest lipid formulation is a lipid solution in which a drug is dissolved in digestible oil, such as vegetable oil or a medium chain triglyceride. Upon oral administration, the triglycerides undergo lipolysis to form a colloidal dispersion within bile salt-lecithin mixed micelles. The lipophilic drug may be solubilized in this mixed micelle at a high concentration, which facilitates passive diffusion along the resulting concentration gradient.[93] Although lipid solutions are easy to formulate, they have limited solvent capacities for most pharmaceutical compounds except those with $\log_{10}P > 4$ or potent drugs.[90] Lipid suspension can overcome the solvent capacity issue by suspending extra drug in lipid vehicles. However, the suspended drug needs to undergo additional dissolution prior to absorbtion.

TABLE 18.8   Physical characteristics of different lipid colloidal systems (modified from Table 18-2 in reference 92)

	Micelles	Microemulsions	Emulsions	Liposome
Spontaneously obtained	Yes	Yes	No	No
Thermodynamically stable	Yes	Yes	No	No
Turbidity	Transparent	Transparent	Turbid	From transparent to turbid, depending on droplet size
Typical size range	$<0.01\,\mu m$	$\sim 0.1\,\mu m$ or less	$0.5-5\,\mu m$	$0.025-25\,\mu m$
Cosurfactant used	No	Yes	No	No
Surfactant concentration	$<5\%$	$>10\%$	$1-20\%$	$0.5-20\%$
Dispersed phase concentration	$<5\%$	$1-30\%$	$1-30\%$	$1-30\%$

Micelle solubilization plays an import role in bio-availability enhancement of class II drugs. Intake of food stimulates secretion of bile salts into the duodenum, increasing bile salts concentration in the duodenum from a typical 1–4 mmol/L in the fasted state to 10–20 mmol/L in the fed-state.[94] It is hypothesized that micelles or mixed micelles formed by bile salts and digested lipids could significantly solubilize hydrophobic drugs, thereby enhancing drug absorption.[95] However, micelles usually have very limited solubilization capacity, which significantly limits their commercial viability.

Emulsions have much higher solvent capacity for hydrophobic materials than micelles, but they are thermodynamically unstable. Unlike emulsions, microemulsions are thermodynamically stable colloidal systems (<100 nm in droplet size), consisting of surfactants/co-surfactants, water, and oil. Construction of a phase diagram helps identify the composition of formulations in regions in which microemulsions can be formed (Figure 18.4[92]). Microemulsions have a reasonably high solubilization capacity, which further enhances their appeal as a promising delivery technology for BCS class II drugs. Because of their thermodynamic stability, microemulsions may have long shelf lives and can form spontaneously with gentle agitation. However, microemulsions are not infinitely stable upon dilution, because dilution changes the composition of the colloidal system.

Self-emulsifying drug delivery systems (SEDDSs) are closely related to microemulsions and emulsions. SEDDSs are isotropic lipid solutions, typically consisting of a mixture of a surfactant, oil, and drug that rapidly disperses to form fine emulsion or microemulsion droplets upon contact with water. As compared to microemulsions and emulsions, SEDDSs offer several advantages:

1. SEDDSs do not contain water, therefore they have smaller dose volumes than microemulsions or emulsions.
2. SEDDSs can be encapsulated into soft or hard gelatin capsules, whereas microemulsions and emulsions have to be dosed by a spoon.
3. Because SEDDSs is an isotropic lipid solution, it does not have common physical stability problems (such as phase separation) associated with emulsions.

Many excellent reviews have captured formulation strategies and clinical advantages of SEDDSs.[89,90,96] A good SEDDS formulation should rapidly and reproducibly self-emulsify into fine dispersions with droplet size less than 1 μm.[97] Small droplets provide a large surface area to facilitate drug absorption. Neoral® is the most notable example where cyclosporine *A* in a microemulsion formulation showed a much higher oral bioavailability, and lower patient variability, after the droplet size was reduced from the original Sandimmune formulation.[98,99] However, measurement of droplet size in an *in vitro* dispersion test may not always predict *in vivo* performance. Sek et al. showed that atovaquone formulated in a crude lipid formulation containing cremophor El, pluronic L121 or a simple lipid solution achieved similar oral bioavailability in beagle dogs as a microemulsion concentrate, despite the former having poor dispersibility.[100] The good *in vivo* performance of the crude lipid formulation and simple lipid solution was attributed to the ability of these formulations to undergo lipid digestion, which helps facilitate absorption of atovaquone *in vivo*. In fact, an *in vitro* digestion test correlated with *in vivo* performance better than the *in vitro* dispersion test for the tested formulations.

Precipitation Inhibition

The majority of formulation technologies for BCS class II compounds aim to maximize drug concentration at sites of absorption, thereby increasing the driving force for the drug to passively diffuse across the intestinal membrane along a concentration gradient. Even though a drug may be solubilized in a dosage form, it may precipitate after oral administration if the drug concentration becomes supersaturated with respect to its solubility in the GI media. For example, a salt of a free base dissolves at low

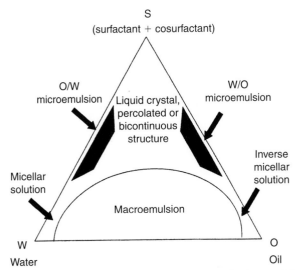

FIGURE 18.4 Hypothetical phase regions of microemulsion systems of oil (O), water (W), and surfactant + consurfactant (S) (copied from Figure 2 in reference 92)

pH in the stomach. As the pH increases in the small intestine, the drug becomes supersaturated, and tends to precipitate as the free base to reach its equilibrium solubility. Supersaturation may also occur with lipid formulations, solid dispersions, and complexation formulations after the dosage form is diluted with GI fluids. Drug precipitation from a supersaturated solution tends to decrease bioavailability, and leads to slower absorption, as demonstrated in several studies.[101,102] Precipitation reduces the free drug concentration at the absorption site, and the precipitated drug may coat the surface of a dosage form to prevent more drug from being dissolved. The rate of drug precipitation/crystallization generally increases with the supersaturation ratio (which is the ratio of drug concentration to its solubility), and decreases with viscosity of the crystallization medium. Certain inert polymers, such as hydroxypropylmethylcellulose (HPMC), and polyvinylpyrrolidone (PVP), are known to prolong supersaturation for certain compounds. For example, PVP has been used to inhibit crystallization of sulfathiazole,[103] phenytoin,[104] oestratiol,[105] and hydrocortisone acetate.[106,107] Cellulose polymers such as HPMC have been used to stabilize the supersaturation of nifedipine,[108] albendazole,[109] hydrocortisone acetate,[110] and ibuprofen.[111] More recently, Gao and his coworkers demonstrated that HPMC may be used in small amounts to inhibit precipitation of paclitaxel from a supersaturable self-emulsifying drug delivery system (S-SEDDS) *in vivo*.[102] Compared to the commercial paclitaxel formulation (Taxol®) and the SEDDS formulation without HPMC, the S-SEDDS containing HPMC had 10-fold higher peak concentration, and five-fold higher oral bioavailability in rats. In another study by Gao and his coworkers,[112] HPMC was also demonstrated to inhibit the precipitation of PNU-91325 from a supersaturable co-solvent (PEG 400 solution containing 20 mg/g HPMC) both *in vitro* and *in vivo*. This led to a five-fold increase in oral bioavailability of PNU-91325, compared to the neat PEG 400 formulation. These polymers may inhibit the crystallization of the drug by increasing the viscosity of crystallization medium, presenting a steric barrier to drug molecules, adhering to the growing crystals, and/or through specific intermolecular interactions such as hydrogen bonding.[113–115]

18.4.4 BCS Class III: High Solubility and Low Permeability

BCS class III compounds have high solubility and low permeability. As shown in Table 18.9,[44] a fair number of marketed products belong to this class. Since passive diffusion is the rate-limiting step for oral absorption of BCS class III compounds, the most effective way to improve absorption and bioavailability of this class of compounds is to increase the membrane permeability of the drug through chemical modification or use of a penetration enhancer. It is much more difficult to modify biological membrane permeability than it is to solubilize a drug. Therefore, delivery technologies targeted for class III compounds are less effective and more variable than those used for class II compounds.

TABLE 18.9 Examples of BCS class III compounds (modified from Table 1 in reference 44)

Drug	Indication	Dose
Abacavir[d]	Antiretroviral	300
Acetylsalicylic acid[a,b,d]	Pain relief	100–500
Acyclovir[d]	Antiviral	200
Allopurinol[d]	Gout	100
Ascorbic acid[c,d]	Vitamin	50 (−1000)
Atenolol	β-blocker	50, 100
Captopril	Antihypertensive	25
Chloramphenicol[d]	Antibiotic	250
Cimetidine	H2-receptor antagonist	200
Sodium Cloxacillin	Antibiotic	500, 1000 (Na-salz)
Codeine[d]	Phosphate antitussive/analgetic	30
Colchicine	Antigout agent	0.5
Ergotamine tartrate[a]	Migraine	1 (tartrate)
Hydralazine[a]	Antihypertensive	25, 50 (hydrochloride)
Hydrochlorothiazide	Diuretic	25
Levothyroxine	Thyroid	0.05, 0.1 (sodium salt)
Metformine[c]	Antidiabetic	500 (hydrochloride)
Methyldopa[a,c]	Antihypertensive	250
Paracetamol[d] (acetaminophen)	Pain relief	100–500
Penicillamine	Chronic polyarthritis	250
Promethazine[d]	Antihistamine	10, 25 (hydrochloride)
Propylthiouracil[d]	Cystostatic	50
Pyridostigmine	Myasthenia gravis	60 (bromide)
Thiamine[c]	Vitamin	50 (hydrochloride)

[a]First pass effect
[b]Degradation in the GI tract
[c]Substrate for active transport
[d]Denotes class III drugs with permeability corresponding to at least 80% absorption

Prodrugs

Most drugs are thought to be absorbed in the small intestine by a passive diffusion process. The membrane permeability largely depends on three interdependent physico-chemical parameters: lipophilicity, polarity and molecular size. Compounds, such as proteins and peptides, have difficulty diffusing across the intestinal membrane, due to their large molecular size, hydrophilicity, and hydrogen bonding potential. In addition, proteins and peptides are susceptible to hydrolysis catalyzed by a variety of enzymes, such as proteases and peptidases, which are present in the intestinal lumen. Prodrug strategies have been successfully employed to improve oral absorption of short-chained peptides by increasing their lipophilicity and protecting them from proteolytic cleavage. A prodrug is a chemical derivative of a parent drug that is designed to overcome limitations posed by poor permeability, solubility, and/or stability of the parent drug. The prodrug is often not pharmacologically active. Once absorbed, it is converted to the active parent drug, either intracellularly or in the systemic circulation. For example, bioreversible cyclization of the peptide backbone reduced the extent of intermolecular hydrogen bonding with aqueous solvents, thus making the cyclized prodrug more readily partition into lipid membranes.[116] In addition, cyclization protects the C-terminal carboxyl group and N-terminal amino group from proteolytic attack, thereby enhancing the prodrug's enzymatic stability.[117] Conjugation of a peptide to fatty acid can significantly increase its lipophilicity, leading to increased epithelial absorption, gastrointestinal stability, and plasma half life of peptide drugs such as calcitonin.[118] Recently, membrane transporter targeted prodrugs have attracted significant interest. For example, PepT1 and PepT2 are two promising peptide transporters that play an essential role in transporting dipeptides, tripeptides, and peptiomimetic drugs such as β-lactam antibiotics.[119] Prodrugs made by attaching the parent drug to a substrate of a peptide transporter can significantly increase the oral absorption through transporter-mediated uptake. PepT1 has been utilized to increase the bioavailability of acyclovir,[120] and cidofovir,[121] through dipeptide prodrug derivatization. In general, synthesis of peptide prodrugs has been limited due to their structural complexity, and the lack of novel methodology. Compared to peptide drugs, prodrugs of small organic molecules are relatively easier to make, and have been successfully employed to increase oral absorption of fosinoprilat,[122] amprenavir,[123] and acyclovir.[120] There are several articles that provide in-depth reviews on prodrugs.[124–126]

An ideal prodrug should have the following characteristics:[124] (1) adequate stability to variable pH environment of the GI tract; (2) adequate solubility; (3) enzymatic stability to luminal contents, as well as the enzymes found in the brush border membrane; (4) good permeability, and adequate $\log_{10}P$, and (5) rapid reversion to the parent drug, either in the enterocyte or once absorbed into systemic circulation. Biotransformation is critical, but often difficult to control. In addition, increasing lipophilicity often reduces aqueous solubility, which may partly negate the benefit of increased permeability. From a regulatory perspective, prodrugs are considered new chemical entities, thus requiring preclinical studies to demonstrate their safety and efficacy. Therefore, utilization of a prodrug strategy really should occur in the early stage of preclinical evaluation, to save time and resources.

Penetration Enhancers

The intestinal cell membrane presents a formidable barrier to polar drugs and macromolecules such as peptides and proteins. Shown in Figure 18.5,[127] intestinal absorptive cells are covered by a mucous gel layer which functions as a defense mechanism against damage. The apical cell membrane has a 1 μm-thick brush border, which is formed by a 10 nm-thick phospholipid bilayer with polar heads facing outwards, and hydrophobic tails facing inward. Cholesterol, which is a major component of this lipid membrane, plays a significant role in regulating membrane structure and fluidity. The membrane proteins are embedded in the membrane or anchored in the peripheral of membranes, and play an important role in carrier-mediated transport. Two adjacent epithelial cells are joined by tight junctions on the apical side (facing the lumen), which prevent entry to most substances except small

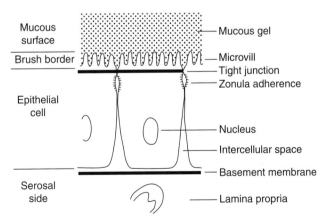

FIGURE 18.5 Schematic diagram of intestinal epithelial cells (copied from Figure 2 in reference 127)

ions and water molecules. Passive diffusion can occur either through the transcellular route (through the lipid bilayer regions and membrane bound protein regions) or the paracelluar route (through the tight junction channels). For class III compounds, passive diffusion through either route is slow and prohibitive. To improve the oral absorption of this class of compounds, penetration enhancers may be used to transiently alter the integrity of the mucosal membrane or open up the tight junctions. Several articles[127–129] have reviewed intestinal absorption enhancers and their mechanisms of action, as shown in Table 18.10.[129]

Long chain fatty acids, such as fusogenic lipids (unsaturated fatty acids such as oleic acid, linoleic acid and monoolein, etc., and their monoglyceride esters), are very effective absorption enhancers in the form of their soluble sodium salts or by the addition of surfactants, such as sodium taurocholate. Studies showed that the mixed micelles of taurocholate and a fusogenic lipid enhanced the oral absorption of gentamycin, streptomycin, fosfomycin, and heparin.[127]

Recently, use of thiolated polymers in combination with reduced glutathione as a penetration enhancer has attracted significant interest.[130] The thiomers/GSH system are made by covalently attaching a thiol group and reduced GSH to poly(acrylic acid) derivatives and chitosan. These polymers have been shown to enhance the oral absorption of calcitonin,[131] insulin,[132] and heparin.[133] The enhanced oral bioavailability is partly due to penetration enhancement, and partly due to the ability of the polymers to protect the peptides from enzymatic degradation.[134] The mechanism of penetration enhancement seems to be attributed to the ability of these polymers to open up tight junctions through their interaction with protein tyrosine phosphate via a GSH-mediated mechanism.

However, use of permeation enhancers to enhance oral absorption of class III compounds does have its limitations. First, the effectiveness of penetration enhancer is significantly reduced *in vivo*, due to dilution with GI fluids after oral administration. Secondly, there are concerns that use of permeation enhancers may cause tissue irritation and damage, especially in chronic therapy. Therefore, until the long-term effects of continued exposure to the enhancer have been assessed, use of permeation enhancers may have significant toxicity ramifications. Currently, the FDA has not approved any excipients as permeation enhancers.

TABLE 18.10   A summary of intestinal drug absorption enhancers and their mechanisms of action (modified from Table 1 in reference 129)

Absorption enhancer	Mechanism of action	Study design
Salicylates		
Sodium salicylate	Increasing cell membrane fluidity, decreasing concentration of non-protein thiols	*In vivo*
Fatty acids		
Medium/long chain glycerides	Paracellular (e.g., sodium caprate dilates tight junctions), and transcellular (epithelial cell damage or disruption of cell membranes)	*In vitro*
Bile salts		
Taurodihydrofusidate, sodium taurocholate, sodium taurodeoxycholate	Disruption of membrane integrity by phospholipids solubilization and cytotic effects, reduction of mucus viscosity	*In vitro*
Surfactants		
Sodium dodecyl sulfate, sodium dioctyl sulfosuccinate	Membrane damage by extracting membrane proteins or lipids, phospholipids acyl chain perturbation	*In situ* and *in vitro*
Chelating agents		
EDTA, EGTA	Complexation of calcium and magnesium (tight junction opening)	*In vitro*
Toxins and venom extracts		
ZOT	Interaction with zonulin surface receptor induces actin polymerization (tight junction opening)	*In vivo*
Anionic polymers		
Poly(acrylic acid) derivatives	Combination of enzyme inhibition and extracellular calcium depletion (tight junction opening)	*In vitro*
Cationic polymers		
Chitosan salts, N-trimethyl chitosan chloride	Combination of mucoadhesion and ionic interactions with the cell membrane (tight junction opening)	*In vitro*

However, excipients (such as surfactants, cyclodextrins, etc.) with known penetration effect on membranes have been used in the marketed products for bioavailability enhancement.

18.4.5 BCS Class IV: Low Solubility and Low Permeability

Class IV compounds exhibit both poor solubility and poor permeability, and they pose tremendous challenges to formulation development. As a result, a substantial investment in dosage form development with no guarantee of success should be expected. A combination of class II and class III technologies could be used to formulate class IV compounds, although the success rate is not expected to be high. Interestingly, some class IV compounds have surprisingly good oral bioavailability. This, in part, may be due to carrier mediated uptake, but in part may be due to the misclassification of these compounds as BCS class IV. The *in vivo* solubility of a class IV compound may be much higher than the aqueous solubility, due to presence of surfactants and other solubilizing agents in the GI fluid.[135] For the class IV compounds that are neither substrates for active transport nor highly soluble *in vivo*, redesigning drug molecules to enhance solubility and/or permeability or searching for a non-oral route may be more likely to succeed. Table 18.11 lists marketed oral drug products of the class IV compounds.

18.4.6 Further Clarifications of the BCS

Traditionally, permeability is defined as the ability of a molecule to penetrate a biological membrane by a passive diffusion process. However, the term "permeability" has a much wider scope in the BCS. The BCS defines permeability by the extent of oral absorption,

which can be influenced by a variety of physiological factors. For example, luminal complexation can reduce the free drug concentration available for absorption. Luminal degradation further degrades compounds, such as proteins and peptides, which are susceptible to intestinal enzymes or microorganisms. Pre-systemic metabolism and active secretion by efflux mechanisms significantly reduces oral bioavailability of drugs, whereas carrier-mediated transport may enhance the oral absorption of poorly soluble and/or poorly permeable drugs. This section will discuss the challenges and opportunities posed by the above factors, and review formulation strategies that potentially address issues posed by these complex physiological processes.

Luminal Complexation and Luminal Degradation

Luminal complexation can significantly limit oral absorption by reducing the concentration of free drug that is available to diffuse across the GI membrane.

For example, it was shown that the bioavailability of norfloxacin was significantly reduced when the antimicrobial drug was co-administered with divalent or trivalent cations in dogs.[136] This study implied that concomitant administration of antacids or vitamin plus mineral products containing aluminum, magnesium, ferrous iron, and copper may decrease oral absorption of antibiotics that are capable of complexing with metal ions.

Luminal degradation can be attributed to chemical decomposition in the aqueous intestinal environment or metabolism by luminal digestive enzymes or luminal microorganisms. Several formulation approaches are available to enhance the stability of acid-labile drugs. For example, tablets or capsules containing the acid-labile drug can be coated with enteric polymers, such as methacrylate polymers, which are only soluble at the higher pH in the small intestine. Acryleze® and Eudragit® are examples of commercially available enteric coating systems, which are formulated to provide strong and pliable enteric films that are resistant to acid. In addition, co-administering an acid-labile compound with anti-acids, such as a proton pump inhibitor, can transiently increase the stomach pH, thereby minimizing acid degradation.

Compared to stabilizing acid-labile drugs, fewer formulation approaches are successful in protecting compounds from degradation by enzymes or microorganisms in the GI tract. Enzymatic degradation and poor permeability pose significant challenges in achieving any meaningful bioavailability for oral delivery of proteins and peptides.[137] Prodrugs may be used to offer some protection to proteins and peptides against enzymatic degradation (see Section 18.4.4).

TABLE 18.11 Examples of BCS class IV compounds (modified from Table 1 in reference 44)

Drug	Indication	Dose
Aluminium hydroxide	Gastrointestinal agent	500
Furosemide[a]	Diuretic	40
Indinavir[a]	Antiviral	200, 300, 400 (sulfate)
Nelfinavir	Antiviral	250 (mesilate)
Ritonavir	Antiviral	100

[a]First pass effect

In addition, lipid vesicles such as water-in-oil micro-emulsions and micelles may shield their encapsulated contents from luminal degradation. For example, micelles were shown to slow ester hydrolysis of ben-zoylthiamine disulfide, resulting in increased *in situ* and *in vivo* absorption.[138] Water-in-oil (w/o) micro-emulsions have also demonstrated some potential in delivering peptides and proteins. The drawbacks of w/o microemulsions are that the encapsulation efficiency is low, and the microemulsions may undergo phase inversion or separation to expose the encapsulated water soluble contents to luminal degradation.[139]

Pre-systemic Metabolism

Before an orally absorbed drug reaches systemic cir-culation, it must first pass through the intestine, and then the liver where drug metabolism known as pre-systemic metabolism may occur. This is known more commonly as the first-pass effect. The first-pass effect cannot only significantly reduce the oral bioavailability of a drug, but can also cause high inter-patient variabil-ity resulting from variation in the expression and activ-ity levels of metabolizing enzymes. The most common reactions of the first-pass effect are phase 1 oxidations mediated by the cytochrome P450 (CYP) enzymes. Historically, presystemic elimination was mainly attrib-uted to hepatic first-pass metabolism, because the liver has a high concentration of metabolizing enzymes. It was only recently discovered that important isozymes of P450—CYP3A4, and CYP2D6—are also present at high concentrations in the intestinal brush border. In addi-tion, the small intestine has much larger surface area and lower blood flow than the liver, which further adds to the significance of intestinal first-pass metabolism.[140]

Many drugs are substrates for CYP3A4. This includes cyclosporine, estradiol, and many protease inhibitors such as saquinavir, ritonavir, indinavir, nelfi-navir, and amprenavir.[141] Since enzymatic reactions typically exhibit saturable kinetics, the bioavailabil-ity of CYP3A4 substrates tends to increase with dose. Another implication from saturable metabolism is that drug–drug interactions may be significant when co-administered drugs are substrates for the same metab-olizing enzyme. Few oral formulation approaches are available to overcome pre-systemic elimination. Co-administration of a drug with an enzymatic inhibi-tor can be used to boost bioavailability of the drug that is susceptible to the same metabolizing enzyme. For example, the bioavailability of cyclosporine was signifi-cantly boosted by CYP3A4 inhibitors, such as ketocona-zole,[142] and reduced by a CYP3A4 inducer rifampin.[143] However, co-administration of another drug may elicit

safety concerns, unless both drugs can be used in syn-ergy therapeutically. For example, the treatment of HIV patients often includes a cocktail of drugs that target dif-ferent stage of viral reproduction. Some HIV drugs may significantly boost oral absorption of others. Dietary components, such as oleic acid and grapefruit juice, have also been reported to significantly improve bio-availability of P-450 substrates, such as propanolol,[144] and midazolam.[145] The bioavailability enhancement effect, at least in the case of grapefruit juice, was attrib-uted to decreased intestinal metabolism, although the mechanism was not clearly understood. Very lipophilic compounds ($\log_{10}P > 5-6$) may enter systemic circula-tion through the lymphatic pathway, thereby bypassing first-pass metabolism to enter the systemic circulation unscathed. Intestinal lymphatics are the major absorp-tion gateway for natural lipids, lipid derivatives, and cholesterol. However, the vast majority of pharmaceuti-cal compounds are not lipophilic enough to have signifi-cant uptake by the lymphatic pathway. When they are, their solubility is extremely poor, such that dissolution or solubility may limit the extent of their absorption. Lipophilic prodrugs may be designed by attaching the parent drug to a lipophlic and/or "functionally based" promoiety to enhance lymphatic uptake. Comprehensive reviews in this area are available.[91,146] In general, the use of lipid prodrugs to target the lymphatic approach is a wide open research area. Much needs to be done before one can assess the practicality of this approach.

P-gp Efflux Mechanism

Enterocyte *P*-glycoprotein (P-gp) is an apically polarized efflux transporter that was first identified in multidrug-resistant cancer cells, but later also found to be present in the intestinal brush border region. P-gp reduces oral absorption by actively secreting absorbed drug from enterocytes back into the intes-tinal lumen. Moreover, P-gp appears to share a large number of substrates with CYP3A,[140,147] and the inter-play between P-gp and CYP enzymes may have sig-nificant impact on oral bioavailability. Wu and Benet proposed that inhibition of efflux transporters (located on the apical side) in the intestine prevents drug recy-cling, resulting in decreased drug access to metaboliz-ing enzymes.[148] In this case, oral bioavailability can be significantly increased, due to a synergistic effect of P-gp inhibition and reduction of intestinal metabo-lism. In contrast to the small intestine, the drug mol-ecule encounters the enzyme prior to the apical efflux transporter in the liver (or kidney). Inhibition of the P-gp increases the drug access to the metabolizing enzymes, therefore boosting the extent of metabolism and maybe decreasing oral bioavailability.

Little is known about how to overcome the absorption barrier posed by the P-gp efflux pump. Certain nonionic surfactants, such as cremophor, have been shown to inhibit the P-gp efflux pump *in vitro*.[149] However, due to GI dilution, a much higher amount of surfactant may be required to achieve a similar effect *in vivo* than *in vitro*. A prodrug approach has been used to reduce P-gp mediated cellular efflux. For example, attaching dipeptides to saquinavir (SQV) can increase cellular permeability of SQV through the peptide transporter, whereas Pg-p-mediated efflux is reduced.[150] Co-administration of a drug with a P-gp inhibitor has also been used to enhance the oral bioavailability of the drug. For example, co-administration of docetaxel, a substrate for P-gp with cyclosporine, which is both a P-gp substrate and inhibitor, increased the bioavailability of docetaxel from 8% to 90% in humans.[151] Although effective, this approach does raise a variety of safety related questions such as:

1. since the P-gp efflux pump and CYP3A share a large number of substrates, what is the effect of administrating a P-gp inhibitor on liver and gut metabolism?
2. if both P-gp and CYP3A are inhibited, what are the implications caused by potential toxic substances that are usually metabolized by CYP3A?
3. is the inhibitory effect transient or long-lasting, reversible or irreversible?
4. what is the effect of inhibitors on inter-subject variability?

Addressing the above questions will help mitigate the safety risk associated with using P-gp inhibitor to improve oral bioavailability.

Carrier-mediated Transport

Although the majority of drugs are absorbed orally through the passive diffusion process, many compounds have been shown to move across cell membranes easily using a specialized carrier-mediated transporter. Transporters play an important role in absorbing essential nutrients, such as sugars, lipids and amino acids, as well as influencing disposition and toxicity of drugs, such as ACE inhibitors, β-lactam antibiotics, etc. Many transporters are located in the brush border membrane in the small intestine, including the peptide transporters (PepT1 and PepT2), amino acid transporters, nucleoside/nucleobase transporters (ENT family), bile acid transporters, and monocarboxylic acid transporters.[126] Recently, transporter-targeted prodrug delivery has attracted significant interest. The rationale underlying this approach is to attach the parent drug to a natural substrate for a transporter. After the prodrug is translocated across the GI tract, the prodrug is biotransformed to release the active moiety, either within the cell or in the systemic circulation. This approach has been successfully used for a number of transporters. For example, attachment to dipeptides was shown to significantly enhance the transport of acyclovir,[120] and cidofovir,[121] via hPepT1-mediated transport, resulting in significantly better oral bioavailability in rats. In another example, acyclovir was conjugated to the native bile acid chenodeoxychloate via a valine linker. The prodrug, which had a good affinity to the bile acid transporter (hSABT),[152] increased the oral bioavilability of acyclovir by two-fold in rats.[153,154] The prodrug approach may also be used for cell-targeted delivery to enhance therapeutic efficacy while reducing toxic side effects. For example, Wu and his coworkers found that asparaginyl endopeptidase (legumain) was expressed at a high concentration in tumor cells.[155] They made a legumain-activated prodrug (LEG-3) by covalently linking an anticancer drug (doxorubicin) to a cell-impermeable substrate for legumain. The prodrug had low permeability to normal cells, but could be activated and chemically modified by legumain in the tumor microenvironment to be cell permeable. Upon administration, there was a profound increase of the end-product doxorubicin in the nuclei of the tumor cells, but little in other tissues. The prodrug had completely arrested the growth of a variety of neoplasms, including multi-resistant tumors *in vivo*. Overall, the areas of transported targeted drug delivery offer exciting opportunities, and may be the future direction for precise and efficient drug delivery of problematic compounds.

18.4.7 Biopharmaceutical Drug Disposition Classification System (BDDCS)

A major limitation of the BCS is that it does not provide an in-depth understanding of how drug metabolism and drug transport may impact the pharmacokinetic performance of drug products. To expand this aspect, Wu and Benet proposed a modified version of classification system—the biopharmaceutical drug disposition classification system (BDDCS)—in their seminal paper published in 2005.[148] After reviewing 130 drugs listed in the WHO Essential Medicines List in terms of their solubility, permeability, and pharmacokinetic parameters, they found a common theme linked the BCS to drug metabolism. The high permeability of BCS class I and II compounds allows ready access to the metabolizing enzymes within hepatocytes. Therefore, compounds in classes I and II are eliminated primarily via metabolism, whereas compounds in classes III and IV have low permeability, and are primarily eliminated unchanged into the urine and bile.

Wu and Benet further suggested that the BCS system could be used to predict transporter effect on oral absorption of drug products. For example, the high solubility and high permeability of class I compounds allows a high concentration in the gut to saturate both the absorptive and efflux transporter. As a result, transporters will not play a significant role affecting oral absorption of class I compounds. The high permeability of class II compounds allows their ready access across the gut membrane, and implies that absorptive transporters will not have an effect on absorption. But their low solubility prevents saturation of the efflux transporter, resulting in the dominant effect of efflux transporters on oral absorption of this class of compounds. The scenario is reversed for the class III compounds. Their low permeability/high solubility indicates that an absorptive transporter will affect the extent of oral bioavailability and rate of absorption of the class III compounds. Applying the same rationale, both the absorptive and efflux transporters could have a significant effect on oral absorption of class IV compounds.

In addition, the BDDCS may provide a useful framework to predict effects of food, enzyme-transporter interplay, and drug–drug interactions on the pharmacokinetic performance of drug products. These predictions were supported by a series of studies investigating the effect of transporter inhibition and induction on drug metabolism listed in Wu and Benet's review article. As shown in Table 18.12,[148] the

authors proposed to use the elimination/solubility criteria for classifying compounds in the BDDCS because it is easier to obtain accurate metabolism data than permeability data. The authors believed that BDDCS could provide a useful framework to predict drug disposition profiles, as well as to expand the number of class I compounds eligible for waiver of *in vivo* bioequivalence study.

18.5 CONCLUDING REMARKS

Successful development of oral drug products is not an easy task. One must understand the physico-chemical properties, mechanical properties, and biopharmaceutical properties of drug products, and how this multitude of factors may influence stability, processability, and bioavailability of drug products. As a new chemical entity is identified for development, formulators need to work with chemists to fully characterize physico-chemical properties of the drug substance through a battery of tests. These typically include screening salts and polymorphs, performing accelerated stability studies, generating solubility/dissolution rate data, measuring membrane permeability using Caco-2 cell lines, etc. Once a salt or polymorph is selected for further development, one needs to understand what the target release profile and desired route of delivery is to achieve therapeutic efficacy of the drug candidate. Most pharmaceutical compounds are small organic molecules to be developed as an immediate-release solid oral dosage form.

The next step is to select a formulation approach, based on understanding of the biopharmaceutical properties of the drug candidate. BCS class I compounds normally do not require special formulation efforts, because their high permeability/high solubility leads to fast and complete oral absorption. As for BCS class II compounds, there are a variety of formulation approaches aimed to enhance solubility and/or dissolution rate of these compounds. It is more difficult to formulate BCS class III compounds, because modification of the permeation characteristics of a drug and membrane is not an easy task. Class IV compounds are expected to have absorption problems, given their poor permeability and low solubility. For these compounds, it is worth considering structural modifications or to use an alternative route to overcome absorption issues. It is important to keep in mind that solubility and permeability are only two pieces of the jigsaw puzzle for the picture of oral bioavailability. A variety of factors, such as luminal degradation, pre-systemic elimination, and transporter effects (both absorptive and

TABLE 18.12 The biopharmaceutical drug disposition classification system (BDDCS) where major route of elimination (metabolized versus unchanged) serves as the permeability criteria (modified from Figure 6 in reference 148)

	High solubility	Low solubility
Extensive metabolism	Class I	Class II
	High solubility	Low solubility
	Extensive metabolism (Rapid dissolution and ≥70% metabolism for biowaiver)	Extensive metabolism
Poor metabolism	Class III	Class IV
	High solubility	Low solubility
	Poor metabolism	Poor metabolism

efflux), may significantly impact oral absorption and disposition of drug products. Although there are no mature formulation strategies to deal with metabolism and transport effects of a drug, new ideas continue to emerge to deliver drugs in an efficient and precise manner. Selection of a good formulation approach is only half of the story in drug product development. The other half lies in developing and scale-up of this formulation so that the drug product can be produced in a reliable and cost effective manner. Integration of physico-chemical, mechanical, and biopharmaceutical properties of a drug candidate enables making science-based decisions to develop a robust and bioavailable drug product that has optimal therapeutic efficacy.

References

1. Martin, A. (1993). *Physical Pharmacy*, 4th edn. Lea & Febiger, Philidelphia, PA. pp. 223.
2. Noyes, A.A. & Whitney, W.R. (1897). The rate of solution of solid substances in their own solutions. Journal of the American Chemical Society 19(12), 930–934.
3. US Pharmacopeia USP29/NF24. (2006). US Pharmacopeial Convention, Rockville, MD, General Chapter <711>. pp. 2675–2679.
4. Food and Drug Administration guidance for industry (1997). *Extended release dosage forms: Development, evaluation and application of in vivo/in vitro correlations.* Food and Drug Administration, Center for Drug Evaluation and Research, Rockville, MD.
5. Leo, A., Hansch, C. & Elkins, D. (1971). Partition coefficients and their uses. Chemical Reviews 71(6), 525–616.
6. Leo, A.J. (1987). Some advantages of calculating octanol-water partition coefficients. Journal of Pharmaceutical Sciences 76(2), 166–168.
7. Leo, A.J. (1995). Critique of recent comparison of *log P* calculation methods. Chemical & Pharmaceutical Bulletin 43(3), 512–513.
8. Mannhold, R. & Dross, K. (1996). Calculation procedures for molecular lipophilicity: A comparative study. Quantitative Structure–Activity Relationships 15(5), 403–409.
9. van de Waterbeemd, H. & Mannhold, R. (1996). Programs and methods for calculation of Log P-values. Quantitative Structure–Activity Relationships 15(5), 410–412.
10. Riggs, D.S. (1963). *The Mathematical Approach to Physiological Problems.* Williams & Wilkins, Baltimore, MD. pp. 181–185.
11. Camenisch, G., Alsenz, J., Van De Waterbeemd, H. & Folkers, G. (1998). Estimation of permeability by passive diffusion through Caco-2 cell monolayers using the drugs' lipophilicity and molecular weight. European Journal of Pharmaceutical Sciences 6(4), 313–319.
12. van de Waterbeemd, H., Camenisch, G., Folkers, G. & Raevsky, O.A. (1996). Estimation of Caco-2 cell permeability using calculated molecular descriptors. Quantitative Structure–Activity Relationships 15(6), 480–490.
13. Lipinski, C.A., Lombardo, F., Dominy, B.W. & Feeney, P.J. (2001). Experimental and computational approaches to estimate solubility and permeability in drug discovery and development settings. Advanced Drug Delivery Reviews 46(1–3), 3–26.
14. Lipinski, C.A., Lombardo, F., Dominy, B.W. & Feeney, P.J. (1997). Experimental and computational approaches to estimate solubility and permeability in drug discovery and development settings. Advanced Drug Delivery Reviews 23(1–3), 3–25.

15. Amidon, G.E., He, X. & Hageman, M.J. (2003). Physicochemical Characterization and Principles of Oral Dosage Form Selection. In: *Burger's Medicinal Chemistry and Drug Delivery*, D.J. Abraham (ed.), 6th edn, Vol. 2, Chapter 18.
16. Byrn, S.R., Pfeiffer, R.R. & Stowell, J.G. (1999). *Solid State Chemistry of Drugs*, 2nd edn. SSCI, West Lafayette, IA.
17. Burger, A. & Grieesser, U.J. (1991). Physical stability, hygroscopicity and solubility of succinylsulfathiazole crystal forms. The polymorphic drug substances of the European Pharmacopoeia. VII. European Journal of Pharmaceutics and Biopharmaceutics 37(2), 118–124.
18. Aguiar, A.J., Krc, J., Kinkel, A.W. & Samyn, J.C. (1967). Effect of polymorphism on the absorption of chloramphenicol from chloramphenicol plamitate. Journal of Pharmaceutical Sciences 56(7), 847–883.
19. Zhang, G.Z., Law, D., Schmitt, E.A. & Qiu, Y. (2004). Phase transformation considerations during process development and manufacture of solid oral dosage forms. Advanced Drug Delivery Reviews 56(3), 371–390.
20. Law, D., Krill, S.L., Schmitt, E.A., Fort, J.J., Qiu, Y., Wang, W. & Porter, W.R. (2001). Physicochemical considerations in the preparation of amorphous ritonavir with poly(ethylene glycol) 8000 solid dispersions. Journal of Pharmaceutical Sciences 90(8), 1015–1025.
21. Law, D., Schmitt, E.A., Marsh, K.C., Everitt, E.A., Wang, W., Fort, J.J., Krill, S.L., Qiu, Y. & Porter, W.R. (2004). Ritonavir-PEG 8000 solid dispersions: *in vitro* and *in vivo* evaluations. Journal of Pharmaceutical Sciences 93(3), 563–570.
22. Pikal, M.J., Lukes, A.L. & Lang, J.E. (1978). Quantitative crystallinity determinations for β-lactam antibacterials. Journal of Pharmaceutical Sciences 67(6), 767–773.
23. US Pharmacopeia USP29/NF24. (2006). US Pharmacopeial Convention, Rockville, MD, General Chapter <905>, pp. 2778–2784.
24. Zhang, Y. & Johnson, K.C. (1997). Effect of drug particle size on content uniformity of low-dose solid dosage forms. International Journal of Pharmaceutics 154(2), 179–183.
25. Yalkowsky, S.H. & Bolton, S. (1990). Particle size and content uniformity. Pharmaceutical Research 7(9), 962–966.
26. Nyström, C., Alderborn, G., Duberg, M. & Karehill, P.G. (1993). Bonding surface area and bonding mechanism. Two important factors for the understanding of powder compactibility. Drug Development and Industrial Pharmacy 19(17–18), 2143–2196.
27. Alderborn, G. & Nyström, C. (1982). Studies on direct compression of tablets. IV. The effect of particle size on the mechanical strength of tablets. Acta Pharmaceutica Suecica 19(5), 381–390.
28. US Pharmacopeia USP29/NF24. (2006). US Pharmacopeial Convention, Rockville, MD, General Chapter <616>, pp. 2638–2639.
29. Haleblian, J. & McCrone, W. (1969). Pharmaceutical applications of polymorphism. Journal of Pharmaceutical Sciences 58(8), 911–929.
30. Ruotsalainen, M., Heinämäki, J., Taipale, K. & Yliruusi, J. (2003). Influence of the aqueous film coating process on the properties and stability of tablets containing a moisture-labile drug. Pharmaceutical Development and Technology 8(4), 443–451.
31. Zografi, G.R., Hollenbeck, G., Laughlin, S.M., Pikal, M.J., Schwartz, J.P. & Campen, L.V. (1991). Report of the advisory panel on moisture specifications. Pharmacopeial Forum 17, 1459–1474.
32. Ahlneck, C. & Zografi, G. (1990). Molecular basis of moisture effects on the physical and chemical stability of drugs in the solid state. International Journal of Pharmaceutics 62(2–3), 87–95.
33. Guidance for industry (ICH Q3B (R2)) (2006). *Impurities in new drug product.* Food and Drug Administration, Center for Drug Evaluation and Research, Rockville, MD.
34. Carstensen, J.T. (1974). Stability of solids and solid dosage forms. Pharmaceutical Sciences 63(1), 1–14.

35. Horikoshi, I. & Himuro, I. (1966). Physicochemical studies on water contained in solid medicaments. III. Character of hydrates of glucoronic acid derivatives. Yakugaku Zasshi 86(4), 319–324.

36. Nystrom, C. & Karehill, P.G. (1995). The Importance of Intermolecular Bonding Forces and the Concept of Bonding Surface Area. In: *Pharmaceutical Powder Compaction Technology*, G. Alderborn, & C. Nystrom, (eds). Marcel Dekker, New York. p. 48.

37. Rowe, R.C. & Roberts, R.J. (1995). Mechanical Properties. In: *Pharmaceutical Powder Compaction Technology*, G. Alderborn, & C. Nystrom, (eds). Marcel Dekker, New York. pp. 288–289, 298–299, 300.

38. Heckel, R.W. (1961). Density-pressure relations in powder compaction. Trans. Am. Inst. Mining, Metallurgical and Petroleum Engineers 221, 671–675.

39. Hiestand, E.N. (1995). Rationale for and the Measurement of Tableting Indices. In: *Pharmaceutical Powder Compaction Technology*, G. Alderborn, & C. Nystrom, (eds). Marcel Dekker, New York. pp. 219–243.

40. Hiestand, E.N. (1991). Tablet bond. I. A theoretical model. International Journal of Pharmaceutics 67(3), 217–229.

41. Amidon, G.L., Lennernäs, H., Shah, V.P. & Crison, J.R. (1995). A theoretical basis for a biopharmaceutical drug classification: the correlation of *in vivo* drug product dissolution and *in vivo* bioavailablity. Pharmaceutical Research 12(3), 413–420.

42. Lennernäs, H. (1995). Does fluid across the intestinal mucosa affect quantitative oral drug absorption? Is it time for a re-evaluation? Pharmaceutical Research 12(11), 1573–1582.

43. Food and Drug Administration guidance for industry (2000). *Waiver of In Vivo Bioavailability and Bioequivalence Studies for Immediate-Release Solid Oral Dosage Forms Based on a Biopharmaceutics Classification System*. Food and Drug Administration, Center for Drug Evaluation and Research, Rockville, MD.

44. Lindenberg, M., Kopp, S. & Dressman, J.B. (2004). Classification of orally administered drugs on the world health organization model list of essential medicines according to the biopharmaceutical classification system. European Journal of Pharmaceutics and Biopharmaceutics 58(2), 265–278.

45. Lieberman, H.A., Lachman, L. & Schwartz, J.B. (1989). *Pharmaceutical Dosage Form: Tablets*, 2nd edn. Marcel Dekker, New York.

46. Bastin, R.J., Bowker, M.J. & Slater, B.J. (2000). Salt selection and optimization procedures for pharmaceutical new chemical entities. Organic Process Research & Development 4(5), 427–435.

47. Berge, S.M., Bighley, L.D. & Monkhouse, D.C. (1977). Pharmaceutical salts. Journal of Pharmaceutical Sciences 66(1), 1–19.

48. Buckton, G. (1995). *Interfacial Phenomena in Drug Delivery and Targeting*. Harwood Academic, London. p. 29.

49. Parrot, E.L. (1986). Milling. In: *The Theory and Practice of Industrial Pharmacy*, L. Lachman, H.A. Lieberman, & J.L. Kanig, (eds), 3rd edn. Lea & Febiger, Philadelphia, PA. pp. 21–46.

50. Aguiar, A.J. & Zelmer, J.E. (1969). Dissolution behavior of polymorphs of chloramphenicol palmitate and mefanamic acid. Journal of Pharmaceutical Sciences 58(8), 983–987.

51. Kahela, P., Aaltonen, R., Lewing, E., Anttila, M. & Kristoffersson, E. (1983). Pharmacokinetics and dissolution of two crystalline forms of carbamazepine. International Journal of Pharmaceutics 14(1), 103–112.

52. Hancock, B.C. & Parks, M. (2000). What is the true solubility advantage for amorphous pharmaceuticals? Pharmaceutical Research 17(4), 397–404.

53. Huang, L.F. & Tong, W.Q. (2004). Impact of solid state properties on developability assessment of drug candidates. Advanced Drug Delivery Reviews 56(3), 321–334.

54. Singhal, D. & Curatolo, W. (2004). Drug polymorphism and dosage form design: a practical perspective. Advanced Drug Delivery Reviews 56(3), 335–347.

55. Yu, L.X., Lionberger, R.A., Raw, A.S., D'Costa, R., Wu, H. & Hussain, A.S. (2004). Applications of process analytical technology to crystallization processes. Advanced Drug Delivery Reviews 56(3), 349–369.

56. Snide, D.A., Addicks, W. & Owens, W. (2004). Polymorphism in generic drug product development. Advanced Drug Delivery Reviews 56(3), 391–395.

57. Raw, A.S., Furness, M.S., Gill, D.S., Adams, R.C., Holcombe, F. O. & Yu, L.X. (2004). Regulatory considerations of pharmaceutical solid polymorphism in Abbreviated New Drug Applications (ANDAs). Advanced Drug Delivery Reviews 56(3), 397–414.

58. Sekiguchi, K. & Obi, N. (1961). Absorption of eutectic mixtures. I. A comparison of the behavior of eutectic mixtures of sulphathiazole and that of ordinary sulphathiazole in man. Chemical & Pharmaceutical Bulletin 9, 866–872.

59. Craig, D.Q.M. (2002). The mechanisms of drug release from solid dispersions in water-soluble polymers. International Journal of Pharmaceutics 231(2), 131–144.

60. Leuner, C. & Dressman, J. (2000). Improving drug solubility for oral delivery using solid dispersions. European Journal of Pharmaceutics and Biopharmaceutics 50(1), 47–60.

61. Breitenbach, J. (2002). Melt extrusion: from process to drug delivery technology. European Journal of Pharmaceutics and Biopharmaceutics 54(2), 107–117.

62. Serajuddin, A.T.M. (1999). Solid dispersion of poorly water-soluble drugs: early promises, subsequent problems, and recent breakthroughs. Journal of Pharmaceutical Sciences 88(10), 1058–1066.

63. Breitenbach, J. (2006). Melt extrusion can bring new benefits to HIV therapy—the example of Kaletra® tablets. American Journal of Drug Delivery 4(2), 61–64.

64. Hersey, A., Robinson, B.H. & Kelly, H.C. (1986). Mechanisms of inclusion-compound formation for binding of organic dyes, ions and surfactants to α-cyclodextrin studied by kinetic methods based on competition experiments. Journal of the Chemical Society, Faraday Transactions 1: Physical Chemistry in Condensed Phases 82(5), 1271–1287.

65. Sella, V.J. & Rajewski, R.A. (1997). Cyclodextrins: their future in drug formulation and delivery. Pharmaceutical Research 14(5), 556–567.

66. Rajewski, R.A. & Stella, V.J. (1996). Pharmaceutical applications of cyclodextrins. 2. *In vivo* drug delivery. Journal of Pharmaceutical Sciences 85(11), 1142–1169.

67. Thompson, D.O. (1997). Cyclodextrins—enabling excipients: their present and future use in pharmaceuticals. Critical Reviews in Therapeutic Drug Carrier Systems 14(1), 1–104.

68. Uekama, K., Hirayama, F. & Irie, T. (1994). Applications of cyclodextrins in pharmaceutical preparations. Drug Targeting and Delivery 3, 411–456.

69. Järvinen, T., Järvinen, K., Schwarting, N. & Stella, V.J. (1995). Beta-cyclodextrin derivatives, SBE4-beta-CD and HP-beta-CD, increase the oral bioavailability of cinnarizine in beagle dogs. Journal of Pharmaceutical Sciences 84(3), 295–299.

70. Betlach, C.J., Gonzalez, M.A., McKiernan, B.C., Neff-Davis, C. & Bodor, N.J. (1993). Oral pharmacokinetics of carbamazepine in dogs from commercial tablets and a cyclodextrin complex. Pharmaceutical Sciences 82(10), 1058–1060.

71. Hostetler, J.S., Hanson, L.H. & Stevens, D.A. (1993). Effect of hydroxypropyl-β-cyclodextrin on efficacy of oral itraconazole in disseminated murine cryptococcosis. The Journal of Antimicrobial Chemotherapy 32(3), 459–463.

72. Shao, Z., Li, Y., Chermak, T. & Mitra, A.K. (1994). Cyclodextrins as mucosal absorption promoters of insulin. II. Effects of

β-cyclodextrin derivatives on α-chymotryptic degradation and enteral absorption of insulin in rats. Pharmaceutical Research 11(8), 1174–1179.

73. Panini, R., Vandelli, M.A., Forni, F., Pradelli, J.M. & Salvioli, G. (1995). Improvement of ursodeoxycholic acid bioavailability by 2-hydroxypropyl-β-cyclodextrin complexation in healthy volunteers. Pharmacological Research 31(3/4), 205–209.

74. Hoon, T.J., Dawood, M.Y., Khan-Dawood, F.S., Ramos, J. & Batenhorst, R.L. (1993). Bioequivalence of a 17β-estradiol hydroxypropyl β-cyclodextrin complex in postmenopausal women. Journal of Clinical Pharmacology 33(11), 1116–1121.

75. Ricevuti, G., Mazzone, A., Pasotti, D., Uccelli, E., Pasquali, F., Gazzani, G. & Fregnan, G.B. (1991). Pharmacokinetics of dipyridamole-β-cyclodextrin complex in healthy volunteers after single and multiple doses. European Journal of Drug Metabolism and Pharmacokinetics 16(3), 197–201.

76. Nakanishi, K., Nadai, T., Masada, M. & Miyajima, K. (1992). Effect of cyclodextrins on biological membrane. II. Mechanism of enhancement on the intestinal absorption of non-absorbable drug by cyclodextrins. Chemical & Pharmaceutical Bulletin 40(5), 1252–1256.

77. Santucci, L., Fiorucci, S., Chiucchiu, S., Sicilia, A., Bufalino, L. & Morelli, A. (1992). Placebo-controlled comparison of piroxicam-β-cyclodextrin, piroxicam, and indomethacin on gastric potential difference and mucosal injury in humans. Digestive Diseases and Sciences 37(12), 1825–1832.

78. Otero Espinar, F.J., Anguiano Igea, S., Blanco Mendez, J. & Vila Jato, J.L. (1991). Reduction in the ulcerogenicity of naproxen by complexation with β-cyclodextrin. International Journal of Pharmaceutics 70(1–2), 35–41.

79. Uekama, K., Horikawa, T., Horiuchi, Y. & Hirayama, F. (1993). *In vitro* and *in vivo* evaluation of delayed-release behavior of diltiazem from its O-carboxymethyl-O-ethyl β-cyclodextrin complex. Journal of Controlled Release 25(1–2), 99–106.

80. Horikawa, T., Hirayama, F. & Uekama, K. (1995). *In vivo* and *in vitro* correlation for delayed-release behavior of a molsidomine/O-carboxymethyl-O-ethyl-β-cyclodextrin complex in gastric acidity-controlled dogs. The Journal of Pharmacy and Pharmacology 47(2), 124–127.

81. Frank, D.W., Gray, J.E. & Weaver, R.N. (1976). Cyclodextrin nephrosis in the rat. The American Journal of Pathology 83(2), 367–382.

82. Olivier, P., Verwaerde, F. & Hedges, A.R. (1991). Subchronic toxicity of orally administered β-cyclodextrin in rats. Journal of the American College of Toxicology 10(4), 407–419.

83. Gerlóczy, A., Fónagy, A., Keresztes, P., Perlaky, L. & Szejtli, J. (1985). Absorption, distribution, excretion and metabolism of orally administered 14C-β-cyclodextrin in rat. Arzneimittel-Forschung 35(7), 1042–1047.

84. Anderberg, E.K. & Artursson, P. (1993). Epithelial transport of drugs in cell culture. VIII. Effects of sodium dodecyl sulfate on cell membrane and tight junction permeability in human intestinal epithelial (Caco-2) cells. Journal of Pharmaceutical Sciences 82(4), 392–398.

85. Swenson, E.S., Milisen, W.B. & Curatolo, W. (1994). Intestinal permeability enhancement: efficacy, acute local toxicity, and reversibility. Pharmaceutical Research 11(8), 1132–1142.

86. Nerurkar, M.M., Ho, N.F.H., Burton, P.S., Vidmar, T.J. & Borchardt, R.T. (1997). Mechanistic roles of neutral surfactants on concurrent polarized and passive membrane transport of a model peptide in Caco-2 cells. Journal of Pharmaceutical Sciences 86(7), 813–821.

87. Dintaman, J.M. & Silverman, J.A. (1999). Inhibition of P-glycoprotein by D-α-tocopheryl polyethylene glycol 1000 succinate (TPGS). Pharmaceutical Research 16(10), 1550–1556.

88. Porter, C.J.H. & Charman, W.N. (2001). Intestinal lymphatic drug transport: An update. Advanced Drug Delivery Reviews 50(1–2), 61–80.

89. Humberstone, A.J. & Charman, W.N. (1997). Lipid-based vehicles for the oral delivery of poorly water soluble drugs. Advanced Drug Delivery Reviews 25(1), 103–128.

90. Pouton, C.W. (2000). Lipid formulations for oral administration of drugs: non-emulsifying, self-emulsifying, and "self-microemulsifying" drug delivery systems. European Journal of Pharmaceutical Sciences 11(Suppl. 2), S93–S98.

91. Charman, W.N. (2000). Lipids, lipophilic drugs, and oral drug delivery. Some emerging concepts. Journal of Pharmaceutical Sciences 89(8), 967–978.

92. Bagwe, R.P., Kanicky, J.R., Palla, B.J., Patanhali, P.K. & Shah, D.O. (2001). Improved drug delivery using microemulsions: Rationale, recent progress, and new horizons. Critical Reviews in Therapeutic Drug Carrier Systems 18(1), 77–140.

93. MacGregor, K.J., Embleton, J.K., Lacy, J.E., Perry, E.A., Solomon, L.J., Seager, H. & Pouton, C.W. (1997). Influence of lipolysis on drug absorption from the gastrointestinal tract. Advanced Drug Delivery Reviews 25(1), 33–46.

94. Singh, B.N. (1999). Effects of food on clinical pharmacokinetics. Clinical Pharmacokinetics 37(3), 213–255.

95. Wiedmann, T.S., Liang, W. & Kamel, L. (2002). Solubilization of drugs by physiological mixtures of bile salts. Pharmaceutical Research 19(8), 1203–1208.

96. Pouton, C.W. (1997). Formulations of self-emulsifying drug delivery systems. Advanced Drug Delivery Reviews 25(1), 47–58.

97. Pouton, C.W. (1985). Self-emulsfying drug delivery systems: Assessment of the efficiency of emulsification. International Journal of Pharmaceutics 27(2–3), 335–348.

98. Mueller, E.A., Kovarik, J.M., van Bree, J.B., Tetzloff, W., Grevel, J. & Kutz, K. (1994). Improved dose linearity of cyclosporin pharmacokinetics from a microemulsion formulation. Pharmaceutical Research 11(2), 301–304.

99. Kovarik, J.M., Mueller, E.A., van Bree, J.B., Tetzloff, W. & Kutz, K. (1994). Reduced inter- and intra-individual variability in cyclosporin pharmacokinetics from a microemulsion formulation. Journal of Pharmaceutical Sciences 83(3), 444–446.

100. Sek, L., Boyd, B.J., Charman, W.N. & Porter, C.J.H. (2006). Examination of the impact of a range of pluronic surfactants on the *in-vitro* solubilisation behaviour and oral bioavailability of lipidic formulations of atovaquone. Journal of Pharmacy and Pharmacology 58, 809–820.

101. Gao, P. & Morozowich, W. (2006). Development of supersaturatable self-emulsifying drug delivery system formulations for improving the oral absorption of poorly soluble drugs. Expert Opinion on Drug Delivery 3(1), 97–110.

102. Gao, P., Rush, B.D., Pfund, W.P., Huang, T., Bauer, J.M., Morozowich, W., Kuo, M.S. & Hageman, M.J. (2003). Development of a supersaturable SEDDS (S-SEDDS) formulation of paclitaxel with improved oral bioavailability. Journal of Pharmaceutical Sciences 92(12), 2386–2398.

103. Simonelli, A.P., Mehta, S.C. & Higuchi, W.I. (1970). Inhibition of sulfathiazole crystal growth by polyvinylpyrrolidone. Journal of Pharmaceutical Sciences 59(5), 633–638.

104. Sekikawa, H., Fujiwara, J., Naganuma, T., Nakano, M. & Arita, T. (1978). Dissolution behaviors and gastrointestinal absorption of phenytoin in phenytoin-polyvinylpyrrolidone coprecipitate. Chemical & Pharmaceutical Bulletin 26(10), 3033–3039.

105. Megrab, N.A., Williams, A.C. & Barry, B.W. (1995). Oestradiol permeation through human skin and stic membrane: Effects of propylene glycol and supersaturation. Journal of Controlled Release 36(3), 277–294.

106. Raghavan, S.L., Trividic, A., Davis, A.F. & Hadgraft, J. (2001). Crystallization of hydrocortisone acetate: Influence of polymers. International Journal of Pharmaceutics 212(2), 13–221.

107. Raghavan, S.L., Kiepfer, B., Davis, A.F., Kazarian, S.G. & Hadgraft, J. (2001). Membrane transport of hydrocortisone acetate from supersaturated solutions; the role of polymers. International Journal of Pharmaceutics 221(1–2), 105.

108. Suzuki, H. & Sunada, H. (1997). Comparison of nicotiamide, ethylurea and polyeythylene glycol as carriers for nifedipine solid dispersion systems. Chemical & Pharmaceutical Bulletin 45(10), 1688–1693.

109. Kohri, N., Yamayoshi, Y., Xin, H., Iseki, K., Sato, N., Todo, S. & Miyazaki, K. (1999). Improving the oral bioavailability of albendazole in rabbits by the solid dispersion technique. The Journal of Pharmacy and Pharmacology 51(2), 159–164.

110. Raghavan, S.L., Trividic, A., Davis, A.F. & Hadgraft, J. (2000). Effects of cellulose polymers on supersaturation and *in vitro* membrane transport of hydrocortisone acetate. International Journal of Pharmaceutics 193(2), 231–237.

111. Iervolino, M., Raghavan, S.L. & Hadgraft, J. (2000). Membrane penetration enhancement of ibuprofen using supersaturation. International Journal of Pharmaceutics 198(2), 229–238.

112. Gao, P., Guyton, M.E., Huang, T., Bauer, J.M., Stefanski, K.J. & Lu, Q. (2004). Enhanced oral bioavailability of a poorly water soluble drug PNU-91325 by supersaturatable formulations. Drug Development and Industrial Pharmacy 30(2), 221–229.

113. Suzuki, H. & Sunada, H. (1998). Influence of water-soluble polymers on the dissolution of nifedipine solid dispersion with combined carriers. Chemical & Pharmaceutical Bulletin 46(3), 482–487.

114. Suzuki, H., Miyamoto, N., Masada, T., Hayakawa, E. & Ito, K. (1996). Solid dispersions of benidipine hydrochloride. II. Investigation of the interactions among drug, polymer and solvent in preparations. Chemical & Pharmaceutical Bulletin 44(2), 372–377.

115. Matsumoto, T. & Zografi, G. (1999). Physical properties of solid molecular dispersions of indomethacin with poly(vinylpyrrolidone) and poly(vinylpyrrolidone-co-vinylacetate) in relation to indomethacin crystallization. Pharmaceutical Research 16(11), 1722–1728.

116. Conradi, R.A., Hilgers, A.R., Ho, N.F.H. & Burton, P.S. (1992). The influence of peptide structure on transport across Caco-2 cells. II. Peptide bond modification which results in improved permeability. Pharmaceutical Research 9(3), 435–439.

117. Mizuma, T., Koyanagi, A. & Awazu, S. (2000). Intestinal transport and metabolism of glucose-conjugated kyotorphin and cyclic kyotorphin: Metabolic degradation is crucial to intestinal absorption of peptide drugs. Biochimica et Biophysica Acta 1475(1), 90–98.

118. Wang, J., Chow, D., Heiati, H. & Shen, W. (2003). Reversible lipidization for the oral delivery of salmon calcitonin. Journal of Controlled Release 88, 369–380.

119. Herrera-Ruiz, D. & Knipp, G.T. (2003). Current perspectives on established and putative mammalian oligopeptide transporters. Journal of Pharmaceutical Sciences 92(4), 691–714.

120. Anand, B.S., Katragadda, S. & Mitra, A.K. (2004). Pharmacokinetics of novel dipeptide ester prodrugs of acyclovir after oral administration: intestinal absorption and liver metabolism. The Journal of Pharmacology and Experimental Therapeutics 311(2), 659–667.

121. McKenna, C.E., Kashemirov, B.A., Eriksson, U., Amidon, G.L., Kish, P.E., Mitchell, S., Kim, J.S. & Hilfinger, J.M. (2005). Cidofovir peptide conjugates as prodrugs. Journal of Organometallic Chemistry 690(10), 2673–2678.

122. Weber, M.A. (1992). Fosinopril: A new generation of angiotensin-converting enzyme inhibitors. Journal of Cardiovascular Pharmacology 20(Suppl. 10), S7–S12.

123. Becker, S. & Thornton, L. (2004). Fosamprenavir: Advancing HIV protease inhibitor treatment options. Expert Opinion on Pharmacotherapy 5(9), 1995–2005.

124. Krise, J.P. & Stella, V.J. (1996). Prodrugs of phosphates, phosphonates, and phosphinates. Advanced Drug Delivery Reviews 19(12), 287–310.

125. Pauletti, G.M., Gangwar, S., Siahaan, T.J., Aube, J. & Borchardt, R.T. (1997). Improvement of oral peptide bioavailability: Peptidomimetics and prodrug strategies. Advanced Drug Delivery Reviews 27(2,3), 235–256.

126. Majumdar, S., Duvvuri, S. & Mitra, A.K. (2004). Membrane transporter/receptor-targeted prodrug design: strategies for human and veterinary drug development. Advanced Drug Delivery Reviews 56(10), 1437–1452.

127. Muranishi, S. (1990). Absorption Enhancers. Critical Reviews in Therapeutic Drug Carrier Systems 7(1), 1–33.

128. Aungst, B.J. (2000). Intestinal permeation enhancers. Journal of Pharmaceutical Sciences 89(4), 429–442.

129. Hamman, J.H., Enslin, G.M. & Kotze, A.F. (2005). Oral delivery of peptide drugs: barriers and development. Biodrugs 19(3), 165–177.

130. Bernkop-Schnürch, A., Kast, C.E. & Guggi, D. (2003). Permeation enhancing polymers in oral delivery of hydrophilic macromolecules: Thiomer/GSH systems. Journal of Controlled Release 93(2), 95–103.

131. Guggi, D., Kast, C.E. & Bernkop-Schnürch, A. (2003). *In vivo* evaluation of an oral salmon calcitonin-delivery system based on a thiolated chitosan carrier matrix. Pharmaceutical Research 20(12), 1989–1994.

132. Caliceti, P., Salmaso, S., Lillie, C. & Bernkop-Schnürch, A. (2003). Development and *in vivo* evaluation on an oral insulin-PEG delivery system. 30th Annual Meeting and Exposition of the Controlled Release Society, CRS. Glasgow, p. 677.

133. Kast, C.E., Guggi, D., Langoth, N. & Bernkop-Schnüch, A. (2003). Development and *in vivo* evaluation of an oral delivery system for low molecular weight heparin based on thiolated polycarbophil. Pharmaceutical Research 20(6), 931–936.

134. Luessen, H.L., De Leeuw, B.J., Pérard, D., Lehr, C., de Boer, A.G., Verhoef, J.C. & Junginger, H.E. (1996). Mucoadhesive polymers in peroral peptide drug delivery: I. Influence of mucoadhesive excipients on proteolytic activity of intestinal enzymes. European Journal of Pharmaceutical Sciences 4(2), 117–128.

135. Hörter, D. & Dressman, J.B. (2001). Influence of physicochemical properties on dissolution of drugs in the gastrointestinal tract. Advanced Drug Delivery Reviews 46(1–3), 75–87.

136. Wallis, S.C., Charles, B.G., Gahan, L.R., Fillippich, L.J., Bredhauer, M.G. & Duckworth, P.A. (1996). Interaction of norfloxacin with divalent and trivalent pharmaceutical cations. *In vitro* complexation and *in vivo* pharmacokinetic studies in the dog. Journal of Pharmaceutical Sciences 85(8), 803–809.

137. Aungst, B.J. (1993). Novel formulation strategies for improving oral bioavailability of drugs with poor membrane permeation or presystemic metabolism. Journal of Pharmaceutical Sciences 82(10), 979–987.

138. Utsumi, I., Kohno, K. & Takeuchi, Y. (1974). Surfactant effects on drug absorption. III. Effects of sodium glycocholate and its mixtures with synthetic surfactants on absorption of thiamine disulfide compounds in rat. Journal of Pharmaceutical Sciences 63(5), 676–681.

139. Constantinides, P.P. (1995). Lipid microemulsions for improving drug dissolution and oral absorption: physical and

biopharmaceutical aspects. Pharmaceutical Research 12(11), 1561–1572.

140. Wacher, V.J., Salphati, L. & Benet, L.Z. (2001). Active secretion and enterocytic drug metabolism barriers to drug absorption. Advanced Drug Delivery Reviews 46(1–3), 89–102.

141. Williams, G.C. & Sinko, P.J. (1999). Oral absorption of the HIV protease inhibitors: A current update. Advanced Drug Delivery Reviews 39(1–3), 211–238.

142. Gomez, D.Y., Wacher, V.J., Tomlanovich, S.J., Hebert, M.F. & Benet, L.Z. (1995). The effects of ketoconazole on the intestinal metabolism and bioavailability of cyclosporine. Clinical Pharmacology and Therapeutics 58(1), 15–19.

143. Hebert, M.F., Roberts, J.P., Prueksaritanont, T. & Benet, L.Z. (1992). Bioavailability of cyclosporine with concomitant rifampin administration is markedly less than predicted by hepatic enzyme reduction. Clinical Pharmacology and Therapeutics 52(5), 453–457.

144. Barnwell, S.G., Laudanski, T., Story, M.J., Mallinson, C.B., Harris, R.J., Cole, S.K., Keating, M. & Attwood, D. (1992). Improved oral bioavailability of propanolol in healthy human volunteers using a liver bypass drug delivery system containing oleic acid. International Journal of Pharmaceutics 88(1–3), 423–432.

145. Kupferschmidt, H.H.T., Ha, H.R., Ziegler, W.H., Meier, P.J. & Krahenbuehl, S. (1995). Interaction between grapefruit juice and midaolam in humans. Clinical Pharmacology and Therapeutics 58, 20–28.

146. Charman, W.N. & Porter, C.J.H. (1996). Lipophilic prodrugs designed for intestinal lymphatic transport. Advanced Drug Delivery Reviews 19(2), 149–169.

147. Aungst, B.J. (1999). P-glycoprotein, secretory transport, and other barriers to the oral delivery of anti-HIV drugs. Advanced Drug Delivery Reviews 39(1–3), 105–116.

148. Wu, C.Y. & Benet, L.Z. (2005). Predicting drug disposition via application of BCS: Transport/absorption/elimination interplay and development of a biopharmaceutics drug disposition classification system. Pharmaceutical Research 22(1), 11–23.

149. Nerurkar, M.M., Burton, P.S. & Borchardt, R.T. (1996). The use of surfactants to enhance the permeability of peptides through Caco-2 cells by inhibition of an apically polarized efflux system. Pharmaceutical Research 13(4), 528–534.

150. Jain, R., Agarwal, S., Majumdar, S., Zhu, X., Pal, D. & Mitra, A.K. (2005). Evasion of P-gp mediated cellular efflux and permeability enhancement of HIV-protease inhibitor saquinavir by prodrug modification. International Journal of Pharmaceutics 303(1–2), 8–19.

151. Malingré, M.M., Richel, D.J., Beijnen, J.H., Rosing, H., Koopman, F.J., Huinink, W.W.T.B., Schot, M.E. & Schellens, J.H.M. (2001). Coadministration of cyclosporine strongly enhances the oral bioavailability of docetaxel. Journal of Clinical Oncology 19(4), 1160–1166.

152. Balakrishnan, A., Sussman, D.J. & Polli, J. (2005). Development of stably transfected monolayer overexpressing the human apical sodium-dependent bile acid transporter (hASBT). Pharmaceutical Research 22(8), 1269–1280.

153. Tolle-Sander, S., Lentz, K.A., Maeda, D.Y., Coop, A. & Polli, J.E. (2004). Increased acyclovir oral bioavailability via a bile acid conjugate. Molecular Pharmaceutics 1(1), 40–48.

154. Balakrishnan, A. & Polli, J. (2006). Apical sodium dependent bile acid transporter (ASBT, SLC 10A2): A potential prodrug target. Molecular Pharmaceutics 3(3), 223–230.

155. Wu, W., Luo, Y., Sun, C., Liu, Y., Kuo, P., Varga, J., Xiang, R., Reisfeld, R., Janda, K.D., Edgington, T.S. & Liu, C. (2006). Targeting cell-impermeable prodrug activation to tumor microenvironment eradicates multiple drug-resistant neoplasm. Cancer Research 66(2), 970–980.

Improving the Oral Absorption of Poorly Soluble Drugs Using SEDDS and S-SEDDS Formulations

Walt Morozowich and Ping Gao

19.1 INTRODUCTION

SEDDS and S-SEDDS are self-emulsifying formulations of poorly soluble drugs that contain both a surfactant and lipid, along with a co-solvent, and they are usually formulated in gelatin capsules. Dilution of SEDDS or S-SEDDS formulations with water results in the generation of a microemulsion with a particle size from <150 nm to as low as 10–20 nm, when properly optimized. SEDDS/S-SEDDS formulations are useful in improving the animal or human oral bioavailability of poorly soluble drugs. S-SEDDS formulations contain less surfactant (and lipid) than the related SEDDS formulations and they create a supersaturated state upon contact with water, when properly optimized. The supersaturated state is maintained for a minimum of ~1–2 hrs and, as a result, S-SEDDS formulations can provide more rapid drug absorption, as evidenced by high C_{max} and shortened T_{max} values, as discussed in the case studies in this chapter, and they have potential for reducing surfactant-induced GI side-effects.

Four poorly soluble drugs are now marketed in lipid–surfactant formulations that are self-emulsifying or SEDDS formulations, with improved oral absorption, and these are: Sandimmune® (cyclosporine),

Neoral® (cyclosporine), Norvir® (ritonavir), Fortavase® (saquinavir), and Aptivus® (tipranavir). The design, development strategy, and improved oral absorption achieved with SEDDS/S-SEDDS formulations of other poorly soluble drugs are described in detail in the case studies, which include paclitaxel and two experimental drugs.

The proposed pathways for the intestinal absorption of poorly soluble drugs via SEDDS/S-SEDDS formulations involves presentation of the drug–microemulsion to the intestinal glycocalyx, with uptake by either the aqueous pathway or equilibrating with or mimicking, the intestinal BA/BAMM (bile acid/bile acid mixed micelle) system.

19.2 OVERVIEW OF SEDDS AND S-SEDDS FORMULATIONS

A SEDDS formulation is defined as a Self-Emulsifying Drug Delivery System that contains a surfactant and usually, but not always, an oil, and a drug. By optimization with various additives, a SEDDS formulation results. Upon contact with water, the SEDDS formulation spontaneously generates an oil-in-water drug microemulsion with a particle size $<\sim$150 nm and, preferably, as low as 10–20 nm. By this definition the term SEDDS includes all other self-emulsify formulations that contain a surfactant and a lipid, such as SNEDDS or SMEDDS. The term, SEDDS, based on the above definition includes "self-emulsifying formulations" or "self-emulsifying," abbreviated as SEF or SE, respectively, and this would also include all self-emulsifying formulations reported in the literature, including various particle sizes (micro-, nano-). This proposal would eliminate the proliferation of alternate labels for "self-emulsifying formulations," and it would centralize the literature.

S-SEDDS (supersaturatable) formulations of poorly soluble drugs (PSDs) are simply SEDDS formulations with a reduced amount of surfactant, with an addition of a crystal growth inhibitor, such as HPMC, other cellulosic polymers or other polymers. S-SEDDS formulations generate a supersaturated drug state upon dispersion with water within the GI tract. The resulting oral bioavailability of a poorly soluble drug in an S-SEDDS formulation can be increased, if formulated properly, and the T_{max} can be shorter than that of the poorly soluble drug in a conventional SEDDS formulation that contains a higher amount of surfactant. In addition to the ability to improve absorption of PSDs, the S-SEDDS formulation with reduced surfactant levels has the potential to reduce the incidence of surfactant induced diarrhea and colitis that can occur with the surfactant-laden SEDDS formulation.

The most common excipients used in a SEDDS/ S-SEDDS formulation are:

1. solvents such as ethanol, propylene glycol, and polyethylene glycol 400 (PEG 400);
2. surfactants such as polysorbate 80, polyoxyl 35 castor oil (Cremophor EL), and polyoxyl hydrogenated 40 castor oil (Cremophor RH40); and
3. lipids such as mono-/di-/tri-olein, Masine, safflower oil, corn oil, MCT, and LCT.

SEDDS/S-SEDDS formulations are usually liquids that can be formulated or encased within a soft gelatin capsule or alternatively, encased in a hard gelatin or an HPMC capsule. Alternate solid SEDDS/S-SEDDS formulations are possible. SEDDS and S-SEDDS formulations can improve the oral bioavailability of poorly soluble drugs (PSDs) by improving the presentation of the drug in the microemulsion to the intestinal mucosal surface glycocalyx, by a process of either simulating the behavior of or equilibrating with the intestinal bile acid mixed micellar (BAMM) system or the bile acid (*BA*) micellar system in the fed and fasted states, respectively, within the intestine.

The objectives of this chapter are:

1. to review scientific literature on the topic of SEDDS and S-SEDDS formulations published from 1998 to 2008, with a few other relevant publications;
2. to provide a detailed summary of the development of the SEDDS and S-SEDDS formulations of poorly soluble drugs, along with the oral bioavailability of the SEDDS/S-SEDDS formulations by us; and
3. to review the underlying mechanism responsible for the improved absorption of poorly soluble lipophilic drugs via SEDDS and S-SEDDS formulations.

19.2.1 Growth in the Number of SEDDS/ S-SEDDS Publications

The first publication containing the words "SEDDS" or "S-SEDDS" was reported in 1992, and by 2007 there were a total of 34 publications with the words SEDDS or S-SEDDS in the title or abstract. Figure 19.1 shows that the cumulative number of SEDDS/S-SEDDS publications dealing with poorly soluble drugs is increasing exponentially.

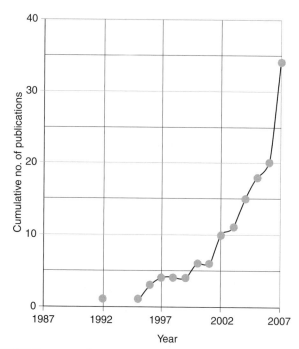

FIGURE 19.1   Growth in cumulative number of annual SEDDS + S-SEDDS publications in PubMed

19.2.2 Marketed SEDDS Formulations

The SEDDS formulation approach has proven the potential of improving the oral absorption of poorly soluble drugs, and it is a new and rapidly expanding area. Four poorly soluble drugs have been marketed in SEDDS formulations, and these are shown below along with their solubility and lipophilicity values, obtained from either the SciFinder (Am. Chem. Soc.), the Drug Bank (NIH) databases or the RxMed database at: http://www.rxmed.com/b.main/b2.pharmaceutical/ b2.1.monographs/CPS-%20Monographs/CPS-%20 (General%20Monographs-%20S)/SANDIMMUNE%20 (CYCLOSPORINE).html

Sandimmune® (Cyclosporine)

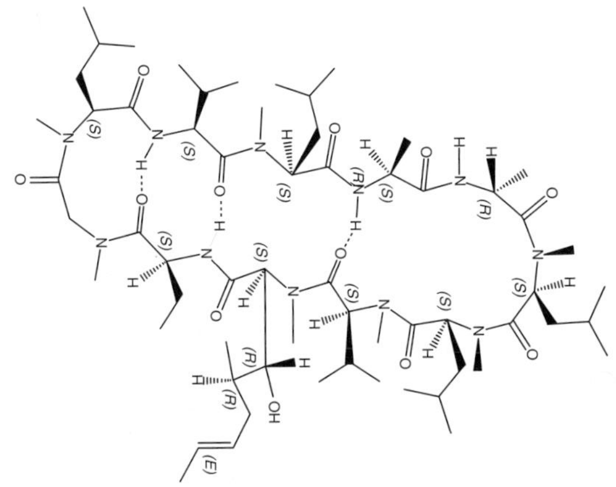

Cyclosporine
Immunosuppressant for organ transplantation:
$MW = 1202.61$
$\log P = 2.92$ Exp.
pKa = non-ionizable
calcS = $9\,\mu g/mL\ H_2O$
Dose = 25–700 mg (2–10 mg/kg).
Marketed Sandimmune formulation and ingredients:
Softgel: 25–100 mg cyclosporine in EtOH, corn oil, Labrafil M 2125 CS, gelatin, glycerol.
Oral Solution: 100 mg/mL in 12.5% EtOH, olive oil, Labrafil M 1944.

Neoral® (Cyclosporine)

Same drug as described above.
Marketed formulation and ingredients:
Softgel: 100 mg cyclosporine/unit. Alcohol (USP dehydrated, 9.5% wt/vol), propylene glycol, corn oil-mono-di-triglycerides, polyoxyl 40 hydrogenated castor oil, DL-α-tocopherol.
Solution: 100 mg/ml. Same ingredients as listed above.

Norvir® (Ritonavir)

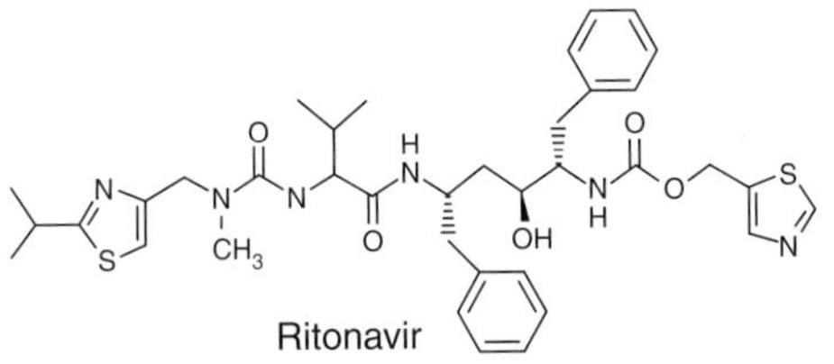

Ritonavir

AIDS drug:
$MW = 720.9$
clog $P = 5.28$
pKa = 3.48 (basic)
calcS = $0.37\,\mu g/mL$ at pH 6, 25°C
Dose = 1200 mg (600 mg BID)
Marketed formulation and ingredients:
Softgel: 100 mg ritonavir, ethanol, oleic acid, polyoxyl 35 castor oil, butylated hydroxytoluene.
Oral Solution: 80 mg/ml drug in ethanol (43% w/v), polyoxyl 35 castor oil, propylene glycol, citric acid.

Fortavase® (Saquinavir)

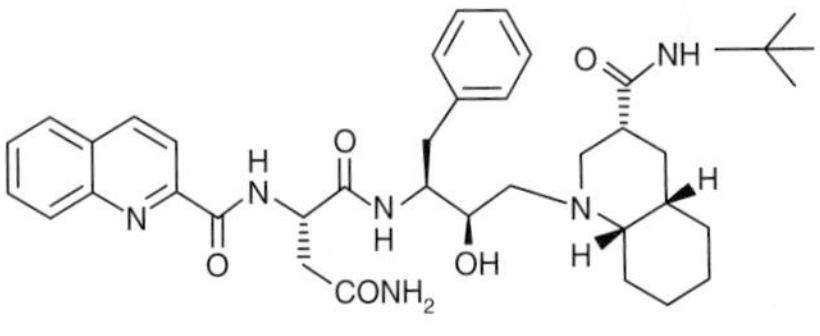

Saquinavir

AIDS drug:
$MW = 670.84$
clog $P = 4.40$
pKa = 7.6
calcS = $5\,\mu g/mL$ at pH 7, 25°C
Dose = 1200 mg
Marketed formulation and ingredients:
Softgel: 200 mg drug in medium chain mono- and di-glycerides, and povidone.

Aptivus® (Tipranavir)

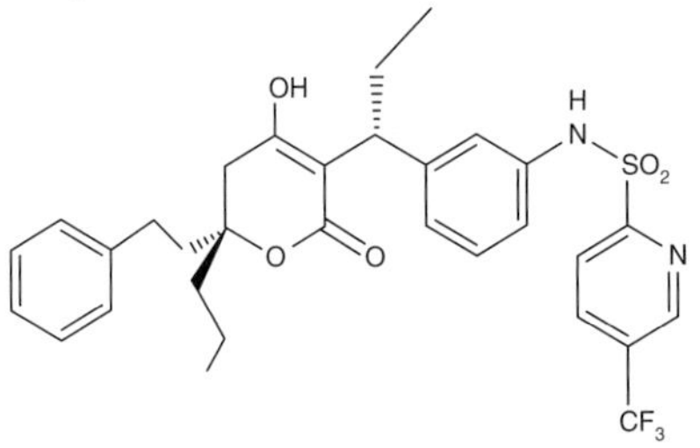

AIDS drug:
$MW = 602.66$
clog $P = 7.2$
pKa = 6.7, 10.2

calcS = 5 μg/mL at pH 6, 25°C

Dose = 1000 mg (with 400 mg Ritonavir) (500 mg BID)

Marketed formulation and ingredients:

Softgel: 250 mg tipranavir. Major inactive ingredients in formulation are 7% dehydrated alcohol, polyoxyl 35 castor oil, propylene glycol, mono-/di-glycerides of caprylic/capric acid.

19.3 REVIEW OF SCIENTIFIC LITERATURE DEALING WITH BOTH THE DEVELOPMENT OF SEDDS/S-SEDDS FORMULATIONS, AND ORAL BIOAVAILABILITY

This section reviews the scientific literature on SEDDS/S-SEDDS formulations over the past ten years from 1998 to 2008, and summarizes the key publications dealing with both:

1. the development and characterization of SEDDS/S-SEDDS formulations; and
2. the determination of the oral bioavailability of the resulting SEDDS/S-SEDDS formulations of poorly soluble drugs in preclinical and clinical studies.

The first citation in PubMed occurred in 1992, and by the end of 2007 the cumulative number of citations was 34 for the search terms "SEDDS" or "S-SEDDS." Most of these citations were also found in a PubMed search for "self-emulsifying formulations," where the total number of citations was 101. However, these search results included many publications that did not deal with both the development of SEDDS/S–SEDDS formulations and oral bioavailability. The 34 citations in the PubMed search for "SEDDS or S-SEDDS" are briefly reviewed chronologically in the following text.

19.3.1 Year 2008: Key Publications on SEDDS Formulations in the PubMed Database, and Related Articles

Using danazol as a model compound, SEDDS formulations were prepared with Cremophor RH40 or Cremophor EL, and a long chain triglyceride. It was concluded that the key design parameters for efficient oral absorption of danazol from lipid based formulations were: (a) rapid dispersibility of the formulation upon dilution with water; and (b) rapid intestinal digestion or hydrolysis of the triglyceride excipients by pancreatic enzymes.[1]

Self-emulsifying delivery systems are useful for improving the absorption of poorly soluble lipophilic drugs. The mechanism for drug absorption was reviewed, and the *in vitro* test methods found useful in formulation design are formulation dispersibility and digestibility of the surfactant and lipid excipients.[2]

SEDDS formulations of alpha-tocopherol containing polysorbate 80, labrasol, EtOH, and Captex 355 were subjected to lipase-catalyzed hydrolysis in biorelevant media to determine the effect of the excipients on the rate and extent of hydrolysis. The authors found that:

> "the excipients influenced each response differently and, therefore, each method can only reveal distinctive characteristics of the SEDDS formulation, and may not be used interchangeably".[3]

Two SEDDS formulations of probucol with the same composition, but with a 100-fold difference in particle size, gave comparable oral bioavailability in fed or fasted minipigs.[4]

19.3.2 Year 2007: Key Publications on SEDDS Formulations in the PubMed Database, and Related Articles

Table 19.1 shows the key surfactant–lipid formulations reported in the literature with poorly soluble drugs.[5] The table shows that many of the drug–lipid formulations, such as the SEDDS formulations, enhance the absorption of a variety of poorly water soluble drugs.

The literature on SEDDS formulations of poorly soluble drugs and oral bioavailability was surveyed, and it was concluded that improved oral bioavailability is best achieved with the aid of screens for dispersibility, lipolysis of triglycerides, and digestion of surfactants.[5]

In a comprehensive review of lipid formulations containing surfactants, such as SEDDS/S-SEDDS, it was stated that the key role of these formulations was to enhance the solubility of the drug in the formulation and in the GI tract.[5a] Figure 19.2 shows that dispersion of a lipid–surfactant SEDDS formulation occurs in the stomach, and this dispersion can equilibrate with the bile salt/phospholipid micelle. Lipid and surfactant hydrolysis products are formed in the intestine by lipolytic pancreatic enzymes.

A decision support tool was developed for orally active poorly soluble compounds, based on the proposed formulation selection process,[6] as shown in Figure 19.3.

TABLE 19.1 Survey of SEDDS formulations and their reported bioavailabilities.[5] Examples of studies describing the bioavailability enhancement of PWSD after administration of SEDDS and SMEDDS formulations

Compound	Formulation(s)	Study design	Observations
Win 54954	SEDDS (35% drug, 40% Neobee M5 (MCT), and 25% Tagat (TO) or PEG 600 solution	Relative BA in dogs	No difference in BA but improved reproducibility, increased C_{max}
Cyclosporin	Sandimmum (SEDDS: corn oil and ethanol) or Neoral (SMEDDS: corn oil glycerides, Cremophor RH40, PG, DL-α-tocopherol and ethanol)	Relative BA in humans	Increased BA and C_{max} and reduced T_{max} from SMEDDS
	Sandimmum (SEDDS) or Neoral (SMEDDS)	Relative BA in humans	Increased C_{max}, AUC and dose linearity and reduced food effect from SMEDDS
	Sandimmum (SEDDS) or Neoral (SMEDDS)	Relative BA in humans	Reduced intra- and inter-subject variability SMEDDS
Halofantrine	5% drug in MCT SEDDS (47% Captex 355, 23% Capmul MCM, 15% Cremophor EL and ethanol), MCT SMEDDS (33% Captex 355, 17% Capmul MCM, 33% Cremophor EL, and ethanol), or LCT SMEDDS (29% Soybean oil, 29% Maisine 35-1, 30% Cremophor EL, and 7% ethanol)	Relative BA in dogs	Trend to higher BA from LCT SMEDDS
Ontazolast	Soybean oil emulsion, drug solution in Peceol, drug suspension or two semi-solid SEDDS comprising Gelucrie 44/14 and Peceol in the ratios 50:50, and 80:20	Absolute BA in rats	BA increases of at least 10-fold from all lipid-based formulations
Vitamin E	SEDDS (Tween 80:Span 80:palm oil (LCT) in a 4:2:4 ratio) or soybean oil (LCT) in solution	Relative BA in humans	BA 3-fold higher from SEDDS
Coenzyme Q_{10}	SMEDDS (40% Myvacet 9–45, 50% Labrasol, and 10% luaroglycol) or powder formulation	Relative BA in dogs	BA 2-fold higher from SEDDS
Ro-15-0778	SEDDS (polyglycolyzed glycerides and peanut oil), PEG 400 solution, wet-milled spray dried powder or tablet of micronized drug	Relative BA in dogs	BA 3-fold higher from SEDDS when compared with other formulations
Simvastatin	SMEDDS (37% Capryol 90, 28% Cremophor EL, 28% Carbitol) or tablet	Relative BA in dogs	BA 1.5-fold higher from SMEDDS
Biphenyl dimethyl dicarboxylate	SEDDS (43% Tween 80, 35% triacetin, and 22% Neobee M-5 (MCT)) or powder formulation	Relative BA in rats	BA 5-fold higher from SEDDS
Indomethacin	SEDDS (70% ethyl oleolate and 30% Tween 85) or powder formulation	Relative BA in rats	BA significantly increased from SEDDS
Progesterone	SEDDS (mono-di-glycerides:polysorbate 80, 50/50 w/w) or aqueous suspension	Relative BA in dogs	BA 9-fold higher from SEDDS
Tocotrienols	Two SEDDS (Tween 80 and labrasol) or LCT solution	Relative BA in humans	BA 2- to 3-fold higher from SEDDS
Danazol	LC-SMEDDS (long chain lipids, Cremophor EL, and ethanol), MC-SMEDDS (medium chain lipids, Cremophor EL, and ethanol) or LCT solution	Relative BA in dogs	BA from LCT solution and LC-SMEDDS 7-fold and 6-fold higher than that from MC-SEDDS
Carvedilol	SEDDS (labrafil M1944CS, Tween 80 and transcutol), and tablet	Relative BA in dogs	BA 4-fold higher from SEDDS
Solvent green 3	Semi-solid SMEDDS (Gelucrine 44/14) or soybean oil emulsion	Relative BA in rats	BA 1.7-fold higher from SMEDDS
Silymarin	SMEDDS (Tween 80, ethyl alcohol, and ethyl linoleate), PEG 400 solution	Relative BA in rabbits	BA approximately 2- and 50-fold higher from SMEDDS than that of PEG 400 solution and suspension

(Continued)

TABLE 19.1   (Continued)

Compound	Formulation(s)	Study design	Observations
Atorvastatin	Three SMEDDS (Cremophor RH40, propylene glycol, and labrafil, estol or labrafac) or tablet	Relative BA in dogs	BA significantly increased from all SMEDDS formulations
Itroconazole	SEDDS (Transcutol, pluronic L64, and tocopherol acetate) or conventional capsule	Relative BA in rats	Increased BA and reduced food effect from SEDDS
Atovaquone	Two SMEDDS (long chain lipids, ethanol, and Cremophor EL or Pluronic L121) or aqueous suspension	Relative BA in dogs	BA 3-fold higher from SMEDDS
Seocalcitol	LC-SMEDDS (sesame oil, Peecol, Cremophor RH40) versus MC-SMEDDS (Viscoleo MCT), Alkoline MCM (medium chain mono- and di-glyceride) and Cremophor RH40	Absolute BA in rats	BA LC-SMEDDS = MC-SMEDDS
PNU-91325	Supersaturable co-solvent (S-co-solvent) and supersaturable SEDDS (S-SEDDS comprising 20% HMPC, 30% Cremophor EL, 18% Pluronic L44, 9% PEG, 6% long chain glyceride lipid, 5% DMA) formulations compared to co-solvent (PG) or Tween 80 solutions	Relative BA in rats	5–6-fold enhancement in oral bioavailability for S-co-solvent, S-SEDDS, and Tween 80 formulations relative to co-solvent
Itraconazole	SEDDS formulation comprising Transcutol, Pluronic L64, and tocopherol acetate versus commercial Sporanox formulation	Relative BA in rats	Increased BA and reduced food effect from SEDDS
7 model compounds including disopyramide, ibuprofen, ketoprofen, and tolbutamide	Comparison of PEG 200 solution and suspension formulations to SEDDS (comprising 25% MCT, 5% diglycerylmonooleate, 45% Cremophor RH40, 25% Ethanol), and liquid microemulsion (comprising 5% MCT, 1% diglycerylmonooleate, 9% Cremophor RH40, 5% Ethanol, and 80% phosphate buffered saline)	Relative BA in rats and dogs	Improved BA relative to the suspension formulations for either or both of the liquid microemulsion and SEDDS formulation in all cases

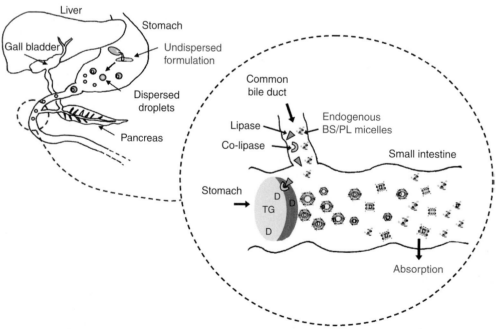

FIGURE 19.2   Cartoon depicting the major physiological and biochemical events occurring with a lipid–surfactant–drug formulation such as a gelatin softgel formulation of a poorly water soluble drug. The lipolytic enzymes (pancreatic lipase) stored in the gall bladder enter the duodenum and they hydrolyze the long chain triglycerides (LCT) to give 2-mono-acyl glycerides. The resulting BA and BAMM particles can equilibrate with the drug–SEDDS microemulsion followed by intestinal absorption of the drug.[5]

Formulation Selection Process

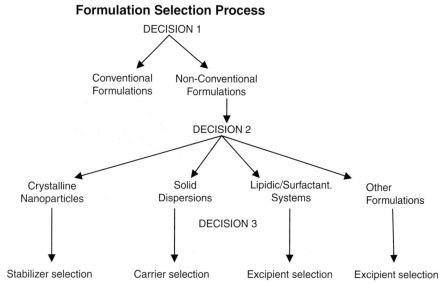

FIGURE 19.3   Decision tree for guiding formulation decisions (Branchu, 2007)

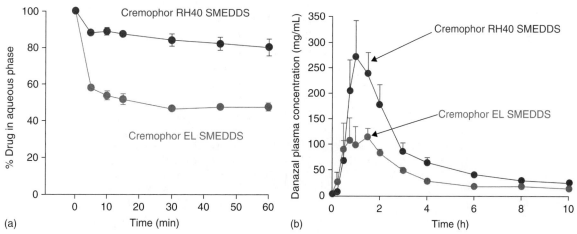

FIGURE 19.4   The effect of lipolytic digestion of the Cremophor RH40 and Cremophor EL formulations of danazol. Left: (a)—the aqueous phase levels of the danazol formulations and right: (b)—the danazol plasma levels of these formulations in the dog. Formulation 1: The Cremophor RH 40 SMEDDS contains 55% w/w Cremophor RH, 37.5% w/w soybean oil/Maisine, 7.5% w/w ethanol. Formulation 2: The Cremophor EL SMEDDS contains 55% w/w Cremophor EL, 37.5% w/w soybean oil/Maisine, 7.5% w/w ethanol. The lower digestibility of Cremophor RH40 results in higher bioavailability.[5]

Figure 19.3 shows the three major decision points in formulation development. The authors concluded that the decision support tool has great potential for improving the efficiency and the predictability of the formulation development process. Figure 19.4 shows that the reported increase in the aqueous solubility of danazol (a) in Cremophor RH40, however, does not result in enhanced oral bioavailability of danazol (b).[5]

In a previous study, increasing the surfactant-to-lipid ratio was found to reduce the oral bioavailability of danazol in dogs.[8] The increase in drug solubilization observed during *in vitro* digestion resulted in increased oral bioavailability of danazol. Interestingly, the oral bioavailability (in beagle dogs) was highest with a soybean–Maisine–Cremophor EL microemulsion generating formulation, and the lowest with a formulation containing Cremophor without soybean–Masine.

A study of the effect of small amounts of lipids on gastric empting and biliary secretion showed that oral administration of as little as 2 gm of glycerol- monooleate (GMO) (in healthy males) resulted in stimulation of biliary secretion of bile and bile acids. The same amount of medium-chain triglyceride (MCT) (Miglyol 810) failed to cause contraction of the gall bladder, and did not result in secretion of bile. The authors pointed out that the amount of lipid, namely, 2 gm of GMO/MCT, is a quantity that "might be realistically expected on administration of 2×1 g soft gelatin capsules." Furthermore, this suggests that administration of 2×1 g of GMO in soft gelatin capsules containing a drug in a clinical study in the fasted state could result in drug absorption that mimics the fed state.[9] The development of lipid-based formulations was reviewed[10] with respect to:

1. major excipient classes (natural product oils, semi-synthetic lipid excipients, fully synthetic excipients, and surfactants);
2. formulation types and modalities (single component lipid solutions, self-emulsifying formulations, and melt pelletization);
3. formulation development and characterization, including drug candidate selection, excipient compatibility, selection of a formulation modality, physico-chemical consideration, biopharmaceutical consideration, *in vitro* characterization, *in vitro* dissolution testing, and role of lipolysis in release testing.

The authors[10] admits that "due to the complex and incompletely understood dynamics of the interaction of formulations with the gastrointestinal milieu," animal bioavailability studies should precede clinical studies. The key advantages of lipid-based formulations are:

1. reduced variability;
2. reduction in the number of formulation-based processing steps;
3. reduction in positive food effect; and
4. the ease of formulation manufacture and scale-up.

The use of lipid-based formulations for enhancing drug absorption was reviewed with respect to the mechanisms responsible for improved oral absorption.[5] The concentration of bile salts in the fasted state in the duodenum/jejunum is ~3–4 mM, while in the fed state the bile salt concentration is ~10–16 mM. This increased concentration of bile salts in the fed state is responsible for increased drug solubilization. With poorly soluble drugs, improved oral bioavailability is often observed in the fed state. The solubilizing property in the fed state is due to the presence of the bile acid mixed micelle (BAMM). The review of the lipid

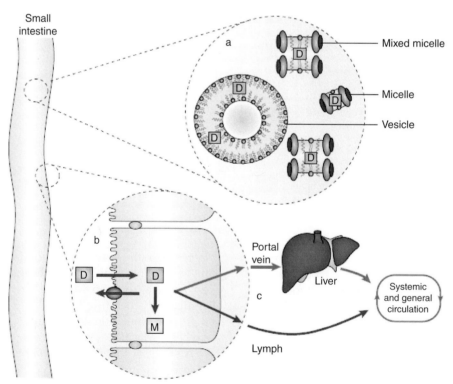

FIGURE 19.5   Cartoon showing that lipid-based drug formulations can improve drug absorption by drug solubilization in the resulting micellar phases, principally the bile acid mixed micelle that arises from bile. Highly lipophilic drugs can undergo lymphatic uptake, thereby, bypassing first pass liver metabolism.[5]

absorption pathway.[5] indicated that highly lipophilic drugs can show significant lymphatics.

The use of surfactants as enterocyte P-gp pump inhibitors (Table 19.2) was reviewed, and improved oral absorption was documented with a number of drugs using this strategy.[11]

The reservation with the use of P-gp inhibitors is that intestinal absorption of undesirable compounds could occur, along with improved absorption of the drug in question.[11] In addition, P-gp inhibitors have pharmacological activity of their own and, therefore, P-gp–drug combinations could result in enhanced side-effects.

The effect of administering a high fat meal (peanut oil) or plain water on the plasma levels of DDT in rats was studied.[12] The resulting plasma profiles for DDT (oral) were much higher after oral administration of peanut oil, compared with oral administration of plain water. The resulting plasma levels of diazepam (oral) were virtually the same after oral administration of peanut oil or water. These data indicate that diazepam is probably not absorbed by the intestinal lymphatics after oral administration, but DDT is, and this is in accord with the literature.[12]

The utility of microemulsion-generating formulations in enhancing the oral absorption of poorly soluble drugs was reviewed. The key considerations in the development of SEDDS formulations capable of generating a microemulsion upon contact with water are: (1) surfactant; (2) co-surfactant; and (3) oils. Using nitrendipine formulations consisting of: (a) medium-chain triglycerides; (b) triglyceride suspension (c) long-chain triglyceride solution, and (d) Tween 80, it was shown that the resulting T_{max} values in a fasted human clinical study were 8, 4, 1.3, and ≥8 hours, respectively. The T_{max} values in the fed state in the same clinical study resulted in T_{max} values of 1.5, 3.5, 1.3, and ≥7hrs.[13] These data are significant, in that the T_{max} of nitrendipine was reduced to 1.5 hours in the fed state, compared to 8 hours in the fasted state.

A nanoemulsion-generating formulation of paclitaxel was developed using 1920 mg of Labrasol plus vitamin E-TPGS (3:1), 80 mg of Labrafil M1944CS, and 20 mg of paclitaxel.[14] Dilution of the formulation with water resulted in formation of a nanoemulsion with a particle (globule) size of 21.58 nm, which is in the range of many microemulsion-generating formulations. The rat oral bioavailability (absolute) of paclitaxel from this nanoemulsion formulation was reported to be 70.25%. The absolute rat oral bioavailability of paclitaxel from the Taxol® IV formulation was only 10.62% and <30% for a S-SEDDS formulation of paclitaxel.

The effect of the fasted (FaSSIF) and fed (FeSSIF-Mod6.5) state (Table 19.3) on the absorption (in dogs) of danazol from a self-emulsifying formulation was found to be in excellent agreement with the higher solubility of danazol in the FeSSIF, as compared to the FaSSIF.[15]

The oral bioavailability of itraconazole in a SEDDS formulation containing transcutol, pluronic, and tocopherol acetate was found to give an AUC (oral) similar to that of the marketed Sporanox® product, however, the T_{max} was 1.3 hours for the SEDDS formulation, and 8 hours for the Sporanox® product.[16]

The oral bioavailability of the naphthalene analog, Ro 15-9778, either in a SEDDS formulation, a PEG 400

TABLE 19.3 Composition of simulated intestinal fluids[17]

	pH	Tauro-cholate	Lecithin	mOsm
Simulated intestinal fluid				
FaSSIF[a]	6.5	3 mM	0.75 mM	270 + 10
FeSSIF[b]	5.0	15 mM	3.75 mM	635 + 10
Simulated intestinal fluid				
FaSSIF-Mod[c]	6.5	3 mM	0.75	311.7 + 0.6
FeSSIF-Mod5.0[d]	5.0	15 mM	3.75 mM	327.0 + 1.0
FeSSIF-Mod6.5[e]	6.5	15 mM	3.75 mM	325.7 + 0.6

[a]FaSSIF: 3.9 gm KH_2PO_4, 3 mM Na TC, 0.75 gm lecithin, 7.7 gm KCl, pH adj. with NaOH to 6.50

[b]FeSSIF: 8.65 gm acetic acid, 15 mM NaTC, 3.75 mM lecithin, 15.2 gm KCl, pH adj. with NaOH to 5.00

[c]FaSSIF-Mod: 3.9 gm KH_2PO_4, 3 mM Na TC, 0.75 gm lecithin, 7.7 gm KCl, pH adj. with HEPES to 6.50

[d]FaSSIF-Mod5.0: 3.9 gm KH_2PO_4, 3 mM Na TC, 0.75 gm lecithin, 7.7 gm KCl, pH adj. with HEPES to 5.00

[e]FaSSIF-Mod6.5: 3.9 gm KH_2PO_4, 3 mM Na TC, 0.75 gm lecithin, 7.7 gm KCl, pH adj. with HEPES to 6.50

TABLE 19.2 Surfactants with P-gp inhibitor activity[11]

Surfactants

C8/C10 Glycerol and PEG Esters, Cremophor, Solutol HS-15, Labrasol, Softigen 767, Aconnon E

Sucrose Esters, Sucrose Monolaurate

Polysorbates, Tween 80, Tween 20

Tocopherol Esters, α-Tocopheryl PEG 100 Succinate (TPGS)

solution, a spray dried powder or a tablet formulation, showed a relative oral bioavailability (in dog) of 389, 100, 35, and 17%, respectively. The self-dispersing SEDDS formulation gave superior oral bioavailability, as compared to the alternate conventional formulations.[18]

In a review of the oral absorption of drugs in SEDDS formulations, it was noted that bioavailability was dependent on the surfactant concentration, and the polarity of the resulting emulsion/microemulsion formed on dilution with water, the droplet size, and the charge.

The rat oral bioavailability of the highly-lipophilic compound seocalcitol was roughly the same in SEDDS formulations and in simple triglyceride solutions, indicating that highly lipophilic drugs may not require SEDDS formulation for maximizing oral bioavailability.[19]

19.3.3 Year 2005–2003: Key Publications on SEDDS Formulations in the PubMed Database, and Related Articles

The mechanism of intestinal uptake of drugs and drug formulations was addressed in a large number of papers by Charman, Porter and coworkers. These publications included the solubilization of poorly soluble drugs in the GI tract after administration of lipid-based drug delivery systems, wherein it was concluded that the digestion and dispersion of the lipidic vehicle provides a solubilization sink that can prevent precipitation of the poorly soluble drug.[20] A study on the factors that dictate lymphatic absorption of poorly soluble drugs showed that the "lymph-lipid pool" is a key determinant of intestinal lymphatic drug transport.[21,22] The physico-chemical properties of halofantrine, such as log D versus pH dependency, were found to explain the extensive lymphatic transport of halofantrine in the fed state. At a pH below 2, the $\log D$ of halofrine is <0, but as the pH is increased to ~7, the $\log D$ is increased to ~3 in aqueous Na taurocholate-lecithin (4:1). The high lipophilicity of halofrine at pH ~7 suggests high affinity for the lymphatic system.[23]

In a review of the lymphatic delivery of drugs, the exceptionally high log P values of itretinate (7.8), and isotretinoin (6.8), are responsible for the extensive lymphatic delivery.[24] The effect of the fatty acid binding protein (FABP) on the enterocyte uptake of fatty acids showed that the FABP can be a determinant of lymphatic drug transport.[22]

A microemulsion-generating formulation was prepared using MCT, DGMO-C, HCO-40, and EtOH, in the ratio of 5:1:9:5 (v/v), and this SEDDS formulation was found to improve the oral absorption of 10 drugs, including ibuprofen, ketoprofen, tamoxifen, testosterone, and tolbutamide, in addition to other new drugs.[25]

An emulsion generating formulation of cyclosporine was developed with an oat galactolipid and MCM (1:1).[26] Dilution of the formulation with water gave a particle size $\sim3\mu$m (an emulsion), whereas dilution of the Neoral formulation of cyclosporine gave a particle size of 10–20 nm (a microemulsion). A clinical study showed that the oral bioavailability of the galactolipid cyclosporine formulation, compared to the Neoral® formulation, was virtually the same, as evidenced by the T_{max} and AUC values. Both formulations showed a T_{max} of ~1.5 hours.

19.3.4 Year 2003–2000: Key Publications on SEDDS Formulations in the PubMed Database, and Related Articles

The Neoral® SEDDS formulation of cyclosporine was the first marketed microemulsion-generating formulation in the pharmaceutical industry. Dilution of the Neoral® formulation with water results in rapid formation of a transparent solution, typical of a microemulsion, with a bluish cast, and a particle size of ~20 nm. Figure 19.6 shows the oral bioavailability of the Sandimmune® emulsion-generating formulation, along with the improved Neoral microemulsion-generating formulation of cyclosporine in a renal transplant patient.[27,28] The Sandimmune® SEDDS formulation contains a long-chain triglyceride, with a surfactant and the lipophilic compound, cyclosporine. The absorption of cyclosporine from the Sandimmune® formulation occurs after partial hydrolysis of the long-chain triglyceride, and this can be a slow process, as shown by the evening dosing blood level curve (SIM p.m.), which shows a peak at 8 hours. The peak blood levels of cyclosporine after morning dosing (SIM a.m.) show a somewhat shorter peak at 4 hours. The Neoral® formulation, however, shows a peak in the blood level curve for cyclosporine at ~1.5 hours in the fasted state, and 1.2 hours in the fed state. The resulting AUC for the Neoral® formulation is larger than that of the Sandimmune® formulation, as shown in Figure 19.6. There is virtually no food effect (AUC = 997, fasting, and AUC = 892, fed) with the Neoral® formulation. The superiority of the new microemulsion-generating Neoral formulation of cyclosporine has been confirmed in expanded clinical studies.[29,30]

It was pointed out that the absorption of poorly soluble drugs can be enhanced in SEDDS formulations

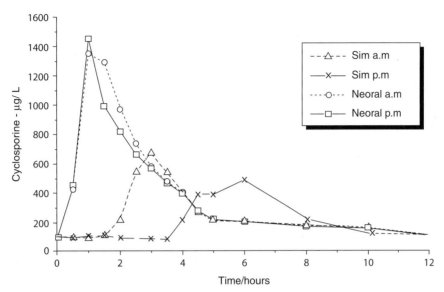

FIGURE 19.6 Representative cyclosporine blood concentration profiles from a renal transplant patient given the currently marketed formulation Sandimmune® (SIM) or the new Neoral® formulation without food (a.m.) or with food (p.m.).[27]

with formulation designed to give a submicron-sized colloidal state upon dilution with water.[2] Knowledge of the efficiency of self-emulsification on contact with water, the susceptibility to digestion of the surfactant excipients, as well as the lipid triglyceride excipients, and the subsequent fate of the drug is useful in optimization of the formulation.[2]

19.3.5 Year 1999–1992: Key Publications on SEDDS Formulations in the PubMed Database, and Related Articles

Studies on intestinal absorption of lipids and, especially, cholesterol, established the key role of the bile acid mixed micelle (BAMM) in the oral absorption of lipophilic compounds.[31–34,7]

There were four papers dealing with SEDDS/S-SEDDS formulations in 1997. The requirements for lymphatic transport were developed, and it was concluded that the log P of the drug should be high (>6), and the drug should be soluble in triglycerides, in order to achieve efficient lymphatic absorption.

The development of SEDDS formulations was reviewed in detail with respect to the factors that influenced ease of emulsification.[35] SEDDS formulations usually contain triglycerides, along with PEG surfactants, with surfactant concentrations greater than 15%.

The first paper found in the PubMed search on "SEDDS or S-SEDDS" was published in 1992, dealing with a SEDDS formulation of the poorly soluble drug, WIN 54954.[35] The particle size of the formulation on dilution with water was <3μm. The SEDDS formulation showed higher AUC in the dog than a PEG 400 solution.

19.4 CASE STUDIES ON THE DEVELOPMENT OF SEDDS AND S-SEDDS FORMULATIONS

The case studies dealing with the development of new SEDDS and S-SEDDS formulations of the poorly soluble drugs, paclitaxel and two experimental drugs, are described in detail in this section, along with emphasis on the key screening tests that were employed in optimizing the SEDDS/S-SEDDS formulations, and the resulting oral bioavailability data. The key *in vitro* screening tests that were applied are:

1. ease of dispersibility of the SEDDS/S-SEDDS formulation in an aqueous medium;
2. particle size upon dispersion; and
3. the free drug concentration in the aqueous medium upon dispersion.

The case studies discussed herein are taken from previous publications.[37–43]

19.4.1 Case Study on the Development of a SEDDS Formulation of Drug X

CASE STUDY

PHYSICO-CHEMICAL PROPERTIES OF DRUG X

The experimental drug is a free acid with two acidic pKas (~6, and ~9), it is highly lipophilic (clogP of ~7), it has a molecular weight of ~600, and it is a poorly soluble drug with an intrinsic aqueous solubility of only ~5μg/ml. A high daily dose of experimental drugs was desired for oral administration in AIDS patients and, as a result, SEDDS formulations with 300mg of the experimental drug per gm of the formulation were explored. The solubility of the experimental drug in various pharmaceutically acceptable excipients is shown in Table 19.4.

The solubility of the drug in surfactants Cremophor EL and Polysorbate 80 was found to be high (~500mg/mL), but the solubility in glycerolipids Capmul MCM and GDO/GMO (glycerol di-olein/glycerol mono-olein) was ~10–20 times lower, suggesting that development of a high dose of the Experimental Drug–SEDDS formulation might be a challenging task.

The SEDDS formulations of Drug X were evaluated and optimized with respect to the key variable, namely, *in vitro* dispersibility and spontaneity of emulsification, particle size upon dilution with water, and the nature of the lipid excipients.

Influence of Dispersibility on Absorption of Drug X–SEDDS Formulation

The effect of the dispersion property (e.g., particle size, dispersion spontaneity) of the 300mg/gm Drug

X–SEDDS formulation on oral bioavailability was evaluated in preclinical studies (rat, dog). These results collectively revealed that the particle size of the 300mg/gm Drug X–SEDDS formulation upon dilution with water is a key factor that dictates the oral absorption of Drug X with a smaller particle size, resulting in improved oral bioavailability.

The ability to generate a microemulsion with the 300mg/g Drug X–SEDDS formulation was explored by adding a small amount of an organic amine. As shown in Figure 19.7, the mean droplet size of the microemulsion/emulsion generated upon dilution of 300mg/gm Drug X formulation with water showed a rapid reduction in particle size as the percentage of diethanolamine (DEA) was increased from 0 to 3%.[37] The presence of a small amount of DEA (~1%) dramatically reduced the particle size of the 300mg/Gm Drug X-SEDDS formulation to about 150nm or less.

The relative oral bioavailability of Drug X in a 300mg/Gm SEDDS formulation with the same composition, but differing only with respect to the presence or absence of DEA, was evaluated orally in rats, dogs, and in humans. The *in vivo* pharmacokinetic results are shown in Figure 19.8.

The relative oral bioavailability of Drug X in rats (non-crossover), dogs (crossover), and humans (crossover) showed that the bioavailability was improved by ~2–3 fold

TABLE 19.4 Solubility of the experimental drug in various formulation excipients[37]

Excipient	Solubility of the experimental drug (mg/gm of excipient)
Ethanol	1950
Propylene glycol	710
PEG 400	670
Glycerol	<10
Polysorbate 80	500
Cremophor EL	430
Capmul MCM	20
GDO/GMO (8:2)	11
Soybean oil	<20
Miglyol 812	20

*Values are the means with the %CV in parenthesis

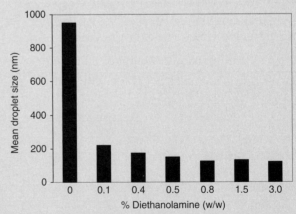

FIGURE 19.7 The mean particle size of the 300mg/gm Drug X SEDDS formulations upon dilution with SIF (dilution factor: 100X) vs. the % diethanolamine (DEA) (w/w) in the formulation. The addition of a small amount of DEA (0.1%) results in a dramatic reduction in particle size from ~950nm to ~200nm.[37]

by the simple addition of 1.5–5.0% of an amine (DEA or Tris) to the corresponding SEDDS formulation of Drug X.

Influence of Lipid Excipients on Absorption of Drug X

To evaluate the effect of the amount of lipid on the oral absorption of Drug X, three SEDDS formulations containing 300 mg/gm of Drug X were evaluated. Drug X–SEDDS formulations were identical in composition (see insert in Figure 19.9), with the exception of the amount of the glycerolipid (an 8:2 mixture of GDO:GMO), which ranged from 50 to 180 mg/gm of formulation.

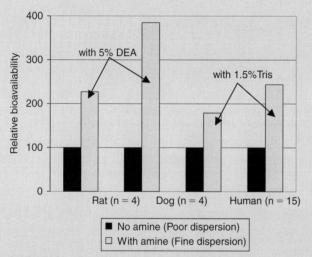

FIGURE 19.8 Plot of the relative oral bioavailability of the 300 mg/gm Drug X SEDDS formulations in the presence and absence of an amine (either DEA or Tris) in the rat, dog (crossover) and the human (crossover).[37]

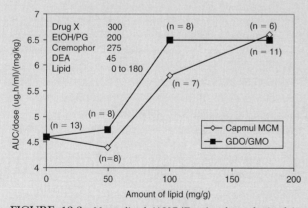

FIGURE 19.9 Normalized (AUC/Dose) values obtained in fasted rats with Drug X SEDDS formulations where the amount of lipid (either GDO/GMO (8:2)) mixture or Capmul MCM) is varied. The number of the rats is given in parenthesis.[37]

A similar SEDDS formulation without GDO/GMO was also administered as a control. In the presence of 45 mg/gm of DEA, the dispersibility of all SEDDS formulations with a wide range of glycerolipid content (0 to 180 mg/gm) was similar, and the dispersion was a microemulsion with a particle size of ~120–150 nm. This observation indicates that: (a) the dispersibility of the formulation is primarily dictated by the presence of an organic amine; and (b) the presence of a substantial amount of glycerolipid in the formulation does not alter the particle size upon dispersing the SEDDS formulation with water.

These formulations were dosed orally as a predispersed emulsion in fasted rats at a dose level of 20 mg/kg. The normalized AUC/dose values for Drug X in four SEDDS formulations containing 0 to 180 mg/g GDO/GMO are plotted in Figure 19.9. A positive dependency is seen for the amount of GDO/GMO in the formula. There is virtually no difference in the AUC/dose ratio when the GDO/GMO concentrations in the SEDDS formulation are low (about 0–50 mg/gm). Both GDO/GMO and Capmul MCM are mixtures of mono- and di-glycerides, but they differ in the chain length of the fatty acids. GDO and GMO consist mainly of oleic acid (C18) glyceride esters, whereas Capmul MCM consists of C8–C10 fatty acid mono- and di-glyceride esters. Three SEDDS formulations with variable amounts of a glycerolipid (Capmul MCM) were similarly evaluated in rats. Their AUC/dose obtained is plotted against the amount of Capmul MCM in the formulation in Figure 19.9, and a positive dependency is seen for the exposure on the amount of Capmul MCM. The AUC/dose values with Drug X–SEDDS formulations containing 180 mg/g of either GDO/GMO or Capmul MCM are essentially the same, indicating that the fatty acid chain length in the glycerolipids does not affect the oral bioavailability of Drug X–SEDDS formulations in rats.

The small difference in the AUC/dose ratio for Drug X between the SEDDS formulations containing 100 and 180 mg/g of either GDO/GMO or Capmul MCM (Figure 19.13) indicates that approximately 100 mg/gm of the mono-/di-glycerides is the minimum quantity required to enhance oral absorption. This implies that a minimum amount of the mono-/di-glyceride of ~100 mg/gm in Drug X–SEDDS formulation is required, in order to increase the oral bioavailability of Drug X.

Influence of Solvent Level on the Emulsification of SEDDS Formulations

The release profiles of Drug X–SEDDS formulations with various ethanol concentrations ranging from

CASE STUDY   (CONTINUED)

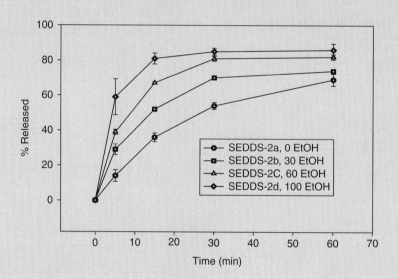

FIGURE 19.10   Effect of EtOH concentration (0–100 mg/g) on the drug release profile from Drug X SEDDS formulations containing 73 mg/g propylene glycol (PG).[37]

0 to 100 mg/gm, while keeping the PG level constant at 73 mg/gm, are shown in Figure 19.10. These *in vitro* drug release profiles indicate little change in the initial percentage of drug released as the PG concentration in the formulation is increased.

The difference in the amount of Drug X released from the SEDDS formulations with varying amounts of PG, from 0 to 75 mg/g (Figure 19.11), is small as compared to the SEDDS formulations with varying amounts of ethanol (0 to 100 mg/gm, Figure 19.10). Thus, the release profile of Drug X from the SEDDS formulations is indicative of the spontaneous emulsification, and it shows a higher sensitivity to the ethanol level than to the PG level.

Preliminary *In Vitro* and *In Vivo* Relationship (IVIVR) with SEDDS Formulations

Three prototype SEDDS formulations of Drug X were evaluated in clinical trial (n = 15, crossover, fasted) at a single dose of 1200 mg with the di-sodium salt of Drug X (filled in hard filled capsules) as a control. The

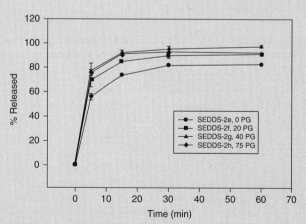

FIGURE 19.11   Effect of propylene glycol (PG) concentration (0–75 mg/g) on the drug release profile from Drug X SEDDS formulation containing 100 mg/g EtOH.[37] The initial slope and the shape of the drug release profiles indicate that an increase in the ethanol concentration in the formulation improves the emulsification spontaneity and the subsequent extent of release. Similarly, the release profiles of Drug X SEDDS formulations with various propylene glycol (PG) concentrations from 0 to 75 mg/gm and a constant EtOH level of 100 mg/gm are shown in Figure 19.10

CASE STUDY   (CONTINUED)

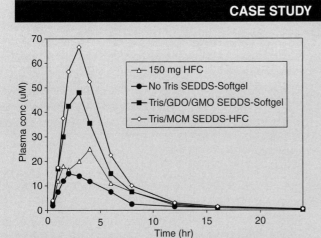

FIGURE 19.12   Pharmacokinetic profiles for three 300 mg/g Drug X SEDDS formulations along with the di-sodium salt of Drug X as a powder formulation in a HFC (control) with a single total dose of 1200 mg of Drug X in fasted human subjects (n = 15).[37]

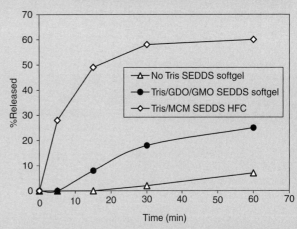

FIGURE 19.13   Drug release profiles from three 300 mg/g Drug X SEDDS dosage forms (i.e., "No Tris" softgel, "Tris/GDO/GMO" softgel, and "Tris/MCM" HFC). The test medium was 900 ml SIF (pH 6.5) with a stirring speed of 50 rpm.[37]

pharmacokinetic profiles observed in humans are shown in Figure 19.12.[37]

The "No Tris" SEDDS softgels showed a lower AUC and C_{max} value, compared to the Tris/MCM SEDDS formulation in gelatin HFC. The di-sodium salt of Drug X was administered as the bulk drug in a capsule and the oral bioavailability was somewhat higher than the No Tris SEDDS softgel. The "Tris/GDO/ GMO" SEDDS softgel showed a two-fold higher C_{max} and AUC value, compared to that of the "No Tris" SEDDS softgel formulation.

As described above, the enhanced absorption of Drug X from the Tris-containing SEDDS formulations appears to be due to the combined effect of better emulsification spontaneity and the smaller particle size upon dilution. Although the Tris/GDO/GMO SEDDS and the Tris/MCM SEDDS formulations of Drug X are very similar in composition, there is a noticeable difference between the release profiles of these two dosage forms (Figure 19.13), as well as their particle size upon dilution with water.

Further investigation indicated that the poor release of Drug X from the Tris/GDO/GMO SEDDS softgel, as compared to the Tris/MCM SEDDS filled in hard gelatin capsule is due to the reduction of the solvent (ethanol and PG) levels in the softgel fill. This was attributed to the solvent migration from the fill material into the gelatin shell, and subsequent evaporation of the ethanol during the softgel drying process. Figure 19.14 shows an IVIVR plot of the *in vivo* AUC values with the three SEDDS dosage forms of Drug X observed in the clinical trial on the percentage of drug released at 60 minuntes in the *in vitro* test.

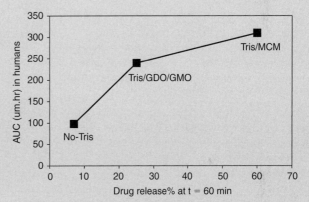

FIGURE 19.14   The IVIVR for the *in vivo* AUC values obtained from the clinical trial are plotted against the *in vitro* percentage drug release using three 300 mg/g Drug X SEDDS formulations at *t* = 60 minutes.[37]

A rank-order correlation was observed between the *in vitro* release and the oral exposure of Drug X among the three SEDDS dosage forms. In addition, there was a rank-order correlation between the oral bioavailability and the population of large particles with a size >1 μm for the three SEDDS dosage forms evaluated in the clinical trial, as shown by the following results. The *in vitro* dispersibility test showed that the "Tris/MCM" SEDDS HFC yielded the smallest amount (~2.3%) of large particles (>1 μm), while the "No Tris" SEDDS softgel showed the highest amount of large particles (~70% > 1 μm) upon dilution with water. The "Tris/GDO/GMO" SEDDS softgel had an intermediate amount of large particles (~12% > 1 μm). These results are in accordance with

19.4.2 Development of Supersaturatable S-SEDDS Formulations

Background on Supersaturated Formulations and the Advantages of Supersaturatable Formulations

The potential for supersaturated drug formulations in improving drug absorption was first proposed by T. Higuchi.[44] Since then, a number of publications have appeared employing supersaturated drug formulations as a means of enhancing the flux (or bioavailability) of drugs in topical formulations,[45] however, the development of supersaturatable drug formulations for improving the oral absorption of poorly soluble drugs has received limited attention. Supersaturated drug formulations can undergo spontaneous crystallization during storage. Supersaturatable drug formulations, on the other hand, become supersaturated only upon contact with water.

Polyvinylpyrrolidone (PVP) and the water soluble cellulosic polymers such as HPMC, methylcellulose, hydroxypropylmethylcellulose phthalate, and sodium carboxymethylcellulose, are useful in generating a supersaturated state with a number of poorly soluble drugs. The cellulosic polymers are excellent crystal growth inhibitors, and they are effective in maintaining the supersaturated state of the drugs at surprisingly low concentrations (<2%).[46,45]

In the initial studies on the development of S-SEDDS formulations, it was found that reducing the amount of surfactant and lipid in a SEDDS formulation, in order to generate a supersaturated state upon dilution of the formulation with an aqueous medium, invariably resulted in rapid precipitation of the poorly soluble drug.[37] However, incorporation of a surprisingly small amount (e.g., ~50 mg/g) of a water soluble cellulosic polymer (e.g., HPMC) into a SEDDS formulation was found to stabilize a supersaturated state, either by preventing or retarding drug precipitation upon dilution with water. These supersaturatable SEDDS (referred as

S-SEDDS), formulations are described in further detail in the following text.

In Vitro Evaluation of the S-SEDDS Formulations

An *in vitro* dissolution/precipitation test was designed to evaluate various prototype S-SEDDS formulations containing poorly soluble drugs with respect to:

1. the kinetics of formulation dispersion, and drug release upon contact with water; and
2. the ability to generate and maintain the supersaturated state under physiologically relevant conditions.

The "biorelevant *in vitro* dissolution/precipitation test" that was developed in our laboratory consisted of simulated gastric fluid (SGF) containing 0.01M HCl and 0.15M NaCl (pH 2.0), stirred at 50–100 RPM at 37°C using a VanKel 7010 dissolution apparatus. The total volume of the biorelevant *in vitro* dissolution medium was 50–100 mL. This volume approached the combined volume of the residual stomach fluid (~20–50 mL) in a fasted state, plus the amount of water (~30–60 mL) administered in either an animal (e.g., dog, monkey) or clinical study in the fasted state.

A unit dose of the S-SEDDS formulation (or related formulation for comparison) was placed into the dissolution fluid, and solution samples were withdrawn from the medium and filtered through a 0.8 μm filter, followed by determination of the drug concentration in the sample filtrate by an HPLC assay. The concentration of drug in the filtrate represented the amount of drug in the aqueous phase plus the amount of drug in the microemulsion/emulsion state with solid particle size <0.8 μm. This *in vitro* dissolution/precipitation test and the resulting drug concentration upon filtration versus time plots were used to guide the development of the S-SEDDS formulations.

CASE STUDY WITH PACLITAXEL

Properties of Paclitaxel and the Marketed Formulations

Paclitaxel (Figure 19.15) is an antitumor agent used in the treatment of advanced breast and ovarian cancer. Paclitaxel has a molecular weight of 853, with a low solubility in water (<1 μg/mL) and in common pharmaceutical vehicles. The currently marketed intravenous (IV) formulation of paclitaxel (Taxol®, Bristol-Meyers Squibb, BMS) contains 6 mg/mL of paclitaxel, 527 mg/mL of Cremophor EL (polyoxyethylenated castor oil), and 49.7% (v/v) of dehydrated ethanol.

The oral bioavailability of paclitaxel using the Taxol® formulation is extremely low (<2%) in rats, and even in humans.[43] The following section describes the development, and the evaluation, of the oral bioavailability of a paclitaxel S-SEDDS formulation in rats.

In Vitro and *In Vivo* Evaluation of a S-SEDDS Formulation of Paclitaxel

In order to examine the applicability of the S-SEDDS technology, paclitaxel was selected as a model drug and prototype S-SEDDS formulations were developed. The *in vitro* and *in vivo* performance of the paclitaxel SEDDS formulations without HPMC, and the resulting S-SEDDS formulations of paclitaxel, prepared with a suspension of powdered HPMC in the SEDDS formulation, were evaluated in comparison with the commercial Taxol® formulation. The *in vivo* oral bioavailability of paclitaxel in the S-SEDDS formulation co-administered with CsA was also assessed in rats, in order to determine the maximal exposure possible, as well as the role of P-gp inhibition when the transporter is exposed to the supersaturated concentration of paclitaxel using an S-SEDDS formulation.

A prototype S-SEDDS solution formulation containing ~60 mg/g of paclitaxel and 5% (w/w) HPMC (Formulation A) was prepared. The apparent paclitaxel solution concentrations in SGF (e.g., 0.01M HCl + 0.15M NaCl, pH 2.0) after dilution of the SEDDS formulation without HPMC (Formulation C) and the S-SEDDS formulation containing 5% HPMC (Formulation A) are shown in Figure 19.16a.

The theoretical concentration of paclitaxel in the test medium with these formulations, differing only in the presence or absence of HPMC, was 1.2 mg/mL based on the dilution factor of 50. Immediately upon dilution of the SEDDS formulation in the SGF medium, an opalescent solution characteristic of a microemulsion was formed. However, turbidity developed by the first sampling time (10 minutes) and crystalline paclitaxel was formed, as determined by microscopy and XPRD, indicating that the dispersion was supersaturated. The apparent paclitaxel concentration in the *in vitro* dissolution test (Figure 19.16a) was

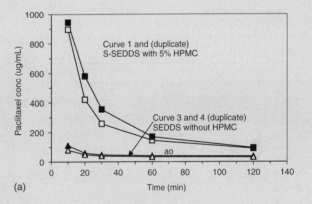

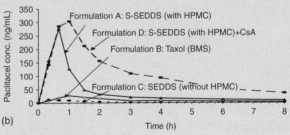

FIGURE 19.16 (a) Apparent concentration–time profiles for paclitaxel observed in the *in vitro* dissolution/precipitation test. (b) Mean plasma concentration–time profiles for paclitaxel in rats after oral administration of the four formulations as indicated, using the S-SEDDS formulation of paclitaxel containing 5% HPMC (Curve 1) and the S-SEDDS formulation with cyclosporine (CsA) (Curve 2), the Taxol® formulation (Curve 3), and the SEDDS formulation of paclitaxel without HPMC (Curve 4)[43]

FIGURE 19.15 Structure of paclitaxel

CASE STUDY   (CONTINUED)

about 0.12 mg/mL at the first sampling point (10 minutes), and the concentration decreased to ~0.03 mg/mL at t = 30 minutes. Similarly, the S-SEDDS formulation with HPMC (Formulation A) initially formed a clear microemulsion, however, the apparent paclitaxel concentration from this formulation was high (~0.95 mg/mL) at t = 10 minutes, and it gradually decreased to ~0.12 mg/mL over 2 hours (Figure 19.16a), indicating supersaturation.

In summary, the S-SEDDS formulation yielded an apparent solution concentration much higher than the aqueous equilibrium solubility of paclitaxel (~0.030 mg/mL) and in the *in vitro* test medium. The comparative *in vitro* study clearly showed that the presence of a small amount of HPMC (5%, w/w) in the S-SEDDS formulation suppressed precipitation of paclitaxel, and generated a supersaturated state that was maintained for longer than 2 hours.

The mean plasma concentration of paclitaxel obtained in rats with the four oral treatment groups (Figure 19.16b) showed that the rank order of the mean $AUC0-\infty$ for the four formulations was:

S-SEDDS + CsA > S-SEDDS > > Taxol® > SEDDS
(Formulation D) (Formulation A) (Formulation B) (Formulation C)

The difference in the pharmacokinetic profiles exhibited by the SEDDS and S-SEDDS (with HPMC) formulations in Figure 19.16b is of great interest, as these two formulations differ only in the content of HPMC, 0% versus 5% respectively. The SEDDS formulation (without HPMC) showed a very low C_{max} of only 13.1 ng/mL, and an oral bioavailability of 0.9%, whereas the S-SEDDS formulation (with HPMC) resulted in a 20-fold increase in C_{max} (~277 ng/mL), and an oral bioavailability of 9.5%. The S-SEDDS formulation with the P-gp inhibitor CsA and HPMC showed similar absorption kinetics, but slower elimination kinetics, resulting in a two-fold increase of the oral bioavailability over that of the S-SEDDS formulation with only HPMC.

The rat bioavailability results indicated that the higher paclitaxel solution concentration generated by the S-SEDDS formulation in the *in vitro* dissolution/precipitation test was the result of supersaturation, which is responsible for the enhanced oral bioavailability of paclitaxel from the S-SEDDS formulation. The failure to provide high oral exposure of paclitaxel with the Taxol® formulation is significant, in that the practice of formulating poorly soluble drugs with high concentrations of surfactants inevitably results in reduction in the free drug concentration or the thermodynamic activity.

CASE STUDY WITH DRUG Y

Drug Y was a candidate under development for preclinical and clinical evaluation. Drug Y has a log p of ~3.5, a water solubility of only ~3 μg/mL in the physiological pH range of 2–7, and it is nonionizable in this pH range. A human oral pharmacokinetic study using Drug Y showed slow and incomplete oral absorption using a powder formulation of the bulk drug in a gelatin capsule. In order to improve the rate and the extent of the oral absorption of Drug Y, an S-SEDDS formulation was developed and evaluated in the clinic.

S-SEDDS Formulations of Drug Y with HPMC

The *in vitro* dissolution/precipitation test using 50 mL of SGF fluid (0.01 M HCl + 0.15 M NaCl, pH 2) was employed in evaluating the performance of 1 gm of the S-SEDDS formulations containing 200 mg of Drug Y filled into two hard gelatin capsules (0.5 g/capsule). Based on a dilution factor of 50, the theoretical concentration of Drug Y in the test medium is 4 mg/mL.

The apparent Drug Y concentration found with the SEDDS formulation (without HPMC) in the *in vitro* dissolution/precipitation test is plotted in Figure 19.17a. The concentration of Drug Y in the medium was about 0.3 mg/mL at the first time point (0.5 hour), and this remained unchanged over the 6 hour test period. In contrast, a markedly higher concentration of Drug Y (~2.7 to 3.5 mg/mL) was observed with the same SEDDS formulation in the same test medium by adding 0.025% w/v of HPMC (Figure 19.17a).

The S-SEDDS formulation of Drug Y containing 40 mg/g HPMC was evaluated. The apparent Drug Y concentration observed is plotted versus time in Figure 19.17a. Little precipitation of Drug Y was observed over the 6-hour test period, and the Drug Y concentration was sustained at ~3–3.5 mg/mL, comparable to the concentrations of Drug *Y* that were observed in the test medium with HPMC. The apparent Drug Y concentration from the S-SEDDS formulation in the test medium was about 10-fold higher than the SEDDS formulation without HPMC in the dissolution medium. The *in vitro* test

CASE STUDY (CONTINUED)

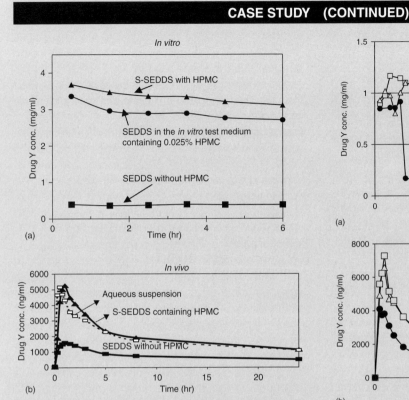

FIGURE 19.17 (a) Apparent concentration–time profiles of Drug Y observed *in vitro* dissolution/precipitation test using the same SEDDS formulation with and without HPMC. All formulations were filled into gelatin hard capsules; (b) Mean plasma concentration profiles of Drug Y in the dogs (n = 6, crossover) using the two SEDDS formulations with and without HPMC as compared to an aqueous suspension formulation[37]

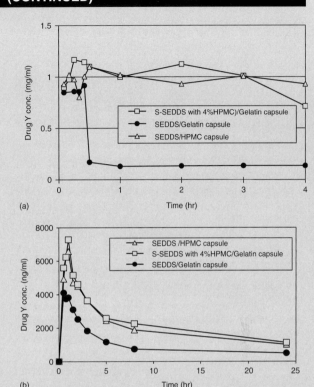

FIGURE 19.18 (a) Apparent concentration Drug Y concentration (obtained by filtration through a 0.8 μm filter) versus time profiles of Drug Y observed in the *in vitro* dissolution/precipitation test using the three formulations with different capsule shells as indicated; (b) Mean plasma concentration profiles of Drug Y in the dogs using the three formulations (n = 6, crossover)[37]

clearly revealed that the presence of a small amount of HPMC could effectively maintain a supersaturated state of Drug Y for at least 6 hours.

The *in vivo* pharmacokinetics of both the SEDDS and the S-SEDDS formulations of Drug Y were evaluated after oral administration in dogs, as compared to an aqueous suspension. Figure 19.17b shows that the mean plasma concentration profile of Drug Y obtained after dosing the S-SEDDS formulation (with 4.4% HPMC) is about three-fold higher in the C_{max}, and the AUC is two and a half times larger, as compared to the same SEDDS formulation without HPMC. This clearly indicates that the S-SEDDS formulation containing HPMC results in an increase in both the C_{max}, and the extent of absorption of Drug Y. The aqueous suspension and the S-SEDDS formulation showed a similar pharmacokinetics profile in dogs.

S-SEDDS of Drug Y in HPMC Capsule

The use of an HPMC capsule was explored as an alternative approach for incorporating HPMC into

an S-SEDDS formulation. Three dosage forms were selected for comparison in the *in vitro* dissolution/precipitation test. The formulations consisted of:

1. the SEDDS liquid formula filled in hard gelatin capsules;
2. the SEDDS liquid formula containing 44 mg of HPMC powder suspended in a hard gelatin capsule; and
3. the SEDDS liquid formula filled into an HPMC capsule.

The SEDDS liquid formula in all three formulations was identical, however, HPMC or an HPMC capsule were employed in 2 and 3. Figure 19.18a shows the apparent drug concentrations of Drug Y as a function of time, obtained with these three dosage forms in the *in vitro* dissolution/precipitation test.

A 1 gm SEDDS formulation of Drug Y containing a suspension of 44 mg of powdered HPMC in hard gelatin capsules showed an almost constant drug concentration of ~1 mg/mL over the entire 4 hour period in the dispersibility test, whereas the concentration obtained with SEDDS

CASE STUDY   (CONTINUED)

formulation of Drug Y without HPMC declined rapidly (Figure 19.18a). The SEDDS liquid filled into an HPMC capsule showed essentially the same Drug Y concentration–time profile as the SEDDS formulation containing suspended HPMC powder filled into gelatin capsules, but the levels of Drug Y were approximately five-fold higher.

The oral bioavailability study was determined in dogs (n = 6, crossover) with the three SEDDS formulations described above. The mean plasma concentration–time profiles of Drug Y are plotted in Figure 19.18b. As expected, the SEDDS formulation in the gelatin capsule showed a low C_{max}, and a low AUC. However, the plasma concentration–time profiles observed for the S-SEDDS formulation (containing HPMC), and the SEDDS formulation filled into HPMC capsules, were almost superimposable, and the resulting C_{max} and AUC values were approximately two-fold higher than that of the SEDDS liquid without HPMC in the gelatin capsule. The *in vivo* behavior of the three formulations is in accord with the *in vitro* test results.

Clinical Evaluation of Drug Y S-SEDDS Formulation

A human clinical trial was designed to evaluate the oral bioavailability of an S-SEDDS softgel of Drug Y, in comparison with two other formulations, namely, the Drug Y powder in a gelatin capsule and an aqueous suspension of Drug Y fine particles. An S-SEDDS formulation of Drug Y containing suspended HPMC was encapsulated in softgels, and these softgels were orally administered to fasted healthy volunteers (n = 23, crossover).

The plasma concentration versus time profiles for Drug Y administered in each of these formulations are shown in Figure 19.19, and the mean C_{max}, T_{max}, and AUC values are reported in Table 19.5. The conventional Drug Y powder formulation in the gelatin capsule showed the lowest mean C_{max} (621 ng/mL), and the aqueous suspension showed a slightly higher mean

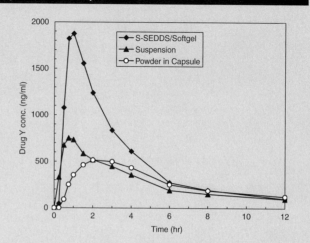

FIGURE 19.19   Human bioavailability study with three formulations of Drug Y formulated as the bulk drug powder in a hard gelatin capsule, an aqueous suspension, and a S-SEDDS formulation (with HPMC) in a softgel (n = 23)[37]

TABLE 19.5   Oral bioavailability of Drug Y in humans administered a 200 mg dose of three different formulations (n = 23, crossover)[37]

Pharmacokinetic parameters	Formulations		
	Drug powder in gelatin capsule	Aqueous suspension	S-SEDDS softgel
C_{max} (ng/mL)	621 (45)	804 (45)	2061 (34)
T_{max} (hr)	2.15 (42)	0.97 (43)	1.03 (36)
AUC ((ng/mL)*hr)	5060 (45)	4892 (45)	7004 (41)

C_{max} (804 ng/mL). In contrast, the S-SEDDS softgel showed the highest C_{max}, and the largest AUC, along with the shortest T_{max} (~1 hour), indicating a more rapid and complete absorption than Drug Y in a capsule or the aqueous suspension.

19.5 PROPOSED PATHWAYS FOR ENHANCED ORAL ABSORPTION OF POORLY SOLUBLE DRUGS WITH SEDDS AND S-SEDDS APPROACH

19.5.1 Drug Absorption Pathway

The enhanced oral bioavailability observed with SEDDS and S-SEDDS formulations of poorly soluble lipophilic drugs, as compared to that of simple aqueous suspension of the drug or the bulk drug powder in a capsule, indicates that SEDDS formulations appear to present the drug more efficiently to the intestinal enterocyte brush border glycocalyx. The enhanced oral bioavailability often seen with the SEDDS and S-SEDDS formulations appears to be due to improved presentation of the poorly soluble drug to the enterocyte brush border membrane.

The pioneering work of Borgstrom et al.,[32–34,47] and others, established that the fed state bile acid mixed micelle (BAMM) and the fasted state bile acid (BA) micelle constitute the endogenous surfactant system that is responsible for the delivery or presentation of poorly soluble highly lipophilic compounds to the enterocyte brush border region, as shown by the following results.

Cholesterol, with a clog$P$ of 12 and a water solubility of ~10 ng/ml is an extremely insoluble and highly lipophilic example of a compound that would not be expected to be absorbed orally but, in fact, it is absorbed orally up to about ~50%. The delivery of cholesterol from the BAMM to the enterocyte surface occurs via collisional transfer.[48–51] Other poorly soluble and lipophilic drugs have been shown to be absorbed more completely in the fed state where the BAMM is present.[52–55] The BAMM system is more effective that the BA system, because of the higher bile acid micellar concentration in the fed (~15 mM), as compared to the BA in the fasted, state (~4 mM). Lipophilic compounds are solubilized by the BAMM or BA particles, and then they are delivered to the enterocyte glycocalyx by collisional contact of the BAMM particle. They are transferred to the glycocalyx:

> "as the ingesta (in the intestinal lumen) is mixed, the bile salt mixed micelles *bump* into the brush border and the lipids, including cholesterol, monoglyceride, and fatty acid (within the bile salt mixed micelles) are absorbed."[52]

Studies on the mechanism responsible for inhibiting crystallization of drugs in aqueous drug solutions containing HPMC suggests that the long HPMC polymer chains could inhibit nucleation of the drug or it could inhibit crystal growth by adsorption of the HPMC polymeric chains onto the surface of the drug nuclei.[56] The cellulosic polymers are useful in inhibiting crystallization in topical and transdermal formulations. Based on this background, Figure 19.20 shows a cartoon of a possible scheme for the presentation of poorly soluble lipophilic drugs in SEDDS formulations to the intestinal enterocyte brush border, followed by uptake by the aqueous pathway or equilibration of the drug with the BA/BAMM pathway or by mimicking the behavior of the BA/BAMM pathway.

The enhanced intestinal absorption and shortened T_{max} values of poorly soluble drugs administered in S-SEDDS formulations is consistent with enhanced uptake by the aqueous pathway in Figure 19.20, due to the higher free drug concentration that is generated by the supersaturated state in the GI tract with the S-SEDDS microemulsion. The shortened T_{max} values seen with the optimized supersaturatable S-SEDDS formulations are consistent with an enhanced uptake by the aqueous pathway, and the enhanced bioavailability seen by the optimized S-SEDDS microemulsion is consistent with enhanced uptake by equilibration with the BAMM pathway or by mimicking the BAMM.

19.5.2 The Enterocyte Absorption of Highly Lipophilic Compounds

A number of highly lipophilic compounds, such as cholesterol, vitamin E, vitamin A, vitamin D, vitamin K, and various carotenoids and phytosterols with log p values >8, are extremely water insoluble, with solubility orders of magnitude less than 1 μg/mL, the value typically ascribed to poorly soluble drugs.[57] These extremely lipophilic and extremely water insoluble compounds are readily absorbed from food sources, and the marketed nutritional supplement products of these compounds are often formulated in simple triglyceride formulations without surfactants. The phytosterols, beta-sitosterol and campesterol, show higher bioavailabilities when administered in emulsified (surfactant plus oil) formulations, as compared to simple soybean oil solutions.

The highly lipophilic drug PNU-74006F with polar substituents is rapidly taken up by the enterocyte apical bilayer, however, the drug is located in (or on) the bilayer and lateral diffusion to the basolaterol region does not occur (Figure 19.21), probably because the polar substituents are capable of H-bonding with the polar phospholipids.[58,59]

19.5.3 Significance of the Glycocalyx in Absorption of Drugs from SEDDS/S-SEDDS Formulations

The glycocalyx is a filamentous structure, with each filament strand about 7 to 15 nm in diameter, consisting of the glycoproteins/glycolipids associated with the enterocyte microvilli that can be visualized by electron microscopy using special sample processing parameters.[60] The glycocalyx filaments are repeatedly branched or anastomosed, and provide an occlusive barrier that prevents direct contact of the enterocyte microvillous bilayer by food particles or other microparticulates (such as SEDDS microemulsions in the intestine, as shown in Figure 19.22).

The tight network of filamenteous chains constituting the glycocalyx, seen in the upper portion of Figure 19.22, are composed of glycolipids and glycoproteins that are firmly anchored (transmembrane) or superficially attached to the surface of the microvilli located on the

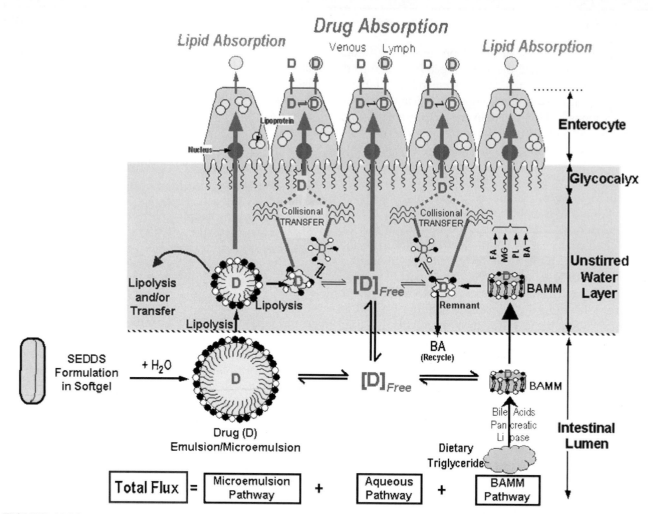

FIGURE 19.20 Cartoon showing proposed pathways for presentation of drugs in SEDDS/S-SEDDS formulations to the enterocyte glycocalyx on apical membrane and uptake of drugs (D) by: (a) the aqueous pathway; (b) the BAMM pathway; and (c) the microemulsion pathway. However, the drug in the emulsion/microemulsion remnant can equilibrate with the free drug in aqueous solution or, in turn, the drug can partition into the BAMM particle. Collisional transfer of the drug to the glycocalyx can occur from the drug–BAMM particle and from the remnant microemulsion particle. The drug in the aqueous media can be taken up by the aqueous pathway. The enterocyte intracellular processing can lead to venous or lymphatic delivery of the drug

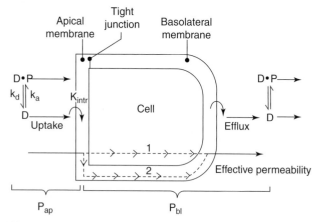

FIGURE 19.21 Cartoon showing the pathway for the uptake of extremely lipophilic drugs (D) by the intestinal enterocyte.[64] Extremely lipophilic compounds with log $P > \sim 8$ with very few polar functionalgroups could be absorbed by diffusion of the compound via the bilayer, through the tight junction and into the basolateral region where the drug could be removed from the basolateral membrane by association

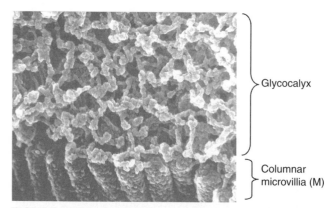

FIGURE 19.22 Scanning electron micrograph (SEM) showing the tightly formed glycocalyx consisting of glycoproteins and glycolipids that are attached to the surface of the columnar microvilli on the lumenal or apical surface of the intestinal enterocyte. The microvilli are seen at the bottom of the SEM with an M scribed on one of the microvilli[59]

apical (lumenal) surface of the intestinal enterocyte. The glycocalyx functions as a physical barrier that prevents direct contact of food particles and microparticulates (including microemulsions) in the intestinal lumen from direct contact with the intestinal microvilli. The cartoon in Figure 19.20 shows that the proposed presentation of a drug in a SEDDS/SEDDS microemulsion particle or remnant thereof, to the glycocalyx, could lead to uptake:

1. by the classical aqueous pathway;
2. by the BA/BAMM pathway; or
3. by simulating the behavior of the BAMM pathway.

The S-SEDDS remnant particles could promote drug uptake by the aqueous pathway through the higher free drug concentration.

19.6 CONCLUSIONS

Table 19.6 shows the water solubility of the compounds in the marketed SEDDS formulations, and the experiment drugs in the SEDDS and S-SEDDS formulations discussed in the case studies. From the data in Table 19.6, the lowest water solubility of 10 drugs formulated in marketed or experimental SEDDS/SEDDS formulations with reasonable oral bioavailability is $0.04 \mu g/mL$, as given by PNU-74006F. The solubility of PNU074006F was determined experimentally in water at pH ~6.5 at room temperature.[37] This is somewhat lower than the publication of another group of 11 marketed and experimental poorly soluble drugs, where the lowest solubility consistent with good oral bioavailability in rats and dogs was reported as "$<3 \mu g/mL$".[25] The solubilities of drugs in a biorelevant fluid that simulates the intestinal fluids would be a better choice than those in water. However, information on the solubilities of drugs in biorelevant fluids is not readily available for the drugs in Table 19.6.

In general, the SEDDS and S-SEDDS formulations are not very useful with drugs with low lipophilicities (e.g., log P or log $D <2$) to improve their absorption. This is because these drugs would not be retained in the resulting microemulsion upon contact with water and the dilution occurring in the stomach and in the small intestine.

We consider that the SEDDS and S-SEDDS approaches are potentially useful for those drugs with key attributes listed below:

1. $MW \leq 600$;
2. clog $P \geq 2$;

TABLE 19.6 Aqueous solubilities of marketed and experimental drugs in SEDDS formulations

No	Drug	Names of Marketed and Experimental SEDDS/S-SEDDS Formulations described in this review	Calc. or Exp. Water Sol. of Drug[a] ($\mu g/mL$)	
1	Cyclosporine	Sandimmune®. Forms a coarse emulsion with H_2O.	9	Calc.
2	Cyclosporine	Neoral®. Forms a microemulsion with H_2O.	9	Calc.
3	Ritanovir	Norvir®.	0.37	Exp.
4	Saquinavir	Fortavase®.	2	Calc.
5	Tipranavir	Aptivus®. Forms a microemulsion with H_2O.	5	Calc.
6	Paclitaxel	Experimental S-SEDDS Formulation.	<0.3	Exp
7	PNU-74006 F	Experimental SEDDS Formulation	0.04	Exp.
8	PNU-91325	Experimental S-SEDDS Formulation.	6	Exp.
9	Drug X	Experimental SEDDS Formulation.	5	EXP
10	Drug Y	Experimental S-SEDDS Formulation.	3	Exp.
11	Danazol	Experimental Formulation. (Charman, 2005)	0.59	Exp.

[a] Calc. = Calculated water solubility using ALogPS in the DrugBank Database (**www.drugbank.com**)

3. do not possess extensive first-pass metabolism;
4. the number of –NH-CO- amide groups ≤ 3;
5. its intrinsic aqueous solubility ≥ 5–$10 \mu g/mL$ (corresponding to a dose of 50–200 mg in human); and
6. shows substantial solubility in pharmaceutically acceptable co-solvents, surfactants, and lipids.

The recognition of the potential of SEDDS and S-SEDDS formulations for improving the gastrointestinal absorption of poorly water soluble drugs has been a major driver of these technologies. Properly designed SEDDS and S-SEDDS formulations provide the formulation scientists with a unique opportunity to the drug absorption profile design the absorption profile of poorly soluble drugs.

ACKNOWLEDGEMENTS

A special acknowledgement is given to the following former colleagues: J. B. Landis, R. D. White, J. W. Skoug, M. J. Hageman, P. R. Nixon, R. J. Haskell, T. Huang, J. B. Bauer, S. L. Douglas, M. T. Kuo, K. J. Stefanski, B. D. Rush, W. P. Pfund, J. R. Shifflet, K. M. Zamora, M. J. Witt, M. E. Guyton, X. He, F. J. Schwende, Q. Lu, and others for their endorsement, development, and evaluation of the bioavailability of the SEDDS and S-SEDDS formulations of paclitaxel, experimental Drug X and Y, as discussed herein.

References

1. Cuiné, J.F., McEvoy, C.L., Charman, W.N., Pouton, C.W., Edwards, G.A., Benameur, H. & Porter, C.J. (2008). Evaluation of the impact of surfactant digestion on the bioavailability of danazol after oral administration of lipidic self-emulsifying formulations to dogs. Journal of Pharmaceutical Sciences 97(2), 993–1010.

2. Pouton, C.W. (2000). Lipid formulations for oral administration of drugs: Non-emulsifying, self-emulsifying and "self-microemulsifying" drug delivery systems. European Journal of Pharmaceutical Sciences 11(suppl. 2), S93–S98.

3. Nazzal, A.H., Zaghloul, A.A. & Nazzal, S. (2008). Comparison between lipolysis and compendial dissolution as alternative techniques for the in vitro characterization of alpha-tocopherol self-emulsified drug delivery systems (SEDDS). International Journal of Pharmaceutics 20, 352(1–2), 104–114.

4. Nielsen, F.S., Petersen, K.B. & Müllertz, A. (2008). Bioavailability of probucol from lipid and surfactant based formulations in minipigs: Influence of droplet size and dietary state. European Journal of Pharmaceutics and Biopharmaceutics. in press.

5. Porter, C.J., Trevaskis, N.L., Charman, (2007). Lipids and lipid-based formulations: Optimizing the oral delivery of lipophilic drugs. Rev. Drug Discov. 6(3), 231–248.

5a. Fatouros, D.G., Karpf, D.M., Nielsen, F.S. & Mullertz, A. (2007). Clinical studies with oral lipid based formulations of poorly soluble compounds. Ther Clin Risk Manag 3(4), 591–604.

6. Branchu, S., Rogueda, P.G., Plumb, A.P. & Cook, W.G. (2007). A decision-support tool for the formulation of orally active, poorly soluble compounds. European Journal of Pharmaceutical Sciences 32(2), 128–139.

7. Humberstone, A.J. & Charman, W.N. (1997). Lipid-based vehicles for oral delivery of poorly soluble drugs. Advanced Drug Delivery Reviews 25, 103–128.

8. Cuiné, J.F., Charman, W.N., Pouton, C.W., Edwards, G.A. & Porter, C.J. (2007). Increasing the proportional content of surfactant (Cremophor EL) relative to lipid in self-emulsifying pid-based formulations of danazol reduces oral bioavailability in beagle dogs. Pharmaceutical Research 24(4), 748–757.

9. Kossena, G.A., Charman, W.N., Wilson, C.G., O'Mahony, B., Lindsay, B., Hempenstall, J.M., Davison, C.L., Crowley, P.J. & Porter, C.J. (2007). Low dose lipid formulations: Effects on gastric emptying and biliary secretion. Pharmaceutical Research 24(11), 2084–2096.

10. Hauss, D.J. (2007). Oral lipid-based formulations. Advance Drug Delivery Reviews 59(7), 667–676.

11. Constantinides, P.P. & Wasan, K.M. (2007). Lipid formulation strategies for enhancing intestinal transport and absorption of P-glycoprotein (P-gp) substrate drugs: In vitro/in vivo case studies. Journal of Pharmaceutical Sciences 96(2), 235–248.

12. Gershkovich, P. & Hoffman, A. (2007). Effect of a high-fat meal on absorption and disposition of lipophilic compounds: The importance of degree of association with triglyceride-rich lipoproteins. European Journal of Pharmaceutics and Biopharmaceutics 32(1), 24–32.

13. Jadhav, K.R., Shaikh, I.M., Ambade, K.W. & Kadam, V.J. (2006). Applications of microemulsion based drug delivery system. Current Drug Delivery(3), 267–273.

14. Khandavilli, S. & Panchagnula, R. (2007). Nanoemulsions as versatile formulations for paclitaxel delivery: Peroral and dermal delivery studies in rats. The Journal of Investigative Dermatology 127(1), 154–162.

15. Dressman, J.B. & Reppas, C. (2000). In vitro–in vivo correlations for lipophilic, poorly soluble drugs. Journal of Pharmaceutical Sciences 11(S2), S73–S80.

16. Hong, J.Y., Kim, J.K., Song, Y.K., Park, J.S. & Kim, C.K. (2006). A new self-emulsifying formulation of itraconazole with improved dissolution and oral absorption. Journal of Controlled Release 10(2), 332–338.

17. Galia, E., Nicolaides, E., Hörter, D., Löbenberg, R., Reppas, C. & Dressman, J.B. (1998). Evaluation of various dissolution media for predicting in vivo performance of class I and II drugs. Pharmaceutical Research 15(5), 698–705.

18. Gershanik, T. & Benita, S. (2000). Self-dispersing lipid formulations for improving oral absorption of lipophilic drugs. European Journal of Pharmaceutics and Biopharmaceutics 50(1), 179–188.

19. Grove, M., Müllertz, A., Nielsen, J.L. & Pedersen, G.P. (2006). Bioavailability of seocalcitol II: Development and characterization of self-microemulsifying drug delivery systems (SMEDDS) for oral administration containing medium and long chain triglycerides. European Journal of Pharmaceutics and Biopharmaceutics 28(3), 233–242.

20. Kossena, G.A., Charman, W.N., Boyd, B.J., Dunstan, D.E. & Porter, C.J. (2004). Probing drug solubilization patterns in the gastrointestinal tract after administration of lipid-based delivery systems: A phase diagram approach. Journal of Pharmaceutical Sciences 93(2), 332–348.

21. Trevaskis, N.L., Porter, C.J. & Charman, W.N. (2006a). The lymph lipid precursor pool is a key determinant of intestinal lymphatic drug transport. The Journal of Pharmacology and Experimental Therapeutics 316(2), 881–891.

22. Trevaskis, N.L., Lo, C.M., Ma, L.Y., Tso, P., Irving, H.R., Porter, C.J. & Charman, W.N. (2006). An acute and coincident increase in FABP expression and lymphatic lipid and drug transport occurs during intestinal infusion of lipid-based drug formulations to rats. Pharmaceutical Research 23(8), 1786–1796.

23. Khoo, S.M., Edwards, G.A., Porter, C.J. & Charman, W.N. (2001). A conscious dog model for assessing the absorption, enterocyte-based metabolism, and intestinal lymphatic transport of halofantrine. Journal of Pharmaceutical Sciences 90(10), 1599–1607.

24. Porter, C.J. & Charman, W.N. (2001). Intestinal lymphatic drug transport: An update. Advanced Drug Delivery Reviews 50 (1–2), 61–80.

25. Araya, H., Tomita, M. & Hayashi, M. (2005). The novel formulation design of O/W microemulsion for improving the gastrointestinal absorption of poorly water soluble compounds. International Journal of Pharmaceutics 305(1–2), 61–74.

26. Odeberg, J.M., Kaufmann, P., Kroon, K.G. & Höglund, P. (2003). Lipid drug delivery and rational formulation design for lipophilic drugs with low oral bioavailability, applied to cyclosporine. European Journal of Pharmaceutical Sciences 20(4–5), 375–382.

27. Lawrence, M.J. & Rees, G.D. (2000). Microemulsion-based media as novel drug delivery systems. Advanced Drug Delivery Reviews 45, 89–121.

28. Holt, D.W., Mueller, E.A., Kovarik, J.M., van Bree, J.B. & Kutz, K. (1994). The pharmacokinetics of Sandimmune Neoral: A new oral formulation of cyclosporine. Transplantation Proceedings 26, 2935–2939.

29. Kovarik, J.M., Mueller, E.A., van Bree, J.B., Tetzloff, W. & Kutz, K. (1994). Reduced inter and intraindividual variability in cyclosporine pharmacokinetics from a microemulsion formulation. Journal of Pharmaceutical Sciences 83, 444–446.

30. Mueller, E.A., Kovarik, J.M., van Bree, J.B., Tetzloff, W., Grevel, J. & Kutz, K. (1994). Improved dose linearity of cyclosporine pharmacokinetics from a microemulsion formulation. Pharmaceutical Research 11, 301–304.

31. Börgstrom, B., Dahlquist, A., Lundh, G. & Sjövall, J. (1957). Studies of intestinal digestion and absorption in the human. The Journal of Clinical Investigation 36, 1521–1529.

32. Borgstrom, B., Patton, J. S. (1991). Luminal events in gastrointestinal lipid digestion. In: Handbook of Physiology, Section 6. The Gastrointestinal System, IV, S. G. Schultz (ed.). The American Physiological Society, Bethesda MD, pp. 475–504.

33. Staggers, J.E., Hernell, O., Stafford, R.J. & Carey, M.C. (1990). Physical–chemical behavior of dietary and biliary lipids during intestinal digestion and absorption. 1. Phase behavior and aggregation states of model lipid systems patterned after aqueous duodenal content in healthy adult human beings. Biochem. 29, 2028–2040.

34. Hernell, O., Staggers, J.E. & Carey, M.C. (1990). Physical–chemical behavior of dietary and biliary lipids during intestinal digestion and absorption. 2. Phase analysis and aggregation states of luminal lipids during duodenal fat digestion in healthy adult human beings. Biochem. 29, 2041–2056.

35. Pouton, C.W. & Charman, W.N. (1997). The potential of oily formulations for drug delivery to the gastro-intestinal tract. Advanced Drug Delivery Reviews 25, 1–2.

36. Charman, S.A., Charman, W.N., Rogge, M.C., Wilson, T.D., Dutko, F.J. & Pouton, C.W. (1992). Self-emulsifying drug delivery systems: formulation and biopharmaceutic evaluation of an investigational lipophilic compound. Pharmaceutical Research 9(1), 87–93.

37. Gao, P. & Morozowich, W. (2007a). Case Studies: Rational Development of Self-Emulsifying Formulations for Improving the Oral Bioavailability of Poorly Soluble, Lipophilic Drugs. In: Oral Lipid-Based Formulations: Enhancing the bioavailability of poorly water soluble drugs, D. Hauss (ed.). Drugs and the Pharm. Sci., 170. Informa Healthcare USA, New York, pp. 275–302.

38. Gao, P. & Morozowich, W. (2007b). Design and Development of Supersaturatable SEDDS (S-SEDDS) Formulations for Enhancing the Gastrointestinal Absorption of Poorly Soluble Drugs. In: Oral Lipid-Based Formulations: Enhancing the bioavailability of poorly water soluble drugs, D. Hauss (ed.). Drugs and the Pharm. Sci., 170. Informa Healthcare USA, New York, pp. 303–328.

39. Morozowich, W., Gao, P. & Charton, M. (2006). Speeding the development of poorly soluble/poorly permeable drugs by SEDDS/S-SEDDS formulations and prodrugs—Part 1. Amer. Pharm. Rev. 9(3), 110–114.

40. Morozowich, W., Gao, P. & Charton, M. (2006). Speeding the development of poorly soluble/poorly permeable drugs by SEDDS/S-SEDDS formulations and prodrugs—Part 2. Amer. Pharm. Rev. 9(4), 16–23.

41. Gao, P., Guyton, M.E., Huang, T., Bauer, J.M., Stefanski, K.J. & Lu, Q. (2004). Enhanced oral availability of a poorly water soluble drug PNU-91325 by supersaturatable formulations. Drug Development and Industrial Pharmacy 30(2), 221–229.

42. Gao, P., Witt, M.J., Haskell, R.J., Zamora, K.M. & Shifflet, J. R. (2004). Application of a mixture experimental design in the optimization of a self-emulsifying formulation with a high drug load. Pharmaceutical Development and Technology 9(3), 301–309.

43. Gao, P., Rush, B.D., Pfund, W.P., Huang, T., Bauer, J. M., Morozowich, W., Kuo, M.S. & Hageman, M.J. (2003). Development of a supersaturable SEDDS (S-SEDDS) formulation of paclitaxel with improved oral bioavailability. Journal of Pharmaceutical Sciences 92(12), 2386–2398.

44. Higuchi, T. (1960). Physical chemical analysis of the percutaneous absorption process. Journal of the Society of Cosmetic Chemists 11, 85–97.

45. Raghavan, R. L., Kiepfer, B., Davis, A. F., Kazarian, S. G. & Hadgraft, J. (2001). Membrane transport of hydrocortisone acetate from supersaturated solutions: The role of polymers. International Journal of Pharmaceutics, 221, 95–105.

45a. Raghavan, S. L., Trividica, A., Davis, A. F., Hadgraft, J. (2001). Crystallization of hydrocortisone acetate: Influence of polymers. International Journal of Pharmaceutics, 212, 213–221.

46. Iervolino, M., Raghavan, R.L. & Hadgraft, J. (2000). Membrane penetration enhancement of ibuprofen using supersaturation. International Journal of Pharmaceutics 198, 229–238.

47. Carey, M.C. & Small, D.M. (1970). The characteristics of mixed micellar solutions with particular reference to bile. The American Journal of Medicine 49, 590–598.

48. Steck, T.L., Kezdy, F.J. & Lange, Y. (1988). An activation-collision mechanism for cholesterol transfer between membranes. The Journal of Biological Chemistry 263, 13023–13031.

49. Lipka, G., Imfeld, D., Schulthess, G., Thurnhofer, H. & Hauser, H. (1992). Protein mediated cholesterol absorption by small intestinal brush border membranes. Structural and Dynamic Properties of Lipids and Membranes 4, 7–18.

50. Thomson, A.B.R., Schoeller, C., Keelan, M., Smith, L. & Clandinin, M.T. (1993). Lipid absorption: Passing through the unstirred layers, brush-border membrane, and beyond. Canadian Journal of Physiology and Pharmacology 71, 531–555.

51. Shiau, Y.F. (1987). Lipid digestion and absorption. In: Physiology of the Gastrointestinal Tract, L.R. (ed.) Johnson,, 2nd edn. Raven Press, New York. pp. 1527–1556.

52. Austgen, L., Bowen, R. A. & Rouge, M. (2004). Pathophysiology of the Digestive System.Colorado State University, http://arbl. cvmbs.colostate.edu/hbooks/contrib.html, see statement: As the ingesta is mixed, the bile salt mixed micelles bump into the brush border and the lipids, including monoglyceride and fatty acids, are absorbed.

53. Mithani, S.D., Bakatselou, V., TenHoor, C.N. & Dressman, J. B. (1996). Estimation of the increase in solubility of drugs as a function of bile salt concentration. Pharmaceutical Research 13(1), 163–167.

54. Bakatselou, V., Oppenheim, R.C. & Dressman, J.B. (1991). Solubilization and wetting effects of bile salts on the dissolution of steroids. Pharmaceutical Research 8(12), 1461–1469.

55. TenHoor, C.N., Bakatselou, V. & Dressman, J.B. (1991). Solubility of mefenamic acid under simulated fed- and fasted-state conditions. Pharmaceutical Research 8(9), 1203–1205.

56. Ziller, K.H. & Rupprecht, H. (1988). Control of crystal growth in drug suspensions. Drug Development and Industrial Pharmacy 14, 2341–2370.

57. Borel, P. (2003). Factors affecting intestinal absorption of highly lipophilic food microconstituents (fat-soluble vitamins, carotenoids and phytosterols). Clinical Chemistry and Laboratory Medicine 41(8), 979–994.

58. Sawada, G.A., Barsuhn, C.L., Lutzke, B.S., Houghton, M. E., Padbury, G.E., Ho, N.F. & Raub, T.J. (1999). Increased

lipophilicity and subsequent cell partitioning decrease passive transcellular diffusion of novel, highly lipophilic antioxidants. The Journal of Pharmacology and Experimental Therapeutics 288(3), 1317–1326.

59. Raub, T.J., Barsuhn, C.L., Williams, L.R., Decker, D.E., Sawada, G.A. & Hom, N.F. (1993). Use of a biophysical-kinetic model to understand the roles of protein binding and membrane partitioning on passive diffusion of highly lipophilic molecules across cellular barriers. Journal of Drug Targeting 1(4), 269–286.

60. Horiuchi, K., Naito, I., Nakano, K., Nakatani, S., Nishida, K., Taguchi, T. & Ohtsuka, A. (2005). Three-dimensional ultrastructure of the brush border glycocalyx in the mouse small intestine: A high resolution scanning electron microscopic study. Archives of Histology and Cytology 68(1), 51–56.

Rational Design of Oral Modified-Release Drug Delivery Systems

Yihong Qiu

20.1 INTRODUCTION

Modified release (MR) drug delivery systems are developed to modulate the apparent absorption and/ or alter the site of release of drugs, in order to achieve specific clinical objectives that cannot be attained with conventional dosage forms. Possible therapeutic benefits of a properly designed MR dosage form include improved efficacy and reduced adverse events, increased convenience and patient compliance, optimized performance, a greater selectivity of activity or new indications. A clinically successful MR product with enhanced medical benefits also offers commercial advantages, such as product differentiation and/or line extension, maximized drug potential and market expansion, and increased cost-effectiveness.[1,2,3] As a result, MR dosage form development has been an important tool of product line extension, and an integral part of product lifecycle management (LCM) strategy that is addressed in Chapter 40.

Drug release modification is a technique or approach by which the delivery pattern of a therapeutic agent is altered via engineering of physical, chemical, and/or biological components into delivery systems for achieving desired/target plasma drug levels defined by clinical pharmacology. According to the United States Food and Drug Administration (FDA), drug release characteristics of time, course, and/or location of an MR system are chosen to accomplish therapeutic or convenience objectives not offered by conventional dosage forms.[4] More specifically, MR solid oral dosage forms include extended-release (ER) and delayed-release (DR) products. A DR dosage

form releases a drug (or drugs) at a time other than immediately following oral administration. An ER dosage form is formulated to make the drug available over an extended period after ingestion, thus allowing a reduction in dosing frequency compared to a drug presented as a conventional dosage form, e.g., a solution or an immediate-release (IR) dosage form. For oral applications, the term "extended-release" is usually interchangeable with "sustained-release," "prolonged-release" or "controlled-release."

The design objective for modifying oral drug release is to alter the rate of drug input (dissolution/ absorption) in the intestinal lumen to achieve a predetermined plasma profile. Common modes of oral MR delivery include:

1. delayed-release (e.g., using an enteric coating);
2. site-specific or timed release (e.g., for colonic delivery);
3. extended-release (e.g., zero-order, first-order, biphasic release, etc.);
4. programmed release (e.g., pulsatile, delayed extended-release, etc.).

Figure 20.1 illustrates some examples of modified release delivery profiles. Significant clinical and scientific advances have been made over the last two decades in delivering therapeutic agents via a non-monotonic pattern at predetermined time intervals as a result of an improved understanding of the relationship between clinical pharmacology, on the one hand, and bodily physiology and biological conditions, on the other. For example, many body functions and diseases follow a circadian rhythm (e.g., daily fluctuations of hormones, gastric secretion and emptying,

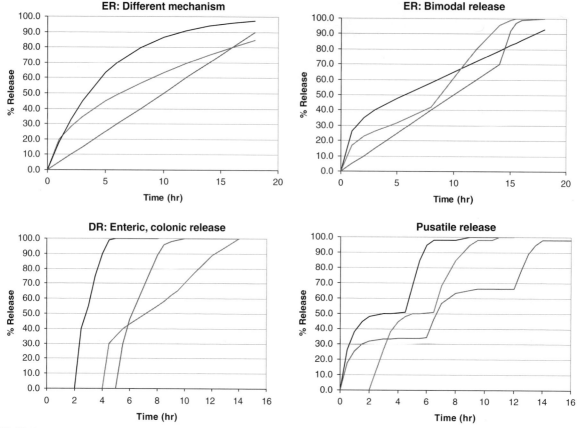

FIGURE 20.1   Examples of oral modified release profiles

bronchial asthma, myocardial infarction, angina, rheumatic disease, ulcer, and hypertension). By timing the administration of a programed release device, therapeutic plasma concentration can be obtained at an optimal time to counter the diurnal nature of certain diseases, such as angina, hypertension, asthmatic attacks or stiffness of arthritic patients during early morning hours, and heart attacks at night. Classic examples of utilizing MR delivery that have achieved significant clinical and commercial successes include modified-release products of Nifedipine, Methylphenidate, Mesalamine, Verapamil, and Diltiazem, to name a few. For example, Procardia® XL is a zero-order release tablet of Nifedipine that not only reduces dosing frequency from t.i.d. to once-daily, but also drastically improves the efficacy-to-safety ratio. Controlling the input rate results in gradual decrease in blood pressure, without the increase in heart rate and syncope associated with t.i.d. administration. Methylphenidate is a compound indicated for attention deficit hyperactivity disorder (ADHD) without patent protection. Several new MR products of methylphenidate were introduced in the 1990s by different developers that offer clear

clinical advantages over the products on the market (e.g., Ritalin®, Ritalin® SR). These products include a bimodal extended-release tablet (Concerta®), capsule (Metadate® CD), and a pulsatile-release capsule (Ritalin® LA,). All of them were designed to produce fluctuation of blood levels over time to overcome acute tolerance associated with a constant rate of delivery, thus enabling dosing convenience of this controlled drug for school children. Asacol® and Lialda™ are delayed-release tablets designed to release mesalamine in the distal ileum and/or colon for ulcerative colitis treatment, while Pentasa® is an extended-release capsule that delivers the same active throughout the gastrointestinal tract.

Hypertension and angina remain two of the most important risk factors for cardiovascular morbidity and mortality. MR products of cardiovascular drugs have been successfully developed to address the pharmacokinetic and circadian challenges to controlling blood pressure and angina by matching drug release to the natural circadian rhythms of the cardiovascular system, i.e., chronotherapeutic drug delivery. Examples of such cardiovascular chronotherapeutic products include Adalat® CC tablets that provide zero-order extended-release followed by delayed immediate release of Nifedipine, as well as Covera-HS® tablets and Verelan® PM capsules, both of which utilize delayed extended-release of verapamil. Following bedtime administration, these products provide a higher concentration of drug in the blood to protect against the early-morning increase in blood pressure and heart rate, while maintaining effective blood pressure reduction for 24 hours. Another classic example is Diltiazem hydrochloride, also a calcium antagonist, for the treatment of hypertension. Three generations of dosage forms were developed with increasing clinical success and commercial competitiveness between the 1980s and 1990s. Annual revenues were approximately $260, $400, and $900 millions for IR tablets (Cardizem®) in 1988, twice-daily ER capsules (Cardizem® SR) in 1991, and once-daily ER capsules (Cardizem® CD) in 1996, respectively. Several years after patent expiry of the active ingredient, another new ER dosage form designed for chronotherapy (Cardizem® LA) was introduced to the market in 2003.

Many compounds are not suitable for MR delivery, due to a variety of reasons, such as undesirable drug properties, dose, lack of pharmacological rationale or technical feasibility. Otherwise, solely for the purpose of convenience one would expect very few marketed drug products with a dosing frequency of more than twice a day. Furthermore, despite many successes with developing oral modified-release products, as many or more failed attempts went unreported in the R&D laboratories of the pharmaceutical industry. Generally, failures in the innovator companies can be partly attributed to the simple fact that the molecule of interest is not feasible for MR delivery. It may also be related to a lack of expertise in rational design and development of a robust MR product. For generic companies, unsuccessful attempts are mostly related to inadequate knowledge and skill in developing MR products and/or overcoming patent hurdles, because feasibility of the active has already been proven by the innovator's product. This chapter provides an overview of current MR technologies and a rational approach to delivery system design. Case studies are used to illustrate how drug property and formulation influence the design and performance of oral MR delivery systems.

20.2 ORAL MODIFIED RELEASE TECHNOLOGIES AND DRUG DELIVERY SYSTEMS

Oral MR drug delivery technology has been applied to new product development for more than 60 years.

Over the past three decades, tremendous progress has been made in the development of theory, mathematical modeling, new rate-controlling materials, and technology platforms, as well as processing technologies. In particular, the emergence of high performance polymers and aqueous-based polymeric dispersions has made conventional processing technology more adaptable to manufacturing MR dosage forms. Today, oral MR technology has become more commonly utilized for in-house development of new products at both innovator and generic companies.

20.2.1 Common Oral Extended-release Systems

Various physical and chemical approaches have been successfully applied to produce well-characterized delivery systems that extend drug input into the GI tract within the specifications of the desired release profile. Today, most proprietary and nonproprietary ER technologies are based on polymeric systems. The fundamental design principles, theoretical considerations, and applications of these systems have been extensively addressed and reviewed.[1,5,6,7] A survey of commercial ER oral solid products indicates that most systems fall into one of three broad categories: matrix, reservoir (or membrane controlled), and osmotic systems (see Table 20.1). Drug release from these ER delivery systems generally involves one or a combination of the following mechanisms: drug diffusion (through pores of a barrier, through tortuous channels or through a viscous gel layer between polymer chains), system swelling (followed by diffusion and/or erosion and dissolution) or osmotic pressure-induced release (drug solution, suspension or wetted mass forced out of the system). Each type of system has its advantages and shortcomings with respect to the performance, applicability, manufacture, control, development time, and cost, etc.

Matrix Systems

In a matrix system, the drug substance is homogeneously mixed into the rate-controlling material(s) and other inactive ingredients as a crystalline, amorphous or, in rare cases, molecular dispersion. Drug release occurs either by drug diffusion and/or erosion of the matrix system. Based on the characteristics of the rate-controlling material, the matrix system can be divided into: (a) hydrophilic; and (b) hydrophobic systems, as shown in Figure 20.2. For practical purposes, the former refers to a matrix system in which the rate-controlling materials are water-soluble and/or swellable, while the latter consists of a water-insoluble inert matrix with minimum swelling. Matrix systems consisting of a mixture of hydrophilic and hydrophobic rate-controlling materials belong to one of the two systems, depending on the dominant mechanism of drug release control. For instance, a matrix containing both types of polymers can be considered a hydrophilic matrix if the release control function and release kinetics (mechanism) remain essentially

TABLE 20.1   Oral extended release systems commonly utilized in commercial products

	Matrix	Reservoir	Osmotic
Systems	Hydrophilic matrix Erosion/diffusion controlled Swelling/erosion controlled Hydrophobic matrix Homogenous (dissolved drugs) Heterogeneous (dispersed drugs)	Membrane controlled Constant activity Non-constant activity Membrane-matrix Combination	Elementary osmotic pump Microporous osmotic pump Layered osmotic pump (e.g., Push-Pull®, Push-Stick®)
Common dosage forms	Monolithic tablet Multi-unit minitablets Layered tablet Compression coated tablet	Multi-unit coated beads Multi-unit coated minitablets Monolithic coated tablet	Coated monolithic tablet Coated layered tablet

unchanged when the insoluble hydrophobic polymer is substituted with a conventional insoluble excipient (e.g., dicalcium phosphate) that does not possess a rate-controlling property. The same holds true for a hydrophobic system, if the hydrophilic polymer is substituted with a soluble excipient (e.g., lactose). The matrix system has been most widely utilized to provide extended delivery of drug substances because of its effectiveness and the capability of accommodating both low- and high-loading of drugs with a wide range of physical and chemical properties. From a product development point of view, it is cost-effective and easy to scale-up and manufacture. In addition, this type of system is also suitable for in-house development, since it is usually manufactured using conventional processes and equipment. However, the release characteristics of a matrix (e.g., kinetics and pH-dependency) are usually determined by the property of the drug substance. To alter release profiles or to achieve unique release patterns (e.g., biphasic or delayed ER), a more complex design and process, such as a layered or compression coated tablet, is sometimes required. Furthermore, a matrix system typically lacks flexibility in offering the multiple strengths that are usually required for phase 1–3 clinical studies in developing a new chemical entity (NCE), because compositionally proportional dosage forms of different strengths usually do not have the same release rate. Thus, additional resources and time are often required for new dosage strengths, except for low dose drugs (e.g., drug loading <5%).

Hydrophilic Matrix Systems

Hydrophilic matrix systems are polymer-based drug delivery systems in which two competing

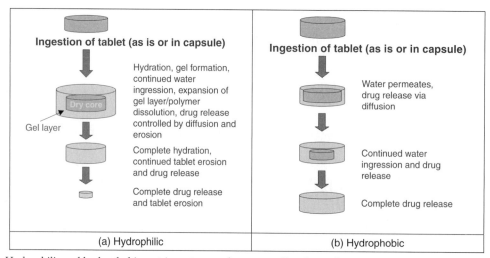

FIGURE 20.2   Hydrophilic and hydrophobic matrix systems and corresponding drug release process

mechanisms are involved in the drug release: Fickian diffusional release, and relaxational release. The primary rate-controlling materials are polymers that hydrate and swell rapidly in an aqueous medium, and form a gel layer on the surface of the system. Diffusion across the viscous gel layer is not the only drug release pathway, as erosion of the matrix following polymer relaxation also contributes to the overall release. The relative contribution of each component to total release is primarily dependent upon the properties of a given drug and matrix composition. For instance, the release of a sparingly soluble drug from hydrophilic matrices involves the simultaneous ingress of water and desorption of drug via a swelling-controlled diffusion mechanism. As water penetrates into a glassy matrix and lowers the polymer glass transition temperature, the polymer swells, slowly disentangles, and eventually dissolves, releasing the undissolved drug. At the same time, the dissolved drug diffuses through this swollen rubbery region into the external releasing medium. This type of diffusion, with concurrent swelling and erosion, generally does not follow a Fickian diffusion mechanism. The continuously changing variables that affect drug release (e.g., diffusion pathlength, viscosity, system dimension, etc.) make obtaining a mechanistic equation or model describing the release profile impossible. Over the past three decades, various models have been explored and developed to achieve a fundamental understanding of drug release from hydrophilic matrices.[6,7,8,9,10,11,12,13,14,15] Among them, a semi-empirical exponent equation that was introduced in the mid-1980s has been widely used to describe drug release behavior from hydrophilic matrix systems:[16,17]

$$Q = kt^n \qquad (20.1)$$

where:

Q is the fraction of drug released in time t
k is the rate constant incorporating characteristics of the macromolecular network system and the drug
n is the diffusional exponent.

This equation has been widely used in this field.[18,19,20,21] It has been shown that the value of n is indicative of the drug release mechanism. For $n = 0.5$, drug release follows a Fickian diffusion mechanism which is driven by a chemical potential gradient. For $n = 1$, drug release occurs via relaxational transport, which is associated with stresses and phase-transition in hydrated polymers. For $1 > n > 0.5$, non-Fickian diffusion behavior is often observed as a result of

contributions from diffusion and polymer erosion. This is also termed "anomalous" release.

In order to describe relaxational transport, Peppas and Sahlin derived the following equation by introducing a second term into Equation 20.1:[19]

$$Q = k_1 t^n + k_2 t^{2n} \qquad (20.2)$$

where k_1 and k_2 are constants reflecting the relative contributions of Fickian and relaxation mechanisms. In the case where surface area is fixed, the value of n should be equal to 0.5. Thus, Equation 20.2 becomes:

$$Q = k_1 t^{0.5} + k_2 t \qquad (20.3)$$

where the first and second terms represent drug release due to diffusion and polymer erosion, respectively. This equation was later successfully applied to describe drug release from hydrophilic matrices.[21,22]

Since the early 1990s, additional models have been investigated in an attempt to enhance the understanding of the matrix delivery systems.[23,24,25,26] One of the examples is the so-called "Spaghetti" model proposed to gain insight into the complex release process from hydrophilic matrix systems. This model treats polymer erosion as diffusion of polymer across an unstirred "diffusion layer" adjacent to the polymer gel layer. Thus, two competitive diffusional processes contribute to overall drug release, i.e., diffusion of drug through the gel layer and diffusion of polymer across the diffusion layer. In addition to the solubility of the drug molecules that defines the diffusion component, polymer disentanglement concentration ($C_{p,dis}$) defined in Equation 20.4 is used to gauge the contribution of polymer diffusion/dissolution:[27]

$$(C_{p,dis})_{eq} = 0.05 \left(\frac{MW_p X_p}{96\,000} \right)^{-0.8} \qquad (20.4)$$

$$M_p \approx kt^1 \qquad (20.5)$$

MW_p and X_p denote the molecular weight and weight fraction of polymer in the matrix, respectively, and M_p is polymer release at time t. Interestingly, the release profile of polymer (Equation 20.5) resembles that for an erosion-controlled system in Equation 20.1. It should be noted that $C_{p,dis}$ is an intrinsic property of the polymer while $(C_{p,dis})_{eq}$ is an "equivalent" $C_{p,dis}$ of polymer in a matrix. One may consider $C_{p,dis}$ as the equivalent "solubility" of polymer, as it defines the concentration at which a polymer detaches from a pure polymer system. Conceptually, the relative contribution of both mechanisms can be characterized by the solubility ratio of the drug, C_s to $(C_{p,dis})_{eq}$:

If $\dfrac{C_s}{(C_{p,dis})_{eq}} >> 1$, then $Q_t = kt^{0.5}$ (release is controlled by drug diffusion)

If $\dfrac{C_s}{(C_{p,dis})_{eq}} << 1$, then $Q_t = kt^1$ (release is controlled by polymer erosion)

Thus, drug release profiles from a hydrophilic matrix vary significantly with formulation design and solubility of the drug. For insoluble compounds, zero-order release is readily attainable as C_s values are generally lower than $(C_{p,dis})_{eq}$. For soluble drugs, release kinetics typically follow the square-root-of-time relationship. To achieve zero-order release, one would need to increase $(C_{p,dis})_{eq}$ in the matrix to lower the ratio of C_s to $(C_{p,dis})_{eq}$, for example, by using polymers of low MW_p or decreasing X_p according to Equation 20.4. However, the practical feasibility of this approach is dependent on the ratio, limited choice of polymer, and the minimum MW_p and/or X_p that is often required to form a robust matrix for extended release.

Hydrophobic Matrix Systems

The hydrophobic matrix system was the earliest oral extended-release platform for medicinal use. In fact, its prototypes can be traced back to the second century BC and the fourth century AD, respectively, when animal fats and wax pills were used to prolong the medicinal effects of Chinese medicines.[28] For example, medical practitioners were instructed to "use wax pills for their resistance to dissolve thereby achieving the effect gradually and slowly."[29,30] In modern medicine, the matrix technology has been successfully applied to many commercial products for many decades. For example, Premarin® tablets, one of the classic examples, have been on the market since 1942. In a hydrophobic inert matrix system, the drug is dispersed throughout a matrix, which involves essentially negligible increase of the device surface or change in dimension. For a homogeneous monolithic matrix system, the release behavior can be described by the Higuchi equation, subject to the matrix-boundary conditions:[31]

$$M_t = [DC_s(2A - C_s)t]^{1/2} \qquad (20.6)$$

where:

Q_t is the drug released per unit area at time t
A is the drug loading per unit volume

C_s is drug solubility
D is the diffusion coefficient in the matrix phase.

Equation 20.6 was derived based on the assumptions that: (1) a pseudo-steady state exists; (2) the drug particles are small compared to the average distance of diffusion; (3) the diffusion coefficient is constant; (4) perfect sink conditions exist in the external media; (5) only the diffusion process occurs; (6) the drug concentration in the matrix is greater than the drug solubility in the polymer; and (7) no interaction between drug and matrix takes place. In the case of $A >> C_s$, Equation 20.6 reduces to:

$$M_t = [2DAC_s t]^{1/2} \qquad (20.7)$$

Thus, the amount of drug released is proportional to the square root of time, A, D, and C_s.

Drug release from a porous monolithic matrix system involves the simultaneous penetration of surrounding liquid, dissolution of the drug, and leaching out of the drug through interstitial channels or pores. The volume and length of the openings in the matrix must be accounted for in the diffusion equation, leading to a second form of the Higuchi equation:[32]

$$M_t = \left[\varepsilon C_s (2A - \varepsilon C_s)\frac{D_a}{\tau}t\right]^{1/2} \qquad (20.8)$$

ε and τ are the porosity and tortuosity of the matrix, respectively, and D_a is the drug diffusion coefficient in the release medium. Tortuosity is introduced to account for an increase in diffusion path length, due to branching and bending of the pores. Similarly, Equation 20.9 can be derived based on pseudo-steady state approximation ($A >> C_s$):

$$M_t = \left[2D_a AC_s \frac{\varepsilon}{\tau}t\right]^{1/2} \qquad (20.9)$$

The porosity, ε, in Equations 20.8 and 20.9, is the fraction of matrix that exists as pores or channels, into which the surrounding liquid can ingress. It is the total porosity of the matrix after the drug has been extracted. The total porosity consists of the initial porosity, ε_a, due to air or void space in the matrix before the leaching process begins, and the porosity created by extracting the drug, ε_d, and the water soluble excipients, ε_{ex}:[33,34]

$$\varepsilon = \varepsilon_a + \varepsilon_d + \varepsilon_{ex} = \varepsilon_a + \frac{A}{\rho} + \frac{A_{ex}}{\rho_{ex}} \qquad (20.10)$$

ρ is the drug density, and ρ_{ex} and A_{ex} are the density and the concentration of water soluble excipient, respectively. When no water-soluble excipient is present in the matrix, and initial porosity, ε_a, is smaller than the porosity, ε_d, Equation 20.10 becomes:

$$\varepsilon \cong \varepsilon_d = \frac{A}{\rho} \qquad (20.11)$$

Hence, Equations 20.8 and 20.9 yield:

$$M_t = A\left[\left(2 - \frac{C_s}{\rho}\right)\frac{D_a C_s}{\tau \rho}t\right]^{1/2} \qquad (20.12)$$

$$M_t = A\left[\frac{2D_a C_s}{\tau \rho}t\right]^{1/2} \qquad (20.13)$$

Similar to Equation 20.7, a square-root-of-time release profile is expected with a porous monolith. In contrast to the homogeneous matrix system, the release from such system is proportional to drug loading, A. It should be noted that: (1) the Higuchi equation was originally derived for planar diffusion into a perfect sink; (2) the square-root-of-time relationship only fits data up to approximately 2/3 of the total release. The fundamental theory and basic derivations of the above equations can be found in Chapter 7.

To describe the general release behavior from hydrophobic matrices in the form of slabs, spheres, and cylinders, a simple semi-empirical exponential relation was introduced by Ritger and Peppas in 1987:[35]

$$Q = \frac{M_t}{M_\infty} = kt^n \qquad (20.14)$$

where:

Q is the fractional release
k is a constant
n is the diffusional exponent.

In the case of pure Fickian release, the exponent n has a limiting value of 0.50 for smooth slabs, 0.45 for smooth spheres, and 0.43–0.50 for smooth cylinders, depending on the aspect ratio. In the 1990s, Wu and Zhou analyzed drug release using the finite element method, and showed the dependence of release kinetics on the initial solute loading, the external volume, and the boundary-layer thickness. The model describes the entire process of diffusional release without the pseudo-steady state assumption.[36,37] It was also used to address a variety of diffusional release problems for slabs, spheres, and cylinders using systematic analysis for Stefan-type problems.[38,39] More recently, Yonezawa et al. published a model that can be used to describe the entire release process of a heterogeneous hydrophobic matrix system made from

a physical mixture of wax, soluble excipients, and the actives by compensating the deviation from the pseudo-steady state approximation (A >> Cs) at the later portion of the release profiles.[40,41,42] In general, hydrophobic matrix systems are not suitable for insoluble drugs, because the concentration gradient is too low to allow complete drug release within a reasonable timeframe, i.e., gastrointestinal (GI) transit time.

Modulation of drug release profile

Historically, constant-rate delivery has been one of the primary target profiles of extended-release systems for maximized coverage and minimized fluctuation in plasma concentrations, especially for drugs with a narrow therapeutic index. In a diffusion-controlled matrix system, the active agent has a progressively longer distance to travel, and smaller releasing surface, as the diffusion front moves inwardly, resulting in decreasing release rate over time, i.e., nonlinear release characteristics. For hydrophilic matrices, the extent of drug release deviation from zero-order kinetics depends on the ratio of C_s to $(C_{p,dis})_{eq}$. Drugs with relatively high C_s typically exhibit a diffusion-controlled release profile. To overcome the inherently non-zero-order kinetics due to decreasing surface area and increasing diffusional pathlength associated with the diffusion-controlled matrix systems, considerable efforts have been, and continue to be, expended on modifying the delivery system. Over the past several decades, many creative designs have been reported that effectively alter the inherent nonlinear release behavior.[23,43,44,45,46,47,48,49,50,51,52,53,54,55,56] For example, non-uniform drug loading was used to offset the decrease in release rate by increasing the diffusional driving force over time. Geometric factors, including cone shape, biconcave, donut shape, hemisphere with cavity, core-in-cup, etc., were utilized to compensate for the decreasing release rate by increasing drug release surface over time. Control of matrix erosion, surface area and swelling, and matrix–membrane combinations have also been shown to be effective in providing zero-order or near zero-order release kinetics. However, many of these designs are more difficult to manufacture or impractical for commercialization.

With the growing need for optimizing clinical therapy, and improved understanding of pharmacokinetics–pharmacodynamics (PK–PD) relationships, additional delivery profiles other than zero-order kinetics are often desired, such as the profiles illustrated in Figure 20.1. These targeted extended-delivery patterns vary with drugs, depending on their respective clinical pharmacology. In order to produce matrix systems having some of these unique drug release patterns or to overcome the inherent limitations such as pH-dependency of drug release, modifications to both hydrophilic and hydrophobic matrices have been investigated. Many of them have been successfully applied to commercial products. Among them are functionally coated matrix, layered tablet, compression coating, combined use of multiple polymers, functional excipients or geometry. For example, TIMERx® and Geminex® (bilayer) matrix systems utilize the synergistic interaction of xanthum gum and locust bean gum in an aqueous environment to form a strong gel with a slowly-eroding core. Matrix systems containing both hydrophilic and hydrophobic rate-controlling materials also offer certain advantages.[57] Below are examples of specific areas in which significant progress has been made over the years in improving matrix delivery systems. Many of the functional enhancements are achieved via utilization of interactions between polymer and drug, polymer and polymer, drug and excipients or polymer–excipients.

pH-independent drug release

Theoretically, pH-independent release is desirable for a more consistent *in vivo* delivery, because pH values in the GI tract vary with location and food intake. Incorporation of buffering agents was investigated to provide constant local pH within a dosage form, and thus pH-independent release profiles.[58,59] However, many buffering agents are soluble small molecules that may leach out of the matrix system at a faster rate than that of the active, losing their intended function. The effectiveness of this approach is highly dependent on buffering capacity, quantity, solubility, and molecular weight relative to the active. Incorporating ionic polymers, such as alginate, anionic polymers containing methacrylic acid or phthalate functional groups, cationic polymers with dimethylaminoethyl methacrylate, etc., in a matrix system is more effective in maintaining a constant local pH environment.[60,61,62] Howard et al., and Zhang et al., showed pH-independent zero-order release of a soluble basic drug (Verapamil HCL) using alginate/HPMC[63] and Alginate/HPMC/enteric polymer,[64] respectively. Qiu et al. investigated combined HPMC/cationic polymer for pH-independent release and altered release kinetics of acidic molecules.[65] When using buffering agents, it is important to determine whether they may interact with either drug molecules or rate-controlling polymers. Such interactions can result in undesired outcomes such as slow drug release or disruption of gel structure.[66] Recently, a so-called self-correcting hydrophilic matrix having strong gels was reported, and shown to be insensitive to both pH and stirring condition.[67,68] This self-correcting

system was based on the incorporation of a high concentration of electrolytes. First, highly concentrated salts help maintain local pH, and thus pH-independent release. Secondly, electrolytes yield salted-out regions that are resistant to erosion and hydrodynamics. However, its potential advantages over a conventional matrix system *in vivo* remain to be confirmed.

Solubility enhancement

Developing ER formulations of poorly soluble drug can sometimes be challenging. Conceptually, certain insoluble drugs may exhibit a "natural" ER behavior when a correct balance between particle size distribution and intrinsic dissolution rate is achieved, such that the slow particle dissolution *in vivo* takes place within the drug particle's transit time through the absorption window in the GI tract. However, using formulation technology to control the release rate is generally more desirable with respect to delivery control, consistency, and completion within GI residence time. Thus, solubilization in a matrix system is sometimes required for this purpose. It may also be needed for the complete absorption of the drug released in the lower bowl due to the limited amount of water available for dissolution. Increased solubility can be obtained through use of amorphous drug or a soluble complex. Rao et al. showed that both enhanced and pH-independent release of insoluble drugs was achieved using cyclodextrin as a complexation agent in an HPMC based matrix.[69] Because of the slow eroding nature of the matrix system, complexation can take place *in situ*. Thus, it does not require a prior formation of the complex using a solution-mediated process. Tanaka et al. recently reported an eroding hydrophobic matrix system containing amorphous solid dispersion of nilvadipine with hydroxypropyl cellulose (L-HPC).[70] Supersaturation was achieved without any recrystallization during dissolution, likely a result of crystallization inhibition by HPC. In addition, the release rate was found to be independent of pH and agitation.

Modification of release kinetics

One of the limitations in controlling the release rate of soluble drugs using a hydrophobic or hydrophilic matrix system is the inherently nonlinear release kinetics. In addition to the use of unique geometry or non-uniform drug loading mentioned above, commercially viable designs have been utilized to achieve zero-order drug release.[71] For instance, layered matrix systems were shown to be effective through control of swelling and surface.[46] Hydrophobic matrices were press-coated with hydrophilic and/or hydrophobic barrier layer(s) to provide delayed drug release from the barrier surface to compensate for the decreasing release rate over time.[72] The same type of design can also be used to effectively control the release rate of highly soluble drugs that are difficult to slow down using monolithic hydrophilic or hydrophobic matrices.[73] Successful use of synergies of polymers for release control of soluble compounds was proven *in vitro* and *in vivo* with the TIMERx® delivery matrix system. In studying a polymer complex between methylcellulose (MC) and carboxyvinylpolymer (CP) on the release characteristics of phenacetin (PHE), Ozeki et al. showed that the release profile of PHE from 20% solid dispersion granules in MC-CP complex can be modulated via altering the MC/CP ratio, and the molecular weight of MC. Contributions of diffusion and polymer erosion to PHE release increased as the molecular weight of the MC increased.[74] The synergistic effect of Starch 1500 in an HPMC-based matrix was recently reported for a soluble drug molecule *in vitro*.[75] However, the underlying mechanism of this observation and *in vivo* performance require further investigation. While the desired outcome of release modification may be achieved by utilizing interactions between polymer and drug or excipients, it is always beneficial to investigate the underlying mechanism of the interactions based on both theoretical consideration and advanced analytical techniques in order to understand the practical utility, application, control, and limitations.[76,77]

Reservoir Polymeric Systems

A typical reservoir system consists of a core containing solid drug or highly concentrated drug solution surrounded by a film or membrane of a rate-controlling material. In this design, the only structure effectively limiting the release of the drug is the polymer layer surrounding the reservoir. Based on Fick's first law of diffusion, the governing one-dimensional release rate of a drug from a reservoir system at steady state is given by:

$$\frac{dM_t}{dt} = \frac{DSK}{L} \Delta C \qquad (20.15)$$

where:

M_t is the total amount of drug released at time t
D is the diffusion coefficient of the drug
S is the effective membrane or barrier surface area for drug diffusion, L is the diffusional pathlength (e.g., thickness of the film)
K is the partition coefficient of drug between the barrier membrane and external aqueous phases
ΔC is the drug concentration gradient between the solubility, C_s, in the reservoir and the drug concentration, C_e, in the external aqueous medium.

Since the membrane coating is essentially uniform in composition and thickness, for a given molecule and system composition, D, S, K, L, and ΔC are constant in Equation 20.15 under sink conditions ($C_s >> C_e$). Thus the amount of drug released as a function of time can be obtained by integration:

$$M_t = \left[\frac{DSK\Delta C}{L}\right] t = kt \qquad (20.16)$$

k is the release rate constant. The driving force of such systems is the concentration gradient of active molecules between reservoir and sink. Thus, the drug release from this type of system follows apparent zero-order kinetics until ΔC is no longer constant, due to complete dissolution of the solid drug in the core. Because the reservoir system relies on ΔC as the driving force for drug diffusion, it is applicable to soluble drugs. For insoluble drugs, the values of C_s may be too low to render adequate driving force, resulting in over-attenuated and incomplete drug release.

In developing oral products based on ER reservoir technology, polymer film-coated beads or tablets and microencapsulates (microparticles, microspheres or nanoparticles) are common dosage form presentations. A polymer membrane that contains the drug also contains a hydrophilic and/or leachable additive (e.g., a second polymer, surfactant or plasticizer, etc.) to give a porous device, offering a predetermined resistance to drug diffusion from the reservoir to the sink. The resistance provided is a function of film thickness, and characteristics of both the film and the migrating species in a given environment. In a real world product, the mechanisms of drug release from the film-coated dosage forms can be categorized into:

1. transport of the drug through a network of capillaries filled with dissolution media ($K = 1$);
2. transport of the drug through the homogeneous film barrier by diffusion;
3. transport of the drug through a hydrated swollen film; and
4. transport of the drug through flaws, cracks, and imperfections within the coating matrix ($K = 1$).[78,79,80]

The key factors affecting drug diffusion are polymers and pore formers in the membrane coat, drug load, and solubility.[81] The preferred reservoir system normally consists of many coated units such as beads, pellets, and minitablets. In fact, most of the marketed products based on the reservoir system are multi-unit dosage forms. Unlike a single-unit tablet, the number of particulates of a reservoir system is often sufficient to minimize or eliminate the impact of any coating defect associated with a limited number of units. An important feature of a multi-unit system is that tailored drug release can be readily obtained by combining subunits with different release characteristics. The multi-unit system is also adaptable to varying dose strengths, without the need of a new formulation. This is highly desirable during the clinical development program of the new drug candidates, where dose levels are frequently adjusted based on the clinical study results.

Similar to matrix systems, drug release from a reservoir system usually varies with pH, unless the solubility of the active is pH-independent. To achieve pH-independent release for drugs with pH-dependent solubility, C_s in the core needs to remain unchanged. Success with incorporating buffering agents to maintain constant pH in the core has been reported. As with the pH-independent matrix system discussed previously, the effectiveness of this approach also depends on the loading, buffering capacity, relative quantity, solubility, and molecular weight of the buffering agent relative to the drug. Finally, the osmotic pressure in the reservoir can become a significant factor in influencing release control depending on loading and solubility of both the active and certain soluble excipients. In some cases, the osmotic components may lead to the undesired coating rupture.

Osmotic Pump Systems

The osmotic pump system is similar to a reservoir device, but contains an osmotic agent that acts to imbibe water from the surrounding medium via a semipermeable membrane. Such a device, called the elementary osmotic pump (EOP), was first described by Theeuwes and Higuchi in 1975.[82] The delivery of the active agent from the device is controlled by water influx across the semipermeable membrane. The drug is forced out of an orifice in the device by the osmotic pressure generated within the device. The size of the orifice is designed to minimize solute diffusion, while preventing the build up of a hydrostatic pressure head that has the effect of decreasing the osmotic pressure and changing the volume of the device.

In an osmotic system, the rate of water imbibition into the system in terms of volume can be expressed as:

$$\frac{dV}{dt} = \frac{Ak}{l}(\Delta\pi - \Delta P) \tag{20.17}$$

where:

dV/dt is the rate of water flow
k is the hydraulic permeability
A is the membrane area
l is the thickness
$\Delta\pi$ is the osmotic pressure difference
ΔP is the hydrostatic pressure difference.

When the device is rigid, the volume of the device remains constant during operation. Thus, the amount of drug released at time t can be expressed by:

$$\frac{dM}{dt} = \frac{dV}{dt}[S] \tag{20.18}$$

$[S]$ is the drug solubility. When the hydrostatic pressure difference is negligible, and there is an excess of solid (saturated solution) in the device, Equation 20.18 becomes:

$$\frac{dM}{dt} = \frac{kA}{l}\Delta\pi[S] \tag{20.19}$$

Therefore, the drug release rate remains constant, delivering a volume equal to the volume of water uptake.

In developing oral products, two types of osmotic pump systems have frequently been used, a one-chamber EOP system, and a two-chamber system (e.g., Push-Pull® and Push-Stick®). A comparison of different types of osmotic devices is provided in Table 20.2. In general, an EOP system is only feasible for molecules with a limited range of solubility, e.g., approximately 50–300 mg/ml, to achieve zero-order and complete release. To overcome such limitations McClelland et al. investigated the conversion of release profiles from first-order to zero-order kinetics for highly soluble (>590 mg/ml) diltiazem hydrochloride released from controlled-porosity osmotic pump devices. By utilizing the common ion effect, the solubility was reduced in the presence of NaCl to 155 mg/ml. As a result, zero-order drug release was achieved over a 14- to 16-hour period. To maintain an effective NaCl concentration within the drug compartment over the release duration, NaCl granules were coated with a microporous cellulose acetate butyrate 381–20 film.[83] In recent years, studies have shown more general application of controlled-porosity osmotic pump system to drugs with different properties.[84,85] For instance, Okimoto et al. described the successful application of a controlled-porosity osmotic pump tablet utilizing (SBE)7m-beta-cyclodextrin as both a solubilizer and an osmotic agent for drugs with varying physical properties, including five poorly soluble and two highly water-soluble drugs.[86] Sotthivirat et al. recently demonstrated that the incorporation of sulfobutylether-cyclodextrin results in the complete and sustained release of a sparingly water-soluble drug, prednisolone from a controlled porosity-osmotic pump pellet dosage form.[87]

The two-chamber device was designed mainly to accommodate less soluble molecules and/or higher drug loading. It consists of a bilayer tablet compressed

TABLE 20.2 Comparison of selected oral osmotic pump systems

Osmotic system	Similarity	Difference
EOP	Osmotic core	Single layer tablet
	Semipermeable membrane controls water flow	One small orifice
		Drug released as a solution
Push-Pull®		Bilayer tablet often latitudinally compressed
		Osmotic agent in both layers
		One or more small orifices
		Drug released as a solution or suspension
Push-Stick®		Bilayer tablet longitudinally compressed
		Osmotic agent in push layer
		One large orifice
		Drug released as a wet mass that requires subsequent disintegration and dissolution
EnSo Trol®		Single layer tablet
		One or more small orifices
		Incorporation of wicking agent and solubility enhancer
		Drug released as a solution
Controlled porosity and single composition osmotic tablet™ (SCOT)		Single layer tablet
		No predrilled orifice
		Drug released as a solution or wet mass through channels or cracks formed *in situ*
L-OROS™		Single softgel capsule
		One small orifice
		Drug released as a liquid

latitudinally or longitudinally, with one push layer containing a highly swellable polymer and a drug layer (Figure 20.3). In the gastrointestinal tract, water is imbibed through the semipermeable membrane into both layers as a result of the osmotic activity gradient established across the membrane by the osmotic excipients. As both the drug and push layers hydrate, a drug suspension (e.g., in Push-Pull®) or semi-solid mass (e.g., in Push-Stick®) is formed *in situ*, and the push layer begins to expand as a result of the hydration and swelling of the hydrophilic polymers. Delivery of the drug substance begins when the volumetric expansion of the osmotic push layer begins to "push" the active in the drug layer through the orifice, which is drilled through the semipermeable membrane on the drug layer side. Since rate control resides within the rate-controlling membrane, drug release is essentially insensitive to environmental effects, such as pH, agitation, and type of apparatus. But this does not apply to the Push-Stick® system, which contains a significantly larger orifice that is required for the delivery

of the high payload. Since the 1990s, new single layer osmotic pump tablets have been designed, and successfully applied to developing commercial products for poorly soluble drugs. The designs are based on the incorporation of solubility enhancement in the tablet core (e.g., EnSoTrol®) or *in situ* creation of larger ports or channels for delivering less soluble compounds (e.g, SCOT™: Single Composition Osmotic Tablet™).

In summary, classic osmotic pump systems offer zero-order release profile that is independent of the drug properties and release environment in most cases. However, fabrication of this type of system often requires specialized equipment and complex processes. This is particularly true with the two-chamber systems, which often translates into higher cost, longer development time, and larger numbers of formulation and processing variables to define and control. Additional drawbacks include: (1) the solvent process required for semipermeable membrane coating; (2) sensitivity of the drug release to variations of device dimension, moisture level, and

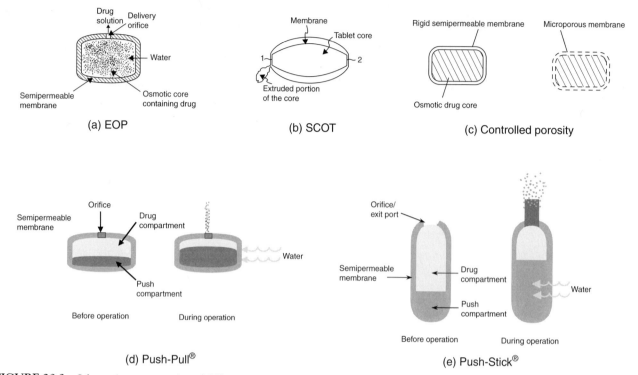

FIGURE 20.3   Schematic representation of different types of osmotic pump systems

membrane uniformity of individual units; and (3) delayed onset of drug release.

Other Extended-release Systems

Additional systems that have been demonstrated to provide extended release are based on formation of less soluble complex or the use of ion-exchange resins,[88] etc. Polysalt flocculates were reported as an effective physico-chemical approach to extending the release of aluminum sulfate through formation of an insoluble complex with sodium carboxymethylcellulose. Drug entrapment was effected by polymeric flocculation, induced by the addition of a physiologically inert electrolyte.[89] More recently, a less soluble interaction product between diltiazem HCl and lambda carrageenan was investigated. Extended release of diltiazem from a compacted tablet was achieved via surface dissolution/erosion. The influence of complex particle size, compression force, pH of the dissolution medium, and compact dimensions on drug release was also evaluated.[90]

Synthetic polymer-based ion exchange resins were a result of advances in polymer chemistry in the middle of the twentieth century. They were first developed for applications in wastewater purification and processing of fermentation products. The utility of these materials for extended delivery of charged drugs

was first suggested by Saunders and Chaudhary.[91] Ion exchange resins are non-absorptive polymeric insoluble particles containing basic or acidic groups in repeating positions on the polymer chain that can form ionic complexes with oppositely charged drugs.[92] The drug is bound to the resin, and released by exchanging with appropriately charged ions in contact with the ion-exchange groups. The interactions are strongly governed by the pH of the medium or by the presence of competing ions. At a particular pH, one of the two entities may become neutralized, depending on their respective pK_a values, thus eliminating the charge. The presence of high ionic strength buffers may reduce electrostatic interactions between the resin and drug, due to a shielding/competitive binding effect. Thus, the resin may carry the drug and release the payload in a certain region of the gastrointestinal tract, due to a pH change or presence of competing ions. Recently, Abdekhodaie et al. developed and experimentally verified new mathematical models for drug release from ion-exchange microspheres.[93,94] The models were successfully applied to investigate the influence of important parameters pertinent to material properties and loading conditions on the kinetics, efficiency, and equilibrium of drug loading to aid the product design. Sriwongjanya and Bodmeier investigated the effect of ion exchange resins when incorporated as release modifiers into the HPMC-based hydrophilic matrix tablets.[95] Two model drugs, propranolol, and diclofenac, were studied. Drug release from matrix tablets containing drug–resin complexes was significantly slower than from the matrix tablets containing drug without resin. Pennkinetic™ technology developed by Pennwalt involves the use of ion-exchange resins in combination with diffusion-controlling membranes to create extended-release liquid dosage forms. Examples of commercial products that utilize ion-exchange resins include Tussionex® Pennkinetic suspension containing hydrocodone and chlorpheniramine, and Codeprex™ extended-release suspension of codeine polistirex/chlorpheniramine polistirex. Additional examples include Duromine, containing the basic drug phentermine forming a complex with an anionic resin, and MS Contin suspension, which uses a polystyrene sulfonate resin. Medical-grade resins are available from a range of suppliers, including Rohm and Haas, and Dow Chemicals. Duolite AP143 is an anionic resin, whereas Amberlite IRP64, Amberlite IRP69, and Amberlite IRP88 are cationic resins marketed by Rohm and Haas.

Drug delivery systems designed to be retained in the upper GI tract have been extensively explored and investigated for targeted and/or extended oral delivery since the 1970s. The primary objective of such systems, especially the gastroretentive devices, is to overcome regional dependency of drug absorption. For ER product, it is intended to prevent a loss of AUC due to truncated absorption of drugs with limited window of absorption. A variety of experimental approaches have been explored, including: (1) utilizing floating (e.g., low density for buoyancy) or settling mechanisms (e.g., high density); (2) bioadhesion; (3) altering motility with active or excipient; and (4) large size to limit gastric emptying, e.g., via expansion by swelling or unfolding.[96,97] The proof-of-concept studies for some of these designs in humans have been reported using direct (e.g., γ-scintigraphy) or indirect (PK) measures. However, none has been shown to function in a reliable and reproducible manner, i.e., consistent performance under fasting conditions with acceptable inter- and intra-subject variability of retention time. In addition, most of the studies were carried out in a limited number of healthy subjects. For oral ER delivery, reproducibility of the gastric retention characteristics is most critical because it directly determines the bioavailability of a product. Therefore, at present there is no credible or reliable gastroretentive technology employed in the marketed products, despite the claims made by some drug delivery companies. However, it is noteworthy that a new expandable system, Accordion Pill™, using the design of a foldable sheet (e.g., ~5 × 2.5 cm × 0.7 mm) has shown promising *in vivo* results based on MRI, γ-scintigraphy, and PK studies. Its prolonged gastric retention with low calorie meals has been demonstrated in healthy volunteers.[98]

20.2.2 Other Common Oral Modified-release Systems

With the improved understanding of an active substance and its clinical pharmacology, various delivery profiles, such as those illustrated in Figure 20.1, are often required for enhanced or more rational and effective clinical therapy. Common examples of these non-monotonic and multi-cargo delivery patterns include delayed drug delivery in the small or large intestines, pulsatile delivery, biphasic delivery (i.e., IR followed ER or ER followed by IR), etc. These drug release profiles can generally be obtained through incorporating a range of immediate-release, delayed-release and extended-release formulation approaches.

Enteric Release

Enteric release is intended to delay the release of the drug (or drugs) until the dosage form has passed through the stomach.[4] The delayed liberation of orally administered drugs has been achieved through a range of formulation approaches, including single- or multiple-unit systems provided with coatings, capsule devices, and osmotic pumps. The earliest physico-chemical approach to delaying drug release is by applying enteric coating to dosage forms as a barrier that controls the release location in the digestive system. Materials used for enteric coating prevent drug release in the stomach, because they are typically acidic polymers that are stable/insoluble at acidic pH. The coatings dissolve rapidly at higher intestinal pH when the dosage forms reach the small intestine, as shown in Figure 20.4. Drugs, such as aspirin, which have an irritant effect on the stomach, can be coated with an enteric film that will only dissolve in the small intestine. Enteric coating is also used to prevent the acidic environment of the stomach from degrading certain acid-labile medications, such as proton pump inhibitors. The common enteric dosage forms include coated tablet or capsule, and coated multi-particulates in a capsule or compressed into a disintegrating tablet.

Colonic Release

Targeting drug delivery to the colonic region of the GI tract has received considerable attention, and is known to offer therapeutic advantages for certain

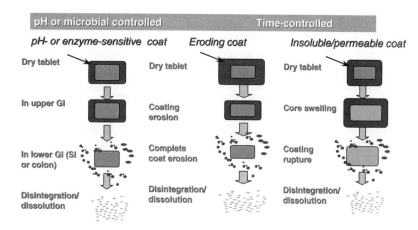

FIGURE 20.4 Examples of different types of delayed-release systems and drug release process

drugs, such as more effective treatment of local disorders of the colon (e.g., ulcerative colitis, Crohn's disease, irritable bowel syndrome, and carcinoma) with reduced incidence of systemic side-effects and lower dosages. Colonic delivery systems are essentially delayed-release dosage forms that are designed to provide either an immediate or sustained release in the large intestine. One of the better-known examples is colonic delivery of mesalazine in the treatment of inflammatory bowel disease. More recently, scientific endeavors in this area have also been driven by the need for a portal for the systemic entry of the active substances, including proteins and peptides that are unstable or poorly absorbed in the small intestine for a variety of reasons (instability, metabolism). For drugs that are well-absorbed throughout the GI tract, sustained delivery in the colon has also been utilized in the treatment of nocturnal asthma or angina, such as the previously mentioned cardiovascular chronotherapeutics products, Adalat® CC and Verelan® PM.

For optimal colonic delivery, the active needs to be protected from the environment of the upper GI tract before being released into the proximal colon. Based on the considerations of the unique features of the colonic environment (pH, transit time, pressure or microflora), various strategies and approaches have been investigated for colon-specific drug delivery. These include coated delivery systems using pH-sensitive or slow eroding polymers, swelling or osmotic controlled systems for timed release, and exploitation of carriers that are degraded specifically by colonic bacteria. Prodrugs have been designed to deliver 5-amino salicylic acid in the colon (e.g., balsalazide, sulfasalazine, olsalazine). Certain plant polysaccharides (such as amylose, inulin, pectin and guar gum), pH-sensitive hydrogels, and microbially degradable polymers, especially azo cross-linked polymers, have

also been studied for targeting drugs to the colon. Among these approaches, coated systems that utilize the transit time and pH differential in the GI tract, as well as prodrugs that rely on colonic bacteria for release, have been utilized in commercial products.

A majority of the marketed colonic delivery products are timed-release systems (see Figure 20.4) that depend on the relatively constant transit time of 3–4 hours in the small intestine. Dosage forms, such as beads or tablets, are coated with enteric polymers that dissolve more slowly at intestinal pH (e.g., Eudragit S). To ensure sufficiently delayed drug release of 3–4 hours following gastric emptying, the weight gain of film-coating is significantly higher than that used in enteric coating. Slowly eroding coating by compression or spraying has also been shown to be effective in timing drug release.[99] The concept of using pH alone as a trigger to release a drug in the colon is based on the pH variations along the GI tract. However, the reliability of this approach *in vivo* is questionable considering (1) the relative small pH difference between small and large intestines, (2) the high inter- and intra-subject variability of intestinal pH, and (3) the impact of disease state on pH. The presence of azo reductase enzymes and glycosidase activity of the colonic microflora is the basis for designing prodrugs or polymers with a triggering mechanism for the release of drug in the colon. Release of drugs from azo-bonded prodrugs or azo polymer-coated dosage forms is supposed to take place after reduction, and thus cleavage of the azo bonds by the azoreductase enzymes present in the colonic microflora. Similarly, natural polysaccharides that remain intact in the upper GI tract may be degraded by polysaccharidases, providing site-specific drug release into the colon. To protect polysaccharides from swelling and dissolving in the stomach and small intestine, chemical cross-linking or use of a protective coat has been used. In principle, exploitation of the most distinctive property of the colon, abundant microflora, offers the best site-specificity and delivery consistency *in vivo*, compared with reliance on transit time or pH. However, applications of these modified polymers or prodrugs in commercial products have been limited, primarily due to the additional resources, cost, and time required for regulatory approval. In recent years, the designs and evaluation of colonic drug delivery systems, as well as manufacturing considerations, have been extensively reviewed in the literature.[100,101,102,103,104]

Pulsatile Release

Pulsatile delivery generally refers to release of a portion of the total payload in a burst, followed by periods of little or no release (lag phase) in a defined temporal pattern. In particular, oral pulsatile drug release pertains to the burst delivery of drugs following a programed pattern from the time of oral administration. For example, Ritalin® LA capsule is a pulsatile delivery system that provides immediate release of 50% of the total dose upon oral ingestion, followed by a burst release of the remaining drug after 4 hours. In the field of modified release, these types of non-monotonic and multi-cargo release profiles have been recognized and/or proven to offer clinical benefits in: (1) optimizing chronotherapy; (2) mimicking natural patterns of endogenous secretion; and (3) providing optimal therapy for tolerance-inducing drugs where constant levels cause receptor down-regulation. Therefore, delivery systems with a pulsatile-release pattern have received increasing interest in new product development.

A variety of pulsatile release systems have been investigated and successfully applied in commercial products. The fundamental system design is based on the combination of a range of formulation approaches, including single- or multiple-unit immediate-release and delayed release systems discussed previously. The delayed release component in pulsatile delivery systems includes site-specific systems in which the drug is released at the desired site within the intestinal tract, or time-controlled devices in which the drug is released after a well-defined time period. Recent literature reviews have provided detailed summaries of design rationale, the prominent design strategies, and various single- and multiple-unit oral pulsatile delivery systems, including Pulsincap®, Pulsys™, and PORT technologies.[105,106,107,108]

Bimodal Release

Among non-monotonic extended release patterns, bimodal (or biphasic) delivery profiles have most commonly been utilized to avoid maintaining a constant plasma level. The usual rationale for such designs includes: (1) providing rapid onset of action by adding an immediate release component to an extended release dosage form; (2) optimizing dosing schedules for chronotherapeutic drugs by incorporating a delayed release component in an extended release dosage form; (3) generating fluctuations of plasma levels to avoid or attenuate the development of acute tolerance due to constant exposure of drug at the receptor site; and (4) overcoming the problems associated with nonlinear pharmacokinetics, extensive first-pass metabolism, idiosyncratic pharmacokinetics or pharmacodynamics resulting in reduced bioavailability or altered drug/metabolite ratios.[109,110,111,112] Since the 1980s, many marketed products with biphasic drug release have been developed for various drugs, such as verapamil, diltiazem, nifedipine, methylphenidate, etc.

As with pulsatile delivery systems, biphasic release profiles are often achieved utilizing a range of formulation approaches, including single- or multiple-unit immediate release, delayed release, and extended release systems based on coating, matrix, and osmotic pump technologies or combinations of these mechanisms. Among common designs that have been applied are mixing systems with varying release rates, using layered tablets or multi-walled coatings, compression-coated tablets with a slow eroding outer layer, combinations of delayed-release coatings with osmotic pumps, etc. For example, Cardizem® CD consists of a rapid-release bead, and an extended-release bead, producing a unique "stair–step release profile."[111] Adalat® CC is a compression-coated matrix tablet that provides zero-order sustained release, followed by a delayed burst release. Lodotra™ also uses press-coated tablets (GeoClock ™) that provide rapid release of prednisone about 4 hours after administration at bedtime, for a more effective treatment of the morning symptoms of rheumatoid arthritis.[113] Tylenol® 8-Hour is a bi-layer caplet designed to provide both fast and long-lasting pain relief. The first layer provides immediate release for fast relief, and the second maintains the blood level of acetaminophen during the dosing interval. A similar design was discussed by Radebaugh et al.[114] Eichel and Massmann described a delayed- and sustained-release system comprising a multi-walled coated drug having an inner wall microencapsular enteric coating, a solid acid either incorporated in the enteric layer or layered over the enteric layer, and an outer microporous membrane wall for release rate control. The solid acid delays drug release by maintaining the enteric polymer in an impermeable state until the acid diffuses out of the drug or is neutralized. The multi-walled coated drug is admixed with an uncoated drug to provide a biphasic release profile.[115]

20.2.3 Materials Used for Modifying Drug Release

Commonly used materials for modifying drug release from oral solid dosage forms can be categorized into long chain substituted or unsubstituted hydrocarbons and polymers. Natural or synthetic long chain hydrocarbons such as fatty acids, fatty acid esters, glyceryl esters, alcohol esters, and waxes were among the earliest materials applied in modifying drug release from matrix systems. The use of waxes for prolonging the medicinal effect of herbal medicines can be traced back to the fourth century AD.[28] Polymers are sourced from natural products (e.g., polysaccharides), chemically modified natural products (e.g., cellulose ethers and esters) or synthetic in nature (e.g., methacrylic ester copolymers). Today, polymers have become the dominating rate-controlling excipients in the modified-release arena, due to their multitude of functionalities and properties that are relatively easy to control from batch to batch. Some of the common materials that are approved for oral administration are briefly discussed in this section, based on their applications in different types of modified-release systems. The list is not intended to be comprehensive, but rather serves as a starting point for the interested reader.

Materials for matrix systems The materials most widely used in preparing matrix systems include hydrophilic and hydrophobic polymers, as well as long chain hydrocarbons. Commonly available hydrophilic polymers include:

1. non-ionic soluble cellulose ethers, such as hydroxypropylmethylcellulose (HPMC, e.g., Methocel K100 LV, K4 M, K15 M, K100 M; Benecel MP 843, MP 814, MP 844; Metolose® 100, 4000, 15000 and 100 000 SR), hydroxypropylcellulose (HPC, e.g., Klucel GXF, MXF, HXF), hydroxyethylcellulose (HEC, e.g., Natrosol 250 HHX, HX, M, G) with varying degrees of substitutions and viscosity grades;
2. nonionic homopolymers of ethylene oxide, such as poly(ethylene oxide), $[H(OCH_2CH_2)_nOH]$ with a molecular weight range of 100 000 to 8 000 000 (e.g., Polyox WSR N-12K, WSR N-60K, WSR-301, WSR-coagulant, WSR-303, WSR-308);
3. water-soluble natural gums of polysaccharides of natural origin, such as xantham gum, alginate, and locust bean gum;
4. water swellable, but insoluble, high molecular weight homopolymers and copolymers of acrylic acid chemically cross-linked with polyalkenyl

alcohols with varying degree of cross-linking or particle size (Carbopol® 71G NF, 971P, 974P and 934P);
5. polyvinyl acetate and povidone mixtures (Kollidon SR);
6. cross-linked high amylose starch; and
7. ionic methacrylate copolymers (Eudragit L30D, FS 30D).

In most cases these polymers can perform qualitatively similar functions, but possess different release-retarding capability and processing characteristics when used at the same level. They are usually available in micronized forms for facilitating the rapid formation of a gelatinous barrier layer on the system surface.

Fatty acids, fatty acid esters, mono-, di-, and triglycerides of fatty acids, fatty alcohols, waxes of natural and synthetic origins with differing melting points, as well as hydrophobic polymers, are used in hydrophobic, non-swellable matrices. Examples include stearic acid, lauryl, cetyl or cetostearyl alcohol, glyceryl behenate, carnauba wax, beeswax, candelilla wax, microcrystalline wax, and low molecular weight polyethylene, to name a few. Insoluble polymers include fine powders of ammoniomethacrylate copolymers (Eudragit® RL100, PO, RS100, PO), ethyl cellulose (Ethocel®), cellulose acetate (CA-398–10), cellulose acetate butyrate (CAB-381–20), cellulose acetate propionate (CAP-482–20), and latex dispersions of the insoluble polymers (Eudragit® NE-30D, RL-30D, RS-30D, Surelease®). However, their application as the sole rate-controlling material in the marketed matrix-based products are still limited.

Materials for reservoir systems The common materials to form a drug release barrier surrounding a core tablet, drug particles, beads or pellets for diffusion-controlled reservoir systems include water insoluble acrylic copolymers, ethylcellulose, and polyvinylacetate. These film-coating polymers had historically been used in an organic solution prior to the 1980s. Today, they are mostly applied as aqueous dispersions that form films by a process of coalescence of submicron polymer particles. Ammoniomethacrylate copolymers (Eudragit® RL 30D, RS 30D) are water permeable and swellable film-formers based on neutral methacrylic esters with a small proportion of trimethylammonioethyl methacrylate chloride. Methacrylic ester copolymers (Eudragit®, NE30D) are neutral esters available as a 30% aqueous dispersion without the need for plasticizers unless increased film flexibility is desired. Ethylcellulose for film-coating is available as an aqueous polymeric dispersion containing plasticizers under the brand name of Surelease®, and as pseudolatex dispersion, Aquacoat® ECD, which requires the addition of plasticizers to facilitate film formation during coating. More recently, a polyvinylacetate aqueous dispersion (Kollicoat SR 30D) has been shown to offer similar functionality, while providing improved resistance to aqueous medium containing alcohol.

Materials for osmotic pump systems Cellulose acetate is the most commonly used polymer that constitutes the semipermeable membrane of an osmotic pump device. Cellulose acetate containing a controlled percentage of acetyl content is often used, together with other pH-dependent or pH-independent polymers to form films of varying water flux and permeability. Polymers used for this purpose include cellulose butyrate, polyurethane, ethylcellulose, poloxamer polyols, PEG, PVC, and PVA. Osmotic agents, such as sodium chloride, are another key ingredient of an osmotic system. In the more sophisticated two-chamber system, a hydrophilic polymer with a very high swelling ratio, i.e., poly(ethylene oxide), is an essential component in the osmotic driving element, the push layer.

Materials for delayed-release systems Materials that have been applied to oral medication for enteric release primarily comprise of: (1) shellac and zein of natural sources; and (2) derivatives of cellulose and methacrylic acid copolymers containing carboxylic functional groups. Technology advances over the past three decades have made synthetic and semisynthetic polymers the most preferred system for enteric film-coating of tablets or particles. At low pH in the stomach, the polymer is impermeable and insoluble, but in the higher pH environment present in the small intestine (e.g., > 5.5), the polymer dissolves and exposes the core tablet for rapid- or slow-release of the actives. Examples of these pH-dependent polymers include cellulose acetate phthalate (CAP), hydroxypropyl methylcellulose phthalate (HPMCP), methacrylic acid and methacrylic esters (Eudragit® L and S, Acryl-EZE®), and polyvinyl acetate phthalate (Sureteric). Some of these polymers (e.g., Eudragit) are often used to obtain predetermined lag times of the delayed release via pH and/or coating thickness control for colonic and pulsatile (later pulses) release. It should be noted that these ionic polymers have also been incorporated into the matrix, reservoir or osmotic pump systems to modify drug release profiles. For delayed-release systems based on slow eroding mechanisms, materials such as those utilized in matrix systems are used in compression-coated tablets that provide pre-determined lag (e.g., Adalat CC).

20.3 RATIONAL DESIGN OF MODIFIED-RELEASE SYSTEMS

The majority of the systems for modifying apparent drug absorption are based on proprietary or nonproprietary polymeric delivery technologies. The ability to achieve the desirable *in vitro* and *in vivo* performance for a given drug substance is highly dependent upon several important factors that include the dose, physico-chemical, biopharmaceutical, pharmacokinetic (PK), and pharmacodynamic (PD) properties of the drug, as well as the proper selection of a delivery technology and formulation design. Each drug substance possesses inherent properties that require considerations specific to both the drug and the delivery system. Thus, successful dosage form development is, in fact, dictated by the properties of a compound in the context of physiological/biological constraints, rather than by the technology platform. This statement is supported by the fact that almost all MR products with expired composition of matter patents have been unable to maintain market exclusivity solely based on delivery technology. There are numerous examples where the performance of the branded products has been matched by their generic counterparts based on similar or different technologies. Notable examples include Procardia® XL, Cardizem® CD, Concerta®, Adalat® CC, Wellbutrin® XL, Ditropan® XL, Glucotrol® XL, Glucophage® XR, Asacol®, Toprol-XL®, to name a few. Therefore, the first stage in designing an MR delivery system should be to integrate a defined clinical rationale with the characteristics of the drug for feasibility evaluation. The second stage is to select an appropriate MR technology, based on the desired dosage form characteristics and practical considerations for *in vitro* and *in vivo* evaluation. More specifically, a rational design process should include the following steps:

1. Identify the clinical need and define *in vivo* target product profile.
2. Conduct a feasibility study through experiments and detailed analysis to assess technical challenges and risk associated with MR delivery based on:
   (a) characterization of the molecule with regard to its physico-chemical and biopharmaceutical properties, dose, regional absorption, and *in vivo* disposition;
   (b) pharmacokinetic simulation to prospectively calculate theoretical drug input rate that corresponds to the desired target plasma profile, based on *in vivo* disposition parameters and certain assumptions.

3. If feasible, select an appropriate MR technology and *in vitro* test methods to design and evaluate formulations with different release rates *in vitro*.
4. Test prototype formulations with profiles that bracket the theoretical target absorption profile *in vivo* in order to:
   (a) identify a formulation with acceptable *in vivo* performance or a direction of formulation refinement if iteration is required;
   (b) explore the *in vitro–in vivo* relationship (IVIVR) or correlation (IVIVC) to aid product development or subsequent rounds of formulation iteration.

In this section, these essential design elements and general considerations are discussed in detail. Case studies are provided to illustrate how drug property, delivery technology, and formulation approach influence the performance of oral modified release delivery systems.

20.3.1 Identification of the Clinical Need and Definition of the *In Vivo* Target Product Profile

The basic clinical rationale of developing an MR product is to achieve optimal drug treatment via programing the input profile, such that the product offers one or more advantages in efficacy, safety, and patient compliance. According to the regulatory directive issued by European Agency for the Evaluation of Medicinal Products (EMEA),[116] development of MR products should be based on a relationship between the pharmacological/toxicological response, and the systemic exposure to the drug/metabolite(s). However, more emphasis has been, in many cases, placed on reducing the dosing frequency or fluctuation of plasma concentrations (PK) associated with IR formulations than on understanding and ensuring an improved pharmacological effect profile (PD). As a result, it is not uncommon to see new drug delivery technologies looking for a suitable drug candidate or projects terminated, due to lack of feasibility or desired outcome. This can be attributed to the often presumed or overly-simplified linear PK/PD relationship, and to the fact that the PK outcomes of drug delivery are generally easy to monitor and quantify.

In reality, the relationship between systemic drug concentration (C), and intensity of effect (E), is very complex because of the vast array of pharmacological mechanisms and physiological processes controlling drug responses. Thus, a variety of models based on the mechanisms of drug actions (reversible, irreversible, and tolerance) have been developed to describe PK/PD, such as sigmoid E_{max}, biophase distribution, slow receptor-binding, turnover, indirect response, signal transduction, and tolerance models.[117] For example, a sigmoidal E_{max} model or the full Hill equation is a four-parameter direct response model:

$$E = (E_{max} C^{\gamma})/(EC_{50}{}^{\gamma} + C^{\gamma}) \qquad (20.20)$$

where:

E is the intensity of the effect
E_{max} is the maximum effect
C is the concentration
EC_{50} is a sensitivity parameter representing C producing 50% of E_{max}
γ is the Hill or sigmoidicity coefficient that reflects the steepness of the E–C curve.

Generally, lower values (<1) will produce broad slopes, higher values (>4) are reflective of an all-or-none type of response. According to this equation, different fluctuations in pharmacological response (ΔE) may result from the same or similar concentration changes (ΔC), depending on the concentration ranges. In addition, the slow and constant mode of drug input often provided by ER dosage forms may have varying therapeutic impacts, depending upon drugs and their PK/PD relationships. Furthermore, the time course of drug effects can be fairly different from the time course of drug concentrations. A short elimination half life does not necessarily indicate short duration of action.

Figure 20.5 shows the sequence of steps between drug administration and clinical response. The importance of efficacy and safety implications of the complex relationship between drug input and pharmacodynamics, and research strategies in guiding the design of drug delivery mode, have been discussed in detail by Bremers and Hoffman.[118,119] For instance, the shape factor (γ), which determines the slope of the E–C curve of the E_{max} model, can have a significant impact on

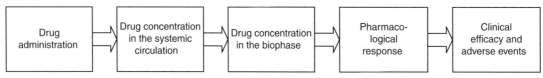

FIGURE 20.5 From drug administration to clinical response

the design of an ER system. A relatively shallow *E–C* profile (small γ) may suggest a lack of pharmacodynamic rationale to develop an ER product, because E is relatively insensitive to even a large change in concentration. When the concentration range required to elicit drug response is very small (large γ), such as for levodopa, the *E–C* profile represents an all-or-none phenomenon. Thus, as long as the drug concentrations remain above the minimum effective concentration (MEC), the drug effect is essentially independent of the fluctuation in plasma levels. It is known that the non-steady state *E–C* curves of certain drugs may exhibit clockwise or counterclockwise hysteresis, due to desensitization or equilibrium delay and formation of an active metabolite.[2] In the former case, either pulsatile or constant rate input may be designed depending upon the desired pharmacological responses of the drugs (e.g. gonadotropin-releasing hormone). On the other hand, a slow input rate may minimize the counterclockwise hysteresis, and thus require lower C_{max} to achieve the desired response.

The impact of input rate on the efficacy and safety ratio is best illustrated by nifedipine. Comparative studies of slow versus rapid input have led to the realization and confirmation that the rate-of-increase of nifedipine concentration, rather than absolute concentration, is the determining factor for the observed haemodynamic effects, i.e., a gradual decrease in blood pressure was observed without side-effects (increase in heart rate) occurring with a slow regimen, while the opposite was observed with a rapid regimen.[118] Methylphenidate represents another classical example where delivery pattern can have a significant impact on the efficacy. To meet the clinical need for a more convenient dosing regimen of this controlled drug, several new MR products with different release modes have been designed, and clinically proven to be effective, since the mid-1990s. The product designs include pulsatile release and biphasic extended-release that provide fluctuations of plasma levels during drug release, thus overcoming the acutely acquired tolerance due to constant level of drug exposure associated with Ritalin® SR, the extended-release version of Ritalin® product lines that had been available for many years. These two examples show that a positive or negative clinical outcome may be rendered by constant PK profiles, depending on the relationship between the kinetics of drug effects and the pattern and timing of drug input. Therefore, the design of release characteristics for an MR product should be based on the desired optimal drug concentration time profile, i.e., target product profile, defined by the quantitative information of the PK/PD relationship.

With increased research and understanding of biomarkers and surrogate end points that reflect underlying mechanism of drug action, it is anticipated that understanding PK–PD relationships will play a more significant role in the establishment of clinical rationale, definition of *in vivo* target product profiles, and early decision in MR product development.

20.3.2 Feasibility Study

In developing MR dosage forms, feasibility assessment is crucial to product design and development success. Once the delivery mode and *in vivo* target product profile are defined, and disposition parameters are available, the corresponding theoretical drug input profile can be obtained by prospective PK simulation, e.g., via adjusting input rate and kinetics to generate *in vivo* PK profiles or by deconvolution of the target plasma profile. With a known therapeutic window or MEC, the required input or absorption duration and kinetics can readily be determined, for instance, by ensuring the plasma levels of the MR design are constantly above the MEC over the dosing interval. When the quantitative PK–PD information is unavailable, the steady state C_{min} of the clinically effective immediate release counterpart may be used as a conservative estimate of the MEC. Figure 20.6 shows an example where a new ER dosage form was designed to maintain the average plasma concentration above the C_{min} ($\sim$100 μg/ml) of a marketed IR dosage form throughout the dosing interval of 24 hours.

Following the completion of the theoretical MR design or paper exercise, the next step would be to do a "reality check," i.e., to evaluate the feasibility of the designed delivery in the GI tract, because favorable and complete drug absorption throughout the GI tract is often an exception rather than a rule. For example, if a predefined plasma profile of a drug corresponds to 16 hours of zero-order drug input, it suggests that the majority of the given dose will have to be absorbed in the large intestine under fasting conditions, because of the limited residence time of solid dosage forms in the small bowel. Thus, understanding absorption characteristics of the individual molecule of interest in the lower GI tract is crucial to the rational design of an MR dosage form. In order to assess technical feasibility and development challenges, it is essential to integrate the drug's physico-chemical and biopharmaceutical properties into the context of the total dose, physiological/biological constraints, and disposition kinetics. Among the key properties of a particular drug substance are solubility, lipophilicity, chemical stability, regional permeability, gut and hepatic first-pass metabolism, whether or not the drug is a substrate of transporters and susceptibility of the drug to metabolism by gut microflora. To help better understand the suitability of a particular drug for

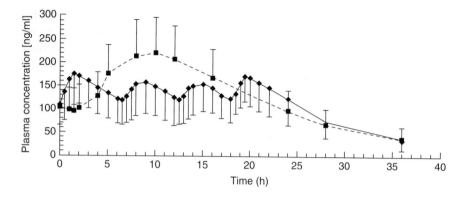

FIGURE 20.6 Mean (±SD) plasma concentration–time profiles of (+)– Tramadol after multiple-dose administration of an immediate release dosage form and a once-daily extended release dosage form in the fasting state. Key: 50 mg IR (◆); 200 mg ER (■). Reprinted with permission from Blackwell Publishing: Malonne, H. et al. (2004). Br. J. Pharmacol. 57(3), 270–278.

TABLE 20.3 Factors affecting the feasibility of developing oral modified-release systems

a. Solubility/dose

Low solubility combined with high dose may limit the suitability for developing a MR system that requires drug delivery in the lower bowel. Drug absorption may be more variable or incomplete when the *in vivo* release occurs past the ileocecal junction where the amount of fluid available for dissolution is progressively limited, and the permeability and surface area are lower. In some cases, apparent absorption of poorly soluble drugs may be inherently prolonged due to the slow dissolution of the drug particles. However, drug release rate and kinetics are usually difficult to control because they vary with surface properties, particle size and size distribution.

b. Stability

Drugs must be stable to pH, enzymes and flora throughout the entire intended delivery regions of the GI tract. For example, a drug subject to degradation by the colonic microflora is not a suitable candidate for MR delivery that requires an *in vivo* absorption beyond approximately 7–8 hours post dosing.

c. Lipophilicity/permeability

Absorption of BCS class III or IV drugs may be limited by permeability that also vary with regions of the GI tract due to difference in available surface area, transporters and enzymatic activities. Altering the release of such drug substances in the lower GI tract typically have little effects on the shape of PK profiles and usually result in truncated absorption.

d. Elimination $t_{1/2}$

The need for ER systems is often a result of short half life. However, other variables (e.g., MEC, volume of distribution, and dose) are also important in determining the ER feasibility. Developing a twice daily (or once daily) system may be possible for one compound, but may not be feasible for another drug having similar half lives.

e. Therapeutic window

One of the important characteristics of oral ER drug delivery is the ability to maintain plasma levels within a therapeutic range with reduced fluctuation. For drugs with relatively short half lives, the lower the MEC and the higher the minimum toxic concentration (MTC), the more likely it is to achieve prolonged drug exposure above MEC using higher doses. However, this will result in greater fluctuation in steady-state plasma levels that is often undesirable for narrow therapeutic index drugs.

f. First-pass metabolism

For drugs with saturable first-pass metabolism (hepatic or gut), bioavailability will be compromised due to slow input if drug absorption from IR dosage form is higher due to transient saturation. No significant impact is expected if drug absorption of both IR and ER is within linear range (i.e., dose proportional).

g. PK-PD relationship

The relationship between drug concentration (C) and the pharmacological effect (E) plays a critical role in determining rationale and need for MR delivery as previously discussed.

MR delivery, some of the important factors and their impact on the product development are summarized in Table 20.3.

Orally administered drugs may be subject to acid or base hydrolysis and other chemical or enzymatic degradation that can influence bioavailability and design of the delivery system. For example, drugs that are unstable in the stomach require delayed onset of drug release until the dosage form enters the small intestine. This may result in shortened total GI residence time for extended absorption. On the other hand, drugs unstable in the lower GI tract due to metabolism by microflora would require complete drug delivery in the small intestine.

The regional absorption characteristics of a compound in the GI tract and residence time of dosage forms are the most important parameters in assessing the suitability of oral MR delivery.[1,120] With significant regional differences in surface area, permeability, secretion, enzymes, transporters, volume of water, etc., a drug substance often exhibits varying apparent absorption in different segments of the GI tract. In general, the transit time of most dosage forms prior to arrival at the colon, a less favorable site for drug absorption, is approximately 4–6 hours, depending on the type of dosage forms, food intake, and composition. This may become a limiting factor for drugs requiring absorption beyond this timeframe after dosing.[121] For certain drugs, favorable absorption in the large intestine can allow continued drug delivery for up to a total of 20–24 hours.[122,123] If drug release is not completed by the time the dosage form passes through the absorption region, a portion of the dose will not be delivered. Hence, it is very important to define the absorption regions or window of a specific compound in the GI tract, before further development proceeds. It should be noted that MR dosage forms designed and tested in adults may not work the same in young children, because of the known differences in GI transit time of the delivery systems between adults and children younger than 3–4 years' of age. With shorter GI residence time in young children, truncation of drug absorption may occur resulting in lower AUC and/or sub-therapeutic plasma levels.[124]

Over the years, many techniques have been utilized to assess regional absorption potential or window of a compound, including *in vitro* or *in situ* models, and site-specific delivery in animal models and human subjects. Permeation characteristics of drugs in different GI segments can be evaluated through *in vitro* permeability of excised tissues or *in situ* perfusion studies in animal models (e.g., rat or rabbit). Site-specific delivery via indwelling access ports in conscious animals (e.g., dog and rat) offers direct comparison of drug absorption in jejunum, ileum, and colon through concurrent monitoring of plasma levels. It can serve as a predictive model for humans, depending on the drug's properties and absorption mechanism. In fact, a reasonably good correlation of regional absorption characteristics has been found between dog and human, particularly for passively transported compounds.[125] For hydrophilic small molecules, in which the paracellular pathway also plays a role in permeation, the dog model usually overestimates the absorption in humans due to the "leakier" canine intestine, especially in the large intestine. To quantify colonic absorption potential, intubation studies have also been used via bolus and/or continuous infusion of a drug solution or suspension into the transverse colon in animal or healthy volunteers. Since the early 1990s, gamma scintigraphic studies have become one of the commonly used techniques in screening drug candidates for oral MR delivery.[126] Regional differences in absorption can be determined by using non-invasive delivery devices, such as the Enterion® capsule of Pharmaceutical Profiles, and the InteliSite® capsule of Scintipharma, Inc. These radiolabeled capsules loaded with a drug solution or powder can be tracked via gamma scintegraphy, and externally activated to release the drug when it reaches the desired location in the digestive tract following ingestion. Another effective method used by the above two companies, and Bio-Images Research Limited, is to administer a radiolabelled MR dosage form, followed by combined analysis of its GI transit characteristics along with location and timing of drug release.[127] A more efficient and often more effective approach is to incorporate feasibility assessment as part of the early product development. By applying interdisciplinary knowledge and integrating the drug's properties (physico-chemical, biopharmaceutical and biological) with regional absorption information in animal models, a decision can often be made initially with regard to proceeding with formulation screening study in humans. This type of screening study typically involves administering prototype formulations with varying *in vitro* release profiles that bracket the target *in vivo* absorption profile by first assuming a wide window of absorption. If bioavailability decreases with slowing drug release, the absorption window can be inferred or approximated by deconvolution or examination of plasma profiles (e.g., using a semi-log plot). For example, the limit of drug release duration *in vivo* normally corresponds to where the observed truncation of apparent absorption occurred. The reliability of the information thus obtained usually depends on the number of the prototypes tested, the *in vitro–in vivo* relationship (IVIVR), and understanding of certain potential confounding factors. This approach is appealing because: (1) the time and cost required for a screening study is similar to that of a "cleaner" scintegraphic study; and (2) with sufficient rationale, knowledge and experience invested in the design of prototypes and *in vitro* screening tools, there is a reasonable chance of identifying a target formulation in the same study or obtaining a rank order of *in vivo* performance which can often be used to guide formulation iteration when necessary. The main drawback of this approach is its potential impact on making a "go/no go" decision when the study result is inconclusive with respect to the absorption window.

The therapeutic window and MEC and their interplays with disposition characteristics of a drug also play a critical role in suitability evaluation for ER delivery. In theory, a lower MEC combined with slower elimination corresponds to a shorter required duration of drug input. Drugs with very short half lives ($t_{1/2}$) and high volume of distribution undergo rapid clearance, which can make extended delivery challenging, especially if the MEC is relatively high or the therapeutic window is narrow. For instance, prolonged absorption is often required to achieve essentially flat plasma profiles for drugs with short half lives and narrow therapeutic indices, since fluctuation of the plasma profiles is determined by the rates of elimination and input duration/kinetics. Therefore, a wide absorption window is often necessary to achieve extended release for this type of drugs. Lastly, it should be noted that a feasibility study is not required for developing generic products, because of the presence of branded products.

20.3.3 Selecting the Modified-release System and Testing System Design

When oral MR delivery is feasible or shows promise, the subsequent logical step is to choose an appropriate MR technology and *in vitro* test method to design and evaluate prototype formulations with different release rates *in vitro*. This decision should be primarily based on drug properties, required dose, types of delivery profiles including release/absorption kinetics, as well as clinical and market needs (e.g.,

type and size of dosage form, number of strengths, etc.). Additional practical considerations include development time, and cost and commercial production factors (e.g., process, equipment, facility, manufacturability, robustness, cost, capacity, environment, etc.). In selecting an MR technology that matches development needs, dose and solubility of the active are often the most important factors to consider. With the size limitation of oral dosage forms, both variables impact the release mechanism and processing behaviors. Generally, there is no technology that is "one-size-fits-all." Nevertheless, it is not uncommon for a drug delivery company to tout a specific technology while downplaying the practicality and viability of technology transformation, such as system and process complexity, and other important development considerations discussed previously. Table 20.4 compares delivery capabilities and limitations of commonly utilized ER systems. From an enablement point of view, different MR systems can be equally effective in achieving the same delivery objective when drug properties and dose are desirable. For example, similar MR performance of verapamil, theophylline, and methylphenidate have been obtained using matrix, reservoir or osmotic pump technologies. Depending on dose and solubility, one type of delivery system may become more-or-less suitable than others for meeting a particular delivery need. Table 20.5 provides a high-level guide to the selection of ER systems on the basis of dose and solubility.

Once an MR system is chosen, *in vitro* characterization of its behavior and attributes is essential prior to

TABLE 20.4 Comparison of commonly used oral extended-release technologies

System	Advantages	Disadvantages
Hydrophilic matrix	Suitable for compounds with a wide range of properties and low to high drug loading	Drug release often sensitive to test conditions
	Generally robust formulation and process when rationally designed	Less flexibility for adjusting dose strengths for single-unit system
	Use of conventional manufacturing equipment and process	Increased formulation/process complexity for tailored drug release (layered or compression coated system)
	Cost effective: shorter development time and lower cost	
	Release kinetics and profiles can be tailored with modification	
	Multi-units possible	
Hydrophobic matrix	Suitable for soluble compounds and low to high drug loading	Not applicable to compounds with low solubility
	Use of conventional manufacturing equipment and process	Non-zero-order release
	Release kinetics and profiles can be tailored with modification	Propensity for incomplete drug release

(Continued)

TABLE 20.4 (Continued)

System	Advantages	Disadvantages
	Multi-units possible	Drug release often sensitive to processing and test conditions
		Less flexibility for adjusting dose strengths for single-unit system
		Increased formulation/process complexity for tailored drug release (layered or compression coated system)
Multi-unit reservoir	Readily tailored release kinetics and profiles (e.g., zero-order, pulsatile, biphasic, colonic)	Only applicable to compounds with relatively high solubility
	Minimized risk of dose dumping and local irritation	Drug release often sensitive to test conditions
	Lower *in vivo* variability (favorable transit property)	Limited drug loading
	More consistent *in vivo* performance	Process development and scale-up more challenging
	Easy dose adjustment: single formulation amenable to multiple strengths	
	Suitable for pediatric/geriatric use	
	Use of conventional manufacturing equipment and process	
Osmotic pump	Applicable to compounds with a relatively wide range of properties	Limited drug loading
		Ghost tablets
	Drug release generally independent of drug properties and test conditions	Delayed onset (1–2 hrs) and/or incomplete drug release
	Zero-order release	Solvent-based process
		Lengthy, complex and inefficient manufacturing processes and control (e.g., layered tablet)
		Specialized equipment, facility
		Highest development and manufacturing cost and time

TABLE 20.5   Guide for MR system selection on the basis of dose and solubility

System	HS/HD	HS/MD	HS/LD	MS/HD	MS/MD	MS/LD	LS/HD	LS/MD	LS/LD
Hydrophilic matrix tablet	0	+	+	+	+	+	+	+	+
Hydrophobic matrix tablet	+	+	+	−	0	+	−	−	−
Hydrophobic matrix pellets	−	−	−	−	+	+	−	+	+
Coated matrix tablet	+	+	+	−	0	+	−	−	−
Coated pellets	−	+	+	−	+	+	−	−	−
Osmotic pump	−	0	0	−	+	+	−	+	+

Note: (1) HS = high solubility; MS = medium solubility; LS = low solubility; HD = high dose; MD = medium dose; LD = low dose
(2) "+" = suitable; "−" = unsuitable; "0" = borderline (may be suitable via system modification)

testing in humans. Factors that often affect the system performance (e.g., dosage form type, size, drug loading, excipients, processing, release mechanism, sensitivity to environmental changes, drug release kinetics, and duration) need to be considered when choosing appropriate *in vitro* test methods. For solid MR dosage forms, a drug release test is the most important among the various mechanical, physical and chemical characterization methods. The USP drug release test (e.g., using Apparatus II or I) is commonly utilized for gauging the likely *in vivo* performance, thus guiding formulation screening despite its undefined relationship with *in vivo* performance at the early design stage. Depending on the drug properties and system design, test parameters including apparatus, agitation, pH, surfactants, additives, ionic strength, mechanical stress, etc., can be varied to better mimic certain GI conditions or to create shear stress on the structure for testing the performance robustness. A detailed discussion of development considerations related to meaningful *in vitro* release tests are provided in Chapter 17.

In designing an MR dosage form, the initial objective is usually to prepare a formulation with an *in vitro* release profile similar to the theoretical *in vivo* absorption profile. Due to unknown IVIVR, additional formulations having *in vitro* profiles that bracket the target profile are useful for identifying a formulation with desired *in vivo* performance when they are tested in humans for the first time. In the event where an iterative study is required, the data from such a screening study provide not only a direction to formulation refinement, but also an opportunity for early exploration of IVIVR or *in vitro–in vivo* correlation (IVIVC). As discussed in Chapter 17, the earlier an IVIVC or IVIVR can be established, the more beneficial it is to the design and development of an MR delivery system. A validated IVIVC offers scientific and regulatory avenues to aid formulation, process development and scale-up, justify specifications, and make changes related to process, equipment, and manufacturing site.

20.3.4 Case Studies: Impact of Drug Property and Formulation Design

The examples discussed in this section are intended to illustrate: (1) the criticality of understanding drug characteristics and feasibility assessment; (2) there is no one-size-fits-all solution to designing an MR product; and (3) insignificance of delivery technology when a drug molecule has desirable properties for MR development.

CASE STUDY 1

METHYLPHENIDATE HCL

Methylphenidate (MPH) is an amphetamine-like central nervous system stimulant commonly prescribed to treat attention-deficit/hyperactivity disorder (ADHD) in children, adolescents, and adults, and also to treat narcolepsy. It is a weak base with pK_a of 8.77, and a log$P$ of 3.19. Its hydrochloride salt is freely soluble in water (18.6 mg/ml), stable, and well-absorbed from the intestinal tract, with a short elimination half life of 3–4 hours.[128] These favorable properties, combined with a low dose, make MPH an ideal candidate for oral MR regardless of technologies applied.

The immediate-release (IR) product (e.g., Ritalin®) that has been on the market since the 1950s is taken two or three times daily with rapid onset of action and demonstrated efficacy. In an attempt to offer more convenient administration and prolonged control of behavior, especially for school children for whom most prescriptions are written, several modified-release formulations have been developed with the objective of maintaining efficacy over the entire school day. This is of particular importance, because it would eliminate the need for repeated administrations of methylphenidate, a Schedule II controlled substance, while the patient is at school. An early MR product, e.g., Ritalin® SR, is a matrix tablet designed to maintain relatively flat plasma drug levels for the required treatment duration. However, the product did not provide equivalent efficacy to the multiple dosing of the IR product during the day, due to the tolerance to the effects of the drug discussed previously, and a delayed onset of action.[129] Other similar ER matrix tablets include Metadate™ ER and Methylin™ ER. It was not until the 1990s that it was demonstrated that varying rate of drug input would overcome the tolerance observed with the formulations with nearly constant delivery rate. Subsequently, a new generation of once-daily MR products were developed that offer the equivalent efficacy of repeated administrations of IR MPH by altering the drug's input profile. The successful commercial products include: (1) ER products generating biphasic release profiles for a rapid onset of action and a prolonged duration of action, such as Metadate® CD capsules consisting of 30% IR and 70% coated ER beads and Concerta® tablets consisting of an ER osmotic pump coated with IR component (Figure 20.7a,b);[130,131] and (2) Pulsatile release products that better mimic PK performance of standard schedules of IR product, such as Ritalin® LA capsules consisting of 50% IR and 50% DR beads that provide IR release 4 hours later (Figure 20.7c).[132,133] This case study shows that all three types of technology are equally effective in achieving a range of *in vivo* delivery performance when the molecule exhibits desirable characteristics suitable for MR design.

CASE STUDY 1 (CONTINUED)

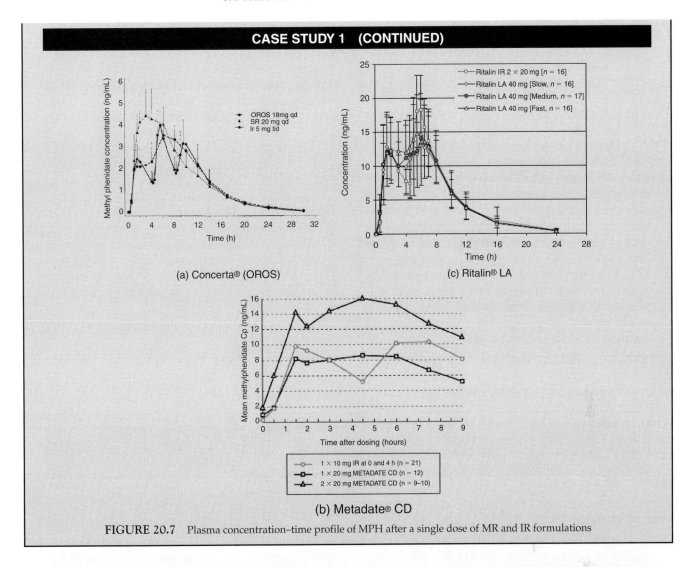

(a) Concerta® (OROS)

(c) Ritalin® LA

(b) Metadate® CD

FIGURE 20.7   Plasma concentration–time profile of MPH after a single dose of MR and IR formulations

CASE STUDY 2

MODEL COMPOUND

The above example shows that favorable absorption characteristics, combined with rapid elimination of MPH, make it possible to achieve the desired PK fluctuation using short pulsing intervals of drug input. To further evaluate the influence of drug's PK properties on the feasibility of oral pulsatile delivery, a model drug molecule was selected based on its physico-chemical and biopharmaceutical properties suitable for extended absorption.[134] It is a weak base with pK_a of 8.99, and solubility of 1.65 mg/ml at pH 6.8. It has a $\log P$ of 2.69, and adequate stability in the intestinal tract. Its disposition parameters available from the literature indicate a terminal elimination rate constant of 0.115 hour^{-1}. PK simulation of the *in vivo* performance of the pulsatile

release designs with varying pulsing intervals was performed by shifting the observed plasma profiles of a single dose study in humans using superposition principle. The basic assumptions for the simulation included: (1) the formulation technology can deliver the exact pulses at predetermined time intervals; and (2) the apparent absorption is uniform over the delivery duration with minimum impact of variable GI transit time, gut metabolism and release/absorption environment. An example illustrated in Figure 20.8 shows that a design of three equally spaced pulses of equal doses over 6 hours hardly generated distinct peaks and troughs in plasma levels corresponding to the input variations. The fluctuations in plasma levels at steady state (not

CASE STUDY 2　(CONTINUED)

shown) were essentially non-existent. Thus, the chance is very low for achieving multiple peaks/troughs at the biophase or site of drug action, which is often the design objective. It should be noted that this type of simulation represents the best case scenario, because the PK profile used for generating the profiles of the subsequent pulse resulted from absorption occurring in the upper intestinal tract with the most favorable absorption environment. In reality, the second and third pulsing doses are expected to produce slower ascending plasma concentrations compared to the first pulse, since they are absorbed in the distal ileum and/or large intestines. This case study illustrates that applying an *in vitro* MR design to obtaining a desired *in vivo* PK and clinical results requires application of multidisciplinary knowledge, and prospective evaluation of *in vitro* and *in vivo* outcomes prior to execution of the experiments. For pulsatile delivery, rapid clearance is essential to achieving distinct PK

fluctuation resulting from pulses of shorter intervals. In addition, the influence of inherently highly variable GI systems on performance of oral dosage forms should also be taken into consideration.

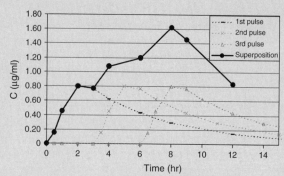

FIGURE 20.8　PK simulation of a pulsatile delivery design by superposition

CASE STUDY 3

DEVELOPMENT COMPOUND A

A development compound in phase 3 clinical trials is a neutral molecule with molecular weight of 236, and favorable log$P$ of 1.44.[135] It is stable and practically insoluble (170 μg/ml). The IR formulation requires a q.i.d. dosing regimen due to rapid elimination in humans ($t_{1/2}$ = 2.5 hours). Based on the MEC of 1 μg/ml, and a total daily dose of 2.4 g, PK simulation indicated that twice-daily administration would require approximately 10 hours of *in vivo* input, suggesting at least 50% of the dose would be released/absorbed in the large intestine for a zero-order delivery system. However, regional absorption data were not available. To investigate technical feasibility of ER delivery, prototype hydrophilic matrix tablets and multi-unit spherical hydrophobic matrix beads were designed as adult and pediatric dosage forms, respectively. Matrix systems were used because of the required high loading of an active with low solubility. *In vitro* studies showed apparent zero-order drug release from the matrix tablet containing the active of low solubility due to the erosion-controlled mechanism. Drug release from the matrix beads more closely followed diffusion-controlled kinetics as a result of combination of high surface area to volume ratio, short diffusion pathlength, and low driving force for drug release. Crossover PK studies

of these formulations with varying release rates were conducted in healthy volunteers. The dosage forms were administered under high fat conditions to increase gastric retention time. Evaluation of the plasma concentration–time profiles showed: (1) decreasing release rates correspond to lower AUCs; and (2) truncated absorption as indicated by the evident slope inflection of the semi-log plot of the terminal phase at approximately 5–6 hours post-dosing. Interestingly, the average truncation time was delayed by about 1–2 hours for the matrix beads, suggesting more favorable GI transit properties of multi-particulate dosage forms. Nevertheless, neither dosage form met the predetermined criteria of maintaining plasma levels above the MEC for approximately 12 hours. Concurrent evaluation of the metabolites showed that the absorption truncation was a result of degradation of the active compound by microflora present in the large intestine, which is consistent with the transit time of dosage forms in the upper GI tract. This case study shows that the *in vivo* delivery window in the GI tract is determined by the inherent property of the drug molecule. Delivery technology is generally ineffective in overcoming feasibility obstacles when there is a large gap between the technology capability and required oral MR delivery need.

CASE STUDY 4

DEVELOPMENT COMPOUND B

A development compound in phase 2 clinical trials is a polar molecule with molecular weight of 284, a pK_a of 8.3, and a $\log D$ of −2.0 at pH 6.8.[136] It is stable and highly soluble (>0.8 g/ml) in the physiological pH range. Low permeability (Caco-2 $P_{app} = 0.27 \times 10^{-6}$ cm/sec) suggests it is likely a BCS class III compound. Phases 1–2 clinical studies used an IR formulation administered every six hours, due to rapid clearance in humans ($t_{1/2} = 4$ hours). Based on the projected MEC of 10 μg/ml, and a total dose of 6 mg, PK simulation indicated that twice-daily administration would require approximately 10 hours of in vivo input, suggesting a significant portion of the dose would be released and absorbed in the large intestine. A preliminary study for assessing the regional absorption in dogs via indwelling access ports to different regions of the intestinal tract showed that AUC values of ileum and colon delivery relative to that of jejunum were 0.94 and 0.67, respectively. In vitro drug release that follows square-root-of-time and near zero-order kinetics were obtained from matrix and ethylcellulose coated multi-unit mini-tablets, respectively. However, a crossover single dose study of three ER formulations with decreasing release rate in healthy volunteers resulted in relative bioavailability values of 50%, 34%, and 29%, respectively. Truncated absorption was observed at approximately 4 hours post-dosing under fasting conditions for all three ER formulations, indicating a lack of absorption in the lower bowel. The result of the dog regional absorption model was considered an outlier, because an extensive database generated had demonstrated the predictive nature of the model. Combined analysis of drug properties, absorption mechanism, and the physiological differences between human performance and the dog model suggests that the favorable absorption characteristics in the dog colon are likely a result of the leakier dog intestine that favors paracellular transport mechanism of a low dose, small polar molecule. This is consistent with previous discussion, and the results of a recent study[126] that used the dog model to predict colon permeability in humans. This study found that the relative bioavailability from administration to the colon of the dog correlated well with that of humans for model compounds of all four BCS classes except for atenolol, a hydrophilic small molecule. This case study illustrates the importance of understanding both the property and transport pathways of a compound in assessing in vivo absorption window for oral MR delivery.

CASE STUDY 5

OXYBUTYNIN HCL

Oxybutynin is an antispasmodic, anticholinergic agent indicated for the treatment of overactive bladder with symptoms of urge urinary incontinence, urgency, and frequency by relaxing bladder smooth muscle. It is a weak base with a pK_a of 9.87, and $\log D$ of 1.83 at pH 7.3. Its hydrochloride salt is freely soluble in water (12 mg/ml), stable, and well-absorbed from the intestinal tract. These favorable properties combined with the low dose (5–15 mg/day) make it an ideal candidate for oral MR, regardless of technologies applied.

For over 20 years, use of IR dosage forms of oxybutynin has been limited by anticholinergic adverse events, such as dry mouth, difficulty in micturition, constipation, blurred vision, drowsiness, and dizziness. These side-effects are dose-related, and sometimes severe. Studies have indicated that oxybutynin metabolism mediated by the cytochrome P450 3A4 isozyme occurs primarily in the proximal gastrointestinal tract and liver. Its primary active metabolite, N-desethyloxybutynin, is also responsible for much of the adverse effects. After administration of the IR formulation, N-desethyloxybutynin plasma levels may reach as much as six times that of the parent drug, substantially affecting the tolerability of the compound within the individual. For instance, in one population studied, after six months more than half of the patients had stopped taking the medication due to side-effects. Another study estimate is that over 25% of patients who begin oxybutynin treatment may have to stop because of dry mouth.

Since the 1990s, ER products have been investigated and developed (e.g., Ditropan® XL, Cystrin® CR tablets) with the aim of allowing once-daily administration and prolonged control of symptoms. Clinical studies have shown that ER formulations not only consistently enhanced patient compliance and efficacy, but also resulted in improved tolerability, including significantly higher continuation rate due to marked reduction of

CASE STUDY 5   (CONTINUED)

moderate/severe dry mouth. The latter was attributed to substantially lower intestinal metabolism, because a majority of the parent drug of the ER dosage form is delivered in the distal intestinal tract where metabolic enzyme activity in the gut wall is lower or absent. As a result, a substantial increase in bioavailability relative to IR formulation was also imparted. More recently, to totally bypass presystemic metabolism, a 4-day transdermal patch (Oxytrol®) was successfully developed with tolerability profile similar to that of a placebo.[136,137,138] This example shows that understanding of a drug's disposition properties, biological, and pharmacodynamic characteristics enables rational development of MR delivery strategy and design with maximized medical benefits.

20.4 SUMMARY

The most important elements of utilizing MR drug delivery design to achieve desired clinical benefits include defining the clinical rationale and understanding the drug molecule. The success of designing a commercially-viable MR dosage form depends on the physico-chemical, biopharmaceutical, pharmacokinetic, and biological properties of the drug candidate, rather than on a particular delivery technology. Today, almost all oral MR delivery needs can be addressed using three broad types of well-established delivery technologies discussed in this chapter. However, there is no "one-size-fits-all" technology. It is more important to select a technology based on technical, practical, developmental, and commercial considerations, because for many compounds with desirable properties for MR delivery, different "sizes" of technologies will fit "one" molecule.

References

1. Qiu, Y. & Zhang, G. (2000). Research and Development Aspects of Oral Controlled Release Systems. In: *Handbook of Pharmaceutical Controlled Release Technology*, D.L. Wise, A.M. Klibanov, R. Langer, A.G. Mikos, N.A. Peppas, D.J. Trantolo, G.E. Wnek, & M.J. Yaszeski, (eds). Marcel Dekker, Inc., New York, NY. pp. 465–503.
2. Qiu, Y. (2007). Design and Evaluation of Oral Modified-Release Dosage Forms Based on Drug Property and Delivery Technology. Proc. CAE/AAPS/CPA/CRS/FIP/APSTJ Conference: Oral Controlled Release Development and Technology. Shanghai, pp. 34–43.
3. Getsios, D., Caro, J.J., Ishak, K.J., El-Hadi, W., Payne, K., O'Connel, M., Albrecht, D., Feng, W. & Dubois, D. (2004). Oxybutynin extended release and tolterodine immediate release. Clin. Drug Invest. 24(2), 81–88.
4. Guidance for Industry. (1997). SUPAC-MR: Modified Release Solid Oral Dosage Forms Scale-Up and Postapproval Changes: Chemistry, Manufacturing, and Controls; *In vitro* Dissolution Testing and *In vivo* Bioequivalence Documentation. US Department of Health and Human Services, Food and Drug Administration, Center for Drug Evaluation and Research.
5. Wise, D.L., Klibanov, A.M., Langer, R., Mikos, A.G., Peppas, N.A., Trantolo, D.J. Wnek, G.E. & Yaszeski, M.J. (eds). *Handbook of Pharmaceutical Controlled Release Technology*, Marcel Dekker, Inc., New York, NY.
6. Robinson, J.R. & Lee, V.H.L. (eds). (1987). *Controlled Drug Delivery: Fundamentals and Applications*, 2nd edn.. Marcel Dekker, Inc., New York, NY.
7. Kydonieus, A. (1980). Fundamental Concepts of Controlled Release. In: *Controlled Release Technologies: Methods, Theory, and Applications*, A.F. Kydonieus (ed.), Vol. 1, p. 7.
8. Narasimhan, B. (2000). Accurate Models in Controlled Drug Delivery Systems. In: *Handbook of Pharmaceutical Controlled Release Technology*, D.L. Wise, A.M. Klibanov, R. Langer, A.G. Mikos, N.A. Peppas, D.J. Trantolo, G.E. Wnek, & M.J. Yaszeski, (eds). Marcel Dekker, Inc., New York, NY. pp. 155–181.
9. Colombo, P., Santi, P., Bettini, R. & Brazel, C.S. (2000). Drug Release from Swelling-Controlled Systems. In: *Handbook of Pharmaceutical Controlled Release Technology*, D.L. Wise, A.M. Klibanov, R. Langer, A.G. Mikos, N.A. Peppas, D.J. Trantolo, G.E. Wnek, & M.J. Yaszeski, (eds). Marcel Dekker, Inc., New York, NY. pp. 183–209.
10. Ford, J.L., Rubinstein, M.H., McCaul, F., Hogan, J.E. & Edgar, P.J. (1987). Importance of drug type, tablet shape and added diluents on drug release kinetics from hydroxypropylmethylcellulose matrix tablets. Int. J. Pharm. 40, 223–234.
11. Lee, P.I. (1983). Dimensional changes during drug release from a glassy hydrogel matrix. Polymer 24(Communications), 45–47.
12. Lee, P.I. & Peppas, N.A. (1987). Prediction of polymer dissolution in swellable controlled release systems. J. Controlled Release 6, 207–215.
13. Lee, P.I. (1985). Kinetics of drug release from hydrogel matrices. J. Controlled Release 2, 277–288.
14. Lee, P.I. (1981). Controlled drug release from polymeric matrices involving moving boundaries. In: *Controlled Release of Pesticides and Pharmaceuticals*, D. Lewis, (ed.). Plenum Publishing, New York, NY. pp. 39–48.
15. Lee, P.I. (1980). Diffusional release of a solute from a polymeric matrix—approximate analytical solutions. J. Membr. Sci. 7, 255–275.
16. Peppas, N.A. (1985). Analysis of Fickian and non-Fickian drug release from polymers. Pharm. Acta Helv. 60, 110–111.
17. Ford, J.L., Mitchell, K., Rowe, P., Armstrong, D.J., Elliott, P.N.C., Rostron, C. & Hogan, J.E. (1986). Mathematical modeling of drug release from hydroxypropyl-methylcellulose matrices: Effect of temperature. Int. J. Pharm. 71, 95–104.
18. Baveja, S.K. & Ranga Rao, K.V. (1986). Sustained release tablet formulation of centperazine. Int. J. Pharm. 31, 169–174.
19. Peppas, N.A. & Sahlin, J.J. (1989). A simple equation for the description of solute release. III. Coupling of diffusion and relaxation. Int. J. Pharm. 57, 169–172.
20. Ranga Rao, K.V., Padmalatha D.K. & Buri, P. Influence of molecular size and water solubility of the solute on its release

from swelling and erosion controlled polymeric matrices. J. Controlled Release, 12, 133–141.

21. Harland, R.S., Gazzaniga, A., Sangalli, M.E., Colombo, P. & Peppas, N.A. (1988). Drug/polymer matrix swelling and dissolution. Pharm. Res. 5, 488–494.

22. Catellani, P., Vaona, G., Plazzi, P. & Colombo, P. (1988). Compressed matrices, formulation and drug release kinetics. Acta Pharm. Technol. 34, 38–41.

23. Lee, P.I. & Kim, C.J. (1992). Effect of geometry on swelling front penetration in glassy polymers. J. Membrane Science 65, 77–92.

24. Lee, P.I. & Kim, C.J. (1991). Probing the mechanisms of drug release from hydrogels. J. Controlled Release 16, 229–236.

25. Ju, R.T., Nixon, P.R., Patel, M.V. & Tong, D.M. (1995). Drug release from hydrophilic matrices. 2. A mathematical model based on the polymer disentanglement concentration and the diffusion layer. J. Pharm. Sci. 84(12), 1464–1477.

26. Ju, R.T., Nixon, P.R. & Patel, M.V. (1995). Drug release from hydrophilic matrices. 1. New scaling laws for predicting polymer and drug release based on the polymer disentanglement concentration and the diffusion layer. J. Pharm. Sci. 84(12), 1455–1463, Dec.

27. Liu, P., Ju, T.R. & Qiu, Y. (2006). *Diffusion-Controlled Drug Delivery Systems in Design of Controlled Drug Delivery Systems*, X. Li & B.R. Jasdi (eds). McGraw-Hill Companies Inc., pp. 107–137.

28. Lee, P. I. (2007). Evolution of oral controlled/modified release dosage forms. Proc. CAE/AAPS/CPA/CRS/FIP/APSTJ Conference, Oral Controlled Release Development and Technology. Shanghai, pp. 22–31.

29. *Recipes for Fifty-Two Ailment*, Mawangdui Medical Manuscript. Dated 168 BC.

30. Ko Hung. (281–341) *Handbook of prescriptions for Urgent Cares.*

31. Higuchi, T. (1961). Rate of release of medicaments from ointment bases containing drugs in suspension. J. Pharm. Sci. 50, 847.

32. Higuchi, T. (1963). Mechanism of sustained release medication, theoretical analysisof rate of release of solid drugs dispersed in solid matrices. J. Pharm. Sci. 52, 1145.

33. Martin, A., Bustamante, P. & Chun, A.H.C. (1993). *Physical Pharmacy*, 4th edn. Lea & Febiger, Malvern, PA. pp. 324–355.

34. Crank, J. (1986). Diffusion in Heterogeneous Media. In: *The Mathematics of Diffusion*, J. Crank, (ed.), 2nd edn. Clarendon Press, Oxford. pp. 266–285.

35. Ritger, P.L. & Peppas, N.A. (1987). A simple equation for description of solute Fickian and non-Fickian release from nonswellable devices in the form of slabs, spheres, cylinders or disk. J. Controlled Release 5, 23–26.

36. Zhou, Y., Chu, J.S., Zhou, T. & Wu, X.Y. (2004). Modeling of drug release from two-dimensional matrix tablets with anisotropic properties. Biomaterials 26, 945–952.

37. Wu, X.Y. & Zhou, Y. (2000). Studies of diffusional release of a dispersed solute from polymeric matrixes by finite element method. J. Pharm. Sci. 88(10), 1050–1057.

38. Zhou, Y. & Wu, X.Y. (1997). Finite element analysis of diffusional drug release from complex matrix systems. I. Complex geometries and composite structures. J. Control. Rel. 49, 277–288.

39. Zhou, Y. & Wu, X.Y. (1998). Finite element analysis of diffusional drug release from complex matrix systems. II. Factors influencing release kinetics. J. Control. Rel. 51, 57–72.

40. Yonezawa, Y., Ishida, S., Suzuki, S. & Sunada, H. (2001). Release from or through a wax matrix system. I. Basic release properties of the wax matrix system. Chem. Pharm. Bull. 49(11), 1448–1451.

41. Yonezawa, Y., Ishida, S. & Sunada, H. (2003). Release from or through a wax matrix system. V. Applicability of the square-root time law equation for release from a wax matrix tablet. Chem. Pharm. Bull. 51(8), 904–908.

42. Yonezawa, Y., Ishida, S. & Sunada, H. (2005). Release from or through a wax matrix system. VI. Analysis and prediction of the entire release process of the wax matrix tablet. Chem. Pharm. Bull. 53(8), 915–918.

43. Hildgen, P. & McMullen, J. (1995). A new gradient matrix, formulation and characterization. J. Contr. Rel. 34, 263–271.

44. Kim, C. (1995). Compressed donut-shaped tablets with zero-order release kinetics. Pharm. Res. 12, 1045–1048.

45. Benkorah, A. & McMullen, J. (1994). Biconcave coated, centrally perforated tablets for oral controlled drug delivery. J. Contr. Rel. 32, 155–160.

46. Conte, U., Maggi, L., Colombo, P. & Manna, A. (1993). Multi-layered hydrophilic matrices as constant release devices (Geomatrix™ Systems). J. Contr. Rel. 26, 39–47.

47. Scott, D. & Hollenbeck, R. (1991). Design and manufacture of a zero-order sustained-release pellet dosage form through nonuniform drug distribution in a diffusional matrix. Pharm. Res. 8, 156–161.

48. Brooke, D. & Washkuhn, R. (1977). Zero-order drug delivery system, Theory and preliminary testing. J. Pharm. Sci. 66, 159–162.

49. Lipper, R. & Higuchi, W. (1977). Analysis of theoretical behavior of a proposed zero-order drug delivery system. J. Pharm. Sci. 66, 163–164.

50. Hsieh, D., Rhine, W. & Langer, R. (1983). Zero-order controlled release polymer matrices for micro and macro-molecules. J. Pharm. Sci. 72, 17–22.

51. Lee, I.P. (1984). Novel approach to zero-order drug delivery via immobilized nonuniform drug distribution in glassy hydrogels. J. Pharm. Sci. 70, 1344–1347.

52. Lee, I.P. (1984). Effect of non-uniform initial drug concentration distribution on the kinetics of drug release from glassy hydrogel matrices. Polymer 25, 973–978.

53. Kuu, W.-Y. & Yalkowsky, S.H. (1985). Multiple-hole approach to zero-order release. Journal of Pharmaceutical Sciences 74(9), 926–933.

54. Kim, C. (2005). Controlled release from triple layer, donut-shaped tablets with enteric polymers. AAPS Pharm Sci Tech. 6(3), E429–E436.

55. Bajpai, S.K., Bajpai, M., Saxena, S. & Dubey, S. (2006). Quantitative interpretation of the deviation from "zero-order" kinetics for the release of cyanocobalamin from a starch-based enzymatically degradable hydrogel. Journal of Macromolecular Science, Part A, Pure and Applied Chemistry 43(8), 1273–1277.

56. Wang, C.-C., Tejwani (Motwani), M.R., Roach, W.J., Kay, J.L., Yoo, J., Surprenant, H.L., Monkhouse, D.C. & Pryor, T.J. (2006). Development of near zero-order release dosage forms using three-dimensional printing (3-DP™). Technology, Drug Development and Industrial Pharmacy 32(3), 367–376.

57. Kshirsagar, R., Joshi, M. & Raichandani, Y. Extended release formulation of levetiracetam. US Patent Application # 20060165796.

58. Delargy, A.M., Timmins, P., Minhom, C. & Howard, J.R. (1989). The optimization of a pH independent matrix for the controlled release of drug materials using *in vitro* modeling. Proceed. Intern. Symp. Control. Rel. Bioact. Mater. 16, 378–379.

59. Ugarkovic, S., Trendovska-Serafimovska, G. & Sapkareva, B. (1996). Controlled release formulation of verapamil hydrochloride tablets. Acta. Pharma. 46, 155–157.

60. Venkatramana, R., Engh, K. & Qiu, Y. (2000). Design of pH-independent controlled release matrix tablets for acidic drugs. Int. J. Pharm. 252(1–2), 81–86.

61. Tatavarti, A.S., Mehta, K.A., Augsburger, L.L. & Hoag, S.W. (2004). Influence of methacrylic and acrylic acid polymers on the release performance of weakly basic drugs from sustained release hydrophilic matrices. J. Pharm. Sci. 93(9), 2319–2331.

62. Tatavarti, A.S. & Hoag, S.W. (2006). Microenvironmental pH modulation based release enhancement of a weakly basic drug from hydrophilic matrices. J. Pharm. Sci. 95(7), 1459–1468.

63. Howard, J.R., Timmins, P. (1988). Controlled Release Formulation, US Patent 4 792 452.

64. Zhang, G. & Pinnamaraju, P. (1997). Sustained Release Formulation Containing Three Different Types of Polymers, US Patent 5 695 781.

65. Qiu, Y., Rao, V. & Engh, K. pH-independent extended-release pharmaceutical formulation, US Patent 6 150 410.

66. Po, L.W., et al. (1990). Characterization of commercially available theophylline sustained- or controlled-release systems, in-vitro drug release profiles. Int. J. Pharm. 66, 111–130.

67. Pillay, V. & Fassihi, R. (2000). A novel approach for constant rate delivery of highly soluble bioactives from a simple monolithic system. J. Contr. Rel. 67, 67–78.

68. Hite, M., Federici, C., Turner, S. & Fassihi, R. (2003). Novel design of a self-correcting monolithic controlled-release delivery system for tramadol. Drug Del. Tech. 3, 48–55.

69. Rao, V., Haslam, J. & Stella, V. (2001). Controlled and complete release of a model poorly water-soluble drug, prednisolone, from hydroxypropyl methylcellulose matrix tablets using (SBE)(7 m)-beta-cyclodextrin as a solubilizing agent. J. Pharm. Sci. 90, 807–816.

70. Tanaka, N., Imai, K., Okimoto, K., Ueda, S., Tokunaga, Y., Ohike, A., Ibuki, R., Higaki, K. & Kimura, T. (2005). Development of novel sustained-release system, disintegration-controlled matrix tablet (DCMT) with solid dispersion granules of nilvadipine. J. Control Release, 58, 108(2 3), 386–395.

71. Shajahan, A. & Poddar, S.S. (2004). A flexible technology for modified release of drugs, multi layered tablets. J. Controlled Release 97(3), 393–405.

72. Qiu, Y., Chidambaram, N. & Flood, K. (1998). Design and evaluation of layered diffusional matrices for zero-order sustained-release. J. Controlled Release 51, 123–130.

73. Qiu, Y., Flood, K., Marsh, K., Carroll, S., Trivedi, J., Arneric, S.P. & Krill, S.L. (1997). Design of sustained-release matrix systems for a highly water-soluble compound, ABT-089. Int. J. Pharm. 157, 43–52.

74. Ozeki, T., Yuasa, H. & Okada, H. (2005). Controlled release of drug via methylcellulose-carboxyvinylpolymer interpolymer complex solid dispersion. AAPS PharmSciTech. 6(2), E231–E236.

75. Levina, M. & Rajabi-Siahboomi, A.R. (2004). The influence of excipients on drug release from hydroxypropyl methylcellulose matrices. J. Pharm. Sci. 93(11), 2746–2754.

76. Bajwa, G.S., Hoebler, K., Sammon, C., Timmins, P. & Melia, C.D. (2006). Microstructural imaging of early gel layer formation in HPMC matrices. J. Pharm. Sci. 95(10), 2145–2157.

77. Kazarian, S.G. & van der Weerd, J. (2008). Simultaneous FTIR spectroscopic imaging and visible photography to monitor tablet dissolution and drug release. Pharm. Res. 25(4), 853–860.

78. Donbrow, M. & Friedman, M. (1975). Enhancement of permeability of ethyl cellulose films for drug penetration. J. Pharm. Pharmacol. 27, 633.

79. Donbrow, M. & Samuelov, Y. (1980). Zero order drug delivery from double-layered porous films, release rate profiles from ethyl cellulose, hydroxypropyl cellulose and polyethylene glycol mixtures. J. Pharm. Pharmacol. 32, 463.

80. Rowe, R.C. (1986). The effect of the molecular weight of ethyl cellulose on the drug release properties of mixed films of ethyl cellulose and hydroxypropyl methylcellulose. Int. J. Pharm. 29, 37–41.

81. Porter, S. & Ghebre-Sellassie, I. (1994). Key factors in the development of modified-release pellets. In: *Multiparticulate Oral Drug Delivery*, I. Ghebre-Sellassie, (ed.). Marcel Dekker, New York. pp. 217–284.

82. Theeuwes, F. & Higuchi, T. (1975). US patent 3 916 899.

83. McClelland, G.A., Sutton, S.C., Engle, K. & Zentner, G.M. (1991). The solubility-modulated osmotic pump, *in vitro/in vivo* release of diltiazem hydrochloride. Pharm Res. 8, 88–92.

84. Makhija, S.N. & Vavia, P.R. (2003). Controlled porosity osmotic pump-based controlled release systems of pseudoephedrine. I. Cellulose acetate as a semipermeable membrane. J. Control Release 14, 89(1), 5–18.

85. Prabakaran, D., Singh, P., Kanaujia, P., Mishra, V., Jaganathan, K.S. & Vyas, S.P. (2004). Controlled porosity osmotic pumps of highly aqueous soluble drug containing hydrophilic polymers as release retardants. Pharm. Dev. Technol. 9(4), 435–442.

86. Okimoto, K., Tokunaga, Y., Ibuki, R., Irie, T., Uekama, K., Rajewski, R.A. & Stella, V.J. (2004). Applicability of (SBE)7 m-beta-CD in controlled-porosity osmotic pump tablets (OPTs). Int. J. Pharm. 286(1–2), 81–88.

87. Sotthivirat, S., Haslam, J.L. & Stella, V.J. (2007). Controlled porosity-osmotic pump pellets of a poorly water-soluble drug using sulfobutylether—cyclodextrin, (SBE)7M—CD, as a solubilizing and osmotic agent. J. Pharm. Sci. 96(9), 2364–2374.

88. Anand, V., Kandarapu, R. & Garg, S. (2001). Ion-exchange resins, carrying drug delivery forward. Drug Discovery Today 6(17), 905–914.

89. El-Menshawy, M.E. & Ismail, A.A. (1976). Polysalt flocculates as a physicochemical approach in the development of controlled-release oral pharmaceuticals. Pharmazie 31(12), 872–874.

90. Bonferoni, M.C., Rossi, S., Ferrari, F. & Caramella, C. (2004). Development of oral controlled release tablet formulations based on diltiazem–carrageenan complex. Pharmaceutical Development and Technology 9(2), 155–162.

91. Chaudhry, N.C. & Saunders, L. (1956). Sustained release of drugs from ion exchange resins. J Pharm. Pharmacol. 38, 975–986.

92. Chaubal, M.V. (2003). Synthetic polymer-based ion exchange resins, excipients and actives. Drug Delivery Technology 3(5).

93. Abdekhodaie, M.J. & Wu, X.Y. (2008). Drug release from ion-exchange microspheres, mathematical modeling and experimental verification. Biomaterials 29, 1654–1663.

94. Abdekhodaie, M.J. & Wu, X.Y. (2006). Drug loading onto ion exchange microspheres, modeling study and experimental verification. Biomaterials 27, 3652–3662.

95. Sriwongjanya, M. & Bodmeier, R. (1998). Effect of ion exchange resins on the drug release from matrix tablets. Eur J. Pharm. Biopharm. 46(3), 321–327.

96. Klausner, E.A., Lavy, E., Friedman, M. & Hoffman, A. (2003). Expandable gastroretentive dosage forms. J. Controlled Release 90, 143–162.

97. Streubel, A., Siepmann, J. & Bodmeier, R. (2006). Gastroretentive drug delivery systems. Expert Opinion on Drug Delivery 3(2), 217–233.

98. Kagana, L., Lapidotb, N., Afarganb, M., Kirmayerb, D., Moora, E., Mardorc, Y., Friedmana, M. & Hoffman, A. (2006). Gastroretentive accordion pill, enhancement of riboflavin bioavailability in humans. J. Controlled Release 113(3), 208–215.

99. Pozzi, F., Furlani, P., Gazzaniga, A., Davis, S.S. & Wilding, I.R. (1994). The TIME CLOCK system, a new oral dosage form for fast and complete release of drug after a predetermined lag time. J. Controlled Release 3, 99–108.

100. Ashford, M. & Fell, J.T. (1994). Targeting drugs to the colon, delivery systems for oral administration. J. Drug Targeting 2, 241–258.

101. Van den Mooter, G. (2006). Colon drug delivery. Expert Opin Drug Deliv. Jan, 3(1), 111–125.

102. Basit, A.W. (2005). Advances in colonic drug delivery. Drugs 65(14), 1991–2007.

103. Chourasia, M.K. & Jain, S.K. (2003). Pharmaceutical approaches to colon targeted drug delivery systems. J. Pharm. Sci. 6(1), 33–66.

104. Shareef, M.A., Khar, R.K., Ahuja, A., Ahmad, F.J. & Raghava, S. (2003). Colonic drug delivery, an updated review. AAPS PharmSci. 5(2), E17.

105. Maroni, A., Zema, L., Cerea, M. & Sangalli, M.E. (2005). Oral pulsatile drug delivery systems. Expert Opinion on Drug Delivery 2(5), 855–871.

106. Arora Shweta, A.J., Ahuja, A. & Baboota Sanjula, Q. (2006). Pulsatile drug delivery systems: An approach for controlled drug delivery. Indian J. Pharm. Sci. 68(3), 95–300.

107. Till, B., Ina, O. & Rolan, B. (2001). Pulsatile drug-delivery systems. Critical reviews in therapeutic drug carrier systems 18(5), 433–458.

108. Anal, A.K. (2007). Time-controlled pulsatile delivery systems for bioactive compounds. Recent Patents on Drug Delivery & Formulation 1(1), 73–77.

109. Eichel, H.J., Massmann, B.D. & Cobb, Jr., J.E. Delayed, sustained-release diltiazem pharmaceutical preparation. US Patent 5 529 790.

110. Hendrickson, D.L., Dimmitt, D.C., Williams, M.S., Skultety, P.F. & Baltezor, M.J. Diltiazem formulation. US Patent 5 286 497.

111. Barnwell, S.G. Biphasic release formations for lipophilic acids. US Patent 5 391 377.

112. Cheung, W.K., Silber, B.M. & Yacobi, A. (1991). Pharmacokinetic principles in the design of immediate-release components in sustained-release formulations with zero-order release characteristics. J. Pharm. Sci. 80(2), 142–148.

113. Buttgereit, F., Doering, G., Schaeffler, A., Witte, S., Sierakowski, S., Gromnica-Ihle, E., Jeka, S., Krueger, K., Szechinski, J. & Alten, R. (2008). Efficacy of modified-release versus standard prednisone to reduce duration of morning stiffness of the joints in rheumatoid arthritis (CAPRA-1), a double-blind, randomized controlled trial. Lancet 371, 205–213.

114. Radebaugh, G.W., Murtha, J.L. & Glinecke, R. Oral sustained release acetaminophen formulation and process. US Patent 4 968 509.

115. Eichel, H.J. & Massmann, B.D. Sustained-release pharmaceutical preparation. US Patent 5 026 559.

116. Points to consider on the clinical requirements of modified release products submitted as a line extension of an existing marketing authorization. European Agency for the Evaluation of Medicinal Products, Committee for Proprietary Medicinal products (CPMP) December, 2003.

117. Mager, D.E., Wyska, E. & Jusko, W.J. (2003). Diversity of mechanism-based pharmacodynamic models. Drug Metab. Dis. 31(5), 510–519.

118. Breimer, D.D. (1996). An integrated pharmacokinetic and pharmacodynamic approach to controlled drug delivery. J. Drug Targetting 3, 411–415.

119. Hoffman, A. (1998). Pharmacodynamic aspects of sustained release preparations. Adv. Drug Delivery Rev. 33, 185–199.

120. Sutton, S.C. (2004). Companion animal physiology and dosage form performance. Advanced Drug Delivery Reviews 56(10), 1383–1398.

121. Bauer, K.H., Lehmann, K., Osterwald, H.P. & Rothgang, G. (1998). Environmental Conditions in the Digestive Tract and their Influence on the Dosage Form. In: Coated Pharmaceutical Dosage Forms, Fundamentals, Manufacturing Techniques, Biopharmaceutical Aspects, Test Methods and Raw Materials. Medpharm GmbH Scientific Publishers, Birkenwaldstr, Stuttgart. pp. 126–130.

122. Abrahamssona, B., Alpstenb, M., Bakec, B., Jonssona, U.E., Eriksson-Lepkowskaa, M. & Larsson, A. (1998). Drug absorption from nifedipine hydrophilic matrix extended-release (ER) tablet-comparison with an osmotic pump tablet and effect of food. J. Controlled Release 52(3), 301–310.

123. Qiu, Y., Cheskin, H., Engh, K. & Poska, R. (2003). Once-a-day controlled-release dosage form of Divalproex Sodium I, formulation design and in vitro/in vivo investigations. J. Pharm. Sci. 92(6), 1166–1173.

124. Vinks, A.A & Walson, P.D. (2003). Developmental Principles of Pharmacokinetics. Chapter 4. In: Pediatric Psychopharmacology, Principles and Practice. A. Martin, L. Scahill, D. S. Charney & J. F. Leckman (eds). Oxford University Press, New York, USA, p. 49.

125. Sutton, S., Evans, L., Fortner, J., McCarthy, J. & Sweeney, K. (2006). Dog colonoscopy model for predicting human colon absorption. Pharmaceutical Research 23(7), 1554–1563.

126. Wilson, C.G. & Washington, N. (2000). Gamma Scintigraphy in the Analysis of the Behaviors of Controlled Release Systems. In: Handbook of Pharmaceutical Controlled Release Technology, D.L. Wise, A.M. Klibanov, R. Langer, A.G. Mikos, N.A. Peppas, D.J. Trantolo, G.E. Wnek, & M.J. Yaszeski, (eds). Marcel Dekker, Inc., New York, NY. pp. 551–566.

127. Stevens, H.N.E. & Speakman, M. (2006). Behaviour and transit of tamsulosin oral controlled absorption system in the gastrointestinal tract. Current Medical Research and Opinion 22(12), 2323–2328.

128. Gualtieri., et al. (1982). Clinical studies of methylphenidate serum levels in children and adults. J. Am. Academy Child Psychiatry 21, 19–26.

129. Pentikis, H.S. & Gonzalez, M.A. (2005). Effect of formulation on methylphenidate release patterns: Clinical implications. Am. J. Drug Delivery 3(1), 47–54.

130. Gonzalez, M.A., Pentikis, H.S., Anderl, N., Benedict, M.F., DeCory, H.H., Dirksen, S.J.H. & Hatch, S.J. (2002). Methylphenidate bioavailability from two extended-release formulations. Int. J. Clin. Pharmacol. Ther. 40, 175–184.

131. Sonuga-Barke, E.J.S., Van Lier, P., Swanson, J.M., Coghill, D., Wigal, S., Vandenberghe, M. & Hatch, S. (2007). Heterogeneity in the pharmacodynamics of two long-acting methylphenidate formulations for children with attention deficit/hyperactivity disorder: A growth mixture modeling analysis. Eur. Child Adolesc. Psychiatry. Published online, 10 December.

132. Markowitz, J.S., Straughn, A.B., Patrick, K.S., DeVane, C.L., Pestreich, L., Lee, J., Wang, Y. & Muniz, R. (2003). Pharmacokinetics of methylphenidate after oral administration of two modified-release formulations in healthy adults. Clin. Pharmacokinet. 42(4), 393–401.

133. Wang, Y., Lee, L., Somma, R., Thompson, G., Bakhtiar, R., Lee, J., Rekhi, G.S., Lau, H., Sedek, G. & Hossain, M. (2004). In vitro dissolution and in vivo oral absorption of methylphenidate from a bimodal release formulation in healthy volunteers. Biopharm. Drug Dispos. 25(2), 91–98.

134. Qiu, Y. (2002). Influence of drug properties and formulation design on in vivo performance of oral modified-release solid dosage forms. AAPS Conference on Pharmaceutics and Drug Delivery, Arlington, VA.

135. Qiu, Y. (2007). Design and evaluation of oral modified-release dosage forms based on drug property and delivery technology. Proceedings of CAE/AAPS/CPA/CRS/FIP/APSTJ Joint Conference, Oral Controlled Release Development and Technology. Shanghai, China. pp. 144–147.

136. Dmochowski, R., Staskin, D. & Kell, S. (2002). Oxybutynin chloride, alterations in drug delivery and improved therapeutic index. Expert Opinion on Pharmacotherapy 3(4), 443–454.

137. Michel, M.C. (2002). A benefit-risk assessment of extended-release oxybutynin. Drug Safety 25(12), 867–876.

138. Dmochowski1, R.R. & Staskin, D.R. (2002). Advances in drug delivery: Improved bioavailability and drug effect. Current Urology Reports 3(6), 1527–2737.

Development of Modified-Release Solid Oral Dosage Forms

Yihong Qiu and Guohua Zhang

21.1 INTRODUCTION

A pharmaceutical dosage form development program generally includes preformulation studies, analytical method development and validation, design, development, scale-up and optimization of formulation and manufacturing process, and stability studies. This chapter will primarily focus on the transformation of technology-based dosage form design discussed in the preceding chapter into commercial modified-release (MR) products that meet patient requirements. The technology transformation process involves design and development of effective manufacturing processes that assure product quality and performance. In addition, regulation, process efficiency, robustness, capability and control, equipment, facility, capacity, development cost and time, environmental impact, market dynamics, etc., must be considered. For MR products, these considerations often have strong implications, not only for developing a reliable dosage form and robust process to ensure a predefined product quality, assure manufacturability and productivity, but also for developing new technologies or marketing the technologies as products.

Solid dosage forms are complex multi-component systems with many solid phases. A majority of components are organic compounds with a very wide range of physical, chemical, and mechanical properties, as opposed to the mostly inert inorganic components used in high technology industries. When combining these different organic solid phases via processing to form a compact mixture system, product performance and/or processability may or may not be acceptable, depending on their chemical, physical or mechanical compatibility. Today's science and technology are unable to model and predict precisely general processing behavior, quality, and performance of the solid mixtures. In addition, the multi-stage batch process used in pharmaceutical manufacturing makes it more difficult to predict and control the process outcome, due to the presence of a multitude of interacting formulation and process variables. For instance, the governing equations of the dynamic flow, stochastic mixing and binding of solid particles having diverse morphology, density and surface properties in the presence or absence of liquid, are either undefined or poorly understood in wet granulation, drying or blending processes, hence limiting our ability to accurately model these unit operations. For a product developed under one set of conditions, even a small incremental change or adjustment of the components or their source, processing condition or equipment often requires investment of extensive resources and time to demonstrate that product quality remains unchanged. This is partly caused by a lack of understanding of the potential impact of such changes, because of the complexity of solid dosage forms, and the current state of science and technology. It is also affected by the conservative philosophy and policy adopted by both sponsors and

Developing Solid Oral Dosage Forms: Pharmaceutical Theory and Practice
ISBN: 978-0-444-53242-8

regulators, since the pharmaceutical industry is one of the most highly regulated industries, and there is generally little margin for error allowed. However, these challenges should not deter scientists from applying principles of multidisciplinary sciences and systematic approach in developing MR dosage forms.

21.2 DEVELOPMENT OF MODIFIED-RELEASE SOLID ORAL PRODUCTS

Because of the complexity of solid dosage forms and the challenges in applying the principles of basic and applied sciences in the pharmaceutical industry, the strategies and approaches that have been, and continue to be, utilized in solid product development vary significantly from company to company, and even across project teams within the same organization. Some groups tend to rely more heavily on empirical studies and personal experiences that can get the job done, but are often inefficient. Some rely on limited past experiences or "gut feelings," that may or may not be valid or applicable. Others take a more rational approach, by systematically applying applicable scientific principles to development. In general, these practices can be divided into three broad categories summarized in Table 21.1.

Adopting a rational development approach with increased level of scientific understanding can result in many benefits for patients, the industry, and regulatory bodies. The advantages include a higher level of assurance of product quality and performance, more robust manufacturing process and process control, increased cost-saving, and improved efficiency through minimized product rejects or recalls and enhanced opportunities for first-cycle regulatory approval. A rational development approach also helps expand risk management strategy, streamline post-approval changes, and offers opportunities for continual improvement post-product launch. In fact, this is the approach the FDA has been advocating as part of its ongoing quality initiative, "cGMPs for the 21st Century," announced in 2002[1] in an effort to enhance and modernize pharmaceutical product quality and manufacturing. Over the past six years, the FDA has collaborated with the International Conference on Harmonization (ICH) and the industry in defining a shared vision, key concepts, and general framework of this initiative. Among the critical concepts is pharmaceutical quality by design (QbD).[2] It is a systematic scientific approach to product and process design and development, to ensure product quality through understanding and controlling formulation and manufacturing variables. In 2006, the principles of QbD were incorporated in the ICH Q8 (Pharmaceutical Development), Q9 (Quality Risk Management) and Q10 (Pharmaceutical Quality System)[3] guidances, which have since been updated. In 2007, the Office of Generic Drugs (OGD) of the FDA officially started implementation of a question-based review (QbR) developed for its chemistry, manufacturing, and control (CMC) evaluation of the abbreviated new drug applications (ANDAs). The QbR is a new quality assessment system that incorporates key elements of QbD. It requires applicants to use the common technical document (CTD) framework to address QbR questions by applying QbD principles.[4]

Under the QbD paradigm, the product is designed to meet patient requirements, the process is designed to consistently meet product critical quality attributes, the impact of starting materials and process parameters on product quality is understood, critical sources of process variation are identified and controlled, and the process is continually monitored and updated to allow for consistent quality over time.[2] Therefore, the merger of scientific, business, and regulatory sensibilities has increased the urgency and begun to propel the adoption of the principles of rational product development in recent years.

21.2.1 Rational Development Approach

Rational product development requires integrated consideration of three essential areas:

1. preformulation investigation;
2. formulation and process studies; and
3. *in vivo* performance evaluation in order to produce a high quality, solid product with predefined delivery and pharmacokinetic performance.

The key to a successful development program is proactively and systematically applying principles of multiple areas of basic and applied sciences, such as pharmaceutical sciences, chemistry, biological sciences, and engineering, mathematics, and statistics, as shown in Figure 21.1.

Development of an MR dosage form starts with defining a target product quality profile, based on the clinical needs discussed in the preceding chapter on MR technology and system design. In addition to the target PK profile, other important criteria include strength, type, size, drug loading, and quality/performance attributes of the dosage form, as well as commercial need, and intellectual property. The second step is to conduct preformulation investigations, to

TABLE 21.1 Comparison of approaches to solid product development

Approach	Characteristics	Likely outcome
Trial-and-error	Ignoring specific characteristics of raw materials and formulation, and scientific principles	Disconnect between data and underlying mechanism
	Trying out various experiments or hypotheses in different directions until a desired outcome is obtained with some degree of reliability	Can often be overwhelmed or misled by data generated from uncontrolled experiments with confounding variables, thus exacerbating problems, and inhibiting innovation
	Over-reliance on past experience and "gut feeling," e.g., copying "recipe" from one compound to another	Inconsistent or non-robust product and process that can often lead to failures during development or post-approval product recalls
	Extensive use of "shotgun" approach	Considerable waste of time, and resources, resulting in poor development efficiency
	Lack of a consistent approach	
Semi-empirical	Combining experience with analysis of abundant data (often retrospectively) to identify trends or build empirical or semi-empirical relationships	Results can be practically useful, but may be unreliable or misleading in certain cases, due to improper design and limitations of experiments and/or lack of comprehensive scrutiny of pooled data, and formulation/process variables involved
	Using best guessed "trial-and-error" approach based on prior knowledge	Lack of fundamental understanding of underlying mechanism
		Lower development efficiency due to time and extensive resources required
Rational	Applying proactively comprehensive knowledge and techniques of multiple scientific disciplines and experience to the understanding of the characteristics of raw materials, delivery system, process, and *in vivo* performance	Enhanced understanding of how material properties, process variables, and product attributes relate to product performance, as well as the interplays between biological system, and the drug substance or dosage form
	Integrating formulation/process design and development by applying systematic approach, and utilizing interdisciplinary scientific and engineering principles	Greater product and process understanding for consistent product quality, improved control, and risk management
		Increased efficiency, decreased cost and product rejects
	Using the "best guessed" approach appropriately by combining prior knowledge with theoretical analysis in experimental designs	Streamlined post-approval changes, and enhanced opportunities for continual improvement
		Conform to quality by design principle under cGMP of the twenty-first century

characterize properties of raw materials including their physico-chemical, biopharmaceutical, and mechanical properties, as well as compatibility, that are discussed extensively in the relevant chapters of this book. Once the quality attributes of the drug substance and excipients are determined, process feasibility and options should be evaluated. There is often more than one way to produce a predefined MR system. An appropriate manufacturing process should be selected, based on technological, economic, and practical considerations, including available technologies and their maturity, development cost and time, process complexity, robustness, scale-up challenges, manufacturability and control, commercial production efficiency, cost and capacity, along with available equipment, facility, and environmental impact.

One of the most critical elements of dosage form development is to apply a unified view of formulation and process development. Integrated formulation and process design will not only result in robust products with predefined quality characteristics, but will also help to ensure optimum productivity, and minimize or avoid potential composition-related processing issues or process-related performance problems. An MR formulation consists of the essential rate-controlling material(s) called for by the chosen system design, and other necessary excipients, such as filler, binder, lubricant, physical or chemical stabilizer, processing aid, etc. Selection of these ingredients requires consideration of their functionality and processing characteristics with respect to the process train, as well as the active ingredient(s).

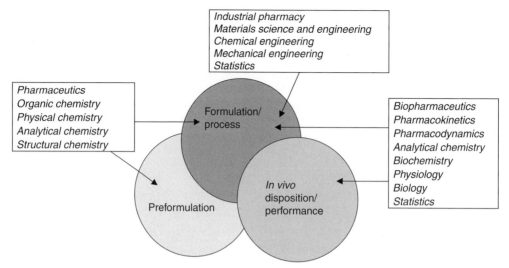

FIGURE 21.1   Integrated scientific disciplines important to rational product development

21.2.2 Preformulation Studies

Preformulation data of a drug substance including solubility, stability, permeability, solid-state properties, and compatibility with excipients, etc., is essential to formulation scientists in developing a stable, safe, effective, and manufacturable dosage form. For an MR product, knowledge and control of the properties of other formulation ingredients, particularly the rate-modifying component, are often equally important. This type of information forms the foundation for rational product and process design, maximizes the chances of success in developing an acceptable product, and ultimately provides a basis for optimizing the quality and performance of the product.

The importance and techniques of a complete physico-chemical characterization in the rational design of a solid dosage form have been discussed in the relevant chapters of this book. The data generated are frequently applied to IR and MR solid products in a similar fashion, as the principles and manufacturing processes of both types of dosage forms are fundamentally the same. For instance, bupropion hydrochloride, an antidepressant, was found to undergo extensive degradation in an alkaline environment, based on preformulation investigation. To develop an acceptable ER dosage form, weak acids or salts of strong acids were incorporated in the formulation (e.g., citric acid, tartaric acid, ascorbic acid, malic acid, tartaric acid, sodium metabisulfate, L-cystine hydrochloride, glycine hydrochloride).[5,6] These stabilizers serve to provide an acidic environment surrounding the active drug that minimizes its degradation. Recently, Oberegger et al. discovered a more

stable bupropion composition for extended-release dosage forms through salt selection experiments.[7]

The potential influence of the solid phase of a drug substance on quality attributes or processing of an ER system has been well-documented. In studying crystalline properties of an insoluble drug, carbamazepine, in a hydrophilic matrix system, Katzhendler et al. found that the rate-controlling polymer, HPMC, not only inhibits the conversion to less soluble dihydrate from the anhydrous form in the hydrated layer, but also induces the formation of the amorphous phase during the drug release process.[8] These types of solid phase transformations may impact swelling and erosion characteristics of the dosage form, as well as *in vivo* drug performance. More recently, Li et al. investigated solid phase transformation of ciprofloxacin during formulation processing using DSC, TGA, PXRD, and powder dissolution.[9] These studies showed that the process-induced phase transition from anhydrate to hydrate could be controlled through proper selection of excipients and processing conditions. Drug release testing of HPMC based ER matrix tablets indicated that phase transformation was significantly inhibited by HPMC in the gel layer of the hydrated tablets.

Many weak bases or weak acids exhibit pH-dependent solubility in the physiological pH range that may affect MR design and drug release, and/absorption in the GI tract. Etodolac, a nonsteroidal anti-inflammatory drug, is very slightly soluble below pH 3. The solubility increases gradually up to pH 5, followed by a 30-fold increase at pH 7. To minimize the dependency of its solubility on pH, a release rate-modifying agent (e.g., dibasic sodium phosphate) was incorporated into the ER tablet formulation to enhance drug release in an acidic environment.[10] However, the effectiveness of this approach is not universal. It often depends on the drug release mechanism, the properties of the drug, and the release-modifying agent, as well as the relative ratio of the two components. For example, in a diffusion-controlled matrix system, a small inorganic molecule (e.g., dicalcium phosphate) soluble at low pH may leach out of the system more rapidly than the active substance, resulting in little change of pH in the matrix over the extended duration of drug release. Thus, it is important to understand the characteristics of the active and the excipient (e.g., solubility, buffering capacity) in relation to the release mechanism, such that the effectiveness of the release-modifying agent is maintained in a delivery device over the entire length of drug release.[11]

21.2.3 Dosage Form Development

Dosage form development involves design and development of a product with a defined target product quality profile, and a defined manufacturing process. The most common options of MR solid dosage forms are single unit tablets, multi-unit beads or mini-tablets in capsules and multiparticulates for reconstitution or sprinkle, manufactured using essentially the same processes as those for the IR dosage forms. Table 21.2 lists dosage forms for different types of MR systems. The general aspects of these dosage forms, related technologies, process development, and in-process control have been extensively addressed,[2,12] and also discussed in detail in the relevant chapters of this book. In general, processes for tablet manufacture include direct compression, wet granulation, dry granulation (e.g., roller compaction, slugging), and melt granulation or thermoplastic pelletizing (e.g., high shear, melt-extrusion, spray-congealing). Processes for producing round solid beads encompass extrusion–spheronization, drug layering of non-pareil seeds, spray granulation/spray drying, and spray congealing. Conventional compression processes are also utilized to prepare mini-tablets, using either small conventional tooling or multi-head tooling (e.g., 2 mm), depending on the tablet size and throughput considerations (Figure 21.2). MR coating of tablets or beads is most often carried out in a pan coater or fluid-bed, depending on the nature of the coating substrate (e.g., size, tensile strength, etc.). Coating by compression (tablet-in-tablet) requires a special compression machine. In most cases, use of

TABLE 21.2 Common dosage forms of different MR systems

MR systems	Dosage form presentation
Matrix ER	Monolithic tablet; layered tablet; multi-units in capsule; compression-coated tablet; multiparticulates for reconstitution or sprinkle
Reservoir ER	Multi-units in capsule; monolithic tablet; multiparticulates for reconstitution or sprinkle
Osmotic ER	Monolithic tablet or capsule; layered tablet; multi-units in capsule
Delayed release	Monolithic tablet; multi-units in capsule; compression-coated tablet; multiparticulates for reconstitution or sprinkle
Pulsatile release	Multi-units in capsule; layered tablet or capsule; compression-coated tablet; multiparticulates for reconstitution or sprinkle

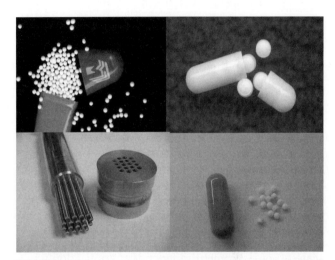

FIGURE 21.2 Examples of beads and mini-tablets prepared with single-head or multi-head tooling

conventional manufacturing processes and equipment is highly preferred. When a more complicated process is required for products of increased complexity, e.g., multi-layered tablets, compression coating, mixed beads, and/or mini-tablets, emphasis should be placed on increased process and product understanding throughout the development lifecycle to ensure successful development from small- to commercial-scale. Compared to the IR counterpart, a higher standard is usually required for the rate-modifying function of the MR product. For example, tighter, and/or additional control of rate-controlling materials or uniformity of functional coat for the reservoir and osmotic pump systems, is often necessary to ensure consistent batch-to-batch product performance.

21.2.4 Product and Process Understanding

A sound dosage form design provides manufacturers with a unique quality product, and helps to ensure optimum productivity and smooth technology transfer. Ideally, the design should be based on a mechanistic understanding of physico-chemical and mechanical transformations of the raw materials that ultimately result in the desired product. However, the diversity and complexity of pharmaceutical ingredients, combined with the unit operation paradigm utilized in pharmaceutical manufacturing, usually make such complete understanding unattainable. In many cases, knowledge gained appears to be material- and equipment-specific (dependent on machine design, geometry, model, manufacturer, etc.), making it challenging to develop universal models for direct application to different scales, processes, and products. Nevertheless, it is both important and possible to apply a systematic approach to dosage form development and experimental designs for in-depth understanding of the process train, sources of variability, and risks to product integrity. For instance, enhanced product and process understanding can be achieved by breaking down unit operations, and applying integrated pharmaceutical theories and engineering principles. Depending on the complexity of the materials and particular unit operation, mechanistic and empirical modeling may be utilized or combined, based on the accumulated scientific knowledge of the system, the theory behind basic unit operations, and the relevant parameters critical to the resulting transformation of the raw materials. Mechanistic models are generally more useful for direct application of scale-up or equipment-independent application when available. In many cases, scientific theories and practical models that describe how the process parameters and material characteristics interrelate can be applied to development or problem-solving. For example, fluidized-bed drying has been shown to be more amenable to mechanistic models compared to high shear wet granulation. More detailed discussions of development and scale-up principles of pharmaceutical manufacturing operations can be found in Chapters 29–37.

In designing a product and manufacturing process, selection of a proper delivery technology, components, and corresponding process options should be based on a comprehensive analysis of information on:

1. target product characteristics (dose, release mode, etc.);
2. preformulation investigations;
3. biopharmaceutics studies;
4. formulation technology;
5. types of equipment and methods utilized to perform unit operations in R&D and production;
6. raw material attributes and potential interactions (e.g., drug–excipient, excipient–excipient);
7. interrelation between materials and unit operations; and
8. how product characteristics dictate the unit operations selected.

This type of information can be used to: (1) guide proper product and process design; (2) anticipate and effectively evaluate the impact of formulation on processing, or vice versa; (3) understand the influence of formulation/processing on product quality and performance; (4) facilitate future technology transfer. For example, multiparticulates offer certain advantages over single unit dosage forms, in that they have minimum risk of dose dumping and exhibit lower *in vivo* variability, due to their more favorable GI transit characteristics. In addition, multi-unit systems can be designed to provide customized release profiles by combining beads with different release rates or to deliver incompatible drugs in the same dosage unit. For MR dosage forms, understanding and control of critical properties and the inherent lot-to-lot variability of rate-controlling materials within or outside USP, and the vendor's specifications are often necessary to minimize their potential impact on processing, drug release, and/or *in vivo* performance. In processing a tablet, components present at high percentages (e.g., drug or polymer) in the formulation often significantly influence or even dominate the processing behavior, be it fluidization, granulation, blending or compaction. Compressibility of a tablet composition depends not only on the deformation and bonding properties of the major components, but also on compression parameters (force, turret speed/dwell time, precompression) or moisture content for predominantly plastically deformed materials. In a drug-layering process, low coating efficiency resulting from drug–excipient interaction can only be resolved by avoiding such interaction, rather than through manipulating processing parameters. Similarly, layer separation of layered tablets caused by incompatibility of the materials should be addressed through a fundamental understanding of the materials (e.g., deformation, bonding, moisture, time-dependency, etc.). In recent years, the potential implication of solid phase changes during processing is an area that has received increased attention.[13] For example, solid phase transition from the stable crystalline to the less stable amorphous drug caused by processing conditions can directly lead to chemical instability of the product.[14] Increased hardening with age (or age-hardening) of tablets may adversely affect the dissolution rate during storage.[15] Depending on the material properties and processing condition, the change of tablet hardness may be attributed to recrystallization of a physically stable phase from a small portion of a metastable or amorphous phase of either the drug substance or excipient (e.g., mannitol) generated during processing. It should be noted that this type of phase transition is often a function of material characteristics, composition, type, and condition of a specific unit operation. Through characterization of the materials and their interplay with the dosage form and process, the solid phase changes can be anticipated and avoided if they are undesirable. They may also be controlled and utilized to enhance product performance (e.g., dissolution).[13]

In building a development strategy, adopting a systematic approach to investigation and process development is essential for a greater understanding of product and its manufacturing process. In addition to the use of prior knowledge and quality risk management, one of the most commonly applied tools is statistical design of experiments (DOE). This is a structured, organized method for determining the relationship between factors (Xs) affecting a process or a system, and the output of the process (Y). For pharmaceutical systems or processes with measurable inputs and outputs, DOE can be used to guide the optimal selection of inputs and analysis of results in formulation screening, problem solving, parameter design, and robustness study. Basic concepts are available in the Experimental Design section of an electronic textbook, *StatSoft*, at http://www.statsoft.com/textbook/stathome.html. The fundamental principles, techniques, and applications of DOE can be found in many books written on this subject.[16] In pharmaceutical development, application of DOE has proven invaluable in maximizing information gained with minimum resources, identifying critical factors among a multitude of variables, solving problems in a complex system consisting of many confounding factors, defining, optimizing, and controlling product and process variables.[17,18,19,20,21] In fact, DOE is so widely applied in today's pharmaceutical R&D and operations that there appears to be a general perception that running statistically designed experiments is equivalent to product and processing understanding. This, in part, is a result of the historical success of using DOE across multiple industries, and partly due to a lack of understanding of the intricacies and pitfalls of designing and executing such experiments in the study of complex pharmaceutical and biological systems. For example, understanding the precision of measurements of inputs versus outputs, and the need for repeat observations or identifying confounding factors, is

not trivial, while putting together an experimental design table is a very simple task. All of the well-known classes of standard statistical experimental designs can be generated automatically by software once the number and nature of input variables and the responses are defined. It should be pointed out that an incorrectly or improperly designed experiment not only results in wasted resources and time, but often generates data that are confusing or misleading. Some common problems associated with designed experiments in dosage form development or investigation include:

1. choosing inappropriate design variables, and, in particular, their ranges;
2. running uncontrolled experiments due to obliviousness to confounding factors;
3. generating unreliable or inconclusive data resulting from inadequately repeated measurements, insufficiently large sample sizes or lack of understanding of the signal-to-noise ratio (SNR).

In building an experimental design it is vital to first acquire a basic knowledge of the studied system, and utilize multidisciplinary principles and expertise (e.g., pharmaceutics, chemistry, engineering, statistics, etc.) to identify factors and define factor levels, as this is the part that requires the most skill. Moreover, a clear understanding of the difference between control and noise factors is also critical. Specifically, it is very important to carefully select a small number of experiments under controlled conditions, and take the following interrelated steps:

1. Define an objective to the investigation, e.g., sort out important variables or find optima.
2. Determine the design variables that will be controlled, and their levels or ranges of variation, as well as variables that will be fixed.
3. Determine the response variables that will be measured to describe the outcome, and examine their precision.
4. Among the available standard designs, choose one that is compatible with the objective, number of design variables, and precision of measurements.

It should be emphasized that DOE is, in most cases, a strategy to gather empirical knowledge, i.e., knowledge based on the analysis of experimental data and not on theoretical models. Thus, it is mainly useful for investigating a phenomenon, not the underlying mechanistic root cause of a problem. Use of experimental design strategy, in conjunction with application of the scientific and engineering theories, techniques and practices presented throughout this book, is essential to the rational and efficient development of robust product and process from laboratory to production scales.

21.3 TECHNOLOGY TRANSFER

In the pharmaceutical industry, "technology transfer" may broadly refer to the processes required for successful progression from drug discovery to product development, clinical trials, and full-scale commercialization. For the development and transfer of knowledge and manufacturing technologies of finished solid dosage forms, it is usually defined as transferring the product out of the development laboratories or the process development pilot plant into full commercial-scale manufacturing facilities. In cases where a secondary commercialization is necessary, it also involves transfer to different facilities in multiple regions or countries. Appropriate technology transfer includes the transfer of scientific information, capability, technological basis of the product and process, and analytical test methods from a knowledge center (donor) to the manufacturing plant (receptor). This process is important to ensure that product quality and performance built in during R&D remain unchanged in full-scale commercial product production.

The establishment of a technology transfer process is a complex process that typically involves multiple functional areas, such as pharmaceutical and analytical R&D, operations, quality, regulatory affairs, and program management. The ultimate goal is to effectively transfer product and specifications, manufacturing and control operations, as well as analytical methods based on sound scientific and engineering principles, while striving for optimization of efficiency, flexibility, and dependability of the process. To maintain production, technology transfer should also be a continuous knowledge/experience transfer and information exchange between parties, rather than a one-time event. Problems often arise at interfaces when the transfer process is not properly planned, communicated, and executed, resulting in a high rate of batch rejections or even a delay in bringing new products to market. Thus, technology transfer has been, and will continue to be, critical to the success of the pharmaceutical industry.

An effective technology transfer should start with planning (e.g., checklists) and establishing success criteria followed by: (1) defining procedures, acceptance criteria, equipment, facility requirements; (2) executing experimental designs; and (3) culminating in qualification and validation. A detailed guide for pharmaceutical technology transfer was published in 2003 by the International Society for Pharmaceutical Engineering (ISPE).[22] This manual presents a clear standardized process for transferring technology between two parties, and recommends a minimum base of documentation in support of the transfer request. The guide consists of three sections:

- Active pharmaceutical ingredients (APIs);
- Dosage forms;
- Analytical methods.

It defines key terms with consistent interpretation that enables the capture and sharing of essential knowledge. It is useful from the earliest phase in a product's lifecycle to post-approval transfers, and provides guidance and insight into the essential activities and documentation required to move a product, process or method from one unit to another. The guide is equally applicable to ethical and generic products, as well as technologies originating from any region around the world. It was published in collaboration with the US FDA and the American Association of Pharmaceutical Scientists (AAPS), with input from the European regulatory authorities, and submission to the Japanese Ministry of Health and Welfare (MHW).

21.4 CASE STUDIES

21.4.1 EXTENDED-RELEASE DOSAGE FORMS OF VERAPAMIL

Verapamil is an L-type calcium channel blocker used in the treatment of hypertension, angina pectoris, and cardiac arrhythmia. Verapamil hydrochloride is a BCS class I compound.[23,24] The strengths of IR dosage forms range from 40 to 120 mg. The favorable dose and solubility indicate that all three types of ER systems are suitable for this compound. Therefore, commercially available once-daily oral ER products include matrix (Isoptin® SR, Calan® SR tablets), reservoir (Verelan® and Verelan® PM Capsules), and osmotic pump systems (Covera-HS® Tablets).

Matrix System
Isoptin® SR and Calan® SR are matrix tablets based on alginate, a pH-dependent gelling polymer.[25] Since

CASE STUDY (CONTINUED)

sodium alginate is insoluble in water at pH below 3, drug release from the matrix tablets is pH-dependent, as shown in Figure 21.3a. At low pH (e.g., pH 1.2), sodium alginate at the tablet surface converts to insoluble alginic acid, and loses the ability to swell and form a viscous gel layer which is critical in controlling drug release. In addition, it was found that stress cracks were created on the tablet surface, allowing undesirable drug diffusion via water-filled cracks. In fact, both Isoptin® SR and Calan® SR tablets need to be taken with food to maintain a narrow peak-to-trough ratio of the plasma profile, due to the significant food effect on oral absorption. To overcome these problems, Howard and Timmins of Squibb designed a new ER matrix system of verapamil, by incorporating a pH-independent polymer in the alginate-based formulation.[26] In an acidic environment (e.g., the stomach), the pH-independent polymer (e.g., HPMC) hydrates to form a gel layer at the surface of the tablet. Drug dissolves in the gel layer, and slowly diffuses into the surrounding aqueous environment. As the pH increases with passage of the tablets from the stomach to the intestinal tract, the alginate in the tablets starts to swell and form a gel layer contributing to the overall

barrier to drug diffusion and matrix erosion. Drug release from this system is independent of pH. A zero-order release profile for up to 80% of the dose was obtained with such a system. To design a more robust pH-independent zero-order ER system, Zhang and Pinnamaraju incorporated an anionic polymer, such as methacrylic acid copolymer, into the matrix system consisting of sodium alginate and a pH-independent polymer, such as HPMC.[27] They demonstrated that drug release from this system is pH-independent and maintains a constant release rate. The results of zero-order release from both types of system designs are shown in Figure 21.3b. A zero-order release profile was obtained for up to nearly 100% of drug release.

Reservoir System

An extended-release capsule of verapamil hydrochloride, Verelan®, is an ER reservoir system that contains a mixture of rapid- and extended-release coated beads[28]. The manufacturing processes for the coated beads include (a) preparation of core beads and (b) film coating of the beads, as follows:

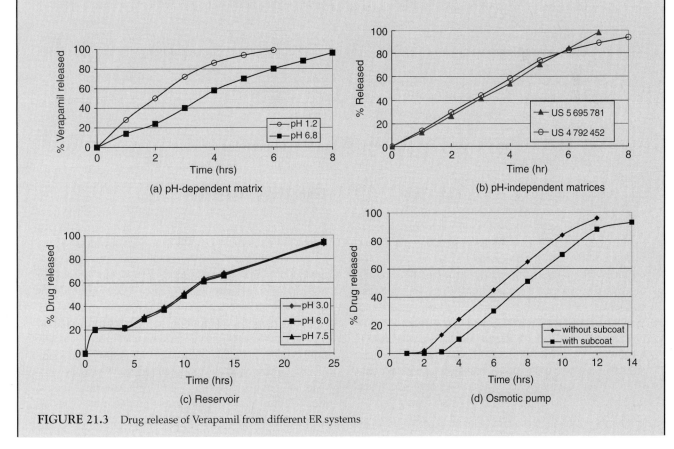

(a) pH-dependent matrix

(b) pH-independent matrices

(c) Reservoir

(d) Osmotic pump

FIGURE 21.3 Drug release of Verapamil from different ER systems

CASE STUDY   (CONTINUED)

(a) Composition and preparation of core beads:

Component	Quantity
Sugar/starch seeds (0.4 to 0.5 mm)	9 kg
Verapamil hydrochloride	30 kg
Malic acid	10 kg
Talc	2.4 kg
Hydroxypropyl methylcellulose suspension in methanol/methylene chloride (60/40)	5%

Preparation of core beads is performed in a coating pan using drug-layering coating technology. The spherical seeds are first thoroughly dampened with sufficient polymer suspension, followed by application of a portion of the powder blend of the active drug, until no more adhesions occur. The coated seeds are allowed to dry after each application of polymer suspension. This step is repeated until all of the powder blend has been applied. The last step involves drying of the coated beads to an acceptable level of moisture content.

(b) Composition and preparation of membrane coating:

Component	Quantity
5% Hydroxypropylmethylcellulose suspension in methanol/methylene chloride (60/40)	2 parts
5% Ethylcellulose in methanol/ methylene chloride (60/40)	8 parts
Talc	5 parts

The membrane coating process is performed in a standard coating pan by spraying the coating solution onto the core beads. The finished capsules contain 20% of the uncoated beads, and 80% of the membrane-coated beads. Drug release profiles in Figure 21.3c indicate that drug release from this system is pH-independent.

The processes described in this example were developed nearly 20 years ago, where the film coating polymers were applied in an organic solution. Significant advances have since been made in polymer coating of solid dosage forms. Today, a majority of membrane coatings for reservoir systems are applied as aqueous dispersions that form films by a process of coalescence of submicron polymer particles. The film-coating process is typically performed in a fluidized-bed with Wurster insert. Coating formulations, as well as processing variables, influence the properties of the resulting functional coating. The drug-layering process is usually carried out in a fluidized-bed. In coating beads, the seeds may first be coated with one layer of active drug, then with one layer of polymer, followed by another active drug layer. The process is repeated until multiple layers are completed to meet the predetermined requirement. The drug substance may be dissolved or dispersed with the coating materials. The details and in-depth discussions of the coating process development are addressed in Chapter 35 of this book.

Reservoir System with Controlled Onset

Verelan® PM is the second-generation reservoir ER system of verapamil approved in 1999. It was developed by applying the science of chronotherapeutics or timing of drug effect with biologic need, to improve clinical outcomes. Verelan® PM is a bead-filled capsule that uses the CODAS™ (Chronotherapeutic Oral Drug Absorption System) technology designed for bedtime dosing by incorporating a 4- to 5-hour delay in the ER drug delivery. The delay is controlled by the type, composition, and level of release-modifying polymers applied to drug loaded beads. The drug release is essentially independent of pH, food intake, and GI motility.

The development of this type of chronotherapeutic MR formulation is based on the well-established relationship of circadian rhythm, and the incidence of cardiovascular events. Heart rate and blood pressure peak during the morning hours, and reach a nadir at bedtime. Thus, the incidence of myocardial infarction, stroke, sudden cardiac death, and myocardial ischemia also increases during the early morning hours.[29] Chronotherapeutic MR formulations, such as Verelan® PM, are specifically designed to deliver the drug in higher concentrations during time of greatest need (e.g., post-awakening period), and in lesser concentrations at night, when heart rate and blood pressure are lowest and cardiovascular events are least likely to occur.

Osmotic Pump System

Covera-HS® tablet is also a chronotherapeutic ER dosage form of verapamil. It is a two-chamber OROS® Push-Pull™ osmotic system that consists of an active drug layer and an osmotic push layer. The device is designed to provide delayed onset of drug release by adding an additional coating layer between the tablet core and the outer semipermeable membrane. Depending on the composition and level of the sub-coat, the onset of drug release can be controlled. The ER drug delivery is independent of pH, GI motility, and food.

The ER osmotic device intended for dosing at bedtime for releasing verapamil to coincide with natural morning rise of blood pressure is prepared with the following steps.[30,31,32]

CASE STUDY   (CONTINUED)

(a) Composition and preparation of active drug layer:

Component	Quantity
Verapamil hydrochloride	600 g
Poly(ethylene oxide)	305 g
Sodium chloride	40 g
Polyvinylpyrrilidone	50 g
Magnesium stearate	5 g

All ingredients except magnesium stearate are granulated with anhydrous ethanol. The dried granules are lubricated with magnesium stearate. This procedure provides granules for the active drug layer.

(b) Composition and preparation of osmotic push layer:

Component	Quantity
Polyethylene oxide	735 g
Sodium chloride	200 g
Hydroxypropylmethylcellulose (Methocel E5)	50 g
Ferric oxide	10 g
Magnesium stearate	5 g

All ingredients except magnesium stearate are granulated with anhydrous ethanol. The dried granules are lubricated with magnesium stearate. This procedure provides granules for the osmotic push layer.

A bilayer core tablet comprising an active layer and a push layer is compressed in a bilayer tablet press to prepare the core tablet. A sub-coat is applied onto the bilayer core tablets using enteric coating material.

Production of layered tablets often faces great challenges, as layered tablets are prone to fracture along the interface, causing layer separation during processing, scale-up or storage, particularly when formulation and process are developed in isolation. Thus, to design a physically robust bilayer tablet with well-adhered layers, prospective assessment of the delamination tendencies of different layers of diverse compositions should be conducted through integrated evaluation of material properties, formulation, and process variables. Knowing the interaction and bonding behavior between different materials during compaction is of vital importance to better understand the compaction behavior, and possible failure mechanisms, of bilayer tablets. For example, the deformation, relaxation, and bonding characteristics of a push layer primarily consisting of polyethylene oxide[33] should be evaluated when the active layer is predominantly deformed by a difference mechanism. Significant mismatch of the physical and mechanical properties between the two layers often leads to difficulties in the development and manufacture of layered tablets. Other parameters important to the development of layered tablets include level and extent of lubrication, granulation characteristics, tamping and compression forces, turret speed, and equipment.[34,35,36]

(d) Composition and preparation of semipermeable membrane:

Component	Quantity
Cellulose acetate	55%
Hydroxypropylcellulose	40%
Polyethylene glycol	5%

All ingredients in the formulation are dissolved in 80% acetone and 20% methanol. The bilayer tablets are coated in a pan coater. Two orifices are drilled on the side of the device containing the active drug. An optional color or clear coat may also be applied.

The most significant drawback of developing osmotic systems is the need for organic solvents in the manufacturing process. Others include tedious and complex processing operations that require extensive process studies and control.

Figure 21.3d shows the *in vitro* drug release profiles of verapamil from the osmotic pump system. The dosage form without and with an enteric sub-coat exhibited a lag time of 1.5 and 3.0 hours in drug release, respectively, followed by zero-order release of verapamil.

21.4 CASE STUDIES

21.4.2 EXTENDED-RELEASE DOSAGE FORMS OF NIFEDIPINE

Nifedipine is also in the class of the calcium channel blockers used in the treatment of hypertension and angina. It is stable, but practically insoluble in water. Oral bioavailability of nifedipine is high, and proportional to the dose (BCS class II). Due to its poor aqueous solubility, the drug substance is usually micronized to increase the specific surface area for enhanced drug absorption. Based on the properties of nifedipine, an ER dosage form can be designed utilizing either eroding matrix or osmotic pressure-controlled mechanisms. Thus, both

CASE STUDY   (CONTINUED)

types of once-daily oral ER delivery systems are available commercially, including matrix tablets (Nifedical® XL, Adalat® CC Tablets, Nifediac® CC, Afeditab® CR), and osmotic pump tablets (Procardia® XL).

Osmotic Pump System

Procardia® XL tablet is an osmotic pump system designed to release drug at a constant rate over 24 hours for once-daily administration. Its delivery technology and principles (Push-Pull™) are essentially the same as those for verapamil (Covera® HS). The main difference is that Procardia® XL tablets release drug suspension formed *in situ*, due to the low solubility of nifedipine compared to the drug solution released from Covera® HS.

Matrix Tablets: Compress-coated System

Adalat® CC tablet contains 30, 60 or 90 mg of nifedipine for once-a-day oral administration. It is a chronotherapeutic ER matrix formulation consisting of an external coat functioning as a slow-release component, and an internal core as a fast-release component. The dosage form is designed to slowly deliver a portion of the dose from the ER coat layer, followed by rapid-release of the remaining dose from the tablet core after complete erosion of the ER layer. When dosed at bedtime, the biphasic drug release profile results in an initial peak at approximately 2.5–5 hours, followed by a second peak or shoulder at approximately 6–12 hours post-dose to coincide with the early morning rise in blood pressure associated with hypertension and angina.[37,38,39] The composition and preparation of the product are described in a granted US patent.[40]

(a) Composition and preparation of IR core tablets:

Component	Quantity
Micronized nifedipine	50 g
Lactose	388 g
Corn starch	150 g
Microcrystalline cellulose	50 g
Magnesium stearate	2 g

All ingredients except microcrystalline cellulose and magnesium stearate are granulated with water. The dried granules are blended with microcrystalline cellulose and magnesium stearate followed by compression into core tablets. An optional enteric coating may be applied to the core tablets.

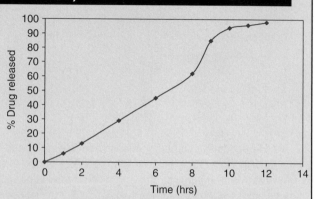

FIGURE 21.4 Drug release profile of Nifedipine from compress-coated tablets

(b) Composition and preparation of controlled release compress-coat:

Component	Quantity
Micronized nifedipine	250 g
Lactose	400 g
Hydroxypropylcellulose	700 g
Citric acid	320 g
Magnesium stearate	27 g

All ingredients except magnesium stearate are granulated with water. The dried granules are lubricated with magnesium stearate. The core tablets from (a) are coated with the compress-coat granules using compress-coating technology.

The resulting tablets with the compress-coats exhibit biphasic dissolution profiles, as shown in Figure 21.4. During the drug release test, hydroxypropylcellulose hydrates to form a viscous gel layer in which a portion of the micronized nifedipine is dispensed. The hydrated layer, with high concentration of water-soluble lactose, erodes and releases nifedipine at a controlled rate for approximately 8 hours. Once the erosion of the compress-coat layer completes, the core tablet is exposed to the aqueous medium, resulting in an immediate release of the remaining dose.

The compression-coating process is performed to enable a compress-coat layer to surround a tablet core (tablet-in-tablet). It involves initial compression of the core formulation to produce a relatively soft tablet, followed by transfer to a larger die for final compression of the compress-coat layer. This type of design can be used to develop an MR product with unique release profiles or formulate two incompatible drugs by incorporating one in the core, and the other in the compress-coat layer. The compress-coat may serve as part of the formulation to provide biphasic release or function as a barrier to delay drug release.

Methylphenidate (MPH) is an amphetamine-like central nervous system stimulant commonly prescribed to treat attention-deficit/hyperactivity disorder (ADHD) in children, adolescents, and adults, and also to treat narcolepsy. It is a weak base with pK_a of 8.77, and a log P of 3.19. Its hydrochloride salt is freely soluble in water (18.6 mg/ml), stable, and well-absorbed from the intestinal tract with a short elimination half life of 3–4 hours.[41] These favorable properties, combined with the low dose, make MPH an ideal candidate for oral MR delivery as discussed in the preceding chapter about MR design. Presently, the technologies utilized in the marketed MR products include ER matrix (Ritalin® SR), reservoir (Metadate® CD), osmotic pump (Concerta®), and mixed beads of IR and DR for pulsatile oral delivery (Ritalin® LA).

Ritalin® LA capsule was developed to mimic PK profiles of standard schedules of IR MPH through releasing the entire dose in two separate IR pulses. The product design is a multiparticulate MR system comprising an immediate-release component and a delayed-release component described as follows.[42]

(a) Immediate-release component:

Ingredient	Amount, % (w/w)
Methylphenidate HCl	13
Polyethylene glycol 6000	0.5
Polyvinylpyrrolidone	3.5
Purified water	83.5

An aqueous methylphenidate solution is prepared according to the above composition, and then coated onto nonpareil seeds to a level of approximately 16.9% solids weight gain using a fluid-bed (Glatt GPCG3, Glatt, Protech Ltd., Leicester, UK) to form the IR particles of the IR component.

(b) Delayed-release component:

Delayed-release particles of methylphenidate are prepared by coating the IR beads with a delayed-release coating solution. The immediate-release particles are coated to varying levels up to approximately 30% weight gain, using a fluid-bed coater.

(c) Drug release testing:

The above pH-independent coated beads (i–v) are tested in vitro in USP Apparatus I (100 rpm) according to the following protocol; the sample is placed in 0.01 N HCl (900 ml), pH 2.0, 37°C.

The pH-dependent coated beads (vi–viii) are tested in USP Apparatus I (100 rpm) according to a modified version of the USP method for enteric protection; the sample is placed for 2 hours in 0.01 N HCl, and then transferred to phosphate buffer pH 6.8 for the remainder of the sampling time points.

The drug release data below show that release characteristics of the DR component can be varied by changing the composition and thickness of the coating applied.

Coating type	Coating solution amount % (w/w)							
	pH-independent					pH-dependent		
Ingredient	(i)	(ii)	(iii)	(iv)	(v)	(vi)	(vii)	(viii)
Eudragit® RS 12.5	49.7	42.7	47.1	53.2	40.6	–	–	25.0
Eudragit® S 12.5	–	–	–	–	–	54.35	46.5	–
Eudragit® L 12.5	–	–	–	–	–	–	–	25.0
Polyvinylpyrrolidone	–	–	–	0.35	0.3	–	–	–
Diethylphthalate	0.5	0.5	0.6	1.35	0.6	1.3	1.1	–
Triethylcitrate	–	–	–	–	–	–	–	1.25
Isopropyl alcohol	39.8	33.1	37.2	45.1	33.8	44.35	49.6	46.5
Acetone	10.0	8.3	9.3	–	8.4	–	–	–
Talc*	–	16.0	5.9	–	16.3	–	2.8	2.25

*Talc is simultaneously applied during coating for formulations in columns (i), (iv) and (vi).

CASE STUDY (CONTINUED)

Coating solution	Coating weight gain (%)	Time (hr)	Active ingredient released (%)					
			1.0	2.0	4.0	6.0	8.0	10.0
(i)	4.0		–	17.0	51.5	75.8	86.0	91.3
(i)	6.0		–	3.3	22.1	46.5	65.5	76.5
(i)	10.0		–	–	–	–	10.2	17.3
(ii)	4.0		8.5	36.9	80.0	92.8	97.5	–
(ii)	6.0		1.3	7.1	40.3	72.4	83.0	–
(ii)	8.0		1.4	3.7	15.1	31.2	47.5	–
(iii)	4.0		6.1	21.3	62.3	82.1	91.3	97.7
(iii)	6.0		3.0	8.2	26.3	52.6	73.0	86.5
(iv)	10.0		3.5	13.4	47.1	80.0	94.8	103.0
(iv)	15.0		0.9	5.4	22.5	52.0	70.3	81.5
(iv)	20.0		1.1	2.9	13.8	36.9	61.0	76.1
(v)	10.0		0.3	6.1	42.4	77.5	92.4	–
(v)	12.5		1.0	2.9	21.2	54.4	76.7	–
(vi)	5.0		33.2	80.6	92.2	93.9	94.3	94.4
(vi)	10.0		0.4	9.8	43.5	61.6	67.5	–
(vi)	15.0		–	–	10.1	29.9	48.4	60.0
(vi)	15.0		–	0.5	44.0	80.2	69.0	–
(vii)	15.0		3.9	52.0	85.0	89.9	91.4	–
(vii)	20.0		0.6	12.4	61.6	75.3	79.6	–
(viii)	20.0		3.8	7.4	43.7	72.4	79.2	79.5
(viii)	30.0		2.1	3.1	8.9	36.9	63.9	73.4

MR formulation	DR coating solution	Coating weight gain (%)	Time (hr)	0.5	1	2	4	6	8	10
				Active ingredient released (%)						
A	(viii)	30		50.2	50.5	51.1	54.3	68	81.8	87
B	(vii)	30		49.7	49.7	49.8	56.1	65.2	72.2	76.6

(d) Preparation of MR capsule and *in vivo* study:
Based on the above investigation, two formulations of multiparticulate MR beads (A and B) were prepared for *in vivo* evaluation in humans in a crossover study. The IR and DR particles are encapsulated in size 2 hard gelatin capsules to an overall 20 mg dosage strength using a capsule machine (Bosch GKF 4000S). The dosage strength of 20 mg MPH consists of 10 mg IR and 10 mg DR beads.

The data below indicate that the MR formulations consisting of IR and DR beads coated with the pH-dependent DR films release MPH in a pulsed manner, in which approximately 50% of the dose was released within the first half hour, followed by release of the remaining dose at about four hours.

MR formulations A and B containing 20 mg MPH were administered to fasted healthy volunteers using

Ritalin® as a reference. The plasma levels of MPH were determined for up to 48 hours after dosing. Figure 21.5 shows the plasma concentration profiles of MPH after oral administration of formulations A and B. Both formulations exhibit two peaks similar to that of the reference control (10 mg dosed twice at a four hour interval). The peak–trough fluctuation of formulation A more

closely mimics that of the twice-administered Ritalin® tablets. Bioavailability is also similar between formulation A and the reference control. It is noted that the development approach adopted in this example was semi-empirical. Thus, significant resource was devoted to achieve the development objective.

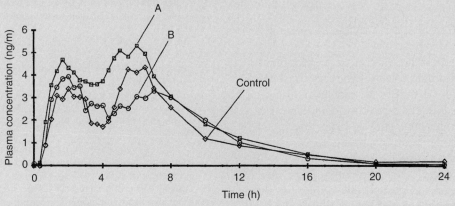

FIGURE 21.5   Methylphenidate plasma profiles following oral administration of three formulations to healthy volunteers; A: 20 mg MR capsule, 30% coating weight gain using coating solution (viii); B: 20 mg MR capsule, 30% coating weight gain using coating solution (vii); Control: two doses of 10 mg RitalinÒ IR tablets administered at times 0 and 4 hours; source: US patent 6 228 398

21.5 INTELLECTUAL PROPERTY CONSIDERATIONS

Intellectual property (IP) rights are central to the pharmaceutical industry, because of high R&D costs, low success rate, and lengthy product testing required before a drug product can enter the market. Beside the most important patents on the composition-of-matter (i.e., chemical entity), an IP portfolio created in developing dosage forms, particularly MR dosage forms, has become a key strategic element in extending product lifecycle. It can often play a significant role by offering differentiated products when the new products, medical needs, and markets are aligned. Over the past two decades many companies have reaped great benefits from this type of IP development. In general, such IP estate may encompass regulatory or legislative exclusivity, trade secrets that are difficult to reverse-engineer, and patents that protect innovations. The patentable subject matter (or statutory subject matter) in dosage form development includes modifications of structure (e.g., new solid phases, salts), formulation (e.g., composition, technology, particle size), method of treatment (e.g., route of delivery, dosing regimen), process, methods of improving bioavailability with

overcoming stability problems, newly discovered clinical benefits (e.g., decreased adverse events, new indication) or performance (drug release profiles, PK or PD outcomes) resulting from MR delivery independent of the delivery technologies applied.[43] One of the successful examples involves development of patents protecting ER products of nifedipine (Procardia XL and Adalat CC). Because the 3-year regulatory exclusivity expired in 1992, the ER products had to rely on the exclusivity provided by patents that claim benefits of ER delivery and controlled particle size for enhancing bioavailability. Among four patents listed in the *Orange Book*,[44] the most critical is US patent 5 264 446 that claims:

> "A solid pharmaceutical composition comprising as the active ingredient an effective amount of nifedipine crystals with a specific surface area of 1.0 to 4.0 m²/g, in admixture with a solid diluent, to result in a sustained release of nifedipine."

As a result, the innovator's products remained free of generic competition for an additional nine years, until the generic competitor utilized finer particle size and amorphous drug disclosed in the US patent 5 455 046.

It should be noted that the above example took place at a time when there were fewer companies with MR development expertise and experience. Because of the increased scientific know-how and technology maturity, as well as more crowded patent landscape in MR oral delivery, formulation and technology-based patents generally have lower hurdles to jump, while process patents are often difficult to enforce. Thus, a robust IP portfolio should be built on continuous development and review of both in-house and in-licensed opportunities throughout product lifecycle. More specifics and examples can be found in Chapters 39 and 40.

21.6 SUMMARY

Following decades of research and development in the area of oral modified-release products, most of the delivery needs can be met by available mature technologies discussed in the preceding chapter for any molecules that are feasible, such as drugs of marketed MR products. The key to developing an MR dosage form with predefined quality attributes and a robust manufacturing process, is to begin with unified view of formulation and process design, and apply a systematic approach throughout the development lifecycle. Rational dosage form development requires application of multidisciplinary knowledge for fundamental understanding of drug substance, excipients, basic unit operations, and delivery technology that matches drug properties, as well as interrelations of these factors.

References

1. FDA unveils new initiative to enhance pharmaceutical good manufacturing practices. (2002). US Department of Health and Human Services, Food and Drug Administration, Center for Drug Evaluation and Research, http://www.fda.gov/bbs/topics/NEWS/2002/NEW00829.html, August 21.
2. Yu, L. (2008). Pharmaceutical quality by design: product and process development, understanding and control. Pharm. Res. 25(4), 781–791.
3. Guidance for Industry. (2006). Q8 Pharmaceutical Development. US Food and Drug Administration, May.
4. Office of Generic Drugs White Paper. (2007). Question-Based Review (QbR) for Generic Drugs: An Enhanced Pharmaceutical Quality Assessment System. US Food and Drug Administration.
5. Ruff, M.D., et al. Pharmaceutical composition containing bupropion hydrochloride and a stabilizer. US Patent 5 358 970.
6. Maitra, A., et al. Pharmaceutical composition containing bupropion hydrochloride and an inorganic acid stabilizer. US Patent 5 968 553.
7. Oberegger, W., et al. Modified release formulations of a bupropion salt. US Patent Application #20070027213.
8. Katzhendler, I., Azoury, R. & Friedman, M. (1998). Crystalline properties of carbamazepine in sustained release hydrophilic matrix tablets based on hydroxypropyl methylcellulose. Journal of Controlled Release 54(1), 69–85.
9. Li, X., Zhi, F. & Hu, Y. (2007). Investigation of excipient and processing on solid phase transformation and dissolution of ciprofloxacin. Int. J. of Pharm. 328(2), 177–182.
10. Michelucci, J.J. Sustained release etodolac US Patent 4 966 768.
11. Rao, V.M., Engh, K. & Qiu, Y. (2003). Design of pH-independent controlled release matrix tablets for acidic drugs. Int. J. Pharm. 252, 81–86.
12. Lieberman, H.A., Lachman, L. & Schwartz, J.B. (eds). (1990). Pharmaceutical dosage forms: Tablets, Vol. 1–2. Marcel Dekker, Inc., New York.
13. Zhang, G., Law, D., Schmitt, E. & Qiu, Y. (2004). Phase transformation considerations in process development and manufacturing of solid oral dosage forms. Adv. Drug Delivery Review 56, 371–390.
14. Wardrop, J., Law, D., Qiu, Y., Engh, K., Faitsch, L. & Ling, C. (2006). Influence of solid phase and formulation processing on stability of ABT-232 tablet formulations. J. Pharm. Sci. 95(11), 2380–2392.
15. Tantry, J.S., Tank, J. & Suryanarayanan, R. (2007). Processing-induced phase transitions of theophylline—implications on the dissolution of theophylline tablets. J. Pharm. Sci. 96(5), 1434–1444.
16. Antony, J. (2003). Design of Experiments for Engineers and Scientists. Elsevier Inc., Burlington, MA.
17. Hwang, R. & Kowalski, D.L. (2005). Design of experiments for formulation development. Pharm. Tech. 12.
18. Hwang, R., Peck, G.R., Besserman, D.M., Friedrich, C.E. & Gemoules, M.K. (2001). Tablet relaxation and physicomechanical stability of lactose, microcrystalline cellulose, and dibasic calcium phosphate. Pharm. Tech. 11, 54–80.
19. Qiu, Y., Garren, J., Samara, E., Abraham, C., Cheskin, H.S. & Engh, K.R. (2003). Once-a-day controlled-release dosage form of Divalproex Sodium II: Development of a predictive in vitro release method. J. Pharm. Sci. 92(11), 2317–2325.
20. Ranjani, V.N., Singh Rekhi, G., Hussainc, A.S., Tillmand, L.G. & Augsburger, L.L. (1998). Development of metoprolol tartrate extended-release matrix tablet formulations for regulatory policy consideration. Journal of Controlled Release 50(1–3), 247–256.
21. Draft Consensus Guideline. (2007). Pharmaceutical Development Annex to Q8. International Conference on Harmonization of Technical Requirements for Registration of Pharmaceuticals for Human Use, November.
22. ISPE Good Practice Guide. (2003). Technology Transfer. International Society for Pharmaceutical Engineering.
23. Vogelpoel, H., Welink, J., Amidon, G.L., Junginger, H.E., Midha, K.K., Möller, H., Olling, M., Shah, V.P. & Barends, D.M. (2004). Biowaiver monographs for immediate release solid oral dosage forms based on biopharmaceutics classification system (BCS) literature data: Verapamil hydrochloride, propranolol hydrochloride, and atenolol. J. Pharm. Sci. 93, 1945–1956.
24. Guidance for Industry. (2000). Waiver of In Vivo Bioavailability and Bioequivalence Studies for Immediate-Release Solid Oral DosageForms Based on a Biopharmaceutics Classification System. US Department of Health and Human Services, Food and Drug Administration, Center for Drug Evaluation and Research.
25. Baiz, E. & Einig, H. (1992). Alginate-Based Verapamil-Containing Depot Drug Form. US Patent 5 132 295.
26. Howard, J.R. & Timmins, P. (1988). Controlled Release Formulation. US Patent 4 792 452.
27. Zhang, G. & Pinnamaraju, P. (1997). Sustained Release Formulation Containing Three Different Types of Polymers. US Patent 5 695 781.
28. Panoz, D.E. & Geoghegan, E.J. (1989). Controlled Absorption Pharmaceutical Composition. US Patent 4 863 742.
29. Sica, D.A. & White, W. (2000). Chronotherapeutics and its role in the treatment of hypertension and cardiovascular disease. J. Clin. Hypertens. 2(4), 279–286.
30. Jao, F., Wong, P.S., Huynh, H.T., McChesney, K. & Wat, P.K. (1992). Verapamil Therapy. US Patent 5 160 744.

31. Jao, F., Wong, P.S., Huynh, H.T., McChesney, K. & Wat, P.K. (1993). Verapamil Therapy. US Patent 5 190 765.

32. Jao, F., Wong, P.S., Huynh, H.T., McChesney, K. & Wat, P.K. (1993). Verapamil Therapy. US Patent 5 252 338.

33. Yang, L., Venkatesh, G. & Fassihi, R. (1996). Characterization of compressibility and compactibility of poly(ethylene oxide) polymers for modified release application by compaction simulator. J. Pharm. Sci. 85(10), 1085–1090.

34. Podczecka, F., Drake, K.R., Newton, J.M. & Haririanc, I. (2006). The strength of bilayered tablets. Eur. J. Pharm. Sci. 29(5), 361–366.

35. Yang, L., Venkatesh, G. & Fassihi, R. (1997). Compaction simulator study of a novel triple-layer tablet matrix for industrial tableting. Inter. J. Pharm. 152(1), 45–52.

36. Li, S.P., Karth, M.G., Feld, K.M., Di Paolo, L.C., Pendharkar, C.M. & Williams, R.O. (1995). Evaluation of bilayer tablet machines: A case study. Drug Dev. Ind. Pharm. 21(5), 571–590.

37. Physicians' Desk Reference. (2007). 61st edn. Adalat CC product monograph.

38. Glasser, S.P., Jain, A. & Allenby, K.S. (1995). The efficacy and safety of once-daily nifedipine: the coat-core formulation compared with the gastrointestinal therapeutic system formulation in patients with mild to moderate diastolic hypertension. Clin Ther. 17(1), 12–29.

39. Granberry, M.C., Gardner, S.F., Schneider, E.F., et al. (1996). Comparison of two formulations of nifedipine during 24-hour ambulatory blood pressure monitoring. Pharmacotherap. 16(5), 932–936.

40. Ohm, A. & Luchtenberg, H. (1990). Press Coated DHP Tablets. US Patent 4 892 741.

41. Gualtieri., et al. (1982). Clinical studies of methylphenidate serum levels in children and adults. Journal of the American Academy of Child Psychiatry 21, 19–26.

42. Devane, J.G. (2001). Multiparticulate modified release composition containing Methylphenidate. US Patent 6 228 398.

43. Qiu, Y. (2005). Intellectual property considerations in pharmaceutical development: basics and examples. Proceedings of CPA/AAPS Short Course: Modern Theory and Practice of Pharmaceutical Sciences in Oral Dosage Form R&D. Shanghai, June 6–10 pp. 316–324.

44. Approved Drug Products with Therapeutic Equivalence Evaluations. US Department of Health and Human Services, Food and Drug Administration, Center for Drug Evaluation and Research, Office of Pharmaceutical Science, Office of Generic Drugs. http://www.fda.gov/cder/ob/

Analytical Development and Validation for Solid Oral Dosage Forms

Xingchun (Frank) Fang, Geoff Carr and Ronald C. Freeze

22.1 INTRODUCTION

A common question that is often asked during drug development is: how much validation of an analytical method is required for the method to be considered appropriately validated? The method validation required prior to the submission of the marketing application is clearly outlined in guidance documents published by agencies such as the ICH[1] and the FDA,[2] but the validation required during the earlier phases of development is a topic open for discussion. In addition to the many guidance documents that discuss method validation, there are several books available that provide a detailed interpretation of the existing regulations, and that also discuss the appropriate techniques for method development and validation.[3,4] This chapter outlines a strategic approach to the development and validation of analytical procedures for solid oral dosage forms from early development to the registration of the marketing authorization, as well as case studies to aid readers in understanding required aspects of method validation and method transfers.

22.2 ANALYTICAL METHOD DEVELOPMENT AND VALIDATION STRATEGY

A strategic approach to development and validation of analytical methods is critical for the efficient operation of a product development group. This strategic approach balances the amount of validation required to ensure that a method is appropriately validated for the phase of development with the need to be cost-effective, and meet tight project timelines.

Existing regulations allow a great deal of flexibility in terms of the amount of data that needs to be submitted during the course of drug development. For clinical studies in the US, the expectations for information to be provided are outlined in 21CRF 312.23(a)(7)(i), and in guidance documents discussing the different IND phases.[5-7] For studies performed in the European Union, similar guidance is provided for Investigational Medicinal Product Dossier (IMPD) content.[8] All of the documents emphasize the graded nature of chemistry, manufacturing, and control (CMC) information needed as development progresses. At all phases, sufficient information should be submitted to ensure the proper identification, strength, quality, purity, and potency of the investigational candidate. The amount of information that will provide that assurance will vary with the phase of the investigational compound, the proposed duration of any planned clinical trials, the dosage form, and the amount of information already available on the compound. It is through developing a defendable strategy for method development and validation that maximizes resources while providing the appropriate assurance of quality that differentiates the most productive R&D analytical groups.

Prior to developing any analytical method for the formulation, the drug substance must be well-understood. At these earliest stages of drug development, it is essential to gather information about the drug substance, such as pKa, solubility in different solutions, sink condition, intrinsic drug dissolution rate (used later for dissolution method development), and UV/Vis characteristics. Another critical part of this early development work will focus on forced degradation studies. The results of these studies will help both in formulation development, and in method development. The first analytical methods that are developed may have minimal validation, but should be sufficient to provide analytical support during early formulation development, such as excipient compatibility, and prototype formulations. The results from these early feasibility studies will determine which of the multiple formulation options are selected for further development and ultimately the clinical study, so the methods should be able to show significant decreases in potency or increases in related substances. These measures will be how the preferred formulations are selected.

In early nonclinical and clinical phases, it is important that the impurity profile observed from each drug substance, and drug product lot, be established for future reference and comparison. If the impurities that are present in the nonclinical studies can be confirmed, even at a later date, the information may support the use of drug substance lots that have certain impurities much later in the development program. To be able to generate an impurity profile in a reliable and repeatable fashion, emphasis must be placed on the related substances method, as well as the assay method that is used for release and stability. In addition to the need to refer back to the impurity profiles, in the early stages of development the first in-house reference standard is normally manufactured and characterized. One key component for calculating purity is to have a specific test that separates all impurities from the compound of interest. An additional key component of this development should establish the stability-indicating capabilities of the methods for drug substances and the selected formulation. Characterization of the impurities can be conducted at later stages of development, and at the earliest stages identification of minor impurities is not critical.

By the time a project enters phase 1, sufficient history with the drug substance and drug product methods should be available to have reasonable confidence in the methodology. At this point, if not already validated, formal validation studies should be conducted. For phase 1, methods should be appropriately validated prior to testing the clinical drug substance lot and the clinical formulation. Partial validation

is normally sufficient for the early stages. Often all parameters, apart from intermediate precision and robustness, are validated at phase 1. Intermediate precision is then completed at phase 2, and robustness is added at phase 3. One validation parameter that isn't necessarily required, but is strongly recommended, is solution stability. By validating a minimum time for which the sample and standard solutions are stable, flexibility in laboratory procedures and the ability to store prepared solutions is achieved. Without validated solution stability, solutions must be prepared freshly before each analysis. Additionally, if significant degradation is observed during the solution stability validation experiments, it may indicate possible degradation during analysis.

An additional reason for a strategic approach to method validation is that the validation studies may need to be repeated multiple times during the drug development stages. This revalidation may be required due to new impurities, changes in formulations or possible improvements in the methodology to utilize new technologies or make methods more appropriate for quality laboratories. The full validation of analytical methods to meet the applicable guidance documents is required by the time of filing the common technical dossier (CTD).[9] Additionally, to avoid confusion, every attempt should be made to have the final methods in place by the time the registration stability studies are started, to avoid the need to discuss method changes during the studies. The strategic approaches for method validation in each phase of drug development are outlined in Table 22.1.

22.3 CATEGORY OF ANALYTICAL METHOD AND METHOD DEVELOPMENT

The reliable analytical method is a key element of a quality system. Methods are used for identification, strength, purity, and quality of products. For the majority of solid oral dosage form drug products, the following tests are required:

- physical appearance;
- identification;
- potency assay;
- related substances assay;
- drug release (dissolution) testing; and
- moisture determination.

During product development other tests may be included, especially if the API has multiple

TABLE 22.1 Phasing approach for analytical method validation in each phase of clinical trail materials

Validation parameters	Pre-clinical	Phase 1	Phase 2	Phase 3
Specificity	Yes	Yes	Yes	Yes
Repeatability	Yes	Yes	Yes	Yes
Intermediate precision	No	No	Yes	Yes
Linearity	Some	Yes	Yes	Yes
Accuracy	Some	Yes	Yes	Yes
Detection limit (DL)	Yes	Yes	Yes	Yes
Quantitation limit (QL)	No	Yes	Yes	Yes
Robustness	No	No	No	Yes
Analytical solution stability	No	Yes	Yes	Yes

polymorphs that have different physical characteristics. These tests could include powder X-ray diffraction, near-infrared, and Raman spectrometry. It is extremely important that the polymorphic form of the actives in products is under control during the manufacturing process and on stability. Additionally, chiral testing may be required during development.

There are four categories that analytical methods fall under, based on the United Sates Pharmacopeia (USP), from highly exacting analytical determinations to subjective evaluation of attributes.[10]

- Category I: analytical methods for quantitation of major components of bulk drug substances or active ingredients (including preservatives) in finished pharmaceutical products.
- Category II: analytical methods for the determination of impurities in bulk drug substances or degradation compounds in finished pharmaceutical products. These methods include quantitative assays and limit tests.
- Category III: analytical methods for determination of performance characteristics (e.g., dissolution, drug release).
- Category IV: identification tests.

The data elements normally required for each of the categories of assays will be listed in Table 22.3. The specific requirement for each individual testing procedure should be taken into consideration, and are discussed in the following text.[2,10]

22.3.1 Identification

As one of the key elements in ensuring the quality of the products, the method intended for identification should be specific for the actives in the drug product. A specific identification test method, such as Fourier transform infrared spectroscopy (FT-IR), is preferred over a chromatography method. FT-IR is often applied to drug substances. For drug products, the extraction of the active and subsequent clean up may be necessary to meet the specificity, due to interference from excipients. If non-specific methods are used, two independent analytical procedures are required at the time of the new drug application. Non-specific methods, such as UV-Vis or chromatographic retention time using thin layer chromatography (TLC) or high performance liquid chromatography (HPLC), are not sufficient in themselves for identification. However, HPLC equipped with a specific detector, such as a diode array detector (DAD) or mass spectrometer (MS), becomes a powerful analytical tool, as it obtains both the retention time and UV-Vis spectra simultaneously, and is considered an acceptable identification technique.[2]

22.3.2 Potency Assay

A specific, stability-indicating procedure should be developed and validated. A fully validated procedure including inter-laboratory precision and specificity, based on stressed studies should be part of the phase 3 method. Reduced validation at earlier phases is applicable as discussed previously.

22.3.3 Impurities[10–13]

Impurities in drug substances and drug products include organic impurities, inorganic impurities, and residual solvents. Organic impurities are generally called related substances, since they are structurally related to a drug substance. These substances may be identified or unidentified degradation products, and can arise from many sources, including the raw materials, starting materials, purchased intermediates, the manufacturing process or during storage of a material. The earlier in drug development that the impurities are identified, the more time there is to address the impurities through process changes or qualification studies. Q3B outlines the identification and qualification thresholds for impurities in drug substances and drug products. During drug development validation of impurity methods for accuracy, detection and quantitation limits, and response factors can be accomplished by spiking the impurities into the drug product or into a placebo mixture.

22.3.4 Dissolution[14–25]

Dissolution or drug release testing is traditionally considered to be a critical quality test for solid oral dosage forms. It is a challenge for scientists to develop a procedure that can not only guide the formulation development process, but can also be used as a regulatory test to detect manufacturing deviation and ensure product consistency at release, and over the product's shelf life. Therefore, the primary goal is to develop a discriminating, rugged, and reproducible dissolution method, which must be able to highlight significant changes in product performance due to small changes in the formulation or manufacturing process. The objective of dissolution testing varies during the lifecycle of a dosage form. During early phase 1, a method is developed to establish the mechanism of *in vitro* drug release. During phase 2 and 3, the objective shifts to identifying a test method that can provide an *in vitro–in vivo* correlation (IVIVC) or other biorelevant information (refer to Chapter 17). By having a method that has a proven IVIVC, significant reduction in the regulatory burden caused by post-approval changes can be achieved. The inclusion of a new chapter in USP 30/NF 25 provides recommendations on how to develop and validate a dissolution procedure.[22]

22.3.5 Blend Homogeneity and Dosage Uniformity

The term "uniformity of dosage unit" is defined as the degree of uniformity in the amount of the drug substance among dosage units. The harmonized compendial chapter on uniformity of dosage units outlines the release criteria to show uniformity. In addition to uniformity at release, it is also important during development to verify the uniformity of blend samples, and also uniformity of dosage units throughout the manufacturing run (lot uniformity). The analytical procedure used for assay can be used to determine the drug content of uniformity samples. In cases where a complicated procedure or long HPLC run time is required for assay, but is not needed for blend uniformity/content uniformity (BU/CU) determinations, a separate testing procedure with short run-time may be developed. BU/CU chromatographic methods may be much shorter than the assay method, because they are not required to be stability indicating. Generating blend uniformity and lot uniformity data is the key to understanding the manufacturing process during the development phases of the product, and is described in the draft guideline for powder blends and finished dosage units stratified in process dosage unit sampling and assessment.[26]

22.3.6 Cleaning Test Method Development

Regardless of the stage of development, if reusable equipment is used during manufacturing, c-GMP requires that cleanness of equipment be validated to eliminate the risk of cross-contamination and ensure that residual material is removed from the equipment after use. The validation of analytical procedures used to determine residual actives from swabbing samples should be conducted as a critical step for cleaning validation (refer to Chapter 25).

In addition to the normal validation required for analytical methods, cleaning methods must also include confirmation of surface recovery. Depending on the equipment, and how cleaning confirmation is performed, surface recovery studies may include rinsing and swabbing, as well as multiple surface types. For many types of equipment, cleaning is performed using large volumes of the appropriate solvent. A portion of the final rinse solvent can be collected and provided for analysis. In this case, confirming recovery based on rinsing is appropriate. For some pieces of equipment, following rinsing the surface is swabbed, and the swabs are provided for analysis. In these cases surface recovery using swabbing is appropriate. Common manufacturing materials include different grades of stainless steel (some of which have very different recovery characteristics), polymers, and glass. Spiking and recovery experiments need to be performed on coupons of the materials that will be used in manufacturing.

There are a number of challenges in validating a cleaning method. To reduce the possible challenges, the laboratory should work closely with the manufacturing group to understand what is required for the method, and eliminate unnecessary hurdles. These hurdles could include the use of kill solutions such as bleach, which destroys the active molecule, but results in degradation products that could have toxic characteristics, cleaning solutions that interfere with the chromatography or degrade the active substance in solution or swabs that have extractables that interfere with the analysis. To reduce the risk of unknown peaks, the same materials that will be used in the manufacturing facility must be used during method development. When possible, pure solvents and pre-conditioned swabs should be used. Solvent selection should be based on the solubility of the active ingredient in the solvent, and the ICH classification of the solvent. The first choice for solvents should be water, isopropyl alcohol (IPA) or a mixture of the two. Minimum recovery requirements can be debated, but recoveries of <50% are difficult to justify. The final analytical method should include an adjustment factor, based on the worst case recovery, to ensure that reported results are a true indication of the amount of residual drug substance left on the surface.

If water and IPA are not viable cleaning solvents, solvents that better solublize the drug substance or cleaning agents may be required. Class 2 solvents should be avoided, and Class 1 solvents should never be used. Additionally, solvents without adequate toxicological data should be avoided. Proposed solvents used as swabbing solvent are listed in Table 22.2 in IHC Guidance Q3C.[12] Depending on the final cleaning solution selected, it may be necessary to do an additional cleaning step, with IPA and/or water, of the areas that were swabbed, to ensure that all other solvents are appropriately removed.

22.3.7 Other Analytical Techniques

Thus far in this chapter we have focused on the key tests required to ensure the key quality attributes of solid oral dosage forms. In addition to the tests described above, many other tests may be required during development, and even as part of the filing, to ensure the quality of the drug product. All methods should be appropriately validated for their intended use, and the amount of validation depends on the type of method and the stage of development. Some of the other methods that may be used include, but are not limited to, near-IR, Raman spectrophotometry, X-ray powder diffraction, GC, optical rotation, and chiral chromatography, which all could also be applied to specific testing.[27–34]

22.4 ANALYTICAL METHOD VALIDATION

Test procedures for assessment of the quality of pharmaceutical products are subject to various requirements. Users of analytical methods described in the pharmacopeias, such as USP/NF, and Phar. Eur., are not required to validate accuracy and reliability of these methods, but merely verify their suitability under actual conditions of use. Recognizing the legal status of the pharmacopeia, it is essential that proposals for adoption of new or revised compendial analytical method or alternate in-house methods be shown equivalent to, or better than, the current method, and

TABLE 22.2 Proposed solvent used as swabbing solvents

No	Solvent	Boiling point (°C)	Relative evaporation rate[1,2]	Remark[3]
1	Isopropanol	82.6	1.7	Class 3
2	Ethanol	78.1	1.95	Class 3
3	0.25% aqueous acetic acid			Pharmaceutical acceptable excipient
4	Acetone	56.2	6.06	Class 3
5	Ethyl acetate	77.3	4.94	Class 3
6	Iso-propyl acetate	85	3.0	Class 3
7	Methanol	64.6	5.91	Class 2
8	Acetonitrile	81.7	2.33	Class 2

[1] All boiling point and relative evaporation rate values were taken from MSDSs

[2] All relative evaporation rates are relative to n-butyl acetate

[3] Classification as per ICH Q3C for residual solvents

be supported by sufficient laboratory data to document their validity.[10,35,36] If there is no compendia procedure, the analytical method must be fully validated prior to use.

22.4.1 Verification of Compendial Methods

A compendial procedure is considered validated if it is published as official text in a pharmacopeia, such as the USP-NF, in a supplement or as an interim revision announcement in the *Pharmacopeial Forum* (PF). When using compendial methods, the full validation is not necessary, but verification of the procedure is very important. Verification ensures that the procedure is suitable for use with a specific ingredient or product, in a specific laboratory, with specific laboratory personnel, equipment, and reagents.[34,35] For example, titrimetric methods for water determination should be verified for accuracy (and absence of possible interference) when used for a new product or raw material. For impurity testing, the suitability of a compendial procedure may be an issue for several reasons (e.g., impurity profile change from different routes of synthesis, composition of formulation, or interference from excipients). It is recommended that the procedure for certification of suitability of the monographs of the pharmacopeia be used.[37–39] Forced degradation may be applied to establish the suitability of the chromatographic condition.

22.4.2 Characterization of Reference Standard

During method validation, a well-characterized standard should be used. A well-characterized reference standard is a critical factor for method validation. For potency assay, the purity of the standard must be assigned. For the impurity assay validation, some impurity standards may not be of high purity, but have to be characterized to confirm their identity. It is important to ensure that any impurities contained in the impurity standard do not interfere with the analysis. If possible, the reference standard (used as primary standard) should always be acquired from a recognized authority, such as the National Institute for Standard and Technology (NIST), USP, EP, etc. For new drugs, this is rarely possible, so an in-house reference standard must be synthesized and characterized. The reference standard should be minimally characterized by the following tests: physical appearance, identification, and purity assignment. The structure should be confirmed using multiple analytical

techniques, such as elemental analysis, infrared spectroscopic analysis, UV-visible spectroscopic analysis, mass spectroscopy, ^{1}H-NMR, and ^{13}C-NMR. Purity assignment can be established by tests for the following items: organic impurity, inorganic impurity, moisture, and residual solvents. The amount of total organic impurities may be determined by HPLC, and/or other chromatographic methods. Moisture and residual solvents may be determined by thermo gravimetric analysis, such as TGA or combined Karl Fischer titration, and GC method. The amount of inorganic residue can be determined using residue on ignition. If the Karl Fischer method for water content and the GC method for residual solvents are used these should be validated (or verified if using a compendial method) prior to use. The in-house standard can be qualified against a primary standard, following a well-defined qualification protocol.

22.4.3 Stability Indicating Method

A stability indicating assay, as required per the ICH guidelines,[40] should be used for any GMP stability program, so that the procedure is able to detect the changes with time in the pertinent properties (e.g., active ingredient, preservative level) of the drug substance and drug product, and should accurately measure the active ingredients without interference from degradation products, process impurities, excipients or other potential system components. It is important that a comprehensive forced degradation study and HPLC co-elution evaluation be conducted, in order to demonstrate the suitability of the procedure to detect any changes that are attributable to degradation.

22.4.4 High Performance Liquid Chromatography Co-elution Peak Evaluation

HPLC with diode array detectors (DAD) or mass spectroscopy (MS) are powerful tools that have the ability to detect even low levels of co-eluting components. These techniques have the ability to evaluate the integrity of chromatographic peaks in HPLC method development and validation, and are widely used in the pharmaceutical industry. Since impurities in pharmaceutical active ingredients, and the actives themselves, often have very similar chemical structures they are also likely to have very similar chromophores and UV spectra. For this reason the software provided with DAD and MS detectors generally includes algorithms that calculate peak purity.

Additionally, during method development, forced degradation studies are performed to generate samples with exaggerated levels of likely impurities. These samples are used to evaluate and identify when co-eluting components are present, at which time the increased level will give the algorithm a greater chance of success. It is important to note that the peak purity check can only prove that the peak is impure or contains a co-eluting component. DAD cannot prove that the peak is absolutely pure.[41]

22.4.5 Forced Degradation Studies

Forced degradation studies (or stress studies), are the main tool used to predict stability issues, develop analytical methods, and identify degradation products or pathways.[42] The forced degradation studies should be performed prior to the other validation parameters (e.g., accuracy, repeatability, intermediate precision, specificity, DL, QL, linearity and range, solution stability, and robustness). An approved protocol is recommended before forced degradation studies can be performed.

For multiple strengths of drug products with the same excipient composition (including different formulation ratios), forced degradation studies can be performed with only one formulation. For multiple strengths or a formulation of drug product with different excipients, each different formulation composition should be evaluated using forced degradation studies.

For IND phase 1 and IND phase 2 applications, the forced degradation studies for the stability-indicating nature of the assay method is method-specific, therefore, if the assay methods for drug substance and drug product have different conditions which can cause changes in selectivity (e.g., different HPLC column, mobile phase composition, gradient program, flow rate, column temperature, etc.), the forced degradation studies should be done for both drug substance, and drug product methods.

If the assay methods for drug substance and drug product have the same conditions, which result in the same selectivity, the forced degradation studies can be done with either drug substance or drug product. It is preferable to do forced degradation studies with drug substance for IND phase 1 projects, and with drug product for IND phase 2 projects.

For IND phase 3 and later phase applications, forced degradation studies should be done for both drug substances and drug products. Additionally, mass balance should be evaluated at phase 3, by adding the related substances detected to the assay results obtained for forced degradation samples. Generally, 5–20% degradation

is optimal for forced degradation studies, although an excessive degradation is acceptable as long as it does not cause failure of peak purity check. The more a sample is degraded, the more likely a loss in mass balance will be observed due to secondary degradation, loss of impurities in the solvent front, and loss of absorption due to ring-opening or other degradation pathways. The forced degradation studies for drug product should be performed before commencing stability studies of registration batches. The stress conditions described below are considered as the extreme conditions. Alternative or less stressful conditions may be applied when excessive degradation or interference is observed. During data acquisition, DAD should be used for HPLC and all spectra of peaks should be collected.

The samples should include drug substance, placebo, and drug product, and may be subject to the following conditions:

Acid/base:	drug substance "as is," 0.1 N HCl/ NaOH at RT for 1 day.
Thermal:	composite sample, 85°C for 10 days.
Thermal–humidity:	composite sample with 0.5 ml D.I. water in crimped vial, 85°C for 10 days.
Photostability:	one layer of composite sample (thickness ≤3 mm, use a petri dish with quartz plate cover, open petri dishes, or dishes covered with parafilm), 3 × ICH option 2 43.
Oxidation:	composite sample, 3% H_2O_2 at RT for 10 days, light-protected.

The following results are required to be included in the report: assay results for parent compound(s), results of co-elution test of parent compound(s), and profile of degradation products and other related compounds. For phase 3 studies the mass balance results should also be described.

22.4.6 Method Validation Parameters

Steps for method validation are as follows:

- The protocols or general SOPs to describe the detailed parameters as per Table 22.3.
- Execution of the protocol in the laboratory.
- Redevelopment and validation if deviation or failure is observed during validation that is attributed to the analytical method.
- Validation report.

TABLE 22.3   Data elements required for analytical method validation

Validation parameters	Identification method	Related substances and residual solvent methods		Assay, dissolution, and preservative methods
		Quantitation	Limit	
Specificity	Yes	Yes	Yes	Yes
Linearity	No	Yes	No	Yes
Range	No	Yes	No	Yes
Accuracy	No	Yes	No	Yes
Precision	No			
• Repeatability		Yes	No	Yes
• Intermediate precision		Yes*	No	Yes*
Detection limit	No	No	Yes	No**
Quantitation limit	No	Yes	No	No**
Robustness	No	Yes	No	Yes

The system suitability should be evaluated for all quantitation methods

*Intermediate precision may be omitted if reproducibility is performed during method validation

**Detection limit or quantitation limit may be required for methods such as determination of absence of active in placebo, dissolution testing of modified release drug products, e.g., acid resistance of enteric coated tablets

Validation parameters are included, but not limited to, linearity, precision, accuracy, robustness, quantitation limit, detection limit, and stability of analytical solution. The analytical parameters, such as system suitability and filter bias, should be evaluated for chromatographic method during method validation.[2,44]

Filter Bias

In modern analytical techniques, the analysis is typically carried out by spectroscopy (UV-Vis) utilizing a chromatographic method (HPLC, GC). Often a filter or centrifuge is utilized to remove particulates that may clog the column or affect absorbance readings. The different types of syringe filters, such as nylon or PTFE with a size of 0.45 or 0.2 μm, should be investigated dependent on the samples. The filter should be validated by filtering a portion of working standard solution through each syringe filter, discarding the first 2–3 mL, and collecting the filtrate for analysis. The result from the filtered solution should be comparable to that of unfiltered solution.

System Suitability

System suitability demonstrates that the system is working properly at the time of analysis. The appropriate system suitability criteria are based on individual technology, and the samples to be analyzed. For all chromatographic procedures, system suitability should include injection repeatability, expressed as RSD of peak responses obtained from five or six consecutive injections of working standard solution, tailing factor, theoretical plate number, resolution, etc.[44] For non-chromatographic methods, system suitability tests are also used to confirm that the system is functioning correctly. For example, titration method should always include a blank titration. For some particle size analysis, the solution with known particle size is used to ensure that the system is functioning as expected.

Since HPLC methods are the most commonly used procedures, the parameters for system suitability are injection repeatability, check standard, USP tailing, theoretical plate number, system drift, and resolution, discussed as follows.

Injection repeatability

The working standard solution will be injected five or six times onto the HPLC column. The mean and RSD for concerned peak response such as area will be calculated as:

$$X \text{ (mean)} = \sum_{i=1}^{n} X_i / n$$

$$\% \text{ RSD} = \sqrt{\frac{(X_i - X)^2}{n - 1}}$$

where:

X_i = peak response of individual injection
n = number of the repeatable injections.

In general, acceptance criteria are as follows, the RSD for peak area of interest from five or six injections of working standard solution should be ≤2.0% for potency assay, ≤10% for impurity testing and residual cleaning testing, and ≤3.0% dissolution testing.

If the product has low strength or S/N of the active peak is less than 50, the RSD of the peak area of the active from the six consecutive injections of ≤3% may be acceptable for potency assay.

Check standard

A check standard is often considered as part of integrated system suitability for potency assay or dissolution assay. The percentage recovery of the active from the check standard is calculated as follows:

$$\% \text{ Recovery} = \frac{A_{CK}}{Wt_{CK}} \times \frac{Wt_{WSTD}}{A_{WSTD}} \times 100$$

where:

A_{CK} is the peak area of the active from the check standard solution
A_{WSTD} is the average peak area of the active from the five or six injections of the working standard solution
Wt_{CK} is the weight of the active used in the preparation of the check standard solution (mg)
Wt_{WSTD} is the weight of the active used in the preparation of the working standard solution (mg).

It is acceptable that the percentage recovery for the check standard solution is in the range of 100.0 ± 2.0. For low dose/strength of drug products, 3.0% difference may be acceptable. Additional standard solutions may be needed in some cases. For example, a quantitation or detection limit solution for an impurity test should be injected to ensure the method is sensitive enough to detect impurities at the required concentration. The sensitivity could vary, based on laboratory, temperatures, columns, and detectors. For a detection limit solution a peak must be observed and integrated. For quantitation limit solutions, the peak area should be compared to the standard peak for recovery. For a quantitation solution the recovery should be between 90% and 110%.

Tailing factor (T)

The tailing factor (T) of active peak from the working standard solution is calculated as follows:

$$T = \frac{W_{0.05}}{2f}$$

where:

$W_{0.05}$ is the peak width at 5% of the active peak height from the baseline
f is the distance from the peak maximum to the leading edge of the peak (the distance being measured at a point 5% of the peak height from the baseline).

The peak is symmetrical if tailing factor is 1.0. It is generally considered to be reasonable if tailing factor is no more than 2.0, but the acceptable tailing factor should be confirmed during robustness experiments since excessive tailing or fronting could impact resolution between peaks.

Theoretical plate number (N)

The theoretical plate number per column (N) for the peak can be calculated from the first injection of the working standard solution as follows:

$$N = 16\left(\frac{t}{w}\right)^2$$

Where t is the retention time of active peak and w is the peak width of the peak, obtained by extrapolating the relatively straight sides of the peak to the baseline. Appropriate requirements for this parameter should be derived from validation data.

System drift

Periodic injections of the working standard solution should be made after a certain number of sample injections and at the end of the run. The percentage recovery of system drift injection can be calculated as follows:

$$\% \text{ Recovery} = \frac{A_{SCK}}{A_{WSTD}} \times 100$$

where:

A_{SCK} is the peak area of the active from the system drifts injection of the working standard solution
A_{WSTD} is the average peak area of the active from the first five or six system suitability injections of the working standard solution.

For system drift, the percentage recovery of system drift injection throughout the run should be within 98–102%. If the system drift meets this requirement, the average peak response from the first consecutive injections can be used for the calculation of the samples, otherwise a bracketing procedure should be used for calculation of the samples. In addition to the peak area, the retention time should also be evaluated. For identification the retention times should not vary by more than 2%.

Resolution (R)

Resolution factor should be calculated to demonstrate that critical pairs of peaks are adequately separated, and therefore independently integrated. The resolution factor from the first injection of the working standard solution can be calculated as follows:

$$R = \frac{2(t_{n+1} - t_n)}{W_{n+1} + W_n}$$

where:

t_n is the retention time of peak n
t_{n+1} is the retention time of peak $n + 1$
W_n is the peak width of peak n
W_{n+1} is the peak width of peak $n + 1$.

The minimum resolution between each identified critical pair of adjacent peaks should be ≥1.5, since this represents baseline separation of two neighboring Gaussian peaks. Resolution can also have an upper limit to make sure that peaks have not drifted too far away, minimizing the risk of co-elution due to significant changes in the retention properties of a column.

Accuracy

The accuracy of the method can be determined by spiking known amounts of the active at suitable levels of the label claimed amount, as shown in Table 22.4, to the corresponding placebo powder (or an amount of placebo mixture containing all the ingredients for the formulation except active), and then calculating the percent recovery of the active. For phase 3 accuracy experiments, triplicate sample preparations are required at each spiking level, and a minimum of three levels should be assessed. Table 22.4 describes the range, and the levels, for each individual testing procedure.

Percentage recovery is calculated by the assayed amount divided by a known amount of analyte spiked in the sample. Typical acceptance criteria are also provided in Table 22.4. Percentage recovery, average recovery from each level and overall levels, and confidence intervals should be evaluated.[45] For potency assays, RSD of recoveries for each spiked level should be no more than 2.0%. For low strength of drug products, e.g., ≤1 mg, wider ranges (3.0% for potency, 5.0% for dissolution) may be applied.

For the dissolution test, drug substance and placebo (or analytically prepared placebo) may be spiked into the dissolution vessel. The mixture of drug substance and placebo may be considered to be useful, if the recovery of the analyte of interest is lower than expected.

TABLE 22.4 Accuracy and acceptance criteria proposed

Test	Accuracy	Acceptance criteria
Cleaning residual	70%, 100%, and 130%	Minimum lowest recovery each level ≥50%
Potency (DS and DP)	70%, 100%, and 130%	Average recovery each level is between 98.0 and 102.0
Dissolution (immediate-release)	50%, 100%, and 120%	Average recovery each level is between 97.0 and 103.0
Dissolution (controlled-release)	20%, 100%, and 120%	Average recovery each level is between 97.0 and 103.0
Dissolution (delayed-release)	Acid stage: 1% and 10% Buffer stage: 50%, 100%, and 120%	Average recovery each level is between 97.0 and 103.0
Related substance (DS and DP)	QL, 100%, and 200% of specification	Average recovery each level is between 90.0 and 110.0 For QL, 80.0–120
Residual solvent	50%, 100%, and 120% of specification	Average recovery each level is between 80.0 and 120.0

However, it could be due to unique characteristics of drug substances in media. For low strength of the drug product, it is not possible to spike drug substance into the dissolution vessel. Drug substances solution with high concentration should be prepared by dissolving in the organic solvent or dissolution medium. The dissolution medium is the first choice. If the medium is not suitable, the organic solvents may be used, but the volume of solvent spiked should not be more than 5% of total the medium volume.

Precision

Precision should be evaluated through repeatability, intermediate precision or reproducibility.

Repeatability

For related substances and residual solvents tests, repeatability can be evaluated by spiking impurities or solvents at the specification limit for the products. In early phases of development little may be known about the impurities, so minimal repeatability data may be generated. For the potency assay, repeatability can be assessed using drug products (tablet or capsules), with a minimum of six determinations, at 100% of the test concentration. The RSD for the percentage label claim of the active should be ≤3.0% for the five or six samples.

Intermediate precision

This is a measure of the method's sensitivity to minor changes in equipment performance, and/or to variation in the operator's technique on any given day. A second analyst should perform the assay, using different equipment, and on a different day to confirm that acceptable results can be obtained. The absolute difference between the mean percentage label claims of the active generated by the two analysts should be <3.0%, but the exact criteria is based on the type of test and ultimate specification (e.g., if the drug substance assay specification is 98–102%, then the difference between laboratories should be <1.5%, but for a drug product with a specification of 90–110% a wider criteria could be used).

Reproducibility

This is a measure of the method's sensitivity to laboratory changes. There could be moderate changes in equipment performance, and/or variation in the operator's technique, and the laboratory environment. Reproducibility is generated by two separate laboratories running the test, and is therefore also called inter-laboratory precision. The absolute difference between the mean percentage label claims of the active generated by the two analysts should be <3.0%, but the exact criteria is based on the type of test, and the ultimate specification (e.g., if the drug substance assay specification is 98–102%, then the difference between laboratories should be <1.5%, but for a drug product with a specification of 90–110% a wider criteria could be used).

The results such as mean, standard deviation, relative standard deviation, and confidence interval should be evaluated and reported for each type of precision.

Linearity

A linear relationship between the concentration and respective response can be obtained by analyzing a series of standard solutions. At least five standard solutions with a specific range, as specified in Table 22.5, should be prepared. One injection of each of the linearity standard solutions may be sufficient. The peak area of the active will be measured at different concentration levels, and plotted against the corresponding

TABLE 22.5 The range in the regression line

Test	Linearity
Cleaning residual	QL to 130%* *consider 200% when specification is very low
Potency (DS and DP)	70% to 130% of LC
Dissolution (immediate-release)	50% to 120% of LC
Dissolution (controlled-release)	20%* to 120% of LC *unless the specification requires lower%
Dissolution (delayed-release)	Acid stage: QL to 10%; Buffer stage: 50% to 120%
Related substance (DS and DP)	QL or reporting level to 200% of specification* If specification is unknown, use 0.5% as specification QL or reporting level to 120% of LC if area percent is reported
Residual solvent	50% to 120%* of specification *consider 200% when specification is very low

concentrations. The correlation coefficient (r), y-intercept, slope of the regression line, and residual sum of squares will be calculated by the method of least squares, and a plot of the data should be recorded.

The correlation coefficient should be not less than 0.999 for potency assay, and not less than 0.99 for other tests. It is very useful to evaluate the difference between estimated value from regression line and actual value. The difference may be defined when applicable. For example, it is acceptable that percentage difference between the calculated value (concentration) from regression line and actual value is no more than 20% at QL level for impurity assay.

In some cases, a combined method for potency and impurity assay is used. It is quite common that impurity standards are unavailable in the early stages of product development. Area percentage or amount of impurity calculated from standard at 100% level of label claim (LC) are typically reported, if it is linear from reporting or the QL level to 120% of label-claimed level of strength. Otherwise, underestimated results may cause some issues later on, if the degradation or impurity approach or exceed qualification/ or identification level as defined in ICH Q3B(R2). If it is nonlinear from the QL to 120% of LC, a diluted standard should be used to minimize bias in the impurity calculation. If impurities are available, impurity standards containing known impurities at respective specification levels should be prepared. By comparing the slope of each impurity to the slope of the main standard, response factors or normalization factors can be established, and a single point standard can be used to quantitate accurately the known impurities.

Specificity

Specificity of the method must be investigated, in order to confirm that an analytical procedure is specific for the analyte of interest in the presence of components such as impurities, degradants, and matrix components (excipients). For an HPLC procedure, specificity can be demonstrated by separation of critical pairs of the two components (the active and impurity or two impurities) that elute closest to each other, by making individual injection of diluent, each impurity, the active, and the placebo (or analytical prepared placebo). In such cases, a diode array detector is useful in detecting co-eluted peaks in the samples spiked with an impurity when impurity is available, and/or in stressed samples.

Stability of Standard and Sample Solutions

It is essential that sample and standard solutions are stable throughout sample preparation and analysis. Proving stability of the standards should be part of the validation process.

The standard solutions should be freshly prepared, and the concentration of the standard solution used as the initial value. Portions of the working standard solutions are stored under refrigeration (5 ± 3°C), and at controlled and monitored room temperatures. These stored portions of standard are assayed at various time points (such as 1 and 3 days, etc.) to determine the concentration of analyte of interest, using freshly-prepared standard solution.

For potency assay, the standard and sample solutions are considered to be stable if the percentage difference between initial values of standard and samples, and those at specific times, is no more than 2.0%, but any downward trend in the data should also be evaluated for possible impact on the analysis.

For dissolution samples, the stability of the samples in the dissolution vessels is also part of the validation process, in addition to standard and sample solutions. The sample in the dissolution vessel should be stable at least up to the final sampling time. The sample solution can be obtained by spiking analyte of interest (either solution in medium or API to be dissolved in medium of vessel within a very short time), and placebo at 37.0 ± 0.5°C.

For impurity assay, the sample solution is considered stable if the following conditions are met:

- If 0.10% ≤ individual related substance <0.50%, the absolute difference between the initial and specific time point values should be ≤0.10%.
- If percentage individual related substance ≥0.50%, the percentage difference between the initial and t-time point values should be ≤20.0%.
- No new degradation product ≥QL of analyte of interest should be detected.

If these conditions cannot be met at any of the time points and storage conditions, then the sample and/or standard solution must be analyzed within the time period in which these conditions do apply. In the worst scenario, the sample solution has to be freshly-prepared prior to each injection to obtain consistent impurity profile results.

Detection Limit (DL), and Quantitation Limit (QL)

As defined in ICH Q2 (R1), the detection limit of an individual analytical procedure is the lowest amount of analyte in a sample that can be detected, but not necessarily quantitated as an exact value. The quantitation limit is the lowest amount of analyte in a sample that can be quantitatively determined with suitable precision and accuracy. The DL and QL are critical parameters of analytical procedure validation for residual solvent and impurity assay. There are several approaches for determining DL and QL, which are described in ICH Q2 (R1) as follows.

Visual evaluation

It is most likely to be used for non-instrumental methods. They can be determined by the analysis of samples with known amounts of analyte, and by establishing the minimum level at which the analytes can be detected (DL) or quantified with acceptable accuracy and precision (QL). For QL determination, six replicate samples may be required to be prepared and tested.

Signal-to-noise ratio approach

The signal-to-noise ratio of peak of analyte of interest in the sample should be at least 3:1 from DL solution, and 10:1 from the QL solution. For chromatographic techniques, the signal of the peak and the baseline noise can be measured manually or using built-in software.

The detection limit and QL of analyte may be determined by serial dilution of a standard solution with diluent, and injecting onto the HPLC system for assay. Then QL and DL will be determined by signal-to noise ratio.

Standard deviation of the response and slope

DL and QL may be expressed in the follows

$$QL = \frac{10\sigma}{S} \text{ and } DL = \frac{3.3\sigma}{S}$$

where:

σ is the standard deviation of the response
S is the slope of the calibration curve.

σ may be estimated based on standard deviation of blank (measurement of the magnitude of analytical background response using six replicate blank samples) or residual standard deviation of regression line or the standard deviation of Y-intercepts.

The reporting threshold for impurity testing is 0.05% level in most cases. The reporting levels are defined as per ICH Q3B(R2), based on daily intake and dose. Therefore, it is prudent that the concentration of the analyte in sample solution is prepared at QL level. The signal-to-noise ratio for the peak of analyte should be more than 10:1. Then, QL solution should be injected as six replicates onto the HPLC system for analysis. The RSD of the peak area of analyte should be ≤10.0%. If the QL level cannot meet any of the above criteria, the 0.10% level will be evaluated. If the 0.10% level still cannot meet any of the above criteria,

the method should be modified to meet all of the above QL criteria.

Robustness

The robustness of an analytical procedure is critical for effective method validation and cost effectiveness later on in routine assay. Robustness of chromatographic conditions will be performed on a sample solution, such as a repeatability sample solution with triplicate injections, by varying the parameters specified in Table 22.6. Only one parameter at a time is altered while the rest of the parameters remain unchanged. The design of experiment (DOE) could also be used to allow multiple parameters to be varied in each experiment, and thus reduce the number of experiments.

The instrument system must be equilibrated under each target and robustness condition. The system suitability requirements should be evaluated in each experiment to ensure the appropriate system suitability criteria are set for the method. Triplicate injections of the sample solution are then made under each condition. The individual determined mean values of analyte and RSD of three injections for each robustness condition are reported. The percentage of target value is calculated for each robustness test condition as follows:

$$\% \text{ of target} = \frac{\text{mean value under test condition}}{\text{mean } \textit{value} \text{ under target condition}} \times 100$$

The percentage of target should be within 98% to 102%. If any of the above robustness parameters fails to meet the acceptance criteria, then a precautionary statement should be included in the method specifying the limitations.

When possible, equivalent studies on different columns (lots and/or suppliers) should be evaluated. For related substances additional evaluation should be made to determine the impact of variations on the specificity of the method.

Sample preparation for potency assay

Robustness of the sample preparation for potency assay will be performed on duplicate sample preparations by varying the parameters specified in Table 22.7. Only one parameter at a time is varied, while maintaining the remaining parameters at target condition. Robustness of the dissolution method will be performed on three tablets (or capsules) by varying the parameters, such as medium pH value

TABLE 22.6 Experimental design for chromatographic parameters

	Parameters	Robustness test condition
	Mobile phase composition	Target ±1% e.g., Target: 50:50 (v/v)
		Test-1: 49:51
		Test-2: 51:49
HPLC	Buffer pH (mobile phase)	Target ± 0.1
	Buffer molarity (mobile phase)	Target ± 10%
	Column temperature	Target ± 3°C
	Wavelength	Target ± 2 nm
GC	Temperature	±5°C
	Flow rate	10% of target

TABLE 22.7 Experimental design for assay sample preparation

Parameters	Test condition
Shaking time*	target ± 20%
Sonication time*	target ± 20%

(±0.1 of target), or concentration of surfactant (±5% of target).

Non-chromatographic Method Validation

Additional tests to control the quality of the drug substances, excipients, and/or drug products, such as particle size distribution, optical rotation, and methodologies such as DSC, PXRD, Raman spectroscopy, and near-infrared spectroscopy should be validated prior to use. The validation parameters may be less extensive than for chromatographic methods, but in general are likely to include repeatability, intermediate precision, and robustness, but specificity and accuracy may also be applicable.

Failure and Revalidation

During method validation, failure to meet validation acceptance criteria may be observed. If this occurs, investigations should be conducted to reveal root causes. If these are attributed to the procedure, the validation will be terminated at this stage, and new method development experiments initiated. The method is then appropriately revised, and all changes are documented prior to revalidation. In case of a failure of comparison during repeatability and intermediate precision, all aspects should be taken into consideration (i.e. chemist skills, lab equipment variation, and sample variation). For any failures during validation experiments, a thorough evaluation is required to ensure that the failure is truly due to the method, and not due to laboratory error or other unexpected issues such as sample homogeneity.

The need to revalidate the method will be evaluated if there are changes, such as column vendor, drug substances route of synthesis, and drug products composition. Some changes may not require revalidation or may only require partial revalidation (e.g., new excipients would require specificity experiments), but the evaluation should always be made, and the justification for not revalidating should be documented.

22.5 METHOD TRANSFERS (MT) AND INTER-LABORATORY QUALIFICATION (ILQ)

22.5.1 Definition

An analytical laboratory which was not a part of the validation process must be qualified to demonstrate that the laboratory executes the analytical procedure in an equivalent fashion to the originating laboratory. The method transfer or ILQ usually occurs between the analytical R&D laboratory and a quality control laboratory. This transfer can be within the same company, but could also be between two different companies or different sites. The qualification can go through method transfer or inter-laboratory qualification. All involved methods must be assessed, in order to determine the status of method transfer and/or ILQ, as necessary.

It is quite realistic or practical to avoid ILQ or MT as a separate study, if a quality control laboratory or receiving laboratory could participate in the initial validation process, such as a reproducibility study. Under certain circumstances, it is very important to decide whether or not the approach of method transfer or ILQ is more appropriate. It might be the case that method transfer is more appropriate in the early phase of drug product development between a CRO and sponsor, and ILQ in a later phase stage.

The following steps will be required for method transfer or inter-laboratory qualification:

- Analytical procedure and testing material including reagent, instrument, and critical parameters should be discussed and understood through technical teams between originating laboratory and receiving laboratory;
- Protocol must be defined and approved regarding parameters, acceptance criteria, time frame, and samples;
- Deviation and investigation may be needed;
- Closure and final report approval.

The method transfer takes the form of a partial revalidation by the receiving laboratory, and may include the following parameters, depending on the analytical procedure: system suitability, linearity, accuracy by recovery study, repeatability, QL/DL for related substance, and residual solvent tests.

For an ILQ, parameters may include system suitability, reproducibility, QL/DL for related substance, and residual solvent tests if QL/DL is not part of system suitability.

22.5.2 Potency

Typically, acceptance criteria for the potency assay in solid oral dosage forms are the same as that for intermediate precision in method validation.

If there is any failure to meet the acceptance criteria, investigation will be conducted. For example, drug product variation may be a cause because the results from two separately taken samples from the same batch are reliable, but not in agreement with each other. It is not unusual for the products, such as active coated tablets. In this case, it is necessary to prepare a composite in one laboratory, and the same composite is analyzed by both laboratories. For "drop" method (prepare a sample by dropping a certain amount of tablets without the grinding process) for potency assay or separate analytical procedure for content uniformity testing, representative samples should carefully be evaluated in order to limit variation of the products. Attention may be paid to the purity of reference standard if pretreatment of the reference standard, such as a drying process, is required. The predefined drying and testing procedure between two laboratories should be addressed.

22.5.3 Related Substance Assay

Typically, acceptance criteria should be followed based on an approved method validation report. During ILQ practices, aging samples such as the stability samples may be selected, so that the samples contain impurities to aid in the evaluation of the data. If such samples are not available, the samples spiked with known impurities, and/or stressed drug substances, may be used where they are analyzed for recovery by both laboratories. To ensure that each laboratory uses the same representative samples, a single laboratory is required to prepare the samples, and the samples are then shipped to the second laboratory in a timely fashion.

22.5.4 Residual Solvent Assay

The acceptance criteria are similar to those defined in the related substance assay, except that samples spiked with solvents at the specification level should be used. It is most probable that the samples spiked with the solvent of interest are prepared by each individual laboratory, and analyzed for recovery study. The absolute difference, as generated by both laboratories, in percentage recovery should be no more than 20%, with 20% RSD for six replicate preparations from each laboratory.

22.5.5 Dissolution or Release Assay

Acceptance criteria should be set up depending upon formulation (e.g., immediate-release or control-/extended-release), and results such as single sampling point or multiple sampling points. For immediate release products, there are at least two early sampling points for which percentage release is less than 85%, and one final sampling point. The 12 units should be tested in each individual laboratory. There are two acceptable approaches, direct comparison, and model independent approach using similarity factor f_2 and difference factor f_1.

In general, percentage mean difference between both laboratories in percentage release should be less than 10% for time points with less than 85% release, and no more than 5% for final sampling point or Q-point.

The model independent approach, using f_2 and f_1, can only be used if criteria for f_1 and f_2 are met. The results are comparable or the receiving laboratory is qualified if f_1 value is within the range 0–15, and f_2 value is within the range 50–100.

As per the FDA guidance for industry,[22] f_1 and f_2 are defined as follows:

$$f_1 = \tau \left\{ \left[\sum_{t-1}^{n} |R_t - T_t| \right] \Big/ \left[\sum_{t-1}^{n} R_t \right] \right\} \cdot 100$$

where:

n is the number of time points
R_t is the dissolution value in percent of the reference (originating laboratory) at time t
T_t is the dissolution value of the test (receiving laboratory) at time t.

$$f_2 = 50 \cdot \log \left\{ \left[1 + (1/n) \sum_{t-1}^{n} (R_t - T_t)^2 \right]^{-0.5} \right\} \cdot 100$$

The criteria to determine difference and similarity are as follows:

- 12 dosage units in each laboratory should be tested.
- Mean dissolution values at each time interval from both laboratories are used.
- Only one measurement should be used after 85% release.
- For mean values used, percentage RSD at the early time point should be less than 20%, and 10% for other time points.

22.6 CASE STUDIES

22.6.1 CASE STUDY 1

Problem

A development phase 1 batch of an API was being analyzed for related substances. The HPLC test method was conducted using external standardization, and using the API as the standard for any unknown impurities. For this purpose, the standard solution included a concentration of API equivalent to 0.10% of the concentration of API in the sample solution. The related substances specification for any unknown impurity was "not more than 0.10%." The method had been validated to phase 1, based on specified, identified impurities, and the quantitation limit was found to be 0.04%.

When one batch was analyzed in one laboratory (Lab 1), it was found to contain an unknown impurity which was estimated at a level of about 0.08%, which met the specification requirement. A sample was then re-analyzed in another laboratory (Lab 2), and this time the reported level of the same impurity was 0.12%, which failed to meet the specification requirement.

Investigation

The out of specification (OOS) investigation conducted at Lab 2 confirmed that there had been no analyst errors, and no assignable causes were identified. Retesting of a new aliquot taken from the same sample confirmed the original result of 0.12%. The investigation was then extended to Lab 1, where again no analyst errors were identified, but again retesting of a new aliquot taken from the same sample confirmed their original result of 0.08%.

The investigation was then extended to closer examination of the chromatograms at both laboratories. Chromatograms were being monitored at a wavelength of around 230 nm, which corresponded to the maximum wavelengths for the API, and also each of the specified, identified impurities. As part of the further investigation, both laboratories repeated the analysis, but using diode array detectors to check the spectra of the API and each impurity. It was verified that the maximum wavelengths for each known component were around 230 nm. For the unknown impurity, the maximum wavelength was around 223 nm, and 230 nm actually coincided with a steep down slope of the spectrum. When both laboratories used 223 nm as the monitoring wavelength for this impurity, they both got results in close agreement with each other.

It should be noted that problems like this can occur when chromatograms are being monitored using detector wavelengths that correspond to the edge of the spectrum for one or more components. The typical instrument specification for UV detectors for wavelength accuracy is ±4 nm. Therefore, if the monitoring wavelength is set at 230 nm, but the true wavelength being monitored varies from this by up to 4 nm, for a component that is being monitored at its absorbance maximum very little difference is likely to be noted, since UV absorbance spectra of organic molecules normally show relatively broad peaks. However, this could lead to very large differences in the recorded absorbance values for any components that are being monitored on the edge of the peak.

To avoid this type of problem, it is recommended that edge-of-peak monitoring be avoided wherever possible.

22.6 CASE STUDIES

22.6.2 CASE STUDY 2

Problem

During a validation study for a related substances test, the recovery was being investigated by spiking with the impurities concerned. For one of those impurities, the recovery was being conducted using a solution at a concentration of 1 μg per mL. Although this should be higher than the detection limit (although this has not yet been verified in this validation study), no peak attributable to this impurity was observed in the chromatogram.

Investigation

The initial investigation verified that the spiking solution had been correctly prepared, all instrumental settings were correct, but no peak was generated by that solution.

Further investigations could lead to various possibilities.

Possibility 1

During method development, there may have been a change of monitoring wavelength to improve method sensitivity for another new component, but the analyst overlooked checking the effect of this on other established components. It is very important during development to consider the impact of any changes on the overall analysis, and in this circumstance it may become necessary to have different monitoring wavelengths for different components, to ensure adequate sensitivity for all components of interest.

It is usually recommended that the detection limit and the quantitation limit determinations be conducted as the first parameter during a validation study, which would have ensured identification of this issue before much work had been completed. In addition, these parameters are often required in order to design other parts of the validation program, which is another good reason to determine them first.

Possibility 2

The sample of impurity or impurity standard that was used during development was from a different batch to that being used in the validation study, and may not have been of the same quality.

It is expected that API batches are synthesized under very controlled conditions in accordance with cGMP requirements. However, the same may not necessarily be the case for impurities that are not synthesis intermediates of the API, and are being specially synthesized. So once an impurity of this type has been identified, it is very important to:

1. ensure that adequate controls are put into place so that we can be confident that we are really manufacturing the same compound each time. It is important to put controls into place for the structural identity for different batches;
2. ensure that the overall purities of different batches are kept reasonably constant.

22.6.3 CASE STUDY 3

Problem

During the precision and accuracy validation of a related substances test for a tablet product, a very broad peak was observed which appeared in chromatograms after about five sample injections, and corresponded to a level of about 1.0%. It made quantitation of impurity peaks very difficult.

Investigation

The initial investigation showed no analytical errors, and the observed additional peaks were genuine. The reason that this had not been addressed during development, and was only observed during validation, was that this was the first time sufficiently long runs were used that would allow a component that eluted after five sample injections to be observed.

This additional component might be due to a tablet excipient, in which case it would not be a problem from the point of view of a new impurity, but would need to be overcome to prevent interferences with this related substances test.

Alternatively, this might be due to a genuine unknown related substance, in which case in accordance with ICH Guideline Q3B(R) it would need to be identified, and then perhaps qualified, which could lead to delays in this product development program.

22.6.4 CASE STUDY 4

Problem

While performing an accuracy experiment for the potency assay for a tablet it was found that the recovery was 10% less than theoretical, although during method development it had been found that the sample extraction procedure had performed quite efficiently.

Investigation

The investigation revealed that a new batch of filters had been purchased for the validation study. Although a filter recovery study had been completed satisfactorily with the previous batch, the new batch did not perform as efficiently. Similar issues have also been experienced with HPLC autosampler vials, when adsorption of an analyte on the surface can occur in some cases.

22.6.5 CASE STUDY 5

Problem

During a tablet stability study, it was observed that the assay values of the samples appeared to be declining for samples stored under accelerated conditions at 40°C/75% RH. There were no increases observed in degradation product peaks in the chromatograms.

Investigation

One possibility could be that the active ingredient degraded to products that were not being detected by the current analytical methodology. Normally it would be expected that such a possibility would have been eliminated by conducting forced degradation (stress) studies prior to commencing the stability study, to ensure that the analytical methodology was suitable for monitoring the formation of tablet degradation products.

In this case, it was subsequently determined that under the accelerated storage condition, the tablet matrix underwent some physical changes that reduced the efficiency of the extraction procedure during the sample preparation stage of the analysis. This type of issue is relatively common during development stages, and it is highly recommended that, as part of an OOS investigation, the efficiency of the procedure for preparing analytical solutions be examined. Even though a method has been fully validated, and the determination of accuracy using recovery studies has been deemed satisfactory, this can still be an issue. Validation studies are typically conducted using either freshly-prepared product or one that has been stored at the correct temperature condition. They are not normally conducted using samples that have been kept under accelerated storage conditions.

22.7 CONCLUSIONS

It is an absolute regulatory requirement that all analytical methods that are used to generate data in a marketing authorization dossier be fully validated. It is generally considered acceptable in the industry to phase this validation as a product progresses through development, and approaches for doing this are discussed in this chapter. During the evolution of analytical methodologies, it is quite likely that methods will need to be applied within laboratories that did not participate in validation, and it is then a GMP requirement to demonstrate that the method functions reliably under such circumstances. The applications of method transfers and ILQs are also discussed in this chapter. Finally, regardless of how thoroughly validations and transfers are conducted, things will go wrong from time to time, and under such circumstances it is very important to conduct very thorough investigations and to be prepared to address a wide variety of root causes.

It is essential that clearly documented studies be conducted according to GMP practices during the development of analytical method as rational validation of inter-laboratory qualification.

References

1. International Conference on Harmonization Q2 (R1) Guideline. (2005). Validation of analytical procedures: text and methodology.
2. US Food and Drug Administration. (2000). Center for Drug Evaluation and Research, August, Guidance for industry: Analytical procedures and methods validation, chemistry, manufacturing, and control documentation.
3. Ermer, J. & Miller, J.H. McB. (2005). *Method validation in pharmaceutical analysis: A guide to best practice.* Wiley-VCH Verlag GmbH & Co., KGaA, Weinheim.
4. Swartz, M.E. & Krull, I.S. (1997). *Analytical method development and validation.* Marcel Dekker, New York.
5. US Food Drug Administration. (2006). Center for Drug Evaluation and Research, January, Guidance for Industry, Investigators, and Reviewers: Exploratory IND Studies.
6. US Food Drug Administration. (1995). Center for Drug Evaluation and Research, November, Guidance for Industry: Content and format of investigational new drug application (INDs) for phase 1 studies of drugs, including well-characterized, therapeutic, biotechnology-derived products.
7. US Food Drug Administration. (2003). Center for Drug Evaluation and Research, May, Guidance for Industry: INDs for phase 2 and phase 3 studies, chemistry, manufacturing, and controls information.
8. European Medicines Agency. (2004). Inspections, December 16, CHMP/QWP/185401/2004, Guideline on the requirements to the chemical and pharmaceutical quality documentation concerning investigational medicinal products in clinical trials.
9. International Conference on Harmonization. (2002). The common technical document for registration of pharmaceuticals for human use: quality M4Q(R1).
10. USP 30/NF 25. (2006). General Chapter <1225> Validation of compendial methods.
11. International Conference on Harmonization, ICH Q3A(R2), Impurities in new drug substances.
12. International Conference on Harmonization. (2006). ICH Q3B(R2), Impurities in new drug products.
13. International Conference on Harmonization. (2005). Q3C(R3), Impurities: guideline for residual solvents.
14. Hauck, W.W., Foster, T., Sheinin, E., Cecil, T., Brown, W., Marques, M. & Williams, R.L. (2005). Oral dosage form performance tests: New dissolution approaches. Pharmaceutical Research 22(2), 182–187.

15. Fortunate, D. (2005). Dissolution method development for immediate release solid oral dosage forms "quick start guideline for early phase development compounds." Dissolution Technologies, August, 12–14.

16. Lagace, M., Gravelle, M., Di Maso, M. & McClintock, S. (2004). Developing a discriminating dissolution procedure for a dual active pharmaceutical product with unique solubility characteristics. Dissolution Technologies, February, 13–17.

17. Qureshi, S.A. (2006). Developing discriminatory drug dissolution tests and profiles: some thoughts for consideration on the concept and its interpretation. Dissolution Technology, November, 18–23.

18. Brown, C.K., Chokshi, H.P., Nickerson, B., Reed, R.A., Rohrs, B.R. & Shah, P.A. (2004). Acceptable analytical practices for dissolution testing of poorly soluble compounds. Pharmaceutical Technology, December, 56–65.

19. Degenhardt, O.S., Waters, B., Rebelo-Cameirao, A., Meyer, A., Brunner, H. & Toltl, N.P. (2004). Comparison of the effectiveness of various deaeration techniques. Dissolution Technologies, February, 6–11.

20. Rohrs, B.R. (2001). Dissolution method development for poorly soluble compounds. Dissolution Technologies, 6–12.

21. Viegas, T.X., Curatella, R.U., VanWinkle, L.L. & Brinker, G. (2001). Intrinsic drug dissolution testing using the stationary disk system. Dissolution Technologies, August, 19–23.

22. USP30/NF25 <1092> The dissolution procedure: Development and validation.

23. Food Drug Administration. (1997). Center for Drug Evaluation and Research. Guidance for industry: dissolution testing of immediate release solid oral dosage forms.

24. USP30/NF25 <711> Dissolution.

25. Gohel, M.C. (2003). Overview on chirality and applications of stereo-selective dissolution testing in the formulation and development work. Dissolution Technologies, August, 16–20.

26. Food Drug Administration. (2003). Center for Drug Evaluation and Research. Guidance for industry: Powder blends and finished dosage units-stratified in-process dosage unit sampling and assessment (draft guidance).

27. Khan, M.A., Kumar, S., Jayachandran, J., Vartak, S.V., Bhartiya, A. & Sinha, S. (2005). Validation of a stability indicating LC method for aminodarone HCl and related substances. Chromatographia 61(11/12), 599–607.

28. Sajonz, P., Wu, Y., Natishan, T.K., McGachy, N.T. & DeTora, D. (2006). Challenges in the analytical method development and validation for an unstable active pharmaceutical ingredient. Journal of Chromatographic Sciences 44, 132–140.

29. Blanco, M. & Villar, A. (2003). Development and validation of a method for the polymorphic analysis of pharmaceutical preparations using near infrared spectroscopy. Journal of Pharmaceutical Sciences 92(4), 823–830.

30. Sokoließ, T. & Köller, G. (2005). Approach to method development and validation in capillary electrophoresis for enantiomeric purity testing of active basic pharmaceutical ingredients. Electrophoresis 26, 2330–2341.

31. Korczynski, M.S. (2004). The integration of process analytical technologies, concurrent validation, and parametric release programs in aseptic processing. PDA Journal of Pharmaceutical Sciences and Technology 58(4), 181–191.

32. Vankiersbick, T., Vercauteren, A., Baeyens, W., Van der Weken, G., Verpoort, F., Vergote, G. & Remon, J.P. (2002). Applications of Raman spectroscopy in pharmaceutical analysis. Trends in Analytical Chemistry 21, 869–877.

33. Moffat, A.C., Trafford, A.D., Joe, R.D. & Graham, P. (2000). Meeting the international conference on harmonisation's guidelines on validation of analytical procedures: quantification as exemplified by a near infra red reflectance assay of paracetamol in intact tablets. Analyst 125, 1341–1351.

34. Blanco, M., Coello, J., Iturriage, H., Maspoch, S. & Pou, N. (2000). Development and validation of a near infrared method for the analytical control of a pharmaceutical preparation in three steps of the manufacturing process. Fresenius Journal of Analytical Chemistry 368, 534–539.

35. Pappa, H., Porter, D. & Russo, K. (2006). Development of a new USP general information chapter: Verification of compendial procedures. Pharmaceutical Technology, 164–169.

36. Krull, I. & Swartz, M. (2001). Determination specificity in a regulated environment. LCGC 19(6), 604–614.

37. EP impurity 5.10.

38. USP 30/25NF <1086> impurities in official articles.

39. International Conference on Harmonization. (1999). Q6A, New Drug Substances and New Drug Products: Chemical Substances (including Decision Trees).

40. International Conference on Harmonization. (2003). Q1A(R2), Stability testing of new drug substances and products.

41. Zhou, W., Yu, K., Fang, F. & Carr, G. Evaluation of HPLC-DAD for determination of co-eluting impurities in pharmaceutical analysis. Submitted for publication.

42. Baertschi, S.W. (2005). Pharmaceutical stress testing predicting drug degradation. Taylor & Francis Group.

43. International Conference on Harmonization. (1996). Q1B, photostability testing of new drug substances and products.

44. US Food Drug Administration. (1994). Center for Drug Evaluation and Research, Reviewer guidance: validation of chromatographic methods.

45. USP30/NF25, <1010> Analytical data-interpretation and treatment.

CHAPTER

23

Statistical Design and Analysis of Long-term Stability Studies for Drug Products

David LeBlond

23.1 INTRODUCTION

This chapter is not intended to reiterate the very detailed and complete information already available in the literature and textbooks on this subject. The literature in this area is vast, and an attempt to repeat it here would be a disservice to the reader. Instead appropriate references are supplied, and the focus is on more recent statistical aspects, approaches, and recommendations that are important and useful, and that are not discussed elsewhere. The material in Sections 23.1 to 23.3 is related to objectives, guidances, test methods, and data management. These sections can and should be profitably read and understood by formulation scientists, analytical chemists, and pharmaceutical development managers who have some understanding of basic principles of experimental design. However, proper design and analysis of stability studies requires specific statistical expertise, much material presented in the remainder of this chapter is technically quite complex, and oriented to meet the needs and interests of professional statisticians.

23.2 STABILITY STUDY OBJECTIVES

The stability of a drug product is defined by the rate of change over time of key measures of quality on storage under specific conditions of temperature and humidity. A stability study should always be regarded as a scientific experiment designed to test certain hypotheses (such as equality of stability among lots) or estimate certain parameters (such as shelf life). Similar to any other scientific process, the outcome of a stability study should lead to knowledge that permits the pharmaceutical manufacturer to better understand and predict product behavior. Thus, a stability study is not merely a regulatory requirement, but is a key component in a process of scientific knowledge-building that supports the continued quality, safety, and efficacy of a pharmaceutical product throughout its shelf life.

Understanding the stability of a pharmaceutical product (or any of its components) is important for proper quality design at many stages of the product lifecycle. Table 23.1 lists some examples of pharmaceutical stability studies/analyses, and their objectives.

Stability is intimately connected to many other key quality aspects of a drug product. For instance, interpretation of the rate of change of a key measure requires knowledge of the associated product release levels, recommended storage conditions, packaging, and stability acceptance limits. Proper interpretation of stability study data requires an understanding of the chemical–kinetic processes, the accuracy and precision of the associated test method, and the statistical limitations of the stability study experimental design. The statistical methodology used to achieve a given objective often depends on the quantity and quality of the data available, and on the lifecycle stage of the product.

Developing Solid Oral Dosage Forms: Pharmaceutical Theory and Practice
ISBN: 978-0-444-53242-8

TABLE 23.1   Applications of stability studies in pharmaceutical development

Product development stage	Objective
Chemical characterization	• Accelerated studies to define degradation pathways
Formulation development	• Establish retest period for active ingredient • Excipient/packaging selection and compatibility studies
Clinical studies	• Verify stability of clinical supplies
Product registration	• Shelf life estimation • Release limit estimation • Determine process capability with respect to release or acceptance limits • Comparison of stability of clinical, development, registration batches
Post-approval commitment	• Shelf life confirmation/extension with long-term studies • Annual stability monitoring
Marketed product	• Determination of predictive model from historical data • Shelf life extension • Assess risk of temperature excursions • Routine trending • Justification of scale-up, process, formulation, dosage strength, manufacturing site, packaging or other post-approval changes • Establish equivalency with new formulations/packages • Annual stability reports

23.3 REGULATORY GUIDANCE

The regulatory aspects of drug product stability are governed by a number of interrelated guidance documents. In the United States, the European Union, and Japan, these guidance documents are provided through the International Conference on Harmonization of Technical Requirements for Registration of Pharmaceuticals for Human Use (ICH). Q1A-E[1,2,3,4,5] govern stability testing of drug substances and products. Q2A-B[6,7] govern the validation of analytical methods used for (among other things) stability testing. Q3A-B[8,9] govern impurity levels in drug substances and products. Q6A-B[10,11] govern acceptance criteria.

One must use caution in interpreting and using such regulatory guidances. Often, their individual scopes are somewhat narrow, and they may not always include the specific objectives of interest to the developer. There is no guarantee that following such guidances will lead to a manufacturable, approvable, high-quality product. Inconsistencies are inevitable, because each of the individual guidances is established by a separate committee. Blind adherence may have undesirable long-term consequences. Some common pitfalls are noted below. A developer must always consider the specific study objectives, and the approach taken should always be scientifically and statistically justified.

23.4 TEST METHODS AND DATA MANAGEMENT

Quantitative, precise, unbiased, stability-indicating test methods are essential components of stability experimentation. All information obtained from a stability study ultimately comes from the test methods used. No amount of statistical sophistication can compensate for a poor measurement system. The following recommendations are meant to promote the use of high quality test methods and data management approaches.

1. Use quantitative test methods that produce a result on a continuous measurement scale. These have higher information content than those that produce binary (yes/no), discrete (1, 2, 3 …), ordinal (low, medium, high), or categorical (A, B, C …) responses.
2. The validity of information obtained from a stability study ultimately depends on the test methods used. Where possible, the test methods used should be thoroughly characterized and validated prior to use. Partial validation may be acceptable for early development studies, but the uncertainties of the test method need to be accounted for in data evaluation. The validation should include determination of bias and imprecision as a function of true concentration level. The sources (components) of variance (replication, instrument, operator, day, lab, calibration run, etc.) should be identified and quantified. Such understanding is important in both study design (e.g., assuring adequate sample size or study power), and analysis (e.g., deciding whether to average replicated test values).
3. Excessive rounding and binning of continuous measured values should be avoided (e.g., conversion of numerically measurable values to "below quantitation" because they are thought

to have "unacceptable" variability or rounding of results for minor components and degradation products to conform to specifications in regulatory guidelines, e.g., ICH Q3A(R2) and Q3B(R2)). Such practices are common when reporting individual analytical results, and may be required for the purposes of conforming to regulatory guidances when used in this manner; however, when values such as stability testing results are used as input for further data analyses, over-rounding and binning of test results lowers the data information content, and distorts the measurement error structure. It should be the decision of the statistician performing the analysis of the data to round results appropriately after all data analysis has been completed. These abuses may limit the statistical procedures available for data analysis, and lead to biased estimates or incorrect conclusions. All information contained in the original measurements should be used for efficient, sound decision making.

4. Storage time should be well-controlled. Regression procedures often assume that storage time is known exactly. Errors in the timescale may introduce bias and uncertainty that undermines the most accurate and precise response measurements. Stability studies typically follow predefined plans, in which sampling times are specified. However, for the purpose of data analysis, only the actual time at which a sample is taken is relevant; this must be accurately reported, especially if it deviates from the time specified in the plan. Company procedures should limit the time between sampling and analysis to as short an interval as possible to prevent additional degradation; ideally, samples should be obtained immediately prior to analysis, even if this requires delaying sampling until after the time specified in the plan. Release test results (obtained at the end of manufacturing) should not be used in place of a true initial (zero-time) test result when the release test date is substantially different from the starting date of a stability study. Storage conditions of manufactured or sampled product should be appropriately controlled.

5. Design stability databases with data analysis in mind. Statistical analyses may lead to approval of a longer shelf life or provide information needed to better manage a product throughout its lifecycle. Often statistical analyses are not performed or included in submissions because hand re-entry of data is required, excessive reformatting must be performed or there may be a delay in obtaining analytical results.

6. As recently advocated,[12] include a trained statistician on the study design and analysis team.

Analytical data are obtained at great expense. The information contained within these data represents a proprietary advantage to the product developer. Thus, the analytical methods used to produce the data, and the computing/statistical methods used to extract information from them, should be of the highest possible quality.

23.5 MODELING INSTABILITY

23.5.1 Stability Study Variables

We will start with shopping lists of key response, experimental, and controlled variables that often appear in drug product stability studies. The lists are by no means exhaustive. Then we will discuss how each is typically incorporated into the kinetic model.

Responses

The response variable that is monitored over time should include, as appropriate, results from the physical, chemical, biological, microbiological, and/or key performance indicators of the dosage form. The potency level of the active ingredient(s), and the levels of related degradants or impurities are always considered. In the case of instability due to degradation, mass balance should be accounted for. Only quantitative variables will generally be amenable to statistical analyses, as described below.

Other critical or key quality attributes also need to be considered if they have acceptance limits. Dissolution may be especially critical for modified-release products or products of poorly soluble compounds where bioavailability may change over time when dissolution is the rate-limiting step for drug absorption. Other responses that may be included in stability studies are color, moisture or solvent level, preservative, antioxidant or pH.

Experimental Fixed Variables

Variables such as storage time, dosage strength, and packaging type are called "fixed" variables because the levels of such variables (e.g., 3 months of storage, 300mg) have specific meaning that is the same whenever that level is used in the study. Typically, except for storage time, "fixed" variables are categorical in nature, and determined in advance by the experimenter.

Storage time is, of course, the primary experimental "fixed" variable always included in a stability study. ICH Q1A[1] recommends testing every 3, 6, and 12 months during the first, second, and subsequent years respectively. Thus, for a typical three-year study, testing would occur at 0, 3, 6, 9, 12, 18, 24, and 36 months. However, although storage times may be "fixed" by the study plan, these are actually measurable. Whenever and wherever possible, the exact measured elapsed time between the start of the study and the removal of a sample for analysis should be accurately reported, at least to the nearest whole day. Every effort should be made to minimize the elapsed time between when a sample is removed for analysis, and the time at which the analysis is actually performed.

Other experimental "fixed" variables (also referred to as "factors" or "predictors") that may be included as part of more complex studies include container type or size, closure type, fill size, desiccant type or amount, manufacturing site, batch size or other covariates.

Experimental Random Variables

Variables such as test result that replicate number or batch number are called "random" variables, because the levels used (say replicate "1," "2" or "3") are not the same whenever they are applied; instead these levels are assumed to represent experimental conditions drawn at random from a hypothetical infinite population of all possible replicates.

The ICH Q1A[1] guidance recommends that stability studies for new product registration include at least three batches of drug product (say batches "1," "2," and "3"). If batch is considered a fixed variable like dosage strength, then the estimated shelf life will reflect only the performance of the three batches in the study. If, on the other hand, batch is considered to be a random effect like replicate, then the estimated shelf life will reflect the hypothetical infinite population of all (future) batches. To properly treat batch as a random variable requires use of a so-called "mixed" regression model, and specialized statistical software such as the MIXED procedure in SAS.[13]

The shelf life estimate will generally be shorter if batch is regarded as random but, since the shelf life specification is meant to apply to all future batches, this may be more realistic. However, in most new product registrations governed by ICH Q1E,[5] where the minimum of three batches are available, batch is treated as a fixed variable, and any inferences are strictly limited to the three batches on hand. This is done, quite simply, because data from only three batches are insufficient to project to the larger population of all future batches. This caveat must be borne in mind when interpreting the results of stability analyses.

Variable Transformations

Sometimes the stability profile of a quality characteristic does not follow a straight line. Examples may include moisture level that approaches equilibrium or an intermediate degradation product that follows a complex kinetic mechanism. In such cases, a nonlinear regression procedure should be considered. A description of nonlinear regression is beyond the scope of this chapter.

When the rate of change in the response measure is nearly constant over time and the change is monotonic, such that a transformation yields a nearly linear stability profile, linear regression (LR) may be used. LR provides a simple description that is easily grasped by non-statisticians, requires few assumptions, and can be executed in widely available software. While the assumptions/approximations of LR are few, they must be satisfied for any estimates, inferences or predictions made using LR to be valid. The assumptions of LR are:

1. The response is linearly related to the storage time.
2. There is no uncertainty in the storage time value.
3. Errors in the response measurements are normally distributed.
4. Errors in the response measurements are mutually independent.
5. The error variance in the response measurement is the same for all measurements.

Various statistical procedures that can be used to verify the above assumptions are discussed in popular statistical texts.[14]

If the kinetic processes of instability are more complex, the profile may exhibit curvature. If a theoretical kinetic model is available, then nonlinear regression approaches (such as with the NLIN procedure of SAS) may be the best way to draw inferences, estimate shelf life, and make predictions from the stability data. In some cases, a nonlinear model can be linearized by transformation. For instance, the first-order kinetic model $y = A\exp(-kt)$ can be rewritten $\log(y) = \log(A) - kt$. Thus, a log transformation of the response, y, may improve conformance to assumption 1 above.

When the kinetic process is not well-understood, various transformations of the response or timescales (or both) may be tried in an effort to allow LR to be used for analysis. It is important that the transformation be valid for all possible response or time values.

For instance, transformations such as $\log(y/(A - y))$ or $\log(t)$ are undefined for $y \geq A$ or $t = 0$, respectively.

Transformation of the timescale can have subtle effects on estimation efficiency, but generally presents few statistical issues. However, transformation of the response scale may fundamentally change the error structure of the response measurements (assumptions 2–5). In favorable cases, a transformation may be found that will improve conformance to all five basic LR assumptions. However, if the transformation does not have a theoretical basis, extrapolations beyond the duration of the study must be made with extreme caution.

Controlled Variables

Temperature and humidity are usually controlled during a stability study. The product label storage condition will dictate the conditions used in studies conducted to estimate shelf life. Table 23.2, taken from ICH Q1A,[1] gives typical conditions used.

For controlled room temperature products susceptible to moisture loss, lower relative humidity storage conditions may be appropriate (40% for long-term and intermediate, and 15% for accelerated conditions). For controlled room temperature products stored in water impermeable containers, ambient RH might be appropriate for different temperature conditions.

While storage temperature and relative humidity are quantitative variables that are often included in drug product stability studies, they are not generally included in a stability model. As specified by ICH Q1E,[5] each storage condition (i.e., long-term, intermediate, accelerated) is evaluated separately. An exception to this is with analysis of accelerated stability studies, as described elsewhere in this text. Inclusion of storage condition variables as predictors in the stability model can be useful in judging the risk of temperature or humidity excursions, which can occur during storage of finished drug products in warehouses or in a patient's environment. Such evaluations will not be discussed in this chapter.

23.5.2 A Statistical Model for Instability

The design and analysis of a stability study requires the specification of a kinetic, predictive model for the instability of each key measure. A model should include mechanistic, experimental, and statistical aspects. That is, the model must take into account the physical or chemical mechanisms that result in changes in level over time. It must account for the fixed effects of variables whose levels are systematically varied as part of the stability study. Further, it must account for the statistical variation introduced by random variables whose levels are not specifically controlled, but vary in the study.

An understanding of the physico-chemical mechanisms of instability of a drug product is an essential component of drug product lifecycle support. Knowing these mechanisms allows a developer to anticipate flaws, design an appropriate formulation and packaging system, and to troubleshoot and support the product throughout its lifecycle. The reader is directed to discussions elsewhere[15] for a discussion of kinetic mechanisms.

As indicated in ICH Q1A,[1] a linearizing transformation or use of an appropriate nonlinear model for the effect of storage time should be considered if the stability profile cannot be represented by a straight line. A thorough discussion of the important topic of physico-chemical mechanisms is beyond the scope of this chapter. The chosen model for the effect of storage time should be scientifically and statistically justified.

Note to reader: The discussion thus far has deliberately been kept at a level accessible to most non-statisticians, but beyond this point good familiarity with complex statistical methods is assumed. The advice of a professional statistician is strongly recommended before using any of the methods described below.

When the key measure changes only a small proportion (say less than 15%) of its initial or potential level over its shelf life, a zero-order kinetic (straight line) model is often found sufficient to describe the relationship between level and storage time. Thus a stability model often takes the form:

$$\mathbf{y} = \mathbf{X}\beta + \mathbf{Z}\gamma + \varepsilon \qquad (23.1)$$

TABLE 23.2 Temperature and humidity control of stability studies

Label Storage	Long-term condition	Intermediate condition	Accelerated condition
Controlled room temperature	25°C ± 2°C/ 60% ± 5% RH	30°C ± 2°C/ 65% ± 5% RH	40°C ± 2°C/ 75% ± 5% RH
Refrigerated	5°C ± 3°C		25°C ± 2°C/ 60% ± 5% RH
Frozen	−15°C ± 5°C		5°C ± 3°C/ Ambient RH
Minimum time period covered by data at submission	12 months	6 months	6 months

where:

y is a column vector of test results

β is a vector of fixed model parameters whose estimate is **b**

γ is a vector of random model parameters whose estimate is **g**. It is typical to assume a multivariate normal distribution for γ

ε is a vector of identically distributed and independent normal deviations with mean zero and true variance σ^2.

We take **X:Z** to be the design matrix for the stability study. **X** will contain a column of 1s for the intercept, a column of month values for storage interval (i.e., the actual storage times, not the planned storage times), and columns of indicators for categorical fixed variables such as packaging or dosage strength. **Z** would contain column(s) of indicators for the levels of random variables, such as batch. If batch is treated as a fixed variable, whose levels are specified in **X**, and there are no other random variables, then the **Z**γ term is omitted.

23.6 LONG-TERM STABILITY STUDY DESIGN

23.6.1 Full and Reduced Designs

When a stability study includes all combinations of dosage strength, packaging, and storage times, the stability design is referred to as a "full-factorial" (or sometimes as just a "full" or "complete") design. Conducting a full design on a new drug product with multiple strengths and packages can be prohibitively expensive, and may stress a company's analytical resources beyond their limits. From a statistical point of view, when the number of study variables is large, a complete factorial may be unnecessary as long as certain assumptions can be made about the stability effects of the variables.

ICH Q1D[4] describes situations in which a "reduced" design can be applied without further justification, and some situations in which further justification will need to be provided. If a design deviates markedly from the principles of ICH Q1D,[4] the protocol must be approved by the FDA or other appropriate regulatory authority, prior to the initiation of stability studies. Some additional clarification is provided in the literature.[16] In a reduced design, only a specific fraction of the possible combinations of dosage strength, packaging, and storage times are actually tested. ICH Q1D[4] refers to two general approaches to reduced designs: bracketing, and matrixing.

23.6.2 Bracketing

In a bracketing approach, the sponsor relies on theory or past experience to identify a small number of variable combinations (say of strength, and packaging) that can be assumed to give "worst case" stability. Often these combinations will be extremes (e.g., of active content, head space, moisture vapor transmission rate), and the sponsor is willing to estimate the product shelf life from a study of these "worst cases" alone. Bracketing assumes that the untested variable combinations will have equal or superior stability, and therefore need not be tested at all. Bracketing requires a thorough understanding of the mechanism(s) of instability from theory or from studies on earlier development or clinical batches. Because bracketing makes strong assumptions about the underlying mechanism of instability, it is not applicable when dosage form formulations or package characteristics differ markedly. In a "pure" bracketing design, the chosen combinations are tested at all time points. Often those combinations not intended to be tested as part of the bracketing design are not even placed on stability.

Bracketing may be applied with no further justification across strength when different strengths have identical or closely related formulations (e.g., capsules of different strength made with different plug sizes from the same powder blend or tablets of different strengths made by compressing varying amounts of the same granulation, formulations that differ only in minor excipients). Further justification should be considered when amounts of drug substance and excipients change in a formulation. When different excipients are used among strengths, generally bracketing is not applied.

Bracketing may be applied with no further justification across packages using the same container closure system, where either container size or fill varies while the other remains constant. Further justification should be considered when the closure systems vary for the same container. Justification could include a discussion of relative permeation rates of the bracketed container closure system.

23.6.3 Matrixing

In a matrixing approach, the sponsor takes advantage of traditional principles of experimental design[17] to reduce study size, without sacrificing statistical power, model structure or parameter estimatability. Matrixing depends on choosing a balanced subset of the full factorial set of combinations that supports a predictive model, including all main effects and critical interactions. Often, all combinations (even those not intended to be tested in the matrix design) are placed on stability in the event there is a need to revert to full testing.

Matrixing with respect to strength may be applied across strengths without further justification when the strength formulations are identical or closely related. Additional justification should be considered when different strengths differ in the drug substance content, excipients change or different excipients are used. Matrixing across batches can be applied when batches are made using the same process and equipment or batches of drug substance. Matrixing across package size and fill is permitted when all packages use the same container closure system. Further justification should be provided when packages use different container closure systems, different contact material, different suppliers or different orientations. Justification should be based on supportive data (e.g., moisture vapor transmission rates or light protection for different containers).

Matrix designs can be complete (all combination of factors are tested) or incomplete (some combinations are not tested at all). In a complex design, combinations of strength and container size are tested, and individual batch of product is not tested in all strength and container size combinations. If design is broken during the course of the study, testing should revert back to full testing through the proposed retest period or shelf life. Where testing exhibits moderate variability and moderately good stability, a matrix should be statistically justified.

Matrixing is not without risks. Highly fractional designs, involving factors other than time, generally have less precision in shelf life estimation, and may yield shorter shelf life than a full design. With large variability and poor product stability, a matrix should not be applied. Techniques are discussed below for comparing and assessing the statistical power of stability designs.

23.6.4 Stability Design Generation

Before a reduced design is considered, assumptions should be assessed and justified. Then, as a starting point, either the design including all possible combinations or an appropriately bracketed subset is taken as the full design. Then reduced designs are obtained by matrixing the full design. The reduced designs may be compared with respect to the following criteria:

1. Probability of justifying the desired shelf life as a function of study duration.

2. Power to detect effects of experimental variables on stability. Any reduced design should retain the ability to adequately detect differences in stability.
3. "Balance" (i.e., each combination of factor levels is tested to the same extent) to assure orthogonality of model parameter estimates.
4. Total number of tests required (or total study cost).
5. Ergonomic spread of testing throughout the study, to optimize analytical resources.

ICH Q1D[4] mandates full testing of all studied factor combinations at the beginning and end of the study, as well as at the time of submission. It also recommends at least three time points for each studied factor combination to be available at the time of submission (nominally at 12 months storage). ICH Q1D[4] provides examples of study designs. These are not the only designs to be considered, but they illustrate many of the principles of balance, as well as the practical constraints. These are discussed below.

Matrixing on Time Points Only

A key principal of fractional factorial design is to maximize testing of extremes of continuous variables. In the case of storage time, this means full testing is required at initial, study completion, and submission (typically 12 months). Thus, reduced testing for a 36-month study can only be considered at five time points: 3, 6, 9, 18, and 24 months. Consider a study with six combinations: two strengths with three batches per strength. Assume a one-third reduction in testing is desired. Which 20 of the $5 \times 6 = 30$ test points should be tested? The principle of balance requires that:

1. each of the 2 strengths be tested 10 times ($2 \times 10 = 20$);
2. each of the 3 batches be tested Z times ($Z \times 3 = 20$);
3. each of the 5 time points be tested 4 times ($5 \times 4 = 20$);
4. each of the 6 strength $\times$ batch combinations be tested Y times ($Y \times 6 = 20$);
5. each of the 10 strength $\times$ time combinations be tested twice ($2 \times 10 = 20$);
6. each of the 15 batch $\times$ time combinations be tested W times ($W \times 15 = 20$).

Note that W, Y, and Z cannot be whole numbers, however, unless the number of tests is evenly divisible by 2 (strength), 3 (batch), and 5 (time) some loss of balance is inevitable. In this case the lowest number of tests that allows balance is $2 \times 3 \times 5 = 30$, which does not allow for any testing reduction at all. Similarly, if a half reduction in testing was desired, which 15 of the

TABLE 23.3   Illustration of use of indicator variable summation to find a matrix design on time points for a product with two strengths

Strength	Batch	S + B + T			
		3 months (T = 0)	6 months (T = 1)	9 months (T = 2)	18 months (T = 3)
Low (S = 0)	1 (B = 0)	0	1	2	3
	2 (B = 1)	1	2	3	4
	3 (B = 2)	2	3	4	5
High (S = 1)	1 (B = 0)	1	2	3	4
	2 (B = 1)	2	3	4	5
	3 (B = 2)	3	4	5	6

TABLE 23.4   Example of a balanced one-half reduction matrix design on time points for a product with two strengths

Strength	Batch	S + B + T mod 2			
		3 months (T = 0)	6 months (T = 1)	9 months (T = 2)	18 months (T = 3)
Low (S = 0)	1 (B = 0)	0	1	0	1
	2 (B = 1)	1	0	1	0
	3 (B = 2)	0	1	0	1
High (S = 1)	1 (B = 0)	1	0	1	0
	2 (B = 1)	0	1	0	1
	3 (B = 2)	1	0	1	0

0 = test, 1 = do not test

30 test points should be tested? Balance would require that the number 15 is evenly divisible by 2 (strength), 3 (batch), and 5 (time). Since 15 is not evenly divisible by 2, full balance is not possible in this case either. In the ICH Q1D[4] examples, the compromise made is to allow more testing on some batch, strength × batch, and batch × time combinations than others. However, the continuous time variable is robust to loss of balance, because of the assumption of a linear change over time. Thus, the inevitable non-orthogonality in the Q1D[4] design examples is probably negligible.

An example illustrating complete and partial balance is as follows. Assume the sponsor desired an analysis at 24 months (perhaps to justify shelf life extension). Then full testing would be required at 24 months, and matrixing would be on the four time points 3, 6, 9, and 18 months only. Thus, the full design would require (2 strengths) × (3 batches) × (4 times) = 24 tests. Since 12 is divisible by 2, 3, and 4, a completely balanced half reduction is possible. A one-third reduction would require 18 tests, however 18 is only evenly divisible by 2 and 3, not by 4. Therefore, only a partially balanced design is possible if a one-third reduction is desired. To identify which of the 12

or 18 tests to include, the mode arithmetic method of Nordbrock[18] can be used. The following steps illustrate this approach.

1. Assign a code of S = 0 or 1 for each strength.
2. Assign a code of B = 0, 1 or 2 for each of the 3 batches within each strength.
3. Assign a code of T = 0, 1, 2 or 3 for the time points 3, 6, 9 or 18 months respectively.
4. For each of the 24 possible strength × batch × time combinations:
   (a) for a half-fold reduction, test only combinations where S + B + T mode 2 = 0.
   (b) for a one-quarter reduction, test only combinations where S + B + T mode 3 = 0 or 1.

Tables 23.3–23.5 show the testing schedule at these time points for these two cases.

In particular, the half or one-third fractions selected in Tables 23.3 or 23.4 are, of course, only one of two or three possible fractions respectively. For instance, one could have decided to test S + B + T mode 2 = 1 in Table 23.3 or S + B + T mode 3 = 0 or 2 in Table 23.4 instead. The sum S + B + T can be generalized

TABLE 23.5 Example of a partially balanced one-third reduction matrix design on time points for a product with two strengths

Strength	Batch	S + B + T mod 3			
		3 months (T = 0)	6 months (T = 1)	9 months (T = 2)	18 months (T = 3)
Low (S = 0)	1 (B = 0)	0	1	2	0
	2 (B = 1)	1	2	0	1
	3 (B = 2)	2	0	1	2
High (S = 1)	1 (B = 0)	1	2	0	1
	2 (B = 1)	2	0	1	2
	3 (B = 2)	0	1	2	0

0 or 1 = test, 2 = do not test

TABLE 23.6 Using mode arithmetic to matrix on time points only for the example of Table 3a of ICH Q1D

Strength	B + S + P mod 3								
	Low (S = 0)			Medium (S = 1)			High (S = 2)		
Package:	A (P = 0)	B (P = 1)	C (P = 2)	A (P = 0)	B (P = 1)	C (P = 2)	A (P = 0)	B (P = 1)	C (P = 2)
Batch 1 (B = 0)	0	1	2	1	2	0	2	0	1
Batch 2 (B = 1)	1	2	0	2	0	1	0	1	2
Batch 3 (B = 2)	2	0	1	0	1	2	1	2	0

0 = use T1, 1 = use T2, 2 = use T3

to $n \times S + B + m \times T$, where n and m are constants other than 1, in an attempt to find a design that achieves the desired balance. The same principles can be extended to more complex situations. The example in ICH Q1D[4] involves a product with 3 strengths, 3 packages, 3 batches, and 5 time points. It is typical to first identify a set of balanced (or approximately balanced) time vectors. Then the various strength × package × batch combinations are then assigned in a balanced (or approximately balanced) way to each of the vectors. The example in ICH Q1D[4] establishes the following testing vectors:

T1: {0, 6,9,12,18,24,36}
T2: {0,3, 9,12,   24,36}
T3: {0,3,6, 12,18,   36}

T1 calls for testing at 7 total time points, but T2 and T3 only 6. However, balance is achieved across the time points 3, 6, and 9. Because of the assumption of linear trend across time, lack of balance does not lead to serious degradation of estimation efficiency. A desirable feature of T1, T2 and T3 above is that each of the time points 3, 6, 9, 18, and 24 is represented twice. Thus if the vectors are evenly spread across the combinations, a one-third reduction of testing at these

time points would be realized. The assignments of the vectors to each of the $3 \times 3 \times 3 = 27$ combinations is illustrated in Table 23.6.

Matrixing on Both Time Points and Other Variables

Continuing the ICH Q1D matrix example, one can further matrix against batch, strength, and package by omitting the testing based on the value of B + S + P mode 3. In the ICH Q1D Table 24.3b example, the criterion for elimination depends on batch as described in Table 23.7.

The resulting approximately balanced matrix provides about a five-ninths reduction in the amount of testing at the 3, 6, 9, 12, 18, and 24 month time points. These examples are provided merely for illustration. Other matrixing designs are possible, and some may well be superior to those illustrated. Once candidate designs are generated by the methods above—or by other standard experimental design techniques—it is best to perform an assessment of their balance and operational feasibility. Those which pass these assessments may be examined further by the statistical methods described in the next section.

TABLE 23.7 Using mode arithmetic to include matrixing against design variables in the example of Table 3b of ICH Q1D

Batch	Do not test if B + S + P mode 3 =
1	2
2	1
3	0

The level of reduction that would be acceptable to a regulatory agency such as the FDA can be addressed by examining the power of the design to detect differences in stability among the different batches, strengths or packages, and/or the precision with which shelf life can be estimated. These characteristics are compared between the candidate matrix design and the full design. If a candidate matrix design sacrifices little relative to the full design, then it should be acceptable from a regulatory point of view.

23.6.5 Comparing Stability Designs

Nordbrock[19] provided a framework for comparing stability designs with respect to their power to detect slope (stability) differences. This same framework can be applied to a comparison of the probability (power) of meeting a desired shelf life claim among competing stability designs.

Review of Preliminary Statistical Concepts

Let R and H be mutually independent random variables with distributions $R \sim N(\delta,1)$ and $H \sim \chi^2(dfe)$. Then, by definition:

$$\frac{R}{\sqrt{H/dfe}} = W \sim \text{nct}(dfe, \delta) \qquad (23.2)$$

where $\text{nct}(dfe,\delta)$ represents a random variable distributed as non-central t with degrees of freedom dfe and non-centrality parameter δ. Further, let $\text{pnct}(Q \mid dfe,\delta)$ be the cumulative distribution of the non-central t random variable W relative to fixed Q, such that:

$$\begin{aligned} \text{Prob}\{W \leq Q\} &= \text{pnct}(Q \mid dfe, \delta) \quad \text{and} \\ \text{Prob}\{W > Q\} &= 1 - \text{pnct}(Q \mid dfe, \delta) \end{aligned} \qquad (23.3)$$

Non-central t distribution functions are present in software packages such as SAS or R. The following approximations may be useful in implementing these

calculations in packages which have a cumulative non-central F (pf()), but not a non-central t:

$$\begin{aligned} \text{pt}(t, dfe, \delta) &= \text{pf}(t^2, 1, dfe, \delta^2) + \text{pt}(-t, dfe, \delta) \sim \\ &= \text{pf}(t^2, 1, dfe, \delta^2) \quad \text{for } \delta \gg 0 \end{aligned}$$

In some software packages, algorithms for non-central t do not converge when δ and/or dfe are large. In those cases, the following approximation may be used:

$$\text{pnorm}(t - \delta) \cong \text{pt}(t, dfe, \delta)$$

with pnorm(z) the standard normal distribution function.

Now consider a linear regression to the fixed model:

$$\mathbf{y} = \mathbf{X}\beta + \varepsilon \qquad (23.4)$$

with fixed model parameters β and $\varepsilon \sim N(0,\sigma^2)$. In applying the concepts below, it is critical to understand the structure of β and $\mathbf{X}$. As an example, consider a stability design that includes measurements (y vector) at a series of time (T) points on 3 batches (B), each of 3 strengths (S), with 3 possible package (P) options. Assume the design will support estimation of all main effects and certain interactions (i.e., others known to be unimportant). In a high level program like SAS, the model might be expressed as:

$$Y = \text{intercept T B S P T*B T*S T*B*S}$$

The column vector β will be composed of one sub-vector for each model term. The length of each sub-vector is 1 for the continuous variables intercept and T. For categorical main effects B, S, and P, the sub-vector length will be number of categorical levels for that variable minus 1; therefore the length will be 2 for each main effect. For interactions, the vector length will be the product of the vector lengths of each of the component main effects in the interaction. Working across in the above model order we see the length of β will be $1 + (1 + 2 + 2 + 2) + (2 + 2) + (4) = 16$. Thus:

$$\begin{aligned} \beta' = (&\beta_{\text{int}}, \beta_T, \beta_{B1}, \beta_{B2}, \beta_{S1}, \beta_{S2}, \beta_{P1}, \beta_{P2}, \beta_{TB1}, \\ &\beta_{TB2}, \beta_{TS1}, \beta_{TS2}, \beta_{TB1S1}, \beta_{TB1S2}, \beta_{TB2S1}, \beta_{TB2S2}) \end{aligned}$$

Each element of β is an effect, attributable to the presence of certain levels or combinations of levels of the variables T, B, S, and P.

The $\mathbf{X}$ matrix in this example will have 16 columns corresponding to each of the coefficients in β, and one row for each result in y. The intercept column in $\mathbf{X}$ will have a "1" in each row, and the T column in $\mathbf{X}$ will have the numerical storage time t at which the corresponding test result in y was obtained. For categorical main effects, the **X** columns corresponding to B, S, and P will contain codes that specify the level of each, corresponding to the respective y test result. A convenient 0/1 coding is shown in Table 23.8, in which the presence of a 0 in the first or second element indicates that the corresponding factor level is not acting to produce the corresponding result. If both the first and second elements are 0, then the third level must be active.

Sub-vector codes for interactions consist of the Kronecker product of the sub-vectors of the component main effects. Thus the 2 T*B columns in **X** corresponding to a y result obtained at 3 months on Batch 2 would be encoded as $3 \otimes (0\ 1) = (0\ 3)$. The four T*B*S columns in **X** corresponding to a y result at 6 months on Batch 1, middle strength would be $6 \otimes (1\ 0) \otimes (0\ 1) = (0\ 6\ 0\ 0)$. In this way, the entire **X** matrix is constructed. Consider the y result corresponding to the 9–month test on Batch 2 of low strength packaged in container type B. The corresponding row of the **X** matrix is then:

$$\mathbf{X} = \left(\begin{array}{c} \cdots \\ 1, 9, 0, 1, 1, 0, 0, 1, 0, 9, 9, 0, 0, 0, 9, 0 \\ \cdots \end{array} \right).$$

The estimates of interest in a stability analysis generally consist of linear functions of the elements of β. Functions of interest might be slopes or differences between slopes for specific combinations of design variables or averages across certain design variables. A linear function of β, say $S = \mathbf{c}'\beta$, will have an estimate $\hat{S} \sim N(S, \sigma_S^2)$ with sampling variance:

$$\sigma_S^2 = \mathbf{c}'(\mathbf{X}'\mathbf{X})^{-1}\mathbf{c}\sigma^2 \qquad (23.5)$$

based on degrees of freedom dfe where:

$$\begin{aligned} dfe = \ & \text{number of rows in } \mathbf{X} \\ & - \text{number of columns in } \mathbf{X} \end{aligned} \qquad (23.6)$$

The dimensions of the contrast column vector **c** will be identical to that of β. The elements of **c** will depend on which of the corresponding elements of β are active in defining a specific linear function of interest.

Finally, note that if $\hat{\sigma}_S^2$ is a sample estimate of σ_S^2 based on dfe degrees of freedom, then its sampling distribution is given by:

$$\frac{\hat{\sigma}_S^2}{\sigma_S^2} \cdot dfe \sim \chi^2(dfe) \qquad (23.7)$$

Power to Detect Slope Differences

Let S represent some slope difference that is of interest, and consider a statistical test of H0: $S = 0$

TABLE 23.8 Coding of design variable levels in the construction of the X matrix

Sub-vector code	B interpretation	S interpretation	P interpretation
(1 0)	Batch 1	Low strength	package A
(0 1)	Batch 2	Middle strength	package B
(0 0)	Batch 3	High strength	package C

against alternative Ha: $S > 0$. H0 will be rejected at the 0.05 level of significance if:

$$\frac{\hat{S}}{\hat{\sigma}_S^2} = \frac{\hat{S}/\sigma_S^2}{\hat{\sigma}_S^2/\sigma_S^2} > qt(0.95, dfe) \qquad (23.8)$$

Now under the assumption that $S = \Delta$:

$$\frac{\hat{S}}{\sigma_S^2} \sim N\left(\frac{\Delta}{\sigma_S^2}, 1\right) \qquad (23.9)$$

Combining Equations 23.2, 23.3, 23.6, 23.7, and 23.8 we may state that:

$$\begin{aligned} \Pr\{\text{H0 rejected} \mid \Delta\} &= \Pr\left\{ \frac{\hat{S}}{\hat{\sigma}_S^2} > qt(0.95, dfe) \mid \Delta \right\} \\ &= 1 - pnct\left(qt(0.95, dfe), dfe, \frac{\Delta}{\sigma_s} \right) \end{aligned} \qquad (23.10)$$

Equation 23.10 may be evaluated as a function of Δ to provide the operating characteristics of the statistical test. Since dfe and σ_S^2 depend, by Equations 23.5 and 23.6, only on **X**, which in turn is determined by the stability design, the operating characteristics can be compared for various designs and storage times as an aid in study planning.

As an example, consider three matrix designs presented in ICH Q1D[4] and the model as described above. Let S be a slope difference between medium and low (medium minus low) strength averaged across all lots. Then the corresponding contrast vector is:

$$\mathbf{c}' = \left(0, 0, 0, 0, 0, 0, 0, 0, 0, 0, -1, +1, -\frac{1}{3}, +\frac{1}{3}, -\frac{1}{3}, +\frac{1}{3} \right)$$

so that:

$$\mathbf{c}'\beta = \beta_{TS2} - \beta_{TS1} + \frac{\beta_{TB1S2} - \beta_{TB1S1} + \beta_{TB2S2} - \beta_{TB2S1}}{3}$$

Assume the stability potency analysis for submission will occur at the 12-month time point. Let $\sigma = 1\%LC$, and let the true slope difference, Δ, vary between 0 and $0.25\%LC/\text{month}$. Figure 23.1 shows the power

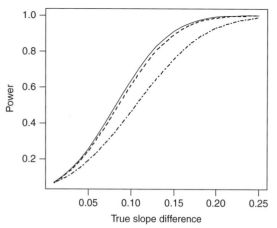

FIGURE 23.1 Comparison of power to detect slope differences at the 12 month time point for three stability designs in ICH Q1D. (Solid line = full design, dashed line = matrix on time points only, dot-dashed line = matrix on both time points and design variables)

as given by Equation 23.10 for various true slope differences. Note that very little power is lost in going from the full design (135 tests required) to the matrix design on time only (ICH Q1D[4] Table 23.3a, 108 tests required). However, considerable power is lost when matrixing includes both time, strength, batch, and packaging (ICH Q1D[4] table 23.3b, 72 tests required).

Probability of Achieving a Shelf Life Claim

Consider a stability-determining test, such as potency, with a lower acceptance limit, L. Let D be the desired shelf life for the product. Further assume that the product will have a true release potency (intercept) of I, a true slope of S and a true analytical standard deviation of σ_S. The regression slope estimate of S, i.e., $\hat{S}$, will have a sampling distribution that can be defined by:

$$\frac{\hat{S} - S}{\sigma_S} + \delta \sim N(\delta, 1) \tag{23.11}$$

Combining Equation 23.11 with Equation 23.7, and comparing with Equations 23.2 and 23.3, we see that:

$$\Pr\left\{ \frac{\dfrac{\hat{S} - S}{\sigma_S} + \delta}{\hat{\sigma}_S/\sigma_S} > Q \right\} = 1 - \text{pnct}(Q, dfe, \delta) \tag{23.12}$$

Now, for a test with a lower limit, the desired shelf life claim will be achieved whenever:

$$I + D \cdot (\hat{S} - \hat{\sigma}_S \cdot qt(0.95, dfe)) > L$$
or
$$\frac{\hat{S} + (I - L)/D}{\hat{\sigma}_S} > qt(0.95, dfe)$$
or

$$\frac{\dfrac{\hat{S} - S}{\sigma_S} + \dfrac{((I - L)/D) + S}{\sigma_S}}{\hat{\sigma}_S/\sigma_S} > qt(0.95, dfe)$$

Comparing this with Equation 23.12, we see that:

Pr{Achieving desired shelflife claim}

$$= 1 - \text{pnct}\left(qt(0.95, dfe), dfe, \frac{((I - L)/D) + S}{\sigma_S} \right) \tag{23.13}$$

Note that a similar derivation in the case of an upper acceptance limit would yield:

Pr{Achieving desired shelflife claim}

$$= \text{pnct}\left(qt(0.05, dfe), dfe, \frac{((I - L)/D) + S}{\sigma_S} \right) \tag{23.14}$$

Equation 23.13 or Equation 23.14 may be evaluated as a function of I, S, and σ_S to provide the operating characteristics of the shelf life estimation goal. Hypothetical I, S, and σ_S may be taken from preliminary stability and analytical studies. Since dfe and σ_S^2 depend, by Equations 23.5 and 23.6, only on $\mathbf{X}$, which in turn is determined by the stability design, the operating characteristics can be compared for various designs and storage times as an aid in study planning.

As an example, consider three matrix designs presented in ICH Q1D and the model as described above. Let S be defined as the slope that represents the stability for Batch 2 of the low strength formulation (and any package). The corresponding contrast vector is then:

$$\mathbf{c}' = (0, 1, 0, 0, 0, 0, 0, 0, 0, 1, 1, 0, 0, 0, 1, 0)$$

so that:

$$\mathbf{c}'\boldsymbol{\beta} = \beta_T + \beta_{TB2} + \beta_{TS1} + \beta_{TB2S1}$$

Assume the stability potency analysis for submission will occur at the 12 month time point. Let: $\sigma = 1\%LC$, the lower acceptance limit for potency, L be 90%LC, the true initial potency level, I be 100%LC, and let the true slope, S, for the combination of interest vary between -0.4 and $-0.1\%LC/month$. Figure 23.2 shows the probability of meeting a shelf life claim of $D = 24$ months, as given by Equation 23.13, for various slopes. Note that very little risk is seen in going from the full design (135 tests required) to the matrix design on time only (ICH Q1D Table 24.3a, 108 tests required). However, considerable risk is encountered when matrixing includes both time, strength, batch, and packaging (ICH Q1D Table 23.3b, 72 tests required).

Implementation in R

The R language[20] provides a good matrix computation and graphics platform for making stability

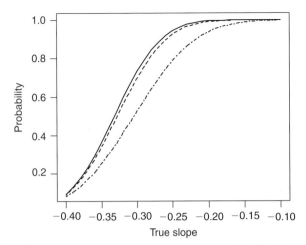

FIGURE 23.2 Comparison of probability of achieving a 24-month shelf life claim at the 12 month time point for three stability designs in ICH Q1D. (Solid line = full design, dashed line = matrix on time points only, dot-dashed line = matrix on both time points and design variables)

design comparisons of power and probability, as described above. The design matrix **X** (up to the time of proposed analysis) may be created manually in an Excel spreadsheet, and imported as a comma separated text file to implement the power and probability calculations illustrated in the following R code.

```
XPXINV<-solve(t(X)%*%X) # information matrix
dfe<-dim(X)[1]-dim(X)[2]
var.e<-1# hypothesized analytical variance
# contrast vector for slope differences
c<-matrix(c(0,0,0,0,0,0,0,0,0,0,-1,1,-0.334,
0.333, -0.334,0.333),ncol=1)
# hypothesized true slope differences
DELTA<-seq(from=0.01,to=0.25, by=0.01)
var.c<-var.e*tI%*%XPXINV%*%c;var.c
# power of detection of a slope difference
power <-1-pt(qt(0.95,dfe),dfe,DELTA/
sqrt(var.c))
# contrast vector for individual combination
slope estimate
a<-matrix(c(0,1,0,0,0,0,0,0,0,1,1,0,0,0,1,0),
ncol=1)
# hypothesized true slopes
S<-seq(from=-0.1, to=-0.4, by=-0.01)
var.a<-var.e*t(a)%*%XPXINV%*%a;var.a
# prob of achieving shelf life goal
I<-100 # Initial potency level
L<-90 # Lower specification for dating
D<-24 # Desired dating (based on 12 month
data)
prob<-1-pt(qt(0.95,dfe),dfe,(S+(I-L)/D)/
sqrt(var.a))
```

23.7 DETERMINATION OF SHELF LIFE

23.7.1 Definition of Shelf Life

A definition of shelf life for a given characteristic that is consistent with ICH Q1E[5] is the longest storage period for which there is at least 95% confidence that the lot mean level of the characteristic remains within its acceptance range. We must translate this definition into a procedure we can apply for estimating the shelf life. The procedure used will depend on the type of data available, and the statistical model employed. When the shelf life is estimated using LR, this definition is consistent with the storage period at which the one-sided upper and/or lower 95% confidence bound for the lot mean level intersects the product acceptance limit.

By this definition, the shelf life is clearly intended to control the mean level of critical characteristics of product lots. Because of analytical variance and content non-uniformity, even when the lot mean level of a characteristic is within a given specification, the measured levels of individual tablets may not be. The occurrence of individual out-of-specification test results in lots tested annual stability monitoring can lead to a costly laboratory investigation. Thus, as part of a shelf life justification, a sponsor may also want to evaluate the probability of individual failures.

Because the above definition of shelf life does not control the spread of individual results, alternative definitions are proposed from time to time, based on prediction or tolerance bounds.[21]

23.7.2 Model Pruning

The first step in shelf life estimation consists of pruning the full model to remove statistically non-significant terms. This process should follow the usual stepwise regression elimination that maintains model hierarchy. Generally, model terms that contain batch variables are eliminated at the $P > 0.25$ significance level, and other terms are eliminated at the more traditional $P > 0.05$ significance level. A good overview of the model building and fitting process is described by Chow and Liu,[22] and by Shao and Chow.[23] The statistical aspects of the analysis for a fixed effects model are discussed by Fairweather,[24] and by Chen and Tsong.[25]

When a mixed effects model is used, the same pruning principles may be employed. Analysis of mixed effects stability models is described by Chen, Hwang, and Tsong,[26] and by Chow and Shao.[27]

A set of SAS macros was made available from the FDA[28] providing analysis of the simple fixed batch case, with no other factors such as strength or packaging. However, this set of macros is not recommended because it is too limited in scope. It is not entirely compatible with the new ICH Q1E[5] guidance, nor with current versions of the SAS package. The MIXED procedure of SAS permits analysis of a mixed model (Equation 23.1), and is an excellent platform for shelf life estimation. Therefore examples of proc MIXED code are provided below.

Simple ANCOVA for the Fixed Batch Case

In the simplest situation, stability data are available for at least three batches of a single strength, stored in a single package type. A good basic reference to ANCOVA is Brownlee.[29] The process begins with preliminary sequential F tests (see Table 23.9) for equality of degradation rates (slopes) and initial values (intercepts) among batches.

Let's call the P-values of the Batch and Month * Batch tests $P(B)$ and $P(M*B)$, respectively. According to ICH Q1E, the final model is selected according to the following rules:

- Select Common Intercept Common Slope (CICS) if $P(B) > 0.25$ and $P(M*B) > 0.25$;
- Select Separate Intercept Common Slope (SICS) if $P(B) < 0.25$ and $P(M*B) > 0.25$;
- Select Separate Intercept Separate Slope (SISS) otherwise.

An aspect of this model selection algorithm that is unique to the ICH Q1E[5] guideline is the use of a critical P value of 0.25 instead of the usual $P = 0.05$. The FDA has indicated that this should be done in order to protect against accidentally obtaining a favorable model (model 1 CICS generally leads to longer product dating) by the statistical accident of getting favorable data, when in fact the real behavior is less favorable.[30] This is still a controversial aspect of the FDA/ICH procedure, but as this has been used for well over 15 years it has become part of industry practice.

The ANCOVA can be implemented simply using the MIXED procedure of SAS, and will be illustrated using the data in Appendix A. Assume the data for batches 4, 5, and 8 are analyzed together (i.e., "pooled" in the drug stability vernacular[31]), and read into a SAS dataset with variables Batch, Month, and Potency. The SAS code below:

```
proc mixed;
class batch;
model Potency = Month Batch
Month*Batch/htype=1;
run;
```

results are shown in the output in Table 23.10.

TABLE 23.9   Simple ANCOVA sequential F tests

Code name for the ANCOVA F-test	What is tested?
Batch	Differences among batch intercepts assuming that batches have a common slope.
Month * Batch	Differences among batch slopes assuming that batches may have different intercepts.

TABLE 23.10   Type 1 tests of fixed effects

Effect	Num DF	Den DF	F Values	Pr > F
Month	1	18	100.99	< 0.0001
Batch	2	18	72.12	< 0.0001
Month * Batch	2	18	1.96	0.1704

The last column gives the $P(B)$ and $P(M*B)$ values on the second and third lines, respectively. Since $P(M*B) < 0.25$, a separate intercept separate slope model is required to estimate the shelf life.

The reader may verify that, for the data in Appendix A, analysis of batches 3, 4, and 5 will lead to the SICS model and analysis of batches 2, 5, and 7 will lead to the CICS model.

Model Pruning for More Complex Studies

Whether a full factorial or a reduced design is used, data should be treated in the same manner as data from a full design study. As an example, if the stability study includes multiple strength and packaging levels, and the design supports estimation of interactions to second order, the following SAS code might be appropriate.

```
Proc mixed;
class batch strength package;
model Potency = Batch Strength Package
Batch*Strength Batch*Package Strength*Package
Month Month*Batch Month*Strength Month*Package
/htype=3;
run;
```

A model pruning procedure similar in spirit to the simple ANCOVA analysis given above should be used (e.g., stepwise regression) to test for statistical significance of model terms containing the various design variables. Model terms are eliminated in a stepwise manner, based on an objective criterion such as their corresponding Type III F test significance. Preliminary statistical tests for terms or interactions involving the batch variable should be conducted at a level of significance for rejection of 0.25. Statistical tests for main effects of matrixed or bracketed variables other than batch should be conducted using the traditional level of significance for rejection of 0.05.

23.7.3 Simple Fixed Batch Case

If the purpose of the stability analysis is to estimate stability parameters or predict performance of only those batches included in the study, the batch variable may be considered a fixed variable. In this case, the $\mathbf{Z}$ matrix in Equation 23.1 is null, and the stability model is the usual fixed linear model:

$$y = \mathbf{X}\beta + \varepsilon \qquad (23.15)$$

where the $\mathbf{X}$ matrix encodes the levels of fixed effects such as batch, strength, packaging, and storage time.

The estimated product shelf life depends on the final stability model. Assuming that model pruning has already been done, $\mathbf{X}$ will include columns only for effects and interactions deemed statistically significant whose estimation can be supported by the data. We consider here the single strength, single package case. Shelf life estimation requires that the upper (or lower) one-sided 95% confidence bound(s) for the mean regression line(s) for each batch be calculated. The SAS MIXED syntax for the SISS model is given below.

```
Proc mixed;
class batch;
model Potency = Month Batch Month*Batch /
Solution alphap=0.1
outpm=outpm;run;
```

In SAS, confidence bounds are easily obtained for time points not studied by including missing values for desired months in the incoming data set. For the other models, the following SAS code should be substituted.

```
SICS: Potency = Month Batch
CICS: Potency = Month
```

The resulting `outpm` SAS data set will contain a listing of the data, as well as the appropriate predicted and confidence bounds for each time point in the incoming data set. Missing values may be included for time points of interest, in order to estimate the shelf life. As an illustration, an analysis of Batches 4, 5, and 8

of the data in Appendix A will provide an "outpm" data set containing the following:

```
batch Month Lower
BATCH4 56 90.8585
BATCH4 57 90.6146
BATCH4 58 90.3708
BATCH4 59 90.1268 ←
BATCH4 60 89.8829
BATCH5 41 90.8015
BATCH5 42 90.5517
BATCH5 43 90.3017
BATCH5 44 90.0518 ←
BATCH5 45 89.8017
BATCH5 46 89.5516
BATCH5 47 89.3014
BATCH5 48 89.0512
BATCH8 25 90.9432
BATCH8 26 90.5079
BATCH8 27 90.0723 ←
BATCH8 28 89.6365
BATCH8 29 89.2004
```

The shelf life for a given batch is the maximum time (rounded to nearest month) during which the upper and lower confidence bounds remain within the acceptance limit. The arrows in the above listing give the maximum month at which the one-sided lower 95% confidence bound for each lot mean remains above an acceptance limit of 90.0%LC.

For the SICS and SISS models, the shelf life must be based on the worst-case batch. ICH Q1E specifies how much extrapolation is allowed. Generally the shelf life is limited to no more than twice the duration of the stability study (assuming that the 95% confidence bound remains within the acceptance specification for this period). In the example above, shelf life is limited to 27 months, based on projections for worst case Batch 8. When limited extrapolation of shelf life is accepted at time of approval, post-approval long-term data must be reported to the FDA to verify the shelf life. Accelerated data are used to justify the temporary excursion of environmental conditions, and support the limited extrapolation of long-term data.

23.7.4 Simple Random Batch Case

If the goal of a stability analysis is to use available stability data to predict stability performance for a future batch of product that (of course) was not studied, then the batch variable should be considered random, and this should be reflected in the stability model and the analysis approach. A prerequisite for such a prediction is the availability of stability data from a reasonably large number of batches (hopefully more than three).

The appropriate predictive model is given by Equation 23.1, where γ is a matrix of batch specific random intercept and slope effect column vectors. The random intercept effect for a given batch may reflect random deviations from a target level of added active ingredient, whereas the random slope effect may reflect random deviations from nominal excipient levels or processing settings.

In this case, Equation 23.1 simplifies to the following form:

$$y_{ij} = a_i + x_{ij}b_i + e_{ij} \tag{23.16}$$

where:

y_{ij} is the observed test result for the ith batch tested at the jth time point

a_i and b_i are the random intercept and slope for the ith batch

x_{ij} is the storage time corresponding to the ith batch tested at the jth time point

$e_{ij} \sim iid\ N(0,\sigma^2)$ reflect measurement variance.

If we assume these batch-specific intercept and slope effects are normally distributed about process mean parameters α and β respectively, and are mutually independent, then we take for the ith batch:

$$\begin{pmatrix} a_i \\ b_i \end{pmatrix} \sim N\left(\begin{pmatrix} \alpha \\ \beta \end{pmatrix}, \begin{pmatrix} \sigma_a^2 & 0 \\ 0 & \sigma_b^2 \end{pmatrix} \right) \tag{23.17}$$

where σ_b^2 and σ_b^2 represent the variances of these random intercept and slope effects among batches. This model may be analyzed using the following SAS MIXED procedure syntax.

```
Proc mixed data=stability;
class Batch;
model Potency = Month /solution
alphap=0.1 outp=outp;
random Intercept Month/ type=vc
subject=Batch;
run;
```

When this code is used to analyze the eight batches of data in Appendix A, the parameter point estimates shown in Table 23.11 are obtained.

TABLE 23.11 Point estimates from Proc MIXED random batch analysis

Parameter	Point estimate
α	101.46
β	−0.2063
σ_b^2	1.4774
σ_b^2	0
σ^2	0.8063

If a "future" lot is included in the incoming data set, whose test results are all missing, then the `outp` data set will contain the estimated one-sided lower 95% confidence bound for potency at the storage times of interest. A partial listing of the `outp` data set is given below.

```
Batch Month Lower
FUTURE 40 90.9427
FUTURE 41 90.7299
FUTURE 42 90.5169
FUTURE 43 90.3038
FUTURE 44 90.0904 ←
FUTURE 45 89.8769
FUTURE 46 89.6632
FUTURE 47 89.4493
FUTURE 48 89.2353
FUTURE 49 89.0210
```

The arrow above indicates that the estimated shelf life for a future lot is 44 months.

23.7.5 Shelf Life Estimation in More Complex Studies

The principles illustrated above also apply when the study includes multiple levels of strength, packaging or other design variables. A good review of model-building aspects in complex cases is provided by Millikin and Johnson.[32]

23.8 RELEASE LIMIT ESTIMATION

The shelf life estimation discussed above depends on the true level at release (i.e., the intercept) being in control. Thus, the true release levels of batches used for shelf life determination are assumed to be representative of those of future lots. Often a process control limit is established to assure good control of the release level. If the measured release level exceeds the limit, the product is not released for sale.

In keeping with the definition of shelf life, a one-sided release limit should ensure with at least 95% confidence that the mean level of a released lot will remain above (or below) a given lower (or upper) stability specification at the end of shelf life. Generally, stability data are available and the objective is to calculate a release limit (RL) from the estimated slope, its standard error of estimate ($\hat{\sigma}_{slope}$), along with established shelf life acceptance limit (SL), the desired shelf life (D), the estimated total analytical standard deviation ($\hat{\sigma}$), and the number of replicates averaged to obtain the reportable release test result (n), then the release limit estimate is given by:[33]

$$RL = SL - \delta \cdot D + t_{p,df} \sqrt{\sigma^2/n + D^2 \cdot \sigma_{slope}^2} \qquad (23.18)$$

where:

δ = min[slope,0] or max[slope,0] for lower or upper RL respectively

$t_{p,df}$ = pth quantile of the t-distribution with df degrees of freedom.

Df = Satterthwaite degrees of freedom determined as described in (3, page 1211)

p = 0.95 or 0.05 for lower or upper RL respectively.

To illustrate application of Equation 23.18, the data from Appendix A will be used. A fixed batch analysis of batches 3, 4, and 5 yields a separate intercept, common slope model. The multiple regression output from a SAS analysis is shown in Table 23.12.

With a stability lower acceptance limit of SL = 90.0%LC, and using the methods shown above, shelf lives of 48, 57, and 43 months are obtained for batches 3, 4, and 5 respectively. As a result, a shelf life of 43 months could be justified for this product. Thus, the development team feels justified in recommending a shelf life for this product of D = 36 months, however, they also decide to establish a lower release limit on the mean of n = 2 replicate tests to assure that no future batch mean will be below 90%LC through 36 months with 95% confidence. From the above SAS output, the following inputs to Equation 23.18 are obtained.

$Slope$ = −0.2131%LC/month
δ = min[slope,0] = −0.2131 (for lower release limit)
$\hat{\sigma}$ = 1.1568 (residual error)
$\hat{\sigma}_{slope}$ = 0.02433

df = 24
p = 0.95 (for lower release limit).

TABLE 23.12 Output from SAS fixed batch analysis

```
Covariance Parameter
Estimates
Cov Parm Estimate
Residual 1.1568


Solution for Fixed Effects
Standard
Effect batch Estimate Error DF t Value Pr > |t|
Intercept 100.82 0.3840 24 262.52 <.0001
Month -0.2131 0.02433 24 -8.76 <.0001
batch BATCH3 1.3556 0.4849 24 2.80 0.0100
batch BATCH4 3.4352 0.5032 24 6.83 <.0001
batch BATCH5 0 . . . . .
```

Application of Equation 23.18 yields a release limit of RL = 99.7%LC for this product.

For a separate intercept, separate slope model, a conservative approach is to take the *slope* estimate from the worst-case batch. In cases where the estimated slope implies a (favorable) divergence over time from the limit of interest, (e.g., negative slope used to estimate an upper RL), the slope should be set to zero, as implied by the δ function above. This provides a worst-case, conservative estimate for the release limit, and ensures that lot mean levels will remain in conformance throughout the storage period, with at least 95% confidence.

When estimates of ($\hat{\sigma}$) and ($\hat{\sigma}_{slope}$) are not obtained from the same regression, then the evaluation of df can be problematic. However, the Satterthwaite[34] approximation may be applied in this case. In principle, a similar approach could be used in the random batch case.

23.9 PROBABILITY OF FUTURE OUT-OF-SPECIFICATION STABILITY TEST RESULTS

The above approaches for estimating product shelf life are meant to control batch mean levels, but give no assurance that individual test results, for lots placed on annual stability, will remain within the stability acceptance limit. Stability failures can result in costly investigations or, in the worst cases, product recall or withdrawal. Thus, after assuring that all regulatory guidance has been followed, it is in a sponsor's interest to predict the probability of out-of-specification stability test results for future batches.

The problem of prediction is fundamentally different than that of hypothesis testing and estimation, and requires a full probability model of the process being simulated. Traditional data analysis methods have yielded ingenious analytical tools, such as tolerance and prediction interval estimates, as aids to risk assessment. However, except in the simplest scenarios, the prediction problem is too difficult to be solved analytically; modern computer simulation approaches are required. Methods such as mixed model regression rely on approximations that may not hold in small samples. Traditional tolerance and prediction intervals do not adequately address estimation uncertainty, and rely on the non-intuitive paradigm of repeated sampling.

The prediction problem can be tackled in a very direct, rigorous, and informative way by taking a Bayesian perspective. Bayesian estimates are directly interpretable as probabilities. Modern tools for implementing the Bayesian approach, such as WinBUGS or the SAS MIXED procedure, are now readily available, and can be used effectively to enhance decision making in the stability arena. Thus, this chapter would not be complete without an illustration of the power of these important methods, by analyzing the data from all eight batches in Appendix A using Gibbs' sampling in WinBUGS.

The central objective of a Bayesian analysis is to estimate $p(\theta | Y)$, the joint posterior distribution of unknown model parameters given the data. From the joint posterior, the distribution of any function of θ or of any quantity that may be predicted from the model can be obtained through Markov Chain Monte Carlo techniques. By sampling iteratively from the posterior distribution, WinBUGS produces a posterior sample of the model parameters, θ from $p(\theta | Y)$.

A sample from the distribution of any predicted quantity (say Zpred) can be obtained by integrating the relevant component distributions in the data model over the posterior as follows:

$$p(Zpred \mid \mathbf{Y}) = \int_{\theta} f(Zpred \mid \theta) \cdot p(\theta \mid \mathbf{Y}) d\theta$$

As with the posterior distribution, the distributions for predicted quantities are obtained within the process of Monte Carlo iterative sampling, and no analytical integration is needed. The example below is practical in nature, and assumes only general familiarity with the Bayesian paradigm. For more depth and discussion of important topics, such as convergence verification, readers are referred to a general text on Bayesian data analysis.[35] For details of WinBUGS operation and syntax the reader is referred to the WinBUGS operator's manual.[36]

23.9.1 Random Batch Model for Prediction

Prediction involving future batches requires a random batch assumption, so the model of Section 23.6.4 will be used with minor modification of symbols and structure. In place of Equation 23.16, we define the true potency, μ_{bi}, for a given lot, b, tested at the ith time, X_i, as:

$$\mu_{bi} = \alpha_b + \beta_b \cdot (X_i - Xbar)$$

where Xbar is the average of the storage period for all non-missing individual measurements in the data set. For the eight batches in Appendix A, Xbar = 9.25 months. This "centering" is used in the model to improve the rate of convergence of the Gibbs' sampler.

Each of the $b = 1, 2 \dots 8$ batches is assumed to have a unique true intercept, α_b, and true slope, β_b. The true slope and intercept for batches are assumed to be independent, and to follow a normal distribution among lots, with the 8 batches on hand representing a random sample from the population of all possible batches. Thus as with Equation 23.17, we have:

$$\begin{pmatrix} \alpha_b \\ \beta_b \end{pmatrix} \sim N\left(\begin{pmatrix} \alpha_c \\ \beta_c \end{pmatrix}, \begin{pmatrix} \sigma_\alpha^2 & 0 \\ 0 & \sigma_\beta^2 \end{pmatrix} \right)$$

The observed potency result, Y_{bi}, for lot b at time point i, will vary about the true value due to analytical variance, and is assumed to follow a normal distribution as follows:

$$Y_{bi} \sim N(\mu_{bi}, \sigma^2)$$

23.9.2 Prior Distributions for Model Parameters

The probability model described above depends on a vector of five model parameters.

$$\boldsymbol{\theta} = \left| \alpha_c, \beta_c, \sigma_\alpha, \sigma_\beta, \sigma \right|$$

A Bayesian perspective considers these parameters to be random quantities, and thus to have a probability distribution. Prior to data collection, the distributions of these parameters are a quantitative expression of the subjective uncertainty about their value. When prior uncertainty is great, it is appropriate to assume prior distributions that are independent, and very broad or non-informative. This was the approach taken here. The following non-informative distributions were used:

$$\begin{aligned} \alpha_c &\sim N(100, 10^{-6}) \\ \beta_c &\sim N(0, 10^{-6}) \\ \sigma_\alpha &= 1/\sqrt{\tau_\alpha} \sim U(0, 100) \\ \sigma_\beta &= 1/\sqrt{\tau_\beta} \sim U(0, 100) \\ \tau_c &= 1/\sigma^2 \sim G(10^{-3}, 10^{-3}) \end{aligned}$$

$U(A,B)$ represents a "flat" uniform distribution with minimum and maximum values A and B respectively. $G(C,D)$ represents a gamma distribution with shape and rate parameters C and D respectively. The parameters for all these distributions are chosen so that the probability density is essentially constant over the likely range of the true parameter values, thus the choice of prior has essentially little or no impact on the final estimation. In cases where substantial prior knowledge and theory on a product or like products are available, it may be appropriate use a more informative prior, but that will not be discussed here.

23.9.3 Predicted Quantities of Interest

The objective of the present analysis is to simulate probability distributions of various predicted quantities that are functions of the original parameters. These consist of posterior or posterior predictive distributions that summarize available knowledge about each predicted quantity.

One quantity of interest is the initial mean potency for the overall manufacturing process, Y_0, where:

$$Y_0 = \alpha_c - \beta_c \cdot Xbar$$

Ideally, Y_0, should be close to 100%LC. If this value is significantly below 100%LC, it may mean that the active ingredient is being lost in the manufacturing process, and an increase in overage is needed to correct this situation.

Certainly it would also be of interest to estimate the distributions for a future batch slope, β_{pred}, and initial potency level, $Init_{pred}$, which can be obtained from the model parameters as follows:

$$\beta_{pred} \sim N(\beta_c, \sigma_\beta^2)$$
$$Init_{pred} = \alpha_{pred} - \beta_{pred} \cdot Xbar,$$
$$\text{where} \quad \alpha_{pred} \sim N(\alpha_c, \sigma_\alpha^2)$$

From these distributions, one can also predict the true mean level, μ_{pred}, and individual potency test result, Y_{pred}, of some future lot after X_{pred} months of storage (for this example we take $X_{pred} = 36$ months). This can be obtained as illustrated in the following sections.

Also of particular interest would be the posterior probability distribution of analytical error, σ, and the predictive posterior distribution of the product shelf life. The shelf life for a given batch will be the storage period during which the true level remains above the stability acceptance limit SL.

$$Shelf.Life = \frac{SL - Init_{pred}}{\beta_{pred}}$$

For this example, we take $SL = 90\%LC$. Some care is needed in the definition of shelf life. Since the distribution of β_{pred} may include non-negative slope values, which could result in inadmissible (negative or infinite) values of $Shelf.Life$. In the WinBUGS code below, $Shelf.Life$ values are truncated in the interval at zero and 100 months.

23.9.4 Implementation in WinBUGS

This application is easily programmed into the freely available[36] WinBUGS software. The WinBUGS code consists of the following three text sections that are placed in a WinBUGS file: Model, Data, and Initial values (to start the Markov Chain Monte Carlo iterations). These are discussed briefly below.

Model

The Model code consists of the following text:

```
model;
{ for( batch in 1 : B ) {
alpha[batch] ~ dnorm(alpha.c,tau.alpha)
beta[batch] ~ dnorm(beta.c,tau.beta)
for( i in 1 : N ) {
mu[batch , i] <- alpha[batch] + beta[batch]
* (X[i] - Xbar)
Y[batch , i] ~ dnorm(mu[batch , i],tau.c)
}
}
# Priors
tau.c ~ dgamma(0.001,0.001)
beta.c ~ dnorm(0.0,1.0E-6)
alpha.c ~ dnorm(100,1.0E-6)
sigma.beta ~ dunif(0,100)
sigma.alpha ~ dunif(0,100)
tau.beta <- 1 / (sigma.beta * sigma.beta)
tau.alpha <- 1 / (sigma.alpha * sigma.alpha)
sigma <- 1 / sqrt(tau.c) # Total analytical SD
# Predicted Quantities of Interest
# Process Initial Target
Y0 <- alpha.c - beta.c*Xbar
beta.pred ~ dnorm(beta.c,tau.beta) # Lot
Slopes
alpha.pred ~ dnorm(alpha.c,tau.alpha)
# Lot Initials
Init.pred <-alpha.pred - Xbar*beta.pred
#Shelf life constrained to [0,100]
Shelf.Life<-max(0,min(100,(90-Init.pred)/
beta.pred))
# Predicted Lot Means at Xpred
mupred <-alpha.pred + (Xpred-Xbar) * beta.
pred
# Individual Prediction at Xbar
Ypred ~ dnorm(mupred,tau.c)
}
```

Data

The potency stability data used for analysis is given in Appendix A. These consist of data from 8 batches. Measurements were taken at up to 11 nominal time points, over a period of 24 months. The WinBUGS code for this data are below.

```
# Data
list(X=c(0, 1, 2, 3, 3, 6, 6, 12, 12, 24, 24),
B=8,N=11,Xpred=36,Xbar=9.25,
```

```
Y=structure(.Data=c(102,NA,NA,101,101,
100.5,100.8,
100.1,99,96.7,97.2,
101,101.3,NA,99.8,99.2,99.5,97.8,97.4,97.2,
96.9,96,
104.8,NA,NA,103,101.2,100.8,99.2,98.6,97.2,
97.6,98,
104,NA,NA,103.2,NA,102.8,103.3,102.4,101.2,
99.1,99.5,
102,101.4,100.8,100.2,99.7,98.8,98.5,98,
97.1,96.6,96.1,
102.7,102,NA,100.6,99.9,99.2,98.5,98.1,97.6,
96.8,96,
101.3,101.5,NA,100.2,99.8,99,98.5,98.5,97.4,
96.6,96.4,
101.6,NA,NA,100,NA,99,NA,97.8,97,NA,NA),.
Dim=c(8,11)))
```

Initial Values

Gibbs' sampling uses Monte Carlo sampling from the various prior, model, and predictive distributions indicated above. The sampling is dependent (not pseudo-random), because the sampling at any iteration depends on the values in the previous iteration; however the sampling procedure is known to converge to the desired posterior distribution. Thus, starting values are needed to initiate the Gibbs' sampling process. Examination of the iterative process showed that convergence to the final distribution was rapid, and that the process did not depend on the initial starting values. However, the results reported here were obtained using the following set of starting values ("0" superscript indicates a starting value for initiating Markov Chain Monte Carlo sampling).

Model parameters:

$$\alpha_c^0 = 100, \; \beta_c^0 = 0, \; \sigma_\alpha^0 = 1, \; \sigma_\beta^0 = 1, \; \tau_c^0 = 1$$

Latent quantities for the 8 lots in the data set:

$$\alpha_b^0 = 100, \; \beta_b^0 = 0, \; b = 1, 2, K18$$

Predicted quantities:

$$\alpha_{pred}^0 = 100, \; \beta_{pred}^0 = 0, \; Y_{pred}^0 = 100$$

Missing potency values in the data set:

$$Y_{bi}^0 = 100 \; \forall \; Y_{bi} = NA$$

The above initial values were specified by the following WinBUGS code.

```
# Initials
list(tau.c=1,sigma.beta=1,beta.
pred=0,beta.c=0,sigma.alpha=1,
alpha.pred=100,alpha.c=100,Ypred=100,
beta=c(0,0,0,0,0,0,0,0),
```

```
alpha=c(100,100,100,100,100,100,100,100),
Y=structure(.Data=c(NA,100,100,NA,NA,NA,NA,
NA,NA,NA,NA,
NA,NA,100,NA,NA,NA,NA,NA,NA,NA,NA,
NA,100,100,NA,NA,NA,NA,NA,NA,NA,NA,
NA,100,100,NA,100,NA,NA,NA,NA,NA,NA,
NA,NA,NA,NA,NA,NA,NA,NA,NA,NA,NA,
NA,NA,100,NA,NA,NA,NA,NA,NA,NA,NA,
NA,NA,100,NA,NA,NA,NA,NA,NA,NA,NA,
NA,100,100,NA,100,NA,100,NA,NA,100,100),.
Dim=c(8,11))
```

Burn-in Period, Sample Size, and Convergence Verification

A "burn-in" period is recommended for Markov Chain Monte Carlo sampling to give the dependent draws a chance to migrate from the initial starting values and approximate the target distribution. A close examination of the sampling process in WinBUGS showed it was very well behaved, and rapidly converged. However, a "burn-in" period of 5000 draws was still used before the samples were used to estimate the distributions of interest. A subsequent sample of 10 000 draws was used for estimation. This large sample size ensured that the Monte Carlo sampling error was insignificant, compared to the variance of the target distributions of all quantities estimated.

The 1000 draw predictive posterior sample was exported from WinBUGS (coda option), and imported as a text file into JMP.[37] The OOS probability was calculated as a percentage of the predictive posterior samples below 95%LC.

23.9.5 Results

The results obtained are illustrated in Table 23.13 and Figure 23.3.

To obtain more specific information on any posterior or predictive posterior sample, it may be exported from WinBUGS and imported into a more general data analysis package such as SAS or JMP to conduct capability analyses or obtain more specific quantiles. The histogram shown in Figure 23.4 was obtained for *Shelf.Life*.

The shaded region identifies the 5% lowest *Shelf. Life* values. The fifth percentile of this distribution was 40.3 months. Thus, 95% of future batches are expected to have a *Shelf.Life* greater than 40 months. Therefore, a shelf life estimate of about 40 months would be consistent with the FDA definition that assures batch means will remain within acceptance limit with 95% confidence.

A process capability analysis (see Figure 23.5) was conducted on *Ypred*.

TABLE 23.13   Posterior and predictive posterior distribution statistics for quantities of interest

Predicted quantity	Distribution mean	Distribution standard deviation	2.5% percentile	Median (50% percentile)	97.5% percentile
$Init_{pred}$	101.5	1.782	97.85	101.5	105.0
Shelf.Life	56.28	11.08	36.32	55.57	81.28
Y_0	101.5	0.6081	100.2	101.5	102.7
Y_{pred}	94.01	2.135	89.81	94.03	98.19
β_{pred}	−0.2068	0.02959	−0.2662	−0.2071	−0.148
μ_{pred}	94.03	1.922	90.1	94.04	97.79
σ	0.9139	0.08429	0.7675	0.9078	1.099

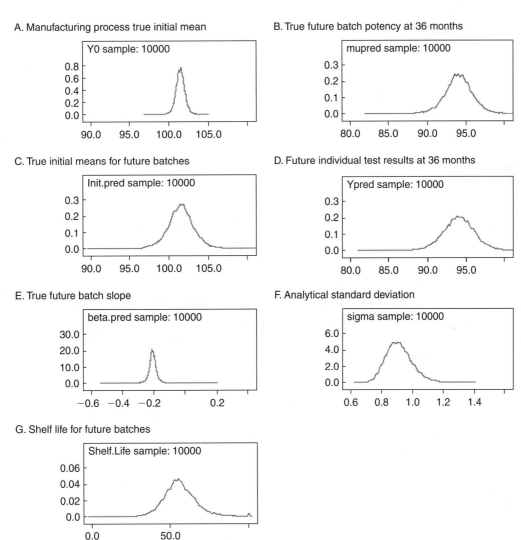

A. Manufacturing process true initial mean

B. True future batch potency at 36 months

C. True initial means for future batches

D. Future individual test results at 36 months

E. True future batch slope

F. Analytical standard deviation

G. Shelf life for future batches

FIGURE 23.3   Kernal density smoothed posterior or predictive posterior distributions of quantities of interest

The area to the left of the acceptance limit of 90%LC contains 2.8% of the predictive posterior distribution. Thus, future lots can expect to have out-of-specification test results at the 36-month time point with a probability of 0.028. In view of this risk, an appropriately shorter shelf life or release limit could be considered, to avoid the cost of investigations or (in the worst case) the disruption of a product recall.

In stability investigations, predictions of future stability test results for a particular batch of interest might

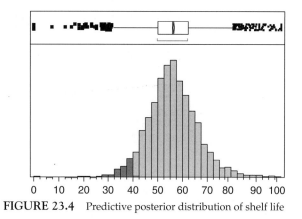

FIGURE 23.4   Predictive posterior distribution of shelf life

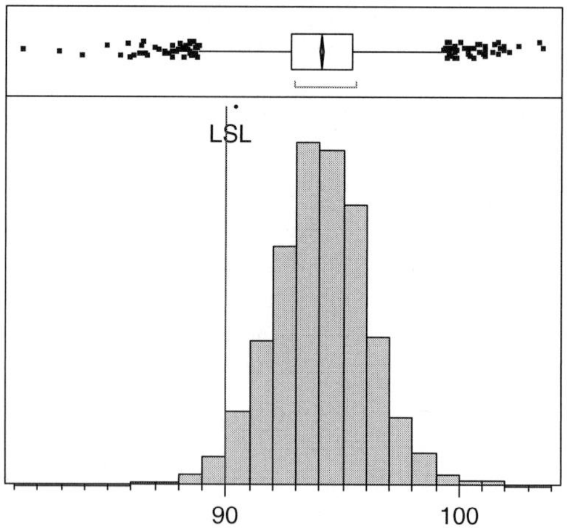

FIGURE 23.5   Process capability of predictive posterior of individual test results at 36 months

TABLE 23.14   Sample data from Shuirmann[38]

Months	Batch 1	Batch 2	Batch 3	Batch 4	Batch 5	Batch 6	Batch 7	Batch 8
0	102	101	104.8	104	102	102.7	101.3	101.6
1	.	101.3	.	.	101.4	102	101.5	.
2	.	.	.	.	100.8	.	.	.
3	101	99.8	103	103.2	100.2	100.6	100.2	100
3	101	99.2	101.2	.	99.7	99.9	99.8	.
6	100.5	99.5	100.8	102.8	98.8	99.2	99	99
6	100.8	97.8	99.2	103.3	98.5	98.5	98.5	.
12	100.1	97.4	98.6	102.4	98	98.1	98.5	97.8
12	99	97.2	97.2	101.2	97.1	97.6	97.4	97
24	96.7	96.9	97.6	99.1	96.6	96.8	96.6	.
24	97.2	96	98	99.5	96.1	96	96.4	.

A '.' indicates test not available.
SAS code for reading these data into a dataset for analysis is given below:

```
data stability;
input Month@;
do batch='BATCH1','BATCH2','BATCH3','BATCH4',
'BATCH5','BATCH6','BATCH7','BATCH8';
input Potency@;output;
end;
cards;
0     102     101     104.8   104     102     102.7   101.3   101.6
1     .       101.3   .       .       101.4   102     101.5   .
2     .       .       .       .       100.8   .       .       .
3     101     99.8    103     103.2   100.2   100.6   100.2   100
3     101     99.2    101.2   .       99.7    99.9    99.8    .
6     100.5   99.5    100.8   102.8   98.8    99.2    99      99
6     100.8   97.8    99.2    103.3   98.5    98.5    98.5    .
12    100.1   97.4    98.6    102.4   98      98.1    98.5    97.8
12    99      97.2    97.2    101.2   97.1    97.6    97.4    97
24    96.7    96.9    97.6    99.1    96.6    96.8    96.6    .
24    97.2    96      98      99.5    96.1    96      96.4    .
                                              run;
```

be useful. In the data set of Appendix A, future values are missing ("*NA*"). In WinBUGS, missing values are treated as predictive quantities to be estimated. Thus, we may directly request predictive posteriors for future (missing) data values that have not yet been obtained.

23.9.6 Bayesian Prediction Using SAS Proc MIXED

The SAS MIXED procedure can provide a posterior sample from a mixed model fit such as the random batch model used with WinBUGS.

```
proc mixed;
class Batch;
model Potency = Month /solution
alphap=0.1 outp=outp;
random Intercept Month/ type=vc
subject=Batch;
prior /out=posterior nsample=10000;
run;
```

By default, non-informative priors are used for both fixed and random parameters. In the above sample code, the posterior data set will contain 10 000 draws from the posterior. This data set may be used to further generate samples of parameter transformations, including predictive posterior for future results as was illustrated in WinBUGS in the previous section.

Sample Data

The following stability data set (Table 23.14) is used as an example in this chapter. It is taken from Shuirmann.[38]

References

1. Q1A(R2). (2003). Stability Testing of New Drug Substances and Products, November.
2. Q1B. (1996). Photostability Testing of New Drug Substances and Products, November.
3. Q1C. (1997). Stability Testing for New Dosage Forms, May.
4. Q1D. (2003). Bracketing and Matrixing Designs for Stability Testing of New Drug Substances and Products, January.
5. Q1E. (2004). Evaluation of Stability Data, June.
6. Q2A. (1994). Text on Validation of Analytical Procedures, October.
7. Q2B. (1996). Validation of Analytical Procedures: Methodology, November.
8. Q3A. (2003). Impurities in New Drug Substances, February.
9. Q3B(R). (2003). Impurities in New Drug Products, February.
10. Q6A. (2000). Specifications: Test Procedures and Acceptance Criteria for New Drug Substances and New Drug Products: Chemical Substances, December.
11. Q6B. (1999). Specifications: Test Procedures and Acceptance Criteria for Biotechnological/Biological Products, August.
12. Tsong, Y. (2003). Recent issues in stability study. Journal of Biopharmaceutical Statistics 13(3), vii–ix.
13. The SAS system for statistical analysis is available from the SAS institute, Inc., Cary, NC, USA.
14. Neter, J., Kutner, M.H., Nachtsheim, C.J. & Wasserman, W. (1996). *Applied Linear Statistical Models*, 4th edn. Irwin/ McGraw-Hill, Inc., Chicago, IL.
15. Carstensen, J.T. (1995). *Drug Stability: Principles and Practices*. Marcel Decker, Inc., New York. Chapters 2–10.
16. Lin, T.Y.D. & Chen, C.W. (2003). Overview of stability study design. Journal of Biopharmaceutical Statistics 13(3), 337–354.
17. Box, G.E.P., Hunter, W.G. & Hunter, J.S. (1978). *Statistics for Experimenters*. John Wiley & Sons, Inc., NewYork.
18. Nordbrock, E. (1994). Design and Analysis of Stability Studies. ASA Proceedings of the Biopharmaceutical Section, 291–294.
19. Nordbrock, E. (1992). Statistical comparison of stability study designs. Journal of Biopharmaceutical Statistics 2(1), 91–113.
20. The R package and associated operators manual are available for download from the following website: http://www.r-project.org/.
21. Kiermeier, A., Jarrett, R.G. & Vebyla, A.P. (2004). A new approach to estimating shelf-life. Pharmaceutical Statistics 3, 3–11.
22. Chow, S.C. & Liu, J.P. (1995). *Statistical Design and Analysis in Pharmaceutical Science*. Marcel Dekker, Inc., New York.
23. Shao, J. & Chow, S.C. (1995). Statistical inference in stability analysis. Biometrics 50, 753–763.
24. Fairweather, W.R., Lin, T.Y.D. & Kelly, R. (1995). Regulatory, design, and analysis aspects of complex stability studies. Journal of Pharmaceutical Sciences 84(11), 1322–1326.
25. Chen, J.J., Ahn, H. & Tsong, Y. (1997). Shelf life estimation for multifactor stability studies. Drug Information Journal 31, 573–587.
26. Chen, J.J., Hwang, J.S. & Tsong, Y. (1995). Estimation of the shelf-life of drugs with mixed effects models. Journal of Biopharmaceutical Statistics 5(1), 131–140.
27. Chow, S.C. & Shao, J. (1991). Estimating drug shelf-life with random batches. Biometrics 47, 1071–1079.
28. Ng, M.J. (1995). STAB Stability System for SAS, Division of Biometrics, CDER, FDA. These SAS macros may be downloaded from the following website: http://www.fda.gov/cder/sas/
29. Brownlee, K.A. (1984). *Statistical Theory and Methodology*. Robert E. Keiger, Malabar, FL.
30. Bancroft, T.A. (1964). Analysis and inference for incompletely specified models involving the use of preliminary test(s) of significance. Biometrics 20, 427–442.
31. Ruberg, S.J. & Stegman, J.W. (1991). Pooling data for stability studies: Testing the equality of batch degradation slopes. Biometrics 47, 1059–1069.
32. Millikin, G.A. & Johnson, D.E. (1992). *Analysis of Messy Data*, Volume III. ANCOVA.
33. Allen, P.V., Dukes, G.R. & Gerger, M.E. (1991). Determination of release limits: A general methodology. Pharmaceutical Research 8(9), 1210–1213.
34. Satterthwaite, F.E. (1946). An approximate distribution of estimates of variance components. Biometrics Bulletin 2, 110–114.
35. Gelman, A., Carlin, J.B., Stern, H.S. & Rubin, D.B. (2004). *Bayesian Data Analysis*. Chapman & Hall/CRC Press, Boca Raton, FL.
36. The WinBUGS package was developed jointly by the Cambridge MRC and the Biostatistics Unit at the Imperial College School of Medicine, London. The software and operators manuals may be downloaded from the following website: http://www.mrc-bsu.cam.ac.uk/bugs/welcome.shtml
37. IMP is a product of SAS Institute, Cary, NC, USA.
38. Shuirmann, D.J. (1989). Current statistical approaches in the center for drug evaluation and research, FDA, Procedings of Stability Guidelines, AAPS and FDA Joint Conference, Arlington, VA, December 11–12.

Packaging Selection for Solid Oral Dosage Forms

Yisheng Chen

24.1 INTRODUCTION

For convenient of handling, use, and for protection purposes, drug products are always packaged in containers for marketing. Stability information of a drug product in containers over the proposed shelf life is part of the quality information required to obtain approval from regulatory agencies to market any drug product, in addition to proof that the product is safe, efficacious, high quality, and made in compliance with cGMP. Product stability is typically demonstrated through real-life formal stability studies under ICH conditions.[1] Study designs and data analysis of long-term studies under ICH conditions have been discussed in Chapter 23. Due to the time-consuming nature of long-term studies, it is very important to select suitable containers to ensure the success of the studies, particularly when packaging protection of products is needed. Product stability may be imparted by formulation design, and proper use of containers. Obviously, formulation design is most critical in developing stable drug products. However, formulation design itself may not be always sufficient to ensure that the product is stable during storage. Due to the vast diversity of drug properties, and their interaction with environmental conditions, some drug products require protection against degrading factors, such as humidity and oxygen. The selection process to identify the proper packaging for the required protection is, therefore, an important part of product development. Although a formal stability study is the unambiguous process to demonstrate the quality of any drug product over its shelf life, conducting a real-life stability study is not the best process for selecting containers, because such studies are empirical, time-consuming, costly, and inefficient, making them unsuitable for screening purposes. Any failure of a formal stability study could delay the time-to-market for the product, diminish the opportunity for providing disease treatment to patients, and lead to significant financial losses for the drug maker. Instead, proper selection of containers can be achieved prior to conducting the formal stability study, using science-based and quality-by-design (QBD) approaches throughout early development stages. Containers can be selected based on material characteristics, and by linking the properties of the drug products with that of the containers. Formal studies can then be conducted to prove that the product is stable in the selected containers. This chapter will focus on the science-based selection of containers and/or packaging materials for protection of solid oral dosage forms.

24.1.1 Definitions

To avoid any possible confusion, several terms related to packaging and containers are defined according to the FDA guidance.[2,3]
- A *packaging component* means any single part of a container closure system.
- A *container closure system* refers to the sum of packaging components that together contain and protect the dosage form. This includes primary packaging components and secondary packaging

Developing Solid Oral Dosage Forms: Pharmaceutical Theory and Practice
ISBN: 978-0-444-53242-8

components, if the latter are intended to provide additional protection to the drug product.

- A *packaging system* is equivalent to a container closure system.

In this chapter, container, container closure system, and packaging are interchangeable.

- *Primary packaging component* means a packaging component is or may be in direct contact with the dosage form, e.g, liners, bottles, desiccant containers in bottles with dosage forms, blister films.
- *Secondary packaging component* means a packaging component that is not, and will not be, in direct contact with the dosage form, e.g., cartons, and over-wraps for blister cards.

24.1.2 General Considerations

Packaging materials used for pharmaceutical products must meet regulatory[2,3] and compendial requirements,[4] provide adequate protection of products against degrading factors, function properly as intended, be compatible with drug products, and be safe for use. In addition, packaging should be elegant for marketing, convenient for use, and low cost for the benefit of patients and product manufacturers.

Containers are used for different types of products for different routes of administration. By routes of administration, pharmaceutical products can be classified as inhalation, injectable, ophthalmic, liquid oral, liquid topical, transdermal, and solid oral dosage forms. Container requirements for different types of products may be different. Concerns for container–drug interaction are the highest for injectable and inhalation products, and lowest for solid oral dosage forms. Therefore, a packaging approved for one type of product cannot be assumed to be approved for another type of product. For detailed information on regulatory requirements for different types of drug products, refer to the FDA guidance Container Closure Systems for Packaging Human Drugs and Biologics.[2]

Proper use of container closure systems can provide protection of solid oral dosage forms from moisture, light, oxygen or other gases, microbial contamination, and mechanical stress, depending on the protection requirements of the product. In general, protection against moisture, light, and oxygen are the most important factors to consider. Resistance to microbial contamination can be readily achieved using well-sealed containers with proper control of materials, manufacturing, and packaging processes under GMP conditions. Protection against physical stress

can be achieved by the use of containers with sufficient strength and minimized headspace, which prevents excess movement of products during handling. Containers normally do not have the capability of protecting products from thermal stress. Heat-sensitive products are typically protected by refrigeration or freezing during storage, shipping, and end use.

As stated above, formal stability studies are not desirable for screening containers for pharmaceutical products. Instead, containers should be selected based on scientific knowledge of the fundamental properties of containers and drug products. Rational selection of containers will minimize the risk of failure in stability studies, increase the efficiency of product development, and reduce the cost for the pharmaceutical industry and patients.

24.2 MATERIAL CONSIDERATIONS

24.2.1 Containers

Containers can be classified by dosage forms for which they are intended, by product contact, by container properties or by purpose of use. Classifications based on dosage forms, such as injectable or solid oral dosage forms, and on product contact, such as primary or secondary packaging, have been given in the introduction section. Alternatively, containers can be classified based on their gas permeability—either as permeable or impermeable containers. In general, polymeric blisters and bottles, such as PVC and PVDC blisters, and PET and HDPE bottles, are permeable to moisture and oxygen, depending on the polymer used in producing the container, while properly sealed glass bottles and aluminum foil/foil blisters can be considered impermeable to gases if there are no imperfections in the bottle seal or pinholes or imperfections in the foil. Containers are also commonly classified as bulk containers and finished containers for use purposes. Bulk containers are used for storage of bulk drug products prior to packaging or for shipping of bulk products to repackagers or contract packagers. Finished containers are the final packages that are used to market and deliver drug products to patients. Finished containers are further classified into unit dose containers, and multiple unit dose containers. Stability data of products stored in the finished containers are the main source of data required by regulatory agencies for approval of shelf life for products.

- *Bulk containers*: for bulk products of solid oral dosage forms, fiber and plastic drums with flexible liners, such as low-density polyethylene (LDPE, or PE) liners, are commonly used. The liners provide a controlled material contact surface for the products, and some protection of products against moisture. Regular fiber drums and PE liners are highly permeable to moisture and other gases. A fiber drum reinforced with aluminum foil may have significantly lower gas permeability than a regular one. Plastic drums or pails, such as high-density polyethylene (HDPE) drums, also have low gas permeability. With the use of heat-sealable laminated foil bags as liners, HDPE drums or fiber drums reinforced with aluminum foil are probably the second-best bulk containers for products that are sensitive to moisture or oxygen. Well-sealed stainless steel containers provide the best barrier for any gases. However, large steel containers are heavy, and hence inconvenient to use.

- *Finished containers*: for finished pharmaceutical dosage forms, plastic bottles (usually HDPE bottles) and flexible packages (such as blisters and pouches) are the most commonly used containers. However, plastic bottles, such as low-density polyethylene (LDPE), high-density polyethylene (HDPE), polyethylene terephthalate (PET) and polypropylene (PP) bottles, and polymeric blisters, such as polyvinyl chloride (PVC), polyvinylidene chloride (PVDC), and polychloro-trifluoroethylene (PCTFE), are permeable to moisture and gases, although permeability varies with materials. Glass bottles are not commonly used, due to safety concerns about broken glasses during handling, and due to heavy weight that can add to shipment costs, even though well-sealed glass bottles can be considered impermeable to gases. Foil/foil blisters or pouches are also impermeable to gases, but they are not commonly used due to the lack of transparency of the material, as well as poor resistance to deformation by external pressure or force.

Container permeability is a critical factor to consider in selecting packaging materials for products that are sensitive to the respective permeants. Moisture and oxygen permeabilities of packaging materials are commonly measured, and reported as moisture vapor transmission rate (MVTR) and oxygen transmission rate (OTR), respectively. Examples of MVTR and OTR data from literature, for some packaging materials, are listed in Table 24.1. Note that the data listed in the table for blistering materials are for flat films. Permeation rate of the formed cavity of blisters will be larger than that of flat films, due to reduced thickness of the formed cavity. The actual dimensions, including surface area and thickness, of any given containers should be accounted for in packaging design and

TABLE 24.1 Moisture and oxygen transmission rates of some packaging materials

Material	MVTR (g.mil/100 in²/day, at 100°F, 90%RH)	OTR (cc.mil/100 in²/day, at 77°F)	Reference
Cold form foil	0.00	0.00	6
Polychlorotrifluoro-ethylene (PCTFE)	0.016	7.00	6
Polyvinyl dichloride (PVDC)	0.1–0.2[a]	0.15–0.90	7
High density polyethylene (HDPE)	0.3–0.4	139–150	6,8
Polypropylene (PP)	0.69–1.0	182	7,9
Low density polyethylene (LDPE)	1.0–1.5	463–500	6
Polyethylene terephthalate (PET)	1.2–2.0	3–5	7
Polyvinyl chloride (PVC)	0.9–5.1	5–20	10
Ethylene vinyl alcohol (EVOH)	1.4–5.4[a]	0.05–0.90	7
Polystyrene (PS)	7–10	350–400	10
Nylon	16–20	1.0	10

[a]Determined at 104°F/90%RH

TABLE 24.2 Barrier thickness of blistering film and resulting moisture vapor transmission rate (MVTR)

Aclar film	Aclar thickness (μm)	MVTR (mg/cm²/day at 38°C, 100%RH)[a]
Rx 160	15	0.042
Rx 20E	20	0.029
SupRx 900	23	0.026
UltRx 2000	51	0.012
UltRx 3000	76	0.008
UltRx 4000	102	0.004

[a]Data from www.gordoncross.com/EXPORT/English/aclar_home.htm

evaluation. Increasing the thickness of the barrier material can reduce the MVTR of both laminated flat films and formed cavities, such as is shown for commercially available laminated film materials Aclar RX 160, SupRx 900, UltRx 2000, UltRx 3000, and UltRx 4000 (Table 24.2) if the dimension of the blister cavity is the same for different films.

Data in Table 24.1 show that materials that have a low MVTR may not have a low OTR. For example, the MVTR of nylon is approximately 1000 times larger than that of PCTFE. However, the OTR of nylon is actually smaller than the OTR of PCTFE. For the purpose of moisture protection, PCTFE is far superior to all other materials listed in the table, except for cold form foil. On the other hand, PVDC and EVOH are better choices for protection against oxygen. Packaging materials should therefore be selected based on the specific need for protection of each individual product. From a material development point of view, data listed in Table 24.1 show that a combination of PCTFE with EVOH can produce a multiple-layer blistering material with excellent barrier properties against moisture and oxygen.

Although aluminum foil may be considered as the ultimate barrier for gases, thin foil (thickness <25 μm) may have pinholes,[5] and the foil may become permeable through the pinholes. Pinholes can be caused either by the presence of organic contaminates in the molten aluminum or by the stress of the rolling process during foil production. The number of pinholes per defined area of the foil increases as the thickness of the foil decreases. This property is important to consider in selecting foil materials, and also in the design of packages using thin foil as a barrier.

24.2.2 Determination of Container Moisture Vapor Transmission Rate

As discussed above, container moisture permeability is an important factor to consider in packaging selection for moisture-sensitive products. Reliable MVTR is critical to ensure the selection of proper materials. Methods for determination of MVTR are currently described in USP Chapter <671>[4] to evaluate the performance of containers. For multiple-unit containers, the USP method uses a single weight gain measurement over a 14-day study period, using control bottles for comparison. Literature data have shown that results obtained by the USP method may be highly variable. For example, the standard deviation of the USP results was higher than the mean weight-gain value[11] in some cases. In one case, the value obtained at 25°C/75%RH was unreasonably higher than at 40°C/75%RH.[11] A high variability in permeability renders the data of little scientific value, either for packaging design or for justification of container post-approval changes. Therefore, an improved method is needed for determination of container MVTR.

For well-sealed plastic containers without gross defects, the mechanism of water ingress into a container is mainly by diffusion of moisture molecules through the container wall,[12] and through the seal. For a relatively large container with a thin wall, the wall can be approximated as a homogeneous planar barrier. If it is assumed that:

1. the diffusion coefficient D of water vapor in the wall is constant at constant temperature;

2. the concentration of moisture at the outside surface is maintained at a constant level of C_0; and

3. the concentration at the inside surface is kept at essentially zero or a "sink" condition; then the initial and boundary conditions for a packaging system can be described as:

$$C = C_i, 0 < x < h, t = 0$$

$$C = C_o, x = 0; C = 0, x = h, t \geq 0$$

where x is the direction of diffusion, h represents the thickness of the wall, C_i indicates the initial moisture concentration in the wall, and t is time.

If the quantity of water diffusing through the wall and entering the "sink" is measured as a result of net diffusion, Equation 24.1 can be used to describe the permeation process.[13]

$$\begin{aligned}
Q_{t,d} = {} & \frac{DC_o}{h}\left(t + \frac{C_i h^2}{2DC_o} - \frac{h^2}{6D}\right) \\
& - \frac{2hC_o}{\pi^2} \sum_{n=1}^{n=\infty} \frac{(-1)^n}{n^2} \exp\left(-\frac{n^2\pi^2 Dt}{h^2}\right) \\
& - \frac{4C_i h}{\pi^2} \sum_{m=0}^{m=\infty} \frac{1}{(2m+1)^2} \exp\left(\frac{-(2m+1)^2 \pi^2 Dt}{h^2}\right)
\end{aligned}$$

(24.1)

where:

$Q_{t,d}$ is the amount of moisture diffused through unit surface area of the wall at time t.

If the amount of water entering the outer surface of the wall material is measured, such as by the measurement of total weight gain (wg) of containers per USP Chapter <671>, the measured quantity per unit surface area by weight gain, $Q_{t,wg}$ includes the amounts of water absorbed by the wall, and the backing material in the closure, and the amount of water diffused through the wall into a "sink" created by desiccants. In this case, Equation 24.2 can be used to describe the permeation process.

$$\begin{aligned}
Q_{t,wg} = {} & \frac{DC_o}{h}\left(t - \frac{C_i h^2}{2DC_o} + \frac{h^2}{3D}\right) \\
& - \frac{2hC_o}{\pi^2} \sum_{n=1}^{n=\infty} \frac{1}{n^2} \exp\left(-\frac{n^2\pi^2 Dt}{h^2}\right) \\
& + \frac{4C_i h}{\pi^2} \sum_{m=0}^{m=\infty} \frac{1}{(2m+1)^2} \exp\left(\frac{-(2m+1)^2 \pi^2 Dt}{h^2}\right)
\end{aligned}$$

(24.2)

Equations 24.1–24.2 show that initial moisture permeation profiles are not linear at the early time, and that the profiles are affected by the initial water concentration in the wall material, regardless of the methods of detection. These equations suggest that the data from the early stage of permeation will vary with the initial conditions. Such dependency on the initial conditions cannot be corrected using control containers, because the driving forces are different for the test and the control containers. Therefore, permeability cannot be determined from early time points by a single weight gain measurement. However, if the permeation process is allowed to proceed for a sufficiently longer time, MVTR can be reliably determined using the simplified forms of Equations 24.1–24.2, regardless of the initial water concentration in the wall and the methods of detection. The effects of initial water concentration on the diffusion profiles, and the advantage of using a steady state method for MVTR can be seen by the following analysis.

For the first method, in which the amount of water diffused into the sink is measured, if $C_i = 0$, and as $t \to \infty$, the quantity of water diffused through the wall in Equation 24.1 can be simplified to a linear function as:

$$Q_{t,d} = \frac{DC_o}{h}\left(t - \frac{h^2}{6D}\right) \qquad (24.3)$$

with a lag time t_L being:

$$t_L = \frac{h^2}{6D} \qquad (24.4)$$

If $C_i = C_0$, and as $t \to \infty$, Equation 24.1 simplifies to:

$$Q_{t,d} = \frac{DC_o}{h}\left(t + \frac{h^2}{3D}\right) \qquad (24.5)$$

with a burst time t_B being:

$$t_B = -\frac{h^2}{3D} \qquad (24.6)$$

Equations 24.3–24.6 show that the initial water concentration in the wall can change the initial diffusion profile to appear either as a lag or as a burst, even though the method of determination remains the same. But the rate of diffusion over steady state is not affected by the initial wall conditions.

For the second method, by which the total weight gain of the entire container is measured, when $C_i = 0$, and as $t \to \infty$, Equation 24.2 can be simplified to a linear function including a burst time as:

$$Q_{t,wg} = \frac{DC_o}{h}\left(t + \frac{h^2}{3D}\right) \qquad (24.7)$$

When $C_i = C_0$, and as $t \to \infty$, weight gain simplifies to a linear function with a lag time in:

$$Q_{t,wg} = \frac{DC_o}{h}\left(t - \frac{h^2}{6D}\right) \qquad (24.8)$$

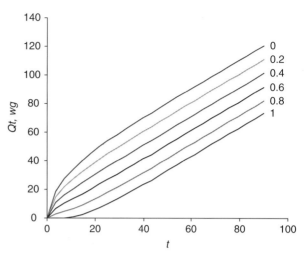

FIGURE 24.1   Simulated weight gain curves of containers filled with desiccants. Numbers at the end of the curves are the values of C_i/C_o

It can be seen from Equations 24.3, 24.5, 24.7, and 24.8 that the permeation rates, which are the slopes of the linear lines, are the same as Equation 24.9 for different methods of detection, as long as steady state permeation is reached.

$$\frac{dQ}{dt} = \frac{DC_o}{h} \qquad (24.9)$$

The constant rate, by different methods for different initial conditions, shows that reliable container permeability can be determined from the steady state permeation data.

The dependence of weight gain profiles on the initial water concentration in the wall, and the advantages of using steady state weight gain data for MVTR, is further depicted in Figure 24.1 for Equation 24.2. The figure simulates the effects of initial conditions, to show that the initial weight gain profiles vary from a burst when the wall is initially dry, to a delay when the wall is initially equilibrated with water, per Equations 24.7–24.8. However, if the permeation process is allowed to proceed for a sufficient time to achieve steady state, rate of weight gain is the same, regardless of the initial water concentration in the wall as long as temperature and the driving force remain unchanged. A similar graph can also be constructed for Equation 24.1, to show that the initial condition has no effect on the rate of permeation through the wall by net permeation if steady state is achieved.

Experimental data for weight gain for two sizes of HDPE bottles containing anhydrous calcium chloride, and closed with induction seal closures with paper backing in the closures, are shown in Figure 24.2. The weight gain profiles agree well with the profiles predicted by theory.

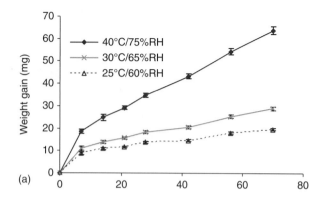

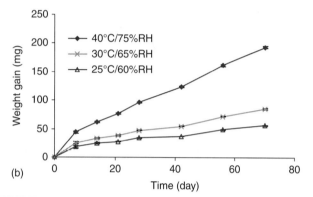

FIGURE 24.2 Weight gain profiles of HDPE bottles containing anhydrous calcium chloride and stored under ICH conditions. Bottle size: (a) 1 oz; (b) 4 oz

the sealed containers. If anhydrous calcium chloride is used, the desiccant must be activated at a temperature higher than 200°C, to remove any potential hydrates on the surface of the desiccant. The moisture sorption capacity of anhydrous calcium chloride in the range below 10%RH at 25°C is actually lower than that of silica gel. Therefore, a large amount of anhydrous calcium chloride must be used to ensure the existence of a sink condition. Alternatively, some other types of desiccant with a higher moisture sorption capacity than calcium chloride at low humidity, such as silica gel or molecular sieve, may be used in a smaller quantity to achieve the "sink" condition.

For high barrier containers, a sensitive balance should be used to ensure that the variability caused by weighing is negligible compared with the measured MVTR. The use of aggressive testing conditions in terms of temperature and humidity is helpful to achieve obvious weight changes over the test duration, and hence minimize the weighing error. Of course, ICH conditions must be used if the MVTR data is intended for prediction of product moisture uptake during shelf life under the same conditions.

MVTRs of some HDPE bottles determined by the steady state permeation method are listed in Table 24.3.[14]

24.2.3 Gas Absorbers

Desiccants and Fillers

Desiccants are commonly used to keep products dry and stable. Dry desiccants can absorb moisture from air either by physical adsorption or by chemical reaction, and thus reduce the humidity in the headspace of sealed containers. Moisture sorption by silica gel is an example of physical adsorption, and sorption by calcium oxide is an example of chemical reaction. Different types of desiccants and their moisture sorption capacities can be found in literature.[15] The most commonly used desiccants for solid pharmaceutical products are silica gel, clay, and molecular sieves.

Silica gel is an amorphous form of silica ($SiO_2 \cdot xH_2O$). It is highly porous. Silica gel particles are composed of an interconnecting network of microscopic pores (capillaries), and therefore have a very large surface area. The mechanisms of moisture adsorption by silica gel include surface adsorption and capillary condensation in the porous network. Silica gel works well at ambient temperature, but at higher temperatures may have decreased adsorption rate and equilibrium moisture content. The moisture in silica gel can be completely removed by drying at 110°C.

Clay is a low cost and efficient desiccant at low temperatures. The primary chemical composition of clay

In practice, water concentration in the container wall is not measured. However, it can be assumed that, at the outer surface, water concentration is proportional to the equilibrium external relative %RH by partition at a given temperature. Taking the container surface area into consideration, it can be shown that MVTR during steady state can be described by Equation 24.10.

$$MVTR = A \frac{d_Q}{d_t} = \frac{ADK \times \%RH}{h} = \frac{AP \times \%RH}{h} \quad (24.10)$$

where A is the surface area, d_Q/d represents the rate of moisture permeation, D and K are the diffusion coefficient and the partition coefficient of moisture in the wall material, respectively, and P represents the apparent moisture permeability of the wall material.

Other factors to consider for ensuring the measurement of reliable container MVTR include maintaining a "sink" condition, balance sensitivity, and test conditions of humidity and temperature. For the weight gain method, a perfect "sink" condition is that an internal relative humidity of 0%RH can be maintained by using a sufficient amount of effective desiccant in

TABLE 24.3 Moisture vapor transmission rate (MVTR) and moisture permeability of some HDPE bottles

Bottle size	MVTR (mg/day, mean ± SD, n = 10)			$P \times 10^6$ (mg·cm/(day·%RH·cm²))		
	25°C/60% RH	30°C/65% RH	40°C/75% RH	25°C	30°C	40°C
40 cc	0.15 ± 0.01	0.26 ± 0.01	0.70 ± 0.02	3.99	6.40	14.67
0.75 oz	0.17 ± 0.01	0.28 ± 0.01	0.71 ± 0.02	3.84	5.88	13.13
1 oz	0.21 ± 0.01	0.34 ± 0.01	0.92 ± 0.01	4.16	6.34	14.71
1.5 oz	0.27 ± 0.01	0.41 ± 0.01	1.02 ± 0.03	4.45	6.30	13.61
3 oz	0.36 ± 0.01	0.53 ± 0.02	1.28 ± 0.02	5.05	6.81	14.36
4 oz	0.59 ± 0.01	0.93 ± 0.03	2.36 ± 0.03	5.19	7.57	16.63
5 oz	0.68 ± 0.02	1.12 ± 0.03	2.82 ± 0.05	5.11	7.76	16.98
175 cc	0.56 ± 0.02	0.94 ± 0.02	2.39 ± 0.04	4.29	6.65	14.70
			Average	4.51	6.71	14.85
			SD	0.53	0.65	1.34

includes silica and aluminum oxide, magnesium oxide, calcium oxide, and ferric oxide. Moisture adsorption capacity may be different for different grades of clay desiccants. Therefore, their moisture adsorption isotherms must be verified during the desiccant selection process. Clay works well at ambient temperature, but at temperatures >50°C it will likely give up moisture rather than absorb moisture. Similar to silica gel, clay can be dried at 110°C.

A molecular sieve is a highly porous crystalline material with precise mono-dispersed pores into which certain sizes of molecules can fit, and hence it can be used to separate one type of molecule from others. These pores are the channels in the crystalline structure of a material such as zeolite. The pore sizes of molecular sieves differ from silica gel, in that the pore size of a molecular sieve is small and precise, while that of silica gel is much larger with a broad distribution. Molecular sieves are available with different effective pore sizes, such as 3, 4, 5, and 10 angstroms. A molecular sieve with a 3 angstroms effective pore size can selectively adsorb water molecules, since the diameter of water molecules is approximately 3 angstroms, while a molecular sieve with 4 angstroms pore size can also adsorb molecular nitrogen and oxygen, in addition to water. Molecular sieve desiccants have a very strong affinity and a high adsorptive capacity for water in an environment of low water concentration. At 25°C/10%RH, molecular sieves can adsorb water to approximately 14% of their own weight. This property makes it possible to create an extremely low humidity environment with a small amount of material. However, at any humidity higher than 50%RH at 25°C, the adsorption capacity of a molecular sieve is smaller than that of silica gel.

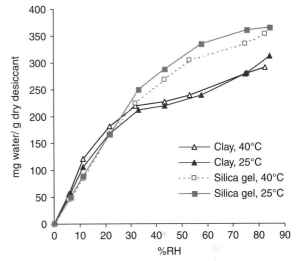

FIGURE 24.3 Moisture sorption isotherms of activated silica gel and Bentonite clay

Moisture sorption isotherms of different types of desiccants can be found in literature.[15] The equilibrium adsorptive capacities of silica gel and clay, for moisture at different temperatures and humidities are shown in Figure 24.3. At humidities lower than 35%RH, moisture sorption capacities are similar for the two desiccants. At higher humidities, silica gel has a higher moisture capacity than clay. It is important to know that different grades of a same type of desiccant may have significantly different moisture sorption capacities. This holds true for clay and zeolite desiccants. Therefore, moisture sorption isotherms of desiccants must be verified for the materials selected. In addition, the moisture sorption capacity of desiccants is a function of temperature. This temperature dependency should be characterized during the selection process, particularly when the isotherm is intended for modeling of packaging design for moisture protection at different temperatures.

The common process for using desiccants is to place a predetermined quantity of activated desiccant into containers with products, and then to seal the containers. The quantity of desiccant to be used is important, since an insufficient quantity will not provide the required protection, while excessive use of desiccant may lead to over-drying and an unnecessary increase in product cost. In many cases, overuse of desiccant is not a problem for product quality. However, over-drying of some hydrates may lead to the formation of unstable amorphous materials, and hence become detrimental to product quality. It is therefore important to understand the product characteristics, the degradation mechanism of the products, and the desired range of humidity for products, before an appropriate quantity of desiccant can be determined. Once the desired range of humidity is determined, a suitable quantity of desiccant to use can be calculated, based on the moisture sorption properties of both the desiccant and the drug product using a modeling method, as discussed later in this chapter.

The environmental conditions and the packaging process for placing desiccants into product containers must be well-controlled in order to maintain the effectiveness of the desiccant, because desiccant may adsorb water vapor quickly when exposed to room air, thus reducing its protection capacity. For example, activated clay, silica gel, and molecular sieves can all absorb approximately 10% of water when exposed to 25°C/75%RH for one hour,[15] leading to a significant loss of protection effect for products. In fact, such an exposure can result in a complete loss of the protection effect of silica gel and clay if the desiccants are intended to maintain humidity lower than 20%RH. Obviously, environmental humidity and exposure time for placing desiccant into containers must be minimized, in order to prevent loss of protection effect of desiccants.

Care should also be taken when desiccants are used for gelatin capsules to prevent brittleness from loss of moisture. Gelatin capsule shells need approximately 12–16% water to maintain physical strength, which corresponds to a relative humidity of approximately 40%–65%RH at 25°C. Humidities lower than 30%RH will likely cause the capsules to become brittle.[16,17]

Fillers such as cotton and rayon are also commonly co-packaged with solid pharmaceutical dosage forms to restrain product movement during shipping. Cotton or rayon can sometimes cause instability problems for drug products. The reasons for this are that these fillers may contain residual oxidative agents that were used

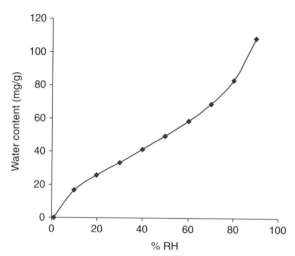

FIGURE 24.4   Moisture sorption isotherm of cotton at 25°C

for processing the fillers, and that fillers can unintentionally act as either a source of water or as a desiccant. The residual oxidative agents can cause degradation of some active pharmaceutical ingredients or result in cross-linking of gelatin capsules or gelatin-coated tablets, if residual formaldehyde exists in the filler, leading to dissolution problems for the drug products. The moisture sorption capacity of cotton is another aspect to consider. The equilibrium moisture content of cotton is shown in Figure 24.4. It can absorb more than 6% of water at humidity higher than 60%RH at 25°C. If dry cotton is used, it can act as a type of desiccant, and absorb water from the co-packaged products. If equilibrated at high humidity during storage prior to use, cotton can be a source of water for the co-packaged dry products, if the products are hygroscopic. Although the amount of cotton used for pharmaceutical products is small, in general the effects of cotton on moisture transfer may still be significant. Quantitative evaluation of the effect of cotton on product moisture content can be carried out using a modeling method, as discussed later in this chapter.

Oxygen Scavengers

When products are sensitive to oxygen in the air, one could choose to either:

1. formulate with antioxidants to stabilize the products;
2. package the products in containers impermeable to oxygen, such as glass or aluminum containers, combined with purging the container headspace using an inert gas, such as nitrogen or argon;
3. use oxygen scavengers in well-sealed containers;
4. combine the techniques of stabilization by formulation and packaging protection.

Stabilization by formulation is a complex subject, beyond the scope of this chapter, and will not be discussed here. Once the product is formulated, appropriate packaging can provide further protection of the product to maximize its shelf life. Normal air contains approximately 21% oxygen, and 78% nitrogen. Purging containers with inert gas can reduce the oxygen level to a range of approximately 0.5–5%. The use of a sufficient amount of oxygen absorbers can reduce oxygen content in the headspace of a sealed container to below 0.1%. Combination of purging to reduce the initial level of oxygen, and the subsequent use of oxygen scavenger in a well-sealed container with low oxygen permeability, is probably the best method for packaging oxygen-sensitive products.

Oxygen scavengers, or oxygen absorbers, are materials which can react with oxygen from the air, eliminating the effects of oxygen when co-packaged with products in closed containers. Oxygen scavengers are commonly used for food products, but are less common for pharmaceutical products. In the food industry, different types of materials are used as oxygen scavengers including:

1. inorganic oxygen absorbers, such as powdered metals or intermediate oxides;
2. organic antioxidants, such as vitamin C or salicylate; and
3. polymer based oxygen absorbers.

The mechanism of product protection by oxygen scavengers is the rapid oxidation of the scavengers with oxygen from the headspace of closed containers, and with the diffused oxygen during storage. According to Grattan and Gilberg,[18] the main reactions for the oxidation of powdered iron with oxygen in the presence of moisture and sodium chloride, as in the commercially available oxygen scavenger Ageless™, can be described by Equations 24.11–24.14.

$$Fe \rightarrow Fe^{2+} + 2e^- \quad (24.11)$$

$$O_2 + 2H_2O + 4e^- \rightarrow 4OH^- \quad (24.12)$$

$$Fe^{2+} + 2H_2O \rightarrow FeOOH + 3H^+ + e^- \text{ (rapid)} \quad (24.13)$$

$$3Fe^{2+} + 4H_2O \rightarrow Fe_3O_4 + 8H^+ + e^- \text{ (slow)} \quad (24.14)$$

The rate of oxidation of powdered iron in air, and hence oxygen reduction in sealed containers, is rapid. It has been shown that, using one packet of Ageless Z-1000 in a 2L sealed container, the oxygen level was reduced from approximately 21% to less than 0.1% in about 20 hours.[19] Due to its effectiveness and low cost, metallic iron is widely used to preserve food and museum items.

There are several disadvantages of using metal iron as an oxygen scavenger.

1. The reaction of metal iron with oxygen requires a water activity as high as 65%–85%RH in the system.[18] In fact, water was included in the form of saturated sodium chloride solution absorbed in molecular sieves as part of the oxygen scavenger, to maintain a critical relative humidity for reaction.[18] A high humidity environment may be detrimental for most solid pharmaceutical products.
2. The reaction is exothermic. The heat released by the reaction may create thermal stress for the co-packaged products.
3. Lastly, the reaction creates a vacuum, due to the elimination of oxygen in the container, which may cause flexible containers to collapse. Therefore, rigid containers will be needed in order to maintain the geometry of packages using this type of oxygen scavenger for products.

Unlike desiccants, oxygen scavengers are not yet well-studied for pharmaceutical products. Therefore, much study, including the characterization of material properties and the oxidation-reduction mechanisms of oxygen scavengers and drug products, needs to be done in evaluating oxygen scavengers for protection of pharmaceutical products. Successful oxygen scavenger candidates for products must be effective, safe to use, clean (so as not to contaminate products), convenient to use, and of low cost.

24.2.4 Drug Products

While there are different types of containers available, selection of containers for product protection clearly depends on the specific protection requirements of any given product. Typically, the protection requirements are identified during the early development stage by accelerated degradation studies using either the active pharmaceutical ingredients (API) or drug products. Details of stability studies have been discussed in Chapters 5–6. Once the drug sensitivity and protection requirements are identified, container design and selection may be made by matching the properties of containers with that of the drug products. If accelerated studies show that the product is not sensitive to moisture and/or other gases, the protection requirements for the product will mainly include the prevention of contamination and physical stress. If a product is sensitive to light, containers with low light transmittance should be the first choice, otherwise, secondary packaging will be needed if transparent primary packaging is used. If a product is sensitive to moisture, containers with low MVTR values are preferred, and desiccant may be used for additional protection.

Different pharmaceutical excipients have different moisture sorption capacities. The same is true for finished pharmaceutical products, since each product contains its own set of excipients. Product moisture sorption capacity is one of the critical factors that determine the rate and extent of moisture ingress into containers during storage. The higher the capacity, the faster the ingression rate will be, assuming other factors to be the same. If desiccants are used for products, it is important to understand the solid-state chemistry of the active pharmaceutical ingredients (API) in the products. Some APIs may exist in different hydrates and/or crystal forms under different humidities. Over-drying by use of excessive desiccants may lead to loss of hydrates, and formation of unstable lower hydrates or amorphous materials. Therefore, drug product properties, including moisture sorption isotherms and the solid-state response to environmental conditions, should be studied. This is particularly important if desiccants are used for quantitative design of packaging to protect moisture-sensitive products. The application of material moisture sorption isotherms and container moisture permeability in quantitative packaging selection for moisture sensitive products are discussed in the following section.

24.3 LINKING PACKAGING PROPERTY WITH DRUG PROPERTY

Traditionally, MVTR is used for classification of containers, and the use of desiccant for products is determined by trial and error. According to USP Chapter <671>, containers are tight containers if not more than one of the 10 test containers exceeds moisture uptake of 100 mg/day/L, and none exceeds 200 mg/day/L. Containers are well-closed containers if not more than one of the 10 test containers exceeds moisture uptake of 2000 mg/day/L, and none exceeds 3000 mg/day/L. This type of classification is very loose, and does not take into account the properties of the products in the containers. As such, this classification is not meaningful in quantitative packaging design for the support of new product development. In product R&D, we need to know if a new container can provide adequate protection of a new product, prior to the use of the container for stability studies. Therefore, vigorous evaluation is needed for container selection. Trial and error for packaging and desiccant selection is of low efficiency, and lacks guiding power. A desirable approach should be science-based, and should allow building

product quality by design (QbD). There are two new methods developed in recent years for evaluating container moisture barrier properties for products. These methods are the use of MVTR/unit dose product,[12] and the modeling approach for prediction of moisture uptake by packaged products during storage.[20] The key element of these two new methods is the linking of packaging property with drug product property, and they are discussed in the following section.

24.3.1 The Use of Moisture Vapor Transmission Rate per Unit Product for Container Comparison

For a given product in different containers, the moisture protection efficiency of the containers for the product can be evaluated using a criterion of "MVTR per unit quantity of product."[12] For solid products, the unit can be a tablet, a capsule or the mass of a product. A smaller value of MVTR/unit product indicates that the container provides better protection for the product from moisture than a container with a larger value. This criterion can be used to rank containers/designs, and to guide packaging selection for new product R&D or it can be used to evaluate the container moisture barrier equivalence for justification of post-approval container changes for a regulatory purpose.

24.3.2 Modeling of Moisture Uptake by Packaged Products

Moisture content of products in permeable containers stored at ICH stability conditions can be predicted by a modeling method[20] if is assumed that:

1. moisture content of a product is a function of the equilibrium humidity;
2. moisture permeation through the container is the rate-limiting step;
3. a quasi-steady state of permeation exists; and
4. moisture permeability of the container is constant at a given temperature.

At quasi-steady state, the rate of moisture permeation through a sealed container at constant temperature and humidity can be expressed using Fick's first law as:

$$\frac{d_Q}{d_t} = k\left(RH_{out} - RH\right) \qquad (24.15)$$

where:

d_Q/d_t is the rate of moisture permeation through the container

k represents the apparent moisture permeability of the container

RH_{out} and RH represent the percentage of relative humidity outside and inside the container, respectively.

If the water content of any unit component in the container is a function of the equilibrium humidity, the total quantity of water, Q, in a sealed package containing n components can be written as:

$$Q = \sum_{i=1}^{i=n} q_i f_i (RH) \qquad (24.16)$$

where q_i and $f_i (RH)$ are the quantity and the moisture sorption isotherm of the ith component in the container, respectively.

Differentiation of Equation 24.16 with respect to relative humidity leads to:

$$\frac{d_Q}{d_{RH}} = \frac{d}{d_{RH}} \left[\sum_{i=1}^{i=n} q_i f_i (RH) \right] \qquad (24.17)$$

By mass balance, the quantity of moisture permeated through the container must equal to the moisture content change in the container, as described by Equation 24.18:

$$k \left(RH_{out} - RH \right) d_t = \frac{d}{d_{RH}} \left[\sum_{i=1}^{i=n} q_i f_i (RH) \right] d_{RH} \qquad (24.18)$$

Rearranging and integration leads to the $t - RH$ profile inside the container as described by Equation 24.19:

$$t = \int_{RH_0}^{RH} \frac{\frac{d}{d_{RH}} \left[\sum_{i=1}^{i=n} q_i f_i (RH) \right]}{k \left(RH_{out} - RH \right)} d_{RH} \qquad (24.19)$$

The water content of each individual component, as a function of time, can be estimated by substituting the RH at time t into the corresponding moisture isotherm of the component, as given by the $t - RH$ profile. Detailed procedures for using this modeling method can be found in literature.[20] Predicted moisture content for a model tablet product in HDPE bottles stored under accelerated and long-term ICH conditions[1] agreed very well with experimental data (Figures 24.5–24.6), demonstrating that this modeling method is highly reliable. The reliability makes it possible to practice a quality by design (QbD) approach to packaging selection for products. Using this modeling method, the effects of any packaging designs and storage conditions on product moisture content can be readily simulated, to select the most suitable packaging for moisture protection. The selected packaging can then be confirmed by real-life stability

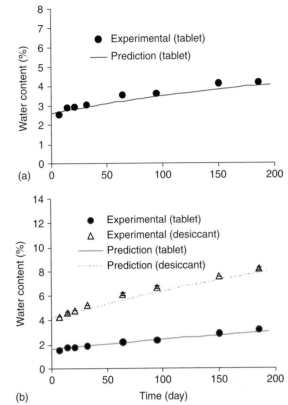

FIGURE 24.5 Experimental and predicted water content of 20 model tablets in sealed 3 oz HDPE bottles and stored at 40°C/75%RH. (a): no desiccant; (b): with 1 g bentonite desiccant

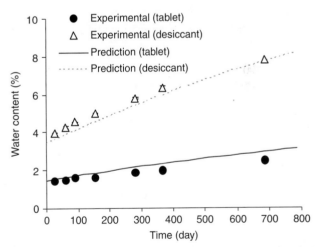

FIGURE 24.6 Experimental and predicted water content of 20 tablets in a sealed 3 oz HDPE bottle with 1 g bentonite desiccant and stored at 25°C/60%RH

study. Suppose it is known that the headspace humidity of a product must not be greater than 30%RH at room temperature over its shelf life, and that desiccant is planned to be used in HDPE bottles for the product. However, it is not known what quantity of desiccant to

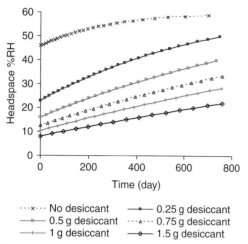

FIGURE 24.7 Simulation of headspace humidity for the same amount of a model product in a 1 oz HDPE bottle with different quantities of silica gel, and stored at 25°C/60%RH

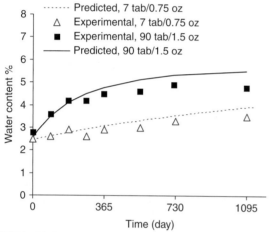

FIGURE 24.8 Predicted and experimental moisture content of tablets in different designs using HDPE bottles and stored at 25°C/60%RH

use or the effect of moisture permeation during the shelf life. With the moisture sorption property of the product, and the container permeability at hand, simulation can be conducted for different amounts of desiccant. The simulation results are shown in Figure 24.7 as examples. Based on the simulation, it can be determined that at least 1 g of the desiccant must be used, in order to maintain the headspace relative humidity and not to exceed 30%RH over two years when stored at 25°C/60%RH. In another case, 7 and 90 tablets were packaged in 0.75 and 1.5 oz HDPE bottles, respectively. Simulation indicated that the moisture content of the tablets in the 0.75 oz bottle would approach an equilibrium value in about one year when stored at 25°C/60%RH, while that of the tablets in the 1.5 oz would not reach the same level of moisture content over three years. The simulated results were confirmed by a formal stability study conducted

under ICH conditions (Figure 24.8). These examples show that the modeling method can be used as a scientific tool to evaluate the moisture protection capability of any proposed packaging design, prior to conducting stability studies for new product development or to evaluate the container equivalence for post-approval container changes. Formal stability studies can then be conducted for confirmation purposes. Modeling is science-based, and can be used as an effective tool for QbD in packaging evaluation for product protection against moisture. Successful application of this method will reduce time and cost for product development.

24.4 POST-APPROVAL PACKAGING CHANGES

Post-approval changes to packaging materials (PACPAC), including a change to a container closure system, to a component of the container closure system, to a material of construction for a component, or to a process involving one of the above, must be reported to the regulatory agency.[2,21] Packaging changes are classified as either major, moderate, or minor, depending on the nature of changes. The categories of changes indicate the regulatory requirements, reporting categories, and hence the levels of burden on the FDA and on the pharmaceutical industry. Major changes require a prior approval (PA) supplement. Moderate changes need a changes being effective (CBE) supplement, while minor changes can be reported to the FDA by the annual report (AR). Categorization of changes depends on the nature of the changes, and the intended use for products, such as for injectable, ophthalmic, liquid oral, solid oral, topical or transdermal dosage forms. It should be understood that the degree of concern for product–packaging interaction, and hence categorization of packaging changes, is different for different types of dosage forms. For example, changes in the size or shape of a container for a sterile drug substance might be considered as a moderate change, while the same changes might be treated as minor changes for solid oral dosage forms. Therefore, a category of PACPAC for one type of product cannot be assumed to be the same category for another type of product.

For solid oral dosage (SOD) forms, there are several questions one needs to answer before proposing post-approval packaging changes. These include:

1. Is the new packaging previously approved by FDA for the same type of dosage form?
2. What type of protection does the product need?

TABLE 24.4 Ranking of moisture vapor transmission rate per tablet and the resulting LOD of a model product

Packaging	MVTR/tablet (mg/tab/day at 25°C/60%RH)	Product lot	%LOD at 25°C/60%RH				
			Initial	6 M	12 M	24 M	36 M
Unit blister	0.078	1	2.7	3.4	3.8	4.5	4.6
		2	2.8	3.5	3.8	4.5	4.6
		3	2.7	3.4	3.8	4.6	4.6
HDPE bottle 1	0.024	1	2.8	3.2	3.5	3.9	4.1
		2	2.7	3.2	3.3	3.9	4.0
		3	2.7	3.3	3.4	3.9	4.1
HDPE bottle 2	0.004	1	2.6	2.7	2.6	2.7	2.7
		2	2.6	2.8	2.6	2.8	2.7
		3	2.8	2.7	2.7	2.9	2.9

3. Does the new packaging provide equivalent or better protection?
4. What type of packaging material information and what type of product stability testing in the new packaging are needed for submission?

Current FDA guidance to industry, Changes to An Approved NDA or ANDA,[21] provides some examples for each category of packaging changes, and a general statement on the potential impact the changes may have on the identity, strength, quality, purity or potency of a drug product as they may relate to the safety or effectiveness of the product. However, the guidance does not list specific requirements on information needed to report to the FDA for the changes. The FDA has been developing a more detailed guidance for post-approval changes for packaging (PACPAC) in recent years. Once finalized and published, the guidance is expected to list specific instructions on what changes to report, and how to report the changes, which will reduce the regulatory burden for the FDA and for the pharmaceutical industry.

The reporting category of packaging changes may be reduced if the new packaging has been approved by the FDA for the same type of dosage form, and if it is demonstrated that the new packaging can provide equivalent or better protection than the existing packaging. Obviously, if it can be demonstrated that a product is not sensitive to environmental conditions, such as moisture or oxygen, then the need for protection equivalency is not applicable for packaging changes. Protection equivalency can be demonstrated either by formal stability studies or by comparative tests. A formal stability study is not preferred for material characterization, because it is time consuming and expensive. Thus, comparative tests are preferred to increase efficiency, and reduce cost. For solid oral dosage forms, container MVTR is commonly used as

one of the criteria to demonstrate the moisture protection equivalency of containers. Two aspects of MVTR that should be taken into account include the reliability of MVTR values, and the correct use of these values. As discussed earlier in this chapter, MVTR for multiple-unit containers determined by the current USP method may be highly variable, and therefore not reliable. Modified methods, such as the steady state sorption method discussed earlier, should be used to ensure the validity of test results and the reliability of comparative evaluation of containers. Obtaining a reliable MVTR value does not yet draw conclusions on container equivalency for product protection. The correct use of the MVTR is more important for drawing meaningful conclusions. Currently, MVTR is reported in a unit of mg/L/day as per USP. This unit has limited utility, because it does not take into account the quantity of products in the container. For example, the USP unit of mg/L/day is not suitable for evaluating the protection equivalency of two different sizes of bottles containing different quantities of the same product. Alternatively, meaningful results can be obtained using a new unit of "MVTR per unit product"[12] proposed by the PQRI container closure working group. According to the studies conducted by the PQRI workgroup, moisture activity, and hence product moisture content in closed containers, is related to the unit of "MVTR per unit product." The lower the "MVTR per tablet" value, the lower the product moisture content, and it does not matter if the container is an HDPE bottle or an Aclar unit blister. Several examples have been reported in the above publication. More examples for using "MVTR per unit product" to rank container moisture protection property and to link it to product moisture content by stability studies are listed in Table 24.4. Tablets of the same lot were packaged in unit blisters, and in two sizes of HDPE bottles, for formal stability study at 25°C/60%RH. The ranking of the MVTR/unit for the three types of packaging are in the order of blister > bottle 1 > bottle 2. At the one-, two-, and three-year time points, significant differences in tablet moisture content were observed in the order of blister > bottle 1 > bottle 2. These data clearly demonstrate that "MVTR per unit product" is a valuable criterion for evaluating moisture protection equivalency of containers.

To summarize, the unit of "MVTR per unit product" links container property with product quality. The unit provides a means of evaluating different types of packaging materials, such as bottles and blisters, as well as a comparison of different quantities of products in varying or the same size of containers. Protection capability is the same or better, as long as "MVTR per unit product" is the same or smaller, regardless of the types of packaging materials and configurations, if moisture protection is the main concern. MVTR per unit product is therefore a science-based criterion for evaluating the moisture protection equivalency, and for justifying post-approval packaging changes.

References

1. ICH Harmonied Tripartite Guideline. (2003). Q1A(R2), Stability Testing of New Drug Substances and Products, November; Q1B Photostability Testing of New Drug Substances and Products, November 1996; Q1C Stability Testing for New Dosage Forms, May 1997.
2. FDA Guidance for Industry. (1999). Container Closure Systems for Packaging Human Drugs and Biologics.
3. FDA Guidance for Industry. (1999). Changes to an Approved NDA and ANDA. November.
4. USP XXX, Chapters <661> and <671>.
5. Hanlon, J.F., Kelsey, R.J. & Forcinio, H.E., (1998). *Handbook of Package Engineering*, 3rd edn. CRC Press, Boca Raton, FL. 101–102.
6. Weeren, R.V. & Gibboni, D.J. (2002). Drug. Del. Tech. 2, 48–53.
7. Armstrong, R.B. (2002). TAPPI PLACE Conference, Boston, MA, September 9–12, pp. 243–269.
8. Kamal, M.R. & Jinnah, I.A. (1984). Permeability of oxygen and water vapor through polyethylene/polyamide films. Polym. Eng. Sci. 24, 1337–1347.
9. Sezi, R. & Springer, J. (1981). Colloid and Polymer Science 259, 1170–1176.
10. Unisource Worldwide, Inc., Specification. http://www.unisourcelink.com
11. Taborsky, C.J. & Grady, L.T. (2001). Water vapor permeation of prescription vials. Pharmacopeial Forum 27, 2417–2427.
12. PQRI Container-Closure Working Group. (2005). Basis for using moisture vapor transmission rate per unit product in the evaluation of moisture-barrier equivalence of primary packages for solid oral dosage forms. Pharmacopeial Forum 31, 262–269.
13. Crank, J. (1986). *The Mathematics of Diffusion*. Clarendon Press, Oxford, pp. 49–51.
14. Chen, Y., Li, Y. & Sanzgiri, Y.D. (2008). Determination of water vapor transmission rate (WVTR) of HDPE bottles for pharmaceutical products. International Journal of Pharmaceutics 358, 137–143.
15. Dobson, R.L. (1987). Protection of pharmaceutical and diagnostic products through desiccant technology. Journal of Packaging Technology 1, 127–131.
16. Kontny, M.J. & Mulski, C.A. (1989). Gelatin capsule brittleness as a function of relative humidity at room temperature. International Journal of Pharmaceutics 54, 79–85.
17. Chang, R.K., Raghavan, K.S. & Hussain, M.A. (1998). A study on gelatin capsule brittleness: Moisture transfer between the capsule shell and its content. Journal of Pharmaceutical Sciences 87, 556–558.
18. Grattan, D.W. & Gilberg, M. (1994). Ageless oxygen absorber: Chemical and physical properties. Studies in Conservation 39, 210–214.
19. Lambert, F.L., Daniel, V. & Preusser, F.D. (1992). The rate of absorption of oxygen by Ageless™: The utility of an oxygen scavenger in sealed cases. Studies in Conservation 37, 267–274.
20. Chen, Y. & Li, Y. (2003). A new model for predicting moisture uptake by packaged solid pharmaceuticals. Journal of Pharmaceutical Sciences 255, 217–225.
21. FDA Guidance for Industry. (1999). Changes to an approved NDA or ANDA.

Clinical Supplies Manufacture: Strategy, Good Manufacturing Process Considerations, and Cleaning Validation

Brian W. Pack, Suchinda Stithit, Lisa Ray, Wei Chen, Jack Y. Zheng and Richard Hwang

25.1 INTRODUCTION

The process of new drug discovery research, development, and commercialization is long, complex, and costly. On the average, it can take more than 10 years, and cost $1 billion or more to bring a new chemical entity to the market. The new drug development process can be characterized into different phases including Phase I, II, III, and IV. The objective for each phase is described in Table 25.1. From Phase I to Phase III, clinical investigation is one of the most important activities to prove the safety and efficacy of a new drug. Obviously, successful supply of clinical materials is the key to assure that clinical studies are conducted as planned, at the right time, with the right dose, and with the right amount of materials. Manufacturing batch sizes of clinical supplies change with demand, availability of drug substances, and study phases. Clearly a strategy needs to be developed to effectively manage the complex clinical supplies manufacturing process.

This includes planning, collaborative communication among the cross-functional team, lean manufacturing, effective training programs, and application of new technologies to facilitate the manufacture of clinical supplies.

Clinical trials are designed to obtain safety and efficacy data for new drug candidates. A primary consideration in these studies is the safety of the clinical trial subjects. Additionally, careful consideration must be given to the quality of the clinical supplies produced, to ensure that there is no unintended consequence on the clinical trial results. Therefore, comprehensive current good manufacturing process (cGMP) controls must be put in place for the manufacture of clinical supplies, to ensure the delivery of quality products. A cleaning verification and/or a cleaning validation program is a key component of the cGMP controls and quality system, and an essential part of any pharmaceutical manufacturing facility. It must be demonstrated, either through cleaning–validation effort, that the cleaning process is under control or, through cleaning verification after each manufacture, that there is no cross-contamination from one lot to the next, such that the safety of product users is assured.

25.2 STRATEGY OF CLINICAL SUPPLIES MANUFACTURE

Over the last few years, there have been major challenges facing the pharmaceutical industry regarding growing regulatory burdens and global clinical trials. More rules and regulations on good clinical practice (GCP) have been implemented or recommended, because of ongoing concerns regarding unreported adverse events, inadequate protection of the clinical trial subjects (especially minors and incapacitated adults), inadequate oversight of clinical trials by Institutional Review Boards (IRBs),[1] unethical use of placebo-controlled trials, and deficient informed consent practices. At the same time, the costs of drug development and discovery have increased substantially. Bringing a new drug to market can cost anywhere between $900 million and $1.7 billion, depending on development and marketing costs. Only approximately one in ten thousand compounds synthesized will pass regulatory approval, and be commercialized, with only a few potential blockbuster drugs. Additionally, the time to bring a new drug to the market is increasing. The time from drug discovery to FDA approval for a new chemical entity (NCE) can be as long as 12 years.

Pharmaceutical companies are being forced to look at how to streamline their manufacturing practices and products.[2] The faster the new drug product is approved by the FDA, the longer the effective life of market exclusivity for the product before its patent expires.

Pharmaceutical manufacturers often rely on various strategies to help keep their new drug pipeline flowing freely. Effective management of clinical supplies delivery prevents it from becoming a rate-limiting step in product development, reduces the time for a new drug going through clinical trials, and ultimately increases the speed to bring a new drug to market. Due to the complexity and long duration of clinical trial programs, success depends on precise timing, monitoring, managing, and coordination of efforts, as well as a smooth flow of information and materials. The primary goal is to help connect clinical trial management teams with clinical supply manufacturing. The proper planning process is crucial to ensure that the project timeline is met. Collaborative communication among the team members, including research and development (R&D) personnel, quality control/quality assurance (QC/QA) personnel, regulatory personnel, medical personnel, clinical investigators, clinical trial material manufacturing personnel, and clinical trial material packaging personnel is essential for the success of the project. An implementation of clinical plan, clinical supplies liaison, a lean manufacturing approach, a cross-functional training program for workers, outsourcing, the use of new technology including modern

TABLE 25.1   Clinical trials in new drug development

Stages	Time	Subject/Study	Study objectives
Clinical trials in phase I	1–2 years	20–80 healthy volunteers Open study	Safety Dose and schedule Pharmacokinetics Pharmacological actions
Clinical trials in phase II	2–3 years	100–200 patients Controlled studies—multicenter	Safety and efficacy Dose, route and schedule Toxicity profile Clinical end points Dose–response curve Short-term adverse effects Pharmacokinetics Pharmacological actions
Clinical trials in phase III	2–4 years	>1000 patients Controlled studies—multicenter	Safety and efficacy in a large population Patient population Product claims Final formulation and product stability Drug related adverse effects
Clinical trials in phase IV	2–4 years	Controlled studies—multicenter	Additional information about the drug's risks, benefits, and optimal use, such as other patient populations, other stages of diseases, over a longer period, extend claims of safety and efficacy

computer technology and new methodologies in drug discovery and development, and process analytical technology (PAT) are among various strategies that can be used to improve clinical trial management. These topics will be discussed later in this chapter.

25.2.1 Clinical Plan

For each new drug candidate targeted for eventual registration, marketing, and distribution, a clinical plan is normally required. The clinical plan provides a detailed listing of clinical trials required for FDA approval, together with duration and the desired timelines.[3] Normally, project plan rationale, workload, and cost are discussed at management meetings or at project team meetings. Planning must include short-term, intermediate-term, and long-term goals with assumptions for bulk drug substance requirements, dose strengths, and quantity of drug product to manufacture. Comparator drug products also need to be

considered. The short-term and intermediate-term planning (1 to 6 months) must include final plans for manufacturing, including the bulk product request with approximately 4-month to 6-month lead time, and packaging requests, which should be received 2 to 3 months before the expected shipping date. Long-term strategic plans can be prepared based on equipment/facility capacity, volume prediction, budget or resources, preferred vendor or contractor relationships, and comparator or drug substance sourcing. There are many challenges in planning for distribution of the clinical trial supplies to multiple investigation centers, especially those in different countries worldwide. Regulations-specific requirements for each country running the clinical trials must be thoroughly understood and considered during the planning.

Long-term strategic planning may be based on workload prioritization, contract arrangements, and inventory management. On the other hand, short-term or immediate-term planning is related more to completing jobs at hand. Clinical plans and process must

TABLE 25.2 Template for phase I clinical trials

Activity name	# of days	Start date	End date	Responsible manager
Clinical protocol development				
• Study objective and rationale				
• Study design and outcomes				
• Subject inclusion and exclusion criteria, and enrollment procedures				
• Study interventions				
• Clinical and laboratory evaluations				
• Management of adverse experiences				
• Criteria for intervention discontinuation				
• Statistical considerations				
• Data collection/site monitoring				
• Adverse experience reporting				
• Subjects/IRB review/informed consent				
Investigator and site selection				
• Investigator's brochure				
• Sponsor–investigator agreement				
Clinical supply vendor/contractor selection				
• Plan and management of vendors				
• Communication plan				
• Vendor quality assurance/cgmp audit				
• Signed agreement				
Clinical trial materials and distribution plan				
• Manufacturing				
• Packaging and labeling				
• Shipment				
Budget/financial aspects				
Regulatory filing / reporting				
Trial master file				
Study site notebook				
Clinical study management /monitoring plan				

(Continued)

TABLE 25.2   (Continued)

Activity name	# of days	Start date	End date	Responsible manager
Case report form (crf)/data management • Database design and setup • Data security and validation				
Quality assurance of clinical trial documents/activities • Site GCP audit				
Risk identification and contingency plan				
Training all personnel involved in the study				
Site management				
Subject recruitment initiation				

be reviewed and updated on a regular basis, to keep the liaison and other team members in the same place with the possible changes for modification of protocols. It is generally a good idea to establish a frame of reference to define how, when, and by whom, to change what—commonly referred to as a "change control" plan. This "change control" should be complementary to the planning process. Planning is the process that requires management to ensure that the project is completed within the timeline. All the risks involved in the project should be identified and assessed during the planning process. The probability of risks occurring, the impact of the risks on the project, and a contingency plan should be incorporated into the planning activities.

A clinical plan template can be developed, since clinical studies usually follow the same basic tasks and flow, regardless what product is being studied. Using the template approach helps to accelerate the project timeline, and bring in best practices learned from past development projects. Table 25.2 illustrates the tasks commonly required in phase I clinical trial studies.

25.2.2 Clinical Supplies Liaison

The clinical supplies liaison (or clinical trials materials manager/team leader, medical coordinator or clinical logistic coordinator) plays an important role in the drug development–clinical trial process. The titles or names for this position may be different, but the tasks that need to be performed are essentially the same. The liaison must understand the project to be able to lead the project successfully, and must effectively communicate and convey the clinical study process and progress to team members, and prioritize task activities and timelines. The liaison should understand team member individuals and their cultures. He or she must be able to organize, manage, negotiate

with, educate, and compromise with multidisciplinary team members to develop the best scenario for all parties involved. A successful liaison must have a strong scientific background, and strong people management skills, i.e., the ability to interact and effectively negotiate with other people. A successful liaison can lead his or her team or customers to achieve a sought-after goal, and eventually push the project through the finishing line in the face of numerous setbacks, delay, adversity, and failures.

25.2.3 Lean Manufacturing

Lean manufacturing is a business management philosophy that seeks to eliminate or reduce waste, and maximize customer value through employee involvement. It evolved mostly from successful Japanese practices in production systems. The lean manufacturing paradigm calls for integration of employee involvement and technological practices. It focuses on the human-centered approach to the design and implementation of advanced manufacturing systems.[4,5] Lean manufacturing is a dynamic system that requires fewer resources, less material, less inventory, less labor, less equipment, less time, and less space. It is intended to eliminate waste, while meeting and exceeding customer requirements and bringing better output, e.g., quality, variety, cost, time, and safety (Figure 25.1).

There are three main approaches in lean manufacturing that lead to better output. First, lean manufacturing involves a new philosophy of manufacturing which focuses on better quality, exceeding customer requirements, and continuous improvement. Secondly, lean manufacturing involves establishment of a new culture and managerial system to incorporate the lean philosophy. The lean team leader and lean steering committee are included in their organizations to

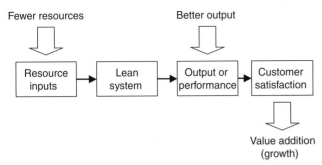

FIGURE 25.1 A lean manufacturing system

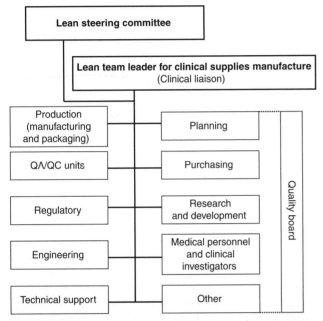

FIGURE 25.2 Implementation of the lean manufacturing system

manage product development, supply chain relations, production operations, and coordination of the overall enterprise toward lean manufacturing. Thirdly, lean manufacturing uses techniques that address specific problems such as just-in-time (JIT), total productive maintenance (TPM), total quality management (TQM), human resource management (HRM), scientific management, six sigma, quality circles, simultaneous engineering, and inventory systems. In a true lean organization, defects or problems are discovered immediately, and solutions are sought right away using whatever techniques are required.

Figure 25.2 shows a model for implementation of lean manufacturing in clinical supplies manufacture in a pharmaceutical firm. The first step occurs when management commits to the lean philosophy illustrated by the three goals:

- Zero Waste is to eliminate what does not belong to the value stream;

- Value Stream Mapping is to identify the scope of activities conforming the value stream; and
- Pull (Kaizen) is to develop workforce capabilities by continuous, gradual, and persistent improvement.

As a new practice of manufacturing, lean manufacturing demands new capabilities from all employees at all levels: problem-solving, focus, teamwork, and creative thinking. Lean manufacturing is not a fixed set of techniques, as has been discussed earlier. As part of the implementation, new techniques unique for each business culture will emerge at each company. However, since businesses share the same interests and join a competitive market, common techniques are likely to appear. The examples of common techniques include:

- Just-in-time (JIT): Just-in-time is a philosophy of manufacturing that focuses on supplying the right materials to the right place in the right quantity just-in-time to achieve perfect work flow, while minimizing waste. It depends on the pull process from the consumer (demand) end, not the push from the production (supply) end. Materials are supplied to the production line only when they are required. JIT can be achieved by using the following techniques: lot size reductions, continuous flow production, pull systems, cycle-time reductions, focused factory production systems, agile manufacturing strategies, quick changeover techniques, bottleneck or constraint removal, and re-engineered production processes.
- Total productive maintenance (TPM): Total productive maintenance is aimed to increase equipment effectiveness, by eliminating the losses due to machine downtime using techniques such as predictive or preventive maintenance, maintenance optimization, safety improvement programs, planning and scheduling strategies, and new process equipment. TPM works on the continuous flow of production. Any interruption to the flow, such as machine breakdown, is considered and treated as waste.
- Total quality management (TQM): Total quality management is designed to improve customer satisfaction and product quality by using several techniques, such as quality systems, quality management programs, process capability measurements, six sigma, competitive benchmarking, and formal continuous improvement programs.
- Human resource management (HRM): Human resource management is designed to effectively use human resources to increase overall performance.

It focuses on leadership, empowerment, communication, and training by using several techniques such as self-directed work teams, cross-functional frameworks, and open communications, in order to bring out the best possible in employees.

Clinical supplies manufacture provides cGMP compliant products at a capability that is designed to deliver on-time clinical supplies, meeting or exceeding customer needs in support of clinical trials. Clinical supplies for the early phase clinical trials (phase I and II) typically need to have acceptable-to-good stability, meet basic dosage form requirements (i.e., assay, impurities, content uniformity) and specific release requirements (i.e., dissolution), and be suitable for small- to intermediate-scale manufacturing (i.e., from hundreds to thousands of units or from several to tens of kilograms). On the other hand, clinical supplies for the later phase clinical trials (phase III) typically need to have good stability, meet all dosage form requirements (including in-process testing requirements) and specific release requirements (i.e., dissolution), be suitable for larger pilot scale manufacturing (i.e., ~50–100 kg), and be scalable to production scale (>100 kg). The numbers of products and volume to manufacture also change as the study phase advances. Typically, the number of products to manufacture, and hence process variety for clinical supplies, decreases and product volume increases with the advancement of clinical trial phases (see Figure 25.3).

The JIT technique can be applied effectively to clinical supplies manufacture for early phase clinical trials, because of the high variety and low product volume for this phase. When clinical trials advance into phase III, lean manufacturing techniques, including just-in-time, total preventive maintenance, total quality management, and human resource management, can be applied to the clinical supplies manufacture, because of the low variety and high volume of the batches.

The lean manufacturing philosophy and methodology can be applied throughout the spectrum of development and manufacturing, from pre-clinical to clinical, from the overall strategic level of the development operation, to the specific and detailed level of the manufacturing processes. Lean manufacturing provides a structured, disciplined, and logical progression for organizations to achieve improvement and breakthrough in quality.

25.2.4 Cross-functional Training

Cross-functional training and education programs are an important consideration in the clinical trial supplies system. All team members should know the system and their roles and contribution to pushing projects through the finishing line. For example, ensuring that all clinical research associates understand why and how to order study medications and comprehend aspects of lead-time is a simple example of instantly recognizable, value-added education and training. Customer orientation and TQM, which are well-known systems in Japanese manufacturing industries, can be used to improve performance within the clinical trial supplies system. Each department should consider how to improve customer satisfaction and the customer relationship. For example, contract manufacturing organizations (CMOs) and third party vendors hired by pharmaceutical manufacturers rely on data about clinical trials and supplies to plan and execute their work. Instead of considering these CMOs as suppliers to deliver the clinical supplies for the clinical trials, the CMOs become customers of the pharmaceutical manufacturer whose drug discovery department delivers bulk active pharmaceutical ingredients (APIs) to them. The bulk APIs, and other related clinical trial data, should be delivered to CMOs before or at least on schedule to satisfy CMOs. Any interruption in the process, such as a delay in the delivery of the bulk drug substance from pharmaceutical manufacturers, can seriously disrupt the timing and success of their work.

25.2.5 Outsourcing of Manufacturing and Packaging

A drug sponsor may want to contract out its clinical supplies manufacturing and packaging for several reasons. Contract manufacturing and packaging

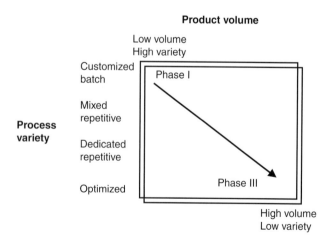

FIGURE 25.3   Relationship of clinical trial phases, process variety, and product volume of clinical supplies manufacture

organizations (CMOs) may provide an expertise or technology required for the project.[6] In addition, contracting out clinical supplies converts the fixed costs of maintaining the personnel and production facilities necessary for manufacturing and packaging the clinical supplies into variable costs of paying CMOs to perform the task, and eliminates the need for a set number of people, facilities, and equipment in-house. However, many drug sponsors choose to manufacture and package their clinical supplies in-house, because they prefer the control and flexibility, and in-house expertise. The question of who will benefit from outsourcing to a CMO might be better asked as why the sponsor cannot or should not do it in-house. The answer is mainly dependent upon just a few factors, such as how a drug sponsor and its board balance risk; whether its product pipeline is full; whether it decides to manufacture and package the commercialized product itself after NDA approval. There are both advantages and disadvantages for contracting clinical trial supplies, as shown in Table 25.3.

In general, small companies (especially small biotech companies) have fewer options, and are most likely to move toward outsourcing. Their limited development pipelines, lack of capacity, and skill deficiency make the decision clear; the risk of investing in capital and experienced staff outweighs the benefit of in-house cGMP pilot or production plants. Mid-tier companies may have the capability to have the cGMP pilot or production plants in-house, but they and their

investors must carefully assess the risks of product failure against their ability to survive such an event. Large pharmaceutical companies can build the capacity in-house, but they also see contract manufacturing as a way to reduce risk in their global manufacturing strategy.

Today, dedicated contractors can provide clinical trial manufacturing services. There are more CMOs offering a wide variety of competencies, reliable service, and competitively high quality. As a result, an increasing number of virtual biotech and large pharmaceutical companies are positioned to exploit CMOs.

25.2.6 New Technology

Integrated clinical trial management software solutions and technologies are currently available to help the pharmaceutical industry meet more stringent compliance challenges. For example, the clinical investigators in multiple countries worldwide can access a database at the same time, using complex planning tools which allow clinical trials at multiple centers in many countries to be coordinated and planned more effectively. Similar technologies are also available for clinical packaging groups to electronically collaborate with clinical investigators, instead of using a paper-based system. New software and technologies allow pharmaceutical companies to more effectively address challenges, and improve their new drug development process.

TABLE 25.3 The advantages and disadvantages of contracting versus in-house production of clinical supplies manufacturing and packaging

Advantages	Disadvantages
In-house	In-house
1. Maintain oversight of quality—reducing risks of production failures	1. High capital costs because facility/equipment may need to be upgraded or acquired
2. More direct control of outcome—reducing risks of bottlenecks	2. May delay another important project
3. Easy to set or change priorities on multiple projects	
4. Lower cost	
5. Easier for technology transfer process	
6. Gain expertise of manufacturing and packaging the new product	
7. Retain intellectual property	
Contract out	Contract out
1. CMOs have expertise and experiences with many companies	1. Resources are needed to manage the CMOs
2. Convert fixed costs into variable costs	2. Difference in culture of the two companies can take more time to work through
3. Save time and cost to upgrade or improve facility/equipment	3. Communication can be more cumbersome
4. Better system in specialized field	4. Less control of project's priority and schedule
5. Can test robustness of the process	5. Confidentiality breach

25.3 GOOD MANUFACTURING PRACTICE (GMP) CONSIDERATIONS IN MANUFACTURING CLINICAL SUPPLIES

25.3.1 Current Good Manufacturing Practice (cGMP) Considerations

The FDA and the pharmaceutical industry have recognized that most early-phase clinical studies are conducted long before the details of product formulation, manufacturing specifications, and production processes are fully defined and validated. Therefore, some of the cGMP requirements are simply not logically applicable to phase I clinical studies. The FDA has expressed a clear recognition of the difference between manufacturing investigational products and commercial products. The agency, however, has a firm commitment to enforce the cGMP requirements, and ensure compliance throughout all phases of development, as stated in the 1991 Guideline on the Preparation of Investigational New Drug Products.[7] In January 2006, the FDA published a draft Guidance for Industry: INDs—Approaches to Complying with cGMP's During Phase 1.[8] The FDA is working toward the goal of advancing public health by improving the product development process and increasing the speed of approval processes for new and better medical treatments. The draft guidance reflects the FDAs current thinking with regard to quality systems and risk management (or hazard control) principles, which is consistent with the FDAs ongoing "cGMP for the 21st Century" initiative.[9]

The Food, Drug, and Cosmetic Act provides that the FDA may approve an NDA only if the methods used in, and the facilities and controls used for, the manufacture, processing, packing, and testing of the drug are found adequate to ensure and preserve its identity, strength, quality, and purity. The FDAs role in the pre-approval process is to review data submitted, evaluate, and approve specifications for the manufacture and control of the drug products based on the submitted data, to ensure cGMP compliance, and to verify the authenticity and accuracy of the data contained in the NDA application.[10]

The cGMPs are not directly concerned with business performance. The FDAs evaluation is usually directed toward compliance issues such as rejects, reworks, and complaints as indicators of inadequately validated production processes, and process deviations as examples of system noncompliance. In fact, the FDA inspection team frequently visits the reject area early in an inspection in order to identify failures. They can then go back into the respective batch records to

evaluate the cause, and to see if adequate remediation has been established and implemented.

FDA inspection teams, highly skilled in drug manufacturing, packaging, and analytical technology, may consist of investigators, analysts, engineers, and/or computer experts, as appropriate. Prior to NDA approval, FDA investigators or inspection teams may perform inspections/data audits, and they will validate/verify the proposed methods.[10] The FDA can conduct pre-approval inspections or audit any processes involved in the NDA submission including, but not limited to, manufacturing of drug substance(s), biobatch manufacturing, raw materials controls, composition and formulation of finished dosage form, container/closure systems, laboratory support of methods validation, product and process controls, product specifications and test methods, product stability, comparison of relevant pre-approval batches and proposed commercial batches, facility–personnel–equipment qualifications, equipment specifications, packaging and labeling controls, process validations, reprocessing, and ancillary facilities (e.g., contract testing laboratories, contract packagers). For example, the FDA may audit biobatch manufacturing batch records to determine if the establishment is in compliance with cGMP requirements. This may include a data audit of the specific batches upon which the application is based (e.g., pivotal clinical studies, bioavailability, bioequivalence or stability batches).

The production of investigational drug products involves added complexity in comparison to marketed or commercial products, due to lack of fixed routines, variety of clinical trial designs, highly specific packaging designs, and needs for randomization and for blinding that increase the risk of product mix-up. It is clear that there may be added risk to clinical trial subjects, compared to patients treated with commercial products. Compliance to cGMP or quality assurance in manufacture of investigational drug product will minimize the risk to the clinical trial subjects. General cGMP considerations on manufacturing of clinical supplies include:

- Quality Management: The investigational clinical trial products or investigational medicinal products (IMP) must be manufactured under controlled processes as per cGMP requirements, and the release of materials should not occur until they meet the predetermined specifications and are released by the quality unit. This ensures that the investigational clinical trial products used for any trial centers have the same or equivalent quality, purity, and safety. The cGMPs are enforced to ensure that there should not be any unsatisfactory manufacturing and packaging processes, which might increase the risk of substandard investigational clinical trial products being given to human subjects during clinical studies. The clinical supplies manufacturer must have a qualified person to verify that the investigational clinical trial products manufactured, packaged, repackaged, and imported conform to the product specifications prior to releasing the batches.

- Manufacturing and Process Control: In many cases, clinical trial runs of a new drug are produced in facilities other than the ones used for full-scale production. The facilities and controls used for the manufacture of investigational clinical trial products, especially the NDA biobatches, should be in conformance with cGMPs regulations. Accurate documentation of batch records is essential, so that the production process can be defined and related to batches used for early clinical, bioavailability or bioequivalence studies of a new drug. Specifications, formulations and manufacturing processes should be as completely defined as possible, based on the current state of knowledge. Critical process parameters should be identified, and the respective in-process controls should be implemented. Specifications, formulations, and manufacturing processes should periodically be reassessed during development, and updated as necessary. There should be sufficient manufacturing and process controls to ensure consistency and reproducibility between clinical trial batches, bio/stability batches used in the same or different clinical trials, and a proposed commercial production process. Any changes from initial manufacturing procedures should be fully documented, and carried out according to written procedures, which should justify and address any implications for product quality, purity, and safety.

- Documentation: The information and knowledge gained from pharmaceutical development studies provide scientific understanding to support the establishment of specifications and manufacturing controls. Therefore, it is essential that all information and knowledge be fully and properly documented. For example, at early stages, the acceptance/rejection criteria may not be as specific; however, these criteria will be more specific and uniform as additional data become available. It is vital that the criteria used and scientific supportive data is fully documented at all stages. The product specifications file (e.g., specifications and analytical methods, manufacturing processes, in-process testing and methods, stability data, and storage and shipment conditions) should be continually updated and documented as development of the product proceeds, ensuring traceability to the previous versions.

- Batch Records: To prevent any potential mix-up or ambiguity, the order in writing for the number of units and/or shipping of the clinical trial product should be received and authorized prior to manufacturing, packaging and/or shipping of the clinical trial batches. The manufacturing batch records for an investigational drug product must be retained for at least five years[11] after the conclusion of the trial or formal discontinuation of the last clinical trial in which the batch was used. During that period the record must be complete and readily available for inspection.

- Laboratory Control: Laboratory equipment and procedures must be qualified and validated. At the early phase of clinical trials, analytical methods performed to evaluate the batches of API used for clinical trials may not yet be fully validated, yet there must be enough control based on scientific information. FDA inspectors will review the authenticity and accuracy of data used in the development of a test method.

- Incoming Materials for Clinical Supplies: When more than one supplier and source of each incoming material, especially the active ingredients, are used during clinical trials, the sponsor should demonstrate that the clinical batches produced from different suppliers, and sources of incoming materials, are equivalent in terms of conformance with established specifications including those stated in the NDA application. The sponsor should undertake due diligence to ensure that the incoming materials meet specifications, and are produced under a state of control.

- Building and Facilities: An addition of any new drug to a production environment must be carefully evaluated as to its impact on other products already under production, and changes that will be necessary to the building and facilities. Construction of new walls, installation of new equipment, and other significant changes must be evaluated for their impact on overall compliance with cGMP requirements. The toxicity, potency, and sensitizing potential may not be fully understood for investigational clinical trial products, and this reinforces the need to minimize all risks of cross-contamination. The risk of cross-contamination can be minimized by using properly designed equipment and facilities, as well as by having in place written comprehensive methods for manufacturing, packaging, inspecting, sampling, testing, cleaning, and sanitizing procedures.[8,12]

- Equipment System: New products, particularly potent drug products, can present cleaning problems in existing equipment. There must be written procedures for sanitation, calibration, and maintenance of equipment, and specific instructions for the use of the equipment and procedures used to manufacture the drug product.[8,12] To prevent the risk of cross-contamination, many companies utilize isolators, as well as single use or dedicated equipment, during the production of investigational clinical trial products.
- Training Program: All personnel involved with investigational products should be appropriately trained in the requirements specific to their duties. Trained, qualified, and experienced persons should be responsible for ensuring that there are systems in place that meet the cGMP requirements. Any training should be documented and kept on file.
- Specifications: Specifications (for starting materials, primary packaging materials, intermediate, bulk products, and finished products), manufacturing formulas, and processing and packaging instructions should be as comprehensive as possible, given the current state of knowledge. They should be periodically reassessed during development, and updated as necessary. Each new version should take into account the latest data, current technology used, regulatory and pharmacopeial requirements, and should allow traceability to the previous document. Any changes should be carried out according to a written procedure, which should address any implications for product quality, such as stability and bioequivalence. "The controls used in the manufacture of APIs for use in clinical trials should be consistent with the stage of development of the drug product incorporating these APIs. Process and test procedure change management should be flexible to provide for changes as knowledge of the process increases and clinical testing of a drug product progresses from pre-clinical stages through clinical stages."[12]

The FDA recognizes that the experimental nature of the drug substance, formulation, and dosage form at an early stage of development has an impact on establishing specifications. At early stages, the acceptance/rejection criteria may not be as specific; however, it is vital that such criteria be scientifically sound, and based upon available scientific data. Specifications used as the basis for approval or rejection of components, container, and closures will be more specific and uniform as additional data become available.[13] The specifications for raw materials and excipients, in-process testing, process evaluation or validation, finished product testing, and stability testing for investigational medical products should be set to ensure that the appropriate quality of the product will be maintained.

- Stability: For phase I clinical trials, it should be confirmed that an ongoing stability program will be carried out with the relevant batch(es) and that, prior to the start of the clinical trial, at least studies under accelerated and long-term storage conditions will have been initiated. When available, the results from these studies should be summarized in a tabulated form. Any supportive data from development studies should be summarized in a tabular overview. An evaluation of the available stability data related to storage conditions stated on the product labels and justification of the proposed period of use, expiration date or retest dates to be assigned to the investigational medicinal product (IMP) in the clinical study should be provided. For phase II and phase III clinical trials, the available stability data should be presented to regulatory agents in a tabulated form. An evaluation of the available data, and justification of the proposed shelf life to be assigned to the IMP in the clinical study, should be provided. Data should include results from studies under accelerated and long-term storage conditions.[14]
- Validation: Non-critical manufacturing processes for clinical trial products are not expected to be validated to the extent necessary for routine production. However, there must be the combination of controls, calibration, and equipment qualification to ensure that the manufacturing processes for clinical trial products are of the same standard as for commercial products.[15]
- Packaging and Labeling Control: Clinical trial supplies are normally packaged in an individual container for each subject in the clinical investigation. The packaging and labeling of investigational clinical trial products are usually more complex than commercial drug products, especially when placebo and active products are packaged with the same appearance and usage label for double-blinded clinical studies. Sufficient reconciliations and proper controls should be in place to ensure the correct quantity of each product required has been accounted for at each stage of processing. Poor labeling control and accountability may have an adverse impact on the firm's ability to ensure that the new drug will always be properly labeled.

"During packaging of investigational medicinal products, it may be necessary to handle different products on the same packaging line at the same time. The risk of product mix-up must be minimized by using appropriate procedures, and/or specialized equipment as appropriate, and relevant staff training must be given."[16]

"Packaging and labeling of medicinal products under investigation are likely to be more complex and more liable to errors (which are also harder to detect) than for marketed products, particularly when blinded products with a similar appearance are used. Precautions against mislabeling, such as label reconciliation, line clearance, in-process control checks by appropriate trained staff, should accordingly be intensified."[16]

- Distribution of Clinical Trial Material: Distribution of clinical trial material to the trial sites must be in accordance with the local laws and regulations specific to the countries of destination. For example, many countries require clinical trial material labels to be translated into the local language. The clinical trial material must be secured and stored under conditions specified in the label.[11]

In a blinded study, a written emergency unblinding method must be established, trained for, and implemented. "Decoding arrangements should be available to the appropriate responsible personnel before investigational medicinal products are shipped to the investigator site."[16]

The investigator is responsible only for drug accountability at the site, and the sponsor is responsible for overall clinical trial materials distributed for use in a trial. Clinical trial material is reconciled at the site level, as well as country/affiliate level. Any discrepancies must be documented and investigated. "The delivered, used and recovered quantities of product should be recorded, reconciled and verified by or on behalf of the sponsor for each trial site and each trial period. Destruction of unused investigation medicinal products should be carried out for a given trial site or a given trial period only after any discrepancies have been investigated and satisfactorily explained and the reconciliation has been accepted. Recording of destruction operations should be carried out in such a manner that all operations may be accounted for. The records should be kept by the sponsor."[16]

"When destruction of investigation medicinal products takes place, a dated certificate of, or receipt for destruction, should be provided to the sponsor. These documents should clearly identify, or allow traceability to, the batches and/or patient numbers involved and the actual quantities destroyed."[16]

25.3.2 A Risk-based Approach

The FDA, the pharmaceutical industry, healthcare professionals, and patients share a common goal of having reliable, high quality, safe, and effective products. There are needs for new products to improve public health. On the other hand, the knowledge about products and processes may not be fully understood for investigational clinical trial products, especially those used in the early phase of clinical study. Through manufacturing science, pharmaceutical firms accumulate knowledge about products, processes, and technology used to manufacture and control these processes, which in turn lay the foundation for a robust quality system. The quality system focuses on critical pharmaceutical quality attributes, including chemistry, pharmaceutical formulation, manufacturing process, product quality, and performance, and their relevance to safety and efficacy. To produce reliable, high quality, safe, and effective products including early phase investigational medicinal products, the desired state of manufacturing is as follows:

- Product quality and performance are achieved and assured by design of an effective and efficient manufacturing process.[17] Quality should be built into the product, instead of relying on testing product alone to ensure product quality. Pharmaceutical firms must continue to move from a compliance mindset to quality by design (building in quality by defining design spaces of product and processes from the development phase and throughout the product's lifecycle). The specifications and process parameters are determined and established by the technical experts, who have a thorough understanding of pharmaceutical science, equipment, facilities, and processes. Any variations in materials and processes that can affect the finished product's identity, purity, and quality should be considered during establishment of the specifications and process parameters.

- Innovative and new technologies are used continuously to improve manufacturing and quality assurance. For example, a common risk associated with a highly potent investigational clinical trial material is cross-contamination during manufacturing of the product. Many pharmaceutical firms choose to use single-use disposable equipment, and components such as disposable bags, tubing, filters, and storage containers to eliminate cross-contamination risk, and to reduce the time spent cleaning and setting up equipment. Proper process design, quality assuring, and component selection are important for the successful implementation of single-use disposable equipment and components. Process analytical technology (PAT) is another example of an advanced technology that can facilitate building the knowledge base and mitigate risk. PAT can be used to aid designing, analyzing, and controlling manufacturing processes. PAT allows a better understanding of processes through timely measurement, and can be used to evaluate quickly changes that impact product quality, thereby reducing risk during manufacturing processes. PAT changes the traditional concepts of process validation, and leads to continuous quality verification strategies.[18]

- Manufacturing science is applied to understand process capability, to ensure that the manufacturing processes are performed in a reproducible manner, and to manage the risk impacting the processes or product quality throughout their lifecycle. Elements of risk should be evaluated, based on the intended use of a product, patient safety, and the availability of drug product supplies. Continuous improvement efforts must be employed to increase process capability and reduce risk.

- Knowledge is shared between pharmaceutical firms and the FDA. The firms should share sufficient knowledge to provide the FDA with process understanding and rationale for the development of specifications and analytical methods. Adequate pharmaceutical development information, including identification of critical quality parameters and attributes, and the justified formulations should be provided to aid understanding the product and processes.

- Risk management review teams and frameworks are used by pharmaceutical firms. Pharmaceutical firms should prioritize activities or actions, based on a risk-assessment, including both the probability of the occurrence of harm, and of the severity of that harm. Based on the level of risk, the firm should apply appropriate manufacturing science and develop control strategies in order to prevent or mitigate the risk of producing a poor-quality product. The firm's risk-based decisions must be made to ensure the identity, purity, potency, and quality as related to safety and efficacy of new drugs throughout their lifecycle (from IND to post-marketing phases).

The desired state of manufacturing discussed above is an objective for the pharmaceutical "cGMPs for the 21st Century: a risk-based approach,"which was announced by the FDA in August 2002 (it aims to ensure that resources are focused on high-risk areas).[19] However, it is the firms' responsibility to ensure that low- and medium-risk areas remain in appropriate states of control, since these lower risk classes will receive less FDA regulatory attention. The FDA has expressed its commitment to modernize the pharmaceutical GMP regulations, and to streamline the clinical development process, to ensure that basic scientific discoveries can be translated more rapidly into new and better medical treatment. In September 2006, the FDA published "Guidance for Industry: Quality Systems Approach to Pharmaceutical cGMP Regulations."[17] The guidance, which was intended to serve as a bridge between the 1978 regulations[3] and the current FDA understanding of quality systems, explains how implementing quality systems can help drug product manufacturers to achieve compliance with current GMP requirements. Although the guidance applies to pharmaceutical finished product manufacturers, it can also be used to guide clinical supply manufacturing.

25.4 CLEANING VALIDATION AND VERIFICATION

The Code of Federal Regulations Part 211—Current good manufacturing practice for finished pharmaceuticals Subpart D—Equipment Sec. 211.67 on equipment cleaning and maintenance states that:

> "Equipment and utensils shall be cleaned, maintained, and sanitized at appropriate intervals to prevent malfunctions or contamination that would alter the safety, identity, strength, quality, or purity of the drug product beyond the official or other established requirements."
> And that "written procedures shall be established and followed for cleaning and maintenance of equipment, including utensils, used in the manufacture, processing, packing, or holding of a drug product."[20]

In accordance with 21 CFR 211.67, the International Conference on Harmonisation (ICH) has issued recommendations on Equipment Maintenance and Cleaning (Q7A, section 5.20–5.26) for compliance and safety which include very similar requirements, with more elaboration on specific details.[21] Again, there is a reiteration that written procedures must be established, and that detailed cleaning agent selection and preparation, responsibilities, schedules, and cleaning acceptance limits be documented with rationales. The purpose is to prevent cross-contamination between different manufactured lots. This cross-contamination concern applies not only to the active pharmaceutical ingredient; it also applies to residual cleaning solvents and detergents.

Even with these seemingly basic requirements outlined above, there have been multiple warning letters issued to pharmaceutical manufacturing facilities since 2002, due to violations of 21 CFR 211.67. Figure 25.4 illustrates the frequency of 483s issued where an infraction against 21 CFR 211.67 was cited (obtained from the CDER Website).[22]

The purpose of this section is to review the approaches for cleaning of equipment used for product

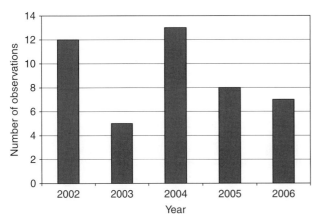

FIGURE 25.4 Frequency of FDA 483 warning letters issued for cleaning violations from 2002 through August 2006

manufacturing. The difference between cleaning validation and cleaning verification is outlined first. An approach is presented to determine the appropriate number and locations of cleaning verification sites (i.e. swabbing locations) used to test for residual product on equipment. Acceptance limit calculations are provided that represent either 1/1000 or 10 ppm product carryover in clinical trial operations. A summary of the current analytical methodologies that have been utilized for cleaning verification assay, along with how to validate a cleaning verification assay, is also presented.

25.4.1 Cleaning Validation Versus Cleaning Verification

Cleaning validation is an extensive, multi-functional program, where the entire manufacturing process is considered from the equipment that will be used to the analytical method that will be used to evaluate cleaning effectiveness.[23] Cleaning validation starts with the preparation of a validation protocol. The validation protocol would include rationales in regard to cleaning agents and procedures,[24] equipment, equipment swabbing locations,[25] safety-based acceptance limits, selection of products used to demonstrate validation,[26,26] and validated analytical methodology. Cleaning verification is a demonstration for each manufacturing run (typically by submission of cleaning swabs to the analytical laboratories) that the active pharmaceutical ingredient has been removed to a level below the pre-established acceptance limit.

When selecting representative products to validate a cleaning program, several approaches have been presented.[26,29] The most conservative approach would be to validate the cleaning procedure for all compounds manufactured. However, this approach is expensive, resource consuming, and thus is impractical. Therefore, manufacturers may choose to validate on a subset of compounds, and examine such parameters as solubility, potency (which drives the acceptance limit), and cleanability. The location and number of swabbing locations for both verification and validation activities are dictated by the product contact surface area (e.g., larger components may require a larger number of swabs), energy dissipation (e.g., roller compaction or tablet pressing regions are more likely to accumulate product), composition of the product contact areas (i.e., polycarbonate versus stainless steel), and cleaning difficulty (tight corners, bends, and hard-to-reach places result in hard-to-clean locations that should be swabbed).[28]

25.4.2 Swab Test Acceptance Criteria

When determining the acceptance limit, a strong scientific rationale with relevant factors generally includes: (1) evaluation of the therapeutic dose of the actives; (2) toxicity of the potential contaminant; (3) solubility of the potential residue; (4) difficulty of cleaning; (5) visual examination; (6) the batch size of the subsequent products on the same equipment; and (7) how the product will be used.[27] Acceptance limit calculations take on the general form where two methods are typically used. Although some authors recommend adjusting the safety factor dependent upon the dosage form,[30] it is most common to utilize the 1/1000th minimum dose and 10 parts per million (ppm) methods.[28,29,30,31,32]

The 1/1000th method assumes that pharmaceuticals are often considered to be non-active at 0.1% of their prescribed therapeutic dosages.[35] The following equation demonstrates how an acceptance limit is calculated utilizing the 1/1000th method:

$$\text{Acceptance Limit}\left(\frac{\mu g}{\text{swab}}\right) = \frac{0.001 \ \frac{\text{Smallest Strength Product A (mg/day)}}{\text{Maximum Daily \# of Dosage Units Product B (units/day)}}}{}$$

$$\times \frac{\text{Lot Size Product B (\# of dosage units)}}{\text{Shared Surface Area (cm}^2 \text{ or in}^2\text{)}}$$

$$\times \frac{\text{Swab area (cm}^2\text{ or in}^2\text{)}}{1 \text{ swab}} \times \frac{1000 \ \mu g}{1 \text{ mg}}$$

$$(25.1)$$

Product A is the product made on the equipment to be cleaned, and product B is the product to be manufactured on the same equipment after it has been used and cleaned for product A.

The second method uses the 10 ppm limit historically used to calculate commercial manufacturing limits. This method allows the maximum carryover of product to be calculated using lot sizes and shared equipment surface area. The formula below shows the method used to develop the 10 ppm acceptance limits:

$$\text{Acceptance Limit}\left(\frac{\mu g}{\text{swab}}\right) = \frac{10\ mg}{1\ kg} \times \frac{\text{Lot Size Product B (kg)}}{\text{Shared Surface Area (cm}^2 \text{ or in}^2)} \times \frac{\text{swab area (cm}^2 \text{or in}^2)}{1\ \text{swab}} \times \frac{1000\ \mu g}{1\ mg}$$

(25.2)

After the two limits are calculated using Equations 25.1–25.2 for each product, the limits are compared. The smaller limit calculated for a product becomes the acceptance limit for the cleaning verification for that product. It is obvious from Equation 25.2 that two variables drive the acceptance limit: lot size of product B, and the shared surface area. For example, if the shared equipment surface area is constant between two products, and the lot size for Product B is 50 kg as opposed to 100 kg, the acceptance limit would be calculated to be half of that of the 100 kg lot size.

25.4.3 Swab Selection

Although swab sampling is different conceptually from both the impurity and potency assay, the same scientific rationale governs the development of these assays. Many of the references listed in Tables 25.4 and 25.5 outline different validation approaches. Seno outlined validation practices in the Japanese pharmaceutical industry for cleaning verification,[33] and Kirsch outlined an approach for swab method validation that is consistent with ICH guidelines for method development.[34] An important aspect of any cleaning verification assay begins with swabbing the surface. Swabs are typically constructed of a polyester knit that will not leave behind fibers after swabbing and that contains minimal extractable materials.[35] Jenkins et al. did an extensive evaluation of swabbing materials as a function of the residual particles left on the surface after swabbing.[36] Quartz wool was found to give excellent recovery of analyte however, it left an excessive amount of particles on the surface. Glass-fiber swabs and cotton swabs also suffered from high levels of residual particles left behind on the surface. Knitted polyester demonstrated the best

balance between recovery, residual particles, and background levels. A guideline for swabbing techniques that discusses swabbing procedures, solvent selection, and recovery as a function of the coupon tested was presented by Yang et al.[37]

25.4.4 Analytical Methodologies

Cleaning verification methods for swabs are typically validated by demonstrating recovery from a "test coupon." This coupon is made of a material that is representative of the manufacturing equipment in regards to material type (e.g., 316L stainless steel), and surface finish. A known amount of an analyte will be spiked onto the coupon; the coupon will be swabbed in a methodical manner illustrated below in Figure 25.5. For example, perform 10 swipes in the vertical direction, rotate the plate and perform 10 swipes in the horizontal direction for a 10 cm × 10 cm coupon. For a larger surface (e.g., 25 cm × 25 cm), 20 swipes in each direction may be required. Some have advocated zigzag patterns, as opposed to horizontal and vertical swipes. It is important to be consistent, and that the validation mimics how the swabs will be collected from the manufacturing equipment. The swab will then be extracted in solvent and analyzed. Depending upon the swab, 5 mL to 20 mL is an appropriate volume of extraction solvent to ensure a reproducible extraction without over-dilution of the analyte, which could ultimately impact analytical detection.

With the advances in analytical technology, it should be a rare exception that the toxicologically-determined cleaning limit cannot be attained from the perspective of determination of the analyte, although it does become more difficult to quantitatively recover low amounts of analytes from surfaces. When selecting the appropriate analytical technique for cleaning verification, several parameters must be considered, such as the safety acceptance limit for the cleaning verification assay, solubility,[38] the molar absorptivity of the molecule or ionization or oxidation potential if alternative detection techniques are an option. In addition, the benefits of requiring a selective assay versus a non-selective assay

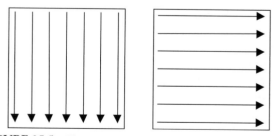

FIGURE 25.5   Illustration of typical swabbing practice

TABLE 25.4 Non-selective analytical techniques for cleaning verification with associated analytes and reported limit of detection (LOD), if available

		Non-selective techniques		
Detection technique	Analyte	Reported/estimated LOD	*Estimated LOQ	Reference
pH	Cleaning agents	200 mg/mL	666 mg/mL	43
Conductivity	Cleaning agents	20–200 mg/mL	67–666 mg/mL	40
Total organic carbon	Sulfacetamide, sulfabenzamide, sulfathiazole	low μg/cm^2	low μg/cm^2	41
	Total carbon	<50 ppb	167 ppb	42
	Detergents	50 ppb	167 ppb	42
	Cleaning agents	0.95 μg/cm^2	3.2 μg/cm^2	43
	Cleaning agents	20 μg/mL–2000 μg/mL	67–6660 μg/mL	43
	Aspirin	3 to 15 ppm	10–50 ppm	44
Visual	Residues	62.5 μg/100 cm^{-2}	208 μg/100 cm^{-2}	45
	Cleaning agents	20 μg/mL–2000 μg/mL	67–6660 μg/mL	43
	Aspirin	>0.1 μg/cm^2	0.3 μg/cm^2	47

*LOQ estimated assuming RSD = 10% and the LOD = 33%.

should be considered. In a non-selective assay, the blank of a rinse and swab blank are determined to ascertain if there is any deviation from the control (i.e., the blank in the same solution). The advantage of this approach is that a variety of residues may be detected which include cleaning agents, excipients, previously manufactured products, degradation products, and active pharmaceutical ingredients. It should, however, be realized that the identity of the contaminant would remain unknown after this assay. The analyst would only know that the equipment had a detectable residue, which may or may not help improve the cleaning process on subsequent manufactures. Many non-selective analytical techniques are outlined in Table 25.4. Within this table the analytes are indicated, and also the reported limit of detection (LOD) for the technique in association with the cleaning assay. The most prevalent of the non-selective assays is total organic carbon (TOC). It has the advantages of good sensitivity, short analysis time, and being capable of detecting all residual carbon—independent of the source.[39] For a selective technique, the target analyte is known before method validation.

Table 25.5 outlines many of the feasible selective analytical techniques. The list is not all-inclusive, because of the multiple detection schemes that can be implemented with high performance liquid chromatography (HPLC). HPLC is commonly used in the pharmaceutical industry. As a result, cleaning verification assays by this approach outnumber all others. Typically, at the time of manufacture, a potency assay has been developed and validated for the drug product. From a conservative standpoint, anything that elutes or co-elutes

at the retention time of the analyte of interest will be attributed to the active. Therefore, the swab method is commonly very similar, if not identical, to the potency method. Characteristic swab assays would most often be isocratic methods with reduced run times. In addition to HPLC with ultra-violet (UV) detection, many other detection schemes are outlined in Table 25.5. The analytical chemist chooses these techniques based upon the chemical properties of the target molecule, and the cleaning acceptance limit, which was previously established based upon dose and equipment surface area considerations. For example, a molecule that does not possess a chromophore and is somewhat potent would pose an interesting analytical challenge. The analyst might consider evaporative light scattering detection, electrochemical detection or mass spectral detection, to name a few possibilities. There are a few examples of analytical techniques listed in Table 25.5 where a specific example for a cleaning verification assay could not be located; however, depending upon the molecular properties of the compound, the cited technique would be a viable option for a cleaning verification assay.

25.4.5 Analytical Method Validation

Regardless of the analytical technique chosen for cleaning verification, there are certain components that are expected of any method validation activity which are outlined in the ICH guidelines on Analytical methods Q2A. For a quantitative impurity test, validation is required for specificity, limits of detection and quantitation, linearity, accuracy, precision (repeatability and

TABLE 25.5   Selective analytical techniques for cleaning verification with associated analytes and reported limit of detection (LOD), if available. When compound not indicated, proprietary listed as analyte

	Selective techniques			
Detection technique	Analyte	Reported/estimated LOD	Estimated LOQ	Reference
HPLC–UV	Amlodipine	0.02 μg/mL	0.7 μg/mL	46
	Ertapenem	0.0006 μg/mL	0.002 μg/mL	47
	Sulfadoxine	0.12 μg/mL	0.4 μg/mL	48
	Acetylsalicylic acid	0.04 μg/mL	0.1 μg/mL	49
	Sumatriptan succinate	0.003 μg/mL	0.01 μg/mL	50
	Losoxantrone	0.005 μg/mL	0.02 μg/mL	51
	Bisnafide	0.004 μg/mL	0.01 μg/mL	52
	Nonoxynol-9	0.06 μg/mL	0.2 μg/mL	53
UV	Any compound with chromophore	Typically higher than HPLC–UV	Typically higher than HPLC–UV	No references for cleaning verification
HPLC–MS	Proprietary	0.00002 μg/mL	0.00007 μg/mL	54
	Proprietary	0.0005 μg/mL	0.002 μg/mL	55
	Proprietary	<0.004 μg/mL	0.01 μg/mL	56
Ion mobility spectrometry (IMS)	Diphenylhydramine	0.0009 μg/mL	0.003 μg/mL	57
	Tamoxifen	0.05 μg/mL	0.2 μg/mL	58
	Proprietary	0.25 μg/mL	0.8 μg/mL	59
Gas chromatography	Methenamine hippurate	Not reported	Not reported	60
HPLC–ELSD	2-amino-bicyclo[3,1,0]hexane-2,6 dicarboxylic acid	0.26 μg/mL	0.9 μg/mL	61
TLC	Chloramphennicol	0.003 μg	0.01 μg	62
OPLC	Steroid hormones	0.03 μg	0.1 μg	63
CE	No reference to compounds	Typically higher than HPLC–UV	Typically higher than HPLC–UV	64
Atomic absorption	Cisplatin	0.0005 μg/mL	0.002	65
HPLC–electrochemical	Clarithromycin	0.3 μg/mL	1.0 g/mL	66
	Isoproterenol sulfate	0.1 ng/mL	0.3 ng/mL	67
Spectroscopy	Proprietary	4 μg/cm^2	13 μg/cm^2	68
	Cleaning agent	Not stated	Not stated	69
	Bovine serum albumin	low μg/cm^2	low μg/cm^2	70
HPLC–fluorescence	Norfloxacin	5 ng	20 ng	71
HP–TLC–fluorescence	Norfloxacin	5 ng	20 ng	74
Ion exchange conductivity	Cleaning agent	0.1 μg/mL	0.3 μg/mL	72
Ion exchange–UV	Cleaning agent	1 μg/mL	3 μg/mL	73
Charged aerosol detection	Mometasone Furoate Albuterol Loratadine	0.6 ng 1.5 ng 1.4 ng	2 ng 5 ng 5 ng	74

intermediate precision, depending upon the phase of development), and range (ICH Q2A).[75] Each of these validation criteria is listed below, with a brief explanation on the applicability to cleaning verification assays. A limit test for cleaning verification assays is often employed during clinical trials. With a limit test, a result of "pass" or "fail" is reported. The limit test significantly simplifies the validation of the cleaning verification assay. In order to validate a limit test, specificity, LOQ, accuracy, and stability must be evaluated at the acceptance limit.

Linearity and range may be excluded. A drawback of the limit test is that the ability for trending the cleaning efficiency (except through failures) for a particular process or compound is eliminated, because a quantitative result is not reported. Due to the fact that the formulation and process are likely to evolve, and the attrition of compounds during development is high, one might argue that trending doesn't provide much value here. However, if the compound makes it to market, a quantitative assay is expected for commercial manufacturing.

Specificity

Specificity should be demonstrated using interferences (i.e. extractables) that arise from the cleaning swabs and/or blank surfaces. Specificity between the excipients utilized in the drug product manufacture is desirable, but not required. If specificity is not achieved it must be assumed that the peak response is from the active pharmaceutical ingredient. If the interference is low enough, it may be acceptable as long as it does not unduly bias the recovery results and/or it can be accounted for appropriately through background subtraction. Significant interference from a surface may indicate compatibility issues for the selected sampling solvent, and may vary (drop) over time as surfaces on equipment are repeatedly cleaned.

Detection and Quantitation Limits

The limit of quantitation (LOQ), as opposed to the limit of detection (LOD), is the most important attribute of the swab method, because it has been previously determined from a safety and cross-contamination standpoint that residual material above the cleaning acceptance limit is of serious concern. The LOQ is defined as a percent relative standard deviation (% RSD) of 10%, and the LOD is defined as a % RSD of 33%. These values are typically determined on low-level injections of the standard. The sensitivity of the method must be low enough to ensure sample responses near the lowest acceptance limit are quantifiable. For typical swab assays, this requirement may necessitate an LOQ of $1\,\mu g/mL$ ($5\,\mu g/swab$ limit, 1 swab into 5 ml of solvent). Larger % RSD values may be acceptable (e.g., 20%), when discussing the acceptable precision for a swab assay (including recovery from surfaces). However, the assay pass–fail limit should be lowered in such a way that this variability is accounted for. For example, if 80% recovery was obtained during validation with a 15% RSD for a $5\,\mu g/swab$ limit, the assay pass–fail limit could be reasonably lowered to 68% to take into account the swabbing variability.

Linearity

Linearity is assessed to cover the full range of acceptance limits required by the method. Linearity has been performed in a couple of different ways. First, linearity has been performed through the preparation of standards that are equal to the resulting swab solution concentration after putting the swab into solvent. The second approach would involve spiking plates at many different levels, and evaluating the recovery at each level. The second approach is problematic, in that recovery is usually observed to decrease as the limit at the spiked level on the surface decreases. Thus, it may be unreasonable to expect linearity over a large range. However, if the range is kept narrow, either approach is suitable.

Accuracy and Recovery

When compared to a typical potency assay, this validation parameter is the most variable.

$$\text{Recovery}(\%) = \frac{\text{spiked amount determined }(\mu g)}{\text{actual spiked amount }(\mu g)} \times 100$$

(25.3)

It is not uncommon to see relative standard deviations of recovery results for cleaning range from 2–10% or higher depending upon the surface. In addition, the recovery of an analyte from the test surface is not expected to be complete. Depending upon the surface's characteristics (e.g., a smooth polished surface versus a rough surface), acceptance limit (e.g., 0.5 mcg/swab versus 100 mcg/swab), and the solubility of the compound, recoveries as low as 20% or lower may be acceptable and accounted for in the method calculations through the use of recovery factors. The minimum sample response (extract concentration) must be not less than the quantitation limit of the assay, to ensure that analyte levels close to the lowest acceptance limit are quantifiable.

Intermediate Precision

With the above-mentioned variability that may be observed during accuracy/recovery determinations, it must be realized that acceptance criteria around intermediate precision must be set accordingly. For example, it is quite likely that if Analyst A could obtain a recovery of 80% for a $5\,\mu g/swab$ limit, Analyst B could obtain a value of only 70% for the recovery. When looking at the residual surface analyte difference between the two analysts, Analyst B would have left only $0.5\,\mu g$ ($0.02\,\mu g/cm^2$ for a $2.5\,cm \times 2.5\,cm$ test coupon) across the tested surface area. It is easy to see that swabbing techniques can play a crucial role in swabbing success when such small amounts are considered. As the compound becomes more potent, the residual differences between Analyst A and Analyst B may be in the nanogram range.

Range

The range of acceptable method performance is based upon the LOQ and the linearity assessment.

Standard and Sample Stability

Stability of the unextracted swabs is determined in order to allow time for transport of the swabs between the swabbing site and the analytical testing site. Standard stability and swab extract stability are determined to facilitate analytical testing. Swab and extract stability must be assessed after contact with each of the product contact surface materials, since sample stability can be affected by surface specific contaminants.

25.4.6 CASE STUDY

Example

The following case study is for a tablet manufactured on a Manesty® tablet press in the clinical trial manufacturing area for a first human dose trial. The compound will be manufactured at doses of 1 mg/tablet, 25 mg/tablet, and 100 mg/tablet, and has a good molar absorptivity. The 1/1000th minimum dose and 10 ppm methods were used to calculate the swab test acceptance limits, assuming an equivalent lot and dosage strength will be manufactured subsequently. The analysis shown below outlines the selection of swabbing locations, acceptance limit calculations, and analytical methodology based upon previously mentioned criteria.

Figure 25.6 is an illustration of the Manesty press. There are magnified views indicating swab locations. All of

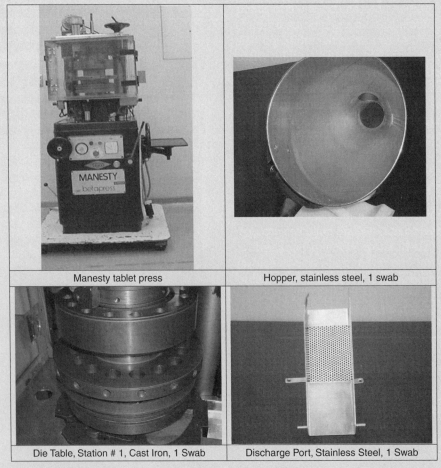

| Manesty tablet press | Hopper, stainless steel, 1 swab |
| Die Table, Station # 1, Cast Iron, 1 Swab | Discharge Port, Stainless Steel, 1 Swab |

FIGURE 25.6   Manesty tablet press with swab locations, material of construction, and number of swabs required per location indicated

CASE STUDY (CONTINUED)

this information (picture, number of swabs, surface areas in Table 25.6, and material of construction) is part of the cleaning master plan, and is generated for each piece of manufacturing equipment, and each swab location. This documentation practice serves as a guide for documenting swab locations and rationales for such locations.

Based upon product contact surface area, outlined in Section 25.4, the surface areas were calculated for each component, and it was determined that three equipment components had large surface areas. In this case, the discharge port, the die table, and the hopper all had significant surface area contributions. In addition, the die table would be considered a high-energy dissipation area, where it is likely that product would accumulate during manufacture. The materials of construction are stainless steel and cast iron therefore, both surface types are swabbed. In turn, an analytical method should be validated where the recovery from stainless steel and cast iron are evaluated. None of the other areas were evaluated to be especially difficult to clean in this example. Thus, no additional swabs were added.

TABLE 25.6 Material of construction and surface area calculations for the product contact surfaces illustrated above

Component	Material	Surface area (cm²)	Surface area (%)	# Swabs
Discharge port	Stainless steel	42.0	5.4	1
Upper punch	Stainless steel	0.6	0.1	0
Lower punch	Stainless steel	1.1	0.1	0
Die	Stainless Steel	0.9	0.1	0
Die table, station 1	Cast iron	126.5	16.3	1
Feeder bowl	Cast iron	145.5	18.8	0
Hopper	Stainless steel	458.9	59.2	1

Acceptance Criteria

Using the 1/1000th minimum dose and 10 ppm methods, Table 25.7 lists the product and equipment characteristics used to calculate the swab acceptance limits for the case study.

1. 1/1000th method:

$$\text{Acceptance Limit} \left(\frac{\mu g}{swab} \right) = \frac{0.001 \times 1 \text{ mg/day}}{5 \text{ units/day}} \text{ Product B}$$

$$\times \frac{\text{Product B (5,000 dosage units)}}{\text{Shared Surface Area 775.5 cm}^2}$$

$$\times \frac{\text{Swab area 25 cm}^2}{1 \text{ swab}} \times \frac{1000 \ \mu g}{1 \text{ mg}}$$

Acceptance limit 5 32.2 mg/swab

2. 10 ppm method:

$$\text{Acceptance Limit} \left(\frac{\mu g}{swab} \right) = \frac{10 \text{ mg}}{1 \text{ kg}} \times \frac{\text{Lot Size Product B 1 kg}}{\text{Shared Surface Area 775.5 cm}^2}$$

$$\times \frac{\text{Swab area 25 cm}^2}{1 \text{ swab}} \times \frac{1000 \ \mu g}{1 \text{ mg}}$$

Acceptance limit 5 322 mg/swab

TABLE 25.7 Lot size and dose strengths for case study

Product	Lowest dose strength mg/tablet	Lot size (kg)	Lot size (units)	Maximum daily dose (units)	Shared surface area (cm²)
A	1	20	10 000	1	
B	10	1	5000	5	775.5

In order to keep the case study simple, only one piece of equipment was used to illustrate selection of swab locations, images included in CT master plan, and calculation of limits. Typically, tablet products are made with several steps, using several pieces of equipment, such as granulator/dryer, mill, blender, press or optional coater. The total product contact surface area of all equipment should be used for calculation of limits. The smallest limit calculated for

a product using all of the calculations becomes the acceptance limit for the cleaning verification of that product. In this case, the acceptance limit would be 32 μg/swab. If product B, the lot to be manufactured next, is unknown at the time of manufacture of Product A, the worse case should be assumed in the calculation. For example, if the smallest lot that has ever been manufactured in the facility is 1000 dosage units or 1 kilogram, those values should be used in the equation to generate a maximum allowable carryover of Product A.

25.5 SUMMARY

This chapter presents a strategy to manage effectively the complex clinical supplies manufacturing process. This strategy includes planning, collaborative communication among the cross-functional team, lean manufacturing, effective training programs, and application of new technologies to facilitate the clinical supplies manufacturing. cGMP considerations to ensure the quality of the clinical materials during the clinical supplies manufacture are also discussed. The comprehensive clinical supply manufacture strategy and cGMP controls prevent clinical supplies manufacture from becoming the bottleneck of a clinical trial program, and consequently reduce the total cycle time of introducing a new drug to the market. In addition, various aspects of cleaning verification and considerations for a cleaning validation program are presented. Such things as acceptance limit calculations, analytical methodology, and validation were outlined to illustrate the vast interest on the topic of cleaning verification in a clinical trial manufacturing facility.

References

1. FDA Guidance for Clinical Investigators. (2006). Institutional Review Boards and Sponsors Process for Handling Referrals to FDA Under 21 CFR 50.54 Additional Safeguards for Children in Clinical Investigations. Draft, May.
2. Carr, D.F. & Cone, E. (2004). Merck Seeks a Cure, Baseline the Project Management Center, June 8.
3. Monkhouse, D.C. & Rhodes, C.T. (eds). (1998). *Drug Products for Clinical Trials: An International Guide to Formulation, Production, Quality Control.* Marcel Dekker, Inc.
4. Paez, O., Dewees, J., Genaidy, A., Tuncel, S., Karwowski, W. & Zurada, J. (2004). The lean manufacturing enterprise: An emerging sociotechnological system integration. Human Factors and Ergonomics in Manufacturing 14(3), 285–306.
5. Womack, J.P. & Jones, D.T. (2003). *Lean Thinking: Banish Waste and Create Wealth for your Corporation,* 2nd edn. Free Press, New York.
6. Broeze, R.J., Macaloney, G. & Parker, S. (2004). Executive roundtable: Cutting costs with contract manufacturing. Next Generation Pharmaceutical Article, September.
7. FDA Guidance for Industry. (1991). Guideline on the Preparation of Investigational New Drug Products (Human and Animal), March.
8. FDA Guidance for Industry. (2006). INDs—Approaches to Complying with cGMP's during Phase 1, Draft January.
9. PQRI/FDA. (2006). Report on the Workshop, "A Drug Quality System for the 21st Century," April 22–24, Washington, DC.
10. FDA Preapproval Inspections (Compliance Program #7346.832).
11. Directive 2003/94/EC Article 13, 2.
12. FDA Guidance for Industry. (2001). Q7A Good Manufacturing Practice Guidance for Active Pharmaceutical Ingredients, August.
13. FDA Guidance for Industry (1995). Content and Format of Investigation New Drug Applications (INDs) for Phase 1 Studies of Drugs, Including Well-Characterized, Therapeutic, Biotechnology-Derived Products, November.
14. Good Manufacturing Practice in Pharmaceutical Production, World Health Organization.
15. FDA Policy Guide. (2004). Process Validation Requirements for Drug Products and Active Pharmaceutical Ingredients Subject to Pre-Market Approval, CPG 7132c.08, March.
16. EU GMP Annex 13.
17. FDA Guidance for Industry. (2006). Quality Systems Approach to Pharmaceutical cGMP Regulations, September.
18. FDA Guidance for Industry. (2004). PAT—A Framework for Innovative Pharmaceutical Development, Manufacturing, and Quality Assurance, September.
19. FDA Guidance for Industry. (2006). Q9 Quality Risk Management, June.
20. CFR 211.67, Code of Federal Regulations PART 211—Current Good Manufacturing Practice for Finished Pharmaceuticals—Equipment cleaning and maintenance, Subpart D—Equipment.
21. ICH Q7A, Good Manufacturing Practice Guide for Active Pharmaceutical Ingredients.
22. US FDA, Center for Drug Evaluation and Research Website. http://www.fda.gov/
23. Garvey, C.R., Levy, S. & McLoughlin, T. (1998). Pharmaceutical Engineering 18(4), 20–26.
24. Hwang, R.-C. (2002). American Pharmaceutical Review 5(3), 42–46.
25. Gerber, M., Perona, D. & Ray, L. (2005). Pharmaceutical Engineering 25(3), 46–54.
26. Agalloco, J. (1992). A publication of the Parenteral Drug Association. Journal of Parenteral Science and Technology 46(5), Sept–Oct., 163–168.
27. Hall, W.E. (1999). Drug Manufacturing Technology Series 3, 269–298.
28. Abco, J.P., Brame, W., Ferenc, B., Hall, W.E., Jenkins, K., LaMagna, J.T., Madsen, R.E., Mullen, M.V., Wagenknecht, D. & Wagner, C.M. (1998). PDA Journal of Pharmaceutical Science and Technology (USA). Vol. 52, Nov–Dec., 1–23.
29. LeBlanc, D.A. (1998). Pharmaceutical Technology 22(10), pp. 136, 138, 140, 142, 144–148.
30. Dolan, D.G., Naumann, B.D., Sargent, E.V., Maier, A. & Dourson, M. (2005). Regulatory Toxicology and Pharmacology, RTP 43(1), Oct., 1–9.
31. Zeller, A.O. (1993). Pharmaceutical Technology Europe (USA) 5, Nov., pp. 18, 20, 22, 24–27.
32. Fourman, G.L. & Mullen, M.V. (1993). Pharmaceutical Technology (USA) 17, Apr. pp. 54, 56, 58, 60.
33. Seno, S., Ohtake, S. & Kohno, H. (1997). Accreditation and Quality Assurance 2(3), 140–145.
34. Kirsch, R.B. (1998). Pharmaceutical Technology 22(2), Suppl., 40–46.
35. Miscioscio, K. & Cooper, D.W. (2000). Journal of the IEST 43(1), 31–37.
36. Jenkins, K.M., Vanderwielen, A.J., Armstrong, J.A., Lesonard, L.M., Murphy, G.P. & Piros, N.A. (1996). PDA Journal of Pharmaceutical Science and Technology 50(1), Jan–Feb., 6–15.
37. Yang, P., Burson, K., Feder, D. & Macdonald, F. (2005). Pharmaceutical Technology 29(1), 84–94.
38. PhRMA Quality Committee. (1997). Max Lazar, Pharmaceutical Technology, Sept., 56–73.
39. Wallace, B., Stevens, R. & Purcell, M. (2004). Pharmaceutical Technology Aseptic Processing, 40–43.
40. Westman, L. & Karlsson, G. (2000). PDA Journal of Pharmaceutical Science and Technology/PDA 54(5), Sept–Oct., 365–372.

41. Bristol, P. (2004). Manufacturing Chemist (England) 75, 37–38.

42. Guazzaroni, M., Yiin, B. & Yu, J.L. (1998). American Biotechnology Laboratory 16(10), 66–67.

43. Biwald, C.E. & Gavlick, W.K. (1997). Journal of AOAC International 80(5), Sept–Oct., 1078–1083.

44. Holmes, A.J. & Vanderwielen, A.J. (1997). PDA Journal of Pharmaceutical Science and Technology/PDA 51(4), Jul–Aug., 149–152.

45. Mirza, T., Lunn, M.J., Keeley, F.J., George, R.C. & Bodenmiller, J.R. (1999). Journal of Pharmaceutical and Biomedical Analysis (England) 19, 747–756.

46. Klinkenberg, R., Streel, B. & Ceccato, A. (2003). Journal of Pharmaceutical and Biomedical Analysis 32(2), Jun., 345–352.

47. Sajonz, P., Natishan, T.K., Wu, Y., McGachy, N.T. & DeTora, D. (2005). Journal of Liquid Chromatography and Related Technologies 28(5), 713–725.

48. Boca, M.B., Apostolides, Z. & Pretorius, E. (2005). Journal of Pharmaceutical and Biomedical Analysis 37(3), Mar 9., 461–468.

49. Nozal, M.J., Bernal, J.L., Toribio, L., Jimenez, J.J. & Martin, M.T. (2000). Journal of Chromatography A 870(1–2), Feb 18, 69–75.

50. Nozal, M.J., Bernal, J.L., Toribio, L., Martin, M.T. & Diez, F.J. (2002). Journal of Pharmaceutical and Biomedical Analysis 30(2), Sept 5, 285–291.

51. Shea, J.A., Shamrock, W.F., Abboud, C.A., Woodeshick, R.W., Nguyen, L.Q., Rubino, J.T. & Segretario, J. (1996). Pharmaceutical Development and Technology 1(1), Apr., 69–75.

52. Segretario, J., Cook, S.C., Umbles, C.L., Walker, J.T., Woodeshick, R.W., Rubino, J.T. & Shea, J.A. (1998). Pharmaceutical Development and Technology 3(4), Nov., 471–476.

53. Shifflet, M.J., Shapiro, M., Levin, C. & DeNisco, R. (2001). LCGC North America 19(3), 312, 314–317.

54. Kolodsick, K.J., Phillips, H., Feng, J., Molski, M. & Kingsmill, C.A. (2006). Pharmaceutical Technology 30(2), 56–71.

55. Liu, L. & Pack, B.W. (2007). Journal of Pharmaceutical and Biomedical Analysis 43(4), 1206–1212.

56. Simmonds, E.L., Lough, W.J. & Gray, M.R. (2006). Journal of Pharmaceutical and Biomedical Analysis 40, 531–638.

57. Payne, K., Fawber, W., Faria, J., Buaron, J., DeBono, R. & Mahmood, A. (2005). The Role of Spectroscopy in Process Analytical Technology, www.spectroscopyonline.com, January.

58. Debono, R., Stefanou, S., Davis, M. & Wallia, G. (2002). Pharmaceutical Technology, April.

59. Munden, R., Everitt, R., Sandor, R., Carroll, J. & Debono, R. (October 2002). Pharmaceutical Technology, 72–78.

60. Mirza, T., George, R.C., Bodenmiller, J.R. & Belanich, S.A. (1998). Journal of Pharmaceutical and Biomedical Analysis 16(6), Feb., 939–950.

61. Risley, D.S., Hostettler, K.F. & Peterson, J.A. (1998). LC-GC 16(6), 562–568.

62. Vovk, I. & (Reprint); Simonovska, B. (2005). Journal of AOAC International 88(5), Sept–Oct., 1555–1561.

63. Katona, Z., Vincze, L., Vegh, Z., Trompler, A. & Ferenczi-Fodor, K. (2000). Journal of Pharmaceutical and Biomedical Analysis 22(2), Mar., 349–353.

64. Fabre, H. & Altria, K.D. (2001). LC-GC Europe 14(5), 302, 304, 306, 308–310.

65. Raghavan, R. & Mulligan, J.A. (2000). Drug development and Industrial Pharmacy 26(4), Apr., 423–428.

66. Rotsch, T.D., Spanton, M., Cugier, P. & Plasz, A.C. (1991). Pharmaceutical Research (USA) 8, Aug., 989–991.

67. Elrod, L. Jr., Schmit, J.L. & Morley, J.A. (1996). Journal of Chromatography A 723, 235–241.

68. Mehta, N.K., Goenaga-Polo, J., Hernandez-Rivera, S.P., Hernandez, D., Thomson, M.A. & Melling, P.J. (2003). Spectroscopy (Duluth, MN, United States) 18(4), 14–16, 18–19.

69. Smith, J.M. (1993). Pharmaceutical Technology (USA) 17, Jun., 88, 90–92, 94, 96, 98.

70. Urbas, A.A. & Lodder, R.A. (2003). NIR news 14(2), 8–10.

71. Simonovska, B., Andrensek, S., Vovk, I. & Prosek, M. (1999). Journal of Chromatography 862, 209–215.

72. Weston, A. (1998). American Biotechnology Laboratory 16(3), 30, 32–33.

73. Shifflet, M.J. & Shapiro, M. (2000). BioPharm 13(1), 51–54, 64.

74. Poster obtained from ESA. Forsatz, B.J., (Schering-Plough Research Institute), Snow, N.H. (Seton Hall University, Department of Chemistry and Biochemistry).

75. ICH Guidelines Q2A, Validation of Analytical Procedures: Text and Methodology.

Specification Setting and Manufacturing Process Control for Solid Oral Drug Products

Wei Chen, Suchinda Stithit, Jack Y. Zheng and Richard Hwang

26.1 INTRODUCTION

The quality of drug products is determined by their design, development, process controls, GMP controls, process validation, and by specifications applied to them throughout development and manufacturing.[1,2] As part of GMP controls the quality of any drug product must be evaluated using methods and criteria listed in its specifications. According to ICH Q6A, a specification is defined as:[1]

> A list of tests, references to analytical procedures, and appropriate acceptance criteria that are numerical limits, ranges or other criteria for the tests described. It establishes the set of criteria to which a drug substance or drug product should conform to be considered acceptable for its intended use. Conformance to specification means that the material, when tested according to the listed analytical procedures, will meet the listed acceptance criteria.

In the pharmaceutical industry, specifications are required by regulatory bodies for any drug substance, intermediates, and finished drug product. Specifications are critical to ensure product quality and consistency, and are an important part of an integrated quality strategy for finished drug products, in addition to following good manufacturing practices (GMPs) (e.g., using suitable facilities, an established/validated manufacturing process, validated test procedures, raw materials testing, in-process testing, and stability testing).[1–3] Specifications for the drug substance, in-process tests, and final product release tests must be based on development information (e.g., batch history, stability, efficacy, and toxicity), and certainly evolve with the cumulative knowledge gained during product research and development. In all cases, specifications either in the clinical trial stages or in the commercialization stage are chosen to confirm the quality of the drug product, and thus must focus on the product characteristics that ensure the identity, strength, and purity of the drug product at release, as well as throughout the duration of clinical trial or the shelf life for commercial products. It is important to have solid rationale and scientific justification for including and/or excluding testing for specific quality attributes, since specifications are used to confirm the product quality rather than to characterize the product.

The following are four fundamental principles that should be taken into consideration during setting specifications for both drug substance, and drug product:

1. Specifications should be based on relevant preclinical development, and clinical study data. These clinical data define the boundaries of key safety and efficacy.

2. Specifications should be related to a manufacturing process. Specifications must be based on data obtained from batches used to demonstrate product performance and manufacturing consistency. Product specifications, especially for process-related degradation products, must be related to the specific manufacturing process.

3. The stability of drug substance and drug product should be taken into consideration for setting specifications. Physical and chemical degradation of drug substance and drug product may occur during storage. These changes could affect product safety and performance.

4. Specifications must be linked to analytical procedures. Critical quality attributes may include characteristics such as assay, impurity profiles, and *in vitro* dissolution. Such attributes can be evaluated by multiple analytical methods to yield different results. During the course of product development, it is common for analytical technology to evolve in parallel with the product. Therefore, analytical data generated during development should be correlated with those generated at the time when the NDA is filed.

For the purpose of this document, early phase development refers to phase 1 or 2 clinical trials, before the start of primary stability studies or pivotal clinical trials. Late phase development refers to phase 3 or pivotal clinical studies. Early phase and late phase specifications refer to specifications established during early phase and late phase development, respectively. The regulatory specification refers to specifications established for the registration and commercial batches.

The specification setting process begins with identification of a set of attributes for testing, development of analytical procedures, and establishment of acceptance criteria that can be used to measure product quality. Specifications are then refined during product development and the commercialization process. Once specifications are set, process controls need to be identified in order to monitor and/or adjust the manufacturing process. The goal of process control is to ensure that an in-process material or the finished drug product meets its respective specifications.

Specifications and specification setting process for drug substances, clinical trial materials, and drug products are described in this chapter. Process controls, particularly in-process material tests, statistical methodology for process controls, and application of process analytical technology (PAT) in-process controls, are discussed. The impact of analytical procedures on the specifications is also discussed.

26.2 SPECIFICATIONS FOR THE DRUG SUBSTANCE

The drug substance, i.e., active pharmaceutical ingredient (API), is the most important component in a drug product. During the early phase of development, the number of API batches is relatively limited, the batch size is usually very small, and manufacturing experience is beginning to evolve. The primary emphasis in setting specifications for a new drug substance is on safety, based on the purposes of clinical studies at this stage. During the later phase of development, as sufficient data and experience become available, product quality becomes the focus for setting specifications based on manufacturing processes and analytical capability, in addition to safety considerations.

ICH guideline Q6A generally applies to products during late stage development, as the guideline specifically states that it is "not intended to apply to the regulation of new drug substance used during the clinical research stage of development."[1] Nonetheless, the main principles of the guideline should be considered carefully throughout development. As discussed above, the primary focus of specifications is safety during the early phase of development. To set specifications at this stage, the tests described in ICH Q6A should be reviewed to determine which tests must have limits, and which tests can be performed "to be monitored." To be monitored tests refer to those that do not have limits or acceptance criteria established. During the early phase of development, some tests can be performed "to be monitored," because whether or not the test is quality-indicating may not yet be known or there may be insufficient data to set a proper limit. During the late phase of development, specifications are gradually developed toward meeting the requirements for registration. Therefore, the late phase specifications should include tests expected at registration, though there may not be enough data available to set appropriate limits until just prior to submission.

The following tests and acceptance criteria are described in ICH Guideline Q6A. An example of early phase and late phase specifications are provided in Table 26.1.

- Description: a qualitative statement about the physical state and appearance of the new drug substance should be provided. For the example in Table 26.1, the acceptance criteria are based on the historical visual appearance data for the drug substance.
- Identification: identification testing should optimally be able to discriminate between compounds of closely related structure that are

TABLE 26.1   Example of specifications for drug substance

Tests	Method	Limits for early phase	Limits for late phase/commercial batches
Description	Visual	White to yellow solid	White to yellow solid
Identity by IR	IR	Spectrum compares favorably with that of the reference standard	Spectrum compares favorably with that of the reference standard
Identity by HPLC	HPLC	N/A	Retention time compares favorably with that of the reference standard
Assay	HPLC	Not less than 93% and not more than 105%	Not less than 93%, and not more than 105%
Related substances	HPLC	Not more than 3%	Not more than 2%
Total related substances			
Individual related substances		Not more than 1%	Not more than 0.7%
Chiral impurities	HPLC		
Form A		Not more than 0.7%	Not more than 0.3%
Form B		Not more than 0.7%	Not more than 0.4%
Residual solvents	GC		
Solvent A		Not more than 2.0%	N/A
Solvent B		N/A	Not more than 0.5%
Water	Karl Fischer titration	Not more than 5.0%	Not more than 2.0%
Residue on ignition	USP	To be monitored	Not more than 0.05%
Heavy metals	USP	To be monitored	Not more than 20 ppm
Particle size	Laser diffraction	To be monitored	N/A
Crystal form	X-ray diffraction	To be monitored	N/A
Microbiological test	Compendial method	N/A	Meet compendial requirements

likely to be present. The test should be specific for the new drug substance such as infrared spectrum (IR). Identification solely by a single chromatographic retention time is not regarded as being specific. However, the use of two chromatographic methods, where separation is based on different principles or a combination of tests into a single procedure, such as high pressure liquid chromatography (HPLC)/UV (ultraviolet) diode array, HPLC/MS (mass spectroscopy) or GC (gas chromatography)/MS is generally acceptable. If the new drug substance is a salt, identification testing should be specific for the individual ions. An identification test that is specific for the salt itself should suffice. New drug substances that are optically active may also need specific identification testing or performance of a chiral assay. For an early phase specification, normally only one identification method is included. A spectroscopic method, such as IR, is generally used. For late phase specifications, two identification methods are typically included (see Table 26.1).

- Assay: this test is used to determine the purity of the drug substance. A specific, stability-indicating analytical method should be included to determine the content of the new drug substance. In many cases, it is possible to apply the same method (e.g., HPLC) for both assay, and quantitation of impurities. Both early and late phase specifications require a proper assay limit, which is commonly expressed as a percentage for new drug substances. The limit usually specifies a correction for water and/or solvent (anhydrous, volatiles-free, or dried). For the example in Table 26.1, the assay method separates all known related substances and degradation products from the drug substance. The lower limit is calculated to allow for related substances and assay variability. The upper limit allows for assay variability. The specification for assay is the same for the drug substances at the early and late phases.
- Impurities: categories of impurities in a new drug substance listed in Table 26.2 include organic and inorganic impurities, and residual solvents.

TABLE 26.2   Classification of impurities in new drug substance

Categories	Physical state	Source	Example
Organic impurities	Volatile Nonvolatile	Manufacturing process Storage	Starting materials By-products Intermediates Degradation products Reagents, ligands, and catalysts
Inorganic impurities	Nonvolatile	Manufacturing process	Reagents, ligands, and catalysts Heavy metals or other residual metals Inorganic salts Other materials (e.g., filter aids, charcoal)
Residue solvents	Inorganic or organic liquid	Manufacturing process	Acetone (class 3) Acetonitrile (class 2) Benzene (class 1)

The identification and qualification threshold is given in Table 26.3.[4]

Organic impurities include starting materials, reaction by-products, process intermediates, degradation products, reagents, ligands, and catalysts. They are process-related, except for degradation products, and may be identified or unidentified, volatile or nonvolatile. Chemical structures of impurities present in the new drug substance at or above an apparent level of 0.1% (e.g., calculated by using the response factor of the drug substance) should be characterized. The early phase specification of new drug substance for organic purities should include limits for total and any unspecified impurity (the largest reported unspecified impurity). Any identified impurity with a potential toxicological risk (e.g., carcinogen, teratogen, mutagen, etc.) should also be included in the early phase specification, with a limit that is acceptable toxicologically without risking human health. A qualitative comparison of impurity profiles, generally an HPLC impurities test, is also performed during the early phase. The impurity profiles of the batches of drug substance to be used in clinical trials must be compared to the batches used in toxicology studies and/or previous clinical trials. The late phase or regulatory specifications of the new drug substance for organic impurities should be consistent with ICH Q3A guideline and include, where applicable, limits for:

- each specified identified impurity;
- each specified unidentified impurity at or above 0.1%;
- any unspecified impurity, with a limit of not more than 0.1%;
- total impurities.

Table 26.1 shows the limit of not more than 1.0% of any individual related substance, and not more than

3.0% of total related substances for the example drug substance during early phase development. The limits in this example are designed to ensure that the clinical trial material will not be significantly different, at a minimum not inferior in terms of impurities, from the material used in toxicological studies. The limits are tightened, based on the process capability and stability data for the late phase specification.

Inorganic impurities can result from the manufacturing process, and are usually known and identified (e.g., reagents, ligands and catalysts, heavy metals, inorganic salts, filter aids, and charcoal). These impurities are normally analyzed using pharmacopeial or other appropriate methods. Limits could be based on pharmacopeial standards or known safety data. The example in Table 26.1 shows that residue on ignition and heavy metals were monitored without specifications established at the early stage of the investigation. The limits at late stage were based on historical data.

Solvents are inorganic or organic liquids used as vehicles for the preparation of solutions or suspensions in the synthesis of a new drug substance. For an early phase specification, a toxicology review of the manufacturing process may be needed to identify the solvents that require limits. Generally, solvents that are used in the final purification step require an appropriate limit. Solvents that are particularly hazardous should be controlled prior to the final drug substance, whenever possible. Solvents that are likely to be or already are carried through to the final drug substance at a level of concern, should be controlled carefully with a proper limit. At the late phase of development, any solvent that may exist in the drug substance should be quantified using appropriate analytical procedures. Control strategy must be in place

TABLE 26.3 Thresholds of impurities in new drug substance

Maximum daily dose[1]	Reporting threshold[2,3]	Identification threshold[3]	Qualification threshold[3]
≤2 g/day	0.05%	0.10% or 1.0 mg per day intake (whichever is lower)	0.15% or 1.0 mg per day intake (whichever is lower)
>2 g/day	0.03%	0.05%	0.05%

[1] The amount of drug substance administrated per day
[2] Higher reporting thresholds should be scientifically justified
[3] Lower thresholds can be appropriate if the impurity is unusually toxic

if the solvents are generally known to be toxic per ICH guideline.[5] Control limits should be based on pharmacopeial standards, ICH safety limits or known safety data with consideration of clinical dose, duration of treatment, and route of administration. For the example in Table 26.1, the drug substance in early phase was recrystallized from solvent A. Material manufactured at the late phase was recrystallized from solvent B. The limits proposed for solvents A and B were based on the projected dose and the relative toxicity of these solvents.

ICH Q6A decision tree #1 shows how to establish an acceptance criterion for a specified impurity in a new drug substance.[1] Any limits to control impurities in the specification are based on the body of data generated during development. It is unlikely that sufficient data will be available to assess process consistency at the time of filing an NDA with the FDA. Therefore, acceptance criteria should not tightly encompass the batch data at the time of filing. Impurities present in the new drug substance, and exceeding the ICH threshold listed in Table 26.3, should be qualified. Qualification is the process to evaluate *in vivo* toxicity of an individual impurity or a given impurity profile at a level specified. After being successfully tested in safety and/or clinical trials, the level of the impurity is considered qualified. Sometimes, higher or lower threshold limits for qualification of impurities may be necessary for some drug categories. If an impurity of a drug or therapeutic class has been known to have adverse effects in humans, qualification threshold limits should be lower than usual. However, when the level of safety concern is based less on patient population, drug class effects, and clinical considerations, a higher threshold limit may be appropriate. The decision tree in attachment 3 of ICH Q3A discusses critical considerations for the qualification of impurities when threshold limits are exceeded. Generally, information from literature should be searched first to qualify an impurity. In many cases, it can be easier to control impurities below the threshold limit during the manufacturing process, than to conduct toxicological evaluation.

To set specification limits of impurities, all data from available stability studies, chemistry development and scale-up studies, and batches for clinical trials should be used to predict potential impurities that may exist in the commercial product. Only impurities that are observed in batches manufactured by proposed commercial synthetic routes will be included in the specification of the new drug substance.

In addition to the universal tests described previously, the following tests may be considered on a case-by-case basis for new drug substances.[1]

- Physico-chemical properties: these are properties such as pH of an aqueous solution, melting point/range or refractive index.
- Particle size and size distribution: the ICH Q6A decision tree #3 provides general guidance on when particle size testing should be considered. Usually, testing for particle size and size distribution should be performed if particle size can have a significant impact on dissolution rates, bioavailability, stability, and manufacturability. Table 26.1 shows that particle size was monitored, but a limit was not established for the drug substance at the early phase of the investigation. The test was removed at the late phase, because particle size did not impact the dissolution rate of the drug substance and drug product, the stability of the drug substance or manufacturability of the drug product. Therefore, no specification needs to be established for particle size distribution.
- Polymorphic forms: different polymorphic forms may affect drug product performance, bioavailability or stability. Polymorphism includes different crystal forms of a new drug substance and its solvates, hydrates, and amorphous forms. Following the ICH Q6A decision #4(1) through #4(3), polymorphism of the new drug substance should be understood, and controlled with appropriate physico-chemical measurements and techniques. These parameters must be controlled

until data show that control is not necessary (i.e., only one form can be generated during polymorph generation studies). Table 26.1 shows that the crystal form of the example drug substance was monitored, but a specification was not established at the early phase of the investigation. The test was removed at the late phase, because polymorphism has not been observed as a result of the current synthetic route, and no specification needs to be established.

- Chiral drug substances present additional technical challenges to pharmaceutical scientists. ICH Q6A decision tree #5 summarizes when, and whether, chiral identity tests, impurity tests, and assays may be needed for both new drug substances and new drug products. For a drug substance developed as a single enantiomer, control of the other enantiomer should be considered in the same manner as for other impurities. An enantioselective determination of the drug substance should be part of the specification. Identity tests should also be capable of distinguishing both enantiomers and the racemic mixture. It is important for a chiral drug substance to control starting materials or intermediates, and enantiomeric impurity, during the manufacturing process. The example in Table 26.1 shows that the limits at early phase are to ensure that lots are not significantly different from the quality of the lots for toxicology studies, and allows for assay variability. The limits at late phase were tightened, based on process capability and stability data available.
- Water content: control of water content is especially important if the new drug substance is hygroscopic or degraded by moisture or when the drug substance is known to be a stoichiometric hydrate.
- Microbial limits: at the early phase, microbial test limits may not be needed for new drug substances used for oral solid dosage forms. At the late phase of development, a microbial limit is generally required, unless a scientific justification can be provided. Appropriate microbial tests and acceptance criteria are based on the nature of the drug substance, method of manufacture, and the intended use of the drug product. Tests may include the total count of aerobic microorganisms, the total count of yeasts and molds, and the absence of specific objectionable bacteria (e.g., *Staphylococcus aureus*, *E. coli*, *Salmonella*, *Pseudomonas aeruginosa*). ICH Q6A decision tree #6 provides additional guidance on when microbial limits should be included in specifications of a drug substance and excipient.

26.3 SPECIFICATIONS FOR CLINICAL TRIAL MATERIALS

In each phase of a clinical investigational program, sufficient information is required to be submitted to the FDA to ensure the proper safety, identification, strength, quality, purity, and potency of the investigational candidate. However, the amount of information to provide varies with the phase and the proposed duration of investigation, and the amount of information previously available. Specification for clinical trial materials is developed based on the following factors:

- compendial standards;
- process development studies; and
- stability of batches used for toxicological/*in vivo* studies.

Often the specification evolves as more manufacturing experience is gained.

26.3.1 Early Development Stage (Phases 1 and 2)

During early development, safety of the drug for use in clinical trials is the most important factor to consider in determining the specifications. When setting the specification limits for the drug substance, the toxicological lots are the benchmark for future lots. Specifications for impurities in early phase clinical trial materials can be based on the quality of materials used in toxicological studies, and the known toxicities of impurities. In addition, intended clinical usage, available clinical data, analytical methods, and process variability should also be considered.

The FDA guideline for phase 1 investigation[7–9] requires quantitative composition of the product, which includes a brief description of test methods to ensure the identity, strength, quality, purity and potency, test results or a certificate of analysis. Specified quality attributes should be monitored based on applicable acceptance criteria. For known safety-related concerns, acceptance criteria should be established and met. For some product attributes, all relevant acceptance criteria may not be known at this stage. It is recommended that an impurity profile should be established, to the extent that future reference, and/or comparison is possible. However, not all impurities of the product need characterization at this stage.

During phase 2 studies, physico-chemical tests and microbiological tests that have been added or deleted from the specifications established for phase 1 studies are required to be reported to the FDA.[10] Physico-chemical tests include identity, assay, content uniformity, degradants, impurities, dissolution, and particle size. Data on the particle size distribution and/or polymorphic form of the drug substance used in clinical trial materials should be included, so that correlations can be established between data generated during early and late phase drug development, and *in vivo* performance. Relaxation of acceptance criteria or any changes that affect safety should also be reported.

26.3.2 Late Development Stage (Phase 3)

As development progresses into phase 3, growing data on batch history, process capability, analytical capability, and stability become increasingly important in specification setting. An updated specification, with a detailed listing of all the tests performed on the product and the tentative acceptance criteria should be provided to the FDA. Test results and analytical data from batch release of representative clinical trial materials should be provided initially, and when any changes are made in the specification. Data on particle size distribution and/or polymorphic form of the drug substance should also be included. Degradation products should be identified, qualified, quantified, and reported. Suitable limits should be established, based on manufacturing experience, stability data, and safety considerations. A dissolution testing program or drug release program should be developed for drug products.

Typical phase 3 specifications for an oral drug product include description, identification, assay, content uniformity of dose units, degradation products, dissolution, water content, and microbiological tests. Additional in-process tests during clinical trial manufacturing of a tablet/capsule dosage form include dimensions, disintegration, and weight (hardness and friability, additionally, for tablet dosage forms). The quality of the product used in these clinical studies will form the basis for product approval, and the quality of the registered product has to reflect that of clinical trial materials.

An example of drug product (capsule) specifications at early phase and late phase development is provided in Table 26.4. The example specifications include description, identification, assay, related substances, water, dissolution, uniformity of dosage unit, and microbiological test. The limit for description is based on historical visual appearance data of the drug product. During early phase development, only an

IR method is used for an identity test. In late phase development two identification methods are used (i.e., IR and HPLC methods). The upper/lower assay limit is calculated to allow for related substances and assay variability. The limit is typical and the same for early and late phases drug product. Related substances (total related substances and individual related substances) are "to be monitored" during the early phase of development. The limits are established for the late phase after more data becomes available. The USP limit is used for the uniformity of dose units test. Limit for dissolution is based on the dissolution study in previous historical batches. At the late phase of development, the limit is set at an earlier time point, based on the data collected during early phase development.

26.4 SPECIFICATIONS FOR COMMERCIAL DRUG PRODUCTS

Specifications for commercial drug products, also known as regulatory specifications, are generally documented in a regulatory submission or in a compendial monograph. Commercial drug product must conform to the regulatory specifications throughout its shelf life. Full compliance with the ICH guideline Q6A is expected for specifications for commercial drug products.

Specifications for commercial drug products are refined from late phase specification, based on analytical capability, process capability, and product stability. These considerations augment the safety requirements. At the time of registration, the number of stability batches representative of the future commercial batches is often limited, and shelf life stability testing has not been completed. Statistical extrapolation of limited stability data to the proposed shelf life is necessary. It is important that specifications are not set too tightly, which could result in unnecessary rejection and time-consuming investigations. On the other hand, controlling patients' risk of using products not meeting requirements should be a top priority. Wessels et al. have proposed a strategy statistically to set an appropriate specification for pharmaceutical products.[11] The authors use linear regression to extrapolate the stability data available at the time of registration. They recommend that a confidence limit of 99% for individual results be used, to determine specifications after batch-to-batch variability is tested according to the ICH guideline on stability testing.[12] Patient risk can be controlled by tightening the specification (e.g., using a confidence limit of 95% instead of 99%).

TABLE 26.4   Example of specifications for a capsule drug product

Tests	Method	Limits for early phase	Limits for late phase
Description	Visual	White capsule	White capsule
Identity	HPLC	N/A	The retention time of the main peak in the chromatogram of the assay preparation corresponds to that in the chromatogram of the reference standard preparation, as obtained in the assay testing
Identity	IR	The IR absorption spectrum of the sample preparation exhibits maxima only at the same wavelengths as that of corresponding reference standard	The IR absorption spectrum of the sample preparation exhibits maxima only at the same wavelengths as that of corresponding reference standard
Assay	HPLC	Not less than 90%, and not more than 110% of label claim	Not less than 90%, and not more than 110% of label claim
Related substances	HPLC		
Total related substances		To be monitored	Not more than 1.0%
Individual related substances		To be monitored	Not more than 0.5%
Water	Karl Fischer titration	To be monitored	5%
Uniformity of dosage units	HPLC	Meet USP<XX>	Meet USP<XX>
Dissolution	USP	Q = 75% at 45 minutes	Q = 75% at 35 minutes
Microbiological tests	Compendial method	N/A	Meet compendial requirements

The following universal tests described in ICH Q6A for drug product specifications are generally applicable to all new drug products:

- Description: a qualitative description of the finished product such as size, shape, and color should be provided.
- Identification: identification testing is able to discriminate between compounds of closely related structure that might be present. Identity tests should be specific for the new drug substance. A single chromatographic retention time, for example, is not deemed as being specific. However, the use of two chromatographic procedures is acceptable if the separation is based on different principles. The combination of tests into a single procedure, such as HPLC/UV diode array, HPLC/MS or GC/MS, is also acceptable.
- Assay: assay methods should determine the drug product strength/content using a specific and stability-indicating method. In cases where use of nonspecific assay is justified, additional supporting analytical procedures should be used to attain overall specificity.
- Impurities: impurities include organic and inorganic impurities, as well as residual solvents. Detailed information can be found in the following

ICH guidelines: "Q3B Impurities in New Drug Products"[15] and "Q3C Impurities: Residual Solvents."[6] Organic impurities that are degradation products of the new drug substance, and process-related impurities from the new drug product, should be monitored. Acceptance limits for individual specified degradation products should be established. The identification and qualification threshold is given in Table 26.5. The emphasis is on impurities arising from drug product manufacture or from degradation. The impurity profiles of batches representative of the proposed commercial process should be compared with the profiles of batches used in development, and any differences should be discussed. The specifications of the new drug product for impurities should be consistent with the ICH Q3B guideline which include, where applicable, limits for:
- each specified identified degradation product;
- each specified unidentified degradation product;
- any unspecified degradation product, with a limit of not more than the identification threshold;
- total degradation products.

The following additional tests described in the ICH Q6A are specific to solid oral drug products.

- Dissolution: dissolution testing measures the rate of release of the drug substance from the drug

TABLE 26.5 Thresholds for degradation products in new drug products

Maximum daily dose[1]	Reporting threshold[2,3]	Maximum daily dose[1]	Identification threshold[2,3]	Maximum daily dose[1]	Qualification threshold[2,3]
≤1 g	0.1%	<1 mg	1.0% or 5 µg TDI, whichever is lower	<10 mg	1.0% or 50 µg TDI, whichever is lower
		1 mg–10 mg	0.5% or 20 µg TDI, whichever is lower	10 mg–100 mg	0.5% or 200 µg TDI, whichever is lower
>1 g	0.05%	>10 mg–2 g	0.2% or 2 mg TDI, whichever is lower	>100 mg–2 g	0.2% or 3 mg TDI, whichever is lower
		>2 g	0.10%	>2 g	0.15%

[1] The amount of drug substance administrated per day
[2] Thresholds for degradation products are expressed either as a percentage of the drug substance or as total daily intake (TDI) of the degradation product. Lower thresholds can be appropriate if the degradation product is unusually toxic
[3] Higher reporting thresholds should be scientifically justified

product using a specific apparatus. Specification of dissolution should be set based on the data of bio-batches. Analysis of the quantity of drug released at a single time point is commonly used for immediate release (IR) formulations when the drug substance is highly soluble. On the other hand, appropriate test conditions and sampling procedures should be established for modified-release formulations. Multiple time point sampling is appropriate for IR products of poorly soluble compounds, and for extended- or delayed-release formulations (see ICH Q6A decision tree 7(1)). In cases where changes in dissolution rate have been demonstrated to significantly affect bioavailability, testing conditions that can discriminate between acceptable and unacceptable bioavailability are desirable (see ICH Q6A decision tree 7(2)). *In vitro–in vivo* correlation (IVIVC) may be used to establish acceptance criteria for extended-release drug products when human bioavailability data are available for formulations exhibiting different release rates. Acceptance criteria should be established based on available batch data when bioavailability data are not available, and drug release is not shown independent of *in vitro* test conditions. The variability in mean release rate at any given time point should not exceed a total numerical difference of ±10% of the labeled content of the drug substance, unless a wider range is supported by a bioequivalency study (see ICH Q6A decision Tree 7(3)).

- Disintegration: disintegration testing can be substituted for dissolution for rapidly dissolving products containing drugs that are highly soluble throughout the physiological pH range.

Disintegration is most appropriate when a relationship to dissolution has been demonstrated or when disintegration is shown to be more discriminating than dissolution (see ICH Q6A decision tree 7(1)).

- Hardness/friability: hardness/friability testing is usually performed as an in-process control. The test should be included in the specification only when the characteristics of hardness/friability have a critical impact on product quality (e.g., chewable tablets).

- Uniformity of dosage unit: testing the uniformity of dosage units includes measurement of both the mass of the dosage form, and the content of the active ingredient in the drug product. Pharmacopeial methods should be used. Often this test is performed as an in-process evaluation.

- Water content: a quantitation procedure that is specific for water is preferred (e.g., Karl Fischer titration). A loss-on-drying procedure may be adequate in some cases. Acceptance criteria should be based on data on the effects of hydration or water absorption on the drug product. Table 26.6 shows a water specification of not more than 7% for an example tablet product. The water in this product is mainly contributed by the water of hydration from excipients. Primary stability data indicate that the packaged tablets absorb water under long-term storage conditions. Based on the stability data, the absolute change through the expiration dating period, and uncertainty in the estimated change, are statistically computed. The water specification of not more than 7% is then established, based on the process capability, change

TABLE 26.6   Example of in-house release and regulatory specification for a tablet product

Tests	Method	In-house release limits	Regulatory limits
Description	Visual	Colored, shaped, and debossed tablet	Colored, shaped, and debossed tablet
Identity by IR	IR	The IR absorption spectrum of the sample preparation exhibits maxima only at the same wavelengths as that of corresponding reference standard	The IR absorption spectrum of the sample preparation exhibits maxima only at the same wavelengths as that of corresponding reference standard
Identity by HPLC	HPLC	The retention time of the main peak in the chromatogram of the assay preparation corresponds to that in the chromatogram of the reference standard preparation, as obtained in the assay testing	The retention time of the main peak in the chromatogram of the assay preparation corresponds to that in the chromatogram of the reference standard preparation, as obtained in the assay testing
Assay	HPLC	Not less than 97% and not more than 106.5% of label claim	Not less than 90% and not more than 110% of label claim
Related substances	HPLC		
Total related substances		Not more than 1.09%	Not more than 2%
Individual related substances		Not more than 0.52%	Not more than 1%
Water	Karl Fischer titration	Not more than 3.8%	Not more than 7%
Uniformity of dose units	HPLC	Meet USP<XX>	Meet USP<XX>
Dissolution	USP	Q = 75% at 30 minutes	Q = 75% at 30 minutes

and uncertainty of the change estimated from the stability data, and the method variation.

- Microbial limits: the type of microbial testing and acceptance criteria used should be based on the nature of the drug, method of manufacture, and the intended use of the drug product. Such testing may not be necessary with acceptable scientific justification (see ICH Q6A decision tree 8).

26.4.1 Product In-house Release Specifications and Regulatory Specifications

Regulatory specifications are legal commitments that a commercial product must conform to throughout its shelf life. In order to meet the regulatory specification, more restrictive in-house release specifications are commonly established for drug products. For examples, tighter assay and impurity (degradation product) in-house release limits can be established to ensure that a product can meet regulatory specifications at the end of shelf life. In Japan and the United States, the concept of release specification may only be applicable to in-house criteria, and not to the regulatory release criteria. In these regions, the regulatory acceptance criteria are the same from release throughout shelf life. However, many companies choose to

have tighter in-house limits at the time of release, to provide assurance that the product will remain within the regulatory acceptance criterion throughout its shelf life. In the European Union, distinct specifications for release and for shelf life are a regulatory requirement.

Degradation of drug product needs to be factored into specification setting, particularly for analytical properties (e.g., potency and impurities) that are affected by the degradation. The in-house release limits for quantitative analytical properties can be calculated from regulatory limits, based on the stability change (increase or decrease), and the measurement variability. The calculated in-house release limits are narrower than regulatory limits, to compensate for measurement variability and/or product instability. The buffer between regulatory limit and in-house limit typically consists of the estimated absolute change through expiration dating period (Change), uncertainty in estimated change (S_{change}), and measurement variation (S_m).

For an analytical property that degrades during storage, the upper and lower in-house limits (UL and LL) can be calculated from upper and lower regulatory limits (URL and LRL) using the following equations. Allen et al. used a similar equation to calculate the setting of in-house limits for a product that degrades during stability storage.[14]

$$UL = URL - t \times \sqrt{S_m^2}$$
$$LL = LRL + Change + t \times \sqrt{S_{change}^2 + S_m^2}$$

where:

t is determined from a t-table using appropriate degree of freedom and level of confidence.

For an analytical property that increases during stability storage, the UL and LL can be calculated from URL and LRL using the following equations.

$$UL = URL - Change - t \times \sqrt{S_{change}^2 + S_m^2}$$
$$LL = LRL + t \times \sqrt{S_m^2}$$

For an analytical property absent of instability, the buffer between in-house limits and regulatory limits typically consists of measurement variability only.

An example of in-house release and regulatory specification for a tablet product is provided in Table 26.6. The assay limits in Table 26.6 are based on the safety, efficacy, process variability, and assay variability. The upper/lower in-house release limits for assay are calculated to protect against exceeding the regulatory limits from stability and assay variability. The regulatory limits of not more than 1% of any individual related substance and not more than 2% of total related substances are the same as for drug substances, because there is no significant degradation observed during the drug product manufacturing process. The upper/lower in-house release limits are calculated based on stability and assay variability, to protect the regulatory limits.

26.4.2 Product Stability and Expiration Date

Once specifications are set, the expiration dating period of a drug product is then established, based on the stability data obtained from long-term stability studies. The FDA guideline[12] requires that at least three batches be tested, to allow for a good estimate of batch-to-batch variability. Stability data from all batches should be combined to estimate an expiration dating period for a drug product. Batch similarity should be tested before all stability data are combined for statistical analysis. Batch similarity is examined by testing the similarity of intercepts and slopes of degradation lines from different batches. If the hypotheses of comparable intercepts and slopes are not rejected at the 0.25 level of significance, the expiration dating period can be estimated based on pooled stability data of all batches. On the other hand, if the hypotheses of comparable intercepts and slopes are rejected

TABLE 26.7 Examples of in-process tests for solid oral dosage forms

Process step	In-process tests	Effects on process and quality attributes
Drying in wet granulation	Loss on drying	• Product stability
Blending/mixing	Blending uniformity	Uniformity of dose unit
Blending/mixing	Particle size distribution	Uniformity of dose unit
Tablet compression	Weight	Uniformity of dose uniformity
Tablet compression	Thickness	Disintegration/dissolution
Tablet compression	Hardness	• Coating quality • Disintegration dissolution
Tablet compression	Friability	• Coating quality • Potency • Shipping
Capsule filling	Weight	Uniformity of dose units
Capsule filling	Joint length	Shipping (Breakage due to improper lock) Packaging (blistering)
Tablet/capsule	Disintegration	Dissolution

at the significance of 0.25, the expiration dating period should be estimated based on the shortest expiration dating period calculated from the worst batch.

Estimate of an expiration dating period is illustrated in the following example. Four different batches (i.e., Lots A, B, C, and D) of a single tablet formulation were placed on long-term stability. Lot B completed 36-month stability. Lots A, C, and D completed 24-month stability. The analysis assumes that zero-order change (linear modeling on the original data scale) is appropriate. Before pooling the data from four lots to estimate the shelf life, a preliminary statistical test was performed to determine whether the regression lines from different lots have a common slope and/or time zero intercept. The statistical model with the effects of Age, Lots, and Age × Lots was used. The probability associated with the interaction term Age × Lots was 0.0063, which is smaller than 0.25. This indicates that there is sufficient evidence that the slopes across lots are statistically different, and the prediction for each lot must be evaluated separately. The individual slope and 95% confidence intervals for each lot are then estimated. The values for both the upper and lower confidence intervals are compared to the regulatory specification of 95% to 105%. The confidence interval with the shortest expiry dating was identified to be Lot A. The projected expiration dating period of Lot A supports the 36-month dating. Therefore, the expiration dating period of the product is set at 36 months.

For more details on shelf life determination, readers are referred to Chapter 24.

26.5 PROCESS CONTROL FOR SOLID ORAL DRUG PRODUCTS

Process control is an all-inclusive term used to describe the controls used during production to monitor and, if appropriate, adjust the process, and/or to ensure that an in-process material with an established specification or the finished drug product will conform to its respective specification.[2] Four types of process controls are as follows:

- Operating parameters: conditions that can be adjusted to control the manufacturing process (e.g., temperature, pH, mixing time, and mixing speed);
- Environmental control: conditions associated with the manufacturing facility (e.g., facility temperature, humidity, clean room classification);
- Process tests: measures used to monitor and assess the performance of the process (e.g., product temperature or exhaust temperature during drying in fluid-bed drier);
- In-process material tests: measures used to assess the quality attributes of an in-process material, and ultimately decide to accept or reject the in-process material or drug product.

Steps in the manufacturing process should have the appropriate process controls identified. All in-process material tests and any of the operating parameters, environmental conditions, and process tests that ensure each critical manufacturing step are properly controlled, and should be established in order to meet the predetermined specifications of final drug product. All critical process controls, and their associated ranges, limits or acceptance criteria should be identified, and justified by experimental data. For critical operating parameters and environmental controls, numeric ranges, limits or acceptance criteria typically can be based on the experience gained during the development of the manufacturing process.

26.5.1 In-process Material Tests and Quality Attributes

In-process material tests are one of the critical components of process controls. They may be performed during the manufacture of drug substance or drug product, rather than as part of the formal battery of tests that are conducted prior to product release.[1] In-process tests that are only used for the purpose of adjusting process parameters within an operating range, e.g., hardness and friability of tablet cores that will be coated and individual tablet weight, are not included in the specifications. Typical in-process material tests for solid oral dosage forms are listed in Table 26.7.

The process material tests directly assess the quality attributes of the in-process materials. Quality attributes are important chemical, physical, and microbiological properties or characteristics of the drug product and intermediate material that must be maintained for proper product performance. Quality attributes of the process are those process parameters that are controlled to ensure that the process reproducibly meets the drug product quality attributes. These attributes are identified during product and process development, and become the basis for ensuring the control of product quality.

During the compression/encapsulation process, in-process material testing is performed on solid oral dosage forms to assure consistency throughout these unit operations. Moisture content is typically performed for granules before tableting and encapsulation. Tablet weights, hardness, thickness, friability, and disintegration testing are typically performed for tablets. Weight testing is performed for capsules. Hardness and disintegration specifications are established during development and bio-batch production. Testing performed during commercial production is to demonstrate both comparability and consistency.

All in-process material tests are critical process controls, because they directly assess the quality attributes of an in-process material, and ultimately lead to a decision to accept or reject the in-process material or drug product. Well-defined proven acceptable ranges (PARs) should be established for these tests, so that the impact on product quality of operating outside the PARs is understood or can be predicted. Data from in-process tests should be routinely evaluated. Statistical tools, such as control charts, can be used to aid the evaluation process.

26.5.2 Powder Blending Uniformity

Powder blending is a fundamental process of mixing for solid dosage forms to ensure content uniformity of final drug products.[15–17] Current GMPs in 21CFR PARTS 210 and 211 state: "Such control procedures should include adequacy of mixing to assure uniformity and homogeneity." In 2003, the FDA issued a guidance document on powder blends and finished dosage units to promote a science-based policy and regulatory enforcement.[18–19] The guidance described the procedure for assessing powder mix adequacy, correlating in-process dosage unit test results with powder blend test results, and establishing the initial criteria for control procedures used in routine product manufacturing.

Powder blend uniformity is a process control (i.e., in-process material test) that critically impacts the uniformity of dosage form. In-process sampling and testing is essential to determine blend uniformity. The sampling technique is crucial to obtain samples that adequately represent the powder mix. The standard sampling device is a thief. However, certain sampling techniques may falsely introduce significant variations. The orientation, angle, and depth of sampling thief insertion, as well as insertion force and smoothness, impact the consistency of the sampling. Potential powder segregation during powder transfer and storage, and powder properties (e.g., flowability, particle size distribution, and density, etc.) also add to the challenge of obtaining representative in-process samples. To address sampling variations, the FDA guideline recommends a stratified sampling scheme. Stratified sampling is the process of collecting a representative sample by selecting units deliberately from various identified locations within a lot or batch or from various phases or periods of a process. By stratified sampling, a sample dosage unit is obtained specifically to target locations throughout the compression/filling operation that have a higher risk of producing failing results in the finished product tests for uniformity of content. This sampling method allows for collection and analysis of powder samples and dosage unit samples. For powder blends, at least 10 sampling locations in the blender should be identified to represent potential areas of poor blending. In tumbling blenders (such as V-blenders, double cones or drum mixers), samples should be selected from at least two depths along the axis of the blender. For convective blenders (such as a ribbon blender), a uniform volumetric sampling should be implemented to include the corners and discharge area (at least 20 locations are recommended to adequately validate convective blenders). At least three replicate samples should be collected from each location. Statistical analysis should be applied to quantitatively measure any variability that is present among the samples. The sample variability can be attributed either to lack of uniformity of the blend or to sampling error. Significant within-location variance in the blend data represents sampling error, while high between-location variance in the blend data can indicate that the blending operation is either inadequate, sampling is biased, or a combination of inadequate mixing and sampling bias.

For the dosage unit production step, samples are collected from 20 locations throughout the compression or capsule filling operation, seven units per location. A product is classified as "readily pass" if the following criteria are met:

- for all individual results (for each batch $n \geq 60$) the RSD $\leq 4.0\%$;
- the mean of each location is within 90% to 110% of target strength;
- all individual results are within the range of 75% to 125% of target strength.

A lot classified as "marginal pass" if RSD $\leq 6.0\%$ ($n = 140$), and "inappropriate" if RSD $> 6.0\%$. Based on the test results of stratified sampling, different controlling criteria are applied for routine manufacturing. Details can be found in the FDA guidance.[20]

26.5.3 Statistical Methodology for Process Control

In-process material testing results can be graphed in a control chart for routine evaluation. A control chart is a line graph displaying the results of repeated sampling of a process over time, together with the control limits statistically established from historical process data. Control charts are commonly used to monitor the quality attributes and process stability. Control charts are one of the most important and effective statistical tools for quality control to monitor the process performance and trend detection. They can be applied for both in-process testing and finished product testing.

Process variability is the result of common cause variation and special cause variation. Common cause variation is a normal and consistent variation, which occurs regularly. It is the random fluctuation expected in testing, and follows a predictable distribution over time. The following are some examples of common cause variations:

- environmental (e.g., humidity, temperature) changes;
- baseline noise caused by regular electric interference;
- normal drift in a balance.

Special cause variation is inconsistent and abnormal variation. It happens infrequently, and is an unexpected event. The only way to reduce special-cause variation is to investigate its cause, and then implement countermeasures to prevent the cause from reoccurring. The following are some examples of special cause variations.

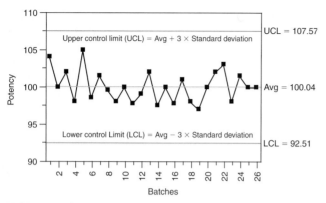

FIGURE 26.1   Example of a control chart

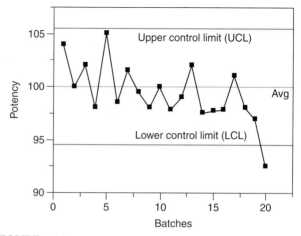

FIGURE 26.2   Example of a control chart with a value outside of the limit

- power outages causing changes in stability chamber storage conditions;
- equipment failure;
- incorrectly prepared stock standard in analysis.

An example of a control chart is provided in Figure 26.1. The centerline of the graph indicates the mean. The control limits typically include mean (μ) and 3 × standard deviation (σ) lines. The control chart limits represent the common variation of a process, and are established from historical data. If process data are approximately normal, about 99.73% of the data will be located within ±3 standard deviations from the process mean. Values falling outside of these limits are alarming signals, because statistically individual values from a normal distribution will be within 3.0 standard deviations of the mean 99.73% of the time. If a process is only subject to common cause variation, a value more than three times the standard deviation is highly unlikely (only 2.7 occurrences per 1000 observations). Therefore, a value outside of control chart limit can be considered as indication of special cause variation. An example of a control chart with a value outside the limit is provided in Figure 26.2.

In addition to a value outside of control chart limits, special cause variation is shown by one or more of the following common out of control alarms:[20]

- seven sequential points are on one side of the mean (a run);
- seven sequential points increase or decrease steadily (a trend).

A run of seven is probably not random statistically, assuming the observed values are from a normal distribution. The probability of seven consecutive values being below the mean is:

$$\left(\frac{1}{2}\right)^7 = \left(\frac{1}{128}\right) = 0.8\%$$

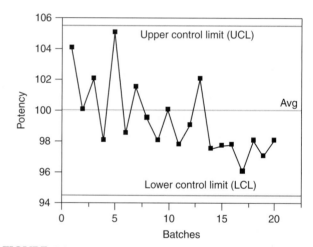

FIGURE 26.3   Example of a control chart with seven or more sequential points on one side of the mean

The occurrence of such an event often suggests that the process should be carefully investigated. An example of a control chart with seven or more sequential points on one side of the mean is provided in Figure 26.3.

The goal of control charting is to separate variability into common-cause and special-cause, with the knowledge that special-cause variability can be addressed and eliminated. When a control chart alarm is observed, an investigation should be performed to identify the assignable cause.

26.5.4 Process Analytical Technology (PAT) and In-process Controls

The FDAs PAT Guidance[21] and 21st Century GMP Initiatives[22] promote a technology-based regulatory environment that encourages the pharmaceutical industry to implement innovative development, manufacturing, and quality assurance practices. The agency is encouraging the industry to utilize science- and engineering-based principles to characterize and understand their processes. With the understanding, a manufacturing process is expected to be more efficient, consistent, and robust, providing the scientific rationales for the development of product specifications. For characterization and control purposes, PAT is a promising technology platform to accomplish our goals.

A PAT platform consists of an automated analyzer system that is integrated with process equipment for operation in a manufacturing environment. The system is capable of generating, analyzing, displaying, and transmitting product and process trend data continuously as a process unit operation is executed. For example, PAT can be used to monitor the critical unit operations of drying and blending, to ensure optimal product dryness and uniformity during blending to allow a homogenous blend for forward processing. This results in a more consistent product quality, faster forward processing, and batch release. Wildfong et al. demonstrated that NIR can be used to monitor the moisture content of granules as they are drying at real-time.[23] Frake et al. showed that continuous inline NIR monitoring of water content and particle size data are suitable means of process control and end point determination for a fluid-bed granulation drying process.[24] Hailey et al. also demonstrated that NIR spectroscopy, interfaced with process equipment and in combination with a fully automated system, can be used for real-time online powder blend homogeneity analysis.[25]

PAT can also be used in finished product analysis. Cogdill et al. developed and validated NIR models for the analysis of API content and hardness of tablets.[26] Spencer et al. demonstrated the feasibility of predicting active drug content in commercial-grade pharmaceutical tablets by NIR spectroscopy.[27] A PAT platform of at-line or inline tablet analysis provides early warning in case of problems. It also offers a near real-time confirmation that the finished product is in compliance with product specifications. More detailed discussions of PAT applications in oral dosage development and manufacturing are provided in Chapter 3 of this book.

26.6 ANALYTICAL PROCEDURES

Analytical procedures evolve in the course of product development. Analytical procedures may also change, as knowledge of process controls (e.g., what the critical impurities are) increase. Comparability of results from changed analytical procedures must be considered during specification setting. It is important to confirm that data generated during development correlate with those generated at the time a NDA is submitted.

An appropriate performance of the analytical procedures is critical for specification setting. For potency assay, the variability of the procedure must be taken into account for the specification setting, in addition to the primary concern of patient safety and batch-to-batch variability. An intermediate precision study may be used as an estimate for the assay variability. For impurity and residual solvent testing, the requirements are outlined in the ICH guidelines.[4,6,13] The testing procedure must be able to determine the levels of impurities with appropriate accuracy and precision. For a specification limit of 0.1% for unknown impurities, the ICH reporting threshold of 0.05% can be used as the required quantitation limit to provide a reliable quantitation at the specification limit. For impurities with potential toxicity, toxicology should be consulted early in the drug development process, to ensure methods with appropriate detection limits are developed and validated.

Analytical procedures must be validated for setting specifications. Since a drug substance or drug product is tested by a set of complementary and supplementary testing procedures, the performance and validation of a particular analytical procedure is influenced by other testing procedures used in setting the specification. It may not be necessary to optimize an individual analytical procedure to its best performance as long as it, together with other testing procedures, adequately tests the drug substance or product.

Validation of analytical procedures is an important part of the registration application for a new drug. Chapter 23 of this book discusses more details with regard to development and validation of analytical procedures.

26.7 CONCLUSIONS

Specifications are based on relevant development data, pharmacopeial standards, test data of drug substances and drug products used in toxicology and clinical studies, and results from accelerated and long-term stability studies. In addition, analytical and manufacturing variability should be taken into consideration. Since specifications evolve through development and commercialization phases, specifications should be evaluated and updated periodically as additional data become available. Rationale for changes to specifications must be scientifically sound, and documented to allow traceability to previous versions.

To ensure specifications are met and product quality attributes are maintained, process controls must be identified, implemented, and effectively controlled during the manufacturing process.

Setting specifications establishes the quality criteria for drug substance and product. The quality of drug product cannot be tested into the product. Instead, quality should be built in by design. Setting proper specifications, and maintaining effective process controls, requires mechanistic understanding of how formulation and process design impact product quality and performance. Using science-based and risk-based approaches, the knowledge gained during different phases of development can be used to justify the tests and criteria in specifications to ensure the safety, efficacy, and quality of drug substances and products.

References

1. FDA. (2000). International Conference on Harmonization; Guidance on Q6A specifications: test procedures and acceptance criteria for new drug substances and new drug products: chemical substances. Federal Register 65(251), 83041–83063.
2. FDA. (2003). Draft Guidance for Industry: Drug Product Chemistry, Manufacturing and Controls Information, January. Available at: www.fda.gov/cder/guidance/
3. FDA. (2001). Guidance for Industry Q7A Good Manufacturing Practice Guidance for Active Pharmaceutical Ingredients, August. Available at www.fda.gov/cder/guidance/
4. FDA. (2003). Guidance for Industry Q3A Impurities in New Drug Substances. ICH, February.
5. FDA. (1997). Guidance for Industry Q3C Impurities: Residual Solvent. ICH, December.
6. FDA. (1999). Guidance for Industry Q6B Specifications: Test procedures and acceptance criteria for biotechnological/biological products, August. Available at www.fda.gov/cder/guidance/
7. Guidance for Industry INDs. (2006). Approaches to Complying with CGMP During Phase 1, January.
8. Guidance for Industry. (2006). Investigators, and Reviewers Exploratory IND Studies, January.
9. Guidance for Industry. (1995). Content and Format of Investigational New Drug Applications (INDs) for Phase1 Studies of Drugs, Including Well-Characterized, Therapeutic, Biotechnology-derived Products, November.
10. Guidance for Industry. (2003). INDs for Phase 2 and Phase 3 Studies Chemistry, Manufacturing, and Controls Information, May.
11. Wessels, P., Holz, M., Erni, F., Krummen, K. & Ogorka, J. (1997). Statistical evaluation of stability data of pharmaceutical products for specification setting. Drug Development and Industrial Pharmacy 23(5), 427–439.
12. ICH guidelines. Q1A (R2) Stability Testing of New Drug Substances and Products.
13. ICH guidelines. Q3B (R2) Impurities in New Drug Products
14. Allen, P.V., Dukes, G.R. & Gerger, M.E. (1991). Pharmaceutical Research 8, 1210.
15. Berman, J. (2001). The compliance and science of blend uniformity analysis. PDA Journal of Pharmaceutical Science and Technology 55(4), 209–222.
16. Venables, H.J. & Wells, J.I. (2001). Powder mixing. Drug Development and Industrial Pharmacy 27(7), 599–612.
17. Geoffroy, J.M., LeBlond, D., Poska, R., Brinker, D. & Hsu, A. (2001). Unit dose sampling and final product performance: An alternative approach. Drug Development and Industrial Pharmacy 27(7), 731–743.
18. FDA. (2003). Guidance for Industry: Powder blends and finished dosage units—stratified in-process dosage unit sampling and assessment, October. Available at www.fda.gov/cder/guidance/
19. Boehm, G., Clark, J., Dietrick, J., Foust, L., Garcia, T., Gavini, M., Gelber, L., Geoffry, J., Hoblitzell, J., Jimenez, P., Mergen, G., Muzzio, F., Planchard, J., Prescott, J., Timmermens, J. & Takiar, N. (2003). The use of stratified sampling of blend and dosage units to demonstrate adequacy of mix for powder blends. PDA Journal of Pharmaceutical Science and Technology 57, 59–74.
20. Gershon, M. (1991). Statistical process control for the pharmaceutical industry. Journal of Parenteral Science and Technology 45(1), 41–50.
21. Guidance for Industry. PAT—A Framework for Innovative Pharmaceutical Development, Manufacturing, and Quality Assurance.
22. FDA. Innovation and Continuous Improvement in Pharmaceutical Manufacturing Pharmaceutical, cGMPs for the 21st Century.
23. Wildfong, P.L.D., Samy, A.S., Corfa, J., Peck, G.E. & Morris, K.R. (2002). Accelerated fluid bed drying using NIR monitoring and phenomenological modeling: Method assessment and formulation suitability. Journal of Pharmaceutical Science 91(3), 631–639.
24. Frake, P., Greenhalgh, D., Grierson, S.M., Hempenstall, J.M. & Rudd, D.R. (1997). Process control and end-point determination of a fluid bed granulation by application of near infra-red spectroscopy. International Journal of Pharmaceutics 151, 75–80.
25. Hailey, P.A., Doherty, P., Tapsell, P., Oliver, T. & Aldridge, P.K. (1996). Automated system for the on-line monitoring of powder blending processes using near-infrared spectroscopy. Part I. System development and control. Journal of Pharmaceutical and Biomedical Analysis, 14, 551–559.
26. Cogdill, R.P., Anderson, C.A., Delgado, M., Chisholm, R., Bolton, R., Herkert, T., Afnan, A.M. & Drennen, J.K. III. (2005). Process analytical technology case study: Part II. Development and validation of quantitative near-infrared calibrations in support of a process analytical technology application for real-time release. AAPS PharmSciTech 6(2), 273-283.
27. Spencer, J.A., Jefferson, E.H., BoClair, T. & Chan, J. (2000). Determination of acetaminophen in tablets by near-infrared reflectance spectroscopy. AAPS Annual Meeting Abstract. October, p. 1775.

Scale-up of Pharmaceutical Manufacturing Operations of Solid Dosage Forms

John Strong

27.1 INTRODUCTION TO SCALE-UP

"Commit your blunders on a small scale and make your profits on a large scale."

—L.H. Baekeland[1]

27.1.1 What is Scale-up?

The development and commercial release of a globally marketed pharmaceutical drug product necessarily begins in the realm of the very small. Drug discovery may focus on the molecular level, and early formulation may deal with only gram quantities of material. It is at the early formulation stage, however, that a tentative sequence of physico-chemical operations is initially proposed and developed to transform the raw materials into a drug product with the desired quality attributes (e.g., potency, dissolution, etc.) At this early stage, these experimental operations are carried out in bench top or small pilot-scale equipment, and the process knowledge in the form of raw data obtained from these experiments is specific to that scale. How does this small-scale data translate to the operation of commercial scale equipment that may be different in design, more than 50 times greater in capacity, and to the quality of the drug product produced at that scale? This is the question that scale-up addresses.

Scale-up is the practice by which process knowledge is developed and formulated in such a way that it can be applied effectively to guide equipment selection, process parameters, process conditions, and process control strategies, irrespective of scale. Under this definition, scale-up need not necessarily be limited strictly to the transfer of knowledge from the small to the large. The same methodology could be used to go from the large to the small or to transfer process technology to equipment of different design.

27.1.2 The Importance of Scale-up in Pharmaceutical Manufacturing

Leo H. Baekeland, the inventor of the world's first synthetic plastic, succinctly summed up in the opening quote a motivating factor for effective scale-up practices: cost. While in principle a process may be designed at the full commercial production scale without small-scale experimentation, the cost of performing empirical studies escalates along with the process scale, as would the cost of the inevitable missteps and errors that may happen during process development. Clearly this would be impractical and prohibitive as an overall strategy for modern drug product development, yet it remains commonplace that a sizeable portion of late-stage drug product development work is still performed at full-scale, in response to recognized gaps in process knowledge remaining after pilot-scale studies have concluded. These gaps may persist due to a lack of scale-up methodology needed to harness knowledge gained at the small-scale, exacerbated by a limited availability of pilot-scale facilities in which to conduct scale-up studies or a rush to meet aggressive project milestones. Filling these gaps at the late stage is much more costly than if

Developing Solid Oral Dosage Forms: Pharmaceutical Theory and Practice
ISBN: 978-0-444-53242-8

they were addressed in pilot studies, and can result in unexpected delays in product development timelines. The establishment of a process design paradigm based on sound, scientifically-based scaling principles can reduce the need for costly late stage full-scale studies, decreasing the risk associated with product development by leveraging knowledge gained in small-scale, inexpensive development studies.

While the bottom line is a motivating factor for any company marketing a product, pharmaceutical companies also have an obligation to produce medicinal products that are efficacious and safe. Product quality does not happen by accident, nor is it acceptable under current regulatory guidelines to use end-product testing to achieve quality by scrapping product that doesn't meet specifications.[2] Rather, quality must be designed into the process, and this can be accomplished only when there is extensive scientific knowledge of the physico-chemical processes that transform the incoming materials into the final drug product. The inability to predict the effects of scale-up is now recognized by regulatory agencies as an area requiring improvement in the current state of pharmaceutical manufacturing, with a general lack of scientific process knowledge identified as a barrier to understanding these physico-chemical relationships.[3]

27.1.3 How is Scale-up Performed?

A manufacturing process may be scaled (albeit inefficiently) by extensive experimentation without any theoretical linkage, to connect that knowledge together to form real process understanding. These less-than-ideal approaches to scaling may employ so-called "rules of thumb," appeals to past experience, and intuition. Conversely, scientific scale-up is achieved by utilizing scientific scaling principles to extract as much information as possible from smaller-scale experiments, in order to guide process development through to the full-scale. If scaling principles are derived from a scientific understanding of the manufacturing process, how is the scientific understanding obtained? Obviously, experimentation is necessary for accumulating raw data, but it is in the analysis of that data that usable knowledge is formed.

There is a popular quote among scientists obtained from the chalkboard of Nobel Prize winning physicist Richard P. Feynmann: "What I cannot create, I do not understand."[4] Perhaps Professor Feynmann was recalling the French philosopher Albert Camus, "That which you cannot explain, you do not understand." A scientist seeks to understand a given natural phenomenon by the creation of a scientific theory, a

theoretical framework of physical knowledge, and mathematical equations against which new discoveries and hypotheses can be tested, accepted or discarded. For the purpose of this text, perhaps another way to rephrase the above quote may be, "That which I cannot model, I do not understand." As explained more fully below, the concept of a model shares many traits in common with scientific theory and, for most intents and purposes, a model can be thought of as a mini-theory. The term "modeling" is intended to mean the application of scientific investigation to understand, mathematically describe, and predict, the behavior of a limited part of the natural world, usually with simplifying assumptions to keep the model compact, understandable, and practically solvable, yet still sufficiently predictive. Regulatory agencies are also recognizing that scientific understanding is obtained through mechanistic modeling,[5] and it is for this reason that much of this text on pharmaceutical scale-up focuses on the topic of models and modeling. Following a technical discussion on how modeling principles can be applied to scale-up, practical strategies for using scale-up methods to improve efficiency and quality are discussed.

27.2 MODELS AND MODELING IN SCALE-UP

27.2.1 Introduction to Models

When a researcher attempts to form an understanding of a physical process or phenomenon, the learning process may be aided by first narrowing down the focus specifically, to the phenomenon of interest, and then forming a simplified representation of that phenomenon. Theoretical models are abstract representations of physical phenomenon intended to aid in understanding and explaining how the world works, and as such they are preliminaries to the formation of scientific theories. Theoretical models are applied to systems, where a system is meant to indicate the specific part of the physical world pertinent to the phenomena of interest. Generally speaking, theoretical models most valuable in scientific research are those that are quantitative, and are expressed in mathematical form.

A model is a simplified representation of the physical world, in the sense that it takes a system that appears too complex to understand as a whole, and strips away the peripheral processes assumed to be unimportant, making the phenomenon of interest more tractable. But, increased tractability may come at the price of potentially omitting relevant aspects of the system that may partially explain its behavior, thus rendering the model inaccurate or incomplete. For example, we may model an ideal gas as if the individual molecules were perfectly elastic billiard balls obeying Newtonian mechanics, and indeed such a model has been tremendously useful in explaining and predicting the kinetic behavior of gases for which it was intended. Yet, it fails when predicting viscosity of gases, and does not account for quantum mechanical effects. Or consider the Rutherford model of the atom as a dense nucleus surrounded by "orbiting" electrons held fast by electrostatic attraction. While this model explained Rutherford's gold foil scattering experiment results, by correctly representing the atom as having a dense central core, the model unfortunately predicts unstable electron orbits, and is untenable as an atomic model in general. A model need only be as complete as necessary to explain the particular phenomenon of interest, and if extended further than what it was developed for, it may fail. However, overcomplication of a model is not a solution either. If a model is made too complex or too encompassing it can become very large and unwieldy, requiring costly estimation of numerous parameters, and sophisticated methods to solve them. If the objective of the pharmaceutical researcher is to reach a workable understanding of a process with a minimum commitment in time and cost, overly complicated models should also be avoided.

The efficient scale-up of a pharmaceutical process depends upon a solid understanding of the behavior of the system(s) in question, which in turn relies upon the formation of models that are sophisticated enough to capture the relevant processes and parameters, yet simple enough to be tractable, and this in turn requires at least some *a priori* knowledge of what physical phenomena may be important to the system behavior, and what may be tentatively ignored. Model development thus tends to be an iterative process, whereby the predictions of the model tell us something about its completeness, and the relevance of its components. If the model fails to be predictive, the parameter list may be expanded to account for processes previously thought to be irrelevant, while parameters that have little impact on the solution are easily identified, and can be omitted.

Models commonly used in scientific research may fall in several categories that differ in their applicability to scale-up.

Scale Models

In everyday parlance, the word "model" usually conveys a literal reproduction of an object at a different scale, such as a model aircraft or a model train. These are physical scaled-down versions of their full-scale counterparts, denoted as "scale models," "prototypes" or "material models," since these models are not theoretical constructs, but actual physical objects that exist in the material world. If the scale model is perfectly geometrically similar to its real-life counterpart, it is then a "true model," and if not it is deemed a "distorted model" (the concepts of true and distorted models bear directly on the concept of similitude discussed in Section 27.3.3). We can see that scale models are similar in appearance, and even move and act very much like the full-size objects they represent, suggesting their potential usefulness for predicting behavior at full-scale. For the pharmaceutical scientist, a familiar example of a scale model may be a pilot-scale high-shear granulator that is a miniature copy of a larger machine used at the commercial scale.

Theoretical Models

Theoretical models, prerequisite as well as complementary to scientific theories, are the scientist's primary tool for gaining a foothold on the understanding of physical phenomena. In contrast to the literal physical existence of scale models, theoretical models are abstractions existing as ideas, and are usually expressed in the form of mathematical equations. There are several types of theoretical models that are commonplace in scientific investigation. For the purposes of scale-up, three general categories of models are described.

Empirical theoretical models

Empirical knowledge is defined as information obtained directly or indirectly from observation and experiment. While it may be argued that all scientific knowledge ultimately comes from such origins, the empirical model, specifically, is a predictive tool built primarily by regressing experimental data to fit a mathematical expression. Empirical models may also be known less formally as curve fits or statistical models. For example, the mean particle diameter of a milled granulation exiting a particular impact mill may be determined and plotted against, e.g., the mill speed, feed rate, screen size, etc. A polynomial regression line may then be fitted to approximate the functional relationship exhibited by the data. This is an example of an empirical model that is commonly used in pharmaceutical research and development.

While such a model may be highly predictive for the system from which the data was collected, the knowledge contained within the model is specific to that system only. Since the empirical model is not explanatory in terms of physico-chemical mechanisms, it is not possible to generalize the model results to systems of different properties. We can consult the aforementioned curve fit to select a mill speed to achieve a desired particle size, but if we apply that curve fit to a different mill to the one from which the original data was obtained, there is no guarantee that it will still be predictive or even that the operating ranges will overlap. In general, purely empirical models are not useful in generating scale-up models.

In addition to curve fits, another example of empirical models is artificial neural networks (ANNs). ANNs are multivariate statistical models that are parameterized by "training" on input and output data sets obtained from experiment. Once trained, the model is ready to generalize predictions based on new data. However, like all statistical methods, ANNs are strong in interpolation, and weak in extrapolation. If the new data is located within the data space that the ANN is already trained on, the ANN can generalize a prediction; however, if the data is outside the ranges that the ANN was trained on, the resulting prediction can be wildly off the mark. As with curve fits the inability to extrapolate makes ANNs unsuitable as scale-up models.

Mechanistic theoretical models

In contrast to the empirical model as primarily a predictive tool, a mechanistic or "first principles" model seeks to explain the behavior of a system by appealing to fundamental physical laws. While the empirical model may be thought of as a "black box" function that provides an output for a given input without reference to the actual mechanisms involved in between, mechanistic models open up the box, and illuminate the relevant processes occurring inside. Hence, they can be thought of as simplified scientific theories. They tell us the how, not simply the what.* Mechanistic models will be discussed in more detail in Section 27.4.

The fact that mechanistic models tell us the how, irrespective of the equipment the process may be taking place in, is what makes them potentially powerful

tools for scale-up. They are constructed from the bottom up; that is, the researcher builds the model upon a foundation of fundamental theory already discovered and established by previous experimental research. For example, if one wants to predict the solidification time of a hot polymer pellet extruded from a twin-screw compounder, a good start to building a model would be the heat diffusion equation, where the temperature at time t can be predicted from the initial temperature and the physical and thermal properties of the material. No matter what compounder we use, or what polymeric material we choose to work with, we can predict the temperature if these properties are known. Moreover, the heat diffusion equation is a model itself. In science, new models are built upon previously established models, as new theories are built upon previously established theories.**

Recalling the milling example from Section 27.2.1, the empirical model that related the observed particle size to observed mill speed contained no information on the nature of this relationship in other systems (i.e., in other mills). However, what if particle attrition was theorized to be controlled by energy input into the material, where energy input could be estimated from fundamental kinetic relationships, the mill operating parameters, and material properties? Such a model is no longer tethered to one particular system, but is generally applicable to any mill where the necessary energy calculations can be made, and the model inputs and material parameters are known. This generalized applicability of mechanistic models allows predictions of system behavior to be made, regardless of the system they are applied to, as long as the properties of the system relevant to the model can be known or estimated.

Semi-empirical theoretical models

Many, if not most, models don't fall neatly under the umbrellas of "empirical" or "mechanistic," but instead possess characteristics of each. In fact, strictly speaking there are no models that are either purely empirical or purely mechanistic. While mechanistic models are built from scientific theory, such theory was ultimately built on empirical evidence, and may be applied to the real world only under a set of assumptions that are likewise empirical. Conversely, empirical models, such as statistical curve fits, have little mechanistic content in the solution, but the

---

*The term "phenomenological model" is also ubiquitous among scientists and philosophers of science, yet its definition seems to be somewhat fluid. Some intend it to mean an empirical model that posits mathematical relationships between observed phenomena, while for others it is meant to convey a mechanistic model that posits physical mechanisms explaining the observed phenomena. To avoid confusion, the terms "empirical model" and "mechanistic model" are used here instead.

**It is this recursive relationship in science, the process by which new research is built upon research that has gone before, that led Newton to state, "If I have seen further it is by standing on ye shoulders of Giants."

choice of input variables influencing the chosen output variables reflects a kind of mechanistic reasoning. For the purposes of this text, however, a model is said to be mechanistic or empirical if either mode of reasoning dominates the model solution. If instead a model contains significant elements of each, it may be termed a semi-empirical model. Sometimes known as "hybrid models," one may find that such models actually outnumber mechanistic models in the literature. In practice, when a researcher is attempting to push back the boundaries of knowledge there is often insufficient or even non-existent theory for estimating key parameters necessary for a solution of the proposed model. Or if sufficient theory does exist, the solution of the model equations may prove intractable. Perhaps the researcher may wish to limit the complexity of a model by estimating a parameter empirically, and thereby avoid unnecessarily convoluted or time-consuming solution techniques.

One example of a semi-empirical model commonplace in pharmaceutical science is the Langmuir isotherm, which was developed on molecular kinetic arguments (see Equation 27.1).

$$\theta = \frac{bP}{1 + bP} \tag{27.1}$$

The Langmuir isotherm model solves for the fraction of adsorbent surface coverage θ by an adsorbate as a function of gas pressure P, with the constant b representing the ratio of adsorption and desorption rate constants. While there is a mechanistic interpretation for the meaning of the constant b, in practice it must be determined empirically, hence the fitted Langmuir isotherm is a semi-empirical model. Some more recent examples of hybrid models in the literature use ANNs empirically to estimate parameters for a mechanistic model or use other ancillary experimental techniques to supply a fitted constant that yields a predictive result.

Semi-empirical models turn out to be highly relevant to scale-up, since they are the type of models produced by dimensional analysis, an elegant methodology used by physicists and engineers for identifying criteria by which one system may scale to another. Incorporating model parameters identified by fundamental scientific knowledge, a mathematical method for manipulating those parameters into relevant dimensionless combinations, and empirical studies to determine how the resulting dimensionless numbers relate to each other, dimensional analysis is a powerful means by which system behavior may be predicted irrespective of scale, even when knowledge of the physical mechanisms at work is incomplete or tentative.

27.3 DIMENSIONAL ANALYSIS: SCALE-UP WITH SEMI-EMPIRICAL MODELING

27.3.1 Introduction to Dimensional Analysis

Scaling-up with Scale Models

The obvious resemblance of the scale model to its full-scale counterpart may suggest that the behavior at the small-scale could be predictive of full-scale phenomena, and qualitatively this is often the case. For example, the model aircraft will pitch and yaw via deflection of its empennage control surfaces, much as a real aircraft will. Likewise, longer high shear wet granulation in the pilot-scale granulator will generally result in greater power consumption, and greater granule densification, just as it will at the larger scale. However, in aerodynamic design, as well as pharmaceutical manufacturing, tight controls on narrow parameter ranges are necessary to yield a predictable and robust result regardless of scale, and mere qualitative descriptions of behavior obtained from observations of a scale model are not sufficient to provide such accuracy. If the scale model is to be used as a predictive tool, quantitative knowledge of how the model behaves needs to be converted into corresponding knowledge at the target scale. This can only take place if there is a theoretical linkage between scales, whereby the pertinent physical phenomena governing the behavior at both scales are themselves quantified. This theoretical linkage that translates the knowledge gained from a scale model to the real world may be obtained through the process of dimensional analysis.

What is Dimensional Analysis?

Dimensional analysis is a method used to identify dimensionless numbers that describe how the behavior of a scaled-down prototype can be interpreted, so that it is predictive of the full-sized process it is intended to model. Scale-up is most easily achieved by keeping these dimensionless numbers constant when changing scale. While the heart of dimensional analysis is purely mathematical, the effective application of the technique cannot take place in a vacuum of scientific knowledge. If dimensional analysis may be likened to an automobile, the engine powering the method is purely mathematical, while the steering is accomplished through the researcher's experience, and familiarity with known fundamental physico-chemical laws. Without this guidance the method is sure to go off course and crash. The rest of this section describes the method of dimensional analysis, but it is intended only as an introduction. The reader may be interested in the excellent text by Zlokarnik for a more thorough treatment of the subject.[6]

What is a dimensionless number?

A physical quantity consists of a pure number and a unit. Simply put, the unit tells you "what" and the pure number tells you "how much of what." If a mass is measured as 5 kilograms, the pure number is 5, and the unit is kilogram. A unit is said to be dimensional if it is expressed in terms of dimensions such as mass [M], length [L], time [T], temperature [Θ] or a combination of these. Obviously, a kilogram unit of mass has the dimension [M]. Velocity units, such as meters per second or miles per hour, would both have the dimensions [L T^{-1}]. Acceleration would have the dimensions [L T^{-2}]. A force unit, recalling Newton's Second Law $F = m \cdot a$, would then have the dimensions [M L T^{-2}]. The celsius unit has the dimension of temperature, and here is given the symbol [Θ].

Dimensionless numbers are those physical quantities that have units in which the dimensions cancel out in the algebraic sense. For example, if we were to divide velocity by the product of acceleration and time, the unit algebra would be:

$$\frac{[\text{L T}^{-1}]}{[\text{L T}^{-2}]\,[\text{T}]} = \frac{[\text{L T}^{-1}]}{[\text{L T}^{-1}]} = 1 \qquad (27.2)$$

The ratio of velocity over the product of acceleration and time is therefore a dimensionless number, however, this is a trivial result since basic Newtonian mechanics tells us that a change in velocity is equal to the product of constant acceleration and elapsed time, and this equality also demands that the dimensions be identical on both sides of the equation. A nontrivial example of a dimensionless number is shown in Equation 27.3:

$$\frac{V\,L\,\rho}{\mu} \rightarrow \frac{[\text{L T}^{-1}][\text{L}][\text{M L}^{-3}]}{[\text{M L}^{-1}\,\text{T}^{-1}]} = \frac{[\text{M L}^{-1}\,\text{T}^{-1}]}{[\text{M L}^{-1}\,\text{T}^{-1}]} = 1 \quad (27.3)$$

where:

V is velocity
L is length
ρ is density
μ is dynamic viscosity.

This ratio is well-known in dimensional analysis as the Reynolds Number (Re), the ratio of inertial forces to viscous forces.

Here are some trickier examples of dimensionality. Angular velocity is often expressed in units of revolutions per minute (RPM). The dimension of the minute unit is [T], but what is the dimension of a revolution? Actually, the revolution unit does not have any dimension at all. A revolution is an angular measurement, as are degrees and radians. An angle is merely the ratio of two lengths, hence angular measurements are dimensionless, and so the dimensions of RPM are [T^{-1}]. Moisture content in a pharmaceutical solid is often expressed as "% w/w" or a percentage based on weight ratios. This unit has no dimension, since percentage is a ratio of weights therefore, the dimensions of mass cancel out.

Dimensions for commonly encountered physical quantities

As illustrated by Equation 27.3, it is not always immediately obvious what dimensions a physical quantity may have. Dimensions for physical quantities commonly encountered in pharmaceutical scale-up are listed in Table 27.1.

Dimensional Analysis Solution Procedure

A. Identify the underlying physics of the phenomena

It may seem that this is putting the cart in front of the horse, since the intent of modeling is to gain an understanding of the process in the first place. However, dimensional analysis shares a trait in common with mechanistic modeling, which is that it is founded on the existence and availability of enough existing scientific knowledge to support the proposed model. If this foundation cannot be laid, dimensional analysis cannot proceed.

B. Assemble relevance list

The relevance list is a list of process and material parameters (e.g., density, viscosity, impeller speed, etc.) that are thought to be important to the behavior of the process. Again, this activity requires an *a priori* insight into the underlying physics of the phenomena, and draws heavily from the researcher's existing experience and knowledge. For example, an engineer should already be aware that viscosity may be ignored for turbulent fluids, but it is important to predicting the behavior of laminar flowing fluids. The choice of parameters in the relevance list ultimately governs the solution obtained hence, this step is the most crucial part of the process.

TABLE 27.1 List of physical quantities, units and dimensions

Physical quantity	Symbol	Typical units[a]	Dimensions
Mass	m	kg, lb_m	[M]
Length	l	m, ft	[L]
Time	t	s	[T]
Temperature	T	K, °C, °F, °R	[Θ]
Linear velocity	v	m/s, ft/s, mph	[L T^{-1}]
Angular velocity	ω	rad/s, deg/s, rpm	[T^{-1}]
Linear acceleration	a	m/s^2, ft/s^2	[L T^{-2}]
Angular acceleration	α	rad/s^2, deg/s^2	[T^{-2}]
Linear momentum	p	kg·m/s, lb_m·ft/s	[M L T^{-1}]
Angular momentum	l	kg·m^2/s, lb_m·ft^2/s	[M L^2 T^{-1}]
Rotational inertia	I	kg·m^2, lb_m·ft^2	[M L^2]
Frequency	ν	Hz	[T^{-1}]
Gravity	g	m/s^2, ft/s^2	[L T^{-2}]
Force	F	N, lb_f/in^2	[M L T^{-2}]
Pressure	P	Pa, lb_f [b]	[M L^{-1} T^{-2}]
Energy	E	J, W·s, BTU	[M L^2 T^{-2}]
Torque	τ	N·m, ft·lb_f	[M L^2 T^{-2}]
Specific[c] enthalpy	h	J/kg, BTU/lb_m	[L^2 T^{-2}]
Power	P	W, J/s, BTU/s	[M L^2 T^{-3}]
Density	ρ	kg/m^3, g/l, lb_m/ft^3	[M L^{-3}]
Dynamic viscosity	μ	N·s/m^2, lb_m·s/ft^2	[M L^{-1} T^{-1}]
Surface tension	σ	N/m, lb_f/in	[M T^{-2}]
Constant pressure specific heat	c_p	J/kg·K, BTU/lb_m·°R	[L^2 T^{-2}Θ^{-1}]
Universal gas constant	$\overline{R}$	J/mol·K, BTU/lbmol·°R	[M L^2 T^{-2} Θ^{-1}]
Specific gas constant	R	J/kg·K, BTU/lb_m·°R, ft·lb_f/lb_m·°R	[L^2 T^{-2} Θ^{-1}]
Thermal conductivity	k	W/m·K, BTU/ft·°R	[M L T^{-3} Θ^{-1}]
Thermal diffusivity	α	m^2/s, ft^2/s	[L^2 T^{-1}]
Heat transfer coefficient	h	W/m^2·K, BTU/ft^2·°R	[M T^{-3} Θ^{-1}]
Heat flux	q	W/m^2, BTU/ft^2	[M T^{-3}]
Mass diffusion coefficient	D	m^2/s, ft^2/s	[L^2 T^{-1}]
Mass flux	J	kg/m^2·s, lbm/ft^2·s	[M L^{-2} T^{-1}]

[a] m = meter, s = second, ft = foot, N = Newton, lb_f = pound force, in = inch, Pa = Pascal, J = Joule, W = Watt, BTU = British Thermal Unit, lb_m = pound mass, kg = kilogram, g = gram, l = liter, °R = degree Rankine, K = Kelvin
[b] The English system of units unfortunately uses pounds (lb) to represent both force and mass
To distinguish between the two, subscripts f and m are used, respectively
[c] The prefix "specific" indicates that the unit is expressed on a per mass basis

C. Identify core matrix and transform into unity matrix

While dimensionless combinations of parameters can be identified by visual inspection for the simplest cases, this will not be practical for typical problems. A general solution strategy requires the simultaneous solution of linear equations arranged in a dimensional matrix, consisting of a core matrix, and a residual. The core matrix is formed by grouping together a set of parameters with units that are linearly independent of each other. The remaining parameters form the residual matrix. The core matrix is then transformed into a unity matrix by a series of linear algebraic operations, while the same transformations are applied to the residual matrix.

D. Form Pi numbers and dimensionless equation

Dimensionless numbers are formed directly from the solution of the core and residual matrices. These numbers, named Pi or Π numbers after the Buckingham Pi theorem of dimensional analysis, constitute a dimensionless equation of the form shown in Equation 27.4, where Π is identically equal to 1. The combination of parameters forming the individual Π numbers on the right hand side of Equation 27.4 are determined by dimensional analysis, but the values of the exponents and the proportionality constant k must be determined empirically. The details are best illustrated by working through an example.

$$\Pi = k \, \Pi_1^\alpha \, \Pi_2^\beta \, \Pi_3^\gamma \, \Pi_4^\delta \dots \qquad (27.4)$$

Example 1: How Does Spraying Rate Scale in Fluid-bed Coating?

Problem   A fluid-bed tablet coating process using an aqueous coating solution has been developed at the pilot scale. It is necessary to know what the spray rate will need to be at the commercial scale, in order to choose the right equipment.

For the sake of illustration, the physical relationship between spray rate and the operating parameters is treated here as an unknown.

Assumptions
1. Local gradients in temperature and density can be ignored.
2. Water is the only volatile component in the spray solution.
3. The system is not limited by saturation (i.e., the outlet conditions are far enough away from 100% relative humidity, such that this constraint can be ignored).
4. Heat loss through system boundaries is not included in the model.
5. The system is in dynamic equilibrium.

Solution procedure
A. Identify the underlying physics of the phenomena

The researcher understands that air can carry heat along with it, and that heat input is required for evaporation of water to occur.

B. Assemble relevance list

Since we are assuming dynamic equilibrium and no temperature gradients, diffusive mass and heat transfer can be ignored. Spray rate is our dependent variable, so that obviously will be part of the

TABLE 27.2   Tentative relevance list

Parameter	Symbol	Dimensions
Spray rate	R	$[\mathrm{M}\,\mathrm{T}^{-1}]$
Air flow	Q_a	$[\mathrm{L}^3\,\mathrm{T}^{-1}]$
Air density	ρ_a	$[\mathrm{M}\,\mathrm{L}^{-3}]$
Air specific heat	$c_{p,a}$	$[\mathrm{L}^2\,\mathrm{T}^{-2}\Theta^{-1}]$
Liquid density	ρ_l	$[\mathrm{M}\,\mathrm{L}^{-3}]$
Liquid specific heat	$c_{p,l}$	$[\mathrm{L}^2\,\mathrm{T}^{-2}\Theta^{-1}]$
Latent heat of evaporation	H	$[\mathrm{L}^2\,\mathrm{T}^{-2}]$
Inlet temperature	T_{in}	$[\Theta]$
Exhaust temperature	T_{ex}	$[\Theta]$

relevance list. In addition, thermal properties of the air and spray liquid are likely to be important. The heat needed to evaporate water is known as the latent heat of vaporization, so that should be a relevant parameter. Operating parameters such as airflow, air temperature, and spray liquid temperature would also appear to be relevant. The coating solution consists of a relatively small percentage of suspended solids in an aqueous mixture, so the actual mass fraction of water in the spray solution is a necessary parameter. However, the mass fraction is a dimensionless number already, and only dimensional numbers are put into the relevance list. Mass fraction instead will appear as dimensionless number Π_1 in the dimensionless equation. A first try at a relevance list might look like Table 27.2.

In general, when there are two or more parameters with identical dimensions remaining in the relevance list, such as $c_{p,a}$ and $c_{p,l}$, ρ_a and ρ_l or T_{in} and T_{ex}, those dimensionally identical parameters are combined to form dimensionless ratios that will appear as Π numbers in the dimensionless equation. All but one of those parameters are then removed from the relevance list (the choice of which ones to remove is actually arbitrary at this point, since the resulting Π numbers can be algebraically recombined as needed to manipulate the final form of the dimensionless equation. Alternatively, parameters with identical dimensions can be combined into one parameter by taking their sum or difference or perhaps a combination of the sum, difference, and division operations may be appropriate. The choice of which form to use depends upon the physical phenomena, and the researcher's prior knowledge. For example, if a chemical reaction or any other phenomena following an Arrhenius dependence is involved, the ratio of absolute temperatures might be an important dimensionless parameter. No chemical reactions are involved in this particular

TABLE 27.3 Revised relevance list

Parameter	Symbol	Dimensions
Spray rate	R	$[M\,T^{-1}]$
Air flow	Q	$[L^3\,T^{-1}]$
Air density	ρ_a	$[M\,L^{-3}]$
Air specific heat	$c_{p,a}$	$[L^2\,T^{-2}\Theta^{-1}]$
Latent heat of evaporation	H	$[L^2\,T^{-2}]$
Temperature difference	ΔT	$[\Theta]$

	ρ_a	Q	H	ΔT
M	1	0	0	0
L	−3	3	2	0
T	0	−1	−2	0
Θ	0	0	0	1

FIGURE 27.1 Core matrix

	Core				Residual	
	ρ_a	Q	H	ΔT	R	$C_{p,a}$
M	1	0	0	0	1	0
L	−3	3	2	0	0	2
T	0	−1	−2	0	−1	−2
Θ	0	0	0	1	0	−1

FIGURE 27.2 Core and residual matrix

example, but it is known that evaporation is an endothermic process that cools the air. Cooling implies a temperature difference, so based on this knowledge the two temperatures are combined into one new parameter ΔT, by taking the difference between them.

Application of experience and fundamental scientific knowledge may further reduce this list. The spray rate is already given in terms of mass per unit time, and since we posit no mechanisms for the importance of spray liquid volume, we omit the liquid density. However, air density is needed, since mass flow of the air cannot be determined without it. In addition, the enthalpy of liquid water is also known to be very small compared to its latent heat of evaporation for typical temperature ranges encountered in a coating process, and since enthalpy is a function of temperature and specific heat, the specific heat of water is also omitted on that basis.

As a rule, if not enough is known about the phenomena to be able to make an informed choice on how to combine dimensionally identical parameters, the relationship between them would need to be explored by preliminary experimentation, before dimensional analysis can be conducted. The revised parameter list is given in Table 27.3.

C. Identify core matrix and transform into unity matrix

The core matrix contains a set of parameters with unit dimensions that are linearly independent of each other. This concept can be best illustrated by constructing a core matrix from the relevance list, as shown in Figure 27.1.

The core matrix contains a row for each dimension present in the relevance list, and an equivalent number of columns, each corresponding to a parameter. Each position in the matrix is filled with the dimensional exponent corresponding to that dimension and parameter. For example, the latent heat of

vaporization has a unit with a temperature dimension to the −2 power, −2 is then inserted into the core matrix as shown in Figure 27.1. The parameters chosen for the core matrix must yield linearly independent rows, such that the core matrix can be transformed into the unity matrix, that is, a matrix consisting of all 0s except for the diagonal filled with 1s. Note that this set of parameters may not be unique, and in general a relevance list contains enough parameters to allow for several combinations yielding a linearly independent core matrix. Fortunately, as long as linear independence is maintained, the choice of parameters isn't important to the results, and algebraic transformations of the resulting Π parameters can be performed to yield the same solution. Since there are at most four rows in the matrix, a set of linearly independent parameters can be chosen by inspection. The core matrix is usually loaded with material properties, while the target parameter and processing parameters tend to be placed in the residual matrix if possible.

It just so happens that the core matrix shown in Figure 27.1 is linearly independent, so the remainder of the parameters in the relevance list will fill the residual matrix. The resulting core and residual matrix are shown together in Figure 27.2.

Linear transformations (e.g., using Gaussian elimination) are now applied to the core matrix to transform it into a unity matrix, and the same transformations are simultaneously also applied to the residual matrix. The transformed matrices are shown in Figure 27.3.

D. Form Pi numbers and dimensionless equation

A dimensionless Pi number can be formed for each column in the residual matrix. As a rule, the number of dimensionless Pi numbers that may be formed from the relevance list is equal to the number of

	Core				Residual	
	ρ_a	Q	H	ΔT	R	$c_{p,a}$
M	1	0	0	0	1	0
L	0	1	0	0	1	0
T	0	0	1	0	0	1
Θ	0	0	0	1	0	-1

FIGURE 27.3 Core unity matrix and transformed residual matrix

dimensional parameters minus the rank of the core matrix, where the rank is simply the number of linearly independent rows. For the present example, we have 6 dimensional parameters, and a rank of 4, leaving $6 - 4 = 2$ dimensionless parameters that can be formed.

Each dimensionless number formed from the core and residual matrices consists of a numerator and denominator. The numerator is simply the residual parameter. The product of the core matrix parameters, each to the power of their respective exponents, where the exponents are the elements of the residual matrix, forms the denominator. This denominator is the same for each of the Π numbers hence, the core matrix parameters are also called the repeating parameters. In our example:

$$\Pi_2 = \frac{R}{\rho^1 \, Q^1 \, H^0 \, \Delta T^0} = \frac{R}{\rho Q} \tag{27.5}$$

$$\Pi_3 = \frac{c_{p,a}}{\rho^0 \, Q^0 \, H^1 \, \Delta T^{-1}} = \frac{c_{p,a} \, \Delta T}{H} \tag{27.6}$$

With the water mass fraction as Π_1, a dimensionless equation relating each of the Π numbers can be put in the form of Equation 27.4. The dimensionless equation can also be expressed where one Π number is a function of the others, such as in Equation 27.7.

$$\Pi_2 = k \, \Pi_3^\alpha \, \Pi_1^\beta \tag{27.7}$$

The dimensionless equation would now take the form shown in Equation 27.8.

$$\frac{R}{\rho Q} = k \left(\frac{c_{p,a} \, \Delta T}{H} \right)^\alpha \phi^\beta \tag{27.8}$$

Discussion   Three dimensionless numbers have been identified as being important in scaling-up the spray rate in a coating process. If Π_3 and Π_1 are both kept constant upon scale-up, then Π_2 must also remain constant, regardless of k, α, and β. To fully understand the relationship between the Pi numbers, however,

empirical studies would need to be carried out in order to determine those constants. While empirical studies take time, materials and effort, fortunately they can be estimated using experiments with the scaled-down prototypes, and then be applied to the full-scale process.

27.3.2 Effective Application of Dimensional Analysis

If the preceding example were to be solved via dimensional analysis by someone knowledgeable and experienced with dimensional analysis and thermodynamic processes, Equation 27.8 would be obtained with a minimum of effort, and after a suitable number of experimental data points had been determined, statistical regression techniques could be used to arrive at the estimates for k, α, and β, after which the scale-up model would be fully defined.

However, we initially assumed for the sake of illustration that the physical relationship between spray rate and the process and material parameters was an unknown. In reality, a researcher familiar enough with thermodynamic theory to understand the concepts of enthalpy, temperature, and latent heat of evaporation, would have been able to solve this particularly simple scale-up problem with a pencil and paper in mere minutes, avoiding the need for dimensional analysis altogether. How? Equation 27.8, with k, α, and β equal to 1, 1, and -1 respectively, can easily be derived from a fundamental energy balance, making a semi-empirical dimensional analysis superfluous. For this simple case it turns out that a first principles mechanistic approach would be the most effective method for arriving at a suitable scale-up model.

When Should Dimensional Analysis be Used?

Dimensional analysis is not the only tool in the researcher's scale-up toolbox and, as the preceding example demonstrates, neither is it always the appropriate tool. The decision whether to use dimensional analysis, to use a mechanistic model or to even attempt to model at all, is highly dependent on the information available to the researcher, as well as the researcher's knowledge and experience.

If there is existing theory where the physico-chemical mechanisms are explained in mathematical form, a dimensional analysis approach is not needed, and would in fact be a waste of time and resources. With a solution already available, a first-principles analysis taking advantage of the known solution would be the

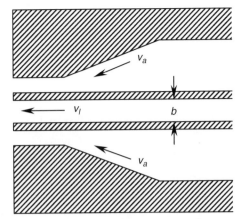

FIGURE 27.4 Cross-section of atomizing nozzle

TABLE 27.4 Tentative relevance list

Parameter	Symbol	Dimensions
Jet diameter	b	[M]
Droplet diameter	d	[M]
Solution spray rate	Q_l	$[L^3 T^{-1}]$
Atomizing air flow	Q_a	$[L^3 T^{-1}]$
Solution density	ρ_l	$[M L^{-3}]$
Atomizing air density	ρ_a	$[M L^{-3}]$
Solution velocity	v_l	$[L T^{-1}]$
Atomizing air flow velocity	v_a	$[L T^{-1}]$
Solution viscosity	μ_l	$[M L^{-1} T^{-1}]$
Air viscosity	μ_a	$[M L^{-1} T^{-1}]$
Solution surface tension	σ	$[M T^{-2}]$

most efficient means of obtaining a scale-up model, such as with the coating scale-up example above.

If no mechanistic mathematical solutions exist, yet the fundamental physico-chemical processes are understood well enough to at least tentatively assemble a relevance list, then dimensionless analysis may be possible. However, the compilation of the relevance list is the crucial step; if a parameter important to the relevant physico-chemical processes is mistakenly omitted from the relevance list dimensional analysis may fail to yield a useful scale-up equation.

If there is no existing theory to make use of, and the underlying physics of the phenomena are not well-understood, the researcher is unfortunately left without a means to scale-up, except by costly experimentation at the target scale, heuristic rules of thumb, intuition, and luck. At this point, a retreat to the lab or pilot plant to gain some physical knowledge would seem to be prudent.

In contrast to Example 1, the following is an example where mechanistic solutions are truly not known to exist.

Example 2: How Does the Spray Droplet Diameter Scale in Fluid-bed Coating?

Problem A fluid-bed tablet coating process using an aqueous coating solution has been developed at the pilot-scale. The coating solution is sprayed through a two-phase atomizing nozzle (see Figure 27.4). It is necessary to know how the mean spray droplet diameter will change when scaling-up to a larger coater utilizing higher capacity spray nozzles.

Assumptions
1. Local gradients in temperature and density can be ignored.
2. Water is the only volatile component in the spray solution.

3. The spray solution is aqueous.
4. Solid particles in suspension are small compared to resulting droplet size.

Solution Procedure
A. Identify the underlying physics of the phenomena

The researcher understands that the break-up of a liquid jet of spray solution into droplets is due to the competing effects of aerodynamic forces, and surface tension of the liquid.

B. Assemble relevance list

Droplet diameter is the target parameter, and is part of the relevance list. Since aerodynamic forces are important, the volumetric flow rate, density, velocity, and viscosity of the air are likely to be important. The volumetric flow rate, density, and velocity of the liquid jet should also affect how the jet breaks up. Surface tension is hypothesized to be important to jet break up, and it is reasonable to assume that the diameter of the jet has an impact on the diameter of the droplets. The water mass fraction of the solution can be omitted, since the density, viscosity, and surface tension describe the overall mechanical behavior of the solution. The tentative relevance list is given in Table 27.4.

Again, the relevance list can be trimmed by recognizing that dimensionless Pi numbers can be formed from dimensionally identical parameters. The dimensionless ratios d/b, Q_l/Q_a, ρ_l/ρ_a, and μ_l/μ_a can be identified as Π_1, Π_2, Π_3, and Π_4, and d, Q_l, ρ_l, and μ_l can be removed from the revised relevance list, since they now are accounted for. Since it is hypothesized that aerodynamic force is the physical mechanism at work, the relative velocity between the atomizing air and the liquid jet would seem to be the physically relevant parameter, hence the two velocities are combined into

TABLE 27.5   Revised relevance list

Parameter	Symbol	Dimensions
Jet diameter	b	$[M]$
Atomizing air flow	Q_a	$[L^3\,T^{-1}]$
Atomizing air density	ρ_a	$[M\,L^{-3}]$
Relative velocity	Δv	$[L\,T^{-1}]$
Air viscosity	μ_a	$[M\,L^{-1}\,T^{-1}]$
Solution surface tension	σ	$[M\,T^{-2}]$

TABLE 27.6   Core and residual matrix

	Core			Residual		
	σ	ρ_a	μ	Q	Δv	b
M	1	1	1	0	0	0
L	0	-3	-1	3	1	1
T	-2	0	-1	-1	-1	0

TABLE 27.7   Transformed core and residual matrix

	Core			Residual		
	σ	ρ_a	μ_a	Q_a	Δv	b
M	1	0	0	-1	1	-1
L	0	1	0	-2	0	-1
T	0	0	1	3	-1	2

one parameter Δv. The revised relevance list is shown in Table 27.5.

C. Identify core matrix and transform into unity matrix

A core matrix and residual matrix can be constructed as shown in Table 27.6. The core matrix is loaded with material property parameters, and all three rows are linearly independent. The processing parameters are located in the residual matrix. Following transformation, the core and residual matrices are as shown in Table 27.7.

D. Form Pi numbers and dimensionless equation

The Pi numbers obtained by transformation of the core matrix are:

$$\Pi_5 = \frac{Q_a\,\sigma_a\,\rho_a^2}{\mu_a^3} \tag{27.9}$$

$$\Pi_6 = \frac{\Delta v\,\mu_a}{\sigma_a} \tag{27.10}$$

$$\Pi_7 = \frac{b\,\sigma_a\,\rho_a}{\mu_a^2} \tag{27.11}$$

The dimensionless equation can now be written as shown in Equation 27.12.

$$\frac{d}{b} = k \left(\frac{Q_l}{Q_a}\right)^\alpha \left(\frac{\rho_l}{\rho_a}\right)^\beta \left(\frac{\mu_l}{\mu_a}\right)^\gamma \left(\frac{Q_a\,\sigma_a\,\rho_a^2}{\mu_a^3}\right)^\delta$$
$$\left(\frac{\Delta v\,\mu_a}{\sigma}\right)^\varepsilon \left(\frac{b\,\sigma_a\,\rho_a}{\mu_a^2}\right)^\varsigma \tag{27.12}$$

Several well-known dimensionless numbers can be identified from the above Pi numbers. Π_6 is the capillary number (Ca), which represents the relative effect of viscous forces and surface tension acting across an interface between a liquid and a gas. Π_7 is the Laplace number (La), which relates the surface tension to the viscous momentum transport inside a fluid. The inverse of the square root of the Laplace number is also known as the Ohnesorge number (Z). Π_5 is not a commonly used dimensionless number however, the ratio Π_5/Π_7 yields the Reynolds number. Finally, $\Pi_6^2\Pi_7$ is the Weber number (We), which is a measure of the relative importance of the inertia of a fluid compared to its surface tension, and figures prominently in theories concerning the formation of droplets and bubbles.

$$We = \Pi_6^2\,\Pi_7 = \frac{\Delta v^2 \rho\, b}{\sigma} \tag{27.13}$$

While Δv in Equation 27.13 would be difficult to measure experimentally, it could be approximated from the known air and solution flow rates, and their respective nozzle orifice dimensions. Researchers in the field of atomization have indeed found that a dimensionless equation in the form shown in Equation 27.14 has been successful in predicting droplet size in atomized sprays.

$$\frac{d}{b} = k(La)^\alpha\,(We)^\beta \left(\frac{Q_l}{Q_a}\frac{\rho_l}{\rho_a}\right)^\chi \tag{27.14}$$

Discussion   No tractable mechanistic theory exists for predicting the diameter of atomized droplets from first principles, yet the mathematical process of dimensional analysis was able to provide criteria by which droplet diameter can be maintained upon scale-up.

This example also serves to illustrate additional benefits of the dimensionless equation:

1. It functions as a guide for experimental design and direction for the researcher when physico-chemical mechanisms are not well-understood.
2. When many parameters are involved, the sheer volume of experimental data can become difficult to manage. Plotting experimental data in terms of dimensionless numbers is a convenient and concise way to display and interpret experimental data.
3. Dimensional analysis reduces the number of functional relationships that need to be investigated.

The mathematical process of dimensional analysis still doesn't provide a complete solution, but it directs the researcher towards which combinations of parameters may be important. However, not all Pi numbers identified through dimensional analysis are necessarily important to the solution. For example, many researchers in atomization have found that the viscosity of air is not an important parameter in determining atomized droplet diameter, thus Π_4 in the above example would not be important to the solution.

Example 3: How Does High Shear Wet Granulation Scale up?

Perhaps the most familiar unit operation to those involved in pharmaceutical manufacturing and development is high shear wet granulation. Because of the many complex physical phenomena involved in granulation that defy a rigorous mechanistic description, granulation scale-up would seem well-suited to a dimensional analysis approach, and many examples of such can be found in the literature. The underlying assumption usually employed is that the wet mass consistency is a direct measure of the quality of the resulting granules, which in turn affects downstream processing. A relevance list for granulation is given in Table 27.8.

It is left as an exercise for the reader to construct and solve the core and residual matrices. The resulting dimensionless numbers are shown in Equations 27.15–27.18.

$$\Pi_1 = \frac{P}{\rho\, N^3\, D^5} = \text{Newton Power Number (N}_P)$$

(27.15)

$$\Pi_2 = \frac{N^2 D}{g} = \text{Froude Number (Fr)} \qquad (27.16)$$

TABLE 27.8 Granulation relevance list

Parameter	Symbol	Dimensions
Bowl diameter	D	[L]
Bowl loading	m	[M]
Impeller speed	N	[T^{-1}]
Impeller power consumption	P	[M L^2 T^{-3}]
Bulk density	ρ_a	[M L^{-3}]
Apparent viscosity	μ	[M L^{-1} T^{-1}]
Gravity	g	[L T^{-2}]

$$\Pi_3 = \frac{\rho\, N\, D^2}{\mu} = \text{Reynolds Number (Re)} \qquad (27.17)$$

$$\Pi_4 = \frac{m}{\rho\, D^3} = \text{fill ratio} \qquad (27.18)$$

While examples of dimensionless analysis applied to granulation are ubiquitous in the literature, limited success has been achieved using this approach. One of the primary difficulties is that dynamic viscosity, μ, is a liquid property, and is not well-defined for a mass of discrete solid particles. Some researchers have approximated μ as an "apparent viscosity," by utilizing a mixer torque rheometer to determine the relationship between torque and shear rate, in which the constant of proportionality is μ/ρ, also known as the kinematic viscosity ν. However, the kinematic viscosity is only a constant for Newtonian fluids by definition, and wet granular materials tend to be non-Newtonian. As shear rate changes with scale, and with radial distance from the impeller axis, the apparent viscosity also changes, which makes calculation of the Reynolds number problematic. Furthermore, measurement in mixer torque rheometry is complicated by the fact that the sample is continuously being compressed and expanded, and instrument geometry, mixing kinetics, shaft speed, and sample weight also have an effect on the measured apparent viscosity. Measurements using mixer torque rheometry may not be reproducible or consistent from one research group to the next, due to these complicating factors.

One solution explored by some researchers is to completely ignore the apparent viscosity, such that the Reynolds number disappears from the list of Pi numbers. The assumption of no long-range interactions (i.e., forces acting over several particle lengths) that impact shear stress may seem a dubious one, but limited success was also achieved with this approach. This example of granulation scale-up emphasizes the fact that dimensional analysis does not dictate one unique solution for a given problem, but rather it provides guidance for the researcher as to how to effectively investigate and scale the phenomena.

27.3.3 Similitude

The concept of similitude or similarity has been previously hinted at in the discussion concerning scale models. Similitude between prototypes of different scale is achieved when the experimental results on one scale are directly applicable to the other. The criteria for achieving similitude are outlined below.

Geometric similitude Geometric similitude requires that the model be the same shape as the full-scale prototype, which in turn requires all ratios of characteristics lengths, all corresponding angles, and all flow directions to be identical. For example, bowl diameter D, bowl height H, fill height h, impeller diameter d, and blade width w all can be identified as characteristic lengths in a granulator bowl. To maintain strict geometric similitude, the ratios D/H, D/h, D/d, D/w, H/h, H/d, H/w, h/d, h/w, and d/w all must be held invariant with respect to scale.

Kinematic similitude Kinematic similitude requires that the ratios of velocities at corresponding points between the model and full-scale prototype are identical, and this is turn depends on geometric similitude being satisfied. The implication of this requirement is that the streamlines of flow are identical regardless of scale. For example, if two geometrically similar granulators are operated, such that the flow pattern in one is "bumping" flow while the other is "roping" flow, kinematic similitude is not satisfied. Geometric similitude is a necessary, but not sufficient, condition to guarantee kinematic similitude.

Dynamic similitude Dynamic similitude requires that the ratios of all forces acting at corresponding points in the model and full-scale prototype are identical, and this is turn depends on both geometric and kinematic similitude being satisfied. For example, dimensional analysis suggests that the ratio of inertial forces to gravitational forces acting on a granule in high shear

granulation should be held constant regardless of scale.

Thermal similitude Thermal similitude is satisfied when the ratios of heat fluxes at corresponding points are identical. Convective heat flow occurs along streamlines hence, thermal similitude is dependent on both kinematic and geometric similitude.

When simplifying the relevance lists in the previous examples, duplicate length parameters were removed, and only one characteristic length parameter was retained. The same procedure was done for velocities, viscosities, etc., with the caveat that the choice of which parameter to retain as the characteristic parameter with those dimensions was arbitrary. Similitude is the underlying principle by which it can be said that the choice is arbitrary. To illustrate why, consider the numerous length parameters that can be identified in granulation scale-up. If the ratios of these parameters are held constant with respect to scale, trivial algebraic manipulations of the Pi numbers can be performed to exchange one length parameter for another, as the researcher sees fit. This would not be possible if geometric similitude was not satisfied, therefore the concept of similitude goes hand-in-hand with dimensional analysis.

In practice, however, it is difficult to achieve strict similitude. This becomes clear when considering all possible length scales occurring within a process. One can hardly scale-up a blending process by keeping the ratio of particle diameter to blender characteristic length constant, for example. In addition, the design and availability of processing equipment can place unavoidable limitations on maintaining similitude. It has been shown that the Collette Gral 10 and 75 are geometrically similar to each other, with the minor exception of chopper placement, but the Gral 300 and 600 deviate significantly from geometric similarity with the smaller models.[7,8] Furthermore, Gral granulators are 2- or 3-speed machines that are designed to maintain constant tip speeds across scales. Although the Froude number is a relevant dimensionless number for granulation, it is not possible to keep the Froude number constant upon scale-up when tip speed is instead maintained. These, then, are examples of distorted models, in which geometric, kinematic or dynamic similitude is violated.

There are ways to deal with distorted models in dimensional analysis. Even though similitude may be violated, the distorted dimensionless number may not be important to the behavior of the system, and can simply be ignored. For example, the ratio of chopper blade diameter to mixer blade diameter is a dimensionless number, yet the literature does not make mention of any observed effects on the behavior of the granular mixture due to distortion of this geometric relationship. However, if the distorted dimensionless ratio is expected to be important, such as the ratio of bowl height to bowl diameter, it can be accounted for by the inclusion of an additional empirically determined distortion coefficient in the model. (If it is unclear why this particular ratio is important, consider that bed depth is a function of this ratio, and that hydrostatic pressure within the bed due to gravitational force is a nonlinear function of depth, according to Shaxby's equation.)

The simplest and quickest way to scale with dimensional analysis is to keep all important dimensionless numbers constant upon scale-up, whenever this is possible. However, scale-up predictions can still be obtained when this is not possible by the construction of a so-called "master curve." For example, researchers have met with success in scaling Gral granulators using the dimensionless analysis shown in Example 3, despite not being able to keep the Froude number constant.[8] The experimental data was plotted in terms of the Power number as a function of the dimensionless product (Re × Fr × fill ratio), which collapsed the data into a single "master curve" for 8 L, 25 L, 75 L, and 600 L bowls. The construction of a master curve was possible despite the geometric distortions noted, however it required the empirically driven solution of the entire dimensionless equation, including exponents and proportionality constant. This example affirms that while distorted models are not ideal, they can still provide for successful scale-up. It should also be noted that the strategy of keeping all important dimensionless numbers constant across scales may fail if it is not clear which dimensionless numbers are important. Physical mechanisms negligible at one scale may dominate at another scale (e.g., electrostatic versus gravitational forces), and therefore the dimensionless numbers most important to modeling the phenomena may also change.

If the phenomena contributing to the behavior of the system can be analyzed separately, it may be possible to tackle a troublesome scale-up problem in parts. For example, if two different physical processes are hypothesized to be important, each one contributing to the net behavior of the system while being independent of each other, the dimensional analysis can be broken into two distinct problems. Mathematically speaking, instead of the dimensionless equation being in the form $\Pi_1 = f(\Pi_2, \Pi_3, \Pi_4, \Pi_5 \ldots)$, it would take the form $\Pi_1 = f(\Pi_2, \Pi_3 \ldots) + g(\Pi_4, \Pi_5 \ldots)$. This strategy could come in handy when it is impossible to maintain similitude for both sub-models simultaneously.

27.4 MECHANISTIC MODELS FOR SCALE-UP

As illustrated in the previous section, dimensional analysis is a powerful procedure for scaling a process, yet there are situations where a mechanistic approach may be better suited. When the phenomena are well-understood in terms of physical mechanisms, and can be expressed as a tractable set of mathematical equations amenable to analytical or numerical solution, dimensional analysis becomes an unnecessary mathematical exercise. Regarding the superiority of modeling from a mechanistic standpoint, a more philosophical argument may be that it transcends the idea of scale-up as only being a process of extrapolation, whereby process equivalence at Scale B is attained by translating knowledge anchored at Scale A. Instead, process knowledge is accumulated on a physico-chemical or mechanistic level, independent of the need to leverage knowledge from some fixed process scale. The real output of a mechanistic scaling model is new physical knowledge and understanding, which is generally applicable to all similar systems.

27.4.1 Mechanistic Modeling versus Dimensional Analysis

In addition to the benefit of providing a fundamental, scale-independent understanding of the physical processes at work, mechanistic modeling is advantageous for several other reasons. It can produce models that generate predictions that are accurate over a greater range of operating conditions than dimensional analysis models that tend to scale-up any experimental error along with the intended process parameters. In addition, it is an ideal tool for the study of specific parameters involved with the phenomena being modeled, since the mechanistic model affords the investigator the opportunity to independently alter any one parameter to study its effects on the model output.

However, these advantages do come at a price. Mechanistic models can be heavily dependent on physical knowledge that may or may not be available or perhaps is only attainable through laborious experimentation requiring a large cost and time commitment. This dependency may be exacerbated by the necessity of increasingly greater computational requirements with more model inputs, often necessitating sophisticated numerical algorithms, and powerful computers, to obtain a solution in a practical length of time. There is little short-term advantage in pursuing mechanistic modeling if the cost of developing and solving the model becomes so large that it is comparable to the cost of simply executing empirical studies at the production scale. After all, the ultimate aim of modeling in a science-based pharmaceutical manufacturing environment is to reduce research and production costs, while maintaining or improving quality.*

A model can be no more accurate than its inputs, and is potentially much more inaccurate, since the output is a function of each input. This is true of all models, but of mechanistic models in particular since they tend to be highly parameterized. The predictive potential of mechanistic models also hinges on a sound understanding of the physical mechanisms at work; if the proposed mechanisms are not formulated well first, the model will not be predictive of experimental data when the time comes to validate the model. This stands in contrast to dimensional analysis models that tend to work in the opposite direction; that is, given a dimensionless equation obtained through dimensional analysis, the unknown constants can be adjusted to conform to the known data, and thus capture the behavior of the system. To compensate for lack of predictive capability, mechanistic models may be modified *ad hoc* by the incorporation of a fitted empirical constant, and therefore become semi-empirical, and in fact this is commonplace in the literature. However, the potential pitfall here is that the explanatory power of the mechanistic model—one of its major benefits—tends to become hobbled if the model must be outfitted with empirically fitted constants for which a mechanistic description is lacking.

Given the above, the reader may be intimidated to even consider mechanistic modeling for scale-up, yet the potential pitfalls above may be avoided. For example, the result of the coating spray rate scale-up example in the last section can be obtained through a mechanistic model that is neither highly parameterized, nor requiring anything more sophisticated than a calculator to solve. The solution of conservation law equations for mass, energy, and momentum can reveal much about scaling relationships, yet models based on these conservation laws are often no more complex than the accounting of inflow and outflows. In general, however, mechanistic models may require at least a modest amount of mathematical/computational effort, and may involve computer simulation, which is the incremental solution of the model equations in subdomains of the system space, discretized in time and/or spatial dimensions.

---

*Quality: the suitability of either a drug substance or drug product for its intended use. This term includes such attributes as the identity, strength, and purity (from ICH Q6A Specifications: Test Procedures and Acceptance Criteria for New Drug Substances and New Drug Products: Chemical Substances).

27.4.2 Developing a Mechanistic Model

Unlike dimensional analysis, there is no clearly defined mathematical procedure for obtaining a mechanistic model. There are myriad physico-chemical phenomena that may be modeled with a variety of specialized mathematical techniques, precluding a simple recipe that is appropriate for all situations. However, a generalized strategy is illustrated in Figure 27.5 and described below.

27.4.3 Definition

A necessary first step to creating a mechanistic scale-up model is to decide what it is that the model will predict. Since the aim of scale-up is to produce material with the same quality attributes, albeit in larger volumes, a quality attribute of the processed material would seem to be the logical choice as the model output. If a tractable theory does not exist which relates the quality attribute of the material to the parameters of the unit operation, mechanistic scale-up modeling may still be useful by instead predicting the conditions imposed upon the material throughout the unit operation. For example, a mechanistic theory relating tablet dissolution to fluid-bed coater parameters is lacking; yet if the fluidized tablet flow patterns, spray characteristics, internal thermodynamic conditions, and applied coating amount can be predicted and kept constant upon scale-up, it would be reasonable to expect that the resulting qualities of the coating that impact dissolution would also remain constant. Note that while multivariate empirical modeling is well-suited to producing models with multiple outputs (and especially so for ANNs), the analytical nature of a mechanistic approach demands that the focus be narrowed to one output, or else the effort is almost sure to collapse under the weight of the resulting complexity and convolution. When multiple quality attributes are of importance in the scale-up of a single unit operation, separate models may be developed for each.

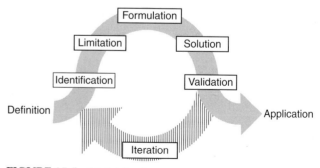

FIGURE 27.5 Model development process

27.4.4 Identification

Given the dependent variable to be predicted, physical phenomena impacting this variable are identified and compiled. While the pharmaceutical scientist may wish to go to the lab or pilot plant and start experimenting to determine what physical phenomena are relevant, it is quite often the case that these relationships are already well-known in the literature, in which case a literature search is time well spent. As with the compilation of the relevance list in dimensional analysis, this is a crucial step in the mechanistic model-building process, since the model will lack predictive power if physical processes important to the behavior of the system are overlooked.

27.4.5 Limitation

In order to arrive at a model that is predictive, yet not so bloated that it is impractical to solve, the scope, sophistication, and level of detail should be kept in accord with the problem definition, and the availability of parameter estimates and solution methods. For example, don't attempt to solve a 3-D Navier Stokes simulation where a simple control volume mass conservation approach will do the trick. While entirely appropriate for academic research, in general it is not likely that the intricate detail provided by such a simulation would be directly applicable to scale-up in a manufacturing environment, nor is it likely that the expense of obtaining such detailed knowledge would be offset by a concomitant realizable cost reduction in development and manufacturing. The number of input parameters increases with the complexity of the model, therefore the cost of experimentally obtaining estimates for these parameters also places a practical limit on the model complexity. Ideally, the cost and effort put into development of the scale-up model will be less than what would otherwise be expended for empirical target scale experiments, in order to realize a short-term benefit, although the long-term benefit of a working process model, and increased mechanistic understanding, will pay off for future projects, regardless.

27.4.6 Formulation

Perhaps the easiest step in the entire development of a mechanistic model is simply writing out the governing equations that need to be solved. If the previous steps have all been completed, formulation of the model equations is a straightforward exercise of adapting general mathematical descriptions of the pertinent physical phenomena to the specific geometry, parameters, and conditions of the system to be modeled. A more generally applicable model may be obtained by non-dimensionalizing the governing equations, so that the results of the model can also be readily applied to other systems. Similar to dimensional analysis, this non-dimensionalization involves the algebraic manipulation of the equation, so that each term is reduced to a non-dimensional form, e.g., dimensionless length ratios replace absolute lengths, dimensionless temperature ratios replace absolute temperatures, etc.

27.4.7 Solution

While the simplest models may require only a calculator to solve, mechanistic models otherwise tend to be cumbersome or even impossible to solve analytically, and require numerical methods to obtain a solution. The selection of a numerical method is specific to the form of the equation(s) to be solved, and a discussion of numerical solutions is outside the scope of this text. However, it is the case that a computer, being a digital machine that deals in "packets" of information, requires an algorithm using a discretized approach, so that the equations can be solved in a step-by-step piecewise fashion. This generally requires a custom computer program (e.g., C++), but spreadsheet programs such as Microsoft Excel®, which includes a powerful macro language that can be used, together with the spreadsheet to automate a solution method, should not be underestimated as powerful numerical solution tools.

27.4.8 Validation

With a working model ready to go, the last step in development is to make sure that the model is actually capable of providing good predictions. This is accomplished by comparing model predictions against a reliable set of experimental data, preferably spanning a range that would normally be encountered in the application of the model. While mechanistic models can be called upon to extrapolate predictions outside the range of validation, and indeed this is one of the advantages of mechanistic modeling, it is always advisable to validate the model over the widest range possible. It may be, for example, that a physical mechanism insignificant over a large part of the validation range (and thus perhaps ignored during model development) could begin to impact or even dominate the solution outside of that range.

27.4.9 Iteration

If the model is not found to be predictive over the validation data set, there may have been an omission or error in the development of the model in which case it may be advisable to go back to the identification step, and double check the procedure. As previously discussed, model building tends to be an iterative process, and it is the rare exception that a model is successful right out of the starting gate. It is more often the case that errors in the solution code, mathematical blunders in the formulated equations or even overlooked physical phenomena keep the model developer going back to the drawing board several times before success is finally achieved.

27.4.10 Application

Finally, the model may actually be put to good use and solved to produce useful scaling predictions. Note that the model development does not necessarily have to be finished at this point. After a history has been developed, there may be a desire to further improve the model to handle different conditions or to take into account new phenomena in order to improve its predictive ability.

27.5 PRACTICAL STRATEGIES FOR PHARMACEUTICAL SCALE-UP

27.5.1 Strategies for Practical Application

With these modeling tools in hand, how should a pharmaceutical manufacturing process be scaled-up to achieve the maximum benefit? First, it is important to know when to begin applying scale-up principles to the development process. One may think that scale-up is an activity that is initiated when a bench-scale or pilot-scale process has been developed, and there is a need to translate that process knowledge to the next larger scale, and often this is exactly how scale-up occurs. Ideally, however, engineers and formulators should begin working together early in the formulation stage, in order to streamline the process for scale-up, and identify potential problems in the small-scale process that might be waiting to erupt on a larger scale. For example, small-scale process development may employ small instrumented tablet presses with narrow diameter turrets, and relatively slow rotation speeds, resulting in low strain rates, and long dwell times compared with commercial scale machines. Potential compression problems such as capping or low hardness may never

arise under those conditions, but once identified at the commercial scale, it would be extremely costly to push back the development timeline, and reformulate once again. If this problem were recognized during formulation, however, it could be addressed quickly with little interruption to the development timeline.

Scale-up principles can effectively be applied early in the formulation by conducting experiments at the small-scale to determine acceptable operating ranges, scaling the unit operations via dimensional analysis or mechanistic modeling to the next larger scale, and confirming that product with the same quality attributes can also be produced in the larger capacity equipment. It is usually the case that the equipment and capabilities of the pilot-scale facility are fixed, and the commercial-scale production facility is already selected early in drug product development, therefore the development process can be guided early on so that the process will translate smoothly from facility to facility upon scale-up. It may be determined in the course of process development that a unit operation may not scale-up well, e.g., the dimensionless numbers governing the behavior of the two respective systems at each scale do not overlap sufficiently to provide for a robust operating parameter space. If this is so, plans can be made for the selection and purchase of new equipment well ahead of time or perhaps the process at the small-scale can be modified in accordance with the capabilities of the existing larger-scale equipment.

When applying scale-up principles, it is important to keep in mind the change in scale between two facilities. There are always errors associated with every scale-up estimate. The magnitude of those errors scale-up along with the process, and the ability to reliably extrapolate process knowledge gained at one scale to another larger-scale is subject to the accuracy of the scale-up model. While formulation may take place at a 5–10 kg batch size or less, commercial production may represent a 30 times or more increase in scale. An optimum jump in scale instead may lie between 5 and 10 times, in order to maximize the predictive accuracy of the scaling models, while minimizing research and development costs. The more intermediate scale steps between the bench top and commercial scale there are, the more financial capital and time that must be expended, yet the less is the risk associated with the resulting commercial-scale production process. Some unit operations may individually require smaller or larger scale jumps, depending on the confidence level associated with that particular unit operation. For example, if geometric similitude cannot be maintained for a fluidized-bed granulation upon scale-up, there is a greater risk associated with that particular unit operation, especially considering that every downstream unit operation is dependent on the quality of granulated material. It may be to the benefit of the overall process to conduct further granulation studies at one or more extra intermediate scales.

While conducting studies at one scale, there should not be a rush to jump to the next scale. A good strategy for scaling-up, contrarily enough, is to postpone it as long as possible! Process knowledge is gained more cheaply and rapidly when the scale is small, which in turn makes process model development more efficient. As long as the experimental studies are scaleable, experiment as much as possible before moving up in size. There is little to be gained from applying scaling principles if the process is not well-understood at the present scale, before jumping up to the next larger-scale. Scaling models may also help to guide the design of experiments. Process variables critical to the behavior of the system can be identified in the course of model development, and can be investigated as factors in design of experiment (DOE) studies. In addition, scaling models can predict how critical variables change throughout the multidimensional variable space, and thereby offer guidance as to where in that variable space experiments should be conducted.

It should also be mentioned that the design of a scalable process might mean the replacement of certain poorly scaleable unit operations with other more scaleable ones, if possible. For example, high shear wet granulation has been the subject of much study using dimensionless numbers as already discussed, yet to date there is still no consensus on any one particular method that works for every formulation. High shear wet granulation tends to be a poorly scaleable unit operation, but it may not be necessary if a better understood dry granulation technique (e.g., roller compaction) or direct compression can be used instead. Moreover, the removal of the wet granulation unit operation also streamlines the downstream process, by removing the need for a granulation drying step. For these reasons, direct compression or dry granulation unit operations should be preferred over wet granulation whenever feasible.

Finally, although this text focuses heavily on process modeling, it should also be mentioned that in certain cases scale-up might be accomplished, not with theoretical models, but with mechanical simulators. The Presster™, manufactured by Metropolitan Computing Corporation (East Hanover, NJ), is a single-station instrumented tablet press that can be configured such that it mimics the punch displacement–time profiles, and strain rates of a variety of actual production presses, while only requiring gram quantities of material. As mentioned above, there may be instances where small-scale equipment cannot operate in the range needed to correspond to the large-scale equipment according to scaling principles. In such cases, the practical application of scale-up modeling is thwarted, and usually the only remaining option is the execution of empirical studies at the larger-scale. If available, a mechanical simulator may provide another option and, being designed for research and development, can usually do so cost-effectively with small quantities. Bear in mind, however, that mechanical simulators usually possess a characteristic in common with theoretical models: they tend to be simplified representations of the actual system being modeled. In the case of the Presster™, the feed material is fed to the punch die via gravity through a tiny hopper, as opposed to being force-fed by a mechanical paddle system used in production presses. If there happen to be problems associated with the mechanical conveyance and agitation of the tablet press feed material (e.g., segregation, attrition, etc.), it will likely go unnoticed using the simulator.

27.5.2 Quality by Design Using Scaling Principles

Science-based Manufacturing

From a regulatory point of view, formulation development has until recently been viewed as a "black box," due to the general inability to reliably predict changes in drug product quality when formulation and process variables are varied.[9] This inability may be at attributed to a lack of scientific understanding guiding the development and control of the manufacturing process, i.e., an over-reliance on empirical studies without a mechanistic interpretation of the data. Without a means of predicting the interrelationships between process variables and drug quality, there is no systematic means by which variability in the process can be handled, except by a narrowing of process parameter ranges to account for the expected maximum variabilities in incoming raw materials and manufacturing conditions. Improvement in quality, reduction in risk, and improvement in productivity are all achievable through a reduction in variability, which is made possible by a physical understanding of the process. Science-based manufacturing is the application of information and knowledge obtained from pharmaceutical development studies and manufacturing experience to generate this physical understanding, which in turn is used to define and support establishment of operating ranges, product specifications, and manufacturing controls.

Science-based manufacturing is today a central concept in the global pharmaceutical product market. Since the 1960s, escalating safety concerns have led to a rapid increase in laws and regulations governing the manufacturing of medicinal products across Europe, the US, and Japan. As pharmaceutical companies began to seek more of a global market, the inconsistencies among the laws and regulations of individual countries became a hindrance to the international marketing of drug products. In response, a joint international effort has been undertaken to harmonize regulatory practices and requirements to ensure that safe, effective, and high quality medicines are developed and registered in the most efficient and cost-effective manner. This effort culminated in formation of the International Conference on Harmonisation of Technical Requirements for Registration of Pharmaceuticals for Human Use (ICH) in 1990. The ICH establishes and publishes guidelines to aid in the harmonization of the registration process, with the objectives of a more economical use of resources, the elimination of unnecessary delay in developing new medicines, and the maintenance of safeguards on quality, safety, efficacy, and regulatory obligations to protect public health. The ICH recognizes the importance of good science in the development of drug products, and that scientific knowledge can even provide for greater freedoms in how drug products are developed and controlled:

> "The Pharmaceutical Development section provides an opportunity to present the knowledge gained through the application of scientific approaches ... to the development of a product and its manufacturing process ... The guideline also indicates areas where the demonstration of greater understanding of pharmaceutical and manufacturing sciences can create a basis for flexible regulatory approaches. The degree of regulatory flexibility is predicated on the level of relevant scientific knowledge provided."[10]

The ICH Q8 guidance on Pharmaceutical Development introduces two key concepts relevant to the application of scientific knowledge to a manufacturing process. The first is the idea of the "design space." The design space is defined as "the multidimensional combination and interaction of input variables (e.g., material attributes) and process parameters that have been demonstrated to provide assurance of quality." In other words, if n is the number of variables in the process, the design space is the n-dimensional volume in which your parameters may vary without impacting the quality of the product. Humans can really only visualize space with $n \leq 3$ dimensions, so it may be more conducive to process development, as well as product registration, to work with multiple independent design spaces of lower dimensionality. From a quality perspective, the key characteristic of the design space is that any movement of the process within the design space is not considered as a process change, and would not initiate a regulatory post-approval change process. The larger the design space,

the more robust (or tolerant to variability) the process is, and the more flexibility there is to accommodate process improvements. Movement to outside of the design space, however, would be considered a process change.

A second concept is quality by design (QbD). Quality should not be "tested into" the products, i.e., the use of end-product testing as an in-process measure to weed out unacceptable product. Rather, QbD refers to the design and development of formulations and manufacturing processes to ensure predefined product quality is met. In other words, quality is built-in or designed-in, rather than tested in. A major player in the QbD concept is process analytical technology (PAT), which is a system for designing, analyzing, and controlling manufacturing through timely measurements (i.e., during processing) of critical quality and performance attributes of raw and in-process materials and processes, with the goal of understanding and controlling the manufacturing process, thereby ensuring product quality. This broad definition of PAT seems to encompass both the application of scientific principles during development, and the use of new analytical technology for real-time process, end point monitoring, and control tools during manufacturing, but the current industry focus seems to be primarily on the latter, which is perceived to currently be a greater need and also a greater paradigm shift. In contrast, the application of science and engineering for the design and scale-up of a manufacturing process is not a new idea, but it remains a very necessary component of QbD that begins with formulation development. Moreover, real-time process monitoring is value added only when the process has already been defined, and this is accomplished by the application of scientific scale-up methods which process monitoring does not address.

Scaling as a Means of Implementing Quality by Design

The output of scale-up modeling is increased process understanding, which in turn is what allows a robust manufacturing process to be designed. The application of scale-up modeling is an opportunity to implement QbD by infusing product quality into the manufacturing process from the very outset of product development. Instead of product quality being merely an observed result of empirical study, the predictive power of scale-up modeling allows quality to become effectively a design principle itself. It is conceivable, for example, that if design space were defined by dimensionless Pi parameters obtained from dimensional analysis, and if dynamic similitude were maintained across scales, the design spaces for

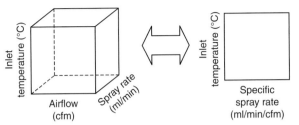

FIGURE 27.6 Absolute design space versus composite design space

a single process at multiple scales would tend to collapse onto each other as one single scale-independent design space. Using this approach it is possible that the commercial scale process design space could be identified even at the formulation stage, subject to the predictive accuracy of the scaling model.*

The idea of defining a design space in terms of the physical processes occurring in the unit operations, and the key dimensionless numbers characterizing those processes, stands in contrast to the more conventional approach of proposing a purely empirical, equipment control-based design space. However, current regulatory opinion seems to favor moving in this more scientific direction, and such an approach would also favor the pharmaceutical manufacturer. Consider a simple example of a design space for a fluidized-bed coating operation. A conventional design space may include the volumetric airflow (cfm), spray rate (ml/min), and inlet temperature (°C) specified as absolute quantities (see Figure 27.6; the design space perhaps may include even more parameters, but for the purpose of illustration the dimensionality here is kept at three). However, applying the lessons learned from Example 1 (Section 27.3.1), it is known that scale-up requires that the spray rate be kept proportional to the volumetric airflow, assuming air density remains constant.

Since spray rate and airflow do not vary independently, the design space is still fully determined if these two parameters are replaced by the ratio of the two, a composite parameter. In doing so, the composite design space is no longer tied to an absolute spray rate range or an absolute volumetric airflow range, which not only imparts scale-independence to the design space (temperature is an intensive quantity hence, already scale-independent), but also provides additional freedom and flexibility for process

changes. Furthermore, determining the design space in terms of composite parameters identified through process modeling results in a reduction in dimensionality, which enhances understanding of the process, increases process control efficiency, and potentially streamlines the product registration.

The application of scientific knowledge gained from scale-up modeling can expand the concept of design space even further. As discussed earlier, the larger the design space the more robust the process can be, since greater variability in process parameters, material properties, and manufacturing conditions can be accommodated. Where variability is difficult to control and design space is tight, robustness suffers. It is here where predictive modeling can be applied to create a dynamic design space, as opposed to the conventional static type. A design space becomes dynamic when one or more of its dimensions is a function of another variable, e.g., a material property such as moisture content or particle size distribution or a process condition such as temperature or humidity. For example, the humidity maintained inside a fluidized-bed granulator can be important to the properties of the resulting granules. For air handling systems where only a chiller is present, seasonal weather variations may result in incoming air humidity fluctuations when the outside air dewpoint temperature nears the chiller temperature. One way to accommodate this source of variability is by determining the design space based on a worst-case humidity, which would have the effect of reducing the size of the design space, and thereby compromising robustness and process flexibility. However, if the humidity inside the granulator can be predicted and controlled by a model incorporating spray rate, inlet temperature, inlet humidity, outlet temperature, etc., the design space is effectively opened back up. The edges of the design space are not fixed in place, but allowed to move and flex according to the source of variability, managing its impact and the risk associated with it. In fact, a dynamic design space of n dimensions can be considered an equivalent reduced form of a static design space of $n + k$ dimensions, where one or more of the remaining n dimensions are functions of the k dimensions associated with the variability.

Process Description in Regulatory Filing

The application of scaling principles can streamline the scientific justification of a drug development process in a New Drug Application (NDA) filing. It is in the best interests of the drug product manufacturer submitting the filing to define the process in such a way as to be no more restrictive than it needs to be, in order robustly to produce a quality product. In keeping

---

*Due to errors extrapolated along with the solution, together with the fact that models can only be approximations to reality, it is reasonable to expect minor modifications to the design space upon scale-up.

with this strategy, it is rarely a good idea to define a process in a way that is specific to a particular brand or model of equipment, since this reduces the flexibility for post-filing changes. Even so, this is often how a process is defined throughout development, since the engineers and pharmacists designing the process are usually developing it with a single target commercial-scale equipment train in mind. When it comes time to describe the process in the NDA irrespective of specific equipment make or model, however, the negative consequences of this approach become apparent. For example, the preparation of a polymeric coating suspension for tablet coating will involve a mixing step that may be defined only by an impeller speed and mixing time, but the number of impeller blades, shape, pitch and diameter, and also the vessel diameter and volume will also probably affect the mixing. Milling feed rate may be defined in terms of a feed screw speed, but this number is meaningless by itself without knowing the feed screw flight depth and pitch. If instead the feed rate is defined in terms of granulate mass per hour, what would be the impact of a change in comminution chamber volume, blade diameter or screen area? If the equipment make and model cannot be specified, the definition of a process in a non-equipment specific way would seem to involve an intimidating number of parameters that tend to be convoluted with each other.

For the description of a batch operation, such as blending or fluidized-bed drying in an NDA, for example, it may be possible to avoid this problem if it is permissible to specify a piece of equipment as being "sized appropriately" for the specified constant batch size, tacitly suggesting that the geometries of any appropriately-sized piece of equipment are not going to vary so much that the proposed process parameters and controls will fail to produce a quality product. For continuous throughput equipment, however, this justification does not hold. Fortunately, this situation can be avoided by the application of scale-up principles, beginning early in process development. Dimensionless Pi numbers introduced in Section 27.3.1 are scale-independent, and therefore they must also be equipment-independent. If the process is developed and defined in terms of dimensionless numbers, the task of describing the process in the NDA is greatly simplified. Returning to the milling feed rate example mentioned above, a dimensional analysis of an impact mill may reveal $R/\rho Av_t$ as an important dimensionless number for defining feed rate, where R is feed rate (MT^{-1}), ρ is granulate bulk density (ML^{-3}), A is perforated screen area (L^2), and v_t is blade tip speed (LT^{-1}). Instead of proposing many

different dimensional parameters to define the feed rate, a reduced set of dimensionless numbers or perhaps even one dimensionless number may fully describe the unit operation in a scale-independent and equipment-independent way.

27.6 CONCLUSION

Building quality into products relies on a solid scientific understanding of the entire manufacturing process—from development to final formulation. It specifically requires that quantifiable, causal, and predictive relationships be established among raw materials, the manufacturing process, and final product quality. While these new flexible modeling approaches to design space determination can play a key role in effectively building quality into a pharmaceutical drug product, thorough scientific knowledge of how the product quality varies over a range of material attributes, manufacturing process options, and process parameters needs to be demonstrated in order to realize this flexibility. Scale-up, in particular the application of scientific principles for modeling and prediction, is a means by which this knowledge can be accumulated, applied, and presented in order to scientifically justify a more sophisticated and effective approach to developing and controlling a manufacturing process.

References

1. Practical life as a complement to university education—medal address. (1916). Journal of Industrial & Engineering Chemistry Research 8, 184–190.
2. ICH Q8.
3. Janet Woodcock, M.D., Deputy Commissioner for Operations, FDA. "Pharmaceutical Quality in the 21st Century—An Integrated Systems Approach" (presentation), October 5, 2005.
4. As quoted in *The Universe in a Nutshell* by Stephen Hawking.
5. Ajaz Hussain, "A Shared Vision for Pharmaceutical Development and Manufacturing in the 21st Century: Contributions of the PAT Initiative" (presentation), CDER, FDA (September 2005).
6. Zlokarnik, M., *Dimension Analysis and Scale-up in Chemical Engineering*.
7. Horsthuis, G.J.B. et al. (1993). Studies on upscaling parameters of the Gral high shear granulation process. Int. J. Pharm, 92, 143.
8. Faure, A., Grimsey, I.M., Rowe, R.C., York, P. & Cliff, M.J. (1999). Applicability of a scale-up methodology for wet granulation processes in Collette Gral high shear mixer-granulators. Eur. J. Pharm. Sci. 8, 85–93.
9. Ajaz Hussain, Proceedings from the Advisory Committee For Pharmaceutical Science, July 19 (2001), Food and Drug Administration, Rockville, MD.
10. ICH Q8.

Process Development, Optimization, and Scale-up: Powder Handling and Segregation Concerns

Thomas Baxter and James Prescott

28.1 INTRODUCTION

Objective of the Chapter

The primary focus of this chapter is to provide guidance in designing bulk solids ("powder") handling equipment to provide consistent, reliable flow, and minimize segregation. The principles discussed in this chapter can be applied to analyzing new or existing equipment designs. The principles can also be used to compare different powders, using the various test methods discussed.

The chapter will focus on the equipment used from the final blend step to the inlet of the press/encapsulation machine used to create the unit dose. This chapter is divided into the following primary topics:

28.1 Introduction: A review of introductory concepts, such a flowability, blending, and segregation.
28.2 Common Powder Handling Equipment: A description of the common handling equipment, and the equipment parameters that affect flowability and segregation.
28.3 Typical Flow and Segregation Concerns: A review of common flow and segregation concerns, and the two primary flow patterns (mass flow versus funnel flow).
28.4 Measurement of Flow Properties: A summary of the flow properties that need to be measured to obtain the equipment design parameters required for consistent, reliable flow.

28.5 Basic Equipment Design Techniques: A review of the basic design techniques for the blender-to-press equipment to provide reliable flow, and minimize the adverse effects of segregation.

At the end of this chapter, you should have a working knowledge of what flow properties need to be measured, how to measure them, and how to apply them to analyze or design handling equipment for reliable flow, and to minimize segregation.

Motivation for the Chapter

Many pharmaceutical processes include powder handling, such as blending, transfer, storage, feeding, compaction, and fluidization. A full understanding of powder flow behavior is essential when developing, optimizing or scaling-up a process. This may include designing new equipment or developing corrective actions for existing equipment. There are several instances where the robustness of a process is adversely affected by flow or segregation problems that develop.

Common flow problems can have an adverse effect upon:

1. Production costs, due to reduced production rates (e.g., tableting rate limitations, required operator intervention), restrictions on raw ingredient selection (e.g., percentage of lubrication used, excipients selected), method of manufacturing (wet granulation versus dry granulation versus

Developing Solid Oral Dosage Forms: Pharmaceutical Theory and Practice
ISBN: 978-0-444-53242-8

637

direct compression), equipment selection (type of blender, bin, press), and overall yield.

2. Product quality, due to variation of tablet properties (weight, hardness, etc.) or segregation and content uniformity concerns.
3. Time to market, due to delays in product/process development, validation or failed commercial batches, since flow problems may not occur until the process has been scaled-up.

28.1.1 Introduction to Flowability

A bulk solid is defined as a collection of solid particles. The term "powder" is often used to describe a fine bulk solid, especially in the pharmaceutical industry. This common term will be used predominantly throughout this chapter. The concepts discussed in this chapter apply to many types of powders with different particle sizes, shapes, and distributions. The powders may include dust, granulations, and granules. The powder could either be a single substance, such as an excipient or active pharmaceutical ingredient (API) or a multi-component blend (final blend). The primary point is that the principles outlined in this chapter can be used to design for all these different types of powders.

A simple definition of "flowability" is the ability of a powder to flow through equipment reliably. By this definition, there is often a tendency to define flowability as a single parameter of a powder, ranked on a scale from "free-flowing" to "non-flowing". Unfortunately, a single parameter is not sufficient to define a powder's complete handling characteristics. In addition, a single parameter is not sufficient to fully address common handling concerns encountered by the formulator and equipment designer. In fact, several design parameters may need to be known for a successful design. The behavior of a powder will depend upon several different parameters or "flow properties." Flow properties are the specific properties of a powder that affect flow that can be measured. Therefore, a full range of flow properties will need to be measured to fully characterize the powder. The measurement of these flow properties is discussed in Section 28.4 of this chapter.

In addition, the "flowability" of a powder is a function of the powder's flow properties and the design parameters of the handling equipment. For example, "poor flowing" powders can be handled reliably in properly designed equipment. Conversely, "good flowing" powders may develop flow problems in improperly designed equipment. Therefore, our definition of "flowability" is "the ability of powder to flow in the desired manner in a specific piece of equipment."

The flow properties of the powder should be quantitative and scalable design parameters. The term "flow properties" often refers to the physical characteristics of the powder that were measured. For example, one might report "the tapped density of a final blend was measured to be 0.6 grams per cubic centimeter." The term "powder flow" often refers to an observation of how the powder flowed through a given piece of equipment. For example, one might report "the powder flow through the press hopper was consistent." In discussing or reporting flowability, both the powder flow properties and the handling equipment must be included. Therefore, the measurement of the powder flow properties can be used to predict behavior in specific equipment during scale-up.

The flow properties that should be measured (Section 28.4), and how to apply the results to a reliable equipment design (Section 28.5), are discussed later in this chapter.

28.1.2 Introduction to Blending

Solid blending processes are used during the manufacture of products for a wide range of industries, including pharmaceuticals. In the pharmaceutical industry, a wide range of ingredients may be blended together to create the final blend used to manufacture the solid dosage form. The range of materials that may be blended (excipients, API), presents a number of variables which must be addressed to achieve products of acceptable blend uniformity. These variables may include the particle size distribution (including aggregates or lumps of material), particle shape (spheres, rods, cubes, plates, and irregular), presence of moisture (or other volatile compounds), particle surface properties (roughness, cohesivity), and many other variables.

The quality of the solid dosage form is dependent on the adequacy of the blend. Producing a uniform mixture of the drug and its excipients is paramount in being able to deliver the proper dose of the drug to the patient. Once an adequate blend is obtained, it is also critical to ensure that it does not segregate in the post-blending handling steps. Millions of dosage units may be created from a single batch, and each and every dose must be of acceptable composition, to ensure the safety and efficiency of the product. Therefore, the homogeneity of pharmaceutical blends and dosage units is highly scrutinized by regulatory bodies throughout the world. Formulation components and process parameters involved with blending operations should be carefully selected, and validated, to ensure uniform blends and dosage units are produced. Blend and dosage unit uniformity data is provided in regulatory submissions, and often examined during pre-approval inspections. This is to ensure that blending processes produce homogeneous blends that do not segregate upon further processing into dosage units. Finally, pharmacopeias require an assessment of content uniformity to be performed on every batch of solid dosage forms manufactured.

The scale of blending operations for the preparation of pharmaceutical dosage forms ranges from the extemporaneous compounding of a few capsules by pharmacists, to large-scale production of batches containing millions of dosage units. The complexity of the blending process can vary substantially. Large-scale production batches often use equipment capable of blending hundreds of kilograms of material. Depending on the dose and characteristics of the drug substance, commercial-scale blending processes can be complex, and may require the preparation of pre-blends or the inclusion of milling operations to achieve acceptable content uniformity. Regardless of the scale of manufacture, the goal remains the same: to prepare a blend that is adequately blended, and can be further processed into dosage units that deliver the proper dose of the drug to the patient.

Blending should not be seen as an independent unit operation, but rather as an integral part of the overall manufacturing process. Blending includes producing an adequate blend, maintaining that blend through additional handling steps, and verifying that both the blend and the finished product are sufficiently homogeneous. Therefore, a complete approach should be used to assess the uniformity of blends, and the subsequent dosage forms produced from them.

A review of the common types of blenders is provided in Section 28.2 of this chapter, but the details of scaling-up common final blending process steps (wet granulation, fluid-bed granulation, roller compaction) are discussed in other chapters.

28.1.3 Introduction to Segregation

"Segregation" can be defined as having particles of similar properties (size, composition, density, resiliency, static charge, etc.) preferentially distributed into different zones within given equipment or processes. Segregation most notably affects the localized concentration of the drug substance. This can result in blend and content uniformity problems. In addition, the segregation of other components of the blend can be responsible for variations in properties such as dissolution, stability, lubrication, taste, appearance, and color. Even if the blend remains chemically homogeneous, variations in particle size can affect flowability, bulk density, weight uniformity, tablet hardness, appearance, and dissolution. Additionally, segregation can create concentrations of dust, which can lead to problems with agglomeration, yield, operator exposure, containment, cleanliness, and increased potential for a dust explosion.

Segregation can occur any time there is powder transfer, such as discharging the final blend from the blender into a bin. Segregation can also occur when forces acting on the particles in the blend, such as air flow or vibration, are sufficient to induce particle movement. This may include handling steps upstream of a blender, including segregation of raw materials at a supplier's plant or during shipment, movement within the blender, during its discharge or in downstream equipment. Of all of these potential instances where segregation can occur, the most common area for problems is post-blender discharge. Therefore, this chapter will focus on segregation of the final blend in the post-blending handling steps.

The current state of understanding segregation is limited to having empirical descriptors of segregation mechanisms (see Section 28.4), and prior experiences with diagnosing and addressing specific segregation behaviors (Section 28.5). Unlike the flow properties tests used to assess how a powder flows though equipment, there are no "first principle" models that describe segregation. Therefore, one cannot currently input the particle properties of the blend components (e.g., particle size and chemical composition of the excipients, and API) into a mathematical model, and obtain a prediction of segregation potential. At best, computational models such as discrete element modeling (DEM) are evolving, and can be tuned to match specific segregation behaviors that are created in physical models. As these models evolve they will become more powerful, and have fewer assumptions and limitations. At the current time, the average pharmaceutical scientist may not be able to use DEM to predict or solve the segregation problems they are likely to encounter. Therefore, when assessing segregation concerns, it is critical to utilize as many resources as possible such as laboratory-scale tests to assess different segregation mechanisms (Section 28.4), and stratified blend and content uniformity data to assess potential segregation trends.

The empirical tests that should be conducted to assess the segregation potential of a final blend (Section 28.4), and how to apply the results to a reliable equipment design (Section 28.5), are discussed later in this chapter.

28.2 COMMON POWDER HANDLING EQUIPMENT

Objective of the Section

The primary objective of this section is to describe the common powder handling equipment used in pharmaceutical processes. This section will also define common terms for powder handling equipment, and provide background for Section 28.3 of this chapter, which will focus upon typical flow and segregation problems.

We will review the common handling equipment and process steps that may affect the flowability and segregation of a powder. In particular, we will review the process steps for the final blend used to manufacture the dosage units, including:

1. processing steps prior to final blending, such as milling, screening, drying and granulation;
2. final blending;
3. discharge from the final blender;
4. intermediate bulk containers ("IBCs," "totes," bins);
5. transfer from the IBC to the press (or encapsulator);
6. feed from the press hopper to the die cavity.

For each of these different process steps, we will review the key equipment parameters that affect the flowability and segregation of a powder. These typical handling steps serve as examples of the concerns with powder handling, but virtually any solids handling application can be analyzed in the same way.

28.2.1 Processing Steps Prior to Final Blending

It is critical to understand the physical properties of the raw ingredients (API, excipients), and how they affect the flowability and segregation of the final blend, when selecting and designing the powder handling equipment. Therefore, the process steps and equipment parameters prior to the final blend step are often critical to the flowability and segregation of the final blend. There are several common pre-blending process steps that may affect the final blend, including:

1. Storage conditions of the raw ingredients, such as the temperature, relative humidity, container dimensions, and days stored at rest (inventory control) can all influence the flowability of the final blend, especially if any of the raw ingredients are hygroscopic.

2. Milling and screening steps that alter the raw ingredients', and thus the final blend's particle size, shape, and distribution. Therefore, milling and screening process parameters, such as the mill type, mill speed, screen size, mill/screen feed method (controlled versus non-controlled feed) may all have an influence on the flowability and segregation potential of the final blend, especially in a dry blending process.

3. Granulation (dry roller compaction, wet granulation, fluid-bed granulation) of the API, together with select excipients, can often have a positive effect on the flowability of the final blend, especially for blends with high active loadings. The granulation parameters, especially those that influence particle size/shape/distribution, will have a significant effect on flowability and segregation potential. For roller compaction, the process parameters that dictate the particle size distribution and shape distribution of the final blend may include the roller compactor speed, roll compactor pressure, mill type, and the screen size. The wet granulation process parameters that affect particle size distribution and shape, as well as the moisture content, are often critical to flowability. Therefore, wet granulation parameters, such as the blade and impeller design/speed, binder addition rate, and method and identification of granulation end point, are critical to flowability, as are the granule milling conditions. Similarly, the fluid-bed granulation parameters that affect the moisture content and particle size, such as the binder addition rate/method, inlet air flow rate and temperature, drying time, end point determination (target moisture, powder temperature, exhaust air temperature), and fluidization behavior for the powder bed are all critical to flowability and segregation. The details of scaling-up different granulation processes are discussed in Chapters 29, 30, and 31.

4. Pre-blending of selected raw materials, such as pre-blending a cohesive powder with a less cohesive powder to reduce the likelihood of flow problems during subsequent handling steps. Pre-blending may also be conducted to achieve a more uniform blend, and reduce the segregation potential.

The measurement of flow properties and the design parameters they provide are discussed in Section 28.4, but they can also be applied to trouble-shooting and developing corrective actions for flow problems in the pre-blending steps if needed.

28.2.2 Final Blending

Final blending may be accomplished on a batch or continuous basis. In the pharmaceutical industry, batch blenders are used almost exclusively. The primary reason for this is that batch blending has historically provided tighter quality control in terms of better uniformity and batch integrity, as compared to continuous blending. Therefore, continuous blenders are not discussed in this chapter.

Batch blending processes consist of three sequential steps: weighing and loading the components, blending, and discharging. Unlike a continuous blender, the retention time in a batch blender is rigidly defined and controlled, and is the same for all of the particles. Batch blenders come in many different designs and sizes, and make use of a wide range of blending mechanisms.

All blenders use one or more of the following mechanisms to induce powder blending: convective blending, shear blending, and diffusive blending.[1,2] Another classification system for blenders is based on their design. This system categorizes blenders into two categories:

- those that achieve blending within a moving vessel; and
- those with fixed vessels that rely on internal paddles or blades to move the materials.

There are many common blenders used in the pharmaceutical industry on a batch basis, including:

1. wet granulators (see Chapter 29 for details);
2. fluid-bed granulators (see Chapter 30 for details);
3. roller compactors (see Chapter 31 for details);
4. tumble blenders (reviewed briefly in this chapter).

Other less-common types of blenders such as pneumatic blenders, extruders, ribbon blenders, planetary blenders, and orbiting screw blenders are not discussed in this chapter.

As a result of the multiple classification systems, a number of terms have evolved throughout the industry to describe families of blenders. Regardless of the terminology used to classify the blender, the important thing is for the pharmaceutical scientist to understand the capabilities and limitations of the equipment when selecting an appropriate blender for a particular product. This is especially important during process scale-up, when equipment of different design and operating principle may need to be used. The optimization and scale-up of the wet granulation, fluid-bed granulation, and roller compaction processes are discussed in Chapters 29 to 31. The optimization and scale-up of tumble blenders is discussed elsewhere in the literature.[3]

Note that some types of tumble blenders, such as bin blenders, serve a dual purpose. In addition to providing the container in which blending is accomplished, bin blenders can also be used to transfer the powder blend to the next unit operation. This is of particular value when manufacturing blends that have the tendency to segregate when discharging the blend onto the compression or filling equipment. This also makes the use of bin blenders desirable during the manufacture of potent drug products that must be processed in high containment facilities. Additionally, by decoupling the blending bin from the drive mechanism, the bin filling, discharge, and cleaning take place at a separate time and location, which increases the efficiency and utilization of equipment.

Discharge from a Blender or Processing Vessel

Powder that has been blended must be discharged from the blender for further processing, including the creation of the unit dose at the press or encapsulator. In many dry blending processes, such as tumble blending, the discharge is driven by gravity alone. As an example, the final blend step may be conducted in a V-blender or a double-cone blender. In these cases, the blender geometry often consists of a converging cross-section to the outlet, through which the powder must be discharged reliably. In these cases, the blender is essentially acting as a "bin," so the equipment parameters of interest are those that are crucial to a bin design. These crucial bin design parameters are discussed in the following section on "intermediate bulk containers," which may also be referred to as "IBC."

For fluid-bed granulation processes, it is not uncommon for a conical "hopper" to be attached to the "bowl" of a fluid-bed granulator, inverted, and discharged to a downstream process step via gravity.

For wet granulators, the final blend may be discharged using mechanical agitation by continuing to operate the plow blade (typically at a lower speed) to discharge the final blend through a central or side outlet. Although the plow blade typically ensures that the blend is discharged from the granulator "bowl" reliably, the design of the transition chute from the blender to the downstream process is also critical. This is especially critical if the equipment below the granulator has a converging cross-section that is full of material, as discussed further in Section 28.5.

When a blender/vessel is discharged manually (hand-scooping), flowability may not be a primary concern, but segregation concerns and other factors (e.g., production rate concerns, operator exposure and safety) may limit the extent to which a blender/vessel can be manually unloaded.

The transfer of the material from the final blender to the downstream equipment, whether it is into an IBC or directly to the press, is critical to the segregation potential. Therefore, parameters such as the transfer method (e.g., manual, gravity, pneumatic), transfer rate, transfer chute height and geometry, venting, and other items will be critical in assessing and minimizing the segregation potential during the blender-to-press transfer steps. Design techniques to minimize segregation during these transfer steps are further discussed in Section 28.5.

28.2.3 Intermediate Bulk Containers

The flowability and segregation potential of the final blend is especially critical during storage and discharge from an intermediate bulk container (IBC). The IBC may be a bin ("tote") or a drum that is used to store and transfer the final blend from the blender to the press. When a drum is used, an attachment such as a conical hopper may be attached to the cone to mate the drum to downstream equipment with a smaller inlet (e.g., press hopper). In both cases, the IBC consists of two primary sections (see Figure 28.1):

1. A cylinder or straight-sided section with a constant cross-sectional area that is often rectangular (with or without radiussed corners) or circular;
2. A hopper section with a changing cross-sectional area that is often a converging conical or pyramidal hopper.

IBCs may be used to store the blend for extended periods of time. During this time, the flowability may deteriorate as the blend is subjected to consolidation pressures, due to its own weight during storage at rest. In addition, IBCs may be used to move the blend from one process step to another, during which time the blend may be subjected to vibration that may adversely affect flowability. Therefore, it is important to determine what consolidation pressures will act on the powder as it is stored and transferred in an IBC.

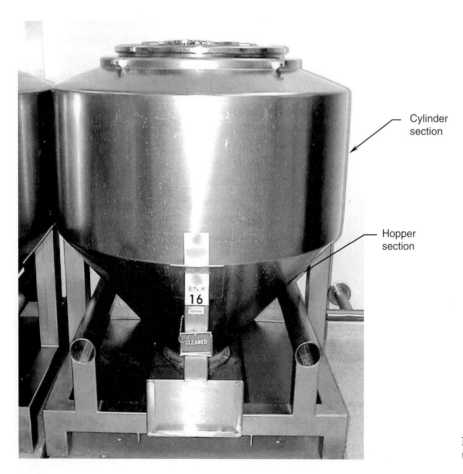

Cylinder section

Hopper section

FIGURE 28.1 Intermediate bulk container ("IBC," "bin," "tote")

The key IBC equipment parameters with respect to flowability and segregation potential include:

1. The cylinder cross-sectional area and height which, along with other parameters such as the fill height, will affect the consolidation pressure acting on the blend.
2. The hopper geometry (planar versus circular) and angles, which will affect the flow pattern that develops during discharge. The flow pattern, discussed in Section 28.3, will also affect the segregation potential.
3. The interior surface finish of the hopper section, which will affect the flow pattern that develops during discharge.
4. The IBC outlet size and shape (slotted versus circular), which will affect whether the blend will discharge reliably without arching or ratholing.
5. General flow impediments, such as upward facing ledges or partially opened valves, that may act as flow obstructions.

The measurement of the flow properties and segregation potential that are used to obtain the key bin design parameters are discussed in Section 28.4 of this chapter. The application of these design parameters to provide reliable flow and minimize segregation from the IBC to the press is discussed in Section 28.5 of this chapter.

Transfer from Intermediate Bulk Containers to the Press/Encapsulator

The flowability and segregation potential of the final blend is also critical during transfer from the IBC to the press/encapsulation machine/etc. This transfer step may be a manual transfer (hand-scooping), in which case flowability may not be a primary concern. The transfer step may also be conducted via pneumatic conveying, in which case the flowability of the blend may not be a primary concern, but equipment and material parameters affecting conveying (conveying gas pressure and flow rate, conveying line diameter and layout, etc.) need to be considered. Pneumatically conveying the final blend may also raise segregation concerns, as further discussed in Section 28.3.

The transfer step may also be conducted via gravity transfer via a single or bifurcated chute (see Figure 28.2), depending on the press configuration. These chutes are often operated in a flood-loaded manner, and may consist of converging sections where the cross-sectional area of the chute is reduced. If this is the case, the chute will need to be designed for reliable flow in a similar manner to the IBCs.

The key transfer chute parameters with respect to flowability and segregation potential include:

1. The chute cross-sectional area and height, which will affect the consolidation pressure acting on the blend, and how it may segregate.
2. Valving and venting of the transfer chute may affect how readily a blend segregates.
3. For converging and non-converging sections of the chute, the chute geometry, angles, and interior surface finish will affect the flow pattern that develops during discharge through the chute.
4. For converging sections of the chute, the outlet shape and size will affect whether the blend will discharge reliably without arching or ratholing.
5. General flow impediments, such as upward facing ledges (mismatched flanges), sight glasses, level probes or partially opened valves may act as flow obstructions.

The measurement of the flow properties and segregation potential that are used to obtain the key chute design parameters are discussed in Section 28.4 of this chapter. The application of these design parameters for equipment from the IBC to the press is discussed in Section 28.5 of this chapter.

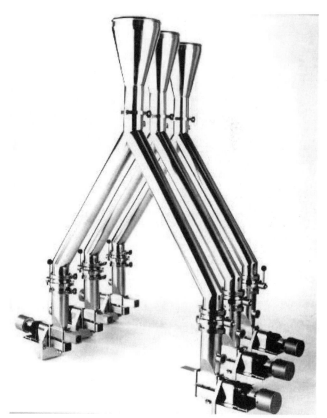

FIGURE 28.2 Bifurcated press feed chute

Feed from the Press Hopper to the Die Cavity

The press feed hopper must also be designed to provide reliable flow, and minimize segregation. Most modern presses consist of a small press hopper that is, in essence, a miniature IBC designed to provide a small amount of surge capacity. The press hopper often consists of a cylinder section and a hopper section similar to a larger IBC. The hopper section may be asymmetric, as opposed to the symmetric hopper designs commonly used for larger IBCs. The press hopper is typically flood-loaded from the IBC/chute above, via gravity feed. However, in some instances, the material level in the press hopper may be controlled via a feeder at the IBC outlet (e.g., rotary valve or screw feeder). Some modern presses do not have press hoppers with a converging hopper, but instead consist of vertical, non-converging chutes from the press inlet to the feed frame inlet.

The key equipment parameters with respect to flowability, which are outlined in the preceding section for IBCs/bins, are also applicable to the press hopper. Since the press hopper outlets are often much smaller than an IBC outlet, flow problems such as arching or ratholing (discussed further in Section 28.3) may be more pronounced at this location. As a result, press hoppers may include mechanical agitators to assist gravity discharge, such as a rotating agitator mounted to a vertical shaft (Figure 28.3).

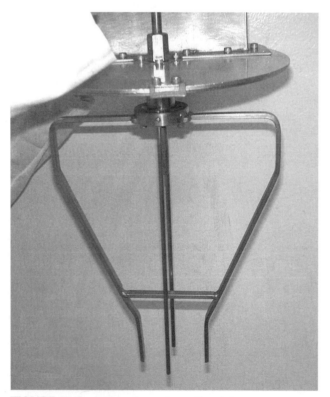

FIGURE 28.3   Agitator for use in small-scale hopper

The same design parameters used for a reliable IBC design (see Section 28.4) can also be used to design a press hopper (see Section 28.5).

28.3 TYPICAL FLOW AND SEGREGATION CONCERNS

Objective of the Section

This section will focus on typical flow and segregation concerns that occur during transfer operations from the final blender to the press. This section will also provide a summary of common flow problems, segregation mechanisms, and the flow patterns that can occur during gravity discharge.

28.3.1 Common Flow Problems

A number of problems can develop as powder flows through equipment such as bins, chutes, and press hoppers. If the powder is cohesive, an arch or rathole may form, resulting in "no flow" or erratic flow. In addition, flooding or uncontrolled discharge may occur if a rathole spontaneously collapses. A deaerated bed of fine powder may experience flow rate limitations or no flow conditions due to the two-phase flow effects between the powder and the interstitial air. Each of these flow problems is discussed in more detail below.

- No flow: no flow from a bin/hopper is a common and significant solids-handling problem. In production, it can result in problems, such as starving downstream equipment, production delays, and the requirement for frequent operator intervention to reinitiate flow. No flow can be due to either arching (sometime referred to as "bridging" or "plugging") or ratholing (also referred to as "piping").

- Arching: occurs when an obstruction in the shape of an arch or bridge forms above the bin outlet, and prevents any further material discharge.
  It can be an interlocking arch, where the particles mechanically lock to form the obstruction, although this is less common with fine pharmaceutical powders. An interlocking arch occurs when the particles are large compared to the outlet size of the hopper. The arch could also be a cohesive arch where the particles pack together to form an obstruction (Figure 28.4). Both of these problems are strongly influenced by the outlet size of the hopper the material is being fed through. Powder

flow properties, discussed in Section 28.4, can be used to determine if these problems will occur and used to address them during scale-up. In particular, the cohesive strength of a powder will dictate what size outlet it can arch over (the greater the cohesive strength, the higher the likelihood of arching).

- Ratholing: can occur in a bin when the powder empties through a central flow channel, but the material at the bin walls remains stagnant and leaves an empty hole ("rathole") through the material, starting at the bin outlet (Figure 28.5). Ratholing is influenced by the bin/hopper geometry and outlet size the material is being fed through. Similar to the problem of arching, this problem will arise if the material has sufficient cohesive strength. In this case, the material discharge will stop once the flow channel empties.

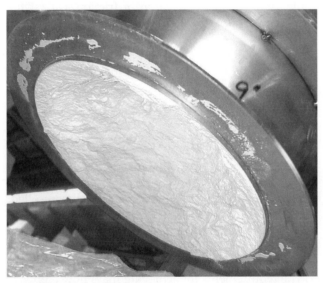

FIGURE 28.4 Cohesive arch

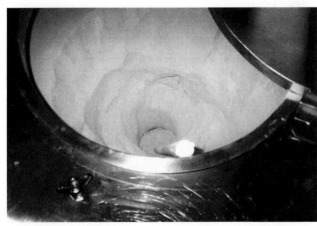

FIGURE 28.5 Rathole

- Erratic flow: erratic flow is the result of obstructions alternating between an arch and a rathole. A rathole may collapse due to an external force, such as vibrations created by surrounding equipment or a flow-aid device, such as an external vibrator. While some material may discharge, falling material may impact over the outlet and form an arch. This arch may then break, due to a reoccurrence of the external force, and material flow may not resume until the flow channel is emptied and a rathole is formed again. This not only results in erratic feed to the downstream equipment (press), but can also result in a non-uniform feed density.

- Fine powder flow concerns (two-phase flow effects): additional flow concerns can arise when handling fine powders, generally in the range below 100 micron in average particle size. These concerns are due to the interaction of the material with entrained air or gas, which becomes significant in describing the behavior of the material. This interaction can result in two-phase (powder/interstitial gas) flow effects. There are three modes that can occur when handling fine powders that are susceptible to two-phase flow effects: steady flow, flooding (or flushing), and a flow rate limitation.[4] These three flow modes are discussed in more detail below.

- Steady flow: will occur with fine powders if the target flow rate (feed rate through the system) is below the "critical flow rate" that occurs when the solids stress is balanced by the air pressure at the outlet. The target flow rate is often controlled by a feeder, such as at the inlet to a compression machine (press feed frame). The critical flow rate and the flow properties tests used to determine it are described in more detail in Section 28.4. At target flow rates exceeding the critical flow rate, unsteady flow can occur by two different modes, described below.

- Flooding: (or "flushing") is an unsteady two-phase flow mode that can occur as falling particles entrain air and become fluidized. Since powder handling equipment often cannot contain a fluid-like powder, powder can flood through the equipment (feeders, seals) uncontrollably. Flooding can also occur when handling fine powders in small hoppers with high fill and discharge rates. In such situations, the powder does not have sufficient residence time to deaerate, resulting in flooding through the feeder. One adverse effect of flooding or flushing may be high variation in the tablet weight and strength.

- Flow rate limitation: is another unsteady two-phase flow mode that can occur with fine powders. Fine powders have very low permeabilities, and are affected by any movement of the interstitial air (air between the particles). This air movement will occur due to the natural consolidation and dilation of the powder bed that takes place as it flows through the cylindrical and hopper geometries. As the material is consolidated in the cylinder, the air is squeezed out. As the powder flows through the hopper and outlet, it dilates and additional air must be drawn in. The air pressure gradients caused as a result of this air movement can retard discharge from a hopper, significantly limiting the maximum achievable rates. This may be observed when the speed of a high-speed press is increased, and the tablet weight variation increases.

During unsteady two-phase flow modes, the material's bulk density can undergo dramatic variations. This can negatively impact downstream packaging or processing operations. Problems can result, such as excessive tablet weight variations, a required reduction in filling speeds, and even segregation. Equipment and process parameters will govern whether such problems occur, and are further discussed in Section 28.5. These parameters include hopper geometry and outlet size, applied vacuum and other sources of air pressure differences (such as dust collection systems), material level, time since filling, and of course the target feed rate.

Material properties, such as permeability and compressibility (discussed in Section 28.4 of this chapter) will also play important roles, as will variations in the material's state of aeration that can occur based on its residence time or degree of compaction from external forces and handling.

One of the most important factors in determining whether a powder will discharge reliably from a hopper is establishing what flow pattern will develop, which is discussed in the section below.

28.3.2 Flow Patterns

Two flow patterns can develop in a bin or hopper: funnel flow and mass flow. In funnel flow (Figure 28.6), an active flow channel forms above the outlet, which is surrounded by stagnant material. This results in a first-in, last-out flow sequence. It generally occurs in equipment with relatively shallow hoppers. Common examples of funnel flow bins include hopper geometries such as asymmetric cones and rectangular-to-round transitions (Figure 28.7).

As the level of powder decreases in funnel flow, stagnant powder may fall into the flow channel if the material is sufficiently free-flowing. If the powder is

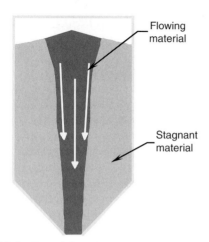

FIGURE 28.6　Funnel flow discharge pattern

cohesive, a stable rathole may develop. Funnel flow occurs if the powder is unable to flow along the hopper walls, due to the combination of friction against the walls and hopper angle. Funnel flow's first-in-last-out flow sequence can also have an adverse effect upon segregation, and result in a non-uniform feed density to the downstream equipment (tablet weight variation).

In mass flow (Figure 28.8), all of the powder is in motion whenever any is withdrawn. Powder flow occurs throughout the bin, including at the hopper walls. Mass flow provides a first-in first-out flow sequence, eliminates stagnant powder, provides a steady discharge with a consistent bulk density, and provides a flow that is uniform and well-controlled. Ratholing will not occur in mass flow, as all of the material is in motion. A mass flow bin design may also be beneficial with respect to reducing segregation (further discussed in Section 28.5).

The requirements for achieving mass flow are:

1. sizing the outlet large enough to prevent arch formation;
2. ensuring the hopper walls are steep and smooth enough to allow the powder to flow along them.

These mass flow design parameters are discussed further in Section 28.4, and their implementation is discussed in Section 28.5 of this chapter.

28.3.3 Common Segregation Mechanisms

The term "segregation mechanism" refers to the mode or motive force by which the components of the blend separate. There are many different segregation mechanisms that can adversely affect uniformity,[5] but three primary segregation mechanisms are of interest

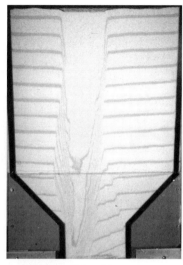
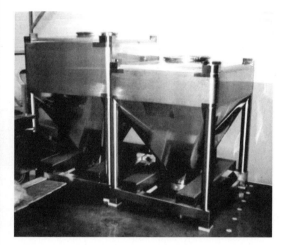

FIGURE 28.7 Examples of funnel flow bins

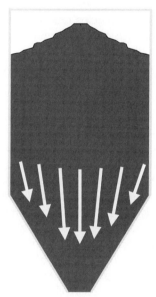

FIGURE 28.8 Mass flow discharge pattern

in typical pharmaceutical blend handling operations. These three primary segregation mechanisms are:

1. sifting segregation (sometimes referred to as "percolation segregation");
2. fluidization segregation (sometimes referred to as "air entrainment");
3. dusting segregation (sometimes referred to as "particle entrainment in an air stream").

The three segregation mechanisms are described in more detail below. These terms are not universally defined, so one must use caution when using them. Segregation may occur as a result of just one of these mechanisms or a combination of several mechanisms.

Material Properties that Affect Segregation

Whether segregation occurs, to what degree, and which mechanism or mechanisms are involved depends on a combination of the properties of the blend, and the process conditions encountered. Some of the primary material properties that influence segregation tendencies include:

1. The mean particle size and particle size distribution of the API, excipients, and final blend: segregation can occur with blends of any mean size, but different mechanisms become more pronounced at different particle sizes, as further discussed below.
2. Particle density: the particle density will affect how the blend components fluidize.
3. Particle shape: rounded particles may have greater mobility than irregularly shaped particles, which can allow more segregation.
4. Particle resilience: this property influences collisions between particles and surfaces, which can lead to differences in where components accumulate during the filling of a bin or press.
5. Cohesive strength of the blend: as a general rule, more cohesive blends are less likely to segregate. However, if enough energy is added to dilate the blend and/or separate particles from one another, even a very cohesive material can segregate.
6. Electrostatic effects: the ability of components to develop and hold an electrostatic charge, and their affinity for other ingredients or processing surfaces, can also contribute to segregation tendencies.

Of all of these, segregation based on particle size is by far the most common.[6] In fact, particle size is the most important factor in the three primary segregation mechanisms considered here, as further described in the following sections.

Sifting Segregation

Sifting segregation is the most common form of segregation for many industrial processes. Under appropriate conditions, fine particles tend to sift or percolate through coarse particles. For segregation to occur by this mechanism four conditions must exist:

1. There must be a range of particle sizes. A minimum difference in mean particle diameters between components of 1.3:1 is often more than sufficient.[6]
2. The mean particle size of the mixture must be sufficiently large, typically, greater than about 100 microns.[7]
3. The mixture must be relatively free-flowing to allow particle mobility.
4. There must be relative motion between particles (inter-particle motion). This last requirement is very important, since without it even highly-segregating blends of ingredients that meet the first three tests will not segregate. Relative motion can be induced in a variety of ways, such as when a pile is formed when filling a bin, vibration from surrounding equipment (such as a tablet press) or as particles tumble and slide down a chute.

If any one of these conditions does not exist, the mix will not segregate by this mechanism.

The result of sifting segregation in a bin is usually a side-to-side variation in the particle size distribution. The smaller particles will generally concentrate under the fill point, with the coarse particles concentrating at the perimeter of the pile (Figure 28.9).

Fluidization Segregation

Variations in particle size or density often result in vertically segregated material when handling powders that can be fluidized. Finer or lighter particles often will be concentrated above larger or denser particles. This can occur during filling of a bin or other vessel or within a blending vessel once the blending action has ceased.

Fluidization segregation often results in horizontal gradation of fines and coarse material. A fine powder can remain fluidized for an extended period of time after filling or blending. In this fluidized state, larger and/or denser particles tend to settle to the bottom. Fine particles may be carried to the surface with escaping air as the bed of material deaerates.

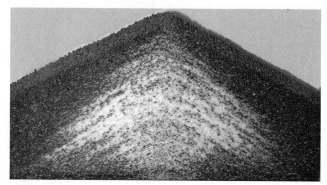

FIGURE 28.9 Example of sifting segregation in a 2-D pile. Note the grey and orange particles are approximately 1200 microns, while the light yellow particles are approximately 350 microns. Photo provided courtesy of Jenike & Johanson, Inc.

For example, when a bin is being filled quickly, the coarse particles move downward through the aerated bed, while the fine particles remain fluidized near the surface. This can also occur after blending, if the material is fluidized during blending.

Fluidization is common in materials that contain a significant percentage of particles smaller than 100 microns.[8] Fluidization segregation is most likely to occur when fine materials are pneumatically conveyed, when they are filled or discharged at high rates, or if gas counter-flow occurs. As with most segregation mechanisms, the more cohesive the material, the less likely it will be to segregate by this mechanism.

Fluidization via gas counter-flow can occur as a result of insufficient venting during material transfer. As an example, consider a tumble blender discharging material to a drum, with an airtight seal between the two (Figure 28.10). As the blend transfers from the blender to the drum, air in the drum is displaced, and a slight vacuum is created in the blender. If both are properly vented, air moves out of the drum and, separately, into the blender. If the bin and drum are not vented, the air must move from the drum to the blender through the blender discharge. In doing so, the fines may be stripped off of the blend, and carried to the surface of the material still within the blender.

Dusting Segregation

Like fluidization segregation, dusting is most likely to be a problem when handling fine, free flowing powders with particles smaller than about 50 microns,[8] as well as a range of other particle sizes. If dust is created upon filling a bin, air currents created by the falling stream will carry particles away from the fill point (Figure 28.11). The rate at which the dust settles is governed by the particle's settling velocity.

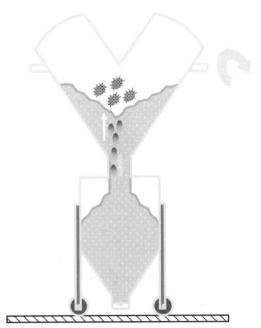

FIGURE 28.10 Example of fluidization segregation from blender to bin

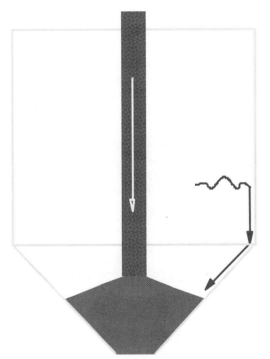

FIGURE 28.11 Example of dusting segregation during filling of bin

The particle diameter is much more significant than particle density in determining settling velocity.

As an example of this mechanism, consider a mix of fine and large particles that is allowed to fall into the center of a bin. When the stream hits the pile of material in the bin, the column of air moving with it is deflected. The air then sweeps off the pile toward the perimeter of the bin, where the air becomes highly disturbed. After this, the air generally moves back up the bin walls in a swirling pattern. At this point, the gas velocity is much lower, allowing many particles to fall out of suspension. Because settling velocity is a strong function of particle diameter, the finest particles (with low settling velocities) will be carried to the perimeter of the bin. The larger particles will concentrate closer to the fill point, where the air currents are strong enough to prevent the fine particles from settling. Dusting segregation can also result in less predictable segregation patterns, depending on how the bin is loaded, venting in the bin, and dust collection use and location.

The empirical tests used to assess these segregation mechanisms are reviewed in Section 28.4, and the application of their results to design equipment to minimize segregation is presented in Section 28.5.

28.4 MEASUREMENT OF FLOW PROPERTIES

Objective of the Section

The primary objective of this section is to provide a description of the different quantitative flow properties that should be measured, as well as the empirical segregation test methods used to assess segregation potential by different mechanisms. This section also reviews the calculation of equipment parameters required for consistent, reliable flow in powder handling equipment for gravity discharge.

The following primary topics are reviewed in this section:

1. Cohesive strength tests: a review of different shear test methods, the Jenike Direct Shear Test method, and the calculation of the design parameters to prevent arching and ratholing.
2. Wall friction tests: a review of the Jenike Direct Shear Test method for measuring wall friction, and the calculation of the design parameters to provide mass flow (mass flow hopper angles).
3. Bulk density test: a review of different bulk density test methods, the compressibility test method, and the application of the compressibility test results.
4. Permeability: a review of the permeability test method, and application of the results (critical flow rate).
5. Segregation tests: a review of two empirical test methods to assess segregation potential.

Note that additional powder characterization methods are discussed in Chapter 9.

28.4.1 Cohesive Strength Tests: Preventing Arching and Ratholing

Dr Andrew Jenike developed his mathematical model of the flow of powders by modeling the powder as a rigid-plastic (not a visco-elastic) continuum of solid particles.[9] This approach included the postulation of a "flow–no flow" criterion that states the powder would flow (e.g., from a bin) when the stresses applied to the powder exceed the strength of the powder. The strength of a material will vary, depending on how consolidated it is. For example, the strength of wet sand increases as the consolidation pressure is increased (e.g., the more one packs it). Therefore, it is critical to be able to measure the cohesive strength of a powder when scaling-up a process and designing equipment.

Test Methods

One of the primary flow problems that can develop in powder handling equipment is a no flow obstruction due to the formation of a cohesive arch or rathole, as discussed in Section 28.3. The required outlet size to prevent a stable cohesive arch or rathole from forming is determined by applying the flow–no flow criterion, and using the results of a cohesive strength test. In order to apply the flow–no flow criterion we need to determine:

1. The cohesive strength of the material as a function of the major consolidation pressure acting on the material: the consolidation pressure acting on the powder changes throughout the bin height, due to the weight of material above it. Therefore, the cohesive strength must be measured over a range of consolidation pressures. The cohesive

strength can be measured as a function of major consolidating pressure using the test methods described in this section.

2. The stresses acting on the material to induce flow: gravity pulls downwards on a potential arch that may form. The stresses acting on the powder can be determined using mathematical models.[9]

To further illustrate the concepts of strength and consolidation pressure, consider an "idealized" strength test, as shown in Figure 28.12. In this idealized test, the cohesive strength of the powder is measured in the following distinct steps:

1. Consolidation of the powder: the powder is consolidated using a prescribed consolidation pressure (P). In the idealized test shown, the sample is contained in a cylinder and the consolidation pressure is applied from the top (Step 1 in Figure 28.12).

2. Fracture of the powder: once the consolidation pressure is applied, the cylinder containing the powder would be removed without disturbing the powder sample (Step 2a in Figure 28.12). After this, the strength of the powder can be measured by applying pressure to the column of powder until it fails or fractures (Step 2b in Figure 28.12). The applied pressure at which the powder failed is referred to as the yield strength (F) (cohesive strength). This idealized test could be repeated several times to develop a flow function (FF), which is a curve illustrating the relationship between the yield strength (F) and the major consolidation pressure (P). An example of a flow function is shown in Figure 28.12.

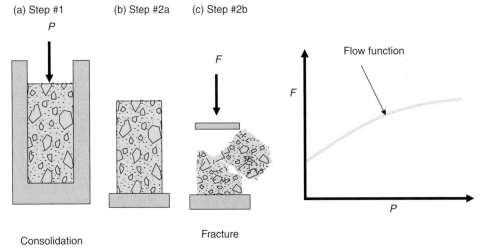

FIGURE 28.12   Schematic of "idealized" strength test: (a) Step#1; (b) Step#2a; (c) Step#2b

This idealized strength test is not possible for the broad range of powders that might be tested. Therefore, several different cohesive strength test methods have been developed. The respective strengths and weaknesses of these different cohesive strength tests are reviewed in the literature.[10,11] Although many different test methods can be used to measure cohesive strength, this chapter focuses specifically upon the Jenike Direct Shear Test method. The Jenike Direct Shear Test method is the most universally accepted method, and is described in ASTM standard D 6128.[12] It is important that these tests be conducted at representative handling conditions, such as temperature, relative humidity, and storage at rest, since all these factors can affect the cohesive strength. An arrangement of a cell used for the Jenike Direct Shear Test is shown in Figure 28.13. The details of the Jenike Direct Test Method are provided in Jenike,[9] including the generation of:

1. Mohr's circle to plot the shear stress (τ) versus the consolidation pressure (σ);
2. Effective yield locus;
3. Flow function.

The data generated experimentally from the Jenike Direct Shear Test can be used to determine the following derived parameters:

1. The flow function that describes the cohesive strength (unconfined yield strength, Fc) of the powder as a function of the major consolidating pressure ($\sigma 1$). The flow function is one of the primary parameters used to calculate the minimum outlet diameter/width for bins, press hoppers, blender outlets, etc., to prevent arching and ratholing. The calculation of the minimum outlet diameter/width is discussed in more detail below.
2. The effective angle of internal friction (δ) that is used to calculate the minimum outlet to prevent arching and the required hopper angles for mass flow (described below).
3. The angle of internal friction for continuous flow or after storage at rest (ϕ and $_t$). The static angle of internal friction (ϕ_t) is used to calculate the minimum outlet to prevent ratholing (described in the following section).

Other testing methods exist that utilize the same principles of consolidation and shearing to determine the cohesive strength of a bulk powder. Annular (ring) shear testers produce rotational displacement between cell halves containing material, rather than a lateral displacement. The loading and shearing operations are more readily adapted to automation, since unlimited travel can be achieved with this type of test cell. The successful use an annular ring shear tester to measure cohesive strength has been discussed in the industry.[13-16]

Calculation of minimum required outlet dimensions to prevent arching (mass flow bin)

The flow behavior of powders through bins and hoppers can be predicted by a complete mathematical relationship. This is very beneficial when scaling-up a process, and designing powder handling equipment. If gravity discharge is used, the outlet size required to

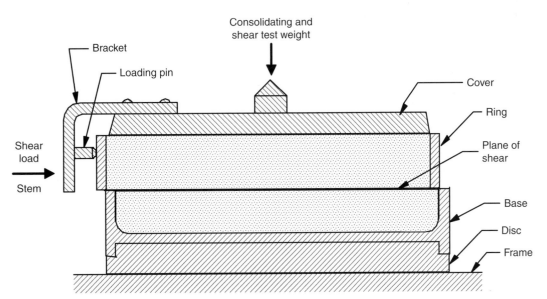

FIGURE 28.13 Jenike Direct Shear Test, cohesive strength test set-up

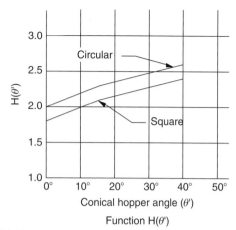

FIGURE 28.14   Plot of derived function H(θ') used to calculate arching dimensions for mass flow bins

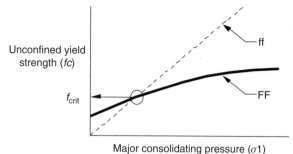

FIGURE 28.15   Example of flow function (FF) and flow factor (ff) intersection, showing f_{crit} at their intersection

prevent a cohesive arch or rathole from forming over a bin outlet can be calculated. The term Bc refers to the minimum outlet diameter for a circular outlet to prevent a cohesive arch from forming in a mass flow bin. The term Bp refers to the minimum outlet width for a slotted outlet (Bp), in which the length:width ratio exceeds 3:1, to prevent arching in a mass flow bin.

The majority of bins used in pharmaceutical processes utilize hoppers with circular outlets. Therefore, we will focus our discussion on the calculation of the Bc parameter. It is worth noting that the outlet diameter required to prevent arching over a circular outlet (Bc) will typically be about two times greater than the required outlet width of a slotted outlet (Bp). The calculation of Bp is provided in Jenike.[9]

For mass flow, the required minimum outlet diameter to prevent arching is calculated in Equation 28.1 below:

$$Bc = H(\theta') f_{crit} / \gamma \qquad (28.1)$$

where:

H(θ') is a dimensionless function derived from first principles (mathematical model) and is given by Figure 28.14. The complete derivation of H(θ') is beyond the scope of this chapter, but is provided in Jenike.[9]

f_{crit} (units of force/area) is the unconfined yield strength at the intersection of the hopper flow factor (ff) and the experimentally derived flow function (FF), as shown in Figure 28.15. The flow factor (ff) is a mathematically determined value that represents the minimum available stress available to break an arch. The calculation of the flow factor (ff) is also beyond the scope of this chapter, but is

provided in Jenike,[9] and is a function of the flow properties and the hopper angle (θ').

γ (units of weight/volume) is the bulk density of the powder at the outlet.

This calculation yields a dimensional value of Bc in units of length, which is scale-independent. Therefore, for a mass flow bin, the opening size required to prevent arching is not a function of the diameter of the bin, height of the bin or the height-to-diameter ratio.

The determination of Bc is especially valuable in making decisions during process scale-up. As a formulation is developed, a cohesive strength test can be conducted early in the development process to determine the cohesive strength (flow function). This material-dependent flow function, in conjunction with Equation 28.1 above, will yield a minimum opening (outlet) size to prevent arching in a mass flow bin. For example, this opening size may be calculated to be 200 mm. This 200 mm diameter will be required whether the bin holds 10 kilos or 1000 kilos of powder, and is scale-independent. In this example, since a 200 mm diameter opening is required, feeding this material through a press hopper or similarly small openings would pose problems with an arch developing over the outlet. This information could then be used early in the development process, to consider reformulating the product to reduce the cohesive strength, and improve flowability.

Calculation of minimum required outlet dimensions to prevent ratholing (funnel flow bin)

If the bin discharges in funnel flow, the bin outlet diameter should be sized to be larger than the critical rathole diameter (Df) to prevent a stable rathole from forming over the outlet. For a funnel flow bin with a circular outlet, sizing the outlet diameter to exceed the Df will also ensure that a stable arch will not form (since a rathole is inherently stronger than an arch). The Df value is calculated in Equation 28.2, and

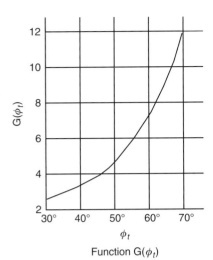

Function G(ϕ_t)

FIGURE 28.16 Plot of derived function G(ϕ_t) used to calculate critical rathole diameter for funnel flow bins

additional details of the calculation are provided in Jenike.[9]

$$Df = G(\phi_t)\, fc(\sigma 1)/\gamma \qquad (28.2)$$

where:

G(ϕ_t) is a mathematically derived function from first principles and is given by Figure 28.16.
$fc(\sigma 1)$ is the unconfined yield strength of the material. This value is determined by the flow function (FF) at the actual consolidating pressure $\sigma 1$ (discussed below).

The consolidation pressure $\sigma 1$ is a function of the "head" or height of powder above the outlet of the bin, and takes into account the load taken up by friction along the walls, as derived by Janssen[20] in Equation 28.3:

$$\sigma 1 = (\gamma\, R/\mu k)\, (1 - e^{(-\mu kh/R)}) \qquad (28.3)$$

where:

γ is the average bulk density of the powder in the bin
R is the hydraulic radius (area/perimeter)
μ is the coefficient of friction, (μ = tangent ϕ'). The value of ϕ' is determined from the wall friction test (discussed in the next section)
k is the ratio of horizontal to vertical pressures. A k value of 0.4 is typically used for a straight sided section)
h is the depth of the bed of powder within the bin.

This relationship in Equation 28.2 cannot be reduced further (e.g., to a dimensionless ratio), as the function $fc(\sigma 1)$ is highly material-dependent.

The application of these parameters (Bc, Df) to design new equipment or develop corrective equipment modifications is further discussed in Section 28.5.

Wall friction: determining hopper angles for mass flow

Test Method The wall friction test is crucial in determining whether a given bin will discharge in mass flow or funnel flow (mass flow and funnel flow are discussed in the previous section). Wall friction is caused by the powder particles sliding along the wall surface. In Jenike's continuum model,[9] wall friction is expressed as the wall friction angle (ϕ'). The lower the wall friction angle, the shallower the hopper or chute walls need to be for powder to flow along them. This coefficient of friction can be measured by shearing a sample of powder in a test cell across a stationary wall surface using a Jenike Direct Shear tester.[9,12] One arrangement of a cell used for the wall friction test is shown in Figure 28.17. In this case, a coupon of the wall material being evaluated is held in place on the frame of the tester, and a cell of powder is placed above. The coefficient of sliding friction (μ, μ = tangent ϕ') is the ratio of the shear force required for sliding (τ) to the normal force applied perpendicular to the wall material coupon (σn). A plot of the measured shear force (τ) as a function of the applied normal pressure (σn) generates a relationship known as the wall yield locus (see Figure 28.18).

The wall friction measured is a function of the powder handled and the wall surface (type, finish, orientation) in contact with it. Variations in the powder, handling conditions (e.g., temperature/RH), and/or the wall surface finish can have a dramatic effect on the resulting wall friction coefficient.[17] The results of the wall friction test are used to determine the hopper angles required to achieve mass flow, as discussed in the following section.

Calculation of recommended mass flow hopper angles

Based upon mathematical models, design charts[9] have been developed to determine which flow pattern is to be expected during gravity discharge from a bin. The design charts use the following inputs for the powder being handled, and the bin design being considered:

1. the hopper angle ("θc" for a conical hopper or "θp" for a planar hopper), as measured from vertical;
2. the wall friction angle (ϕ'), as measured from the wall friction tests;
3. the internal friction angle (δ), as measured from the cohesive strength tests.

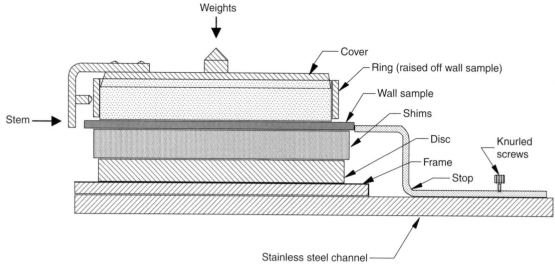

FIGURE 28.17   Jenike Direct Shear Test, wall friction test set-up

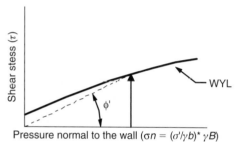

FIGURE 28.18   Example of wall yield locus generated from wall friction test data

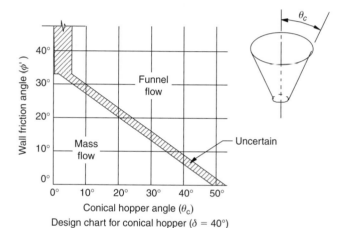

Design chart for conical hopper ($\delta = 40°$)

FIGURE 28.19   Mass flow/funnel flow design chart for conical hopper handling a bulk solid with an effective angle of internal friction (δ) of 40°

This chapter will focus on the calculation of the recommended mass hopper angles for a conical hopper (θc), since the majority of pharmaceutical processes utilize bins with a conical hopper. The methods to calculate the recommended mass hopper angles for a planar hopper (θp) with a slotted outlet are similar in approach, and are outlined in Jenike.[9] It is worth noting that the recommended mass flow angles for planar hopper walls (θp) can often be 8° to 12° shallower than those for a conical hopper (θc), for the same sized opening.

An example of such a design chart for a conical hopper is shown in Figure 28.19. The design chart shown is specifically for a powder with an effective angle of internal friction (δ) of 40°; the design charts will be different for different values of δ.[9] Hopper angles required for mass flow are a function of δ, since flow along converging hopper walls involves interparticle motion of the powder. For any combination of ϕ' and θc that lies in the mass flow region, mass flow is expected to occur. If the combination lies in the funnel flow region, funnel flow is expected. The "uncertain" region is an area where mass flow is expected to

occur based on theory, but represents a 4° margin of safety on the design, to account for inevitable variations in test results and surface finish.

As an example of using the design chart, a bin with a conical hopper angle (θc) of 20° from vertical is being used. Wall friction tests are conducted on the hopper wall surface, and a wall friction angle of 35° is measured for the normal pressure calculated at the outlet. Based upon the design chart, this bin would be expected to discharge in funnel flow. In that case, the designer would need to find another wall surface, with a wall friction angle that is less than 20°, to ensure mass flow discharge.

The wall friction angle (ϕ') is determined by the wall friction tests described above. The value of ϕ' to use for the hopper design charts will be selected for the expected normal pressure (σn), against the surface at the location of interest in the bin (e.g., the hopper outlet). For many combinations of wall surfaces and powders, the wall friction angle changes, depending on the normal pressure. When mass flow develops, the solids pressure normal to the wall surface is given by the following relationship:

$$\sigma n = (\sigma'/\gamma b) * \gamma B \qquad (28.4)$$

where:

$(\sigma'/\gamma b)$ is a dimensionless parameter that can be found in Jenike;[9]
B (units of length) is the span of the outlet: the diameter of a circular outlet or the width of a slotted outlet;
γ is the bulk density at the outlet.

Generally, ϕ' increases with decreasing normal pressure (σn). The corresponding normal pressure to the wall (σn) is the lowest at the outlet where the span (B) is the smallest. Therefore, it is at the outlet where the wall friction angle (ϕ') is the highest for a given design, provided the hopper interior surface-finish and angle remain constant above the outlet. As a result, if the walls of the hopper are steep enough at the outlet to provide mass flow, mass flow is to be expected at the walls above the outlet (regardless of total bin size).

The hopper angle required for mass flow is principally dependent on the outlet size selected for the hopper under consideration. The hopper angle required for mass flow is not a function of the flow rate, the level of powder within the bin or the diameter or height of the bin. Since the wall friction angle generally increases with lower normal pressures, a steeper hopper is often required to achieve mass flow for a bin with a smaller outlet.

28.4.2 Bulk Density

The bulk density of a given powder is not a single or even a dual value, but varies as a function of the consolidating pressure applied to it. There are various methods used in industry to measure bulk density. One prominent method is utilizing different sized containers that are measured for volume after being loosely filled with a known mass of material ("loose" density), and after vibration or tapping ("tapped density"), such as the USP Chapter <616> method.[18] These methods can offer some repeatability with respect to the conditions under which measurements are taken. However, they do not necessarily represent the actual compaction

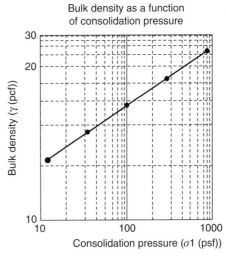

FIGURE 28.20 Example of bulk density versus consolidation pressure plot from compressibility test data

behavior of a powder being handled in a bin, chute or press hopper. Therefore, it is necessary to measure the bulk density over a range of consolidation pressures, via a compressibility test,[9,19] for design purposes. The results of the compressibility test can often be plotted as a straight line on a log–log plot (see Figure 28.20). In powder handling literature, the slope of this line is typically called the "compressibility" of the powder.

The resulting data can be used to determine capacities for storage and transfer equipment, and evaluate wall friction and feeder operation requirements. As an example, when estimating the capacity of a bin, the bulk density based upon the average major consolidation pressure in the bin can be used. For the calculation of the arching dimensions (Bc), and recommended mass flow hopper angles (θc), the bulk density based on the major consolidation pressure at the bin outlet can be used.

28.4.3 Permeability

The flow problems that can occur due to adverse two-phase (powder and interstitial gas) flow effects were reviewed in Section 28.3. These problems are more likely to occur when the target feed rate (e.g., tableting rate) exceeds the "critical flow rate," based on the powder's physical properties. The results of the permeability test are one of the primary flow properties used to determine the critical flow rate. The permeability of a powder is a measurement of how readily gas can pass through it. The permeability will have a controlling effect on the discharge rate that can be achieved from a bin/hopper with a given outlet size. Sizing the outlet of a piece of equipment or

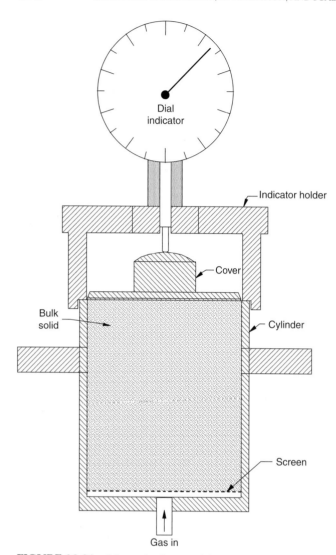

FIGURE 28.21   Schematic of permeability test set-up

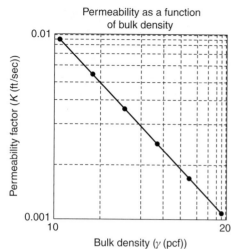

FIGURE 28.22   Example of permeability versus bulk density plot from permeability test data

choosing the diameter of a transfer chute should take into consideration the target feed rate.

Permeability is measured as a function of bulk density.[19] A schematic of the permeability tests is provided in Figure 28.21. In this test set-up, gas is injected at the bottom of the test cell through a permeable membrane. During the test, the pressure drop and flow rate across the powder are measured. The method involves measuring the flow rate of air at a predetermined pressure drop through a sample of known density and height. The permeability is then calculated using Darcy's law. The permeability of a powder typically decreases as the bulk density increases, so the test is conducted over a range of bulk densities.

Once the permeability/bulk density relationship is determined (see Figure 28.22), it can be used to calculate the critical flow rates that will be achieved for steady-flow conditions though various outlet sizes. The critical flow rate is dependent upon the permeability, bin geometry, outlet size, and consolidation pressure. The details of calculating critical flow rates are outside the scope of this chapter, but mathematical models have been developed for these calculations.

Higher flow rates than the calculated critical flow rate may occur, but may result in non-steady or erratic feed and resulting adverse effects, as discussed in Section 28.3. Permeability values can also be used to calculate the time required for fine powders to settle or deaerate in equipment.

28.4.4 Segregation Tests

When developing a product or designing a process, it is beneficial to know whether the blend will be prone to segregation. If the blend is prone to segregation, it is beneficial to know what segregation mechanism(s) will occur, since this information can be used to modify the material properties (e.g., excipient selection, component particle size distribution, etc.) to minimize the potential for segregation. An understanding of the potential for segregation can alert the equipment or process designer to potential risks that may then be avoided during the scale-up process. In some cases, significant process steps, such as granulation, may be required to avoid potential segregation problems.

There are two ASTM standard practices on segregation test methods.[21,22] These tests are designed to isolate specific segregation mechanisms, and test a material's tendency to segregate by that mechanism. A brief description of these test methods follows.

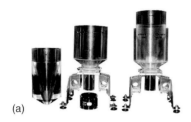

(a)

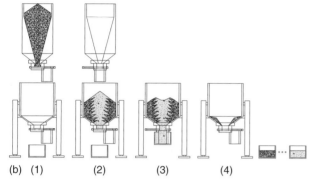

(b) (1)   (2)   (3)   (4)

FIGURE 28.23   Sifting segregation testers (a); and sifting segregation test sequence (b). Photo provided courtesy of Jenike & Johanson, Inc.

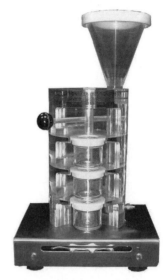

FIGURE 28.24   Fluidization segregation tester (controls not shown). Photo provided courtesy of Jenike & Johanson, Inc.

Sifting segregation test method

The sifting segregation test (Figure 28.23a) is performed by center-filling a small funnel flow bin, and then discharging it while collecting sequential samples. If sifting segregation occurs either during filling or discharge, the fines content of the discharging material will vary from beginning to end. Samples are collected from the various cups (i.e., the beginning, middle, and end of the discharge). These collected samples can then be measured for segregation by particle size analyses, assays, and/or other variables of interest.

The sequence for performing the sifting segregation test is depicted in Figure 28.23b, and is as follows:

1. the blend is placed in mass flow bin;
2. the material is discharged from a fixed height, dropping into a funnel flow bin. This transfer of material will promote segregation if the material is prone to segregate due to sifting;
3. the material is discharged from the funnel flow bin. The discharge pattern will cause material from the center to discharge first, and material from near the walls to discharge last;
4. the collected samples are then measured for segregation.

Fluidization segregation test method

The fluidization segregation test (Figure 28.24) is run by first fluidizing a column of material by

injecting air at its base. After the column is thoroughly fluidized, it is held near a minimum fluidization velocity for a predetermined period of time. The air is then turned off, and the material is allowed to deaerate. The column is then split into three equal sections (top, middle, and bottom) and the resulting samples are measured for segregation.

Several other researchers and companies have developed various segregation testers, including methods that induce vibration,[23,24] shearing in a cell,[26] and methods that capture material from a pile after it has formed.[25,26,27] Improvements and variations to the ASTM test methods have also been made. A new fluidization segregation tester that utilizes a different mechanism to fluidize the bed has been developed.[28] It uses a smaller test sample, and provides unit-dose samples for analysis. An alternate way to run the sifting segregation test involves cycling the blend multiple times to strengthen the segregation "signal."[29]

Segregation tests are useful for identifying the:

1. segregation mechanism(s) that might be active for a given blend;
2. general segregation trend that may be observed in the process;
3. comparisons between different formulas, variations of the same formula, etc.

However, the test results have limitations. Most notably, the segregation results are not scaleable, and cannot be tied quantifiably to the process. The segregation tests do not necessarily mean that a highly segregating material cannot be handled in a manner that prevents content uniformity problems. Therefore, the segregation test methods are primarily used as a stress test, to identify the dominant segregation mechanism(s) expected to occur. This information enables the equipment designer to take the appropriate precautionary measures during scale-up or make corrective actions to existing equipment. Design techniques to minimize the potential for segregation are outlined in Section 28.5.

28.5 BASIC EQUIPMENT DESIGN TECHNIQUES

Objective of the Section

The primary objective of Section 28.5 is to review basic design techniques for the bin-to-press feed system, to provide consistent, reliable flow for gravity feed, and minimize segregation. In particular, we will review the following basic design techniques:

1. reliable funnel flow bin design;
2. reliable mass flow designs for bins, transfer chutes, and press hoppers;
3. minimizing adverse two-phase flow effects (e.g., feed/tableting rate limitations, flooding);
4. minimizing segregation during blender to press transfers.

For each of these different design concerns, we will review the key equipment design parameters. Regardless of whether the equipment being designed is a bin, transfer chute or press hopper, a crucial first step in designing a reliable feed system is determining the flow pattern, and designing the equipment accordingly. The wall friction tests and design charts used to determine if a hopper will discharge in mass flow or funnel flow were discussed in Section 28.4.

28.5.1 Reliable Funnel Flow Design (Preventing a Rathole)

Funnel flow occurs when the hopper walls are not smooth and/or steep enough to promote flow at the walls. Funnel flow bins can be prone to ratholing if the material is cohesive enough. A funnel flow bin design can be considered if all of the following design criteria are met:

1. Segregation of the final blend is not a concern. Since a funnel flow bin will discharge in a first-in-last-out flow sequence, any side-to-side segregation that occurred as the bin was filled will often be exacerbated in funnel flow discharge.
2. The final blend has low cohesive strength so the formation of a stable rathole is not a concern.

This can be checked by comparing the bin outlet diameter/diagonal length to the critical rathole diameter (Df) for the estimated major consolidation pressure ($\sigma 1$) for the bin design in question as per Equations 28.2 and 28.3 (see Section 28.4). If the outlet diameter is less than Df, ratholing is a concern.

3. Flooding due to a collapsing rathole is not a concern. Flooding can result in highly aerated (low density) powder being fed from the bin to the press, which may have an adverse effect on the tablet properties (weight, hardness, dissolution variation), and can result in segregation.
4. A non-uniform feed density is not a concern. Since tablet presses operate as volumetric feeders, variation of the feed density into the press feed frame can result in tablet weight variation.

If all of these design criteria are met, a funnel flow bin design can be considered. If a funnel flow bin design is acceptable, the first concern is checking that the outlet diameter is greater than the critical rathole diameter (Df), to ensure that a stable rathole will not form. If the diameter of the funnel flow bin is not greater than Df, the following steps can be considered to reduce the likelihood of ratholing:

1. Enlarge the bin opening: this may require using a slotted outlet, which would require a feeder capable of feeding uniformly across the entire outlet (e.g., mass flow screw feeder) or a valve capable of shutting off such an outlet. Using a larger outlet diameter may not be a practical modification, since the opening may need to be increased to be larger than standard valve or feeder sizes.
2. Reduce the material level in the bin: the critical rathole diameter typically decreases with a reduction in the major consolidation pressure ($\sigma 1$), which is a function of the fill height.
3. Use an internal, mechanical agitator: an internal, mechanical agitator, such as an agitator with "arms" that rotate about a central vertical shaft, may be a practical modification on a small scale for a press hopper. A bin with a discharge valve (e.g., Matcon discharge valve) could also be considered as a means of failing a stable rathole, but may need to be assessed via full scale trials to determine the operating parameters required (valve "stroke" setting, etc.).
4. Use external vibrators: the effectiveness of external vibrators to collapse a stable rathole would need to be assessed via full-scale trials prior to installation, since vibration may actually increase the strength on the blend in the bin and increase the likelihood

of ratholing. Trials would be required to assess the optimum vibrator type (high-frequency/low-amplitude versus low-frequency/high-amplitude), number of vibrators required, location, frequency settings, and other design considerations.

There are several adverse effects of using a bin that discharges in funnel flow (first-in-last-out flow sequence, non-uniform feed density, exacerbation of segregation). In addition, the potential options to prevent a rathole are often limited or impractical. Therefore, a common design technique for preventing ratholing is to redesign the bin for mass flow. The design techniques for mass flow are discussed in the following section.

28.5.2 Reliable Mass Flow Designs for the Bin, Chute, and Press Hopper

Mass flow discharge from a bin occurs when the following two design criteria are met:

1. The bin walls are smooth and/or steep enough to promote flow at the walls;
2. The bin outlet is large enough to prevent an arch.

The wall friction tests and design charts used to determine if a bin will discharge in mass flow or funnel flow were discussed in Section 28.4. This section focuses on design techniques for mass flow bins, but these techniques may also be extended to obtaining mass flow in a transfer chute and press hopper. These techniques may be applied to designing new equipment or modifying existing equipment to provide mass flow.

When designing the bin to provide mass flow, the following general steps should be taken:

1. Size the outlet to prevent a cohesive arch: the bin designer should ensure that an arch will not form by making the outlet diameter equal to or larger than the minimum required outlet diameter (Bc, see Figure 28.25). If a slotted outlet is used (maintaining a 3:1 length:width ratio for the outlet), the outlet width should be sized to be equal to or larger than the minimum required outlet width (Bp, see Figure 28.25). The outlet may also need to be sized based upon the feed rate and two-phase flow considerations, as discussed below. If the outlet cannot be sized to prevent an arch (e.g., press hopper outlet that must mate with a fixed feed frame inlet), an internal mechanical agitator or external vibrator could be considered, as discussed in the preceding section.
2. Make the hopper walls steep enough for mass flow: once the outlet is sized, the hopper wall slope should be designed to be equal to, or steeper than, the recommended hopper angle for the given outlet size, and selected wall surface. For a conical hopper, the walls should be equal to, or steeper than, the recommended mass flow angle for a conical hopper (θc, see Figure 28.25). If the bin has a rectangular-to-round hopper, the valley angles should be sloped to be equal to or steeper than, θc. For planar walls, the walls should be equal to, or steeper than, the recommended mass flow angle for a planar hopper (θp, see Figure 28.25).
3. Pay careful attention to the interior wall surface finish: when conducting the wall friction tests, it is beneficial to conduct tests on several different finishes (e.g., #320 grit finish, #2B cold rolled finish, #2B electro-polished finish, etc.). This will provide the bin designer with a range of design options for the bin. Testing multiple wall surfaces will also enable the designer to assess the sensitivity of the wall friction results to different finishes. It is not sufficient to simply test a 304 or 316 stainless steel with no regard to the interior finish. The wall friction of the blend may vary significantly from finish to finish. The orientation of directional finishes, such as a mechanical polish, is also critical to assess and control during fabrication. In addition, it cannot be assumed that an interior surface finish with a lower average roughness (Ra) will provide the best wall friction properties.
4. Consider velocity gradients: even when a bin is designed for mass flow, there still may be a velocity gradient between the material discharging at the hopper walls (moving slower) versus the center of the hopper (moving faster), assuming a symmetric bin with a single outlet in the center. Depending upon the application, the bin designer may want to increase the velocity gradient to enhance blending between vertical layers of material in the bin. Or, the bin designer may want to reduce the velocity gradient to enhance blending on a side-to-side basis. The decision to increase or decrease the velocity gradient will be depend upon the segregation that occurs upon filling the bin, and its effect upon content uniformity. The velocity gradient is reduced by making the hopper slope steeper, with respect to the recommended mass flow hopper angle (θc). The velocity gradient is increased by making the hopper slope closer to (but still steeper than) the recommended mass flow hopper angle. Changing the interior surface to reduce friction or using an insert (discussed more below) are other methods used to control the velocity gradient. Asymmetric

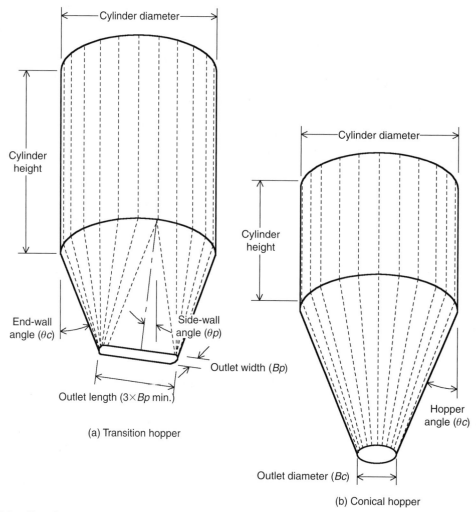

FIGURE 28.25   Mass flow design parameters (Bc, Bp, θc, θp)

hoppers, which are common for press hoppers, are especially prone to velocity gradients since the material will move faster at the steeper hopper wall. In addition, a velocity gradient cannot be completely eliminated, especially as the material level in the hopper empties. Velocity profiles, and their effect on blending material, can be calculated *a priori*, given the geometry of the bin (θc) and measured flow properties that were discussed in Section 28.4 (i.e., ϕ', δ, ϕ).

5. Avoid upward-facing lips/ledges due to mismatched flanges (e.g, see Figure 28.26), level probes, view ports, partially opened valves, etc., especially in the hopper section. Ideally, interior protruding devices should be located in the straight-sided, (non-converging) section of a bin/press hopper if possible, where they will be less detrimental in upsetting a mass flow pattern.

If the bin designer is modifying an existing funnel flow bin to provide mass flow, several different options can be considered, including:

1. Using a different interior surface finish with better wall friction properties (i.e., lower wall friction). The bin designer should conduct wall friction tests on alternative wall surfaces, to assess if changing the surface finish (e.g., electro-polishing an exiting #2B finish) will convert the bin from funnel flow to mass flow. This is often one of the most cost-effective modifications to obtain mass flow.
2. Using a flow-controlling insert such as a Binsert® (Figure 28.27) to obtain mass flow within the same bin. A properly designed insert can change the stresses that develop in the bin during discharge, so that mass flow can be obtained at a wall where the material was previously stagnant.

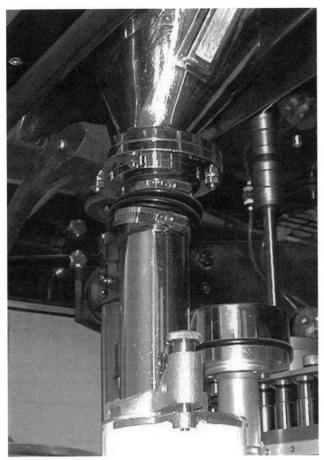

FIGURE 28.26 Example of an upward-facing ledge at a flange connection

3. Modifying the hopper geometry. Use a different geometry that is more likely to provide mass flow (e.g., conical instead of a rectangular-to-round hopper with shallower valley angles). If the hopper is modified to have a slotted outlet, it is crucial that the feeder the hopper mates to withdraws material across the entire outlet.

In addition to these design techniques for bins, there are several additional design techniques for designing transfer chutes for reliable mass flow including:

1. For converging sections that have a full cross-section (i.e., hoppers), use the same design criteria discussed above for a mass flow bin.
2. For non-converging sections of the chute, the chute should be sloped to exceed the wall friction angle (ϕ') by a least a 10° margin of safety. As an example, if the measured wall friction angle for the given wall surface (from the wall friction test results) is 40° from horizontal, the recommended chute angle for the non-converging portion of the chute would be at least 50° from horizontal.

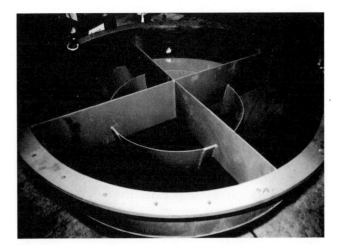

(a)

Example of a "closed" Binsert® design

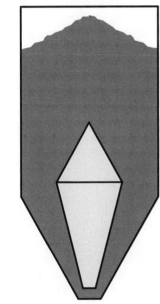

(b)

FIGURE 28.27 (a) Example of an "open" Binsert® design; (b) Example of a "closed" Binsert® design

3. If a bifurcated chute is used, the sloping chute legs should be symmetric, to prevent velocity gradients and the possibility of stagnant material in the shallower leg.
4. Use mitered joints between sloping and vertical sections.

28.5.3 Minimizing Adverse Two-phase Flow Effects

The primary focus in preventing adverse two-phase flow affects is to ensure that the powder handling equipment is designed so that the critical flow rate through a given outlet is greater than the target feed rate. The critical flow rate is determined using mathematical models, with permeability and compressibility test results as primary inputs. The critical flow rate is also a strong function of the outlet size, and increases as the outlet size increases. The target feed rate is often set by the required maximum tableting rate for the process. Adverse two-phase flow effects are typically most pronounced at the press feed hopper, since it often has the smallest outlet in the entire press feed system. Therefore, the press hopper will typically have the lowest critical flow rate.

When designing the powder handling equipment to minimize adverse two-phase flow effects, the following general design techniques are beneficial:

1. Design the equipment for mass flow: mass flow will provide consistent feed and a more uniform consolidation pressure acting on the powders. In addition, having a first-in-first-out flow sequence will allow the material more time to deaerate before being discharged through the outlet. This will reduce the likelihood of flooding. Mass flow will also prevent collapsing ratholes that can result in the powder aerating and flooding as it falls into the central flow channel. It is worth noting that mass flow can result in a lower critical flow rate than funnel flow, but will be more stable. Therefore, simply using a mass flow bin design may not be the only corrective action required if a flow rate limitation occurs. However, designing the equipment for mass flow is often the first step in addressing adverse two-phase flow effects.

2. Use larger outlets for the handling equipment: the critical flow rate is a strong function of the cross-sectional area of the outlet. Therefore, increasing the outlet can often be highly beneficial in reducing two-phase flow effects. The goal would be to increase the outlet size until the critical flow rate for the selected outlet size exceeds the target flow rate. Since this may not be feasible for a press feeder hopper, in which the outlet size is fixed to mate with the press feed frame inlet, additional design techniques are discussed below. Computer software can be used to model the two-phase flow behavior to assess the effect of changing the outlet diameter.

3. Reduce the fill height in the handling equipment: the critical flow rate through a given outlet increases as the major consolidation pressure ($\sigma 1$) decreases. Therefore, reducing the fill height will be beneficial, but will be much less effective than increasing the outlet size.

4. Reduce the target feed rate: if possible, reducing the target feed rate (tableting rate) to be less than the critical flow rate will be beneficial, but is often impractical since it will result in decreased production rate.

5. Consider gas pressure differentials: a gas pressure differential can have a beneficial or adverse effect upon two-phase flow effects. A positive gas pressure differential at the outlet (i.e., bin at a higher gas pressure than the equipment downstream) may be beneficial in overcoming a feed rate limitation. In this case, the air pressure is forcing the material in the direction of flow. Conversely, a negative gas pressure differential at the outlet can further reduce the critical flow rate, since the negative gas pressure acts to further retard the flow rate.

6. Add air permeation: air permeation may be added to the system actively via an air injection system or passively through a vent. In particular, adding judicious (often very small) amounts of air at the location in the press feed system where the interstitial gas pressure is lowest can often be beneficial. However, this can be very unstable for small systems and/or very low permeability materials.

7. Changing the particle size distribution of the powder: the permeability of a powder is a strong function of its particle size distribution (PSD). Powders with a finer PSD are often less permeable and, therefore, more prone to adverse-two phase flow effects. Even a reduction in the percentage of fines can often be beneficial in increasing the permeability of a powder, and decreasing the likelihood of adverse two phase-flow effects.

The key to implementing any corrective actions designed to reduce adverse flow-effects will be using a mathematical two-phase flow analysis to assess the effects on the bulk solids stresses and interstitial gas pressure. This analysis would need to use inputs such as key flow properties (permeability, compressibility), and equipment/process parameters (tableting rate, bin/hopper geometry, and gas pressure gradients) to assess the effect of the potential corrective actions outlined above.

28.5.4 Minimizing Segregation in the Blender-to-Press Transfer Steps

It may be a challenging process for a designer to determine which segregation mechanism(s) is dominant, and develop appropriate corrective actions. This requires knowledge of the material's physical and chemical characteristics, as well as an understanding of the segregation mechanisms that can be active. One must identify the process conditions that can serve as a driving force to cause segregation. Flow properties measurements (wall friction, cohesive strength, compressibility, and permeability) can help to provide understanding of the behavior of the material in storage and transfer equipment. Consideration should be given to the fill/discharge sequence, including flow pattern and inventory management, which gives rise to the observed segregation. Testing for segregation potential (see Section 28.4) can provide additional insight about the mechanisms that may be causing segregation. Sufficient sampling is required to support the hypothesis of segregation (e.g., blend samples and final product samples, samples from the center versus periphery of the bin). Finally, one must consider the impact of analytical and sampling errors specific to the blend under consideration, as well as the statistical significance of the results, when drawing conclusions from the data.

From the previous discussion about segregation mechanisms, it can be concluded that certain material properties, as well as process conditions, must exist for segregation to occur. Elimination of one of these will prevent segregation. It stands to reason, then, that if segregation is a problem in a process, one should look for opportunities to either: (1) change the material or (2) modify the process equipment or conditions. This chapter focuses on the equipment and process design techniques to minimize segregation.

Some generalizations can be made when designing equipment to minimize segregation. The complete details on how to implement these changes correctly are beyond the scope of this chapter. However, all equipment must be designed based on the flow properties and segregation potential of the blends being handled.

Primary equipment and process design techniques to minimize segregation during the final blender-to-press transfer include:

1. Minimize the number of material transfer steps. The tendency for segregation increases with each transfer step and movement of the bin. Ideally, the material would discharge directly from the blender into the tablet press feed frame, with no additional handling. In-bin blending is as close to this as most firms can practically obtain. This assumes that a uniform blend can be obtained within the bin blender in the first place.
2. Storage bins, press hoppers, and chutes should be designed for mass flow. In mass flow, the entire contents of the bin are in motion during discharge. In funnel flow, stagnant regions exist.
3. Minimize transfer chute volumes to reduce the volume of displaced air, and the volume of

potentially segregated material. However, the chute must remain large enough to provide the required throughput rates.
4. Use a storage bin with a larger height:diameter aspect ratio. A mass flow bin with a tall, narrow cylinder will minimize the potential for sifting segregation, compared to that of a short, wide bin. A downside is that taller drop height may exacerbate other segregation mechanisms.
5. Bins and blenders should be vented to avoid gas counter-flow. Air in an otherwise "empty" bin must be displaced out of the bin as powder fills it. If this air is forced through material in the V-blender, it can induce fluidization segregation within the blender. A separate pathway or vent line to allow the air to escape without moving through the bed of material can reduce segregation.
6. Velocity gradients within bins should also be minimized. The hopper must be significantly steeper than the mass flow limit to achieve this. A steeper hopper section may result in an impractically tall bin. Alternate approaches include the use of inserts (discussed previously). If an insert is used, it must be properly designed and positioned to be effective. Asymmetric bins and hoppers should be avoided if possible, and symmetrical ones should be used whenever possible.
7. Dust generation and fluidization of the material should be minimized during material movement. Dust can be controlled by way of socks or sleeves, to contain the material as it drops from the blender to the bin, for example. Some devices are commercially available. An example of this is a solids decelerator shown in Figure 28.28.
8. Drop heights should be minimized where possible. Drop heights may aerate the material, induce dust, and increase momentum of the material as it hits the pile. This will increase the tendency for each of the three segregation mechanisms to occur.
9. Valves should be operated correctly. Butterfly valves should be operated in the full open position, not throttled to restrict flow. Restricting flow will virtually assure a funnel flow pattern, which is usually detrimental to uniformity.
10. Use a symmetrical split whenever a process stream is divided. A symmetrical split, such as a bifurcated chute to feed two sides of a press (a Y-branch), will eliminate potential differences in the flow between the two streams. Consideration must be given to any potential for segregation upstream of the split. Even seemingly minor details, such as the orientation of a butterfly valve prior to a split, can affect segregation. Proper

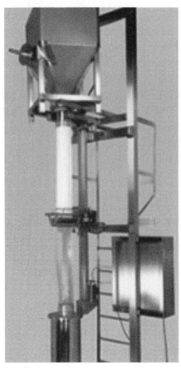

FIGURE 28.28   Example of a solids deceleration device. Photo provided courtesy of GEA Process Engineering

designs should be utilized for Y-branches to avoid stagnant material and air counter-flow.

Other specific solutions may be apparent once the segregation mechanism has been identified. As an example, mass flow is usually beneficial when handling segregation-prone materials, especially materials that exhibit a side-to-side (or center-to-periphery) segregation pattern. Sifting and dusting segregation mechanisms fit this description.

It is important to remember that mass flow is not a universal solution, since it will not address a top-to-bottom segregation pattern. As an example, consider the situation in a portable bin where fluidization upon filling the bin has caused the fine fraction of a blend to be driven to the top surface. Mass flow discharge of this bin would effectively transfer this segregated material to the downstream process, delivering the coarser blend first, followed by the fines.

In summary, when addressing segregation concerns it is crucial to know your process, and how the blend will segregate before implementing equipment designs or corrective actions.

References

1. Rippie, E.G. (1980). Powders. In: *Remington's Pharmaceutical Sciences*, A. Osol, G.D. Chase, A.R. Gennaro, M.R. Gibson & C.B. Granberg, (eds), 16th edn. Mack Publishing Company, Easton PA. pp. 1535–1552.
2. Venables, H.J. & Wells, J.I. (2001). Powder mixing. Drug Dev. and Ind. Pharm. 27(7), 599–612.
3. Alexander, A.W. & Muzzio, F.J.(2006). Batch Size Increase in Dry Blending and Mixing. *Pharmaceutical Process Scale-Up*, 2nd edn. Taylor & Francis, (2006). pp. 161–180.
4. Royal, T. A. & Carson, J.W. (2000). Fine Powder Flow Phenomena in Bins, Hoppers and Processing Vessels. Presented at Bulk 2000. London.
5. Bates, L. (1997). User guide to segregation. British Materials Handling Board.
6. Williams, J.C. (1976). The segregation of particulate materials: A review. Powder Technology 15, 245–251.
7. Williams, J.C. & Khan, M.I. (1973). The mixing and segregation of particulate solids of different particle size. Chemical Engineer January, 19–25.
8. Pittenger, B.H., Purutyan, H. & Barnum, R.A. (2000). Reducing/eliminating segregation problems in powdered metal processing. Part I: Segregation mechanisms. P/M Science Technology Briefs 2(1), March. 5–9.
9. Jenike, A.W. (1964, Revised 1980). Storage and flow of solids. Bulletin 123 of the Utah Engineering Experimental Station 53(26).
10. Schulze, D. (1996). Measuring powder flowability: A comparison of test methods Part I. Powder and Bulk Engineering 10(4), 45–61.
11. Schulze, D. (1996). Measuring powder flowability: A comparison of test methods Part II. Powder and Bulk Engineering 10(6), 17–28.
12. Standard Shear Testing Method for Powders Using the Jenike Shear Cell. (2006). ASTM Standard D6128-06, American Society for Testing and Materials.
13. Bausch, A., Hausmann, R., Bongartz, C. & Zinn, T. (1998). Measurement of Flowability with a Ring Shear Cell, Evaluation and adaptation of the Method for Use in Pharmaceutical Technology. Proc. 2nd World Meeting APGI/APV, Paris, May, pp. 135–136.
14. Hausmann, R., Bausch, A., Bongartz, C. & Zinn, T. (1998). Pharmaceutical Applications of a New Ring Shear Tester for Flowability Measurement of Granules and Powders. Proc. 2nd World Meeting APGI/APV, Paris, May, pp.137–138.
15. Nyquist, H. (1984). Measurement of flow properties in large scale tablet production. International Journal of Pharmaceutical Technology and Product Manufacturing 5(3), 21–24.
16. Ramachandruni, H. & Hoag, S. (1998). Application of a Modified Annular Shear Cell Measuring Lubrication of Pharmaceutical Powders. University of Maryland, Poster presentation at the AAPS Annual Meeting. San Francisco.
17. Prescott, J.K., Ploof, D.A. & Carson, J.W. (1999). Developing a better understanding of wall friction. Powder Handling and Processing 11(1), January/March, 27–35.
18. The United States Pharmacopeia. (2002). Chapter <616> Bulk and Tapped Density. US Pharmacopeial Forum 28(3).
19. Carson, J.W. & Marinelli, J. (1994). Characterize powders to ensure smooth flow. *Chemical* Engineering 101(4), April, 78–90.
20. Janssen, H.A. (1895). "Versuche uber Getreidedruck in Silozellen", Verein Deutcher Igenieure, Zeitschrift, V. 39, Aug. 31, 1045–1049.
21. Anonymous. (2003). Standard Practice/Guide for Measuring Sifting Segregation Tendencies of Bulk Solids. D6940-03, ASTM International.
22. Anonymous. (2003). Standard Practice for Measuring Fluidization Segregation Tendencies of Powders. D6941-03, ASTM International.
23. Ahmed, H. & Shah, N. (2000). Formulation of low dose medicines—Theory and practice. American Pharmaceutical Review 3(3), 9–15.

24. Globepharma's Powdertest ™ http://www.globepharma.com/html/powertest.html (accessed September 2006).

25. Massol-Chaudeur, S., Berthiaux, H. & Doggs, J. (2003). The development and use of a static segregation test to evaluate the robustness of various types of powder mixtures. Trans IchemE 81(Part c), June, 106–118.

26. Johanson, K., Eckert, C., Ghose, D., et al. (2005). Quantitative measurement of particle segregation mechanisms. Powder Technology 159(1), November, 1–12.

27. De Silva, S.R., Dyroy, A. & Enstad, G.G. (1999). Segregation Mechanisms and Their Quantification Using Segregation Testers In: *Solids Mechanics and Its Applications*, Volume 81, IUTAM Symposium on Segregation in Granular Flows. pp. 11–29.

28. Hedden, D.A., Brone, D., Clement, S.A. et al. (2006). Development of an improved fluidization segregation tester for use with pharmaceutical powders. Pharmaceutical Technology, 30(12), December, 54–64.

29. Alexander, B., Roddy, M., Brone, D. et al. (2000). A method to quantitatively describe powder segregation during discharge from vessels. Pharmaceutical Technology, Yearbook, 6–21.

Process Development and Scale-up of Wet Granulation by the High Shear Process

Lirong Liu, Michael Levin and Paul Sheskey

29.1 INTRODUCTION

Wet granulation is widely applied in pharmaceutical manufacture. Many studies were conducted to better understand the complexity of the process. Recently, emerging innovative technologies are being developed to improve the wet granulation process, process control, and process robustness. These efforts are evolved to meet the changing environment of the twenty-first century globalization dynamics, and emerging changes in regulatory demands. However, in many cases the process development, scale-up, and critical to quality (CTQ) of wet granulation could be challenging, and somewhat formulation-dependent. Best practices (Section 29.17) and detailed considerations (Section 29.10) for formulation and process design and development are the key factors for successful development of a robust wet granulation process.

29.2 PRINCIPLES OF WET GRANULATION AND PROCESS CONSIDERATION

Wet granulation refers to a process involving granulating the powder with liquid (aqueous,

non-aqueous, hot-melt … etc.) to achieve the desired properties for subsequent processes (Section 29.3). During the initial formulation development, the simplicity of future manufacturing processes should be one of the key considerations. If all other things are equal, the design of the dosage form should consider a dosage form that is simple to manufacture consistently in future production. For example, if a product can be directly compressed, and the resulting product meets all the design requirements, then dry or wet granulation may not add value to the quality or the performance of the product. Similar concepts should be applied for designing the granulation process to maximize the process robustness with available technology and resources.

29.3 PURPOSE OF WET GRANULATION

1. Densification
2. Improve flowability
3. Improve compressibility
4. Improve uniformity
5. Improve wettability
6. Easier to disperse or transfer.

Developing Solid Oral Dosage Forms: Pharmaceutical Theory and Practice
ISBN: 978-0-444-53242-8

29.4 COMMON WET GRANULATION EQUIPMENT USED FOR MANUFACTURE

Based on the principles of operation, commonly seen wet granulation equipment includes:

1. V-blender
2. Double-cone blender, ribbon blender
3. Low-shear mixer
4. High shear granulator
5. Fluid-bed granulator
6. Spray-dry granulator
7. *In situ* granulation
8. Rotor processor
9. Rotating disk processor
10. Foam granulation process.

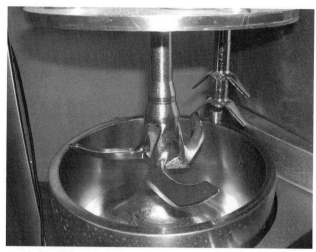

FIGURE 29.3   Top-drive high-shear mixer/granulator with vertical chopper

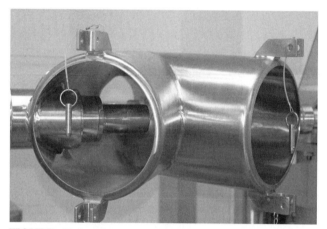

FIGURE 29.1   V-blender can be used for wet-granulation by infusing the liquid through center intensified bar or nozzles

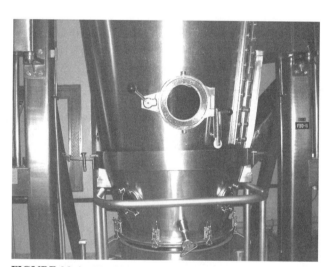

FIGURE 29.4   Fluid-bed granulator

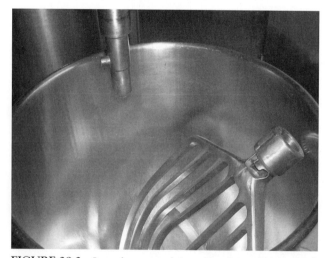

FIGURE 29.2   Low-shear granulator with agitator disassembled

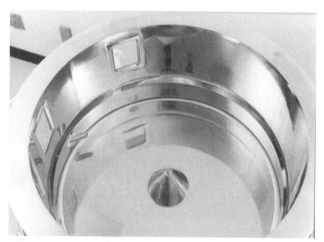

FIGURE 29.5   Rotor granulator

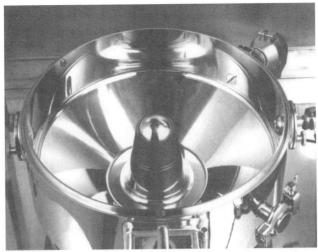

FIGURE 29.6 Rotating disk processor (Granurex®, Vector Corporation)

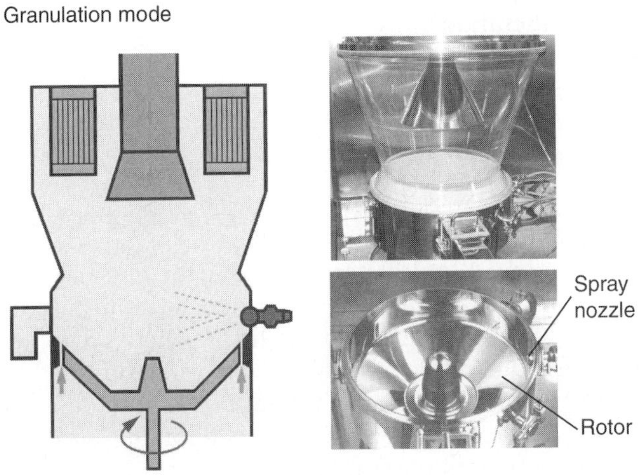

Granulation mode

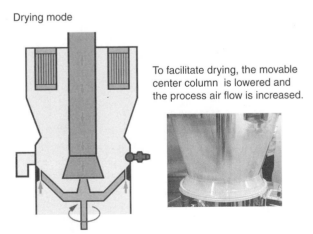

FIGURE 29.7 Graphic display of rotating disk processor in granulation mode

Drying mode

To facilitate drying, the movable center column is lowered and the process air flow is increased.

FIGURE 29.8 Graphic display of rotating disk processor in drying mode

29.5 EQUIPMENT SELECTION CONSIDERATIONS

For a well-designed formulation, wet granulation can be effectively performed and controlled by using different types of equipment. However, some formulations may be benefited by using one specific process. Common factors include:

1. API properties (size, structure, density, solubility, porosity, stability … etc);
2. Flowability of final granules;
3. Degree of densification required;
4. Better size control/reproducibility;
5. Moisture control/reproducibility of final granules;
6. Limitations of rotary compression process design (short feeder time, short dwell time, limited filled depth … etc.);
7. Process issues: sticking, lubrication, dust deposit, heat … etc.;
8. Manufacture cost improvement (acceptable process time, including granulation and drying if needed);
9. Availability of equipment;
10. Use of process analytical technology (PAT) application.

Traditionally, high shear granulators are widely used in the pharmaceutical industry for wet granulation, due to relatively short process time when compared to other earlier equipment. However, as more products may require special attention to meet the twenty-first century regulations and changing global economy, one should consider "Best Practices" (Section 29.17) for proper design and selection of the formulation, process, and equipment.

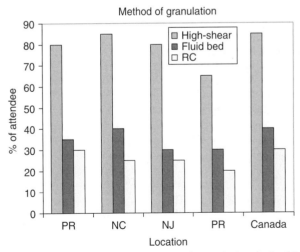

FIGURE 29.9 Survey of preference of granulation method by location

Equipment consideration	HS	FB	RD
Density	+++	+	++
Shape	+	+	++
Pt distribution	++	++	+++
Stability	−	++	++
Cost and time	+++(FB)*	++	++

HS: Highshear process, FB: Fluid-bed process,
RD: Rotating disk process

*Note FB is used as dryer

FIGURE 29.10   Consideration of equipment

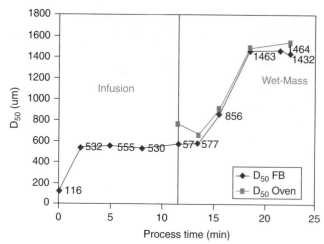

FIGURE 29.11   The particle size change in a typical wet-granulation process

29.6 INTRODUCTION TO THE WET GRANULATION PROCESS

29.6.1 Granule Growth Stages

Based on the interactions between the powder and granulation agents, the wet granulation process can be described by the following four steps.

1. Pendular;
2. Capillary;
3. Funicular;
4. Droplet.

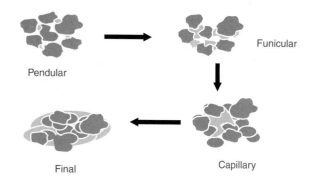

29.6.2 Granule Size Change Mechanism during Granulation Process

1. Nucleation;
2. Coalescence;
3. Layering;
4. Abrasion.

29.6.3 Process Considerations for Particle Size Growth

1. Identify the minimum moisture content required to form desired size;
2. Evaluate the size distribution of end point granules at manufacture scale;

3. Include the down stream processes in considerations;
4. Formulation limitation/formulation characterization;
5. Measurements and correlation of measurement to process robustness.

During the granulation, the particle size will increase as the liquid and energy are applied to the powders in the chamber. A typical particle size change is shown in Figure 29.11. As granules reach the end point, use of a chopper in the high shear granulator may break the large agglomeration into smaller pieces. In production equipment, the increasing weight of the granules will also enhance the size growth of the granules circulating at the bottom portion.

Comparison of Considerations of Process Parameters in High Shear and Fluid-bed Granulation

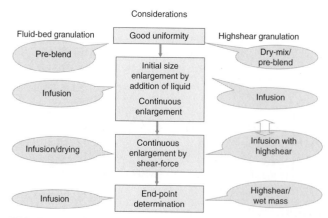

FIGURE 29.12   Considerations of process design for wet granulation

29.7 OVERALL CONSIDERATION FOR PROCESS PARAMETERS

29.7.1 Pre-blend Stage

Design Preference

- Blade at low-speed, no chopper to avoid excess dust;
- Blade at high-speed, chopper on-off for uniformity;
- Protect or remove nozzle(s) if possible;
- Typical 3–15 minutes at various scales.

Key Focus

- Proper set-up including filter, seal, and spray device position if so equipped.
- Not over-purging the chamber to avoid segregation.
- Recollect dust from filter, lid, inside wall, for low dose product.

Common Issues

- Excess dust;
- Heat accumulation;
- Segregation;
- Fluidization followed by settlement.

29.7.2 Infusion Stage I

Design Preference

- Set blade/impeller at low speed or, low speed initially, then increase the speed;
- Adjust spray distance, atomization, spray zone location (infused before chopper);
- Establish relationship between amount of spray, spray rate, tip speed, and amount of load;
- Monitor temperature variation of infusing liquid between sub-batches;
- Load comprises 50–75% of total volume;
- Typically 5–15 minutes at various scales.

Key Focus

- Type of high shear granulator: top drive design versus bottom drive design;
- Position of chopper and style of chopper;
- Dynamic change of granule bed height;
- Dynamic change of granule bed shape;
- Temperature may decrease due to liquid infusion.

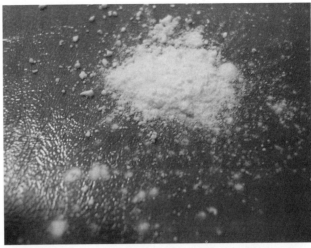

FIGURE 29.13   Example of granules at Infusion Stage I

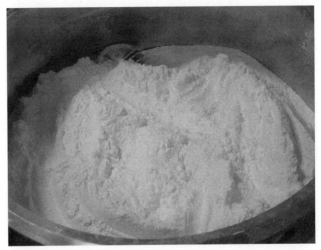

FIGURE 29.14   Example of chamber appearance after Stage I

Common Issues

- Droplet uniformity;
- Sticking on peripherals (underneath the blade/impeller and bottom).

Granule Behavior

- Average size: around 50–100 μm;
- Some unwetted particles can be observed (5–30%);
- No major lumps appear yet;
- Watch for accumulation spots;
- Bed densification by 20–40%.

Chamber Appearance

- No major power sticking on side;
- Relatively clean chamber and blade/impeller;
- No wet spot on the lid.

29.7.3 Infusion Stage II

Design Preference

- Blade at high speed with or without chopper at high speed;
- Keep uniform spray before chopper position;
- Typical 3–12 minutes at various scales.

Key Focus

- Observation of significant granule size growth;
- About 50–80% of all granules reach target size;
- Cascading motion from side to center observed;
- Temperature increases slowly;
- Moderate densification;
- Acoustic sound may change.

Common Issues

- Poor uniformity in size, and less than 1–2% of lumps appear;
- Some fine granules observed 1–5% ("fine" granules will not survive the fluid-bed drying process).

Granule Behavior

- Average size: around 100–400 μm;
- Some lumps appear 1–2%;
- No more than 5% of fine particles allowed after this stage;
- Watch for shape of granules;
- Granules are forming at variety of stages and sizes.

Chamber Appearance

- No major power sticking on side;
- Little or some sticking of granules on side wall and blade/impeller;
- Some wet spot/sticking of granules on the lid;
- Some granules may stick on spray gun(s).

29.7.4 Wet Mass Stage

Design Preference

- Blade/impeller at high speed and chopper at high speed;
- Typically a few minutes at various scales until desired end point;
- Large lumps may require size reduction at full manufacture scale;
- End point should consider downstream process impact.

Key Focus

- >90% of granules reach targeted particle size;
- 2–10% granules may be significantly oversized;
- Temperature may increases significantly;
- Cohesive behavior (see Granule Cohesion Test);
- Condensation moisture may appear on lid or side wall;
- Clean swept path may appear;
- Some lumps in 4–8 inches are normal if heavy granules are desired.

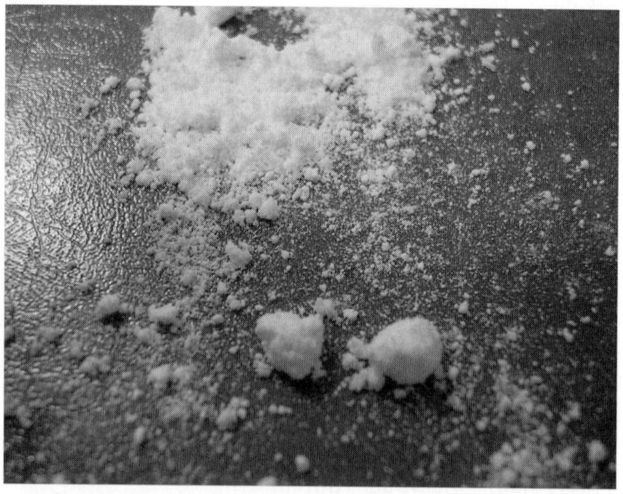

FIGURE 29.15   Example of granules at Infusion Stage II

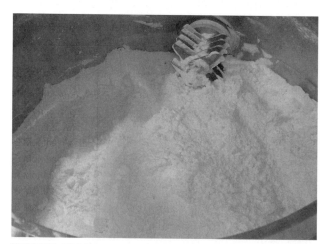

FIGURE 29.16   Example of chamber appearance after Infusion Stage II

Common Issues

- Selection of robust method of end point determination;
- PAT consideration;
- Last 1–2% fine is difficult to grow to desired size;
- Consistency;
- Reproducibility;
- Change of raw material properties;
- Fear of over-granulation.

Granule Behavior

- Average size: around 200–1500 μm;
- Some large lumps appear, but less than 0.5% is acceptable;
- No more than 1% of fine particles allowed after this stage;
- Watch for shape of granules: smooth, somewhat round appearance with few irregular shapes and rough edges;
- Granules are forming at variety of stages and sizes, even at end point.

Chamber Appearance

- No major power sticking on side;
- Some sticking of granules on side wall and blade/impeller;
- Some wet spot/sticking of granules on the lid;
- Some granules stick on spray gun(s).

Granules can be observed at different sizes and stages, even at the end point with best equipment and process.

The chamber should show a relatively clean surface, without excess residuals after discharge (residuals on center and edge may require scraping in between batches).

29.7.5 Popular End Point Observations

Cohesion Test 1

1. cohesion lumps form after squeezing by hand;
2. can be easily separated into individual granules.

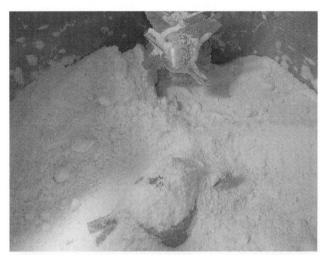

FIGURE 29.18 Example of chamber appearance after wet mass stage

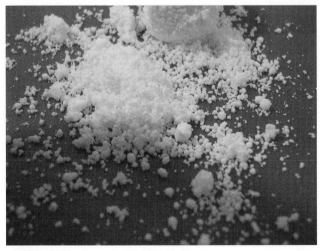

FIGURE 29.17 Example of end point granules at wet mass stage

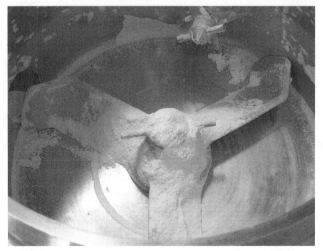

FIGURE 29.19 Example of a typical chamber surface after discharge

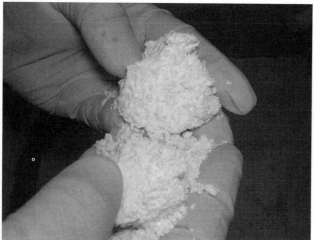

FIGURE 29.20   Cohesion Test 1

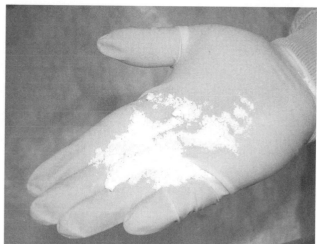

FIGURE 29.22   Cohesion Test 2 Step 3

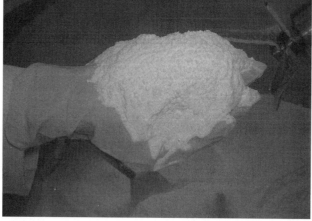

FIGURE 29.21   Cohesion Test 2 Step 1–2

29.7.6 Example: Typical Considerations for a High Shear Granulation Process

TABLE 29.1   Example of process design at manufacture scale

 Example: Typical considerations in high shear process

High shear granulator Zanchetta 900-L

Formulation: IR oral tablets, medium dose, low solubility API

Batch size: 150 kg

Pre-blend	Infusion I	Infusion II	Wet mass
5 minutes	10 minutes	5 minutes	1–3 minutes
Blade slow	Blade slow	Blade high	Blade high
No chopper	No chopper	Chopper high	Chopper high
	Spray at 1 kg/m in per nozzle (×3)	Spray at 1 kg/m in per nozzle (×3)	End point by amperage 24–26 amp.

29.8 COMPLEXITY OF WET GRANULATION

Wet granulation can be performed by using different methods and equipment. The basic design of the process generally includes some or all of the following steps:

1. Pre-mix;
2. Infusion I: spray the granulation agent while operating the equipment to distribute the liquid into the blend;

Cohesion Test 2

1. withdraw handful of granules;
2. shake off large granules and look for fine granules (no more than 1–2% fine granules exist);
3. discharge most granules off hand, and examine the amount and shape of the fine particles sticking to the glove;
4. look for condensation moisture on lid.

Step 1: Look for percentage of desired and fine granules;

Step 2: Look for percentage and shape of fine granules sticking to the glove.

3. Continue to Infusion II: spray to a predetermined condition; and/or
4. Wet mass to a predetermined end point (e.g., low or high shear granulator);
5. Discharge and continue to drying or sizing process.

From blend (dry solid powder) to the wet end point granules, the granulation process involves the following mechanisms:

1. Once the API and the other excipients are in contact with the granulation agent, they may be partially dissolved or wetted by the liquid. Different materials may compete with each other for the infused liquid. Even at end point, the degree of granulation varies in size, density, and shape.
2. Many physical properties of the starting materials such as viscosity, density, and heat capacity are constantly changing during the infusion and wet massing.
3. For granulation by using a high shear granulator, the materials are rotated at a speed around 8–12 m/sec. Due to the friction between the particles and particle-to-equipment, the temperature of the granules may increase as the process progresses. This phenomenon may accelerate the liquid uptake process for some formulations or dry off the liquid in other cases, depending on the formulation, and the degree of completion of the granulation process.
4. During the wet mass, the shear forces applied to the granules are quite different from location to location. The granules at the tip of the blade/impeller are exposed to more forces than the granules at the center. This difference can be significant at production scale equipment.

Due to the complexity, it is sometimes difficult to come up with one fixed process parameter that can be applied to wet granulation at all scales and at all times. Good knowledge of scale-up can overcome the potential challenge for most of the current equipment.

With the use of PAT, process controls that can automatically compensate for variation or change in material or equipment can be used to sustain a consistent result (Section 29.17). There is also new emerging granulation equipment that does not proportionally increase its dimension when output is significantly increased, this equipment may reduce the need for scale-up.

29.9 COMMON ISSUES

Most common issues for scale-up and routine manufacture are:

1. Variation in the performance of granules (e.g., flowability, compressibility, and dissolution);
2. Inconsistent process (e.g., end point variation, particles size change, moisture variation … etc.);
3. Difficulty of scale-up;
4. Stability issues;
5. Other process related issues (e.g., sticking, filming).

To design a robust process is one of the common challenges in wet granulation. With new technology and better understanding of old technology, one can reduce, or avoid, future failure if proper considerations are incorporated into the design during formulation and process development.

29.10 CONSIDERATIONS OF PROCESS DESIGN

1. Identify the impact of API and raw materials;
2. Proper selection of which type of equipment should be used;
3. Understand the impact of process parameters;
4. Select designs that can reduce the sensitivity of end point determination;
5. Utilize the contribution from each step from beginning to end, and balance the design based on the overall process.

29.10.1 Identify Impact from Active Pharmaceutical Ingredient (API) and Other Raw Materials

Formulation has significant impact on the behavior and the degree of challenge of the wet granulation process.

For example, if the majority, e.g., 80% or higher, of the ingredients (including APIs) in a formulation have a strong affinity or good solubility to the granulation agent, the end point determination may be challenging for some formulations. Extra efforts in formulation design and optimization may be needed. A good way to reduce unexpected events is to establish an earlier measurement of how material will interact with the granulation agent at an early stage and, if possible, at relatively small-scale (10–00 g).

CASE STUDY

Situation

An immediate-release formulation containing 30% of a silicate-based excipient is granulated using a 900-L Zanchetta high shear granulator. Production reports a significant change in the particle size of the final granules when a new lot of this silicate-based material is used.

Resolution

After an investigation, a method related to water absorption by using a small-scale rheometer was developed to identify the maximum capability of absorption water. From the six-sigma approach, a control space related to this property was established. Based on this new information, the supplier could now provide a more consistent material within the control space.

29.10.2 Proper Selection of Which Type of Equipment to be Used

Wet granulation can be performed in many ways. Proper selection of equipment will maximize the success of wet granulation, even with limitations from API or formulation. A good example would be choosing between a fluid-bed granulator and a high shear granulator. If formulation has a very narrow end point window or potential stability issue due to moisture exposure, selection of a process using fluid-bed granulation may be of benefit. Fluid-bed granulation may also provide granules with enhanced compressibility for some formulations. However, if higher densification and time/cost factors are the major considerations, then a high shear granulator may be preferable. In some cases, the granules manufactured by fluid-bed may show a slightly faster release and a higher bioavailability. The selection of type of wet granulation process should be examined.

There could be a variety of equipment based on the same principle, but with significant difference in their design. For example, there are different varieties of high shear granulators available. Based on the location of the main impeller/blade (top drive or bottom drive), and the configuration of the chopper/granulators (side mounted or vertical mounted), there are quite a few designs available for the pharmaceutical industry. A brief description of the impact of bottom drive versus top drive will be discussed in the following sections.

29.10.3 Understand the Impact of Process Parameters

There are numerous process parameters that may have an impact on the granulation. The following is a list of some common parameters for high shear granulation.

1. Amount of granulation agent infused;
2. Amount of shear force applied;
3. Rate of infusion;
4. Rate of shear force applied;
5. Additional shear force contributed by chopper/granulator;
6. Method of infusion;
7. Temperature of granulation agent;
8. Temperature of granulation chamber;
9. Surface cleanness of the blade and chamber.

Depending on the characteristics of the formulation there could be more factors. Understanding and control of the above parameters will provide a minimum control to avoid unexpected events in daily manufacture (Section 29.11).

29.10.4 Select a Design that Reduces the Sensitivity of End Point Determination

There is no universal definition of how the granules should look at the end of wet granulation. There is also no "right" or "wrong" end point, as long as the process meets or exceeds the expectation of the design. In many case, the definition of end point granules may vary from company to company or project to project. The formulators or process scientists/engineers could intuitively select the end point based on scientific justification, their prior experience, and sometimes, the culture of the company. However, proper selection of the end point should be based on overall consideration of the whole process.

For granules design to be dried in a fluid-bed dryer, the end point design should produce granules strong enough to survive the fluid-bed drying process. However, excess densification may include a higher percentage of larger granules or even lumps that may create problems for the following drying (e.g., case-hardening) or milling (e.g., excess fines or significant increase in milling temperature).

On the other hand, for granules that are designed to be dried in an oven-tray dryer, the formulator or process scientist/engineer can take advantage of oven-drying, and design for smaller granules at the end point that may also reduce the drying time, and avoid potential issues during milling.

Some formulations are limited to a very narrow window for end point determination. The formulator or process scientist/engineer can purposely add sufficient water to slightly over-wet the granules. Then the wet-granules pass through one or multiple steps of milling for proper size selection. However, this technique should not be used if there is a stability or granule performance issue.

For some formulations, large/heavy granules may create a relatively narrow window for end point determination. Selection of small to medium granules for these formulations may expand the end point window, and reduce over-granulating. For some formulations, selection of small to medium granules at the end point may exhibit a constant ratio of power consumption to load weight when scale-up from experimental scale to commercial-scale occurs.

As a general consideration, unless there is a special requirement, small to medium end point granules, with a D_{50} around 200–1000 μm before sizing, may mitigate the inherent variations in manufacture and scale-up.

29.10.5 Utilize the Contribution from Each Stage and Maintain a Balanced Design

Some manufacturing issues are due to a biased design that may expect too much from wet granulation. For example, if the design calls for heavy end point granules, this could create problems downstream. Commonly related issues are wide distribution of end point particle size, uneven fluidization in the fluid-bed dryer or over-heating/clogging of the mill due to excess chunks of granules.

During process development many efforts are made to understand the granulation process. However, in some cases, little effort may be applied to the subsequent processes that may turn out to be critical to the performance of the granules.

A good example is the impact on the *in vitro* dissolution behavior of the porosity of a tablet of an immediate-release formulation. There are many factors that may contribute to the dissolution profile. Some of these factors are highly influenced by the process after granulation. (e.g., inter-granule porosity after compression and the amount of moisture … etc.)

The manufacturing process after wet granulation may have major impact on the dissolution outcome. Process design for such formulations should consider the overall contribution of each step. To fully understand this type of process, identification of the critical to quality (CTQ) stages of the manufacturing process after granulation are equally as important as granulation itself.

Some formulations require a very heavy end point granule, and in this case the process may be better controlled by targeting over-granulation on purpose, and following a well-designed sizing process. This design will produce consistent dense granules.

29.10.6 Consideration of the Design of the Equipment

Equipment based on the same principle, but different in design, may create variation in manufacture. High shear granulators are commonly used for wet granulation. Based on the location of the main blade/impeller and the position of the chopper/granulator, there could be some difference in the outcome of the granulation.

A study (Section 29.11) is performed to compare the impact of the design of the two common configurations: bottom drive high shear with side chopper versus top drive high shear granulator with vertical chopper.

For a formulation with end point determination that is sensitive to the amount of liquid added, the top drive granulator may bring some advantage by slightly enlarging the window for end point determination. However, for formulation that requires a rapid densification, the bottom-drive granulator may be a better choice.

29.11 IMPACT OF PROCESS PARAMETERS FOR THE HIGH SHEAR PROCESS

29.11.1 Function of Parameters

TABLE 29.2 Functions of process parameters for the high shear process

Parameter	Function
Amount of granulation agent	Agglomeration
Extent of wet mass time	Energy
Peripheral tip speed	Energy
Temperature of granulation agent	Hydration rate
Method of infusion/spray rate	Uniformity/hydration
Design of equipment	Mechanical
Different dry/mill method	Attrition
Chopper application	Energy
Residue heat and materials in multi-batches	Energy
Volume of load	Mechanical

29.11.2 Amount of Granulation Agent

CASE STUDY A

1. Starch-based IR formulation;
2. Vector GMX high shear granulator;
3. Amount of granulation agent used at five different levels;
4. Other parameters: constant.

Focus: In general, the more granulation agent added, the heavier the granules become.

Focus: There is an optimal density related to the amount of granulation agent added. Excess granulation agent may not further increase the size or densification.

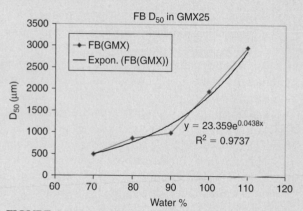

FIGURE 29.23   Case Study: impact on the particle size by the amount of granulation agent

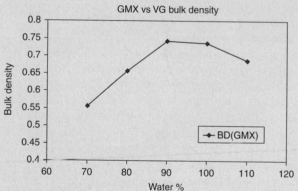

FIGURE 29.24   Case Study: impact on the bulk density by the amount of water added

CASE STUDY B

IR formulation

High shear Granulator: Lodige MGT-75

Observation: More water → smaller granules.

Investigation

Geometry of the blade changes due to materials attached on blade. The blade loses granulation ability, and additional water does not increase the size.

Lesson learned

- Adjust the spray pattern;
- Properly position the spray zone;
- Consistent infusion;
- Avoid processes that require adding granulation agent all the way to the end point (specially for hydrophilic modified-release formulation with heavy end point granules);
- Apply wet mass to end point without spraying.

29.11.3 Extent of Wet Mass Time

General trend: the more energy applied the larger the granules become.

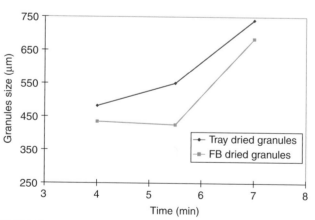

FIGURE 29.25   Case Study: impact on the granule size by the wet-mass time.

CASE STUDY A

High shear Granulator: Niro-Fielder PP-1

Amount of Granulation Agent Used: 26%

Granulated for 4, 5.5, and 7 minutes

Focus:

- Fear of overgranulation—when to stop;
- Sensitivity of exciepient variability;
- Formulation limitation;
- Impact from infusion quantity and rate of infusion.

CASE STUDY B

High shear granulator Vector GMX-600;

Hydrophilic polymer system: 30%;

Amount of granulation agent used: 24%;

Granulated for 3, 7, 9, and 11 minutes.

Observation: Wet massing does not increase the granule size. This phenomenon is sure to (1) most increase size during infusion stages, (2) formulation contains high absorption capacity of granulation agents, (3) temperature significantly increases during wet mass.

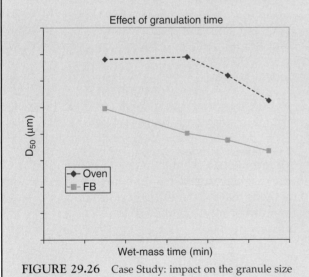

Effect of granulation time

FIGURE 29.26 Case Study: impact on the granule size by the wet-mass time

CASE STUDY

High shear granulator: Niro-Fielder PMA-25;
Formulation: hydrophilic MR tablets;

Granulation	A	B	C
Time (min)	6	4.8	4
Speed (rpm)	400	500	600 (560, max out).

FIGURE 29.27 Case Study: impact on granules size by impeller speed

Focus:

- Formulation: high percentage of excipient that changes viscosity significantly during wet massing;
- Type of equipment selected;
- Change in bed dynamic;
- Temperature increases;
- Reproducibility of end point.

29.11.5 Temperature of Granulation Agent

General trend: the warmer the granulation agent is, the larger/faster the granules grow. When will the temperature of the granulation agent have an impact on the granulation outcome?

1. Site transfer between different climate zones:
   Tropic area versus temperate area;
   Keep temperature of granulation agent constant.
2. Multi sub-batches in the same day:
   Morning batch versus afternoon batch.
3. Overnight temperature decrease may impact the early morning batch.

29.11.4 Peripheral Speed/Tip Speed

General trend: the faster the energy is applied, the larger the granules become. A typical high shear granulator will have a peripheral speed/tip speed around 8–12 meters/second.

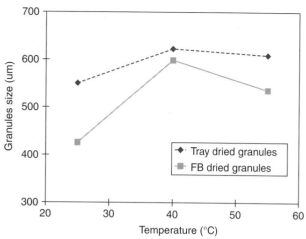

FIGURE 29.28   Case Study: impact on granule size by the temperature of granulation agent

---

29.11.6 CASE STUDY

SPRAY RATE/GUN TO BED DISTANCE POSITION OF NOZZLE(S)

1. Consideration of balance between wet mass speed/time and spray rate;
2. The nozzle to bed distance may require adjustment if bed height is significantly reduced during processing

Focus:

1. Some formulations may significantly reduce bulk volume. Chopper at a position that is higher than the bed may lose its function;
2. Chopper is not in the optimal position: side mounted chopper versus vertical chopper;
3. Spray by pressure versus by air atomization;
4. Over-atomization;
5. Hydrophilic matrix formulation may significantly increase its bulk volume after Infusion II stage.

CASE STUDY A

Equipment: Zanchetta high shear granulator, 900 L;

Infusion rate: adjust from 3 kg to 2 kg with same total amount;

Result: larger granules due to more energy input.

CASE STUDY B

Equipment: Zanchetta high shear granulator, 900 L;

Observation: poor uniformity in end point granules;

Result: bed height significantly decreases after Infusion I stage;

Improvement: adjust the nozzle to maintain similar spray zone.

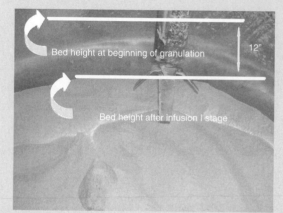

FIGURE 29.29   Case Study: change in bed height in a high shear granulator

29.11.7 Method of Infusion

Impact from different method: spray versus pump/pour.

General trend:

- For formulations with a majority of ingredients that are soluble in the granulation agent, different infusion methods may have an impact on granulation outcome.
- For formulations containing ingredients that can absorb a high degree of granulation agent, different methods may not have a significant impact.
- Poor uniformity may derive from bad selection of infusion method.
- Consider the "snow ball effect" from lumps larger than few inches.

Special process considerations:

- Avoid potential sensitivity to infusion method and apply granulation process that may be less sensitive. Go for fluid-bed granulation, rotor process or others.
- Multi-nozzles with constant nozzle to bed distance may reduce the sensitivity.
- Select light end point granules instead of heavy granules.

CASE STUDY A

Hydrophilic formulation with water as granulation agent.

Focus: significant difference in end point particle size distribution at end point. Infusion by spraying produces smaller granules.

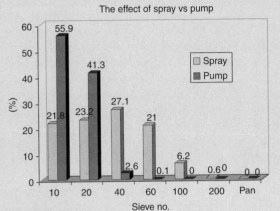

FIGURE 29.30   Case Study: effect of different infusion method

CASE STUDY B

Hydrophobic formulation with water as granulation agent.

Focus: no significant difference in end point particle size distribution at end point.

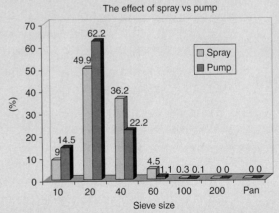

FIGURE 29.31   Case Study: effect of different infusion method

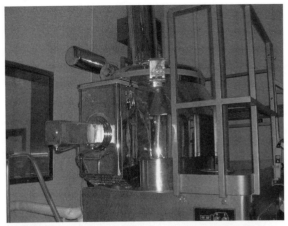

FIGURE 29.32   Example of a bottom-drive granulator

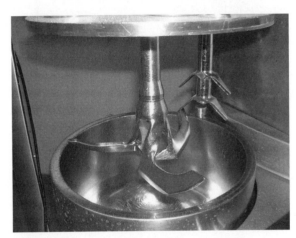

FIGURE 29.33   Example of a top-drive granulator

29.11.8 Design of Granulation Equipment

TABLE 29.3   Common high shear granulators

Common high shear granulators in the United States

Blade	Chopper	Manufacture
Top-drive	Vertical	Gral (Gea)
	·	Vector Gmx
Bottom-drive side		Tk Fielder (Gea)
		Powrex (Glatt)
		Lodige
Bottom-drive	Vertical	Zanchetta

What are the Differences?

- Difference in blade/impeller function: top drive versus bottom drive;
- Difference in chopper function: side chopper versus vertical chopper;
- Difference in geometry of chamber.

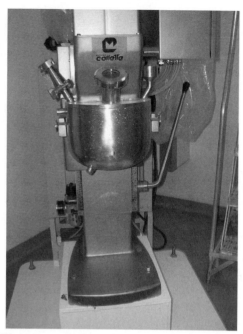

FIGURE 29.34 Example of top-drive granulator with vertical chopper at development scale

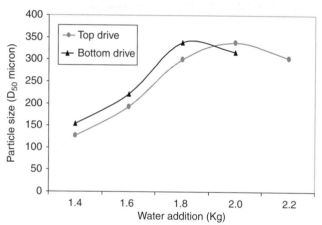

FIGURE 29.35 (a) impact by different design

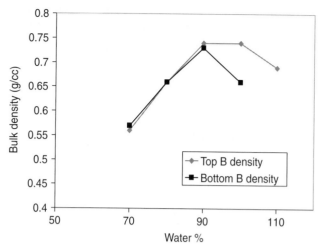

FIGURE 29.35 (b) impact by different design on bulk density

Impact by design on bulk density at various percentages of granulation infused.

29.11.9 Different Drying Methods

General trend:

Drying process by using a fluid-bed dryer may have an impact on the size of the final dried granules.

CASE STUDY

Formulation: hydrophilic HPMC-based MR formulation;

Wet granulation process: wet granulated by high shear process and by fluid-bed process;

Drying process: dry by oven-tray-drying or fluid-bed dryer.

Result:

Size (D_{50})	By oven tray dryer	By fluid-bed dryer
High shear process	430.4 μm	381.7 μm
Fluid-bed process	227.4 μm	164.7 μm

CASE STUDY A

Focus:

1. Granulation using a bottom drive granulator may need relatively less water and energy to produce granules with similar size;
2. Side chopper may be more effective than vertical chopper when chopper location is out of the path of granule movement.

Impact on particle size distribution of end point granules with different levels of granulation agent added.

29.11.10 Difference in Chopper Application

General trend: formulation containing extremely effective binder may not be benefited by application of certain chopper design.

CASE STUDY

Formulation: hydrophilic Xanthan gum-based MR formulation granulated with enteric polymer suspension.

Wet granulation process: wet granulated by high shear process with same parameters except one process with the application of chopper and the other one without the chopper;

Drying process: dry by fluid-bed dryer with same parameters;

Equipment: Gral 75 Liter.

Process parameters and result:

	Process time (minutes)	
Process parameter	**With chopper**	**Without chopper**
Pre-mix	3	3
Infusion I	5	5
Infusion II	7	7
Wet mass	3	3
End point granules, (D_{50}, μm)	510.8	541.3

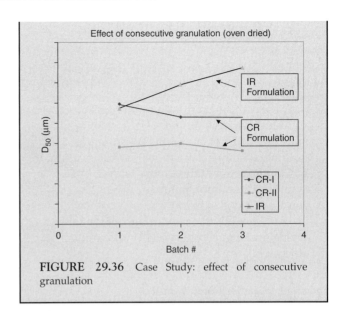

FIGURE 29.36 Case Study: effect of consecutive granulation

29.11.11 Impact by Residue Heat and by Residual Materials in Multi-batch Consecutive Process

General trend: many manufacturing processes will granulate multi-batches consecutively with 1–2 hours in between batches. For some formulations, residual heat and residual material inside the chamber may impact the granulation outcome.

CASE STUDY A

IMPACT BY RESIDUAL HEAT

Design: granulate three batches consecutively with one hour in between sub-batches.

Formulation: two hydrophilic polymer-based CR formulations and one IR formulation.

Equipment: Vector GMX High shear granulator.

Wet granulation process: wet granulated by high shear process with the same parameters.

Drying process: dry by fluid-bed dryer with same parameters.

Result: the granule size (D_{50}) shows an increasing trend for IR formulation. The CR formulations show no significant impact by the residual heat.

CASE STUDY B

IMPACT BY RESIDUAL MATERIAL

Formulation: IR formulation;

Equipment: Zanchetta high shear granulator;

Wet granulation process: multiple infusion stage followed by infusion to end point determined by amperage;

Drying process: dry by fluid-bed dryer until end point by moisture content

Observation: residual material underneath the impeller creates high friction, and invalidates the instrumentation end point determination by amperage.

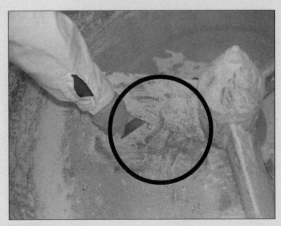

FIGURE 29.37 Case Study: impact by residual from previous sub-batches

29.12 END POINT DETERMINATION

29.12.1 Consideration of End Point

1. Even with the best formulation, best process, and best equipment, the end point will consist of granules that have different sizes, shapes, different moisture contents, and different strengths.
2. Evaluate the impact on the performance of final dosage by different design of end point. For example: dissolution failure due to heavy end point for IR dosage form.
3. The process should consider impact for subsequent drying, milling, compression, and coating processes.

Enlarged Image for Final Granules

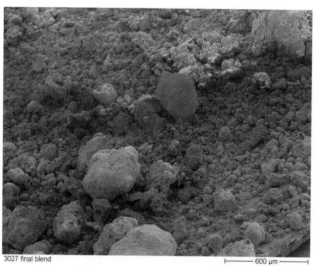

FIGURE 29.38   Example of final granules under SEM

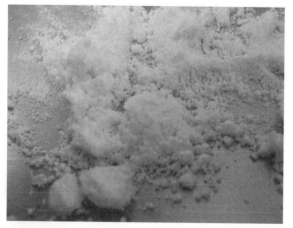

FIGURE 29.39   Appearance of typical medium granules manufactured at large scale

29.12.2 Common Methods for End Point Determination in Production

TABLE 29.4   Common methods for end point determination

Method for end point	Advantage	Disadvantage
Wet-mass time	Low cost	Excipient variation sensitive
Amount of granulation agent	Low cost	Excipient variation sensitive
Moisture content	Relative low cost	Indirect measurement
Torque	Technology mature	May not be sensitive enough
Kw	Technology mature	May not be sensitive enough
Amp	Technology mature	May not be sensitive enough
Digital imaging	Direct measurement	Relatively new
NIR	Wide selections	Indirect measurement
Acoustic sound	Low cost	Indirect measurement
Effusivity	Pseudo-direct	New technology

29.12.3 Manufacturing Considerations

1. Unless required by performance of final dosage, avoid end point of extremely heavy granules that may unnecessarily challenge the reproducibility of future manufacture.
2. Consider light to medium or medium granules as the end point. This may augment future scale-up and daily production.
3. Define and monitor the change in API, and other raw materials. For example, go beyond moisture content and poor size distribution specification.
4. Consider the impact from following processes such as drying, milling, blending … etc.
5. For formulation with poor flow or compression, end point particle size distribution may be tied in with the size of the resulting tablet/capsule size (for example, avoid extremely fine granules for a large tablet).
6. Equipment reliability. They are not all the same.

Equipment Reliability: Drift of Instrumentation

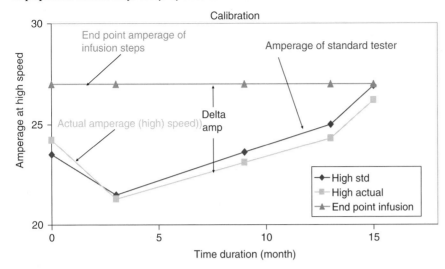

FIGURE 29.40 Drift of instrumentation used to measure the amperage in a high shear process

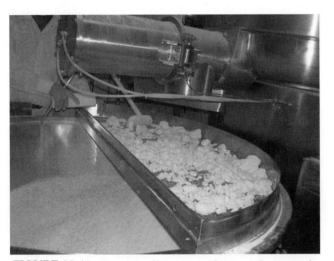

FIGURE 29.41 Example of heavy granules at production scale

29.13 APPLICATION OF PROCESS ANALYTICAL TECHNOLOGY (PAT)

A variety of methods to control the end point have been explored. A brief summary of commonly considered methods to control the end point are listed below.

1. moisture content;
2. torque;
3. power consumption;
4. NIR;
5. digital imaging;
6. effusivity.

Torque and power consumption have commonly been used for routine manufacture for the past two decades.

In recent years, additional methods based on process analytical technology (PAT) have been applied for end point determination, and successful end point controls have been reported.

Another use of PAT in the wet granulation area is to identify critical to quality (CTQ) factors. For example, the NIR image of a tablet with faster dissolution may show more domains of API than a tablet with slower dissolution. As more PATs are being developed and applied in pharmaceutical industry, tighter control of the over-granulation process, rather than just the end point determination, will be more common (Section 29.17).

29.14 DESIGN OF EXPERIMENT (DOE)

Design of experiment (DOE) is an excellent tool to identify the critical steps in wet granulation. However, due to the complicated nature of the granulation itself, the approach should consider the following factors:

1. perform a screening study to identify critical factors;
2. the factors and response should be science-based, and risk-evaluated;
3. consider a design with a resolution higher than level IV. For a process with a narrow window, consider level V or full design.

29.15 STATISTICAL AIDS FOR PROCESS CONTROL

Statistical aids have been implemented for better understanding of process limitation and improvement of product quality. Common methods such as process capability index (Cpk), performance capability index (Ppk), and six sigma can provide good statistical analysis of the robustness of the process. They also provide reliable statistical measurements to compare or control the variation of the process.

Many companies have implemented these programs to better understand and improve their manufacturing process, e.g., Right-First-Time (Pfizer Inc.), and others. These tools should be applied as upstream as possible in the product development process.

29.16 SCALE-UP AND PROCESS MEASUREMENT OF GRANULATION

The particle size of granulates is determined by the quantity and feeding rate of the granulating liquid. Wet granulation is used to improve flow, compressibility, bioavailability, and homogeneity of low dose blends, electrostatic properties of powders, and stability of dosage forms. Due to rapid densification and agglomeration that are caused by the shearing and compressing action of the impeller in a high shear single pot system, mixing, granulation, and wet massing can be done relatively quickly and efficiently. The dangers lie in a possibility of over-granulation, due to excessive wetting and producing low porosity granules, thus affecting the mechanical properties of tablets. As the liquid bridges between the particles are formed, granules are subjected to coalescence, along with some breakage of the bonds. It stands to reason that mean granule size depends on the specific surface area of the excipients, as well as the moisture content, and liquid saturation of the agglomerate.

During the wet massing stage, granules may increase in size to a certain degree, while the intragranular porosity decreases. However, heating and evaporation may also take place, leading to a subsequent decrease in the mean granule size, especially in small-scale mixers.

Load on the main impeller is indicative of granule apparent viscosity and wet mass consistency. The following forces act on the particles: acceleration (direct impact of the impeller), centrifugal, centripetal, and friction. The interplay of these forces affects all stages of the granulation process. While binder addition rate controls granule density, impeller and chopper speed control granule size and granulation rate, and the end point controls the mix consistency, and reproducibility.[6] Other factors that affect the granule quality include spray position and spray nozzle type, and, of course, the product composition. Such variables as mixing time and bowl or product temperature are not independent factors in the process, but rather are responses to the primary factors listed above.

Numerous attempts to quantify the granulation process include measurements of motor current, motor voltage, capacitance, conductivity, vibration, chopper speed, impeller shaft speed, motor slip, diffraction of a laser beam, blade tip speed, and swept volume. Most of the early attempts to monitor granulation have only historical value. Motor current and/or voltage are still used by some OEMs as an indicator of the load on the main motor, but these measurements have little predictive value.

Product and jacket temperature are usually measured by thermocouples. These response variables are controlled by a variety of factors notably, the speed of the main impeller, and the rate of binder addition.

Granulation process signatures obtained with acoustic emission sensors to monitor changes in particle size, flow, and compression properties are one of the emerging technologies that should be mentioned.[2,25] Use of a refractive NIR moisture sensor for end point determination of wet granulation was described by several authors.[21,22] There are technological challenges associated with this approach, as the sensor can only measure the amount of water at the powder surface. Several attempts were made to evaluate the use of a focused beam reflectance measurement (FBRM) particle size analyzer for granulation end point determination.[16,18,9] A major disadvantage of the FBRM method is that measured distribution depends on optical properties, and shape of the particles, as well as the focal point position, solids concentration, and probe location.

In the mixing process, changes in torque on the blades and power consumption of the impeller shaft occur as a result of changes in the cohesive force or the tensile strength of the agglomerates in the moistened powder bed.

The most popular measurements are direct and reaction torque, and the power consumption of the main motor. Power consumption of the impeller motor for end point determination and scale-up is widely used because the measurement is inexpensive, it does not require extensive mixer modifications, and it is well-correlated with granule growth. The problem with power consumption is that this measurement reflects the overall mixer performance and mixer motor efficiency, as well as the load on the main impeller. Up to 30% of the power consumption of a motor can be attributed to no-load losses due to windage (by cooling fan and air drag), friction in bearings, and core losses that comprise hysteresis and eddy current losses in the motor magnetic circuit. Load losses include stator and rotor losses (resistance of materials used in the stator, rotor bars, magnetic steel circuit), and stray load (current losses in the windings). Attempts to use no-load (empty bowl, or dry mix) values as a baseline may be confounded by a possible nonlinearity of friction losses with respect to load. As the load increases, so does the current draw of the motor. This results in heat generation that further impacts the power consumption. A simple test might be to run an empty mixer for several hours, and see the shift in the baseline. Also, as the motor efficiency drops with motor age, the baseline most definitely shifts with time. Motor power consumption is nonlinearly related to the power transmitted to the shaft, and the degree of this nonlinearity can only be "guestimated."

Impeller power consumption (as opposed to motor power consumption) is directly proportional to torque, multiplied by the rotational speed of the impeller. The power consumption of the mixer motor differs from that of the impeller by the variable amount of power draw imposed by various sources (mixer condition, transmission, gears, couplings, motor condition, etc.).

Direct torque measurement requires installation of strain gauges on the impeller shaft or on the coupling between the motor and impeller shaft. Since the shaft is rotating, a device called a slip ring is used to transmit the signal to the stationary data acquisition system. Impeller torque is an excellent PAT inline measure of the load on the main impeller and was shown to be more sensitive to high frequency oscillations than power consumption.

29.16.1 End Point Determination

Granulation end point can be defined by the formulator as a target particle size mean or distribution.

It has been shown that once you have reached the desired end point, the granule properties and the subsequent tablet properties are very similar, regardless of the granulation processing factors, such as impeller or chopper speed or binder addition rate. This can be called "the principle of equifinality."

The ultimate goal of any measurement in a granulation process is to estimate viscosity and density of the granules, and, perhaps, to obtain an indication of the particle size mean and distribution. One of the best ways to obtain this information is by measuring load on the main impeller, as power consumption or torque.

Mixing and agglomeration of particles in wet granulation has been studied extensively. The optimal end point can be thought of as the factor affecting a number of granule and tablet properties, such as mean particle size, disintegration, friability, and hardness.

The classical power and torque profiles (Figure 29.42) start with a dry mixing stage, rise steeply with binder solution addition, level off into a plateau, and then exhibit an over-granulation stage. The power and torque signals have similar shape, and are strongly correlated. The pattern shows a plateau region where power consumption or torque is relatively stable.

Based on the theory of Leuenberger,[1,3,4] useable granulates can be obtained in the region that starts from the peak of the signal derivative with respect to time, and extends well into the plateau area. The peak of the derivative indicates the inflection point of the signal. Prior to this point, a continuous binder solution addition may require variable quantities of liquid. After that point, the process is well-defined and the amount of binder solution required to reach a desired end point may be more or less constant.

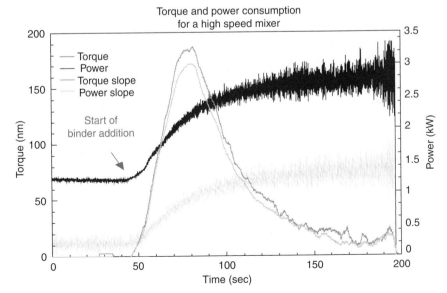

FIGURE 29.42 Typical power consumption and torque signals obtained from a high shear mixer-granulator. Note the slope of the signals (first derivative with respect to time)

The torque or power consumption pattern of a mixer is a function of the viscosity of both granulate and binder. With increasing viscosity, the plateau is shortened and sometimes vanishes completely, thereby increasing the need to stop the mixer at the exact end point. At low impeller speeds or high liquid addition rates, the classic S-shape of the power consumption curve may become distorted, with a steep rise leading into over-granulation. The measurements are also affected by the method of binder addition.

29.16.2 End Point Scale-up

A proper scientific approach to scale-up of any physical process requires application of dimensional analysis and a modeling theory.

Imagine that you have successfully scaled-up from a 10 liter batch to a 300 liter batch. What exactly happened? You may say: "I got lucky." Apart from luck, there had to be similarity in the processing of the two batches. According to the modeling theory, two processes may be considered similar if there is a geometrical, kinematic, and dynamic similarity. Two systems are geometrically similar if they have the same ratio of linear dimensions. Two geometrically similar systems are kinematically similar if they have the same ratio of velocities between corresponding points. Two kinematically similar systems are dynamically similar when they have the same ratio of forces between corresponding points. For any two dynamically similar systems, all the dimensionless numbers necessary to describe the process have the same numerical value.[5] Thus, the process of scale-up from any system to a similar system on a larger scale, when described in dimensionless terms, does not require any scale considerations. One should be careful, however, to apply this approach to all mixers. It was shown, for example, that Collette Gral 10, 75, and 300 are not geometrically similar, and thus corrections for dissimilarities should be made in any scale-up attempt.

The so-called "π-theorem" (or Buckingham theorem) states: every physical relationship between n dimensional variables and constants can be reduced to a relationship between $m = n - r$ mutually independent dimensionless groups, where r = the number of dimensional units, i.e. fundamental units, such as length, mass, and time.

Dimensional analysis is a method for producing dimensionless numbers that completely describe the process. The analysis should be carried out before the measurements have been made, because dimensionless numbers essentially condense the frame in which the measurements are performed and evaluated.

TABLE 29.5 Dimensionless numbers useful in high shear process scale-up. Notation is followed by basic dimensional units of M (mass), L (length) and T (time)

$Ne = P/(\rho n^3 d^5)$	Newton (power)
$Fr = n^2 d/g$	Froude
$Re = d^2 n \rho/\eta$	Reynolds

P: power consumption [ML^2T^{-5}]
ρ: specific density of particles [ML^{-5}]
n: impeller speed [T^{-1}]
d: impeller diameter [L]
g: gravitational constant [LT^{-2}]
η: dynamic viscosity [$ML^{-1}T^{-1}$]

It can be applied even when the equations governing the process are not known.

Dimensional analytical procedure was first proposed by Lord Rayleigh.[23] Dimensionless representation of the process is independent of scale, and thus can be easily scaled-up. Scientific scale-up procedure using dimensional analysis is a two-step process: (1) describe the process using a complete set of dimensionless numbers, and (2) match these numbers at different scales. This dimensionless space, in which the measurements are presented or measured, will make the process scale invariant.

Dimensionless Reynolds numbers, relating the inertial force to the viscous force, are frequently used to describe mixing processes, especially in chemical engineering.[24]

Froude numbers have been extensively applied to describe powder blending, and have been suggested as a criterion for dynamic similarity and a scale-up parameter in wet granulation.[15] The mechanics of the phenomenon were described as interplay of the centrifugal force (pushing the particles against the mixer wall), and the centripetal force produced by the wall, creating a "compaction zone." We have seen that there exists a sort of a "principle of equifinality" that states: "an end point is an end point is an end point, no matter how it was obtained." The rheological and dimensional properties of the granules are similar. This means that the density and dynamic viscosity are constant, and the only two variables that are left are impeller diameter, and speed. It is therefore seen appropriate to characterize and compare different mixers by the range of the Froude numbers they can produce. A matching range of the Froude numbers would indicate the possibility of a scale-up, even for the mixers that are not geometrically similar.

We have attempted to compute Froude numbers for mixers of different popular brands, and the results are

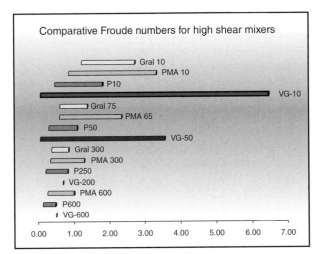

FIGURE 29.43 Comparative Froude numbers for high shear mixers. Explanations in the text

presented in Figure 29.43. Such representation allows some comparison between otherwise noncomparable devices. Obviously, such comparison should not be used in absolute terms. Rather, its use and relative usefulness will be evident during scale-up and technology transfer between various stages of product development.

Looking at the chart, we can notice that both the minimum and the maximum Froude numbers tend to decrease with mixer scale. This, essentially, is a restatement of the fact that laboratory scale mixers tend to produce higher shear and intensity of agglomeration, having relatively more powerful motors. As was shown by Horsthuis et al.,[15] it is possible to match dynamic conditions of Collette Gral 10 and 75 or Gral 75 and 300, but not between Gral 10 and 300. The Fielder PMA mixers exhibit essentially the same pattern of Froude number distribution as the Grals. The popular Diosna P-series and Powrex VG-series mixers show a distribution pattern of Froude numbers similar to those of other brands. Again, we notice a tendency of larger mixers to have smaller Froude numbers in both extremes and ranges. It is then understandable why scaling-up the process quantified on a 10 liter mixer is sometimes so difficult to apply to a large production scale—it is virtually impossible to match Froude numbers for a comparable set of dynamic conditions. The impeller speed is the governing factor in Froude representation because it is squared. The geometrical dimensions of the blades are of secondary significance.

A word of caution: in addition to matching Froude numbers, certain corrections may be needed to account for geometric dissimilarity of vessels in machines of different size. Once again, formulators should be encouraged to experiment with low speeds,

in an attempt to simulate dynamic conditions that exist in production mixers.

The rationale for using Froude numbers to compare different mixers may be found in the fact that, at any desired end point (as defined by identical particle size mean and distribution), viscosity and density of the wet mass are similar in any mixer, regardless of its brand and model, and the Newton power number, Ne, will depend solely on the diameter d, and speed n, of the impeller.

The dimensional analysis starts with a list of all variables thought to be crucial for the process being analyzed (the so-called "relevance list"). To set up a relevance list for a process, one needs to compile a complete set of all dimensionally relevant and mutually independent variables and constants that affect the process. The word "complete" is crucial here. All entries in the list can be subdivided into geometric, physical, and operational. Each relevance list should include only one target (dependent "response") variable. Many pitfalls of dimensional analysis are associated with the selection of the reference list, target variable or measurement errors (e.g., when friction losses are of the same order of magnitude as the power consumption of the motor). The larger the scale-up factor the more precise the measurements of the smaller scale have to be.[26,27]

Dimensional analysis can be simplified by arranging all relevant variables from the relevance list in a matrix form, with a subsequent transformation yielding the required dimensionless numbers. The dimensional matrix consists of a square core matrix, and a residual matrix. The rows of the matrix consist of the basic dimensions, while the columns represent the physical quantities from the relevance list. The most important physical properties and process-related parameters, as well as the "target" variable (that is, the one we would like to predict on the basis of other variables) are placed in one of the columns of the residual matrix. The core matrix is then linearly transformed into a matrix of unity, where the main diagonal consists only of 1s, and the remaining elements are all 0. The dimensionless numbers are then created as a ratio of the residual matrix and the core matrix, with the exponents indicated in the residual matrix. For more information on the applications of this approach to end point scale-up, see Levin.[20]

The end result of the dimensional analysis of the high shear granulation process under the assumed condition of dynamic similarity is a dimensionless expression of the form $Ne = f(Re, Fr, h/d)$, where h/d is a dimensionless geometric factor, usually referring to bowl height/blade diameter or a fill ratio. The actual form of the function f can be established empirically.[10,11,12,13,17,18,19,21]

29.16.3 Practical Considerations

To scale-up a granulation end point, it is advisable to run a trial batch at a fixed speed, and with a predetermined method of binder added (for example, add water continuously at a fixed rate to a dry mix with a water-soluble binding agent).

Before adding the liquid, measure the baseline level of motor power consumption P_0 or impeller torque τ_0 at the dry mix stage. During the batch, stop the process frequently to take samples and, for each sample, note the end point values of power consumption P_e or impeller torque τ_e. For each of these end points, measure the resulting wet mass density, ρ. As a result, you will be able to obtain some data that will relate the end point parameters listed above with the processing variables in terms of net motor power consumption $\Delta P_m = (P_e - P_0)$ or net impeller power consumption $\Delta P_i = 2\pi \cdot (\tau_e - \tau_0) \cdot n$, where n is the impeller speed [dimension T^{-1}].

Once the desired end point is determined, it can be reproduced by stopping the batch at the same level of net power consumption ΔP (for the same mixer, formulation, speed, batch size and amount/rate of granulating liquid). To account for changes in any of these variables, you have to compute the Newton power number Ne for the desired end point:

$$Ne = \Delta P/(\rho n^3 d^5)$$

In other words, if you have established an end point in terms of some net impeller or motor power ΔP, and would like to reproduce this end point on the same mixer at a different speed or wet mass density, calculate the Newton power number Ne from the given net impeller power, ΔP, impeller speed n, blade radius d, and wet mass density ρ (assuming the same batch size), and then recalculate the target ΔP with the changed values of speed n or wet mass density, ρ.

Wet mass viscosity η can be calculated from net impeller power ΔP, blade radius d, and impeller speed n, using the following equations:

$$\Delta P = 2\pi \, \Delta\tau * n$$

$$\eta = \varphi * \Delta\tau/(n * d^3)$$

where:

$\Delta\tau$ is the net torque required to move wet mass
n is the speed of the impeller
d is the blade radius or diameter
φ is mixer specific "viscosity factor" relating torque and dynamic viscosity.

Note: the correlation coefficient φ can be established empirically by mixing a material with a known

dynamic viscosity, e.g., water. Alternatively, you can use impeller torque τ as a measure of kinematic viscosity, and use it to obtain a non-dimensionless "pseudo-Reynolds" number, based on the so-called "mix consistency" measure, that is, the end point torque, as described in the case studies.

Fill ratio **h/d** can be calculated from a powder weight, granulating liquid density ($1000\,kg/m^3$ for water), rate of liquid addition, time interval for liquid addition, and bowl volume V_b. The calculations are performed using the idea that the fill ratio **h/d** (wet mass height to blade diameter) is proportional to V/V_b, and wet mass volume V can be computed as:

$$V = m/\rho$$

where:

m is the mass (weight) of the wet mass
ρ is the wet mass density.

Now, the weight of the wet mass is computed as the weight of powder plus the weight of added granulating liquid. The latter, of course, is calculated from the rate and duration of liquid addition and the liquid density. Finally, you can combine the results obtained at different end points of the test batch or from different batches or mixer scales (assuming geometrical similarity) into one regression equation. Given wet mass density ρ, wet mass viscosity η, fill ratio $h/d \sim m\,V_b/\rho$, set-up speed n, and blade radius or diameter d, you can calculate the Reynolds number **Re** (or the "pseudo-Reynolds" number), and the Froude number **Fr**. Then you can estimate the slope, a, and intercept, b, of the regression equation:

$$Ne = b \cdot (Re \cdot Fr \cdot h/d)^a$$

or

$$\log Ne = \log b + a \cdot \log(Re \cdot Fr \cdot h/d)$$

And, inversely, once the regression line is established, you can calculate the Newton power number Ne (which is the target quantity for scale-up) and net power ΔP (which can be observed in real-time as a true indicator of the target end point) for any point on the line.

29.17 BEST PRACTICES

29.17.1 Consideration of Robust Process

The best practices are to design a robust manufacture process that will (1) consistently produce a safe and effective product, and (2) its performance will meet or exceed the original design. Best practice should begin with consideration of formulation, process, and equipment. Tools involved are described in

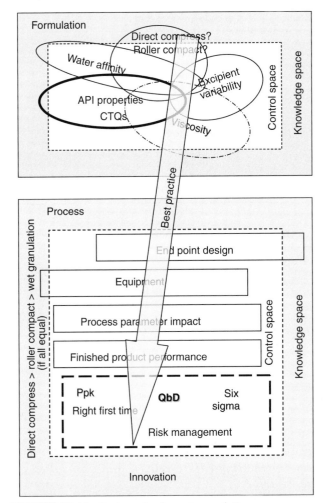

FIGURE 29.44   Best practice for wet-granulation process

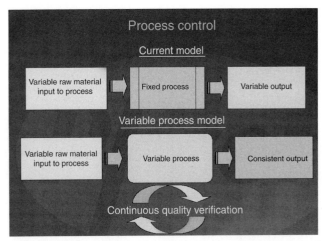

FIGURE 29.45   Advanced process control system (courtesy of Dr. Steve Hammond, Pfizer Inc. "Advanced Control Systems to Improve Efficiency of Pharmaceutical Manufacturing Processes," presentation at NJPhAST Innovation Workshop, March, 2008)

variation and deviation may produce more consistent product. With emerging process feedback control technology, a variable process that compensates for the inevitable variation and deviation is becoming popular, with the aid of PAT.

29.18 PRINCIPLES AND SCALE-UP OF FOAM GRANULATION

29.18.1 Introduction

The concept and application of foam granulation technology was initially published externally from Dow Chemical in 2004. The scale-up of conventional wet granulation processes involving solid dosage forms, and the issues surrounding these activities have been documented in the pharmaceutical literature. In this section, an initial evaluation of the scalability of foam granulation technology (FGT) was conducted in high shear granulation equipment at the laboratory (10-L), pilot (150-L), and full-manufacturing (600-L) scales. Immediate-release (IR) and controlled-release (CR) model formulations were used in the study. The laboratory scale trials were conducted at Larkin Laboratory at The Dow Chemical Company, Midland, MI. The pilot and full-manufacturing scale trials were conducted at the Perrigo Company in Allegan, MI. The variables studied were lot size, main-blade tip speed in the granulator, and delivery rate of the foam to the granulator equipment. Granulation and processing variables were scaled linearly from laboratory to manufacturing-scale. Testing conducted on each trial

Sections 29.13, 29.14, and 29.15. Additional considerations include application of PQRI, Ppk, knowledge space/control space, and risk management.

Due to the complexity of modern delivery systems, understanding of factors related to physical and chemical properties of granules, Biopharmaceutical Classification System (BCS), scale-up and post-approval change (SUPAC), GI tract behaviors of dosage forms, and in vivo–in vitro correlation (IVIVC) may add values to better understand the CTQs, and effectively understand the process robustness. Innovation with emerging technologies may significantly improve the process robustness, and should be included in best practices.

29.17.2 Emerging Concept of Process Design and Control

A robust process should include the consideration of material variation and process normal deviation (Common Cause). A process that can allow such

included physical testing of the prepared granules and finished tablets, as well as drug dissolution.

29.18.2 Experimental

Scale-up Plan

Laboratory scale: 10-L, vertical high shear granulator (Glatt Air Techniques, Ramsey, NJ), and laboratory-scale foam generator (Corrosion Fluids Inc., Midland, MI).

↓

Pilot scale: 150-L, top-drive high shear granulator (model GMX-150, Vector Corporation, Marion, IA), and laboratory-scale foam generator (Corrosion Fluids Inc., Midland, MI).

↓

Manufacturing scale: 600-L Gral, top-drive high shear granulator (GEA Niro Pharma Systems, Columbia MD), and production-scale foam generator (Hansa Industrie-Mixer GmbH & Co., Stuhr-Heiligenrode, Germany).

Table 29.6 shows the protocol used for the immediate-release and controlled-release scale-up trials. The variables were scaled linearly, so that reasonable comparisons could be made. The authors determined that the maximum liquid flow rate of the 7% METHOCEL E5PLV binder solution that could be sustained using the Hansa foam generator (Hansa Industrie Mixer, Stuhr-Heiligenrode, Germany) at the 135 kg manufacturing scale was 1.52 liters per minute. To maintain linear scaling, flow rates of 0.40 liters per minute at the 35.5 kg pilot scale, and 0.017 liters per minute at the 1.5 kg laboratory scale were used.

Table 29.7 shows the model immediate-release (IR) formulation used in the scale-up trials. Table 29.8 represents the model controlled-release (CR) formulation. Both formulations used a foamed 7% wt/v METHOCEL E5PLV aqueous solution as the binder system.

TABLE 29.6 Protocol for immediate-release and controlled-release scale-up trials

Variable	10-L	150-L	600-L
Lot size (kg)	1.5	35.5	135
Main blade (tip speed), rpm	420	145	95
Chopper blade, rpm	1500	1500	1500
Foam (liquid) delivery rate (mL/min)	17	400	1520
Method of drying	Tray	Fluid-bed	Fluid-bed

TABLE 29.7 Model immediate-release (IR) formulation

% w/w per tablet	Ingredients
44.0	Naproxen sodium, USP: 110 mg
1.78	METHOCEL E5PLV, USP (foamed binder, 7% solution): 4.45 mg
20.0	Microcrystalline cellulose, NF (PH-102 grade): 50 mg
30.72	Fast Flo Lactoce-316, NF: 76.8 mg
3.0	Croscarmellose sodium, USP: 7.5 mg
0.5	Magnesium stearate, NF: 1.25

TABLE 29.8 Model controlled-release (CR) formulation

% w/w per tablet	Ingredients
20.0	Naproxen sodium, USP: 100 mg
30.0	METHOCEL K4MP, USP: 150 mg
1.78	METHOCEL E5PLV, USP (foamed binder, 7% solution): 8.9 mg
15.0	Microcrystalline cellulose, NF (PH-102 grade): 75 mg
32.72	Fast Flo Lactoce-316, NF: 163.6 mg
0.5	Magnesium stearate, NF: 2.5 mg

Granulation Sequence (Continuous Method) Used for the Immediate-release and Controlled-release Trials

- Powders, except magnesium stearate (see Tables 29.7 and 29.8), were charged into the granulator (Figure 29.46), and premixed for 1 minute at laboratory scale, and 5 minutes at pilot-scale and full-scale to achieve a uniform mixture before the agglomeration step.
- Foamed binder solution was incorporated at a continuous rate (Table 29.6) onto the moving powder beds in the high shear granulators. Figure 29.47 shows the equipment hook-up for the foam addition from the foam generator to the high shear granulator. Only the manufacturing scale equipment is shown in this report. The laboratory and pilot-scale high shear equipment is similar in configuration, but smaller in size.
- After the addition of the foamed binders, the laboratory-scale trials were mixed for an additional 30 seconds. The pilot-scale and full-scale trials were mixed for an additional five minutes. This is common practice in the pharmaceutical industry when using conventional spray techniques, and is called the wet massing phase of a wet granulation. The purpose of the wet massing phase is to distribute the liquid/binder system evenly throughout

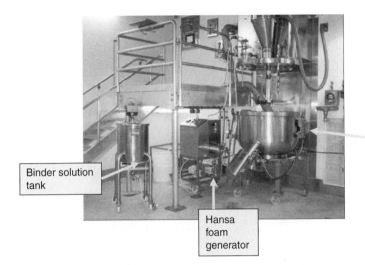

Binder solution
tank

600-L, full
scale high
shear granulator

Hansa
foam
generator

FIGURE 29.46 600-L Gral high shear granulator used in manufacturing-scale study

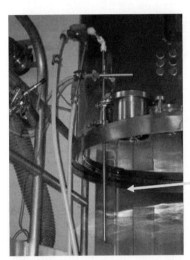

Foam delivered to
powders in granulator
bowl via tube
(No nozzles required)

FIGURE 29.47 Foam generator showing foam delivery hook-up used in the 600-L Gral

the powder mass. However, it is the opinion of the authors of this report that when using foam technology, this step is not necessary, because foam is capable of spreading among powder particles, and distributing much quicker and more efficiently than current conventional spray techniques.

- After granulation, the laboratory scale trials were wet milled using a CoMil, model 197 (Quadro Inc., Millburn, NJ). The pilot-scale trials used a CoMil model 196, and the manufacturing scale trials used a CoMil model U30. All were equipped with a similar square-hole screen opening of 0.5-inch, and a square-edge impeller.

Granulation Sequence (Batch Method)

Only one batch process trial was conducted. It was a controlled-release formulation, and only at the manufacturing-scale. Identical quantities of ingredients, including

the foamed binder, were used as in the manufacturing-scale continuous trial, so that direct comparisons could be made between the two processes. The batch process allows wet granulations to be prepared by adding foamed binders to static powder beds. This innovation simplifies the wet granulation process even further than the continuous foam addition process and, in addition, may help reduce worker exposure to potent APIs.

Powders were added to the granulator, and premixed in the same fashion as the continuous process. Then the mixer blades were turned off. Foam was pumped into the granulator on top of the static powder bed at a rate of 2.0-L/minute. The inlet tube shown in Figure 29.2 was reconfigured, so that the foam would be broadcast evenly across the surface of the static powder bed to promote its even distribution. Half of the quantity of the foam (19.3 kg) was added to the static powders. The granulator bowl was dropped to allow for the taking of a photograph (Figure 29.48). The mixer was turned on, and mixed for 5 minutes to distribute the foam. The mixer blades were then turned off, and the remaining portion of the foam (19.0 kg) was pumped onto the static powder mass. The mixer was again turned on and mixed for 5 minutes to fully incorporate the foam into the powders. Finally, the granulator bowl was dropped and the high quality, wet granulation was examined (Figure 29.49). In hindsight, after the completion of the batch process trial, it was obvious to the authors that there had been enough head space between the pre-mixed powders and the internal side of the top of the granulator that the entire quantity (38.3 kg) of the foamed 7% METHOCEL E5PLV solution could have been pumped into the granulator initially, and then undergone the 5 minute wet massing phase.

After milling, granulations were dried in trays for laboratory-scale, and in a fluid-bed dryer (Figure 29.50) for pilot and manufacturing scales. The dried

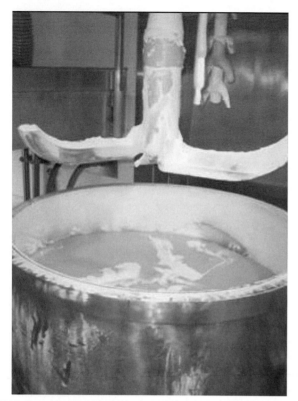

FIGURE 29.48   600-L Gral containing 38.3 kg of foamed 7% wt/v METHOCEL E5PLV binder solution that had been dispensed onto the surface of the 135 kg of powders within the bowl of the granulator prior to the wet massing step

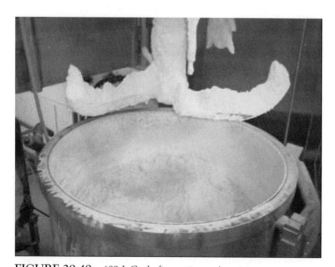

FIGURE 29.49   600-L Gral after wet massing step

granulations were sized using CoMil grater-type screens with same size opening and impeller tip speeds (laboratory scale: 2A062G037, 1307 rpm; pilot and manufacturing scale: 2F062G037, 500 rpm).

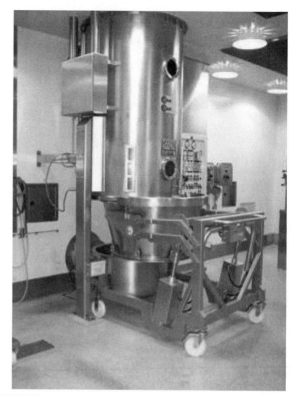

FIGURE 29.50   Glatt WSG 120 fluid-bed granulator/dryer

Tablet Preparation

Tablets were prepared from the milled granulations on an instrumented 16-station Manesty Betapress (Thomas Engineering, Inc., Hoffman Estates, IL) modified by Team Pharmaceuticals, Inc. (Martin, MI), and equipped with 9/32-inch (7.14 mm), round, standard concave tooling for preparation of the immediate release tablets, and 13/32-inch (10.3 mm), round, flat-faced, bevel-edged tooling for preparation of the controlled-release tablets. The tablet press data acquisition and analysis system was from Binary Applications (Midland, MI). Final compression forces of 2000 lb (8.9 kN), and 6000 lb (26.7 kN), were applied during the preparation of tablets. Target tablet weights of 250 mg and 500 mg were used for the immediate-release and controlled-release tablets respectively.

Powder/Granule Testing

The milled granules were analyzed for density, compressibility (CARR) index (CI), flow, and particle size distribution. The density of a 40-g sample of each granulation was tested using a Vanderkamp tap density tester (model 10700, VanKel Industries, Edison, NJ). A volume measurement was taken before tapping (apparent density), and after 500 taps (tap density). The compressibility index was calculated using Equation 29.1 below:

$$\% \text{ compressibility} = \frac{100(T - B)}{T} \qquad (29.1)$$

where:

T = tapped (packed) density (g/cm^3)
B = bulk (apparent) density (g/cm^3).

A 40-g sample of each granulation was shaken for 5 minutes on a RoTap® sieve shaker (Model B, W.S. Tyler, Gastonia, NC) equipped with a series of five screens and a pan. The amount of material retained on each screen size was measured, and a particle size distribution was calculated.

Tablet Property Testing

Tablets were tested for friability, thickness, crushing strength, and drug dissolution. The friability of 20 randomly chosen tablets from each trial was measured by tumbling them for 6 minutes in a Vanderkamp (Model 10801) friabilator (VanKel Industries, Edison, NJ), and then measuring the percentage weight loss. The crushing strength of 20 randomly chosen tablets from each trial was tested using a Key (Model HT500) hardness tester (Key International, Englishtown, NJ). Tablet thickness was measured using an Absolute Digimatic caliper (Series No. 500) (Mitutoyo Corp., Japan) on 10 tablets of the 20 randomly chosen tablets. The weight of each of the 20 tablets was measured, and the percentage weight variation was calculated.

Dissolution testing of six individual tablets sampled from each of the trials was performed using a Varian (Model VK7025) dissolution system (Varian, Inc., Cary, NC). The dissolution method used was as follows:

- Medium: DI water, 900 mL, 37.5°C.
- Apparatus 2: 50 rpm.
- Time/tolerance (IR): not less than 80% of the labeled amount dissolved in 45 minutes.
- Time/tolerance (CR): not less than 80% of the labeled amount released within 8–10 hours.

29.18.3 Results and Discussion

IR Scale-up Study

Bulk and tap density measurements, as well as the tablet crushing strength values of the IR granulations, were very similar from laboratory to pilot to manufacturing scale (Table 29.9). All friability results were less than 0.42% weight loss, 6 minutes testing. PSD testing showed good correlation between the three process

TABLE 29.9 Tablet and granule testing results for the immediate-release trials

Test	Laboratory-scale	Pilot-scale	Full-scale
Bulk density (g/mL)	0.622	0.620	0.655
Tap density (g/mL)	0.748	0.792	0.862
Compressibility index (%)	17	22	24
Tablet crushing strength (kp) 2 M lb (8.9 kN, SD)	8.1 (1.1)	8.6 (1.1)	11.5 (1.6)
Tablet crushing strength (kp) 6 M lb (26.7 kN, SD)	10.6 (0.8)	9.5 (1.1)	10.8 (1.4)
Tablet friability (6 min.) 2 M lb (8.9 kN)	0.22	0.42	0.35
Tablet friability (6 min.) 6 M lb (26.7 kN)	0.16	0.06	0.07

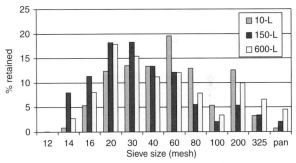

FIGURE 29.51 Particle size distribution testing results for the immediate release trials

scales (Figure 29.51). Results of IR drug dissolution testing showed a minimum of 80% drug released within 30 minutes for all tablets (Figure 29.52).

CR Scale-up Study

Bulk and tap density measurements of the CR granulations showed good similarity from laboratory to pilot to manufacturing scale (Table 29.10). The crushing strength results reflected good tablet quality for all three scales with the pilot-scale trials showing the highest values. All friability results were less than 0.35% wt. loss, 6 minutes testing. PSD testing showed good correlation between the three scales (Figure 29.53). Dissolution curves were similar for tablets from all three scales (Figure 29.54).

Comparison of Batch Versus Continuous Foam Addition

Figure 29.55 and Figure 29.56 show the results of the particle size distribution and drug dissolution testing, respectively. The results show a high degree of

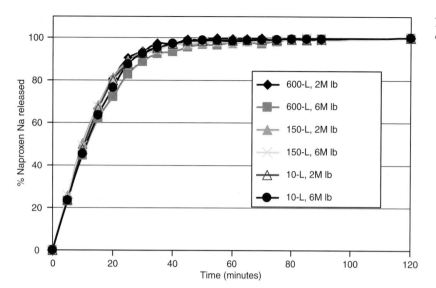

FIGURE 29.52   Drug dissolution testing results of the immediate release trials

TABLE 29.10   Tablet and granule testing results for the controlled-release trials

Test	Laboratory-scale	Pilot-scale	Full-scale
Bulk density (g/mL)	0.497	0.458	0.499
Tap density (g/mL)	0.622	0.620	0.719
Compressibility index (%)	20	26	30
Tablet crushing strength (kp) 2 Mlb (8.9 kN, SD)	9.5 (1.1)	15.1 (0.8)	10.8 (0.8)
Tablet crushing strength (kp) 6 M lb (26.7 kN, SD)	20.8 (0.8)	30.2 (0.9)	24.8 (0.9)
Tablet friability (6 min.) 2 M lb (8.9 kN)	0.35	0.33	0.33
Tablet friability (6 min.) 6 M lb (26.7 kN)	0.07	0.27	0.27

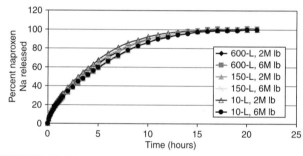

FIGURE 29.54   Drug dissolution testing results for the controlled-release trials

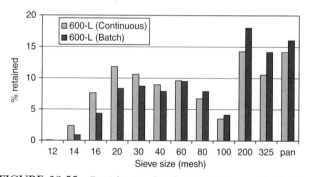

FIGURE 29.55   Particle size distribution testing results for the controlled-release batch versus continuous process

similarity between the two foam addition techniques. The results also show the processing flexibility inherent in the foam technology. The fact that the foam did not over-saturate the powders that it was in close contact with, even though it had been in contact for several minutes. This could not happen if conventional spray techniques were being used.

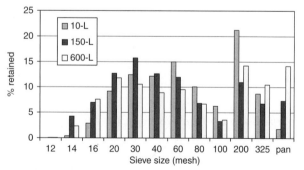

FIGURE 29.53   Particle size distribution testing results for the controlled-release trials

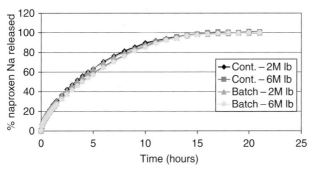

FIGURE 29.56 Comparison of drug dissolution testing results for the batch versus continuous process

29.18.4 Conclusion of Foam Granulation Study

Results from the trials using the continuous addition of foam showed that the foam granulation technology itself scaled easily with similar granule and tablet characteristics between scales. The results of the trials comparing continuous addition of foam versus batch addition of foam at the manufacturing scale, showed the process flexibility inherent in foam granulation technology.

29.19 BOTTOM LINES

The complexity of wet granulation is better understood by emerging technologies and approaches. With proper considerations during the design of the manufacturing process, a more robust process can be achieved.

Incorporation of the understanding of control space and risk assessment of the API, ingredients, process, and equipment can better control the outcome. Selection of the end point should be based on the overall process considerations. If possible, select an end point that will enlarge the end point window, and add the advantage of process robustness. Reducing the sensitivity of end point determination can avoid future unexpected manufacturing events.

1. Know your design space and your process capability: identify CQAs/KQAs and CPPs/KPPs, and establish necessary controls of API, key ingredients, measurement of process parameters, and equipments. Keep in mind that: (a) quality by design (QbD), and (b) formulation and process are two sides of the same coin.
2. Select proper equipment to maximize the success of daily production. Avoid "we always do it like this."
3. Target a proper end point, with consideration to maximize process robustness and prevent

regulatory burdens. Always look into details, and extended the considerations downstream, see both the forest and the trees.
4. Apply PAT technology, and use statistical tools (DOE, sixsigma, FMEA, Gage R&R ... etc.) for continuous success.
5. Explore new technology for future manufacturing process, such as continuous WG process, innovated process with less or no burden of good flowability, compressibility ... etc.
6. Prepare for unexpected events, and OOSs. Set up an escape door.

References

1. Bier, H.P., Leuenberger, H. & Sucker, H. (1979). Determination of the uncritical quantity of granulating liquid by power measurements on planetary mixers. Pharm. Ind. 4, 375–380.
2. Belchamber, R. (2003). Acoustics—a process analytical tool. Spec. Eur. 15(6), 26–27.
3. Betz, G., Bürgin, P.J. & Leuenberger, H. (2003). Power consumption profile analysis and tensile strength measurements during moist agglomeration. Int. J. Pharm. 252(1–2), 11–25.
4. Betz, G., Bürgin, P.J. & Leuenberger, H. (2004). Power consumption measurement and temperature recording during granulation. Int. J. Pharm. 272(1–2), 137–149.
5. Buckingham, E. (1914). On physically similar systems: Illustrations of the use of dimensional equations. Phys. Rev. NY 4, 345–376.
6. Cliff, M.J. (1990a). Granulation end point and automated process control of mixer-granulators: Part 1. Pharm. Tech. 4, 112–132.
7. Cliff, M.J. (1990b). Granulation end point and automated process control of mixer-granulators: Part 2. Pharm. Tech. 5, 38–44.
8. Dilworth, S.E., Mackin, L.A., Weir, S., Claybourn, M. & Stott, P.W. (2005). In-line techniques for end point determination in large scale high shear wet granulation. 142nd British Pharmaceutical Conference.
9. Macias, K. & Carvajal, T. (2008). An assessment of techniques for determining particle size during high shear wet granulation. Tablets and Capsules 6(1). January.
10. Faure, A., Grimsey, I.M., Rowe, R.C., York, P. & Cliff, M.J. (1998). A methodology for the optimization of wet granulation in a model planetary mixer. Pharm. Dev. Tech. 3(3), 413–422.
11. Faure, A., Grimsey, I.M., Rowe, R.C., York, P. & Cliff, M.J. (1998). Importance of wet mass consistency in the control of wet granulation by mechanical agitation: a demonstration. J. Pharm. Pharmacol. 50(12), 1431–1432.
12. Faure, A., Grimsey, I.M., Rowe, R.C., York, P. & Cliff, M.J. (1999). Applicability of a scale-up methodology for wet granulation processes in Collette Gral high shear mixer-granulators. Eur. J. Pharm. Sci. 8(2), 85–93.
13. Faure, A., Grimsey, I.M., Rowe, R.C., York, P. & Cliff, M.J. (1999). Process control in a high shear mixer-granulator using wet mass consistency: The effect of formulation variables. J. Pharm. Sci. 88(2), 191–195.
14. Faure, A., York, P. & Rowe, R. (2001). Process control and scale-up of pharmaceutical wet granulation processes: a review. Eur. J. Pharm. Biopharm. 52(3), 269–277.
15. Horsthuis, G.J.B., van Laarhoven, J.A.H., van Rooij, R.C.B.M. & Vromans, H. (1993). Studies on upscaling parameters of the Gral high shear granulation process. Int. J. Pharm. 92, 143.

16. Ganguly, S. & Gao, J.Z. (2005). Application of On-line Focused Beam Reflectance Measurement Technoy in High Shear Wet Granulation. AAPS General Meeting, Contributed Paper.

17. Landin, M., York, P., Cliff, M.J., Rowe, R.C. & Wigmore, A.J. (1996). The effect of batch size on scale-up of pharmaceutical granulation in a fixed bowl mixer-granulator. Int. J. Pharm. 134, 243–246.

18. Landin, M., York, P. & Cliff, M.J. (1996). Scale-up of a pharmaceutical granulation in fixed bowl mixer granulators. Int. J. Pharm. 133, 127–131.

19. Landin, M., York, P., Cliff, M.J. & Rowe, R.C. (1999). Scaleup of a pharmaceutical granulation in planetary mixers. Pharm. Dev. Technol. 4(2), 145–150.

20. Levin, M. (2006). Wet Granulation: End point Determination and Scale-Up. In: Encyclopedia of Pharmaceutical Technology, Swarbrick, J. (ed.), Taylor & Francis, New York.

21. Miwa, A., Toshio Yajima, T. & Itai, S. (2000). Prediction of suitable amount of water addition for wet granulation. Int. J. Pharm. 195(1–2), 81–92.

22. Otsuka, M., Mouri, Y. & Matsuda, Y. (2003). Chemometric evaluation of pharmaceutical properties of antipyrine granules by near-infrared spectroscopy. AAPS Pharm. Sci. Tech. 4(3). Article 47.

23. Rayleigh, L. (1915). The principle of similitude. Nature, 95(2368), March 18, 66–68.

24. Reynolds, O. (1883). An experimental investigation of the circumstances which determine whether the motion of water shall be direct or sinuous, and of the law of resistance in parallel channels. Philos. Trans. R. Soc. London 174, 935–982.

25. Rudd, D. (2004). The use of acoustic monitoring for the control and scale-up of a tablet granulation process. J. Proc. Anal. Tech. 1(2), 8–11.

26. Zlokarnik, M. (1991). Dimensional analysis and scale-up in chemical engineering. Springer Verlag.

27. Zlokarnik, M. (1998). Problems in the application of dimensional analysis and scale-up of mixing operations. Chem. Eng. Sci. 53(17), 3023–3030.

28. Keary, C.M. & Sheskey, P.J. (2004). Preliminary report of the discovery of a new pharmaceutical granulation process using foamed aqueous binders. Drug Dev. Ind. Pharm. 30(8), 831–845.

29. Hlinak, T. (2000). Granulation and scale-up issues in solid dosage form development. American Pharmaceutical Review 3(4), 33–36.

30. Yasumura, M. & Ashihara, K. (1996). Scale-up of oral solid dosage forms. Pharm. Tech. Japan 12(9), 1279–1289.

31. Russo, E. (1984). Typical scale-up problems and experiences. Pharm. Tech. 8(11), 46–48, 50–51, 54–56.

32. Ashihara, K. & Yasumura, M. (1996). Scale-up for solid drugs as illustrated by scale-up of a granulation process. Kagaku Kogaku 60(3), 180–182.

33. Sheskey, P., Keary, C. & Clark, D. (2006). Foam Granulation: Scale-up of Immediate Release and Controlled Release Formulations from Laboratory Scale to Manufacturing Scale. Poster presented at the 2006 Annual Meeting and Exposition of the American Association of Pharmaceutical Scientists, San Antonio, Texas, USA, Oct. 29–Nov. 2.

34. Liu, L. (2002). The effect of process parameters and scale-up of wet granulation. Invited Speaker, Tablet and Capsule Manufacturing 2002, May 14–15. Atlantic City, NJ.

35. Smith, T.J., Sackett, G.L., Maher, L., Jian Lee, McCarthy, R., Shesky, P. & Liu, L. (2002). The Comparison of Wet Granulation by Top-Drive and Bottom-Drive High Shear Granulator. AAPS 2002 Annual Meeting, November 10–14, Toronto, Canada.

36. Smith, T.J., Sackett, G.L. & Liu, L. (2002). The Direct Comparison of Wet Granulation by High Shear Granulator and an Innovative Rotor Processor. AAPS 2002 Annual Meeting, November 10–14. Toronto, Canada.

37. Liu, L. (2001). The Optimization of Process Parameters and Scale-Up of Wet Granulation. Invited Speaker, "Tablet Manufacturing CANADA 2001", November 13–14, Toronto, Canada.

38. Smith, T.J., Sackett, G.L., Maher, L. & Liu, L. (2001). The Change in Particle Size of Immediate Release and Controlled Release Formulations During High Shear Wet Granulation Processes. AAPS 2001 Annual Meeting, Oct. 21–25. Denver, CO.

39. Liu, L. (2001). Troubleshooting and Process Development of Controlled Release Dosage Form-Case Study. Invited Speaker, "Troubleshooting Solid Dose Manufacturing 2001", September 11–12. Raleigh, NC.

40. Liu, L., Shlyankevich, A., Orleman, J., Quartuccio, C. & McCall, T. (2001). The Osmolarity of The Standard FDA High Fat Meal and Its Effect on the In Vitro Performance of A Novel Controlled Release System. AAPS 2001 Annual Meeting, October 21–25. Denver, CO.

41. Shlyankevich, A., Liu, L., Lynch, P. & McCall, T. (2001). Comparison of USP Apparatuses 2 and 3 in Dissolution Testing of Immediate Release/Controlled Release Bi-layer Tablets. AAPS 2001 Annual Meeting, October 21–25. Denver, CO.

42. Liu, L. (2001). The Effect of Process Parameters and Scale-Up of Wet Granulation. Invited Speaker, Tablets Manufacturing Technology 2001 Conference, April 10–11. Atlantic City, NJ.

43. Smith, T.J., Sackett, G.L., Goldsberry, T., Maher, L., Whiting, T. & Liu, L. (2001). Comparison of End Point Determination by Wet Mass Time, Product Temperature Change, and Power Consumption for Scale-Up of High Shear Granulation of Immediate and Controlled Release Formulations. Pharmaceutical Congress of America, March 24–29. Orlando, FL.

44. Liu, L. (2000). Optimization of Process Parameters and Scale-Up of Wet Granulation. Invited Speaker, Tablet Manufacturing Puerto Rico, TechSource, November 7–8. San Juan, Puerto Rico.

45. Liu, L. (2000). How to Optimize the Scale-Up Process for Pharmaceutical Tablets-The Challenge of Scale-Up and Process Optimization of Wet Granulation. Invited Speaker, The 7th Annual Pharm Tech, Puerto Rico Conference & Exposition, June 26–28. Puerto Rico.

46. Liu, L., DeBellis, M., Lynch, P., Orleman, J., Shlyankevich, A. & McCall, T. (2000). The Effect of Tip-Speed and Thermal Behavior on Wet Granulation Process Under Constant Numbers of Rotations of a Novel Controlled Release System. AAPS 2000 Annual Meeting and Exposition, October 29–November 2. Indianapolis, IN.

47. Liu, L., Sackett, G.L., Smith, T.J. & Goldberry, T.J. (2000). The Effect of Load Volume on a Novel Controlled Release System in a High Shear Granulator. AAPS 2000 Annual Meeting and Exposition, October 29–November 2. Indianapolis, IN.

48. Sackett, G.L., Smith, T.J., Goldberry, T.J. & Liu, L. (2000). The Effect of Load Volume on Particle Size and Temperature Rise of Wet Granulation in a High Shear Granulator. AAPS 2000 Annual Meeting and Exposition, October 29–November 2. Indianapolis, IN.

49. Liu, L. & Giambalvo, D. (1999). The Effect of Process Parameters of a Fluid-Bed Granulation of a Novel Controlled Release Polymeric System. AAPS 1999 Annual Meeting, November 14–18. New Orleans, LA.

50. Liu, L. (1998). High Shear Granulation and Impact on Solid Dosage Form Performance-Case Study. Invited Speaker, Pharmaceutical Unit Processes and Solid Dosage Form Development: Industry and Regulatory Perspectives, May 18–21. Duquesne University, Pittsburgh, PA

51. Liu, L., McCall, T. & Diehl, D. (1998). The Effect of Process Variables on a Wet Granulation by High Shear Mixer and Fluid-Bed Granulator of a Novel Hydrophilic Matrix System. Controlled Release Society Annual Meeting, June 21–24. Las Vegas.

52. Liu, L., DiNicola, D., Diehl, D., Garrett, D., Bhagwat, D. & Baichwal, A. (1998). The Comparison of Wet Granulation Performed By Top-Drive and Bottom-Drive High Shear Granulator of a Novel Controlled Release Polymeric System. AAPS 1998 Annual Meeting. San Francisco, CA.

53. Liu, L. & Giambalvo, D. (1998). The Effect of Process Variables on Coating Efficiency of an HPMC-Based Film Coating Using a Perforated Coating Pan. AAPS 1998 Annual Meeting. San Francisco, CA.

54. McCall, T., Liu, L. Diehl, D., DiNicola, D. & Baichwal, A. (1998). The Effect of Speed of Main Blade and Use of Chopper in the Wet Granulation By High Shear Granulator of a Novel Controlled Release Polymeric System. AAPS 1998 Annual Meeting. San Francisco, CA.

55. DiNicola, D., Liu, L., McCall, T., Fitzmaurice, K. & Bhagwat, D. (1998). Evaluation of Physical Characteristics and Functional Performance of Controlled Release Granulations. AAPS 1998 Annual Meeting. San Francisco, CA.

56. Diehl, D., Liu, L. & McCall, T. (1998). Effects of Mill Screen Size on Particle Size and Dissolution Rate. AAPS 1998 Annual Meeting. San Francisco, CA.

57. Liu, L. (1997). Scale-Up of a Hydrophilic Matrix System-Case Study. 39th Annual International Industrial Pharmaceutical Research and Development Conference (June Land O'Lakes), June 2–6. Merrimac, WI.

58. Liu, L., McCall, T., Labudzinski, S. & Baichwal, A. (1997). The Temperature Change and Power Consumption During the Wet Granulation Process of Three Hydrophilic Matrices Containing Water-Soluble and Water-Insoluble Drugs. AAPS 1997 Annual Meeting, Nov. 2–6. Boston, MA.

59. Liu, L., McCall, T., Labudzinski, S., Baichwal, A. & Bhagwat, D. (1997). The Compressibility and the Effect of Compression Force on the *In-Vitro* Dissolution Performance of a Novel Hydrophilic Matrix System. AAPS 1997 Annual Meeting, Nov. 2–6. Boston, MA.

60. Diehl, D., Liu, L., Fitzmaurice, K. & Bhagwat, D. (1997). Effects of Granulation Parameters on the Bulk Manufacture of a Novel Controlled Release System. AAPS 1997 Annual Meeting, Nov. 2–6. Boston, MA.

61. Diehl, D., Liu, L., Fitzmaurice, K., Bhagwat, D., McCall, T. & Baichwal, A. (1997). Reproducibility of the Physical Parameters and Dissolution Performance in the Scale-Up of a Novel Controlled Release System. AAPS 1997 Annual Meeting, Nov. 2–6. Boston, MA.

62. DiNicola, D., McCall, T., Liu, L., O'Toole, K., Fitzmaurice, K., Bhagwat, D. & Kondrat, K. (1997). Stability of a Controlled-Release Hydrophilic Matrix System Under Accelerated Environmental Conditions. AAPS 1997 Annual Meeting, Nov. 2–6. Boston, MA.

63. DiNicola, D., McCall, T., Liu, L., Bhagwat, D. & Baichwal, A. (1997). Development of Controlled Release Formulations Using Either High Shear or Fluid-Bed Granulation Techniques. The 24th International Symposium on Controlled Release of Bioactive Materials, June 15–19. Stockholm, Sweden.

Process Development, Optimization, and Scale-up: Fluid-bed Granulation

Ken Yamamoto and Z. Jesse Shao

30.1 OVERVIEW OF THE FLUID-BED GRANULATION PROCESS

One commonly used strategy to improve undesirable powder characteristics of the active pharmaceutical agent (API) is to granulate the API with other excipients. There are two widely used methods to make granules: dry granulation, which involves mechanical compaction (slugging or roller compaction) followed by a dry sizing process, and wet granulation using a liquid binder (low shear wet granulation, high shear wet granulation or fluid-bed granulation). While separate drying equipment is required following a low shear or high shear wet granulation process, fluid-bed wet granulation is a one-pot process which can blend, wet granulate, and dry all in one piece of equipment.[1]

A typical fluid-bed wet granulation sequence consists of dry blending, wet granulation, and drying steps. Raw materials are first fluidized by hot inlet air for blending. Granulation fluid is then sprayed onto the pre-blended material, until the desired moisture content or granule size is achieved. At this point, drying begins until a predetermined product temperature is reached. Binder solution is commonly used as a granulation fluid however, it can also be added as a dry ingredient into the powder bed. Granules produced using the fluid-bed process have advantages of being homogeneous, free-flowing, and less dense. Generally speaking, these granules require lower pressure to compress into tablets than granules made by other granulation methods.

The amount of solvent removed during fluid-bed wet granulation and drying steps can be calculated using heat and mass transfer theory. By taking process variables, such as spray rate, dew point, volume of inlet air, and powder characteristics of raw material into consideration, a robust manufacturing process can be developed for a variety of formulation compositions and manufacturing scales.

Being a self-enclosed system, the fluid-bed is a preferred technology for highly potent compounds requiring containment. When coupled with a clean-in-place (CIP) system, fluid-bed becomes the preferred granulation method for such potent compounds.

30.2 EQUIPMENT DESIGN

30.2.1 Batch-wise Models

Among the three well-established batch fluid-bed methods, top spray is commonly used for granulating purposes, due to its ability to produce highly porous particles with better dispersibility and compressibility for downstream compression. The bottom spray design (Wurster) is very popular for layering of active component and coating to modify drug release, due to its good film formation in such units. Drug-layering on sugar beads using Wurster inserts is widely reported in literature. Tangential spray (rotary) methods are mostly used in pelletization and coating of the formed pellets. The operating mechanisms are shown in Figure 30.1. Design and operational details for the three methods are described below.

Top Spray

The main components for a top spray processor are:

1. An air-handling unit optionally equipped with humidification and dehumidification for dew point control;
2. A product container;
3. An expansion chamber;
4. A spray system containing single or multiple nozzles;
5. An exhaust system with a filter and, optionally, an explosion suppression system.

Glatt expansion chambers come in models known as tall conical GPCG design or the shorter and wider WSG design. GPCG machines are suitable for top spray and bottom spray granulation, while the WSG design is suited for drying of wet granules, and occasionally for top spray granulation processes.

Top spray has a simple set-up, offers a high capacity, and is typically used for either granulating powders or spray drying. When a binder solution is sprayed through the nozzles, the droplets produced bind to fluidizing powder particles, forming agglomerates. There are cases when water is sprayed into the powder bed, which contains a dry binder, to form granules. Granulation with water is also referred to as instantizing, and is mostly used in the food and diagnostic industries. Granules formed by instantizing are generally more loosely formed and friable. Controlling inlet air dew point and bed temperature is important for batch-to-batch consistency.

A top spray fluid-bed can also be used as an alternative to the traditional spray drying process using hot air. Since the air volume in a fluid-bed can be increased easily, it does not demand a high temperature to dry sprayed droplets. This is especially attractive to protein formulations, which can be denatured if the processing temperature is too high. Particles formed through a top spray fluid-bed method are larger in size, due to the effect of layering. Flowability of these particles is generally better, as a result of larger particle formation with narrow size distribution.

Since the particles formed are very porous, the top spray method is not suitable for coating of beads and fine particles for controlled-release products. One exception is hot-melt coating, where molten materials are sprayed onto fluidized particles. Jones and Percel[2] used all three methods to produce sustained-release chlorpheniramine maleate pellets by spraying molten partially-hydrogenated cottonseed oil, and found that the top spray method resulted in a smooth surface, and a decreased dissolution rate.

Bottom Spray

Bottom spray, originally developed by Dale Wurster in the late 1950s, is most commonly used in coating of particulates and tablets. There are several unique features with a Wurster-type column design. First, the nozzle is mounted at the bottom of the product container, and above the air distribution plate. Secondly, the air distribution plate has larger holes in the middle than on the outer rim. This allows more air flow through the middle portion of the plate. Lastly, an insert (partition) is placed above the plate. This configuration ensures particles are fluidized upward in the insert, fall outside the insert, pass under the insert, and are lifted again inside the insert. The region inside the insert is commonly referred to as the up-bed region, while that outside the insert is known as the down-bed region. Particles are sprayed in the up-bed, and dried in the down-bed many times, until the desired film thickness is achieved.

Since coating solution is sprayed from the bottom, coating efficiency is typically much higher than by top spray. Mehta and Jones[3] have demonstrated that bottom spray produced a much smoother coating compared to top spray, especially when organic solvent-based solution was sprayed. Top spraying solvent-based solution leads to flash evaporation and more spray drying, resulting in a rough surface formation.

Tangential Spray

The tangential spray process involves a variable-speed rotating disk inside the product bowl. The spray nozzle is mounted at the side (near the bottom)

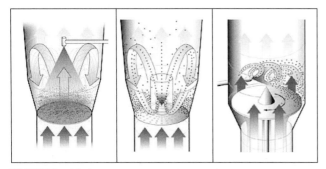

FIGURE 30.1 Top spray, bottom spray, and tangential spray mechanisms used in batch fluid-beds. Courtesy Glatt Air Techniques, Inc.

of the bowl, and is buried in the batch during processing. The gap between the disk and bowl wall can be adjusted, to allow varying amounts of air through. During granulation, the rotating disk imparts a centrifugal force to the material, forcing the particles to move to the outer part of the disk. The air flow then provides a lifting force. These two forces, along with natural gravity, make the material travel in a spiraling helix form. This motion results in the compaction of the material, to produce uniform and dense granules, thereby enabling the manufacture of high-dose loading products. An added advantage is that further coating of the formed pellets can be done in the same processor, without having to discharge the pellets. Disk speed and air volume need to be reduced, compared to the granulation stage, in order to avoid film breakage potentially caused by abrasion.

30.2.2 Semi-continuous Design

The best known case of implemented semi-continuous fluid-bed technology is the Glatt MultiCell,[4,5] which combines high shear granulation and fluid-bed drying (Figure 30.2). Typically, three fluid-bed dryers are set up side-by-side along with a horizontal high shear granulator and a wet sieving mill. After wet granulation, the wet mass is wet screened and loaded in the first fluid-bed for partial drying (pre-drying). Partially dried granules are then pneumatically conveyed to the second fluid-bed unit for continued drying (final drying), then to the third unit for final drying, and equilibration (cooling). The dried granules are then conveyed to a dry mill for milling.

The three fluid-bed units are designed for different air temperature and humidity conditions, with the first one typically set at high temperature (60°C), and the last cell at ambient temperature and humidity.

GEA Niro Pharma Systems (Columbia, MD) recently demonstrated a new version of a semi-continuous fluid-bed coater, the SUPERCELL™.[6,7] This device is capable of automatically pre-weighing small batches of tablets (typically 30–40 g) into the coating chamber, coating them rapidly (typically <10 minutes), and finally pneumatically conveying them out of the chamber. The ability of SUPERCELL to rapidly and uniformly coat tablets and capsules is claimed to be due to uniquely patented designs, i.e., a special gas distribution plate, and a two-fluid spray nozzle located below it.

The atomizing gas is mixed with low-pressure drying gas, thereby reducing the momentum of the atomizing air. Attenuation of the spraying momentum, along with a very short processing time, is expected to reduce tablet wear-and-tear, thereby improving tablet appearance. Conceivably, friable or hygroscopic tablets can also be processed in such a unit, due to its rather short coating time. A vendor-sponsored study of coating an enteric film on aspirin tablets confirmed good acid resistance for tablets coated with >9% weight gain. No tablet edge defects after coating were found. A prototype model is shown in Figure 30.3. Acceptance and use of this device by the pharmaceutical industry is yet to be seen.

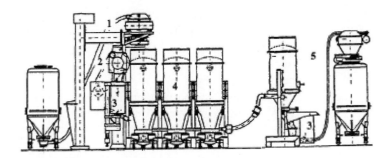

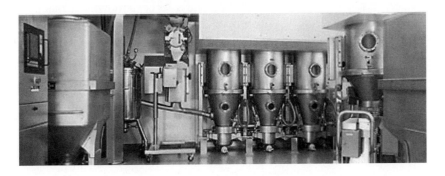

FIGURE 30.2 Semi-continuous fluid beds, glatt multicell. 1. Dosing unit; 2. High shear granulator; 3. Sieve; 4. Fluid-bed; 5. Pneumatic transport system. Courtesy Glatt Air Techniques, Inc.

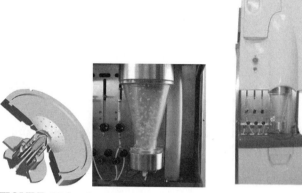

FIGURE 30.3   Cutaway view of the liquid nozzle and gas distribution plate, tablet movement inside the coating chamber, and the SUPERCELL coater general appearance. Courtesy Glatt Air Techniques, Inc.

30.2.3 Continuous Models

Glatt developed various continuous fluid-bed models with the GF and AGT units shown in Figure 30.4. In the GF model the inlet air plenum is divided into multiple chambers, each with adjustable temperature and air flow control. By this means, spray agglomeration, drying, and cooling can all be done in this single unit. By controlling air flow in the various chambers, the overall powder flows in a plug fashion toward the discharge port.

In the 1980s, Glatt commercialized the AGT technology which has a discharge pipe right in the middle of the bottom screen. Air velocity in this pipe determines what size particles can be discharged. Heavy particles with sinking velocity greater than the air velocity inside the pipe will be discharged, while smaller particles are blown back to the fluidized-bed and are exposed to layering again.

Continuous processors are typically used in the chemical, food, and agricultural industries.

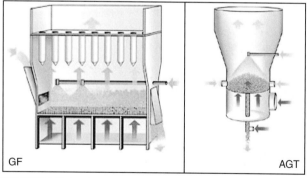

FIGURE 30.4   Continuous fluid beds, Glatt GF and AGT units. Courtesy Glatt Air Techniques, Inc.

30.3 FLUID-BED HYDRODYNAMICS

30.3.1 Product Temperature and Moisture Content Profiles through Fluid-bed Processing

A fluid-bed wet granulation process consists of dry blending, wet granulation, and drying steps. A typical example of product temperature and moisture content profiles through fluid-bed processing is that product temperature initially increases during the blending step. It then decreases after spraying starts, and eventually bottoms out. Assuming that there is no heat loss from the equipment surface, and that the materials are well mixed by fluidization air, product temperature could reach:

1. Wet bulb temperature of the inlet air when the spray rate is greater than the drying capacity of the inlet air. In this case, product temperature is kept constant at the wet bulb temperature, even after drying begins. This continues until water levels in the wet mass become less than the drying capacity, at this time the product temperature rises.
2. Between the inlet air temperature and the wet bulb temperature of the inlet air, if the spray rate is lower than the drying capacity of the inlet air. In this case, the product temperature starts increasing immediately after spraying is stopped.

Once product temperature starts rising, a good correlation between the moisture content of granules and product temperature can be established. Product temperature becomes a good indicator for predicting the drying end point.

Following moisture level changes through fluid-bed processing yields more information than monitoring product temperature. Moisture level of starting materials first decreases during the blending step, then it increases when spraying starts, and then keeps increasing until spraying stops. The accumulation of moisture depends on processing parameters (inlet air and spraying conditions). A good correlation between moisture content and size of wet granules can also be established. When the spraying step is completed, accumulated moisture within the wet mass starts to be removed. It has also been demonstrated that a good correlation between moisture content and size of dry granules exists.

30.3.2 Moisture Mass Balance during the Fluid-bed Process

Moisture profiling throughout the process can not only be used as a fingerprint for the formulation and process, it is also useful for process development and trouble shooting purposes. When wet granules contact the hot inlet air, the hot inlet air exchanges its heat for moisture. The temperature of the air drops, due to evaporative cooling, and exits from the process chamber as exhaust air. Water in wet granules is vaporized instantly by heat at this temperature. Since the granules are suspended into fluidization (inlet) air, and contact surface area between air and wet granules is considered to be huge, heat and mass transfer reach equilibrium instantaneously.

The Drying Process

Figure 30.5 shows moisture balance during fluid-bed operation. In the drying process, moisture in wet granules is removed by dry inlet air. During wet granulation, there is another source of moisture, which is sprayed binder solution.

As shown in Figure 30.6, moisture removed (M_r) during the drying process can be calculated from moisture contents of inlet (M_{in}) and outlet air (M_{out}) as:

$$M_r = M_{out} - M_{in}$$

M_{in} and M_{out} can be determined by monitoring temperature and relative humidity of inlet and outlet air. Using moisture content (M_{end}) and weight (W_{end}) of wet granules at wet granulation end point, the moisture content of wet granules during the drying process can be calculated:

$$M_g = \frac{(M_{end} - M_r)}{W_{end} - M_r} \times 100$$

The Wet Granulation Process

To predict moisture balance during the wet granulation process, there are two parameters that need to be taken into consideration, i.e., moisture removed (M_r), and moisture accumulated in the wet granules (M_A) for the wet granulation process (Figure 30.5). Since the binder solution is sprayed onto the powder bed during this process, moisture in the sprayed binder solution (M_s) needs to be built into the equation, in order to calculate the moisture level accumulated in wet granules:

$$M_A = M_s - M_r = M_s - (M_{out} - M_{in})$$

Moisture content of wet granules can be calculated using initial conditions which include batch size (W_{ini}), and initial moisture content of powder bed (M_{ini}):

$$M_g = \frac{M_{ini} + M_A}{W_{ini} + M_A} \times 100$$

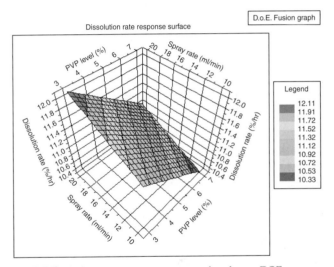

FIGURE 30.6   Dissolution response surface from a DOE

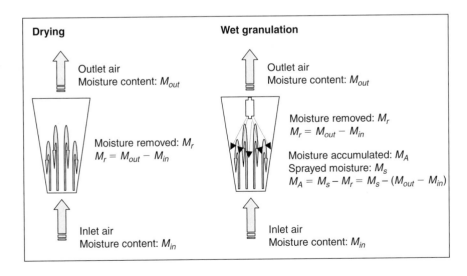

FIGURE 30.5   Moisture mass balance during fluid-bed process

Prediction of Moisture Profile During the Fluid-bed Process

By taking air factors, including air volume per unit time and specific volume, into consideration, the moisture profile during fluid-bed operation can be predicted. Briefly, a given inlet air drying capacity is expressed as:

$$DC = H_{inwb} - H_{indb}$$

$H_{in\,wb}$ and $H_{in\,db}$ are the absolute moisture content of the wet bulb and the dry bulb temperature of inlet air, respectively.

The rate of moisture removal (X_r) is expressed as:

$$X_r = \left(H_{inwb} \times \frac{V_{in}}{VH_{spout}} \right) - \left(H_{indb} \times \frac{V_{in}}{VH_{spin}} \right)$$

where:

V_{in} is inlet air volume per unit time

$VH_{sp\,in}$ and $VH_{sp\,out}$ are specific volume of the inlet air and outlet air, respectively.

Then moisture content for drying is expressed as:

$$M_g = \frac{M_{ini} + (X_s - X_r) \times t}{W_{end} + (X_s - X_r) \times t} \times 100$$

And the moisture content for wet granulation process is expressed as:

$$M_g = \frac{M_{ini} + (X_s - X_r) \times t}{W_{ini} + (X_s - X_r) \times t} \times 100$$

X_s and t are spray rate and running time, respectively.

Watano et al. described an empirical method to calculate the heat transfer coefficient (hp) and rate of moisture removed.[21]

30.4 MECHANISMS OF AGGLOMERATION

30.4.1 Phases in Granule Growth

The main objective of the granulation process is to improve undesirable powder characteristics of raw materials (poor powder flow, fluffiness, segregation, etc), therefore the specific needs must first be identified. Granulation properties after the process are likely different, depending on the target of the process.

Moisture content of wet granules can be controlled by process parameters. If there is a target moisture range in mind, it can generally be achieved through process controls (air and spray conditions). At the beginning of the process, the powder bed is assumed to be dry, with no aggregation. Following binder spraying, the powder bed becomes wet, then aggregation starts, and granule size increases with the spraying of more binder solution. Granule growth rate during the wet granulation process can vary from slow progress in the beginning, to rapid growth exceeding the desired end point. To develop a robust wet granulation process the basic concept of granule growth, and its influencing factors, need to be understood.

30.4.2 Bonding Mechanisms

Rumph[8] classified particle–particle bonding mechanisms into five categories:

1. solid bridges;
2. interfacial forces and capillary pressure in movable liquid surfaces;
3. adhesion and cohesion forces in bonding bridges which are not freely movable;
4. attraction between solid particles, such as van der Waals forces, electrostatic forces or magnetic type interactions; and
5. form-closed bonds, such as particles interlocking or entangling.

Category 1 is the moisture-mediated bonding mechanism, with interfacial and capillary forces between particles playing important roles to form particle–particle bonds during the wet granulation process. Particle–particle bonds are classified into four categories, based on the phase of interaction between liquid and particles: pendular, funicular, capillary, and droplet, according to Newitt and Conway-Jones, and Barlow.[9,10] Assuming a binder solution is used as the granulation fluid which is sprayed into fine droplets, liquid bridges between particles can be viscous and adhesive. Formed solid bridges will remain after drying.

Upon spraying binder solution onto the powder bed, moisture content increases, and the surface of powders becomes self-adhesive due to coalescence of binder solution. During the coalescence, water may be absorbed into particles resulting in high void saturation with increased deformation capability (plasticity) which helps to bind particles together (see Huang and Kono,[11,12] and Abberger[13]). Once liquid bridges start to be formed between particles (nucleation), the progress of granule growth is determined by a balance of cohesive and adhesive forces between particles (viscosity of liquid bridge), and impact from collision of particles during the wet granulation process.[14] Since two or more particles are held together with liquid bridges, granule size could be regulated by number, size, and viscosity of the liquid bridges. If the liquid bridge size is small or less viscous, then the bridge can hold only small particles or breakage may occur. If the liquid bridge size is large and/or viscous, the liquid bridges could hold heavier and larger particles, as well as granules, together.

30.5 FORMULATION AND PROCESS VARIABLES AND THEIR CONTROL

Like many other unit operations, many variables can impact manufacturability and product quality in the fluidized-bed wet granulation process. In order to develop a robust process, it is necessary to evaluate the effects of these variables at an early stage. These variables can be classified into three groups, i.e., equipment related, formulation related, and process related variables. Performance of a fluidized-bed wet granulator depends on equipment related variables, such as equipment size (dimensions) and shape, position of spray nozzle (top, bottom, tangential), number of spray guns, etc. These variables need to be assessed during the scale-up activity from one scale to another. This aspect is treated in Section 30.6 of this chapter.

Due to the basic mechanism of granule growth during the wet granulation process, particle size and its distribution, density, wettability, solubility, and hygroscopisity of starting materials impact product quality (bioperformance, content uniformity, chemical stability, etc.), and manufacturability of the formulation. It is also well-known that cohesiveness and static charge of raw material can cause undesirable homogeneity and low-yield problems after the wet granulation process. On the other hand, inlet air conditions (relative humidity of dew point, temperature, air volume or velocity), and spraying conditions (spraying rate, atomizing air pressure, spray gun position), are key variables to make a consistent quality product batch after batch (reproducibility).

30.5.1 Formulation Variables

There are a variety of excipients commercially available for fluid-bed formulation development, and each excipient has different material properties. It is important to understand excipient functionality and its behavior during processing. Since multiple excipients are put into a formulation, it then becomes complicated to understand the impact of all these excipients on manufacturability, and the final product quality.

Schaefer and Worts investigated the influences of starting material property and its mixing ratio in the fluid-bed granulation process, using crystalline lactose and starch as raw materials. It was shown that the granule size depended on the ratio of lactose and starch, with higher lactose content generating larger granule size. It was also indicated that the higher the surface area of starting materials, the smaller the granule size obtained after granulation.[15] Wan et al. also demonstrated that, after fluidized-bed wet granulation, the granule size of lactose, a water-soluble excipient, is larger than the granule size of corn starch, a water-insoluble excipient.[16] Since different excipients have different particle sizes, and interact differently with water, processing conditions will need to be different in order to obtain similar granule properties.

A binder is an essential component of the granulation process, which provides binding ability in the formulation after drying. The binder can be added either as powder or sprayed as solution to the powder bed during the wet granulation process. Wan et al. reported that larger granule size and higher density is obtained when the binder is added as a powder, rather than by spraying as a solution.[16] Schaefer et al. demonstrated that droplet size of the binder solution is influenced by viscosity of the binder solution. However, it was also shown that viscosity is not the sole factor to affect granule size.[17] The type of binders, and the binder concentration, could be critical variables when the binder solution is sprayed using a nozzle system. Binders such as hydroxypropylcellulose, polyvinylpyrollidone, hydroxypropylmethylcellulose, and pre-gelatinized starch are commonly used for fluid-bed wet granulation with a range of 2–5%W/W solution.[20]

30.5.2 Key Process Variables

As discussed in the previous section, there are three major factors influencing the fluid-bed wet granulation process, namely air conditions, spray conditions, and equipment related factors. The equipment related factors are, for example, design of equipment, bag filter, distributor, shape of bowl and/or extension chamber, shaking mechanisms, position and number of spray nozzles. These factors need to be carefully evaluated when batch size is changed, and/or a formulation is transferred from one site to another.

Inlet Air Conditions

Air conditions including temperature, dew point (or absolute humidity), and inlet air volume are the three key factors influencing drying and wet granulation. Since moisture from wet granules is evaporated and removed as exhaust air during the wet granulation and drying process, exhaust air contains a higher amount of moisture than inlet air. As described in Section 30.3.2, the amount of moisture inlet air can remove (DC) is:

$$DC = H_{inwb} - H_{indb}$$

Absolute moisture values are inlet air dependent, and this is the reason why dew point of inlet air and inlet air temperature are the critical factors for the wet granulation and drying process. The same inlet air temperature and inlet air volume could result in a different DC value, due to a different dew point. If there is no dew point controller and/or dew point monitoring system available, it is recommended inlet air relative humidity and temperature are measured to make the DC consistent (manufacturing process reproducible). These absolute moisture values can be obtained from the psychometric chart.

The powder bed is fluidized by inlet air, and it is important to keep sufficient fluidization throughout the process, otherwise the bed may collapse. It may be necessary to adjust inlet air volume during the wet granulation and drying process, because of weight change of wet versus dry materials. Inlet air volume needs to be reduced in order to minimize attrition during the drying process. Amount of moisture removed per unit time is expressed as:

[Amount of moisture removed/min]
= DC × air volume/min

When inlet air volume is adjusted, the amount of moisture removed per unit time will change.

Spray Rate, Droplet Size, and Spray Pattern

Since formation of liquid bridges among particles is the main mechanism of granule growth, it is reasonable to expect that spray rate and droplet size significantly impact the wet granulation process, and influence granule size and size distribution. The effects of spray rate and droplet size on fluid-bed wet granulation are not much different from those for the high shear wet granulation process. If the spray rate is too fast, rapid granule growth occurs, and the process could be sensitive to subtle changes of raw material and process conditions. Water-soluble components may be dissolved into binder solution, which accelerates granule growth. If the spray rate is too slow, it takes a long time to reach the desirable end point, and in worst cases this results in no granule growth. Large droplet size tends to produce larger and denser granules, while a fine mist may result in spray drying

the binder solution. Spray pattern and atomizing air influence droplet size. Shaefer et al.[17,18] reported that a broad spray pattern creates insufficient air and liquid mixing, which causes droplet size to become larger (Table 30.1). Small changes of air and liquid flow ratio (air-to-liquid mass ratio) influence droplet size changes (Table 30.2).

The effect of droplet size and powder material particle size on granule size after fluid-bed melt granulation using PEG 3000 was examined by Abberger et al.[19] It was concluded that the mechanism of agglomeration depended on the ratio of the binder droplet size to the particle size of the solid powder. When the solid powder particle size is smaller than the binder droplet size, immersion of the solid particle in the surface of the binder solution is the main mechanism of nucleation. Distribution of the binder solution to the solid particle makes the solid particle's surface sticky and deformable. When the solid particle size is greater than the binder droplet size, these sticky and deformable wet particles stick together, and this becomes the dominant nucleation mechanism.

30.5.3 Granule Growth under Drier Conditions (Low Moisture Content of Wet Granules during the Granulation Process)

AbuBaker et al.[20] investigated the effects of processing conditions on granule properties using a $2^{5-1} + 2$ factorial design of experiment (DOE), using a fluid-bed

TABLE 30.1 Influence of spray angle on droplet size (d50, μm)

Air dome setting		
2	5	1.2
(ca 30°)	(ca 40°)	(ca 60°)
56 μm	89 μm	100 μm

Data from reference 17. Binder solution: gelatine 4%, 40°C; liquid flow rate: 150 g/min; air flow rate: 10 Nm³/h.

TABLE 30.2 Influence of liquid flow rate and air-to-liquid mass ratio on droplet size (d50, μm)

Mass ratio	Liquid flow rate (g/min)		
	100	150	200
1.15	129 μm	99 μm	98 μm
	123 μm	113 μm	98 μm
1.43	106 μm	90 μm	79 μm
	102 μm	86 μm	88 μm

Data from reference 17. Binder solution: gelatine 4%, 40°C.

granulator/dryer. The factors evaluated were fine and coarse drug particle size, binder solution concentration (11% and 16%), spray rate (70 and 110 g/min), atomizing air pressure (1 and 3 bar), and inlet air dew point (−5 and 15°C). Statistical analysis from the study indicated that the spray rate and atomization air pressure ratio significantly influence granule size. Due to the very low moisture content (less than 2%) of granules, distribution of binder solution to solid particle surface makes the particle surface ready for aggregation, which is likely to be the main mechanism of granule growth. In this case, factors such as the spray rate and atomization pressure (liquid-to-air) ratio, which controls the droplet size of binder solution, become dominant factors for granule growth. The level of moisture content in wet granules may not be a good parameter to monitor, due to a very small change of the moisture level during the process.

30.5.4 Granule Growth under Wetter Conditions (High Moisture Content of Wet Granules)

When moisture is accumulated in wet granules more liquid bridges are formed, which increases the contact surface area between particles. As a result, the bonding capability of wet particles becomes higher than that for drier particles. It was reported that granule size is proportional to the humidity level inside the fluid-bed,[21] thus granulation size could be monitored by measuring moisture content of the wet mass. Watano et al.[22,23,24] introduced an IR sensor to monitor moisture level during fluid-bed granulation, and established a good correlation between moisture content and granule size.

30.6 SCALE-UP CONSIDERATIONS

Scale-up of fluid-bed processes from small laboratory units to large commercial machines has been a continuing activity in the chemical and pharmaceutical industry for over half a century. In spite of this, fluid-bed scale-up is still not an exact science, but remains a mix of mathematics, engineering, and personal judgment. There are many simplifications, approximations, and educated guesses involved in fluid-bed granulation and drying. Better data, more realistic models, and more exact equations are always sought after in this field. The secret to successful fluid-bed scale-up lies, however, in the recognition and management of uncertainties, rather than finding out its exact attributes.[25] Generally speaking, equipment

variables, such as the type and size of the equipment, and key process variables, such as spray rate, atomization pressure, and inlet air temperature, all affect the product quality attributes. Control of such parameters, to yield a consistent product at a large batch size (scale), thereby constitutes a successful scale-up strategy. Equally important is the consistent quality of incoming raw materials (API and excipients). A change in particle size distribution of the API is known to impact granulation characteristics, and ultimately compressibility.

Among the three steps involved in fluid-bed agglomeration (dry mixing, spray agglomeration, and drying), the spray agglomeration stage is the most critical phase to monitor. During this phase, dynamic granule growth and breakdown takes place, along with solvent evaporation. Schaefer and Worts[21] demonstrated that granule size is directly proportional to bed humidity during granulation. Therefore, controlling bed humidity becomes critical. Gore et al.[26] studied various processing parameters, and concluded that air temperature, spray nozzle location, spray rate, and atomization pressure can all affect granule characteristics. If one has to limit the number of process parameters to control for scale-up purposes, bed humidity and atomizing air pressure would be chosen. Atomization pressure affects granule growth through its effect on droplet size and spray pattern. Maintaining binder droplet size, when performing scale-up activities, is regarded as key to scale-up success. Along with atomization pressure, nozzle atomization air volume should also be recorded.

The primary consideration in scaling-up the fluid-bed process is to maintain drying efficiency between laboratory and production equipment. In a larger unit, inlet air temperature may need to be lowered, due to its higher air volume, in order to maintain the same drying efficiency as in smaller units. Otherwise, spray drying of binder solution can occur. Another commonly used method is to maintain bed temperature, which can be achieved by balancing air temperature, dew point, air flow, and spray rate.

An additional consideration during scale-up is material handling procedures and transfer methods. While hand-scooping into and out of the bowl is convenient for small-scale processors, it is physically demanding, and may not even be acceptable from a worker safety perspective. Vacuum transfer becomes a preferred option, and a common practice. This is achieved through the creation of negative pressure inside the unit, by running the blower with the inlet air flap minimally open and leaving the outlet flap fully open. Ingredients can be charged one-by-one via vacuum, then the mixing and granulation phases can be started. For granule discharge, the product can be vacuum transferred, bottom discharged by gravity or side discharged into another intermediate bulk container (IBC) for further mixing and compression. Fully contained IBCs aided by vacuum transfer are commercially available that can be linked to the discharge port of the fluid-bed processor. These units eliminate bowl opening during product discharge, and are typically used for potent compounds. If the fluid-bed is equipped with clean-in-place cleaning nozzles, it can then be washed down before the bowl disengages from the expansion chamber.

30.6.1 Batch Size and Equipment Selection

Scale-up from small laboratory sized fluid-bed machines can be made much easier if the same line of equipment is to be used. Manufacturers generally keep scale-up issues in mind when designing their line of processors. However, if equipment from a different manufacturer is to be used at the commercial site due to availability limitations, efforts will need to be spent on modifying process parameters. This is because of differences in air flow pattern, expansion chamber geometry, gun spray pattern, etc.

Minimum and maximum batch size within selected top spraying equipment can be approximated using the following equations:

$$S_{min} = V \times 0.5 \times BD$$

$$S_{max} = V \times 0.8 \times BD$$

where:

S is batch size in kilograms
V is the product bowl working volume in liters
BD is the bulk density of finished granules in g/cc.

Linear scale-up can be used as a rough estimate in the beginning. Assuming that 6 kg scale batches have been made in a 22 L bowl at 60% volume, and that the next scale-up will be done in a 100 liter bowl, a starting batch size of 30 kg is then recommended. It must be kept in mind that, as the batch size increases in the larger units, the powder bed will become more compacted, resulting in a higher bulk density in the bowl. Jones[27] predicted that approximately 20% higher bulk density should be factored in when comparing larger units to smaller ones.

For tangential-spray in a rotary fluid-bed granulator, minimum and maximum batch sizes can be determined as follows:

$$S_{min} = V \times 0.2 \times BD$$

$$S_{max} = V \times 0.8 \times BD$$

Rotor granulation is amenable to a wider range of batch size changes in the same bowl, although one should keep in mind that a larger batch load typically produces denser granulation, due to increased mass effect. Similar to a top spraying model, a good starting point would be for the finished product to occupy 60% of the working capacity or volume of the rotor product chamber.

For bottom spraying in a Wurster-type of equipment, the minimum and maximum batch size can be calculated using the following expressions:

$$S_{min} = \frac{1}{2}(\pi R_1^2 H - N\pi R_2^2 H) \times BD$$

$$S_{max} = (\pi R_1^2 H - N\pi R_2^2 H) \times BD$$

where:

R_1 is the radius of the chamber
R_2 is the radius of the partition
N is the number of partitions
H is the length of the partition.

30.6.2 Spray Rate Scale-up

Spray rate scale-up is determined by the drying capacity of the equipment, rather than by the increase in batch size. In other words, spray rate change should be based on similarities in fluidization patterns at different scales. However, one should keep in mind that, at a given atomization pressure and air flow volume, change in liquid spray rate affects droplet size which in turn impacts particle agglomeration.

Two methods can be used to determine spray rates. If air volume can be read out directly from the equipment, spray rate can be simply calculated:

$$S_2 = S_1 \times \frac{V_2}{V_1}$$

where:

S_1 is spray rate in the laboratory scale equipment
S_2 is spray rate in the scaled-up equipment
V_1 is air volume in the laboratory scale equipment
V_2 is air volume in the scaled-up equipment.

If there is no direct air volume readout on the equipment, cross-sectional areas of the product bowl screens can be used for approximation as follows:

$$S_2 = S_1 \times \frac{A_2}{A_1}$$

where:

A_1 is cross-sectional area of the laboratory scale equipment
A_2 is cross-sectional area of the scaled-up equipment.

Using a 22 L bowl as the starting point, scale-up and scale-down factors have been tabulated for ease of use as listed in Table 30.3.

Recently, AbuBaker et al.[20] proposed that the ratio of spray rate/atomization pressure is the most important factor controlling the droplet size of the spray. The authors reached this conclusion while working on scaling-up an eroding tablet formulation with a high drug load. By maintaining a constant ratio, scale-up from 8 kg to 70 kg was successful, despite differences in drug particle size, granulator geometry, and number of nozzles used.

The authors have further devised a new process parameter termed "driving force," which is the product of spray rate, binder concentration, and droplet size, then normalized by batch size. Granule growth rate was shown to correlate well with calculated driving force.

$$Drivingforce = \frac{\begin{array}{c}SprayRate \times BinderConcentration \\ \times DropletSize\end{array}}{BatchSize}$$

Conceivably, if driving force is maintained constant at different scales, scale-up can be done with ease, resulting in granules with the same particle size.

30.6.3 Rotary Disk Speed Scale-up

A simple way to scale-up disk speed is by maintaining radial velocity (V) constant as the diameter of the disk increases.

$$N_2 = N_1 \times \frac{d_1}{d_2}$$

TABLE 30.3 Approximate scale-up factors for fluid-bed granulators

Unit volume (L)	Screen diameter (mm)	Spray rate scale-up factor	Run time scale-up factor
1.75	100	0.21	0.38
4.50	150	0.47	0.44
22	220	1.0	1.00
45	350	2.5	0.82
100	500	5.2	0.87
215	730	11.0	0.89
420	900	16.7	1.14
670	1000	20.7	1.47
1020	1150	27.3	1.70
1560	1250	32.3	2.20
2200	1750	63.3	1.58
3000	1740	62.6	2.18

where:

N is the disk speed (rpm)
d is the diameter of the disk (m)
Subscripts 1 and 2 represent the first and second set of conditions.

Radial velocity (V, m/sec) can be calculated from:

$$V = \frac{\pi d N}{60}$$

Alternatively, radial acceleration can be held constant, in order to maintain the centrifugal force acting on the bed steady. Since radial acceleration equals to $2 \times V^2/d$, the following scale-change equation can be derived:

$$N_2 = \sqrt{\frac{N_1^2 d_1}{d_2}}$$

Assuming that a disk speed of 200 rpm was used in a 485 mm rotor, the scaled-up disk speed for the 780 mm rotor would be:

Using radial velocity method:

$$N_2 = \frac{200 \times 0.485}{0.780} = 124 \; rpm$$

Using radial acceleration method:

$$N_2 = \sqrt{\frac{(200)^2 \times 0.485}{0.780}} = 158 \; rpm$$

Known equipment parameters for the Glatt RSG and GRG rotor granulators are listed in Table 30.4.

Scale-up in a rotor granulator can also be done by maintaining centrifugal force (Fc) constant for different sized rotors or the same rotor with different amounts of material loading. Horsthuis et al.[28] used the Froude number for scale-up in high shear Gral compounders. Chukwumezie et al.[29] modified the Froude number method to maintain centrifugal force (Fc) in rotor granulation. By maintaining a centrifugal force of 41 667 Newtons for a 1 kg batch in a 12-inch rotor at 500 rpm, these authors were able to scale the process up to a 10 kg load in a 19-inch rotor at 200 rpm.

$$Fc = \frac{W \times V^2}{R}$$

where:

W is the batch weight
V is the radial velocity
R is the plate radius.

Typical batch size ranges for the GPCG, RSG, and GRG lines of machines are listed in Table 30.5.

TABLE 30.4   Glatt RSG and GRG rotor parameters

Model	Disc diameter	Radial velocity (m/sec)	Speed (rpm)	Air volume (m³/hr)	# of nozzles
RSG 1/3	295	0–27	0–1800	80–580	1–2
RSG 5/15	485	0–30	0–1200	120–750	1–3
RSG 15/30	620	3.7–22	113–680	200–1500	2–4
RSG 60/100	780	4.4–22	108–540	600–3000	2–4
GRG 100	1000	5–25	100–500	800–4500	3–6
GRG 200	1400	5–25	70–340	1000–6000	3–6
GRG 300	1600	5–25	60–300	1400–8000	4–8

TABLE 30.5   CPCG, RSG, and GRG batch size ranges

GPCG	RSG	GRG	Disk (mm)	Maximum working volume (L)	Typical batch size range (kg)
1 & 3	1	N/A	300	4.5	0.5–3.0
5 &15	5	N/A	500	30	3–20
30 & 60	30	30	620	60	5–40
60 & 120	60	60	780	105	10–75
N/A	N/A	100	1000	180	25–125
N/A	N/A	200	1400	430	50–300

30.6.4 Rational Scale-up

Due to the large numbers of interrelating parameters affecting product attributes, scale-up efforts can be significantly improved by employing rational approaches, such as design of experiments (DOE). DOE allows the scientist to narrow down the most critical formulation and process parameters to monitor during scale-up trials. Full factorial designs afford the identification of factor-to-factor interactions that cannot be revealed by the one-parameter-at-a-time method.

As an example, a controlled-release formulation was granulated in a small-scale GPCG-3 top spray granulator in the authors' laboratory. A $2^3 + 2$ design (three factors, two levels, with two center points) was utilized in this study, with the factors being polyvinylpyrollidone (PVP) level, spray rate, and hydroxypropylmethylcellulose (HPMC) viscosity variation (within the same commercial grade). Resulting granulations were compressed into tablets and tested for dissolution. The response surface plot is shown in Figure 30.6. While there were no significant effects of spray rate and HPMC viscosity on dissolution, PVP level did appear to be a statistically significant factor. Controlling PVP levels in the formulation is therefore important, although how PVP affects HPMC gelation during dissolution still remains unclear.

Process analytical technology (PAT) also proves to be a valuable tool in process monitoring. Among well-established PAT methodologies is the near-infrared (NIR) spectroscopy technique via fiber optic probes placed inside the bowl of the granulator. Since a wide spectrum (1100–2500 nm) of signal is captured in real-time along the granulation process, it can then be processed to reflect water and particle size changes. Frake et al.[30] installed an inline NIR system in a Glatt GPCG 30/60. The second derivative changes in absorbance at 1932 nm were used to correlate with moisture, while the zero-order absorbance at 2282 nm was selected to reflect particle size increase during granulation. This continual inline NIR monitoring has been demonstrated to provide a suitable means of end point determination for a top spray granulation process.

Rantanen et al.[31] employed a multichannel NIR detector in a Glatt WSG-5 unit to monitor moisture level during granulation and drying of blends and pellets. Moisture detection was performed at 1990 nm throughout the mixing, spraying, and drying phases. Together with bed temperature measurements, NIR moisture monitoring provides a value-added tool for better process understanding.

Watano et al.[32] utilized an IR moisture sensor for a laser scattering spray size analyzer for their work with agitation fluid-beds. They recommended that if the ratio of spray area to vessel cross-sectional area is kept constant, localized over-wetting can be prevented. By means of moisture control, drying efficiency during wetting and agglomeration phases can be maintained constant among the different sized vessels. In a follow-up article,[33] these researchers further correlated the relationship between IR absorbance and granule moisture content. Except for very dry conditions, such as low spray rate or high air temperature, there appears to be excellent correlation between measured moisture level (by offline drying) and IR absorbance.

Another method in monitoring real-time granule growth is by image analysis. Watano et al.[34] developed an image processing system by coupling a particle image probe (CCD camera), and an image processing unit. A close agreement in granule size between image process and the traditional sieve analysis was obtained. The authors further automated this system, to make it capable of controlling the spray rate at the end of the granulation phase or in order to avoid excessive agglomerate formation.[35] Modulation of spray rate was accomplished via fuzzy logic, a linguistic algorithm employing if-then rules, and a process lag element. Good control of granule growth was reported.

30.6.5 Scale-up via Semi-continuous (Batch-continuous) Processing

The principle of using continuous processing to improve cost-efficiency is well-established in the food and bulk chemical industries. The pharmaceutical industry has been rather slow in adopting such a strategy, due to relatively high profit margins, constant product changeover at the manufacturing site, and equipment qualification concerns. Semi-continuous processes, however, offer several advantages over traditional batch-wise processing. The most important of these is the ability to manufacture small and large volumes in the same equipment set-up, thereby eliminating scale-up needs. Other advantages include ease of automation, and less product risk in case of batch failure.[36]

Betz et al.,[37] using the Glatt MultiCell and two placebo formulations, demonstrated that consistent yield (discharge from the high shear granulator), compression profiles, and tablet disintegration can be generated throughout many subunits manufactured. This method has been extensively tested by Roche Basel, with over 30 marketed products. It was postulated that 600 subunits can be manufactured to constitute a large "batch" of 4200 kg.[37] One other such subunit set-up has been installed in Pfizer's Freiburg, Germany, facility.

30.6.6 Scale-up via Continuous Processing

True continuous fluid-bed processing equipment is rarely used by the pharmaceutical industry, although suitable equipment lines are available. The primary applications are the chemical and food industries. An example is the Glatt GF series, which were developed over a decade ago in order to improve throughput of fluid-bed processes. Originally designed for drying solids, today various models are available for granulation, coating, pelletizing, drying, and cooling applications.

The design feature of the GFG (granulator) is its inlet air plenum, which is divided into multiple chambers, thereby enabling the introduction of air with different temperatures and velocity in each chamber. Together with the correct placement of spray nozzles above each chamber, it is possible to create quite different conditions in different sections of the process chamber. Agglomeration, drying, and cooling therefore, can be done as the product travels from chamber-to-chamber all in the same unit.

30.7 SUMMARY

Fluid-bed granulation is a widely used and well-characterized unit operation in the pharmaceutical industry. With proper selection of equipment design, operating conditions, and suitable excipients, it has been shown that this technology can be scaled-up from the laboratory to commercial production. Although the wet granulation process can vary from formulation to formulation, it is important to understand basic concepts of equipment design and fundamental granulation theory, in order to develop robust and scalable formulations and processes. Application of PAT and DOE can help establish a design space for the fluid-bed process, as well as serving as great tools for scale-up and technology transfer. When a formulation and process are optimally developed using fluid-bed technology, the granules will ultimately impart superb quality to the end product (tablet, capsule, etc.).

Acknowledgements

The authors thank Miss Stephanie Sobotka for her valuable assistance during the preparation of this chapter.

References

1. Rubino, O.P. (1999). Fluid-bed technology. Pharmaceutical Technology 23(6), 104–113.
2. Jones, D.M. & Percel, P.J. (1994). Coating of Multiparticulates Using Molten Materials: Formulation and Process Considerations. In: *Multiparticulate Oral Drug Delivery*, Ghebre-Sellassie, (ed.), Vol. I. Marcel Dekker, New York. pp. 113–142.
3. Mehta, A.M. & Jones, D.M. Coated pellets under the microscope. Pharmaceutical Technology 9(6), 52–60.

4. Leuenberger, H. (2001). New trends in the production of pharmaceutical granules: Batch versus continuous processing. European Journal of Pharmaceutics and Biopharmaceutics 52, 289–296.

5. Betz, G., Junker-Burgin, P. & Leuenberger, H. (2003). Batch and continuous processing in the production of pharmaceutical granules. Pharmaceutical Development and Technology 8, 289–297.

6. Birkmire, A.P., Walter, K.T., Liew, C.V. & Tang, E.S.K. (2004). Tablet coating in the novel SUPERCELLTM coater: Evaluation of color uniformity. Poster presented at the 2004 AAPS Annual Meeting and Exposition. Baltimore, MD.

7. Felton, L., Sturtevant, S. & Birkmire, A. (2006). A novel capsule coating process for the application of enteric coatings to small batch sizes. Poster presented at the 2006 AAPS Annual Meeting and Exposition. San Antonio, TX.

8. Rumpf, H. (1962). Agglomeration. John Wiley & Sons Inc, New York. p. 379.

9. Newitt, D.M. & Conway-Jones, J.M. (1958). A contribution to the theory and practice of granulation. Trans. Instn. Chem. Engrs. 36, 422–442.

10. Barlow, C.G. (1968). Granulation of powders. Chemical Engineering 220, CE196–CE201.

11. Huang, C.C. & Kono, H.O. (1988). The granulation of partially prewetted alumina powders—a new concept in coalescence mechanism. Powder Technology 55, 19–34.

12. Huang, C.C. & Kono, H.O. (1988). A mathematical coalescence mode in the batch fluidized bed granulator. Powder Technology 55, 35–49.

13. Abberger, T. (2001). The effect of powder type, free moisture and deformation behaviour of granules on the kinetics of fluid-bed granulation. European Journal of Pharmaceutics and Biopharmacetics 52, 327–336.

14. Ennis, B.J., Tardos, G. & Pfeffer, R. (1991). A microlevel-based characterization pf granulation phenomena. Powder Technology 65, 257–272.

15. Schaefer, T. & Worts, O. (1977). Control of fluidized bed granulation IV. Effects of binder solution and atomization on granule size and size distribution. Archiv for Pharmaci og Chemi Scientific Edition 5, 14–25.

16. Wan, L.S.C. & Lim, K.S. (1989). Mode of action of polyvinylpyrrolidone as a binder on fluidized bed granulation of lactose and starch granules. STP Pharma Pratiques 5, 244–250.

17. Schaefer, T. & Worts, O. (1977). Control of fluidized bed granulation I. Effects of spray angle, nozzle height and starting materials on granule size and size distribution. Archiv for Pharmaci og Chemi Scientific Edition 5, 51–60.

18. Schaefer, T. & Worts, O. (1977). Control of fluidized bed granulation II. Estimation of droplet size of atomized binder solutions. Archiv for Pharmaci og Chemi Scientific Edition 5, 178–193.

19. Abberger, T., Seo, A. & Schaefer, T. (2002). The effect of droplet size and powder particle size on the mechanism of nucleation and growth in fluid bed melt agglomeration. International Journal of Pharmaceutics 249, 185–197.

20. AbuBaker, O., Canter, K., Ghosh, S., Hedden, D.B., Kott, L., Pipkorn, D., Priebe, S., Qu, X. & White, C. (2003). Development of a novel scale up parameter to optimize and predict fluid bed granulation using experimental design (DOE). AAPS PharmSci. 5(4). Abstract T3295.

21. Shaefer, T. & Worts, O. (1977). Control of fluidized bed granulation III. Effect of inlet air temperature and liquid flow rate on granule size and size distribution. Control of moisture content of granules in the drying phase. Archiv for Pharmaci og Chemi Scientific Edition 6, 1–13.

22. Watano, S., Fukushima, T. & Miyanami, K. (1996). Heat transfer and granule growth rate in fluidized bed granulation. Chemical & Pharmaceutical Bulletin 44, 572–576.

23. Watabe, S., Morikawa, T. & Miyanami, K. (1996). Methematical model in the kinetics of agitation fluidized bed granulation. Effects of moisture content, damping speed and operation time on granule growth rate. Chemical & Pharmaceutical Bulletin 44, 409–415.

24. Watabe, Takahashi, H., Sato, Y., Yasutomo, T. & Miyanami, K. (1996). Measurement of moisture content by IR sensor in fluidized bed granulation. Effects of operating variables on the relationship between granule moisture content and absorbance of IR spectra. Chemical & Pharmaceutical Bulletin 44, 1267–1269.

25. Matsen, J.M. (1996). Scale-up of fluidized bed processes: Principle and practice. Powder Technology 88, 237–244.

26. Gore, A.Y., McFarland, D.W. & Batuyios, N.H. (1985). Fluid bed granulation: Factors affecting the process in laboratory development and production scale-up. Journal of Pharmacy Technology 9, 114–122.

27. Jones, D.M. (1985). Factors to consider in fluid bed processing. Journal of Pharmacy Technology 9, 50–62.

28. Horsthuis, G.J.B., van Laarhoven, J.A.H., van Rooij, R.C.B.M. & Vromans, H. (1993). Studies on upscaling parameters of the Gral high shear granulation process. International Journal of Pharmaceutics 92, 143–150.

29. Chukwumezie, B.N., Wojcik, M., Malak, P. & Adeyeye, M.C. (2002). Feasibility studies in spheronization and scale-up of ibuprofen microparticulates using the rotor disk fluid-bed technology. AAPS PharmSciTech 3, article 2, 1–13.

30. Frake, P., Greenhalgh, D., Grierson, S.M., Hempenstall, J.M. & Rudd, D.R. (1997). Process control and end-point determination of a fluid bed granulation by application of near infra-red spectroscopy. International Journal of Pharmaceutics 151, 75–80.

31. Rantanen, J., Lehtola, S., Rämet, P., Mannermaa, J.-P. & Yliruusi, J. (1998). On-line monitoring of moisture content in an instrumented fluidized bed granulator with a multi-channel NIR moisture sensor. Powder Technology 99, 163–170.

32. Watano, S., Sato, Y., Miyanami, K., Miyakami, T., Ito, T., Kamata, T. & Oda, N. (1995). Scale-up of agitation fluidized bed granulation. I. Preliminary experimental approach for optimization of process variables. Chemical & Pharmaceutical Bulletin 43, 1212–1216.

33. Watano, S., Takashima, H., Sato, Y., Yasutomo, T. & Miyanami, K. (1996). Measurement of moisture content by IR sensor in fluidized bed granulation. Effects of operating variables on the relationship between granule moisture content and absorbance of IR spectra. Chemical & Pharmaceutical Bulletin 44, 1267–1269.

34. Watano, S. & Miyanami, K. (1995). Image processing for on-line monitoring of granule size distribution and shape in fluidized bed granulation. Powder Technology 83, 55–60.

35. Watano, S., Sato, Y. & Miyanami, K. (1996). Control of granule growth in fluidized bed granulation by an image processing system. Chemical & Pharmaceutical Bulletin 44, 1556–1560.

36. Vervaet, C. & Remon, J.P. (2005). Continuous granulation in the pharmaceutical industry. Chemical Engineering Science 60, 3949–3957.

37. Betz, G., Junker-Bürgin, P. & Leuenberger, H. (2003). Batch and continuous processing in the production of pharmaceutical granules. Pharmaceutical Development and Technology 8, 289–297.

31

Development, Scale-up, and Optimization of Process Parameters: Roller Compaction

Timothy J. Smith, Gary Sackett, Paul Sheskey and Lirong Liu

31.1 HISTORY

As with many technologies used in the pharmaceutical industry, roller compaction processes and equipment were adapted and modified from other industries. The basic principle of passing material between two counter-rotating rolls was utilized in the nineteenth century in the mining industry, to crush rock for the purpose of making it easier to extract the desired precious material. Some of the first reported work of using roller compactors to compress pharmaceutical powders occurred in the mid-twentieth century. Equipment improvements in the areas of feed-screw/roll design and instrumentation have continued to bring the equipment and process to today's twenty-first century technology.

31.2 GENERAL OPERATIONAL PRINCIPLES

Typical roller compaction processes consist of the following steps:

- convey powdered material to compaction area (normally with screw feeder);
- compact powder between two counter-rotating rolls with applied forces;
- mill compact (sheet, flake or briquette) to desired particle size distribution.

Milled, roller compacted particles are typically dense, with sharp-edged profiles as shown in Figure 31.1.

31.3 REASONS TO USE ROLLER COMPACTION

There are several reasons for using roller compaction technology:

- no or low dust, increased safety when working with toxic or explosive materials;
- improved flow characteristics;
- no segregation of components;

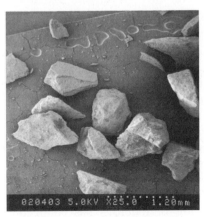

FIGURE 31.1   SEM photo of milled, roller compacted particles

Developing Solid Oral Dosage Forms: Pharmaceutical Theory and Practice
ISBN: 978-0-444-53242-8

- increased bulk density;
- increased particle size.

31.4 ADVANTAGES AND DISADVANTAGES OF ROLLER COMPACTION

31.4.1 Advantages

- simple process (no wetting or drying steps);
- moisture-sensitive products can be processed;
- heat-sensitive products can be processed;
- drug and color migration do not occur;
- shorter disintegration times can be obtained (if no binder is used);
- less equipment, cost, and space are required;
- continuous process.

31.4.2 Disadvantages

- dissolution can be adversely affected, due to densification;
- powders must be compressible (if primary product powder is not compressible, then a compressible component must be added to the formulation);
- usually requires the addition of a lubricant to minimize sticking to the rolls.

31.5 FEED SYSTEM

Over the years different manufacturers have employed vertical, horizontal, tapered, and angular screw mechanism (or various combinations) to convey the product to the compaction zone, as shown in Figure 31.2. In addition to conveying the product, the feed mechanisms are also designed to facilitate the removal of entrained air from the product.

31.6 ROLL DESIGNS

Different roll designs are utilized, depending on the equipment manufacturer, and the type of processing or product desired. Roll surfaces typically are smooth, serrated or pocketed. Roll shape may be flat or straight-sided cylinders or may have a flanged-type outer edge (known as "concavo–convex" or "D" and "P") shaped rolls. Some examples are illustrated in Figure 31.3.

In addition to the shape and texture of the rolls, the mounting of the rolls has changed over time.

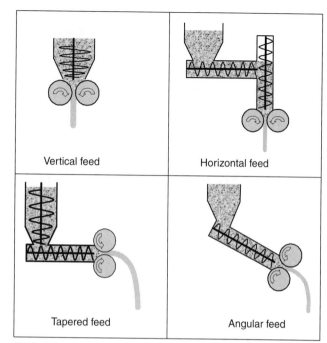

FIGURE 31.2   Roller compaction feed systems

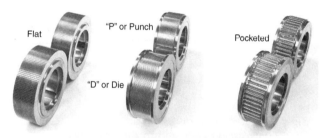

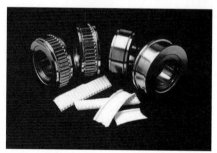

FIGURE 31.3   Roll designs

Originally, the rolls were mounted between two bearing mounts. To make the rolls easier to remove for cleaning, the mounting design has changed to a cantilevered design.

31.7 COMPACTION THEORY

As the powder is compacted, it passes through three different regions or zones, as shown in Figure 31.4.

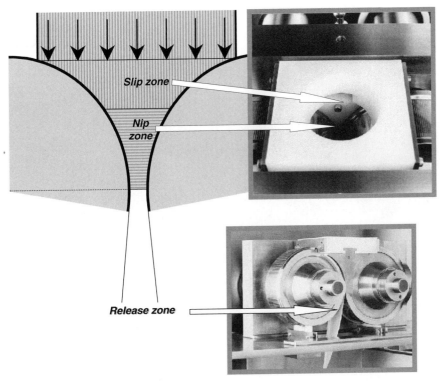

FIGURE 31.4 Compaction process

Compaction process details (illustrated in Figure 31.4)

Slip zone	Deaeration of the powder occurs in this region.
	Powder is forced into the gap between the rolls via a sliding motion that results from the rotation of the feed screw and roll surfaces.
	Internal friction coefficient of powder determines the size of the slip zone (larger coefficient = smaller slip zone = longer compaction time).
Nip zone	Defined by the nip angle (a) which is determined theoretically by the compression factor, roll/powder friction angle, and the internal friction angle.
	Starts where no slippage of powder occurs at the roll surface.
	Powder is carried into the roll gap at the same speed as the roll surface.
	To achieve acceptable compaction, the nip angle must be large or residence time in the nip zone must be increased to permit particle bonding to occur.
Release zone	Elastic recovery (expansion) of the compacted sheet occurs as it is released from the rolls.
	Expansion of the compact is a function of the physical characteristics of the material, roll diameter, and roll speed.
	More effective deaeration of the powder reduces the expansion due to improved bond formation (conversion to plastic deformation as opposed to elastic).

31.8 DEAERATION

Sometimes the powder being compressed needs to have more air removed than the feed system and roller compactor can achieve on its own. A deaeration section just prior to the rolls is then utilized. The section consists of a sintered metal or screen that permits air to be removed via a vacuum device.

31.9 CONTROL MECHANISMS

Various control schemes have been implemented to better understand and control the compaction process. Independent, variable speeds for feed screw and rolls are utilized, in addition to monitoring the electrical current/power and/or torque applied to the screws/rolls. Typically hydraulic pressure is used to apply

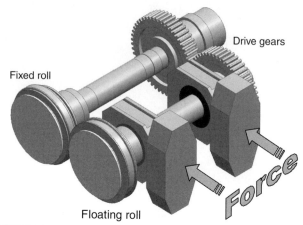

Drive gears

Fixed roll

Floating roll

FIGURE 31.5   Control mechanisms

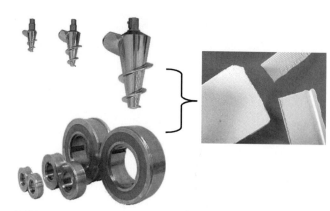

FIGURE 31.6   Scalable roller compaction

the force to the rolls—the force (hydraulic pressure) is either set at a predetermined level or is modulated via control feedback to maintain the proper roll force (Figure 31.5). Some systems have also instituted a roll gap measurement or control, to assist in maintaining the proper compaction conditions.

31.10 SCALE-UP

Roller compaction equipment comes in various sizes, as shown in Figure 31.6, but the product remains consistent as the device scale is increased, if processing parameters are adjusted appropriately.

31.10.1 Scale-up Throughput Calculations

Step 1:	
Using data from pilot scale equipment calculate the compacted sheet density.	$\gamma = \dfrac{Q \times 1000}{\pi \cdot D \cdot W \cdot t \cdot N \times 60}$ D = Roll diameter (cm) W = Roll width (cm) t = Sheet thickness (cm) γ = Sheet density (g/cc) N = Roll speed (rpm) Q = Throughput (kg/h)
Step 2: Using the computed sheet density, compute the projected throughput for the larger roll compaction unit. Note: The throughput in the roll compactor is directly related to the powder feed rate.	$Q = \dfrac{\pi \cdot D \cdot W \cdot t \cdot \gamma \cdot N \times 60}{1000}$ D = Roll diameter (cm) of large unit W = Roll width (cm) of large unit t = Sheet thickness (cm) from small unit γ = Calculated sheet density (g/cc) N = Roll speed (rpm) from small unit

Scale-up throughput calculations

31.10.2 Scale-up for Achieving Consistent Sheet Density

1. Determine the force applied per linear inch of the compaction roll width. Use this as the starting point for processing on larger units.
2. For initial scale-up, use the same linear roll velocity.
3. Adjust the screw speed as necessary, to achieve the desired compact thickness.

Note: the screw speed may not scale directly from laboratory size roll compactor to the production size.

31.11 CASE STUDIES

31.11.1 SCALE-UP CASE STUDY

A matrix, controlled-release tablet formulation containing theophylline 50%, METHOCEL K4MP CR (hypromellose 2208 USP) 30%, anhydrous lactose 19.75%, and magnesium stearate 0.25% was scaled-up from laboratory-scale to production-scale, using a roller compaction granulation process (see Table 31.1).

Figure 31.7 shows the similarity of the particle size distribution testing results of milled ribbons manufactured using pilot-scale and production-scale roller compaction equipment.

Figure 31.8 shows the similarity in the drug dissolution results of tablets prepared from the controlled-release

TABLE 31.1 Roller compaction scaling factor

		Trial #		
		1	2	3
Scale from:		TF-156	TF-156	TF-156
Scale to:	TF-156	TF-3012	TF-3012	TF-3012
Roll setting:	Actual	Direct scale	2 × scale	4 × scale
Pressure setting:	Direct	Direct	Direct	Direct
Roll speed (rpm):	8	4	8	16.01
Roll linear velocity (in/min):	148.5	148.5	297	593.9
Screw speed (rpm):	10.4	5.2	10.4	20.8
Roll force (tons):	5.3	10.8	10.8	10.8
Screw/roll ratio:	1.3:1	1.3:1	1.3:1	1.3:1
Force (tons) per linear inch:	3.1	3.1	3.1	3.1

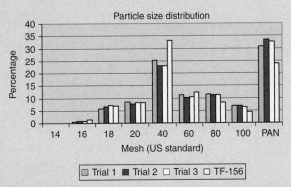

FIGURE 31.7 Particle size distribution results comparing material generated using pilot-scale and production-scale roller compaction equipment

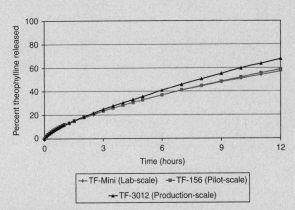

FIGURE 31.8 Drug dissolution results for all three scales of manufacturing studied

CASE STUDY   (CONTINUED)

study using different roller compaction equipment manufacturing scales.

Table 31.2 shows the tablet physical testing results of tablets prepared using different scales of manufacturing using roller compaction granulation. Data show good similarity between scales of manufacturing. The results also show that the speed at which the roller compactor equipment was operated at did not influence tablet crushing strength values.

Stability Testing of Scale-up Study

Formulation theophylline 50%, METHOCEL K4MP CR (2208 USP) 30%, anhydrous lactose 19.75%, and magnesium stearate 0.25%.

TABLE 31.2   Results of tablet physical testing

Trial description	Tablet crushing strength (kp, sd)	Tablet thickness (mm)	Tablet weight (mg, sd)
TF-mini (laboratory)	17.3, 1.9	5.77	401.5, 8.3
TF-156, 1 × speed (pilot)	17.9, 1.6	5.82	402.1, 6.6
TF-156, 4 × speed (pilot)	20.6, 1.1	5.82	398.8, 3.6
TF-3012, 1 × speed (production)	21.2, 1.1	5.72	400.1, 3.6
TF-3012, 4 × speed (production)	21.6, 1.3	5.79	401.2, 3.6

TABLE 31.3   Effect of storage time and conditions on physical properties of hydrophilic controlled-release matrix tablets using a Vector TF-3012 production-scale roller compactor

Stability sample (time, condition)	Crushing strength (kp, sd)	Thickness (mm)	Average tablet weight (mg, sd)
Initial	21.8, 1.0	5.7	401, 2
Ambient (21°C/50% RH)			
1 month	20.8, 2.1	5.7	402, 9
2 months	19.3, 1.8	5.8	400, 5
3 months	18.5, 1.0	5.9	403, 4
6 months	17.0, 1.0	5.8	403, 4
9 months	19.3, 1.3	5.9	401, 5
12 months	18.9, 1.1	5.7	403, 5
Accelerated (40°C/75% RH)			
1 month	18.7, 1.5	5.7	405, 7
2 months	17.4, 1.1	5.9	404, 4
3 months	17.4, 0.9	5.9	400, 4
6 months	15.5, 0.9	5.8	402, 4
9 months	11.3, 0.8	6.0	404, 6
12 months	13.4, 0.9	6.0	413, 6

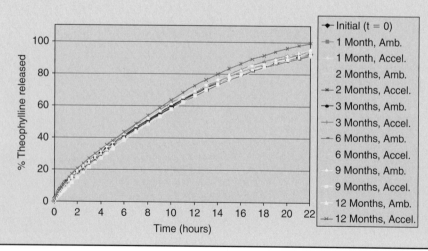

FIGURE 31.9   Drug dissolution testing of stability samples from production-scale (Vector model TF-3012) roller compaction granulations

31.11.2 Bulk Densities of Various Materials Before and After Roller Compaction

Material	Before	After	% Change
Acetaminophen	0.360	0.567	57.5
Aminobenzoic acid	0.334	0.491	47.0
Calcium carbonate, precipitated	0.267	0.657	146.1
Dibasic calcium phosphate, dihydrate	0.695	0.943	35.7
Dicalcium phosphate, granular	0.890	0.939	5.5
Lactose, hydrous	0.633	0.697	10.1
Magnesium carbonate, light	0.152	0.460	202.6
Sulfadiazine	0.296	0.592	100.0
Sulfisoxazole	0.368	0.610	65.8

Bulk densities of various materials before and after roller compaction

31.11.3 Effect of Compaction Pressure on Bulk Density

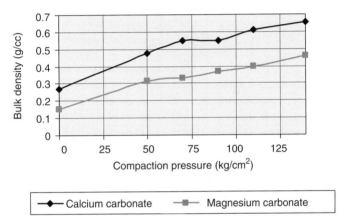

Effect of compaction pressure on bulk density

31.11.4 Compaction of Aspirin

Material: Aspirin

Before roll compaction:
Particle size: Less than 44 micron
Bulk density: 0.282 g/cc

After roll compaction:
Bulk density: 0.639 g/cc

Microns	US mesh	Percent retained	Cumulative percent
1190	16	14.50	14.50
840	20	22.60	37.10
420	40	43.20	80.30
250	60	5.90	86.20
177	80	3.90	90.10
149	100	2.10	92.20
<149	PAN	7.80	100.00
Total		100.00	

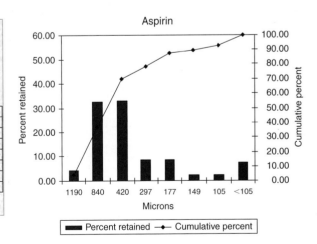

Compaction of aspirin

31.11.5 Troubleshooting

Problem	Possible cause	Remedies
Sticking to compaction rolls	Insufficient lubricant level	Add lubricant; typically 0.2–0.5%
	Excessive moisture	Reduce moisture content Dehumidify environment
	Poor scraper adjustment	Decrease clearance between rolls and scrapers Replace worn scrapers
	Excessive force	Decrease roll force
	Melting of product	Cool rolls to decrease temperature; use water or nitrogen
	Improper roll configuration	Use smooth rolls, or grooved rolls
Soft compact/friable granulation	Improper formulation	Increase compressible binder Decrease lubricant level
	Compaction force too low	Increase compaction force
	Compaction (dwell) time too short	Decrease roll speed
	Excess blend time for powder and lubricant	Decrease blend time
	Raw material variation	Monitor key raw material specifications
Excessive fines	Air entrapment	Use deaeration system
	Leakage of powder	Tighten seals (top/side) Replace worn seals
	Poor powder compressibility	Increase compressible binder Screen/sieve product to desired particle size
	Improper granulator/mill screen	Use coarser screen for milling compacts
	Improper granulator/mill speed	Slow mill speed down
	Low compaction force	Increase roll force
Low bulk/tap density	Compaction force too low	Increase roll force
	Particle size too large	Use finer screen/plate to mill the compacts
	"Challenging material"	May need to pass material through roller compactor several times
Poor flow characteristics	Too many fines	See remedies for "Excessive fines"
	Particle size too small	Use coarser screen/plate to mill the compacts
Poor granule dissolution	Compaction force is too high	Decrease roll force
	Improper formulation	Add a disintegrant (i.e. starch; MCC)
Drug release profile – too slow	Poor formulation – slow release	Increase % hydrophilic polymer Use polymer with lower MW Decrease % lubricant
Drug release profile – too fast	Poor formulation – fast release	Increase hydrophilic polymer (i.e. HPMC) Use polymer with greater molecular weight (MW)
Low throughput/production rate	Feed rate too slow to compaction zone	Increase screw/roll speed ratio
	Improper screw design	Use an alternate screw (double flight)
	Air entrapment	Use a deaeration system
Poor product stability/ discoloration	Heat generation during compaction or milling	Decrease compaction force Use water-cooled rolls Use nitrogen cooling
Improper sheet thickness	Poor scalability of the screw/roll speed ratio	Increase screw/roll speed ratio to Increase thickness Decrease screw/roll speed ratio to decrease thickness
	Improper roll gap setting	Adjust roll gap to desired thickness
Compaction in hopper/top seal	Improper screw/roll speed ratio	Increase roll speed or Decrease screw speed
	Improper screw/hopper clearance	Increase clearance between the screw feeder and side walls of the hopper
Mottled (spotted) tablet appearance	Overcompaction of powder	Decrease compaction force
	Material sticking to rolls	Follow remedies for "Sticking to compaction rolls"

Troubleshooting

31.12 APPLICATION OF PROCESS ANALYTICAL TECHNOLOGY TO ROLLER COMPACTION

Process analytical technology (PAT), e.g., NIR, effusivity … etc., are being used to monitor and control the modern roller compaction process.

31.12.1 CASE STUDY

Use of effusivity as a non-destructive method to determine the effects of compression forces on the thermal property changes in the products from two pharmaceutical compaction processes.

Method

Formulation (A) contained 30% hydroxypropyl methylcellulose, 69% lactose Fast-Flo®, and 1% magnesium stearate. The mixture was blended in a high shear mixer, and compressed by a hydraulic press (Carver press) at 1250, 2500, 3750, 5000, 7500, and 10000 psi for 10 seconds.

A similar formulation (B) with 0.3% of magnesium stearate was blended in a v-blender, and compressed into ribbons using a roller compactor (Vector Model TF-156) equipped with 6cm wide smooth rolls at 500, 750, 1000, and 1500 psi. The ratio of screw speed to roll speed was kept constant for all compression levels. The thermal effusivity of the compacts and ribbons were analyzed using Mathis Instruments Thermal Effusivity Sensor (Model ESP-01), with 315g of weight applied on the top of the ribbon.

Formulation (B) was used to study the impact of the roll design. Ribbons were manufactured using two different roll types, smooth surface, and serrated surface. The thermal effusivity of both sides of the ribbons was analyzed with same effusivity sensor, and 500g of weight applied.

Effusivity

$$Effusivity = \sqrt{k \rho c_p}$$

where:

k = thermal conductivity (W/m · K)
ρ = density (kg/m^3)
c_p = heat capacity (J/kg · K)

Result: Effect of Pressure by Hydraulic Press Process

The effusivity results of the compacts manufactured with a Carver press at different pressures are shown in Figure 31.10.

Result: Effect of Pressure by Roller Compactor Process

The effusivity results of ribbons manufactured with the roller compactor (smooth rolls) at different pressures with 315g of weight applied to the sensor are shown in Figure 31.11.

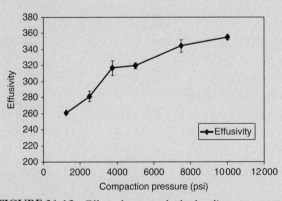

FIGURE 31.10   Effect of pressure by hydraulic press process

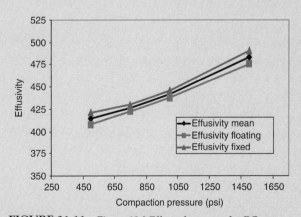

FIGURE 31.11   Figure 12.2 Effect of pressure by RC process

CASE STUDY   (CONTINUED)

Result: Effect of Different Roll Surface Design

The effusivity results from ribbons manufactured using smooth rolls and serrated rolls at different pressures with 500 g of weight applied to the sensor are shown in Figure 31.12 and Figure 31.13.

Conclusions

As the compaction pressure increases, a general trend of increase in thermal effusivity is observed. This is due to the significant change in density and/or porosity of the compacted tablet or ribbon.

Comparing the effect of the smooth roll to the serrated roll, there is a significant difference in thermal effusivity. The variation in thermal effusivity was greater for the ribbon produced using the smooth rolls. This may be due to increased slippage at the roll/powder interface. The roll serrations reduce slippage, thus producing more consistent compact density/thermal effusivity results.

Differences in thermal effusivity measurements from the floating to fixed roll side may be due to variability in the pressure distribution or curvature of the compacted ribbon affecting the contact with the effusivity sensor.

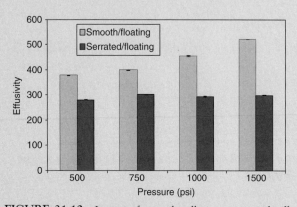

FIGURE 31.12 Impact of smooth roll versus serrated roll measured on floating roll side of the ribbon

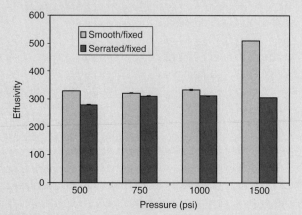

FIGURE 31.13 Impact of smooth roll versus serrated roll measured on fixed roll side of the ribbon

31.13 ROLLER COMPACTOR SUPPLIERS

ALEXANDERWERK AG
Kippdorfstr. 6–24, 42857 Remscheid/Germany.
Telephone: +49 (0) 2191/7 95-0.
www.alexanderwerk.com.

FITZPATRICK
832 Industrial Drive, Elmhurst, IL 60126 USA.
Business telephone: 630-530-3333; Fax: 630-530-0832.
www.fitzmill.com.

GERTEIS MASCHINEN + PROCESS
ENGINEERING AG
Stampfstrasse 74, Postfach 2138, CH-8645 Jona, Switzerland.
Telephone: +41 55 222 55 22; Fax: +41 55 222 55 23.
www.gerteis.com.

VECTOR CORPORATION
675 44th Street, Marion, IA 52302-3800 USA.
Business telephone: 319-377-8263 Fax: 319-377-5574.
www.vectorcorporation.com (ISO 9001 Certified).

References

1. Sheskey, P.J., et al. (2000). Effect of process scale-up on robustness of tablets, tablet stability, and predicted *in vivo* performance. Pharmaceutical Technology 14, November 30–52.
2. Parrott, E.L. (1981). Densification of powders by concavo-convex roller compactor. Journal of Pharmaceutical Sciences 70(3), 288–291.
3. Sackett, G., Liu, L., Smith, T. J., Roy, Y., Natoli, D., Qiu, R., Mathis, N. & Sheskey, P. (2005). Application of Thermal Effusivity as a Non-Destructive Method to Evaluate the Impact of Compression Forces. 2005 American Association of Pharmaceutical Scientists Annual Meeting. Nashville, TN, USA.

Development, Optimization, and Scale-up of Process Parameters: Tablet Compression

Dale Natoli, Michael Levin, Lev Tsygan and Lirong Liu

32.1 INTRODUCTION

Compressing pharmaceutical tablets is one of the most efficient processes for producing a single dose of medication. Tablets are accepted and trusted by professionals and consumers alike, they are easily administered and simple to dose.

Compressing powders into a solid form dates back thousands of years. It wasn't until the early 1800s that tablet compression was automated, in the sense that the hand crank was replaced by a leather belt and a steam driven power bar. Early single station tablet presses produced an average of 100 tablets per minute (TPM), while maintaining uniformity requirements for tablet hardness, thickness, and weight. Soon after, single station presses were fading and making room for a new technology, the rotary tablet press. Introduced in the mid-1800s, the rotary tablet press boasted speeds capable of compressing 640 tablets per minute, compared to high speed presses today which are capable of compressing up to 24 000 tablets per minute.

32.2 OPERATIONAL PRINCIPLES OF COMPRESSION BY ROTARY PRESS

Modern rotary presses usually include the following components:

Name of component	Function (s)
Hopper	Containing powder
Feeder (gravity, forced, centrifugal/die feed)	Distribute power into die cavity Provide additional mixing
Turret	Position and progress the punch and die
Punch, lower and higher	Accept powder from feeder Contain powder until compression occurs Densify and compress the powder Eject the compressed tablet
Feed cam	Lower the lower punch to allow powder to come in
Cam pressure rolls upper/lower	Force upper and lower punch to compress
Ejection cam	Lift the lower punch and push tablet above the turret
Ejection plate	Remove tablet off turret
Hydraulic	Provide hydraulic pressure
Instrumentation	Monitor force, speed, distance … etc.
Air handling	Provide exhaust.

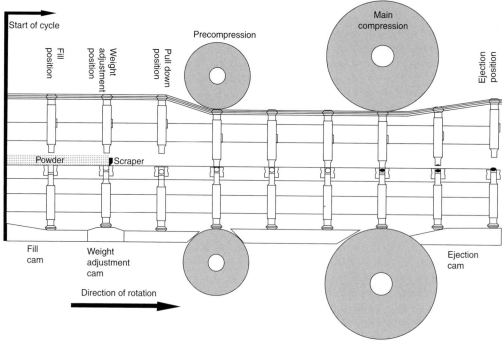

FIGURE 32.1   Rotary tablet press cycle

32.3 BEST PRACTICE

FIGURE 32.1   Continued

32.4 TOOL DESIGN

Good granulation is important for compressing quality tablets. If the granulation is poor, the long-term results will also be. A proper tablet granulation will have good flow, compressibility, and release properties. Tablet compression tooling is equally responsible for the success of a tableting program. Tooling must be engineered to withstand the stresses associated with tablet compression, provide satisfactory service life, and maintain physical tablet uniformity. A proper tablet design is also critical. Pharmaceutical marketing departments feverishly attempt to design unique tablets, anticipating the design will quickly become branded, and trusted in the eye of the consumer. A proper tool design is essential for putting that innovative design into the sight of the consumer.

The basic knowledge of tablet compression tooling and tablet design can save literally millions of dollars, prevent product loss, and reduce unnecessary equipment downtime. Understanding the basic physics of tablet compression will greatly enhance the ability to compress quality tablets more efficiently, and provide better knowledge to troubleshoot and identify potential pitfalls before they occur, and they will.

Communication is important with any tableting campaign. Marketing, R&D, engineering, production, and the tooling supplier must be in accord, and communicate new product-design and production requirements. The ideas and responsibilities of these departments may vary, but they share the common goal of manufacturing a quality tablet, efficiently and productively.

32.4.1 Terminology

To communicate properly and understand the following material it is important to have a basic understanding of the terminology used in this industry. Although these terms are most common and accepted, some terms may vary slightly between countries. This article deals with the terminology and general information related to the most commonly used rotary press tooling, the "TSM," "B," "D," "Euronorm" 19 mm, and 24 mm configurations.

TABLE 32.1   Common tooling terminology

Term	Definition
Tooling set	A complete set of punches and dies to accommodate all stations in a tablet press
Tooling station	The upper punch. lower punch, and die which accommodate one station in a tablet press
Head	The largest diameter of a common punch which contacts the machines cams and accepts the pressure from the pressure rollers
Head flat	The flat portion of the head which makes contact with the pressure rollers and determines the maximum dwell time for compression
Top head angle	Angle from the outside head diameter to the top head radius; it allows for sufficient head thickness and smoother camming
Top head radius	The radius on the top of the head which blends the top head angle to the head flat. Some head configurations may consist of only the head radius without the head angle. This radius makes the initial contact with the pressure roll and allows a smoother transition into the compression cycle
Head back angle	Sometimes referred to as the inside head angle. Located underneath the top head angle or the top head radius which contacts the machine camming for vertical movement of the punch within the punch guides
Neck	Located below the head and provides clearance as the punch cycles through the machine cams
Barrel or shank	The vertical bearing surface of a punch which makes contact with the punch guides in the machine turret for vertical guidance
Barrel chamfer	Chamfers at the ends of the punch barrel, eliminate outside corners
Barrel-to-stem radius	The radius that blends the punch barrel to the stem
Stem	The area from the barrel to the edge of the punch tip
Tip length	The straight portion of the punch stem
Tip straight	The section of the tip that extends from the tip relief to the end of the punch tip; it maintains the punch tip size tolerance
Land	The area between the edge of the punch cup and the outside diameter of the punch tip; this adds strength to the tip to reduce punch tip fracturing
Tip face or cup	The portion of the punch tip that determines the contour of the tablet face; it includes the tablet embossing
Cup depth	The depth of the cup from the highest point of the tip edge to the lowest point of the cavity
Tip relief	The portion of the punch stem which is a undercut or made smaller than the punch tip straight; most common for lower punches to aid in reducing friction from the punch tip and die wall as the punch travels through the compression cycle; the area where the punch tip and relief meet must be sharp to scrape product from the die wall as the lower punch travels down for the fill cycle
Key	A projection normally of mild steel which protrudes above the surface of the punch barrel. It maintains alignment of the upper punch for reentry into the die; mandatory on upper punches with multiple tips and all tablet shapes other than round; commonly used with embossed round tablet shapes when rotation of the punch causes a condition known as double impression
Key position	The radial and height position of a key on the punch barrel; not found in all presses
Punch overall length	The total length of a punch, other than flat-face tablet configurations, that is normally a reference dimension which consist of a combination of the working length and the cup depth dimensions
Working length	The dimension from the head flat to the lowest measurable point of the tip face, responsible for the consistency of the tablet overall thickness
Anneal	A heat-treating process used on fragile punch tips to decrease the hardness of the punch cups reducing punch tip fracturing
Bakelite tip relief	An undercut groove between the lower punch tip straight and the relief; it assures a sharp corner to assist in scraping product adhering to the die wall; normally a purchased option for lower punches
Major axis	The largest dimension of a shaped tablet
Minor axis	The smallest dimension of a shaped tablet
End radius	The radius on either end of a capsule or oval-shaped tablet

TABLE 32.2   Tablet terminology

Term	Definition
Major axis	The largest dimension of a shaped tablet
Minor axis	The smallest dimension of a shaped tablet
End radius	The radius on either end of a capsule or oval-shaped tablet
Side radius	The radius on either side of an oval or modified shaped tablet
Band	The center section of a tablet between the cup profiles; of the die profile
Compound cup	A cup profile which consists of two or more radii
Embossed	The raised identification on a tablet or a punch face; an EMB punch tip results in an engraved tablet
Engraved	The depressed identification on a tablet or a punch face; an engraved punch tip results in an embossed tablet

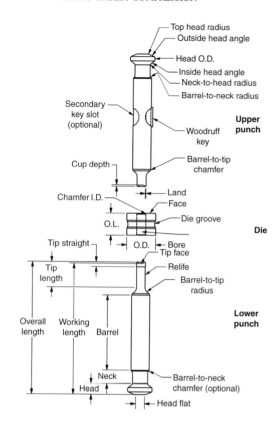

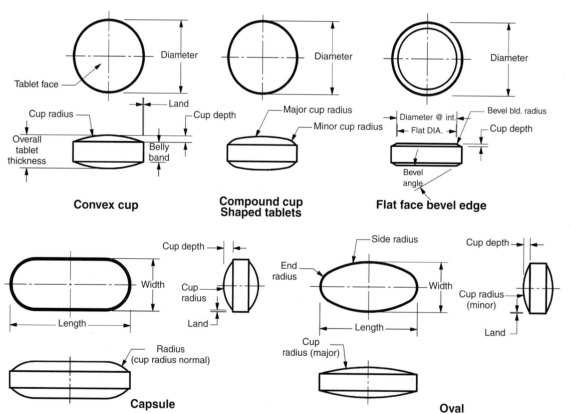

FIGURE 32.2

32.4.2 Common Tooling Standards

Internationally there are two recognized standards for tablet compression tooling, the "TSM" and the "EU" standards. Both TSM and EU standards identify the physical tool configuration for B and D type tablet compression tools, their critical dimensions and associated tolerances ensure tablet quality, and an efficient tablet press operation.

The TSM tooling standard is recognized in the Americas, and is considered exclusive to the United States. TSM is the acronym for the *Tableting Specification Manual*, which is published, revised, and distributed by the American Pharmacist Association in Washington DC. The TSM standards, once known as the IPT standards, were originally developed in 1968 by a committee consisting of major pharmaceutical companies in the United States. The motivation was an attempt to maintain standardization for B and D tablet compression tooling, which provides interchangeability between tablet presses. The TSM provides engineered drawings that are a valuable reference for troubleshooting and tool inspection. Today, the TSM committee consists of professionals from the tablet press, tooling, and tablet manufacturing industries. The TSM also includes useful information such as standard cup configurations for round tablets and a reference to common bisects for breaking tablets into multiple uniform dosages.

The EU tooling standard is internationally recognized, and is more widely used than its counterpart, the TSM standard. EU (the acronym for Eurostandard and Euronorm) is considered the European standard for interchangeable B and D type compression tools. The EU standards are authored by Mr Trevor Higgins with the attempt to establish a tooling norm that provides tool interchangeability with the most common B and D type European tablet presses. The EU standard is printed and distributed by I Holland Ltd, Nottingham, England.

32.4.3 EU, TSM, B, and D Type Punches

The TSM and EU standards manuals provide mechanical drawings and technical information for B and D type tools, which constitute a majority of the tool configurations used today. The B type configuration has a nominal punch barrel diameter of 0.750″ (19 mm). The B type has two different die sizes. The larger B dies have a diameter of 1.1875″ (30.16 mm), and the smaller BB dies have a 0.945″ (24 mm)

diameter. The D type has a larger nominal barrel diameter of 1″ (25.4 mm) and a die diameter of 1.500″ (38.10 mm.) The B and D tool designation identifies the physical tooling size, and was coined by engineer Frank J. Stokes in the late-1800s.

Mr Stokes resided in Philadelphia, Pennsylvania when he developed the first commercially available rotary tablet press in the United States, the Stokes B1 Rotary. The B1 rotary press was extremely successful, and most wanted by pharmaceutical companies nationwide. Mr Stokes, realizing the need for compressing larger and heavier tablets, developed the Stokes D3 rotary tablet press. The D3 tablet press uses slightly larger punches and dies, increasing the overall capacity to compress larger and heavier tablets.

During the second industrial revolution, Mr Stokes expanded manufacturing capabilities, and operated a facility in England for international distribution. Stokes soon became the world's leading tablet press manufacturer, and sold tablet presses and tooling in nearly every industrialized country. The designation B and D quickly became the international standard for identifying a tablet press capacity and a tool configuration, as it still is today.

At the brink of World War II, Stokes left England and focused all manufacturing activities in Pennsylvania. Stokes left behind trained engineers and qualified manufacturing personnel, who soon realized the potential of the tablet press market, and began manufacturing tablet presses and tooling, under the name Manesty. As a marketing strategy, Manesty re-engineered the punches and tablet press cams, to enhance tooling life and provide better performance. The Manesty punch is similar to the original Stokes design, but is exclusive to Manesty presses and not interchangeable with the more popular Stokes tablet presses. Manesty called their tablet presses the Manesty B3B, and the larger Manesty D3A.

Manesty soon became a major supplier in the compression equipment industry, and successfully competed against Stokes in the global market. In the mid-1980s the tablet press industry exploded, and press manufacturers were competing with tablet press output and innovation. Accommodating newer and higher-speed tablet presses, the original Manesty tooling standard was refined to provide better interchangeability with the most common B and D tablet presses, identified by the Eurostandard, often referred to as the EU standard and the EU norm.

There are various models of tablet presses that do not conform to the standard B and D tool configuration,

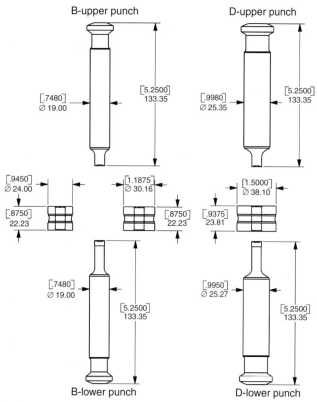

FIGURE 32.3   Punch and die terminology

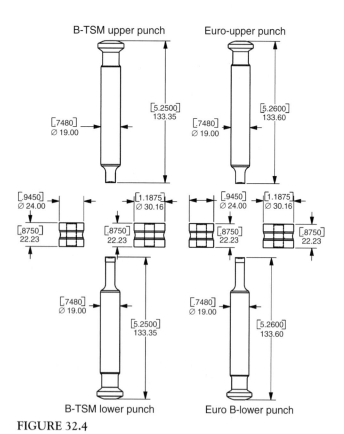

FIGURE 32.4

that are engineered to be exclusive to a particular make and model of tablet press. Some of the more common configurations were designed in the early 1900s, and are still used on tablet presses today. These unique tablet presses are generally larger, and engineered to compress larger tablets more effectively. Kilian Gmbh, a division of IMA in Milan, Italy, is a major European manufacturer of tablet presses using the most common unique tool configuration. The Kilian style upper punch does not use the common punch head configuration to guide the punches through the press cams instead, the upper punch is guided by a machined cam angle located on the side of the upper barrel. The Kilian design provides a larger head flat, therefore, increasing the compression dwell time over the more popular B and D type tools.

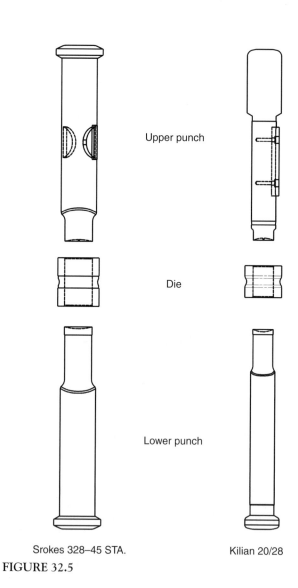

FIGURE 32.5

32.4.4 Recent Innovations

New technology continues to introduce innovative tool configurations in the effort to provide better efficiency of tablet press speed, product yield, cleaning and safety.

In 1997, IMA introduced a line of unique tablet presses called the IMA Comprima. The IMA Comprima models use an innovative approach with tool design and granulation delivery. Unlike traditional tablet presses using a gravity feed frame or force feeding mechanism to fill the die with granulation, the Ima Comprima feeds the granulation through the die table, taking advantage of the centrifugal force created by the rotating turret for a rapid and uniform die fill. Unlike traditional presses, the IMA Comprima ejects the compressed tablet through the bottom of the die, and uses gravity to eject the tablet from the press. Traditional tablet presses eject the tablet at the top of the die, requiring a mechanical stop or a take-off bar to physically contact the tablet and knock it from the lower punch face. The IMA Comprima press is engineered to improve product yield, while providing a dust free environment for a cleaner operation and a safer environment for the operator.

The most recent innovation with tablet press and tooling technology is developed by Fette GmbH, located in Schwarzenbek, Germany. The new technology was introduced in 2005, and is being favored by high-volume tablet manufacturers. The technology does not use traditional compression dies, instead Fette developed die segments. Die segments provide an advantage over traditional dies by combining the tablet press turret die table and dies into three, five or seven integral segments. Die segments are much easier and quicker to install than individual dies and die locks, dramatically reducing tablet press set-up time. Because the concept does not require the use of dies, more space is available around the turret circumference to increase the number of punches, resulting in more tablets compressed per revolution than traditional presses of the same size.

Tablet press technology has recently brought attention to the steel used for punches and dies with "wash in place" tablet presses. "Wash in place" tablet presses are becoming more common, and are available from most major tablet press suppliers. To reduce the possibility of tool discoloration and corrosion, it's important that the tools are immediately removed and dried, if the tools cannot be confirmed dry in the tablet press turret.

32.4.5 Cup Depth, Overall Length, and Working Length

These are the most critical dimensions in any tooling program that relate directly to final tablet thickness, weight, and hardness. The overall length (OL) is a reference dimension, therefore, does not have a specified tolerance. A reference dimension is defined by the *Machinery Handbook*[2] as:

> A dimension, usually without a tolerance and used for information purposes only. It is considered auxiliary information and does not govern production or inspection operations. A reference dimension is the repeat of a dimension or is derived from other values shown on the drawing or on related drawings.

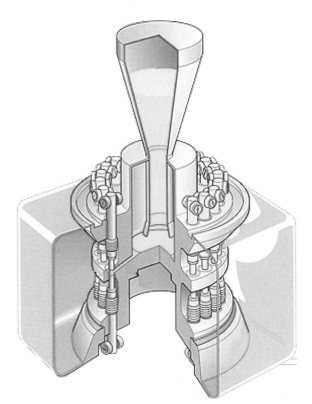

FIGURE 32.6   IMA press and tools

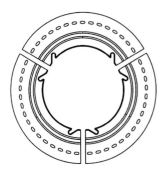

Fette 2090 die segments

FIGURE 32.6A   Continued

The two dimensions making up the punch overall lengths are the working length and the cup depth, with the exception of flat-face tip configuration, which does not have a cup and is used to compress a wafer type tablet. The two dimensions are the working length dimension, with a tolerance of ±0.001", and the cup depth, tolerance ±0.003". Combining the two tolerances that affect the OL of a punch, the calculated tolerance would be ±0.004". The major concern with these dimensions is to maintain consistency within a set of punches in order to maintain tablet weight, hardness, and thickness. The more critical of the two dimensions is the working length (WL). The working length needs to be inspected as a single dimension, and preferably for consistency within the given working-length tolerance, not for a number formulated from the cup depth subtracted from the overall length. A set of punches should be separated into uppers and lowers, and inspected for variances as such. For example, all of the upper punches are checked for length consistency, and then all of the lower punches are checked as a separate unit. As long as both upper and lower punches fall within the desired tolerance range, tablet thickness, hardness, and weight will be consistent. Although the cup depth is not responsible for tablet thickness, it should be confirmed within the given tolerance to maintain tablet overall consistency, it should also be inspected as single dimension.

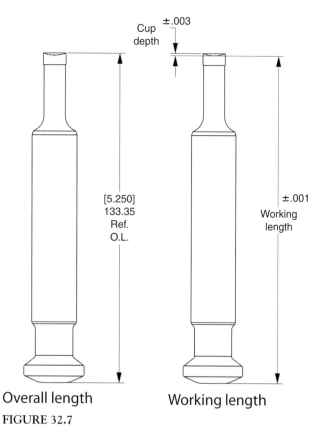

Overall length　　　　Working length

FIGURE 32.7

32.4.6 Tooling Options

During the 1980s, the tablet compression industry was introduced to higher speed and more automated tablet presses, ensuring interchangeability with the TSM standard tool configurations. Although the standard tool configuration may be compatible, in some cases it was not optimal and required minor modification to achieve expected performance. Also, the standard tool configuration may not be desirable for compressing certain products. All products are different and have unique characteristics, and likewise may require slight tooling modifications. Tablet manufacturers need to be informed of available options to achieve the best possible performance from the tablet press and tooling. A description of tooling options that can be a benefit on both high-speed and standard presses follows.

Common Tooling Options

Domed heads

The domed head configuration is adaptable to both the upper and lower punch, and maintains the identical top head radius and head flat as the Eurostandard. It is an option only for the TSM head configuration, is compatible with the American TSM cams, and should be considered for all high-speed tablet presses. As the speed of the tablet press continues to increase, tablet manufacturers are coming to realize the advantage of the domed-style head with the larger top radius. The domed head style has several advantages over the standard TSM head profile. The larger 5/8" radius on the domed head reduces the enormous stress, which is more common with the smaller 5/16" radius on a standard head when the punch makes initial contact with the pressure roller. This stress can cause a condition called head pitting, which is identified by voids on the head flat. This form of pitting is detrimental to the life of the punches and pressure rollers. The domed head configuration provides a smoother transition into the compression cycle of the tablet press, reducing stress and premature wear of the pressure rollers.

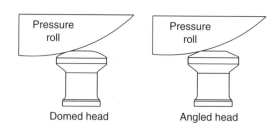

Domed head　　　　Angled head

FIGURE 32.8

Extended head flat

Some tool manufacturers will provide a head profile with a larger head flat. The advantage of the larger head flat is to increase the tablet press output and/or to increase the dwell time of compression. The disadvantage of the extended head flat is the possibility of head fracturing. Head fracturing can occur if the pressure roller makes contact with the head outside of the neck diameter. The initial contact of the pressure roller to the head should always be within the diameter of the neck to provide support.

Rotating heads

The rotating punch head is a two-part punch configuration, the head is separate from the punch barrel and tip, allowing the head to be removed and replaced as the head wears. When compressing round tablets, the punches will rotate as they are pulled around the cam track through the various stages of the tablet compression. As the punches rotate, the wear and stress on the back angle of the head is distributed around the entire back angle bearing surface. When compressing tablet shapes other than round, the punches do not rotate, causing the wear to be concentrated at a single point, resulting in premature head wear. Because the rotating head configuration allows the head to rotate when compressing non-round tablet shapes, the wear is distributed along the entire surface of the back angle. This helps to decrease head wear, and prolong the life of the punches.

Mirror finished heads

Some high-speed tablet presses use heavy metal cams, such as bronze and bronze alloys. This material is good for eliminating premature head wear and prolonging tool life, but it has a negative effect by contaminating the lubrication and turning it to a black or dark green color. The typical finish of a punch head is done with fine emery or fine abrasive pads. This finish leaves fine radial lines on the contact surfaces of the heads, and has a filing effect on the softer cams, causing discoloration of the lubrication and premature cam wear. Polishing the punch heads with a soft cotton wheel and fine polishing compound to a mirror finish, helps to keep the lubrication cleaner, and prolongs cam life.

Bakelite relief and double deep relief

It is important to maintain a sharp edge around the lower punch tip relief. A sharp edge assists with the pull-down cycle of the lower punch after tablet ejection. If residual product is adhered to the die wall, the sharp lower punch tip relief will help scrape the die clean, as well as cutting through the product to reduce the possibility of product becoming wedged and recompressed between the punch tip and die wall. Product wedged between the punch tip and die wall may cause excessive heat, and thermal expansion of the punch tip. This could result in punch binding and/or seizure, premature head wear, tablet discoloration or burning, and dark specks contaminating the tablet. A bakelite relief assures a sharp edge to assist with removing product adhered to the die wall, allowing the punch tip to move freely in the die. A "double deep relief" increases the depth of the lower punch relief, and provides the same results as the bakelite relief; both designs ensure a sharp edge at the punch tip. The bakelite relief is an added cost option for punches, whereas the double deep relief is generally a no-charge option.

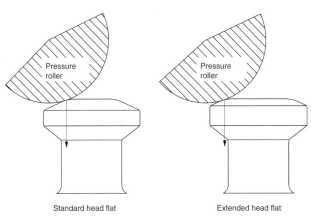

FIGURE 32.9

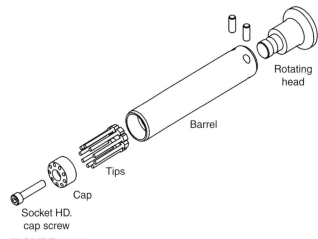

FIGURE 32.10

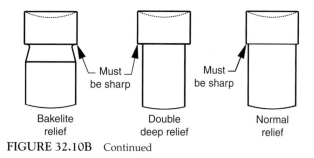

FIGURE 32.10B   Continued

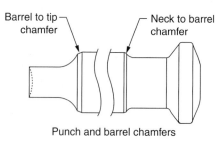

Punch and barrel chamfers

FIGURE 32.11

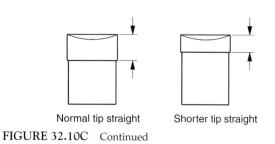

FIGURE 32.10C   Continued

Short lower punch tip straight

The lower punch tip creates a tremendous amount of friction as it travels the full length of the die through the various stages of tablet compression. When compressing sticky products or products with a low melting point, the friction created by the lower punch tip can cause lower punch binding. Reducing the bearing surface of the lower punch tip will reduce friction, allowing the punch to travel easier in the die and reducing operating temperatures.

Punch-barrel chamfers

Punch-barrel chamfers are required on punches used with presses fitted with rubber or plastic guide seals. The barrel chamfer has an advantage over the common break edge for these press models. The absence of a chamfer on the tip end of the punch can create difficulties while installing punches. Forcing the punch past the seal can cause damage to the seals, resulting in seepage of lubrication from the upper-punch guides, causing product contamination. Damaged lower guide seals can allow product seepage into the lower punch guides and mixing with the lubrication, causing tight punches and possibly press seizure. A barrel chamfer on the head end of the punch can reduce wear of the punch guides caused from the punches being cocked from the torque of rotation as the punch travels vertically in the guides.

Key types and positions

Punch barrel keys are mandatory for upper punches when compressing non-round tablets. The upper punch key maintains alignment of the tip for re-entry into the die for compression. Keys are not generally required for lower punches, as the lower punches do not leave the die during the compression cycle, so maintaining alignment is not required. Keys may also be required when compressing round tablets with embossing, to eliminate the punch from spinning after compression, causing damage to the embossed tablet and reducing the likelihood of a "double impression" on the tablet face. The punches may also require keys when the orientation of the embossing for the top and bottom of the tablet is required to be constant.

Keys fitted to the upper punches are available in two configurations: (1) the standard Woodruff key, sometimes referred to as the pressed-in key, and (2) the feather or flat key, often referred as the European key. The Woodruff key, often referred to as the half-moon key because of its shape, is available in two styles, the standard and the Hi-Pro. The Hi-Pro key has a tab on each side of the exposed top section, and rests on the barrel. The tabs keep the key secure by eliminating the rocking action common to the standard Woodruff key. To obtain maximum security for high-speed presses, the Woodruff key is fastened into the barrel using screws. Because the Woodruff key is pressed into position, it can swell the barrel at the position of the key slot, causing excessive drag, and sometimes galling of the upper punch and punch guide.

The feather key is a longer flat key, and comes in a variety of lengths, depending on the tablet press. Unlike the pressed-in Woodruff key, the feather keys fit into a milled slot and are secured into position using machine screws.

The height and radial position of a key is critical to obtain maximum press performance. Unfortunately, no standard has been established, due to the particular requirements of the many styles of tablet presses. If the key is placed too low or is too long, it can interfere

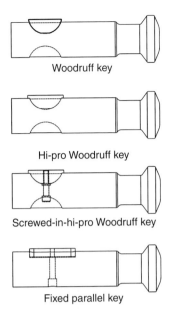

FIGURE 32.12

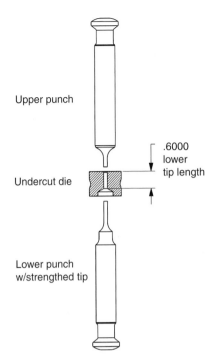

FIGURE 32.13

with the upper punch guide seal, and cause damage and/or seepage of lubrication, resulting in product contamination. If the key is too high, it can travel out of the key slot at the top of the punch guide, resulting in severe damage to the punches and press.

32.4.7 Tool Configuration for Small and Micro Tablets

It's common to experience difficulties maintaining tablet hardness, thickness, and weight while compressing small and micro tablets. Compression force is sensitive and will generally require minimum forces. In some cases the tablet is compressed by the weight of the punch. Excessive tonnage can distort the punch tip, and alter the critical working length, making tablet consistency virtually impossible. Tip breakage is also frequent, and can damage additional punches and the tablet press, most commonly the feed frame. A special tool configuration is recommended for compressing tablets smaller than 0.125″ (3 mm). This configuration modifies the punches and dies, and is used in conjunction with a shallow fill cam that is fitted on the press to minimize lower punch travel in the die. The punch modification involves shortening the punch tips, and eliminating the lower punch relief. Shortening the tip straights to their minimum length will strengthen the tip, increasing the maximum compression force considerably. The lower punch tip relief is removed to reduce the clearance between the tip stem and the die bore, providing additional support to the tip stem, decreasing distortion. Reducing the tip

length increases the barrel length; therefore the bottom of the die is undercut to accept the longer barrel for tablet ejection.

32.4.8 Tapered Dies

A tapered die has numerous advantages. A die can be tapered on one or on both sides, with the advantage of turning the die over and doubling its life. The biggest advantage of a tapered die is to exhaust trapped air in the product as the upper punch enters the die at the beginning of the compression cycle. This is especially helpful for deep-cup punches, fluffy granulation, and high-speed presses. A tapered die provides the ability to compress a harder tablet with the same amount of pressure as required with a straight die. It is helpful in reducing capping and laminating. Taper will allow the tablet to expand at a slower rate as it is being ejected from the die, reducing stress that can cause lamination and capping. Taper decreases the ejection force, prolonging the life of the lower punch heads and ejection cam, thus reducing friction and allowing the press to operate at a lower temperature. Tapered dies help align the upper punch tip upon entering the die, eliminating premature tip wear; this is especially helpful for presses with worn upper punch guides. A standard taper on a BB or D die is 0.003″ × 3/16″ deep. Die taper can be tailored to meet special requirements. Although there are numerous advantages with using taper, there are disadvantages as well. Because the

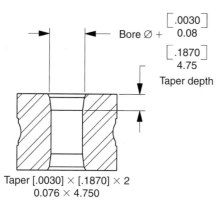

FIGURE 32.14

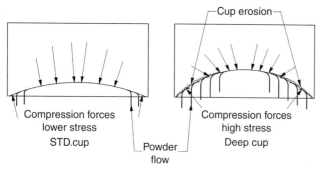

FIGURE 32.15

taper is conical, with the largest area at the top, the upper punch can wedge in between the punch tip and die wall as it is pressed into the die. Excess product can migrate between the punch tip and die bore, due to the additional punch tip to die bore clearance as a result of the taper. If the upper punch is wedged and sticks in the die, it will be evident by spotty tablets and/or premature wear at the back angle of the upper punch.

32.5 TABLET DESIGNS

Proper punch face contour is essential for tooling life and tablet quality. The compression force should be determined during the R&D phase of a new product. If heavy compaction forces are required, then shallow or standard cup configurations should be considered to ensure satisfactory tooling life and tablet quality. If the compaction force is to remain light to standard, a variety of configurations may be considered. Compression force has a lateral force that can expand the sides of the punch cup outward toward the die wall.

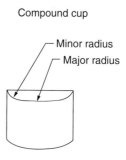

FIGURE 32.16

Excessive pressure can permanently distort and cause premature failure of the punch tip. For a high compaction force the cup may be strengthened by:

1. increasing the land area on the punch tip to provide additional strength;
2. reducing the hardness of the punch tip, allowing the tip to flex without breaking;
3. increasing the cup radius or decreasing the cup depth to eliminate the damaging effect of flexing and abrasion to the inside of the cup.

The flat-face bevel edge (FFBE) tablet configuration is subjected to the same lateral force. These edges can be strengthened by steps 1 and 2, and by increasing the radius between the flat and the bevel, which is normally 0.010–0.015″. The flat-face radius-edge (FFRE) configuration provides a stronger punch tip than the flat-face bevel edge, and can eliminate edge chipping by reducing sharp corners on the tablet face. Another common cup configuration is the compound cup. The compound cup has two radii which make the tablet roll better during the coating process, eliminating tablet edge erosion. The compound cup design generally has more cup volume, and is the optimum tablet design for heavy tablets, as it generally reduces the tablet band, giving the tablet a thinner appearance. However, the compound cup is one of the weakest tablet designs, due to the stresses created at the intersection of the two cup radii and the steep cup which causes excessive abrasion during compression, shortening the tool life.

Elaborate three-dimensional cup configurations are becoming more common in the candy and vitamin industry. Because of the high and low cup designs, it is critical that compaction forces are determined during the R&D phase and results provided to the tooling manufacturer.

The concavity standards for round punch tips are published in the *Tableting Specification* manual (TSM). These standards (Table 32.3) include cup depths for shallow, standard, deep, extra deep, modified ball, flat-face bevel edge (FFBE), and flat-face radius edge

TABLE 32.3 Examples of tooling standard

TABLET DIAMETER													
INCHES [MILLIMETERS]	SHALLOW CUP DEPTH		STANDARD CUP DEPTH		DEEP CUP DEPTH		EXTRA DEEP CUP DEPTH		MOD. BALL CUP DEPTH		F.F.B.E./ F.F.R.E. CUP DEPTH	
1/8 [3.175]	0.005	[0.127]	0.017	[0.432]	0.024	[0.610]	0.030	[0.762]	0.040	[1.016]	0.007	[0.178]
5/32 [3.970]	0.007	[0.178]	0.021	[0.533]	0.030	[0.762]	0.036	[0.914]	0.049	[1.245]	0.008	[0.203]
3/16 [4.763]	0.008	[0.203]	0.029	[0.737]	0.036	[0.914]	0.042	[1.067]	0.059	[1.499]	0.009	[0.229]
7/32 [5.555]	0.009	[0.229]	0.026	[0.635]	0.042	[1.067]	0.048	[1.219]	0.069	[1.753]	0.010	[0.254]
1/4 [6.350]	0.010	[0.254]	0.031	[0.787]	0.045	[1.143]	0.050	[1.270]	0.079	[2.007]	0.011	[0.279]
9/32 [7.142]	0.012	[0.305]	0.033	[0.838]	0.046	[1.168]	0.054	[1.372]	0.089	[2.261]	0.012	[0.305]
5/16 [7.938]	0.013	[0.330]	0.034	[0.864]	0.047	[1.194]	0.060	[1.524]	0.099	[2.515]	0.013	[0.330]
11/32 [8.730]	0.014	[0.356]	0.035	[0.899]	0.049	[1.245]	0.066	[1.676]	0.109	[2.769]	0.014	[0.356]
3/8 [9.525]	0.016	[0.406]	0.036	[0.914]	0.050	[1.270]	0.072	[1.829]	0.119	[3.023]	0.015	[0.381]
13/32 [10.318]	0.017	[0.432]	0.038	[0.965]	0.052	[1.321]	0.078	[1.981]	0.128	[3.251]	0.016	[0.406]
7/16 [11.113]	0.018	[0.457]	0.040	[1.016]	0.054	[1.372]	0.084	[2.134]	0.133	[3.378]	0.016	[0.406]
5/32 [11.905]	0.020	[0.508]	0.041	[1.041]	0.056	[1.422]	0.090	[2.286]	0.148	[3.759]	0.016	[0.406]
1/2 [12.700]	0.021	[0.533]	0.043	[1.092]	0.059	[1.499]	0.095	[2.413]	0.158	[4.013]	0.016	[0.406]
17/32 [13.493]	0.022	[0.559]	0.045	[1.143]	0.061	[1.549]	0.101	[2.565]	0.168	[4.267]	0.016	[0.406]
9/16 [14.288]	0.024	[0.610]	0.046	[1.168]	0.063	[1.600]	0.107	[2.718]	0.178	[4.521]	0.016	[0.406]
19/32 [15.080]	0.025	[0.635]	0.048	[1.219]	0.066	[1.676]	0.113	[2.870]	0.188	[4.775]	0.016	[0.406]
5/8 [15.875]	0.026	[0.660]	0.050	[1.270]	0.068	[1.727]	0.119	[3.023]	0.198	[5.029]	0.016	[0.406]
11/16 [17.463]	0.029	[0.737]	0.054	[1.372]	0.073	[1.854]	0.131	[3.327]	0.217	[5.512]	0.020	[0.508]
3/4 [19.050]	0.031	[0.787]	0.058	[1.473]	0.078	[1.981]	0.143	[3.632]	0.237	[6.020]	0.020	[0.508]
13/16 [20.638]	0.034	[0.864]	0.061	[1.549]	0.083	[2.108]	0.155	[3.937]	0.257	[6.528]	0.020	[0.508]
7/8 [22.225]	0.037	[0.940]	0.065	[1.651]	0.089	[2.260]	0.167	[4.242]	0.277	[7.036]	0.020	[0.508]
15/16 [23.813]	0.039	[0.991]	0.069	[1.753]	0.094	[2.388]	0.179	[4.547]	0.296	[7.518]	0.020	[0.508]
1 [25.400]	0.042	[1.067]	0.073	[1.854]	0.099	[2.515]	0.191	[4.851]	0.316	[8.026]	0.025	[0.635]

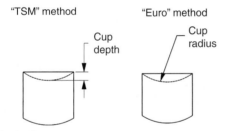

FIGURE 32.17

(FFRE). For radius cup designs, the TSM identifies the cup by the cup depth, whereas the European tableting industry identifies the cup by the cup radius.

32.5.1 Tablet Shapes

There are as many tablet shapes as there are applications, which are endless. Tablets are used in automobile air bags, batteries, soaps, fertilizers, desiccants, and buttons just to name a few. Historically, round tablets were most common, uncomplicated, and easy to set-up and to maintain. Special-shape tablets are tablet shapes other than round, and include shapes such as capsule, oval, square, triangle, etc. Exotic shape tablets are more unique than round or special shapes. Exotic shaped tablets include animal and heart-shaped tablets, and other unique tablet shapes requiring an internal radii or angle.

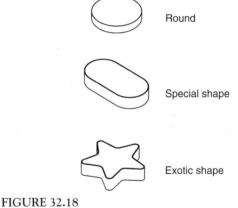

FIGURE 32.18

A unique tablet shape will provide better tablet identification, helping to maintain consumer interest and loyalty. The most common special shapes in the pharmaceutical industry are the capsule, modified capsule, and oval shapes. These shapes typically accommodate more volume, and are more unique than standard rounds. A film-coated tablet is better to use with a modified capsule rather than a capsule shape, to eliminate twinning during the coating process. A modified capsule shape can be designed to have the appearance of a capsule shape with the advantage of a radius on the major axis, reducing the contact surface area during the coating process.

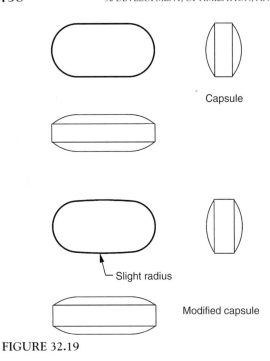

FIGURE 32.19

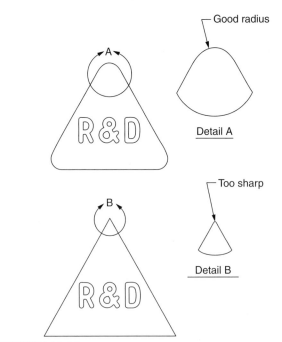

FIGURE 32.20

32.5.2 Tablet Face Configurations

Tablet shapes are virtually infinite, as are tablet face configurations. The tablet face configuration is commonly referred to as the "cup" of the punch. The cup is the area at the tip end of the punch that is responsible for the configuration of the top and bottom of a tablet. The TSM provides cup depth standards for the six most common cup configurations for round tablets. The TSM defines the cup depth of single radius tablet configurations by the depth of the concavity, and differs from the EU configurations which use the cup radius value. The cup radius is more difficult to check and to set internal limits for reworking.

A single radius cup is the strongest cup configuration, and is the most common configuration for round tablets. Adding another radius to the cup changes the cup configuration to a compound cup or a dual radius cup. The compound cup has the advantage of having more volume than the single radius cup. Increased volume to the cup will reduce the size of the "Belly Band," making the tablet appear to be thinner and easier to swallow. The configuration of the compound cup is better for film-coating. The rounded edges tend to roll better in the coating pan, reducing the possibilities of edge erosion. There are several disadvantages to using the compound cup design. The intersection of the two cup radii becomes a high stress point which is prone to failure under extreme loading, and therefore has a much lower maximum compression force rating than the single radius shallow and standard cup. Extreme loading is

not uncommon with the compound cup configuration. The compound cup has more volume therefore, as the upper punch cup enters the die, it fills the die with air, which then must be extracted before compression. Because of this, the compound cup commonly requires slower press speeds or higher compression force than a single radius shallow or standard cup. The compound cup sidewall is steep, and receives high abrasion as the tablet is being compressed, wearing the tip, and weakening the cup. The tip land is critical to the punch tip strength, and should be checked often for wear. If the land wears thin it will cause a condition known as "J hook" which is a common cause of capping and laminating. The land is easily refurbished, using 400 grit sharpening stones and a large cotton buff wheel. The compound cup design has a smaller window or available space for engraving and printing than the single radius shallow and standard cup.

Three-dimensional cup configurations are common with vitamins and candies. The three-dimensional cup configuration provides raised features on the tablet surface, providing the opportunity to sculpt features and character details.

32.5.3 Undesirable Shapes

A tablet shape too close to round may cause a condition known as punch-to-die binding or self-locking. These shapes need to be avoided in order to provide maximum tablet output and satisfactory tool life.

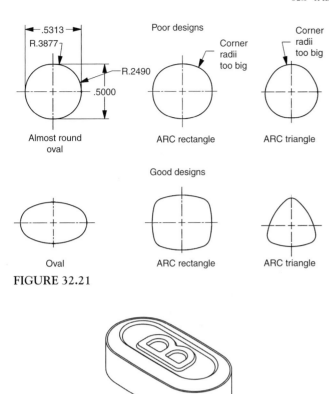

FIGURE 32.21

FIGURE 32.22 Raised embossing in panels

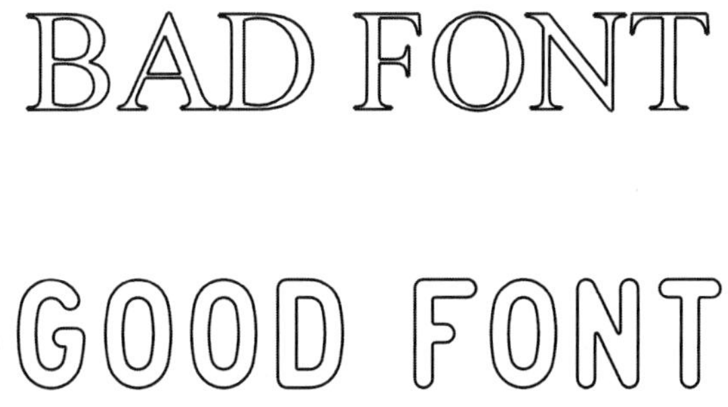

BAD FONT

GOOD FONT

FIGURE 32.23

The corner radius of a special shape, such as a square or triangle, is critical for maintaining the strength and integrity of the die. A corner radius less than 0.032" can cause excessive stress and failure, as the die is locked into position with the die lock and subjected to the shock of tablet compression.

32.5.4 Tablet Identification

There are two basic methods for identifying a tablet, printing and engraving; the latter is the most common. There are two styles of engraving, embossed and debossed. With debossing, the identification is raised on the cup face and engraved into the tablet, while embossed identification is cut into the cup face and raised on the tablet. These two styles can be used in conjunction with each other.

To ensure product identification, many companies engrave their corporate logos on their product line. As tablet size decreases, the legibility of the identification tends to diminish, eventually reaching the point at which it is no longer legible. For this reason, tablet manufacturers should consider the entire range of tablet size when considering the format of a logo for better legibility. As a tablet decreases in size, the logo and drug code are subject to picking (product sticking in or around the identification). Because some products are more prone to picking than others, formulation data and product history, if available, should be provided to the tooling manufacturer so that they may engineer an engraving style and format to help minimize picking and sticking. A company that engraves or embosses most or all of their tablets should consider maintaining a character font. The font should be designed to eliminate sharp corners whenever possible, and open closed-in areas of a character as much as possible.

For sticky products, the engraving style can be designed to pre-pick the islands of a character, for example, filling in the centers of the B, R, 0, 8, etc. The pre-pick character can be difficult to film-coat, and is prone to fill in and bridging therefore, for film-coated tablets the characters can be partially pre-picked. A partial pre-pick is generally preferred, and only removes a percentage of the island instead of removing the island completely. A ramped engraving style, which is also referred to as a tapered peninsula, provides the same advantages as a pre-picked style, and is used at the outside corners and open areas of a character. It provides a lower depth of these areas, and then tapers the tablet surface (Figure 32.24).

The radius at the top of an engraving cut at the tablet surface can be a main contributor to picking and tablet erosion. A general guide for the value of the radius is approximately one third of the engraving cut depth. For example, if the engraving cut depth is 0.012", then the radius at the top of the engraving should be 0.003"/0.004". The angle of a standard engraving cut for a non-coated tablet is 30°. If sticking occurs, it is recommended to increase the angle to 35–40°, which is the angle recommended for film-coated tablets. The wider engraving angle may diminish legibility of the engraving cut by allowing more light into the bottom of the cut, but has a better draft angle which provides improved product release (Figure 32.25).

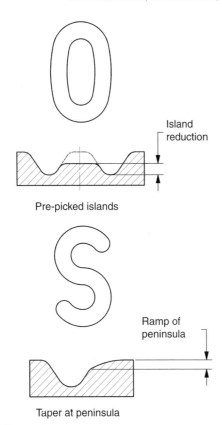

FIGURE 32.24

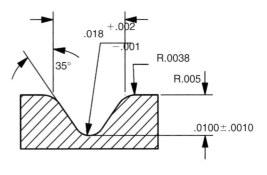

Engraving cut

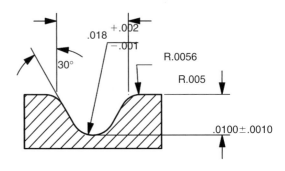

Engraving cut for ffbe

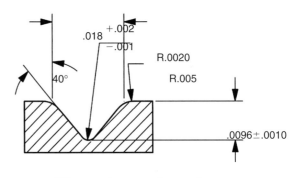

Film coat engraving cut

FIGURE 32.25

Incorrectly placing an engraving cut too close to the tablet edge or too close to the secondary radius for compound cups can result in punch tip fracturing. Although tooling manufacturers generally maintain certain guidelines for the layout and configuration of the engraving, they must consider the amount of engraving in relation to the tablet size, tablet configuration, and product characteristics before releasing the final tablet design for approval.

32.5.5 Bisects

Bisects, commonly known as a score or break line, are available in a variety of styles (Figure 32.26). The purpose of a bisect is to break the tablet into a predetermined dosage, most commonly two equal parts. Breaking a tablet into prescribed dosages should give the consumer a certain degree of confidence that they are receiving the proper dosage. Bisects should be placed on the upper punch whenever possible. Placing the bisect on the lower punch can create problems when the take-off bar removes the tablet from the lower punch. The depth of the bisect is generally deeper than the engraving cut, therefore making it

difficult to slide the tablet across the punch face at the ejection cycle.

The standard TSM bisect has two different configurations for concave tablets, protruding and cut flush. The protruding bisect style follows the curvature of the cup, and extends past the tip edge of the punch. This style helps break the tablet into equal parts, because the extended bisect is pressed into the tablet band. The problem with this style is that the protruding bisect may run into the tip edge of the lower punch if they become too close during tablet press set-up or if the tablet press continues to cycle after the hopper has been emptied. Hitting the bisect into the

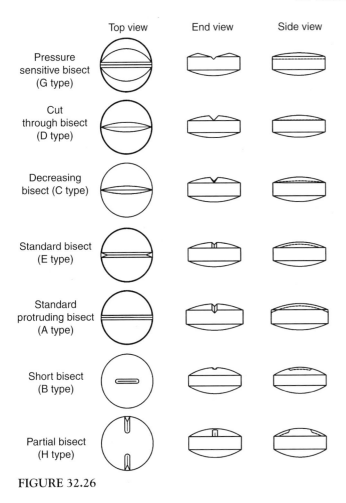

| | Top view | End view | Side view |

Pressure sensitive bisect (G type)

Cut through bisect (D type)

Decreasing bisect (C type)

Standard bisect (E type)

Standard protruding bisect (A type)

Short bisect (B type)

Partial bisect (H type)

FIGURE 32.26

lower punch edge will leave deep impressions, while smashing and swelling the protrusion of the bisect on the upper punch. This is the reason the standard cut-flush bisect has become more popular (Figure 32.26).

A cut-through bisect, also known as a European-style bisect, can only be used on radius cup designs. It has an advantage over the standard bisect, allowing the consumer to break the tablet easily into equal dosages. The cut-through bisect is wider at the center of the tablet than the standard bisect, which reduces the available engraving space on the tablet face. The height of the cut-through bisect is generally the same as the cup depth.

32.5.6 Steel Types

Choosing a steel type is generally left up to the tooling manufacturer, unless a specific type has been requested. The criteria for selecting a steel type includes the quantity of tablets to be produced, the abrasiveness or corrosiveness of the granulation, the pressure required for compression, and the cup configuration.

There are two basic categories of steel common to the tablet tooling industry, standard and premium. Although the categories may imply that one is superior in quality to the other, this is not the case. Standard steel is the most commonly-used grade, whereas the premium grades are generally used for abrasive products and special applications. The cost is generally higher for premium steels, due to the quantity of material purchased by the tool manufacturer and the steel composition. Premium steels also tend to be harder and more difficult to machine. Because premium steels are harder, they can also be more brittle and prone to fracturing under excessive pressure. Commonly used standard steel grades are S-5, S-7, S-1, and 408, and premium steel grades are D-2, D-3, 440-C, stainless steel, and 0-1. Table 32.4 shows the toughness-wear relationship.

32.5.7 Inserted Dies

Dies are normally manufactured from D-3 premium steel. D-3 steel is superior for wear, but due to the high carbon and high chromium content does not provide toughness. Dies are not subjected to the same stresses or shock as the punches, and therefore can be manufactured from harder and better wearing steels.

The most common die for compressing abrasive granulation is the carbide-lined die. The carbide-lined die has a carbide insert which is inserted into a steel sleeve, which provides a cushion to reduce the possibility of chipping and fracturing the carbide insert. Carbide dies are more expensive than steel dies, but this is easily justified with the extended die life (die life is easily increased by 10 times in most cases). Because the carbide die is much harder, it is more brittle and subject to fracturing under excessively heavy compression forces.

If the carbide insert is too thin at its narrowest point due to the tablet size, the carbide insert can fracture due to die lock pressure and stresses of tablet compression. This is also true for the steel sleeve. The tooling manufacturer should be consulted to determine if a tablet size is acceptable for a carbide liner.

Ceramic-lined dies are becoming more widely used as tougher grades become available. The most common ceramic grade used for compression dies is currently partially stabilized zirconia (PSZ). Dies lined with PSZ have the same general wear characteristics and require the same precautions as carbide-lined dies, but have an advantage in reducing the friction coefficient during the fill and ejection cycles.

When inserting carbide or ceramic dies into the die pocket, a die driving rod fitted with a nylon tip should be used to prevent carbide fracturing. Die lock pressure should also be reduced by 10%.

TABLE 32.4   Shows the toughness–wear relationship

Punch tip diameter	Max. compression force by cup depth (Kilonewtons)						
	Shallow concave	Standard concave	Deep concave	Extra-deep concave	Modified ball	F.f.b.e.	F.f.r.e
1/8	12.5	4.4	2.7	1.8	1.0	3.7	4.9
5/32	18.0	7.0	4.2	3.1	1.6	5.3	7.6
3/16	27.0	9.6	6.1	4.7	2.2	7.2	11.0
7/32	37.0	14.0	8.3	6.7	3.0	9.3	14.9
1/4	49.0	20.0	12.5	10.5	3.9	11.5	19.5
9/32	60.0	27.0	18.5	14.5	5.0	14.0	25.0
5/16	75.0	37.0	26.0	18.0	6.1	16.5	30.0
11/32	92.0	48.0	34.0	22.0	7.4	19.0	37.0
3/8	107.0	61.0	44.0	26.0	8.8	22.0	44.0
13/32	127.2	73.0	55.0	30.0	10.5	25.0	51.0
7/16	149.0	87.0	67.0	35.0	13.5	29.0	60.0
15/32	168.0	104.0	79.0	40.0	14.0	33.0	68.0
1/2	192.0	120.0	92.0	47.0	16.0	38.0	78.0
17/32	219.0	137.0	107.0	53.0	18.0	43.0	88.0
9/16	242.0	159.0	123.0	59.0	20.0	48.0	99.0
19/32	271.0	179.0	139.0	66.0	22.0	53.0	110.0
5/8	302.0	200.0	157.0	73.0	24.0	59.0	122.0
11/16	363.0	246.0	195.0	88.0	30.0	63.0	147.0
3/4	436.0	296.0	238.0	104.0	36.0	75.0	175.0
13/16	509.0	356.0	284.0	122.0	42.0	89.0	206.0
7/8	587.0	417.0	331.0	142.0	48.0	103.0	238.0
15/16	679.0	482.0	286.0	163.0	56.0	118.0	274.0
1	770.0	552.0	445.0	185.0	63.0	119.0	311.0

32.5.8 Multi-tip Tooling

Normally, one punch compresses one tablet, the exception is found in multi-tip tooling. Multi-tip tools are more common to Europe, and have only recently been accepted in the United States. The multi-tip tool configuration is engineered to compress more than one tablet at a time, with the total number of tablets per punch dictated by the punch size and tablet size.

There is a tremendous advantage in using multi-tip tooling when considering production, operating efficiency, and overall capacity. Increasing production by the multiple of punch tips can be achieved, but typically should not be expected. Using the formula:

Tablets currently produced
    × number of punch tips × 0.9
    = number of tablets expected
will provide a more accurate estimate of the tablets per minute rate.

Multi-tip punches are available in two configurations, as a solid punch or an assembly with multiple parts. Because the solid punch design does not have multiple parts it is easier to clean, unfortunately if only one tip is damaged the entire punch is unusable and discarded. The multiple part punch design separates the punch tips from the punch body. The punch tips are fixed in place using a cap and/or set screws. If a punch tip is damaged, it can be simply removed and replaced, putting the punch back into service. To properly clean the multiple part design, the tool is required to be disassembled, cleaned, and dried thoroughly before reassembly. This procedure can require substantial labor.

Tablet compression and ejection force most likely will increase as will the operating temperature. To reduce the potential of product sticking in the punch face it is suggested the tablet press and tooling operating temperature are monitored. If the compression

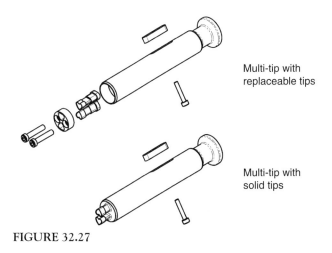

Multi-tip with
replaceable tips

Multi-tip with
solid tips

FIGURE 32.27

TABLE 32.5 Particle consolidation mechanisms

Material	Reversible	Time dependent
Elastic (rubber)	yes	no
Plastic (avicel)	no	yes
Brittle (emcompress)	no	no
Visco-elastic (starch)	partly	yes
Brittle-plastic (lactose)	partly	yes

and/or ejection force becomes too great, the punches may show premature wear on the head flats and back angles, and excessive wear on the tablet press cams. The rotating head option for the lower punch is recommended. The rotating head will reduce punch in die friction by allowing the punch head to spin freely as it takes the torque stress away from the punch tips in the die. The lower punch will be able to move more easily through the cycles of tablet compression.

32.5.9 Punch Tip Pressure Guide

Punch tip pressure is calculated by tablet press manufacturers, and is dictated by the tablet configuration and steel type. With the assistance of computer aided design (CAD) and finite element analysis (FEA) software, tooling manufacturers have become more accurate with the maximum tonnage for round and shaped tablet designs. Table 32.5 gives the cup configurations with the corresponding maximum tonnage force for round punch tips. This guide has been calculated from the computer-generated procedure "Finite Element Analysis," and is the most accurate guide available.

Calculating the maximum compression force for shaped tablets (i.e., capsule, oval, etc.) can be difficult and confusing. Contacting the tooling supplier to request these values is recommended. The maximum tonnage for round and shaped tablets should be provided on the engineered tablet drawing provided by the tooling supplier, along with the cup volume and surface area. It is important that these values have a strong presence with R&D, and are used when formulating a new product. The tonnage requirement should be acceptable before the product reaches the production phase. If tool failure is experienced at the R&D phase, the tablet can be redesigned to accept the required tonnage.

32.6 CARE OF PUNCHES AND DIES

Punches and dies are precision instruments and can damage easily, so great care must be taken when cleaning, transporting, and storing them. Upon receiving punches, they should be cleaned and dried thoroughly prior to use. If standard operating procedures require incoming inspection, then the tools should be inspected immediately, and any concerns or discrepancies reported to the supplier before the tools are used and/or put into storage for future use. Following inspection, the tooling should be lightly oiled, packed in a protective container, and stored in a dry place.

When tooling needs to be shipped, they should not be shipped in storage containers. Most storage containers are not designed to support the weight of the tooling through the handling practices of commercial freight companies. Tooling should be returned in their original individual plastic or cardboard shipping containers, and packed tightly to avoid movement. Because punch tips are extremely fragile, they should be protected at all times from contacting each other or other hard surfaces. A dent or nick on a punch tip can keep the punch from fitting properly into the die. To avoid damage to the die during tablet press set-up, a proper driving rod should be used when inserting the die in the die table. A mild steel rod with the same diameter as the punch guide, fitted with a nylon tip, is recommended. To prevent damage to the die, die table, and die lock, the die lock pressures indicated by the tablet press manufacturer's operator's manual should be observed. Excessive die lock pressure can distort the die bore, and cause punch tightness, fracture the die, and even crack the die table costing thousands of dollars to repair.

32.7 TOOLING INSPECTION

Tooling inspection programs are becoming more common and are performed as a precautionary measure to ensure critical dimensions and embossing details are correct. Confirming critical dimensions will also confirm clearances between the punch and mating parts of the tablet press. Most tooling suppliers will provide a detailed inspection report or a Certificate of Conformance to assure tablet manufacturers that a specific set of tooling is within the specified tolerance, and capable of producing consistent and quality tablets. The inspection area should be an atmospherically controlled environment, well-lit for visual inspection, and equipped with calibrated measuring equipment instruments and gauges. The tooling inspection program should be divided into two sections, incoming inspection, and in-process inspection.

The incoming inspection program is for new tools, and confirms adherence to critical dimensions. Tools that are supplied with a detailed inspection report should be verified by checking a small percentage of tooling to verify the suppliers inspection report. A confirmation of the checked dimensions should be recorded, and maintained for future reference.

The in-process inspection procedures are recommended for determining the wear subjected on critical dimensions responsible for tablet quality and press operation. The most important dimension affecting tablet hardness, weight, and thickness consistency is the working length of the punches. It is not critical to inspect the working length for a calculated dimension, but to inspect for consistency within the set. During the inspection process it is good practice to determine if the punches and dies are in need of polishing and/or light reworking.

The outer dimensions of the punch tip are also critical for inspection and examination. Unfortunately, a worn punch tip is difficult or nearly impossible to inspect using traditional measuring instruments such as a micrometer or an indicator. The punch tip wears at the edge of the cup, and can only be measured accurately using an optical comparator. Dies should be visually checked for wear rings in the compression zone, and replaced if worn. The severity of a die wear ring can be checked with an expanding indicator. The expanding indicator will not provide the actual die size, only the depth of the wear ring. The expanding indicator is also capable of measuring the amount and depth of the die taper. The results of the working length inspection should be documented, noting tool wear and polishing or reworking if performed. When tooling wear exceeds the new tool specification, it is not generally considered unusable or out-of-new punch specification.

32.8 TOOLING REWORKING

If considerable reconditioning of the punches and dies is necessary, the tools should be returned to the manufacturer for evaluation. Extensive reworking of the tooling should only be performed by skilled personnel, to assure conformance to strict tolerances providing tablet consistency and proper press operation.

Polishing the cup is the most common procedure of punch maintenance performed by the tablet manufacturer, it can easily be performed with proper training. Improper or excessive polishing can reduce the cup depth, and diminish the height of the embossing, thus reducing legibility and the ability to film-coat. There are three common procedures in polishing the cup: (1) a large soft cotton wheel fitted to a bench grinder motor; (2) a dremel tool using nylon brushes and polishing paste; and (3) drag finishing, a process that drags the punch through a fine media of walnut shells or plastic pellets infused with polishing compound. The most effective method is using the large cotton wheel. Polishing the cup with a large soft cotton wheel is the only method that polishes the cup and restores the critical land at the same time. Restoring the land can increase tool life, strengthen the punch tip, and reduce the likelihood of capping and laminating. Polishing the punch cups with nylon brushes or using a drag finisher is the simplest method of polishing, but will not restore the tip edge or refurbish the tip land which removes the hooked edge commonly referred to as a "J hook" that is common to capping and laminating. It is not advisable to polish or restore the punch head flat as this can alter the critical working length, resulting in inconsistent tablet hardness, thickness, and/or weight.

32.9 PRESS WEAR

Tablet press wear can sometimes be the reason for tooling failure, it is often overlooked. As the tolerances of punches and dies are constantly monitored, the critical tolerances of a tablet press should also be. For example, if tablet overall thickness is inconsistent the working length of the punches should be checked first; in most cases this dimension is the easiest to check. If the working length of the punches is acceptable, the tools are usually put back into service, but frequently

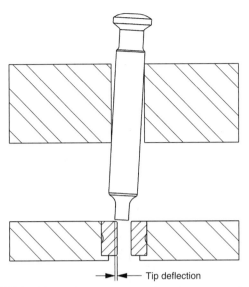

FIGURE 32.28 Deflection of punches indicates excessive wear in turret guides

experience a reoccurrence of the initial problem. If the pressure roller is out of round, out of concentricity or worn with severe pitting or flat spots, the result will be inconsistent tablet thickness, as would be expected with improper punch working lengths.

Figure 32.28 shows the correct way to check the turret guide for wear. A new turret may have approximately 0.003" tip deflection. A turret guide considered worn has a tip deflection of 0.012–0.014", and should be sleeved or replaced.

Problems in tableting often have a domino effect. It is important to identify and remedy a problem before it affects other areas of the press, the tooling, and tablet quality.

32.10 PURCHASING TABLET COMPRESSION TOOLING

Considering all the available tooling options and steel types, it can be confusing and complicated purchasing tablet tooling. Before making the final purchase it is advisable to request a tool and tablet drawing for approval. Most tooling manufacturers can submit a sample tablet made of copper or a special grade of plastic for further approval. The following list is a guideline for information that is needed by the tooling manufacturer to properly custom manufacture tooling meeting the requirements of the product and tablet press.

- The size, shape and cup depth of the tablet to be compressed (a sample tablet or sample tools would be sufficient if this information is not available).
- Drawing number of the tablet if a drawing exists, if not, request a drawing for future reference.
- Hob number, if the order is a replacement.
- Press type, model number, and number of stations required.
- Steel type if other than standard.
- Historical data referencing tablet problems such as capping, sticking, picking, high ejection forces, etc.
- If the tablet has a core and will be coated.
- Special options such as tapered dies, domed heads, key type, etc.
- Special shipping instructions.

32.11 CONSIDERATION OF TOOLING

Choosing the proper tooling options is critical for a smooth operation. It is recommended to utilize all available industry resources such as tablet press and tooling manufacturers for assistance with these choices. Chances are they have resolved similar difficulties for other customers and have the expertise to recommend the correct options. Recording and maintaining tableting problems are important and should be communicated to the tooling manufacturer. Remember, without the knowledge of common tableting problems the tooling manufacturer can only continue to supply standard tooling.

CASE STUDY

Objective

To develop the compression process parameters and control space for a bi-layer tablet by applying RFT (right-first-time)/six sigma approach.

Methods

The overall approach following the RFT/six sigma is shown in Figure 32.29. The applied RFT/six sigma tools include failure mode and effects analysis (FMEA),

---

CASE STUDY   (CONTINUED)

process mapping, cause and effect analysis, design of experiment (DOE), control plan … etc.

A bi-layer tablet is used for this development. The key ingredient of the formulation includes a water-soluble active pharmaceutical ingredient (API), compressible sugars, flavors, flow-aid, lubricant, and other ingredients. The manufacturing process includes blending, milling, and compression using an instrumented rotary press. Failure modes and effects analysis (FMEA) is used to identify critical process parameters (CPPs). The CPPs include compression force at first station (pre-compression), compression force at second station (main compression), and turret speed. The critical quality attributes (CQA) include potency, content uniformity, and lamination. Two designs of experiments (DOEs) are used to understand the knowledge space, and identify control space and operation parameters.

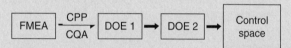

FIGURE 32.29   The overall approach following the RFT/six sigma. FMEA: failure mode and effect analysis; DOE: design of experiment; CPP: critical process parameters; CQA: critical quality attribute

DOE Design

Study I
Goal: establishes the preliminary compression parameters.
Design: three factors at two levels (3 × 2).
Factor 1: main compression.
Factor 2: pre-compression.
Factor 3: speed.

Study II
Goal: identified optimal process parameters.
Design: two factors at three levels (2 × 3).
Factor 1: main mompression.
Factor 2: speed.
(Sampling plan: PQRI driven).

Results

Laminations are shown in Figure 32.30 and 32.31. Based on these results, the operation ranges for compression are optimized as: (1) pre-compression 0.15–0.3 Kp; (2) main compression 6–7 Kp; and (3) turret speed at 18–20 rpm.

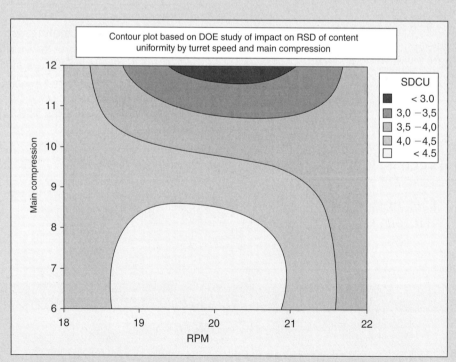

FIGURE 32.30   Impact on RSD of content uniformity by turret speed and main compression force

CASE STUDY   (CONTINUED)

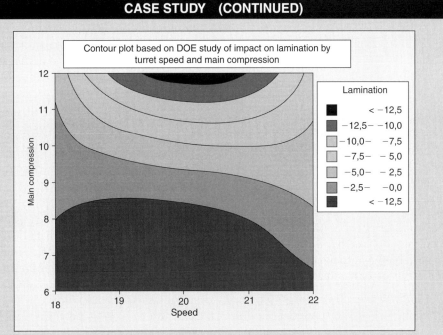

FIGURE 32.31 Impact on lamination by turret speed and main compression force. Note: lamination index > 0 = meets requirement

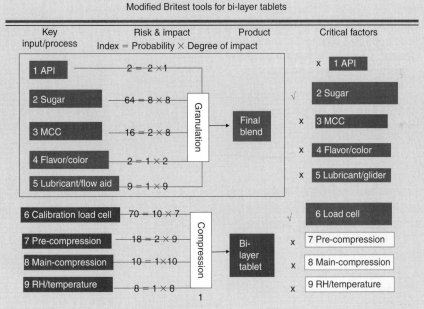

FIGURE 32.32 Application of Britest tool in troubleshooting

Conclusions

Optimization of compressing of a bi-layer tablet could be difficult due to: (1) the confounding interaction of powder-filling of two layers that may have different flowability; and (3) separation/lamination of two layers. However, by applying the RFT/six sigma approach and utilization of these process characteristic tools, the optimal process parameters and control space can be effectively identified.

(2) competition of compression force between two layers;

32.12 SCALE-UP OF COMPRESSION

In this section we will examine press speed as a major factor in tableting, and review measures and functions of tableting speed, such as dwell time, contact time, consolidation time, and decompression (relaxation) time.

The importance of dwell time in compaction has been a subject of discussion for the last 30 years, and yet there is still confusion about how to measure or even define it. Moreover, other important time segments of the compaction event have been neglected, mostly because they depend on press geometry and are difficult to quantify. We have taken a comprehensive approach to calculations of such time events, and got press efficiency factors as a byproduct. In order to evaluate press or tableting efficiency, we need to consider such important factors as feed time, ejection time, and total tableting time.

32.12.1 Compaction and Compression

Tablets are made of powder compressed in a die by punches. On a rotary tablet press the die table, along with many punches, rotates and pushes each set of upper and lower punches between compression rollers (Figure 32.33). This causes the punches to move inside the die and compress the powder. Two processes

take place when the tablet is made: compaction and compression. During tableting, both processes occur simultaneously (Figure 32.34).

By definition, compaction is the increase in mechanical strength of powder under force due to consolidation of particles. Thus, compaction is related to particle consolidation and bonding, which has a direct effect on the tablet hardness and friability.

Compression, on the other hand, is defined as a reduction in bulk volume of the powder under force due to displacement of air between particles. Compression results in a reduction of void space between solid particles, which means a decrease in the porosity of a tablet. It is a known fact that porosity, along with the pore size and distribution, affects total surface area, disintegration, and dissolution time.

Several variables are useful in describing the compaction process. Tablet hardness, or breaking force, of a cylindrical tablet can be converted into tensile strength $\sigma = (2 \cdot F/(\pi \cdot d \cdot h)$, where F is the crushing force, d is tablet diameter and h is the tablet thickness (tensile strength is better than hardness because it is normalized with respect to tooling size and shape). A quantity known as "solid fraction," or relative density, is defined as SF = $w/(\rho \cdot v)$, where w is tablet weight, ρ is true density, and v is tablet volume.

Three types of graphs are required to represent and characterize compaction adequately: tabletability (tensile strength versus applied compaction pressure), compressibility (solid fraction versus applied pressure), and compactibility (tensile strength versus solid fraction). If the graphs coincide for any two items, then formulations are essentially identical with respect to the compaction process. This information can be extremely useful in scale-up.

There are three major mechanisms of particle consolidation: elastic, plastic and brittle fracture (Table 32.5). Any deformation of elastic materials under stress is temporary, it disappears when the pressure is removed (rubber may provide a typical example). Plastic materials, such as avicel, are deformed permanently even at small pressures. For some materials (such as emcompress), powder particles undergo fragmentation under applied pressure. Such deformation is called "brittle fracture."

No material deforms by a single mechanism. There is always a combination of either elastic and plastic or brittle and plastic behavior, and usually one of the mechanisms predominates. The so-called "visco-elastic" materials deform elastically at low pressures, but as the pressure increases, at some point ("yield point"), the deformation becomes irreversible. Likewise, there are materials, such as lactose, which initially show some fragmentation, but then may exhibit plastic flow

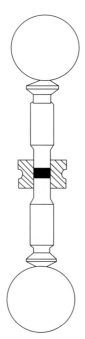

FIGURE 32.33   Punch and die set

TABLETING PROCESS

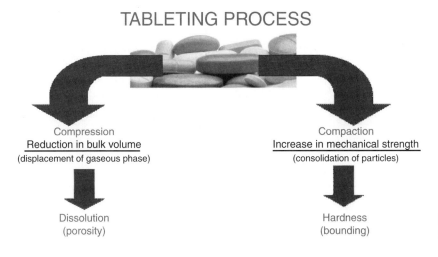

Compression
Reduction in bulk volume
(displacement of gaseous phase)

Compaction
Increase in mechanical strength
(consolidation of particles)

Dissolution
(porosity)

Hardness
(bounding)

FIGURE 32.34 Compression and compaction as two simultaneous processes in tableting

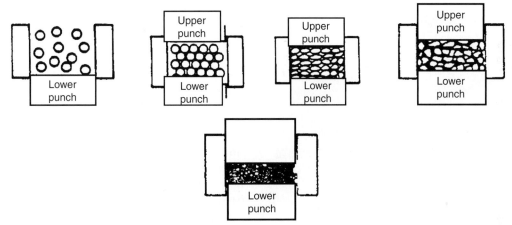

FIGURE 32.35 Consolidation stages with plastic flow

under increased pressure. Plastic flow is time-dependent, and decreases as pressure rises (due to decrease in porosity). Thus, plastic and visco-elastic materials exhibit what is called "strain rate sensitivity," that is, they are sensitive to the speed of tableting.

As powder particles consolidate, they go through several stages of consolidation (shown in Figure 32.35 for plastically deforming material). The main events are: reduction in the volume of air between solid particles, particle rearrangement, particle deformation, plastic flow into the interparticulate voids, and formation of interparticulate bonds due to plastic deformation.

32.12.2 Tableting Failure

Most scale-up problems in tableting are speed related, as the product is moved from a relatively slow

R&D press to high-speed production machines. Such problems are: capping, lamination, cracks, picking, and chipping. Other general problems relate to flowability of powders (feeding issues), underlubrication (may cause sticking), and temperature sensitivity (some powders, such as ibuprofen formulations may even melt in the die during long batches as the in-die temperature increases).

Capping is a stratification phenomenon that results in a horizontal dislocation of a tablet layer (Figure 32.36). Capping tendency increases with compression force and tableting speed,[14,15,18,19] with precompression force,[6] and with punch penetration depth and tablet thickness.[26] Capping occurs due to increase of elastic energy under high speed compaction, compared to a lesser increase in plastic energy. It may also be a result of expansion of air trapped in pores of the tablet, although this assumption has been

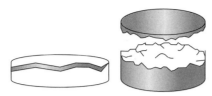

FIGURE 32.36   Tablet capping

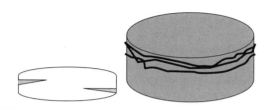

FIGURE 32.37   Lamination

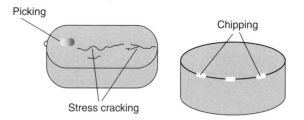

FIGURE 32.39   Picking, chipping and stress cracking

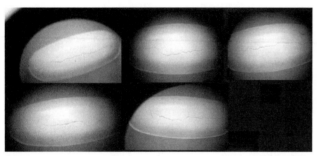

FIGURE 32.38   Crack on the upper side of tablets due to stress relaxation

disputed in literature. Press speed is a major factor contributing to capping due to slow process of stress relaxation.

Lamination (Figure 32.37) occurs when the tablet splits apart in single or multiple layers. Lamination is often blamed on over compressing—too much compression force flattens out the granules, and they no longer lock together. Lamination can also occur when groups of fine and light particles do not lock together. The tendency of tablets to laminate increases with speed, compression force, and precompression force.[6,7] It is a fact that the consolidation part of the compaction cycle (during the "rise time" of the force–time profile) is 6–15 times more important than the decompression part as a factor contributing to capping and lamination.[20,30]

Elastic recovery during decompression can cause stress cracking due to elastic recovery during ejection (Figure 32.38). This is clearly a strain rate (speed) related phenomenon. Chipping may be caused by inadequate (brittle) formulation, take-off misalignment, sticking, while picking/sticking to punch faces is formulation dependent (Figure 32.39).

32.12.3 Main Factors of Tableting

The major factors of a tableting process are force and speed of compaction. The compression force is the dominant factor of the tableting process. As the compression force increases, tensile strength (hardness) of tablets increases, and then may level to a plateau or even decrease as evidenced by numerous studies. Increased force may cause lamination and capping. Also affected are friability, disintegration times, and dissolution profile.

As the punch speed increases, so does the porosity of tablets,[2] and their propensity to capping and lamination. The tensile strength of compacts tends to decrease with faster speeds, especially for plastic and viscoelastic materials, such as starch, lactose, avicel, ibuprofen, or paracetamol (there have been numerous studies, e.g., Fell and Newton;[13] Rees and Rue;[24] Armstrong and Blundell;[4] Roberts and Rowe;[27,28] Holman and Leuenbarger;[17] Armstrong;[3,5] Garr and Rubinstein;[14,15] Marshall, York and MacLaine;[21] Monedero et al [22]). Speed also affects the compact temperature in the die, and its mechanical integrity. With increase in porosity, one should expect a drop in disintegration and dissolution times, but the interplay of the force–speed relationship may confound the effect. Although the energy absorbed by the tablet may not change, the power expended in the compaction process may differ greatly with speed, and this, in turn, may have an effect on tablet properties.

The third important factor is the force profile, which is directly related to the diameter of compression roll. Larger rolls will provide larger contact times, and with all other factors being equal, this may translate into an increase in tablet hardness (Figure 32.40 and Table 32.6).

Numerous other factors may affect the scale-up process. Among them is the quality of the measurements, variation in tooling, powder properties, and tablet weight.

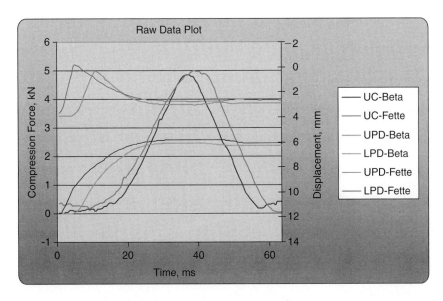

TABLE 32.6 Larger hardness for larger roll diameter at approximately the same dwell time (linear speed)

	Material: Avicel PH101	
Press:	Betapress	Fette 2090
Stations	16	36
Wheel, mm	177.8	300
Speed, RPM	113	58.2
Dwell time, ms	9.3	10.2
Hardness, kP	24.4	36.2

- Feeding time, Tf: time when the die is fed with powder.
- Contact time, Tc: time when both punches are moving, with their tips in contact with the material that is being compacted, and their heads in contact with the pressure rolls (Tc = Ts + Td + Tr).
- Consolidation (solidification) time, Ts: the portion of contact time, Tc, when punches are changing their vertical position in reference to the rolls, decreasing the distance between the punch tips.
- Dwell time, Td: the portion of contact time, Tc, when punches are not changing their vertical position in reference to the rolls.
- Decompression (relaxation) time, Tr: the portion of contact time, Tc, when punches are changing their vertical position in reference to the rolls, increasing the distance between the punch tips before losing the contact with the rolls.
- Compression time, Tp: the portion of contact time, Tc, before the decompression period begins, Tp = Ts + Td.
- Ejection time, Te: time when the tablet is being ejected from the die.
- Total time, Tt: time required to produce one tablet on a press (including time between tablets).

32.12.4 Compaction Event

A typical compaction event is represented in Figure 32.41 in terms of pressure (force divided by punch tip area) versus time. The event can be broken into three parts: consolidation, dwell, and relaxation times. We can see that compression reaches its peak well before the punches are vertically aligned with the center of the compression roll (middle of dwell time). The time between the peak of compression and the middle of dwell time is called peak offset time.[12,16] This phenomenon is due to plastic flow in the material being compressed; this flow relieves the pressure causing the force decrease. Thus, the shape of the compression–time form depends on the plasticity of powder.

32.12.5 Tableting Time Definitions

Let us informally define all discernable time events of the compaction cycle that can be calculated on the basis of geometrical parameters.

Note that all times are defined by punch position relative to compression roll. Thus, all calculations can be done on the basis of press geometry, without any reference to product properties or punch displacement measurements. Once the optimal processing parameters have been established on a research press, the scale-up can be optimized with the help of relatively simple calculations by matching the most important time events.

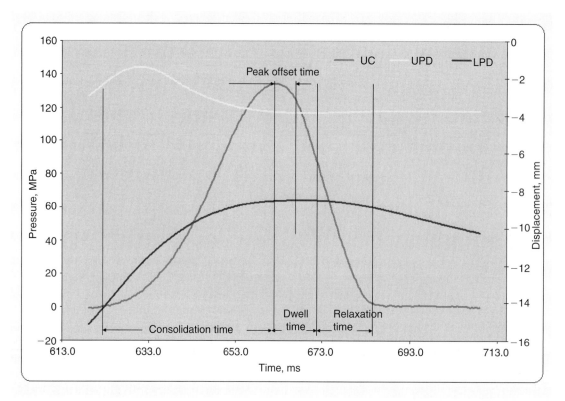

FIGURE 32.41   A compaction event. UC: upper compression; UPD: upper punch displacement; LPD: lower punch displacement

32.12.6 Dwell Time and Contact Time

As we already know from the above definition, contact time is the time when punch head is in contact with the compression roll, while dwell time is when the flat portion of punch head is in touch with the compression roll (Figure 32.42).

Dwell time is defined as a portion of the contact time when punches are not changing their vertical position with respect to the rolls, that is, when a flat portion of the punch head is in contact with the rolls. Note that dwell time, unlike contact time, as defined does not depend on the roll diameter. The notion of dwell time is largely misused or misunderstood. In fact, it should be used as a yardstick, a measure of linear (that is, tangential or angular) velocity, and therefore it will depend on the punch head geometry. The speed comparisons based on the dwell time assume that the punch has a flat head. The velocity, then, is the length of that flat portion divided by the dwell time. For the same linear velocity, the smaller the punch head flat, the smaller the dwell time. To everyone's surprise, dwell time for dome-shaped punch heads is practically zero by definition, regardless of press linear velocity or RPM. That is why, compared to dwell time, linear velocity is a better measure of press speed.

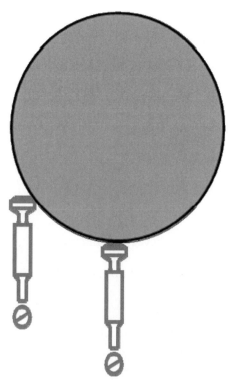

FIGURE 32.42   Geometry of contact time and dwell time

Any attempt to calculate dwell time from compression–time traces (e.g., as a duration of 90% of the peak) is doomed to failure, because such a curve depends on the material properties of the powder being compressed. Plastic flow and elastic recovery distort the "ideal" shape of the force–time profile.

A "classic" simple formula of dwell time does not take into account trajectory curvature:

$$DT \ (msec) = (L \cdot NS \cdot 3,600,000)/(\pi \cdot PCD \cdot TPH)$$

where:

L is **L**ength of a flat portion of the punch head (mm)
NS is **N**umber of **S**tations
π is 3.14159265
PCD is **P**itch **C**ircle **D**iameter of the turret (mm)
TPH is press speed in terms of **T**ablets **P**er **H**our.

Dwell time is historically used as a sort of "yardstick" to measure compaction speed (Figure 32.43).

As you can see, Manesty Betapress is ideally positioned within the range of production speeds of the fast-speed presses. That is probably why this press is often used for R&D work. On the other hand, small presses, such as the Korsch PH106 or Piccola, do not even come close to benchmark production speeds of

6–15 ms in terms of dwell time. In fact dwell time, as defined, depends on tooling geometry (it is zero for a punch with round head, for example). A linear (tangential) speed of the turret is a better way to represent press speed independent of punch head geometry (Figure 32.44). In the following text, we will present the comprehensive set of formulas representing all tableting events that can be derived from press and tooling geometry.

32.12.7 Tableting Geometry

Press speed is a major factor in tableting, and yet the commonly used measures of press speed (such as RPM, tablets per hour, dwell time, linear speed, etc.) do not take into account significant differences in press and tooling geometry, press deformation, tablet thickness or depth of fill.

Let us introduce a tableting notation that will enable us to generate formulas for exact calculation of the compaction time events (Table 32.7). In order to visualize some of the variables with respect to press geometry, let us look at the sketch in Figure 32.45.

Based on the above considerations, the following formulas can be derived (Table 32.8). The above algorithms and formulas are based on an extensive list

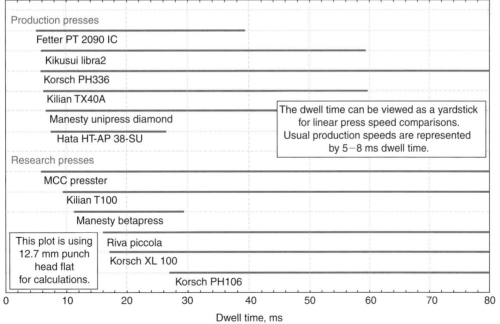

FIGURE 32.43 Dwell time ranges for rotary tablet presses

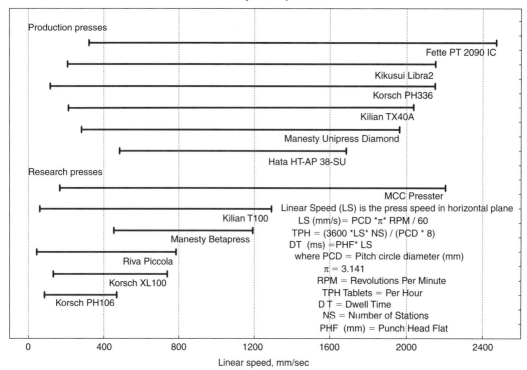

FIGURE 32.44 Linear speed ranges for rotary tablet presses

TABLE 32.7 Notation used in formal calculations of compaction time events

A	angular displacement of punch axis from vertical plane through roll axis, rad;
Ae°	angle of slope of ejection ramp, deg.
Af°	central angle of turret occupied with feed frame, deg.;
d	rate of total press deformation, mm/kN;
Ee	ejection efficiency factor; Ee = Te/Tt
Ef	feeding efficiency factor; Ef = Tf/Tt
Es	consolidation efficiency factor; Es = Ts/Tt
F	compression force, kN;
Hf	depth of fill, mm;
Hi	in–die tablet thickness, mm;
Ht	out–of–die tablet thickness, mm;
Lf	length of feed frame on pitch circle, mm;
Ns	number of stations;
R1	radius of compression roll, mm;
R2	radius of punch head curvature, mm;
R3	radius of punch head flat, mm;
R4	radius of turret pitch circle, mm;
r	frequency of turret rotations, 1/min;
T1	time of turret rotation by angle A1, ms;
T2	time of turret rotation by angle A2, ms;
Tc	contact time, ms; Tc = Ts + Td + Tr;

(Continued)

TABLE 32.7 (Continued)

Td	dwell time, ms;
Te	tablet ejection time, ms;
Tf	die feeding time, ms;
Tr	decompression, or relaxation, time, ms;
Ts	consolidation time, ms
Tt	time to produce one tablet on a press, ms;
Va	angular velocity of press turret, rad/s;
Vh	linear horizontal velocity of punches, mm/s;
Vv	average vertical speed of compaction during consolidation time (compaction rate combined for both punches), mm/s;
Xs	horizontal travel of punch during consolidation time, mm (in direction perpendicular to vertical plane through roll axis);
X1	horizontal distance of punch axis from vertical plane through roll axis, mm;
Z	vertical displacement of upper punch from axis of pressure roll, mm;
Zr	vertical travel of punch during relaxation time, mm; Zr = (Ht–Hi)/2
Zs	vertical travel of punch during consolidation time, mm;
Zu	upper punch penetration, mm;

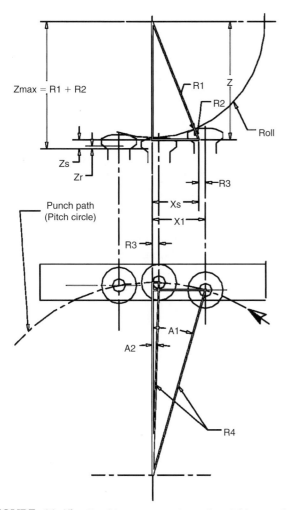

FIGURE 32.45 Graphic representation of variables used in calculation of compaction time events

of published papers, and on our own investigations into the geometry and dynamics of tableting.

Calculation of consolidation time, Ts, is based on geometrical parameters such as roll diameter, pitch circle diameter, punch geometry, depth of fill, and in-die tablet thickness. Calculation of Ts takes into account a correction for press deformation, if the rate of deformation is known. Other calculation formulas are based on the analysis of Rippie and Danielson[25] and represent an extension of work by Muños-Ruiz et al.[23] Calculation of vertical punch displacement, Zs, during consolidation time is based on depth of fill, Hf, and in-die thickness, Hi. A new, more accurate expression for dwell time calculation takes into account the rotational motion of the punches. A proper formula to calculate decompression (relaxation) time, Tr, is used for estimation of all periods of the compaction events and the entire contact time, Tc.

32.12.8 Tableting Scale-up

In order to replicate any process adequately on a different scale, one has to make sure that on both scales the processes are similar. There are three similarity principles in the general theory of modeling: matching geometric, kinematic, and dynamic ratios of characteristic variables. Geometric considerations in simulating compression on a rotary press would require matching die and punch set, and compression rolls. Unlike many other pharmaceutical unit operations, scale-up of tableting process from R&D to production does not involve increase of volume: the die size does

TABLE 32.8 Formulas for tableting times, velocities, and press efficiencies

$$(17)\ Ts = \frac{\arcsin\dfrac{\sqrt{(R1+R2)^2 - \left(R1+R2 - \dfrac{Hf - Hi + d{*}F}{2}\right)^2} + R3}{R4}}{\dfrac{2{*}Pl{*}r}{60000}} - \arcsin\frac{R3}{R4}$$

$$(18)\ Tr = \frac{\arcsin\dfrac{\sqrt{(R1+R2)^2 - \left(R1+R2 - \dfrac{Ht - Hi + d{*}F}{2}\right)^2} + R3}{R4}}{\dfrac{2{*}Pl{*}r}{60000}} - \arcsin\frac{R3}{R4}$$

$$(19)\ Td = \frac{60000{*}\arcsin\dfrac{R3}{R4}}{Pl{*}r} \qquad (20)\ Vh = \frac{2{*}Pl{*}R4{*}r}{60} \qquad (21)\ Tt = \frac{60000}{Ns{*}r}$$

$$(22)\ Es = Ns\ \frac{\arcsin\sqrt{\dfrac{(R1+R2)^2 - \left(R1+R2 - \dfrac{Hf - Hi}{2}\right)^2} + R3}{R4}}{2{*}Pl} - \arcsin\frac{R3}{R4}$$

$$(23)\ Te = \frac{60000{*}(Ht + Zu)}{2{*}Pl{*}R4{*}r{*}\tan(Ae° {*} Pl/180)} \qquad (24)\ Ee = \frac{Ns{*}(Ht + Zu)}{2{*}Pl{*}R4{*}\tan(Ae° {*} Pl/180)}$$

$$(25)\ Tf = \frac{60000{*}Lf}{2{*}Pl{*}R4{*}r} \qquad (26)\ Ef = \frac{Ns{*}Lf}{2{*}Pl{*}R4} \qquad (27)\ Vv = \frac{1000{*}(Hf - Hi + d{*}F)}{Ts}$$

not increase. Moreover, it is easy to match the compression force. The most critical factor of tableting scale-up is the rate of compaction, i.e., punch speed.

A new class of single station tablet presses, generally called "compaction simulators" was introduced in 1980s. They were designed to simulate punch movement on a rotary press at high speed to enable making one tablet at a time for formulation development. The classic hydraulic simulator is using theoretical equation for punch movement, as developed by Rippie and Danielson.[25] Another type of machine, called Presster, is using the principles of similarity to replicate the actual process of making tablets on a rotary press (Figure 32.46). Yet another product, called Parcus, introduced recently as a material sparing device, can also be used to make single tablets at high production speeds, with the goal of eliminating scale-up problems. Useful information on practical use of compaction simulators and their applicability to scale-up can be found in numerous publications.[8,9,10,11,29,31,1]

Scale-up of tableting process involves shorter die feeding times (can affect tablet weight), smaller consolidation times (may lower compactibility), and faster ejection (can create cracks or lamination). At the same production rate, duration of tableting events depends on roll diameter, pitch circle diameter, number of stations, punch geometry, length of feed frame, and the angle of ejection ramp. On the other hand, the speed of various tableting events becomes a limiting factor in press productivity. However, matching consolidation time Ts or a sum of Ts and Td, will, most probably, ensure the same tablet quality or at least, bring the process to a close proximity of the target.

To properly scale-up a formulation based on consolidation time, one should:

1. Evaluate the minimum consolidation time Ts (or Ts + Td) at which tablets of a satisfactory quality can be produced (i.e. the maximum compaction speed) during formulation development. If possible, use a compaction simulator, Presster or a high-speed rotary press equipped with Parcus to establish optimal Ts, or Ts + Td to match those in production.
2. Calculate at what speed (RPM) different production presses can offer the established

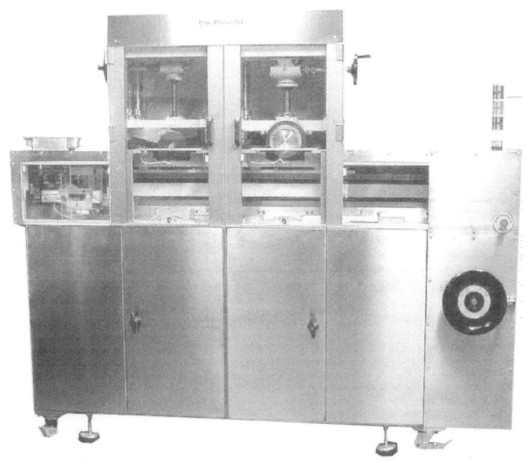

FIGURE 32.46 Presster™ Rotary Tablet Press Replicator. Photo courtesy of MCC: Metropolitan Computing Corporation, East Hanover, New Jersey, USA

minimum satisfactory consolidation time, and what tablet output can be expected from different presses at that speed.

Now that we know how to calculate time events, we can apply this information to practical problems of scale-up. In the following example, we will try to scale-up "a perfect formulation," by matching consolidation time Ts, and dwell time, Td.

Let us say that we have a wet granulation of a low-dose of brittle API, mixed with Avicel PH102, and 0.5% magnesium stearate. On all presses we will use TSM B 3/8" round flat tooling, with 10 mm depth of fill, 300 mg target tablet weight, and out-of-die target thickness of 5 mm, corresponding to 10 kN of compression force. Let us further assume that tablets were made in R&D on a 16-station Manesty Betapress at 50 RPM. Our objective is to move this product to production, where we have a choice of a 36-station Korsch PH336, a 36-station Kikusui Pegasus 1036 or a 37-station Fette P3000 tablet press.

Calculation of Ts and Td yields the results shown in Table 32.9.

We see that both the Korsch and Kikusui presses can match the Ts + Td = 57.6 ms, but Fette cannot, even at the slowest speed of 30 RPM. If, however, we increase the Betapress speed to 60 RPM, we are able to match Ts + Td = 48.1 for all presses under consideration (Table 32.10). Obviously, given a choice, Fette P3000 is preferred because of its high consolidation efficiency factor (Es = 1.36).

Another example involves scale-up of a formulation from a 10-station Riva Piccola tabletop R&D press to a 14-station Riva Compacta, a 36-station Kikusui Libra 2 or a 61-station Fette PT3090. Let us say that all formulation, tooling, and processing parameters are the same as in the previous example. For 50 RPM, Riva Piccola achieves Ts + Td = 78.1 ms (Table 32.11). It is too slow for the other three presses to match. Piccola has to be run at at least 56 RPM (Table 32.12) to be matched with the other presses at slow speeds (e.g., Fette has to be run at a mere 15.6 RPM).

TABLE 32.9   Consolidation time Ts and dwell time Td for production tablet presses matching Betapress run at 50 RPM. Es is the consolidation efficiency factor as defined above

Tablet press	Stations	RPM	TPH	Ts, ms	Td, ms	Ts + Td, ms	Es
Manesty Betapress	16	50.0	48 000	42.1	15.5	57.6	0.56
Korsch PH336	36	33.4	72 169	44.6	13.0	57.6	0.89
Kikusui Pegasus 1036	36	34.8	75 230	42.6	15.0	57.6	0.89
Fette P3000	37	30.0	133 200	36.7	11.7	48.4	1.36

TABLE 32.10   Matching Ts + Td for Manesty Betapress, Korsch PH336, Kikusui Pegasus 1036, and Fette 3090

Tablet press	Stations	RPM	TPH	Ts, ms	Td, ms	Ts + Td, ms	Es
Manesty Betapress	16	60.0	57 600	35.1	13.0	48.1	0.56
Korsch PH336	36	40.1	86 603	37.2	10.8	48.0	0.89
Kikusui Pegasus 1036	36	41.8	90 277	35.5	12.5	48.0	0.89
Fette P3000	37	30.2	134 112	36.4	11.6	48.0	1.36

TABLE 32.11   Ts and Td for Riva Piccola run at 50 RPM

Tablet press	Stations	RPM	TPH	Ts, ms	Td, ms	Ts + Td, ms	Es
Riva Piccola	10	50.0	30 000	54.1	24.0	78.1	0.80

TABLE 32.12   Matching Ts + Td = 69.6 ms for Riva Compacta, Riva Piccola, Kikusui Libra 2, and Fette PT3090 rotary tablet presses

Tablet press	Stations	RPM	TPH	Ts, ms	Td, ms	Ts + Td, ms	Es
Riva Compacta	18	40.0	43 200	50.0	19.6	69.6	0.60
Riva Piccola	10	56.0	33 612	48.3	21.4	69.7	0.80
Kikusui Libra 2	36	23.9	51 664	51.3	18.3	69.6	0.74
Fette PT3090	61	15.6	114 000	52.7	17.0	69.7	1.67

TABLE 32.13   Comparison of Ts + Td for Fette PT3090 at 60 RPM, Kikusui Libra 2 at 92.2 RPM and Riva presses at maximum speed

Tablet press	Stations	RPM	TPH	Ts, ms	Td, ms	Ts + Td, ms	Es
Fette PT3090	61	60.0	439 400	13.7	4.4	18.1	1.67
Kikusui Libra 2	36	92.2	199 120	13.3	4.8	18.1	0.74
Riva Compacta	18	100.0	108 000	20.0	7.9	27.9	0.60
Riva Piccola	10	100.0	60 000	27.0	12.0	39.0	0.80

If the production manager and the marketing considerations demand that the product be run on the Fette press (because of its high efficiency and production rate), then we can do the analysis backwards to see if the research press can match Ts + Td of Fette at, say, a mid-range speed of 60 RPM. Table 32.13 shows that while Kikusui Libra can match that target speed, Riva presses cannot.

References

1. Amidon, G.E. (2008). Powder Compaction and "Simulation." Arden House Conference, February, 308.
2. Armstrong, N.A. & Palfrey, L.P. (1989). The effect of machine speed on consolidation of four directly compressible tablet diluents. The Journal of Pharmacy and Pharmacology 41, 149–151.
3. Armstrong, N.A. (1989). Time-dependent factors involved in powder compression and tablet manufacture. International Journal of Pharmaceutics 49, 1–13.

4. Armstrong, N.A. & Blundell, L.P. (1985). The effect of machine speed on the compaction of some directly compressible tablet diluents. Pharmacology 37, 28P.

5. Armstrong, N.A. (1990). Considerations of compression speed in tablet manufacture. Pharmaceutical Technology 9, 106–116.

6. Bateman, S.D., Rubinstein, M.H. & Thacker, H.S. (1990). Pre- and main compression in tableting. Pharm. Tech. Int. 2, 30–36.

7. Bateman, S.D., Rubinstein, M.H. & Wright, P. (1987). The effect of compression speed on the properties of ibuprofen tablets. The Journal of Pharmacy and Pharmacology 39, 66P.

8. Bateman, S.D. (1988). High speed compression simulators in tableting research. Pharmaceutical Journal 240, 632.

9. Bateman, S.D. (1989). A comparative investigation of compression simulators. International Journal of Pharmaceutics 49, 209–212.

10. Bateman, S.D., Rubinstein, M.H., Rowe, R.C., Roberts, R.J., Drew, P. & Ho, A.Y.K. (1989). A comparative investigation of compression simulators. International Journal of Pharmaceutics 49, 209–212.

11. Celik, M. & Marshall, K. (1989). Use of a compaction simulator system in tableting research. Part 1: Introduction to and initial experiments with the system. Drug Development and Industrial Pharmacy 15(5), 759–800.

12. Dwivedi, S.K., Oates, R.J. & Mitchell, A.G. (1991). Peak offset times as an indication of stress relaxation during tableting on a rotary tablet press. The Journal of Pharmacy and Pharmacology 43, 673–678.

13. Fell, J.T. & Newton, J.M. (1971). Effect of particle size and speed of compaction on density changes in tablets of crystalline and spray-dried lactose. Journal of Pharmaceutical Sciences 60, 1866–1869.

14. Garr, J.S.M. & Rubinstein, M.H. (1991a). An investigation into the capping of paracetamol at increasing speeds of compression. International Journal of Pharmaceutics 72, 117–122.

15. Garr, J.S.M. & Rubinstein, M.H. (1991b). The effect of rate of force application on the properties of microcrystalline cellulose and dibasic calcium phosphate mixtures. International Journal of Pharmaceutics 73, 75–80.

16. Ho, A.Y.K. & Jones, T.M. (1988). Punch travel beyond peak force during tablet compression. The Journal of Pharmacy and Pharmacology 40, 75P.

17. Holman, L.E. & Leuenberger, H. (1989). Effect of compression speed on the relationship between normalized solid fraction and mechanical properties of compacts. International Journal of Pharmaceutics 57, R1–R5.

18. Mann, S.C., Roberts, R.J., Rowe, R.C. & Hunter, B.M. (1982). The influence of precompression pressure on capping. The Journal of Pharmacy and Pharmacology 34, 49P.

19. Mann, S.C., Roberts, R.J., Rowe, R.C., Hunter, B.M. & Rees, J.E. (1983). The effect of high speed compression at sub-atmospheric pressure on the capping tendency of pharmaceutical tablets. The Journal of Pharmacy and Pharmacology 35, 44P.

20. Mann, S.C. (1987). An investigation of the effect of individual segments of tableting cycle on the capping and lamination of pharmaceutical tablets. Acta Pharmaceutica Suecica 24, 54–55.

21. Marshall, P.V., York, P. & MacLaine, J.Q. (1993). An investigation of the effect of the punch velocity on the compaction properties of ibuprofen. Powder Technology 74, 171–177.

22. Monedero, M., Jime Nez-Castellanos, M.R., Velasco, M.V. & Muñoz-Ruiz, A. (1998). Effect of compression speed and pressure on the physical characteristics of maltodextrin tablets. Drug Development and Industrial Pharmacy 24(7), 613–621.

23. Muñoz-Ruiz, A. et al. (1992). Theoretical estimation of dwell and consolidation times in rotary tablet machines. Drug Development and Industrial Pharmacy 18(9), 2011–2028.

24. Rees, J.E. & Rue, P.J. (1978). Time-dependent deformation of some direct compression excipients. The Journal of Pharmacy and Pharmacology 30, 601–607.

25. Rippie, E.G. & Danielson, D.W. (1981). Viscoelastic stress/strain behavior of pharmaceutical tablets: Analysis during unloading and postcompression periods. Journal of Pharmaceutical Sciences 70, 476–482.

26. Ritter, A. & Sucker, H.B. (1980). Studies of variables that affect tablet capping. Pharm. Tech., 57–62.

27. Roberts, R.J. & Rowe, R.C. (1985). The effect of punch velocity on the compaction of a variety of materials. The Journal of Pharmacy and Pharmacology 37, 377–384.

28. Roberts, R.J. & Rowe, R.C. (1986). The effect of relationship between punch velocity and particle size on the compaction behaviour of materials with varying deformation mechanisms. The Journal of Pharmacy and Pharmacology 38, 567–571.

29. Rubinstein, M.H. (1992). Applications of compaction simulators. Pharm. Manuf. Int. 168, 177–182.

30. Ruegger, C.D. (1996). An investigation of the effect of compaction profiles on the tableting properties of pharmaceutical materials. PhD Thesis, Rutgers University.

31. Tye, C.K., Sun, C. & Amidon, G.E. (2005). Evaluation of the effects of tableting speed on the relationships between compaction pressure, tablet tensile strength, and tablet solid fraction. Journal of Pharmaceutical Sciences 94(3), 465–472.

Development, Optimization, and Scale-up of Process Parameters: Pan Coating

Stuart Porter, Gary Sackett and Lirong Liu

33.1 INTRODUCTION

In the modern pharmaceutical industry, film-coating is generally referred to as a process by which a thin continuous layer of solid is applied onto the surface of a dosage form or its intermediate. The purpose of film-coating includes aesthetic enhancement, increase of shelf life, taste masking, moderating the release profile of active pharmaceutical ingredient (API), trademarking, and protection of intellectual property ... etc.

The thickness of the film is generally less than a hundred microns. The composition of the film may include a mixture of inert excipients, as well as an API.

33.1.1 Theory of Film-coating

Film-coatings can be applied by different methods, such as spraying a liquid, dipping into a liquid, precipitating from supercritical fluids or depositing a powder using an electrostatic technique.

Spraying a liquid is the most widely used process for film-coating and typically includes three basic steps:

- spraying an atomized liquid on the target surface that is in continuous movement;
- maintaining a controlled balance between spray and evaporization, by applying heated air flow in contact with the target surface;
- continuing the process until the desired amount of coating is applied.

33.1.2 Evolution of Pharmaceutical Coating Technologies

Application of coatings to medicinal products can be traced back by more than a century. However, a uniform and consistent film-coating process that meets the minimum requirements imposed by today's regulatory requirements has only been available for the past few decades.

Sugar-coating in a smooth bowl-shaped container, originally with an external heat source, probably represents one of the earliest processes used as a pharmaceutical coating process. Film-coating emerged as an alternative to the sugar-coating process to reduce process time, and minimize exposure to high temperature and excessive moisture. The evolution in design of equipment has progressed from an open system to one that is completely enclosed, and self-contained. Liquid delivery and air handling systems have also improved, as demand for precision and accuracy became more of a regulatory requirement. The efficiency and accuracy of heat exchange has been improved by routing air flow in and out of the perforated area on the side of wall of the coating pan, while various types of instrumentations are used to monitor the key process parameters (KPP).

At the end of the last century, film-coating had evolved to such a degree that it might not be recognized by an operator performing the task of coating just 50 years earlier. Another development has been the implementation of process analytical technology (PAT) in order to monitor and control the uniformity of the spraying process, and determine the end point of the process. Other innovative approaches to film-coating have emerged at the beginning of the twenty-first century. These approaches include online ink-jet processes, powder electrostatic coating, precipitation from supercritical fluid, and small footprint continuous coating process.

33.1.3 Coating Equipment: Introduction

Based on the coating chamber, coating pans can be classified as solid pans (Figure 33.1), fully-perforated pans (Figure 33.2), partially-perforated pans (Figure 33.3), and coating pans based on the other mechanisms.

Based on the type of process, the coating pan can be classified as batch process coating pan, continuous coating pan, or off-press continuous coating pan (Figure 33.4). The selection of type of coating pan will be based on the needs for the desired coating. For example, a continuous coating pan can be used for product that calls for high output, and low manufacturing cost.

33.2 FILM-COATING FORMULATIONS

33.2.1 Overview of Types of Film-coating Formulations

Film-coating systems are usually defined by the way the coating materials are formulated into a liquid coating system, and typically take the form of:

- polymers applied as organic–solvent-based solutions (today, typically reserved for modified-release applications);

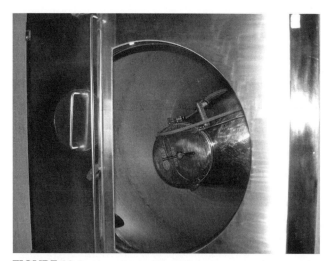

FIGURE 33.1　A modern solid coating pan at manufacture scale

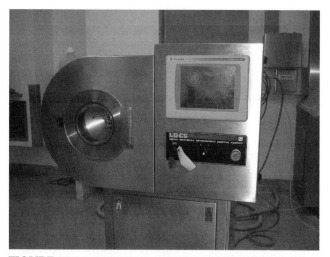

FIGURE 33.3　An experimental-scale partially perforated pan

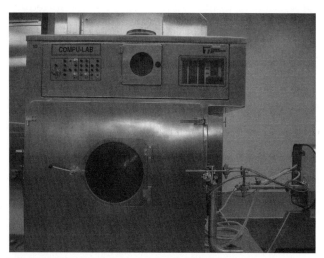

FIGURE 33.2　Example of a pilot-scale fully perforated pan

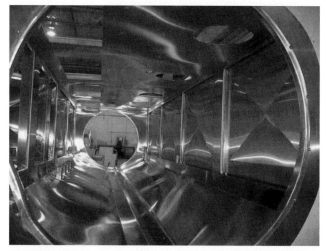

FIGURE 33.4　Chamber of a continuous coating pan. Courtesy of O'Hara Inc.

- polymers applied as aqueous solutions (most commonly used for immediate release film-coatings);
- polymers applied as aqueous dispersions (mainly used for modified-release applications);
- various materials applied as hot-melts (typically used for modified-release and taste-masking applications).

The transition to aqueous processes has been driven by a genuine desire to avoid:

- the hazards associated with using both flammable and potentially toxic solvents;
- dealing with the environmental issues that are associated with using organic solvents;
- the additional costs associated with the aforementioned issues.

Water is not however, a panacea, and there are often potential problems (that are associated with the use of aqueous systems) that need to be resolved.

Potential problems to be faced when using aqueous coating systems include:

- the possibility that processing times will be increased;
- the potentially negative impact on drug stability, if water is not effectively removed during processing;
- the increased likelihood that the harsher process conditions used may affect drug dissolution characteristics.

Aqueous coating formulations can take two forms, namely:

- aqueous solutions of polymers, which are typically reserved for immediate-release coating applications;
- aqueous dispersions (latexes) of polymers, which are typically used in modified-release coating applications.

When it comes to forming coatings from polymer solutions, the process generally involves the conversion of a viscous liquid into a visco-elastic solid as a result of continual solvent evaporation, through a series of stages:

- rapid evaporation of solvent from finely-atomized droplets of solution which are deposited onto the surface of the substrate to begin the process of build-up of coating material;
- continued solvent evaporation (now at a slower rate) from the coating that is forming on the substrate surface.
- immobilization of polymer molecules (at the so-called "solidification point"), such that continued

solvent loss now leads to the development of shrinkage stresses within the coating;
- continuation of solvent loss (usually throughout the life of the product) at extremely slow rates.

In contrast, the formation of coatings from aqueous polymer dispersions (see Figure 33.5), while still involving a process of evaporation, is radically different from that involving a polymer solution.

The polymer dispersion, containing the polymer as discrete "particles," must undergo a process of coalescence where the dispersed polymer particles must flow together. For this process to occur, a critical pressure must develop within the film structure, and the particles of polymer must soften sufficiently to permit flow. The pressure develops as a result of water evaporation whereby, as the porosity of the membrane is reduced during evaporation, a capillary network is formed within the structure of the coating, such that movement of water during the evaporation process causes capillary forces to develop. The ability of the polymer particles to soften sufficiently is dependent on two factors, namely:

- appropriate heat provided by the coating process; and
- the glass transition temperature of the formulated coating system.

The glass transition temperature of the coating system (dictated by the properties of the polymer, and the properties and concentration of the plasticizer, where needed) determines the minimum film-forming temperature (MFFT) of the system. The product temperature within the coating pan must exceed the MFFT for film coalescence to occur.

While it is common for many coating formulations to contain a plasticizer (see later discussion), polymer dispersions may require the presence of a plasticizer

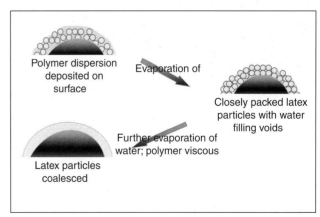

FIGURE 33.5 Schematic of film formation from aqueous polymer dispersions

to facilitate film formation. Generally, it is necessary to use plasticizers with polymer dispersions when:

- the polymer on which the dispersion is based has a high glass transition temperature (such as ethyl cellulose), such that the minimum film-forming temperature (MFFT) of the system exceeds the product temperatures experienced in the process;
- if the flexibility of the resultant film-coating needs to be improved.

Unnecessary or excessive use of plasticizers should always be avoided otherwise excessive tackiness will be experienced.

The typical ingredients used in film-coating formulations are:

- polymer;
- plasticizer;
- colorants;
- solvent/vehicle.

When designing coating formulations, there are several important issues to consider. These generally involve the need to optimize:

- the visual characteristics of the final product;
- the functional characteristics of the coating;
- the "processibility" of the coating system (e.g., issues relating to preparation and application of the coating liquid, as well as those associated with processing time and costs).

Film-coatings are applied to pharmaceutical oral solid dosage forms for a number of purposes, often leading to coatings being categorized on the basis of their intent with regard to influencing drug release. Thus, two main categories of film-coatings have evolved, namely:

- Immediate-release coatings, which although often used for aesthetic purposes, may also be used to:
  - improve product stability;
  - facilitate product identification;
  - affect an improvement in product organoleptic characteristic (such as taste and odor).
- Modified-release coatings, which can be subdivided into two further categories, namely:
  - delayed-release (enteric) coatings;
  - extended-release (sustained- or controlled-release) coatings.

33.2.2 Overview of Types of Materials Used in Film-coating Formulations

Polymers

Polymers are the main building blocks of coating formulations, providing the main characteristics for the final coating formulation, and are usually characterized in terms of:

- Chemistry, which will mainly influence:
  - solubility of coating system;
  - rheology of coating liquid;
  - mechanical properties of coating;
  - permeability characteristics of coating.
- Molecular weight (or molecular weight distribution), which is likely to influence:
  - mechanical properties of coating;
  - rheology of coating liquid.

Unlike that of inorganic materials, the molecular weight of a polymer is much more difficult to define. Any given sample of polymer will consist of a broad distribution of molecular weights.

In order to characterize the molecular weight of a polymer, we usually measure this molecular weight distribution (using techniques such as gel permeation chromatography), and then express the molecular weight in terms of a statistically defined average, as shown in Figure 33.6, where two measured parameters are indicated:

- weight average molecular weight, M_w;
- number average molecular weight, M_n.

A derived parameter that is often useful is the polydispersity function, which is defined as:

$$\text{Polydispersity} = M_w/M_n$$

The influence of molecular weight on the mechanical properties of polymers is shown in Figure 33.7. Generally, an increase in molecular weight has these effects:

- tensile strength increases;
- elastic modulus increases;
- adhesion decreases.

Polymer molecular weight can, as stated earlier, affect coating solution viscosity. In absolute terms, the relationship between polymer molecular weight and solution viscosity is governed by the Mark–Houwink equation:

$$[\mu] = kM^\alpha$$

where:

$[\mu]$ is the *intrinsic viscosity* of the polymer
M is its molecular weight
k and α are constants relating to the solvent system used and the solution temperature.

For more pragmatic reasons, we often prefer to use the term *nominal viscosity*, where:

$$\text{Molecular weight} = k(\text{nominal viscosity})^n$$

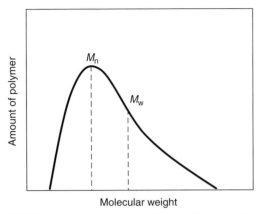

FIGURE 33.6 Typical molecular weight profile for a polymer

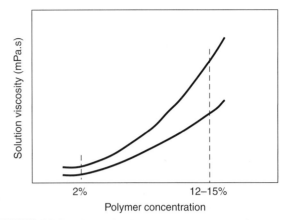

FIGURE 33.8 Effect of polymer concentration on the viscosity of aqueous polymer solutions

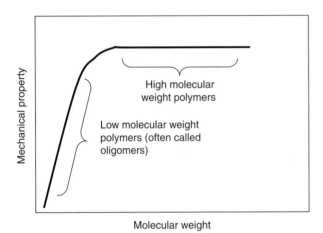

FIGURE 33.7 Effect of molecular weight on the mechanical properties of polymers

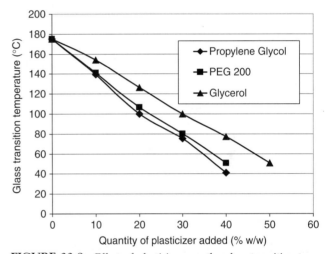

FIGURE 33.9 Effect of plasticizers on the glass transition temperature of HPMC

Nominal viscosity is usually measured in water at 25°C, using a solution containing 2% w/w polymer.

Not only does polymer molecular weight influence solution viscosity, but so does polymer concentration, as illustrated in Figure 33.8. As stated previously, nominal viscosity, a term usually assigned to a particular grade of polymer, is measured for dilute solutions of polymer. No particular batch of polymer will conform exactly to the nominal viscosity value for that grade. Hence, the manufacturers (and usually the compendia as well) will set a specification range. As can be seen from the Figure 33.8, at the 2% solids concentration (usually used for setting the nominal viscosity specification), the batch-wise variation in solution viscosity is usually quite small (often only ±2 cP or mPas). However, as we increase the solids content of the solution, not only does the viscosity increase exponentially, but the difference in solution viscosity from batch-to-batch increases dramatically, so that

we may actually experience batch-wise variation in solution viscosity (depending on the solids contents of our coating solutions) in the order of ±200–300 cP.

Plasticizers

Plasticizers are another common ingredient added to coating formulations. They are typically used to:

- reduce the glass transition temperature, T_g (see Figure 33.9);
- increase flexibility.

Most polymers that we use in film-coating are essentially amorphous materials and, as such, exhibit a reasonably well-defined glass transition temperature (a fundamental characteristic of polymers that has a profound effect on polymer properties that can also influence film formation, especially when using aqueous polymer dispersions). This transition does not represent a change in state (as we see with melting point), but rather is indicative of a point where there is a dramatic increase molecular mobility. At this point, the polymer changes from a tough, rigid, inflexible, and brittle material into one that is softer, and more pliable. These latter properties are of great value in film-coating, and thus it is beneficial to match the glass transition temperature of the final coating system to the coating conditions that will be used.

For most coating systems, it is desirable that the glass transition temperature of that system be optimized for the coating process conditions used. For aqueous polymer dispersions (or latexes), it is critical that such optimization is achieved, otherwise appropriate coalescence of the coating will not occur.

A list of common plasticizers used in coating formulations is shown in Table 33.1, and their effects on film mechanical properties are shown in Figure 33.10.

When it comes to selecting a suitable plasticizer for a coating formulation, some key issues to consider are:

- Efficiency: this defines how much plasticizer must be added to produce the desired effect.
- Compatibility: this indicates how effectively the plasticizer interacts with the polymer, and the level up to which that interaction occurs.
- Permanence: this relates to both plasticizer–polymer compatibility, and plasticizer volatility (see Figure 33.11 for an example of poor plasticizer permanence).

The common general effects of plasticizers when used in film-coating formulations are shown in Table 33.2.

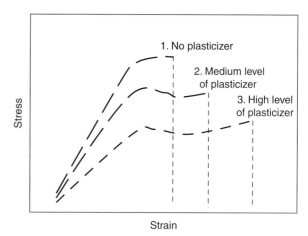

FIGURE 33.10   Effect of plasticizers on the mechanical properties of film coatings

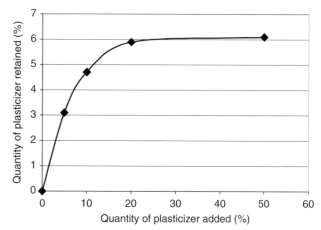

FIGURE 33.11   Example of lack of plasticizer permanence (loss of propylene glycol from HPMC films)

TABLE 33.1   Common Plasticizers Used in Film-Coating Formulation

Class	Examples
Polyhydric alcohols	• Propylene glycol • Glycerol • Polethylene glycols
Acetate esters	• Glyceryl triacetate (Triacetin) • Triethyl citrate • Acetyl triethyl citrate
Phthalate esters	• Diethyl phthalate
Glycerides	• Actetylated monoglycerides
Oils	• Castor oil • Mineral oil

TABLE 33.2   Summary of common effects of plasticizers

Property	Effect of increased plasticizer concentration
Tensile strength	Reduced
Elastic modulus	Reduced
Film adhesion	Variable, but increased under optimal use conditions
Viscosity of coating liquid	Usually increased, with effect being greater as plasticizer molecular weight is increased
Film permeability	Variable, depending on physico-chemical properties of plasticizer
Glass transition temperature (T_g) of film	Reduced, with magnitude of effect being influenced by compatibility with polymer

Colorants

Colorants are typically used in film-coating formulations to:

- improve product appearance;
- aid in product identification;
- improve product stability.

A list of common colorants used in coating formulations is shown in Table 33.3. While it is possible to use either water-soluble colorants (dyes) or water-insoluble colorants (pigments), as shown in the table, the use of pigments has several advantages, since:

- by replacing some of the polymer, pigments allow the solids content of film-coating formulations to be increased, while still maintaining a sprayable viscosity;
- being a solid inclusion in the final dried coating, pigments allow the moisture barrier properties of the coating to be improved;
- pigments tend to be more light stable than water-soluble colorants;
- pigments are less prone to color migration as the coatings dry;
- by excluding light, pigments can improve the stability of photo-labile drug substances.

In order to exert these properties effectively, it is desirable that the colored film coating is able to completely mask the substrate. The ability to achieve this goal is usually expressed as the hiding power (or contrast ratio) of the coating. The consequences of poor hiding power include the fact that:

- higher coating levels will have to be employed to get uniform appearance from tablet-to-tablet, and from batch-to batch;

TABLE 33.3 Common types of colorant used in film-coating formulations

Type	Examples
Water-soluble dyes	• FD&C yellow #5 • FD&C blue #2
FD&C lakes	• FD&C yellow #5 lake • FD&C blue #2 lake
D&C lakes	• D&C yellow #10 lake • D&C red #30 lake
Inorganic pigments	• Titanium dioxide • Iron oxides
"Natural" colorants	• Riboflavin • Beta-carotene • Carmine lake

- if the tablets are intagliated (i.e., have a logo), higher levels of coating can cause increased risk of logo bridging;
- the contrast ratios of film coatings colored with selected pigments are shown in Table 33.4.

Generally, the main factors that can influence the hiding power of a particular film-coating are:

- the quantity of light reflected at the polymer–pigment interface (which, in turn, is influenced by the refractive index of the colorant, see Figure 33.12);
- the wave length of light absorbed by the colorant;
- the amount of light absorbed;
- the concentration of the colorant in the coating (see Figure 33.13);
- the thickness of the coating (see Figure 33.13).

The ability of film coatings to improve product stability is generally related to:

- the influence of pigments on coating permeability (generally, as pigment concentration is increased, up to a critical level called the critical pigment volume concentration, film permeability to

TABLE 33.4 Typical contrast ratio values for coating colored with selected pigments

Pigment	Contrast ratio
None	33.3
Titanium dioxide	91.6
Red iron oxide	99.5
Yellow iron oxide	98.4
Indigo carmine lake	99.5
Tartrazine lake	66.7

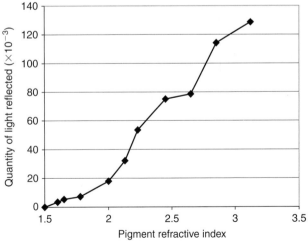

FIGURE 33.12 Hiding power and influence of pigment refractive index

environmental gases, such as water vapor and/or oxygen are reduced); decreased permeability can lead to improved product stability;

• the ability of the coating to exclude light, an important issue when coating products containing photo-labile APIs (such as nifedipine, as shown in Figure 33.14).

In summary, the general effects of pigments on the properties of film-coatings are shown in Table 33.5.

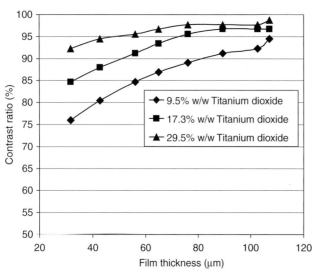

FIGURE 33.13 Effects of pigment concentration and coating thickness on the contrast ratios of colored film coatings

Other Additives

While polymer, plasticizers, and colorants constitute the major ingredients in film coating formulations, other materials that might be used for a variety of reasons include:

• anti-adhesive agents, especially when the polymer is somewhat tacky;
• flavoring agents (typically in nutraceutical applications);

TABLE 33.5   General effects of pigments in film-coatings

Property	Effect of increased pigment concentration in film
Tensile strength	Reduced (but effect may be minimized by effective pigment dispersion in film)
Elastic modulus	Increased
Film adhesion	Generally, little effect
Viscosity of coating liquid	Increased, but usually not substantially
Film permeability	Reduced, unless critical pigment volume concentration (CPVC) is exceeded
Hiding power	Increased, but effect is dependent on refractive index, and light absorption characteristics, of pigment

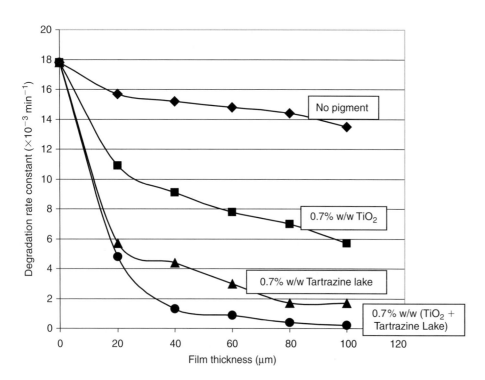

FIGURE 33.14 Photostabilization of Nifedipine using pigmented film coatings

• surfactants (to facilitate the wetting of insoluble materials dispersed in the coating formulation);
• pore-forming agents (especially in extended-release film-coating formulations).

Solvents/Vehicles

Currently, most coating formulations that are applied to oral solid dosage forms are liquids. Thus, the key additive that is used to render the coating formulation a liquid is a solvent (the term vehicle is used to describe the situation where an aqueous polymer formulation is preferred). A list of common solvents used in coating formulations is given in Table 33.6.

Quite clearly, in modern film-coating practices, water is often the preferred solvent to be used. Nonetheless, water is a compromise solvent for these reasons:

• Water has higher latent heat of vaporization (see Table 33.7), thus requiring more energy input to the coating process to ensure that effective drying takes place (thus often precluding the use of conventional coating equipment).
• Aqueous coating systems have higher surface tensions than their organic solvent-based counterparts (see Table 33.8), thus impacting

wetting and adhesion (see Table 33.9) on many types of pharmaceutical tablets (e.g., vitamins).
• Aqueous coating systems are more viscous than organic solvent-based systems (see Table 33.10), thus having some impact on pumping and atomization efficiency.

In some cases, these potential challenges that need to be faced when using aqueous coating formulations have necessitated the continued use of organic solvents, especially when:

• the coating process will not accommodate the use of water (i.e., drying is poor);
• the adhesion achieved with aqueous systems is unacceptable;
• certain critical ingredients (e.g., polymer) are neither water-soluble, nor available as a latex system;
• exposure to an aqueous process would cause stability problems for the product being coated.

TABLE 33.6 Examples of common solvents used in film-coating formulations

Class	Examples
Water	–
Alcohols	Methanol
	Ethanol
	Isopropanol
Esters	Ethyl acetate
	Ethyl lactate
Ketones	Acetone
Chlorinated hydrocarbons	Methylene chloride
	1:1:1 Trichloroethane
	Chloroform

TABLE 33.7 Latent heats of vaporization of common solvents

Solvent	Latent heat of vaporization (kJ kg^{-1})
Methylene chloride	556.7
Methanol	1967.1
Water	2260.4

TABLE 33.8 Surface tension values of common solvents

Solvent	Surface tension (mN m^{-1}) at 20°C
Acetone	23.7
Chloroform	27.1
Ethyl alcohol	22.8
Methyl alcohol	22.6
Water	72.8

TABLE 33.9 Adhesion values of HPC coatings deposited from various solvents

Solvent system	Adhesion value (kPa)
Methylene chloride: methanol (9:1)	29.8
Ethanol: water (95:5)	23.9
Acetone: water (9:1)	20.2
Chloroform	14.4
Water	7.1

TABLE 33.10 Influence of solvents on the viscosity of HPMC-based coating solutions

Solvent	Polymer concentration (% w/w)	Solution viscosity (mPa s) (cP)
60:40 methylene chloride–methanol	5.0	40
80:20 ethanol–water	5.0	70
Water	10.0	450

33.2.3 Film-coating Formulations Used for Immediate-release Applications

Characteristics of Polymers Used

Polymers used in immediate-release film-coating formulations are generally water soluble. Polymers are selected for their ability to:

- form strong, flexible films;
- adhere strongly to tablet surfaces;
- form elegant films;
- facilitate ease of processing (pumping, spraying, atomization, and lack of tackiness);
- permit rapid drug release from dosage forms.

A typical dissolution profile for a product coated with an immediate-release film-coating is shown in Figure 33.15.

Examples of Types of Polymers Used

Examples of polymers used in immediate-release coating formulations are shown in Table 33.11.

Cellulosic polymers

Cellulosic polymers, especially HPMC, have long been the mainstay of film-coating formulations, with a popularity that stems from their:

- common usage from the early days of film-coating when organic solvents were always used;
- global regulatory acceptance;
- ready availability from a number of vendors;
- ability to form coatings generally having acceptable properties (such as good film strength and aqueous solubility).

Vinyl pyrrolidone polymers

The most common vinyl polymer used in the pharmaceutical industry today is, of course, poly (vinyl pyrrolidone). While this polymer has been primarily used as a wet binder in granulation processes, it has certain utility in film coatings (because of its potentially high film adhesion characteristics), although uses are somewhat limited because:

- It forms extremely tacky films (both during application of the coating and on final coated product).
- It creates coatings that tend to be somewhat brittle.

In contrast, poly (vinyl pyrrolidone)-poly (vinyl acetate) copolymer potentially has greater utility because:

- its films are much less tacky than the homopolymer;
- its films exhibit good adhesion characteristics;
- it produces coating solutions with low viscosities.

Vinyl alcohol polymers

Poly (vinyl alcohol) has gained popularity recently because of its good film properties, and the relatively low viscosity of coating solutions made with this polymer. Typical properties of coatings made with this polymer include:

- formation of coating solutions that can be somewhat tacky;
- creation of strong films that can adhere strongly to tablet surfaces;
- creation of films that are claimed to have good barrier properties, especially with respect to moisture and oxygen;

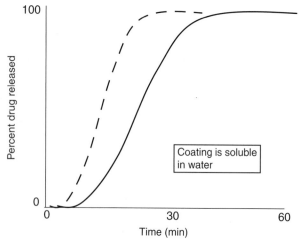

FIGURE 33.15 Typical drug release profile for products coated with immediate-release coatings

TABLE 33.11 Examples of common polymers used in immediate-release coating formulations

Polymer class	Examples
Cellulosic	• Hydroxypropylmethylcellulose • Hydroxypropylcellulose • Hydroxyethylcellulose
Vinyl	• Poly (vinyl pyrrolidone) • Poly (vinyl alcohol) • Poly (vinyl pyrrolidone), poly (vinyl acetate) copolymers • Poly (vinyl alcohol), poly (ethylene glycol) copolymers
Glycols	• Poly (ethylene glycol)
Acrylics	• Amino alkyl methacrylate copolymers
Other carbohydrates	• Maltodextrins • Polydextrose

development of films that may, under certain circumstances, delay dissolution of APIs that are relatively water-insoluble to begin with.

Poly (vinyl alcohol)-poly (ethylene glycol) is a copolymer, designed specifically to overcome some of the shortcomings of the homopolymer, and typically produces:

- films that are less tacky than the homopolymer;
- films that exhibit good adhesion characteristics;
- films that are very flexible;
- coating solutions that have low viscosity.

Acrylic polymers

The acrylic polymers that are typically used in IR film-coating applications are:

- not water soluble, per se (the polymer tends to dissolve readily at low pH);
- traditionally used to create film-coatings with improved taste masking capabilities, since the pH in the mouth is usually alkaline (i.e., above that where the coating will dissolve in water);
- usually applied as solutions in organic solvents, although special polymer grades that allow aqueous polymer suspensions to be prepared are now available.

Formulation Strategies Used

Traditionally, immediate-release film-coatings have utilized relatively simple formulation strategies, typically combining a single polymer in combination with other ingredients, such as plasticizers and colorants. The introduction of aqueous coatings created a major challenge for formulators, especially with regard to managing the viscosity of the coating formulation, and achieving acceptable adhesion of the coating to the surface of the tablets being coated.

Such challenges have typically been met, over the course of time, by utilizing polymer mixtures, such as blends of:

- different molecular weight grades of the same polymer (such as a mixture of HPMC 6 cP and HPMC 3 cP);

- similar polymers (such as HPMC + HPC);
- cellulosic polymers with other carbohydrate materials (such as HPMC with maltodextrins, polydextrose, or lactose).

The properties of some typical polymer blends are shown in Table 33.12.

33.2.4 Film-coatings Used for Modified-release Applications

As described earlier, film coatings used for modified-release applications can be subdivided into two main categories, namely:

- delayed-release (or enteric) coatings;
- extended-release coatings.

Delayed-release (Enteric) Coatings

Enteric coatings are primarily used for the purpose of:

- Maintaining the stability of APIs that are unstable when exposed to the acidic conditions of the gastric milieu. Such APIs include erythromycin, pancreatin, and the class of proton pump inhibitors, such as omeprazole.
- Minimizing the side-effects (e.g., nausea, gastric irritation and bleeding) that can occur with certain APIs, such as aspirin and certain non-steroidal inflammatory compounds.
- Creating opportunities for "night-time dosing" strategies, where the intent is to allow the dosage form to be consumed at bed-time, to permit effective blood levels of the API to be attained just prior to waking.
- Facilitating colonic drug delivery.

The functionality of enteric coatings is, for the most part, mediated by a change in pH of the environment to which the enteric-coated product is exposed. That said, such functionality can be greatly affected by many factors, such as:

- the nature of the API contained in the dosage form; this is especially true when that API possesses distinct pH effects of its own;

TABLE 33.12 Film properties of various polymer blends

Polymer	Tensile strength σ (MPa)	Elastic modulus, E (GPa)	σ/E value ($\times 10^{-2}$)	Film adhesion (kPa)
HPMC blend	31.74	2.25	1.41	250.5
HPMC/HPC blend	17.68	0.99	1.79	253.5
HPMC/lactose blend	13.53	2.34	0.58	500.6

- the quantity of coating applied; insufficient coating can result in ineffective gastric resistance, while too much applied coating can seriously delay drug release when the dosage form passes into the small intestine;
- the presence of imperfections in the coating (e.g., cracks, "pick marks," etc.) that can also lead to reduced gastric resistance;
- the chemistry of the polymer used (especially dissolution pH, and dissolution rate at a given pH);
- the influence of the *in vitro* test conditions used (such as pH and ionic strength of the test medium, as well as the agitation rate used in the test).

Enteric film-coating polymers are essentially poly-acids (see Figure 33.16), and typically only dissolve in water above pH = 5.0 to 6.0. These polymers are selected for their ability to:

- form tough films;
- adhere strongly to tablet surfaces;
- facilitate ease of processing (pumping, spraying, atomization, and lack of tackiness);
- permit rapid drug release from the dosage form once it passes from the stomach into the small intestine (see Figure 33.17).

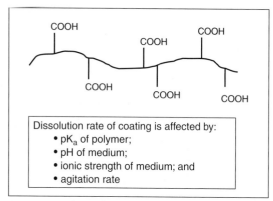

FIGURE 33.16   Structure of enteric-coating polymers

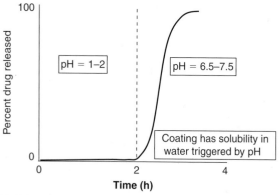

FIGURE 33.17   Typical drug release profile from products coated with enteric coatings

A list of commonly-used enteric-coating polymers is given in Table 33.13, and these form the basis of enteric-coating formulations used in either organic solvent-based or aqueous coating formulations. A breakdown of coating systems especially designed for aqueous coating applications is shown in Table 33.14.

While enteric-coated products have conventionally taken the form of tablets, more recently a preference has been shown for coating multiparticulates, because

TABLE 33.13   Examples of common polymers used in enteric coating formulations

Polymer	Comments
Cellulose acetate phthalate	Hydrolysis potential – high**
Cellulose acetate trimellitate	Hydrolysis potential – medium**
Polyvinyl acetate phthalate	Hydrolysis potential – low**
Hydroxypropylmethylcellulose phthalate	Hydrolysis potential – medium**
Hydroxypropylmethylcellulose acetate succinate	Hydrolysis potential – low**
Poly (MA – EA)* 1:1	–
Poly (MA – MMA)* 1:1	Relatively high dissolution pH
Poly (MA – MMA)* 1:2	Relatively high dissolution pH

*MA = Methacrylic acid; EA = Ethyl acrylate; MMA = Methyl methacrylate
**When exposed to conditions of elevated temperature and humidity

TABLE 33.14   Examples of aqueous enteric coating systems

Product	Form	Polymer
Eudragit L30D*	Latex dispersion	Poly (MA–EA)**
Eudragit L100-55*	Spray-dried latex	Poly (MA–EA)**
HP-F	Micronized dry powder	HPMCP
Sureteric	Formulated, dry powder system	PVAP
Acryl-Eze	Formulated, dry powder system	Poly (MA–EA)
Advantia Performance	Formulated, dry powder system	Poly (MA–EA)
Aquateric	Spray-dried pseudo latex	Poly (MA–EA)
Aquacoat ECD	Pseudo latex dispersion	CAP
Aqoat	Dry powder	HPMCAS
CAP	Dry powder	CAP
CAT	Dry powder	CAT

*Competitive acrylic products now available from BASF, Eastman, & Sanyo
**MA = Methacrylic acid; EA = Ethyl acrylate

of the more consistent GI transit characteristics of this type of dosage presentation. Enteric-coated capsules (especially one-piece softgels containing garlic or fish oils used in nutraceutical applications) have also become quite commonplace.

Extended-release Coatings

Extended-release coatings are typically those that are completely insoluble in water, and permit the release of the API by some manifestation of diffusion through an intact coating membrane. Polymer selection, and the general formulation strategies employed in this category will very much depend on a number of factors, including a desire to:

- create a specific type of drug-release characteristic;
- minimize the risk of dose-dumping;
- utilize processing methodologies that already exist within the company;
- prepare a unique dosage form that enables the manufacturer to take a proprietary position with respect to dosage form presentation.

In order to meet these requirements, critical objectives include the need to:

- Achieve the target drug-release characteristics in a reproducible manner.
- Ensure that drug-release characteristics are insensitive to expected variations in raw materials and coating-process conditions.

- Confirm that the coating formulations (and associated coating processes) are essentially uncomplicated, and facilitate scale-up from the laboratory into production.
- Ensure that the final product is stable, and does not exhibit time-dependent changes in drug-release characteristics.

When it comes to designing extended-release products, these may take a number of forms, namely:

- Tablets, prepared as:
  - film-coated tablets;
  - film-coated mini-tablets;
  - compacted, film-coated particulates.
- Capsules, prepared as:
  - encapsulated, film-coated particulates;
  - film-coated capsules.

Because of the desire to minimize dose dumping and facilitate more consistent gastrointestinal transit times, coated multiparticulates often form the basis for extended-release products where an applied coating is the main mediator of drug release. Such coated multiparticulates (see Figure 33.18) often take the form of:

- drug-loaded pellets (non-pareils);
- granules (irregularly-shaped granules or granules that have been spheronized);
- drug crystals;
- drug/ion-exchange-resin complexes.

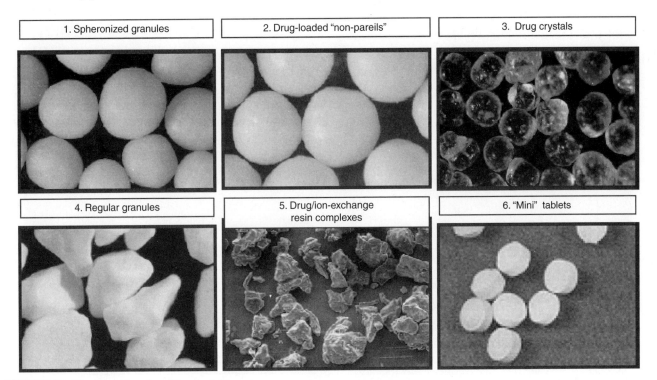

FIGURE 33.18   Examples of multiparticulates

In terms of designing extended-release coating formulations, the types of polymers used are often selected for their ability to:

- form tough films;
- adhere strongly to tablet surfaces;
- facilitate ease of processing (pumping, spraying, atomization, and lack of tackiness);
- permit drug to be released slowly, and at a consistent rate, throughout the GI tract.

A typical drug release profile is shown in Figure 33.19.

A list of common polymers used for extended-release coating applications is shown in Table 33.15, while examples of aqueous coating systems are shown in Table 33.16.

The performance of extended-release coating formulations is contingent on a number of issues that include the:

- Nature of polymer used, especially in terms of its chemistry (which can greatly influence coating permeability), and molecular weight (which has a significant effect on coating robustness).
- Presence of additives, such as:
  - plasticizers (which can greatly influence coating robustness, as well as the extent of film formation when using aqueous polymer dispersions);
  - anti-adhesive agents (which are often used to reduce agglomeration in the case of multiparticulates, as well as reduce imperfections in the coating caused by picking and sticking);
  - colorants which, although used for identification purposes, can influence film permeability;
  - water-soluble pore-forming agents, which are typically added to the formulation as a deliberate strategy to modify the permeability characteristics of the applied coating.

- Coating thickness which is, in turn, influenced by the:
  - surface area to be covered;
  - quantity of coating applied;
  - uniformity of distribution of coating;
  - coating process efficiency.

TABLE 33.15 Examples of common materials used in extended-release coating formulations

Coating material	Membrane characteristics
Fats and waxes (beeswax; carnauba wax; cetyl alcohol; cetostearyl alcohol)	• Permeable and erodible
Shellac	• Permeable and soluble (at high pH)
Zein	• Permeable and soluble (at high pH)
Ethylcellulose	• Permeable and water-insoluble
Cellulose esters (e.g., acetate)	• Semi permeable and water insoluble
Acrylic ester copolymers	• Permeable and water insoluble

TABLE 33.16 Examples of aqueous extended-release coating systems

Product	Polymer used	Comments
Surelease	Ethylcellulose	Plasticized aqueous polymer dispersion. Addition of lake colorants should be avoided
Aquacoat	Ethylcellulose	Pseudo-latex dispersion. Plasticizer must be added to facilitate film formation
Eudragit NE 30D*	Acrylic copolymer	Latex dispersion. No plasticizer needed unless it is necessary to improve film flexibility
Eudragit RL 30D*	Acrylic copolymer	Aqueous polymer dispersion. No plasticizer needed unless it is necessary to improve film flexibility
Eudragit RS 30D*	Acrylic copolymer	Aqueous polymer dispersion. No plasticizer needed unless it is necessary to improve film flexibility

*Also available as Kollicoat Systems

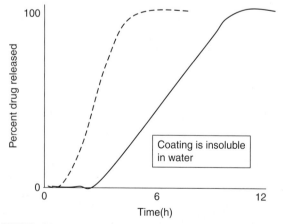

FIGURE 33.19 Typical drug release profile from products coated with extended-release coatings

While extended-release coating formulations have typically been designed as polymer solutions in organic solvents, there has been significant interest over the last 20 years in using aqueous coating systems. Irrespective of the formulation approach used, it is critical that:

- The formulation of the coating enables the appropriate drug release characteristics to be achieved in a consistent manner.
- The membrane obtained is structurally sound.
- The coating systems are readily adaptable to existing coating process technology.
- The coating formulation and processes are sufficiently optimized to prevent time-dependent changes in drug-release characteristics occurring.

Meeting these objectives can be more challenging when using aqueous polymer dispersions, since it is necessary to ensure that:

- Coalescence of the coating during film formation proceeds to an end point where membrane porosity is eliminated.
- This completeness of coalescence is either achieved during the coating process or by means of a short curing step performed at the conclusion of that process.
- Further gradual coalescence, over an extended period of time, is avoided.

Thus, the coating formulation used must be suitably optimized in terms of its ability to achieve completeness of film coalescence in the particular coating process to be employed. This usually means that the minimum film-forming temperature (which is closely related to the glass transition temperature of the polymer employed, either in its natural state or as modified by the presence of a plasticizer) is matched to the typical temperature conditions used in the process. In addition, the coating process conditions employed must also be optimized to ensure that they enable the correct temperature conditions to be achieved (to facilitate film coalescence).

33.3 DESIGN AND DEVELOPMENT OF THE FILM-COATING PROCESSES

33.3.1 General Introduction to Coating Processes and Equipment

Overview

A film coating is usually applied onto tablets until they reach a targeted weight range. Alternatively, the quantity of film coating may be expressed as a percentage weight gain. A typical weight gain for an aesthetic coating is 2 to 4%, whereas for clear coatings, the weight gain may be as little as 0.5 to 1.0%. For controlled release applications, the quality of the film is directly related to its thickness. A thickness of 30 to 50 microns (this translates to 4 to 6 mg polymer/cm^2 of tablet surface) is usually sufficient to provide a satisfactory enteric coating. Since a batch of smaller tablets contains a greater total tablet surface area, it will require a greater weight gain to achieve a controlled release film of a suitable thickness.

The reasons for selecting film-coating are essentially the same, regardless of whether the process is performed in a perforated coating pan or by the fluid-bed coating process. In general, the major criterion for deciding between whether to use the coating pan or fluid-bed coating is the size of the product substrate. A rule of thumb is that if the product is approximately 6 mm or less in diameter, then the preferred equipment for coating is the fluid-bed coater. When coating small particles in a perforated coating pan (with air flow that is drawn down through the tablet bed), the pressure drop across the product bed drastically reduces the process air volume, a factor which will reduce the evaporative capacity of the pan. This, coupled with the close contact of the product in the spray zone, makes the coating of small particles in the coating pan less desirable. For the coating of large product substrates, the relatively rough product movement experienced in the fluid-bed makes it less desirable. Additionally, it may be difficult to achieve an acceptable product movement with large irregular shaped tablets in a fluidized-bed coater.

Batch-coating Systems

Batch-coating requires some type of container in which the product to be coated is placed and then heated. Coating pans are manufactured in a variety of styles. Each of them can perform coating when used properly. Typically the container for the product will be cylindrical, and rotate on a horizontal axis. A coating material will be sprayed onto the product using some type of dispersion device, typically a spray gun. Droplets from the spray gun are composed of a solution (or suspension) which is a mixture of a liquid carrier and solids. The principle of this type of coating is to apply the solution in such a manner that a droplet from the spray gun will land on the product and spread. The temperature of the product will then rapidly evaporate the liquid from the suspension, leaving only the dried solids. The suspension viscosity must be such that any evaporation that occurs between the

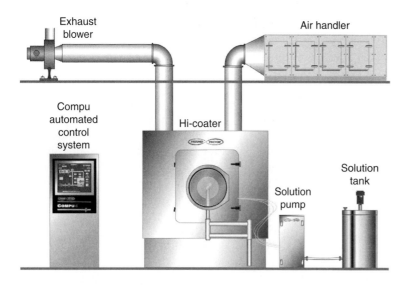

FIGURE 33.20 Example of a coating system for batch processing

spray gun and the product will allow the droplet to spread before the carrier evaporates. This will leave a dry coating, consisting of the solids that were in the solution, on the surface of the product.

Each tablet must have an equal probability of passing through the spray, in order to produce a uniform coating. The drums typically have some type of mixing baffle that forces the product to not only tumble, but to move back and forth on the cylindrical wall of the coating pan. The coating pan must provide a means for conditioned process air to pass through or over the product for heat transfer. A means for mounting spray guns must also be provided inside the coating pan.

The coating pans referenced in this section will be those that are considered as closed-operation pans (opening to the pan is closed during operation). Coating can be performed in open pans, but at a loss of efficiency. The function of the coating drum is to provide a space where product can reside, and be moved in such a manner that all surfaces of the product are exposed for an equal amount of time to the spray.

The challenge of film-coating is to apply the spray droplets uniformly, and for all of the droplets to dry at the proper evaporative rate. The spray droplets must contain the proper level of liquid when they strike the tablet surface. If the spray droplets contain too much liquid, over-wetting of the substrate will occur. If the droplets are too dry, they will not spread or coalesce to form a smooth film. While it sounds fairly easy, a number of variables (at sometimes seeming almost infinite) can cause difficulties in the pursuit of an acceptable coating.

Continuous Coating Systems

A continuous coating system differs from the batch system in that the tablets, once they are heated, are coated with the total amount of coating material in one pass through the spray. The systems and equipment for the two types of coating are very similar, except for the operation of the coating pan unit.

System Components

The peripheral equipment for a coating system, for either the batch system or the continuous coating system, will be very similar. Figures 33.20 and 33.21 show equipment components typically used with batch and continuous coating systems. Some systems may not require all of these components, depending on the source for the process air.

Overview

Process air is drawn in through an air handler where it will be heated, dehumidified (or humidified), and filtered before going to the coating pan. The process air goes through some type of perforated coating pan, and is exhausted through duct work to a dust collector and a blower. Finally, the exhausted air is returned to the source for the process air. Solvent systems will require a solvent recovery unit or an incinerator before the process air can be exhausted back to the source of the process air. Some solvent systems may be a closed-loop system, where the outlet process air becomes the source for the inlet process air. This type of system has to be designed for some loss of air after the solvent recovery unit, because compressed air will be added to the process air if pneumatic spray guns are utilized. A closed-loop system has the advantage of using process air which is conditioned for the operating parameters, thus it requires less energy to operate the system, but it is more difficult to make operational.

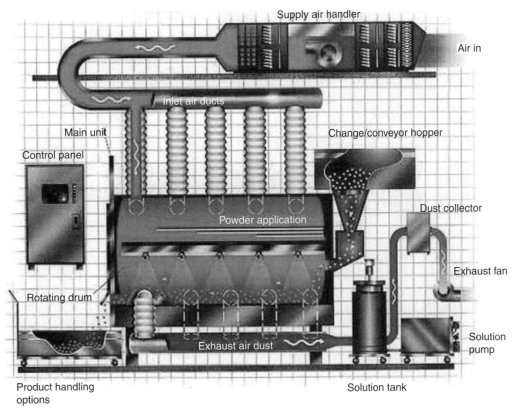

FIGURE 33.21 Example of a coating system for continuous process

33.3.2 Pan Units

Comparison of Batch-type Coating Pans

The coating drum can be either fully or partially perforated around the cylindrical surface, which allows process air to be drawn through a product placed in the coating pan. An example of a partially perforated coating drum is shown in Figure 33.22, which shows integrated exhaust plenum on the outside of the drum. A fully perforated drum is shown in Figure 33.23, which does not have integrated plenums.

The coating drum rotates and the product tumbles in the drum, always remaining near the bottom of the pan. Partially-perforated coating pans are constructed with exhaust plenums onto the outside of the pan. Process air enters the coating pan through a mouth ring at the front opening of the pan or through the back of the pan, and is drawn out through the exhaust plenums built onto the exterior of the cylindrical portion of the drum (see Figure 33.24). The perforations in the coating pan are located over these plenums. This arrangement forces all of the process air to travel through the tablet bed. Because of the plenum system and the tablets, there is greater pressure drop in the path of the process air (compared to the fully-perforated pan). The path of the process air through the fully perforated pan is shown in Figure 33.25.

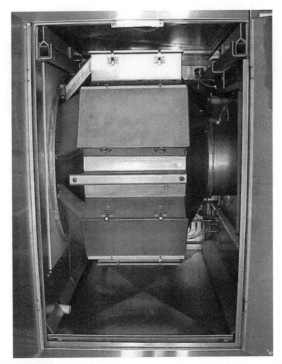

FIGURE 33.22 Exhaust plenum on the exterior of a partially perforated coating drum

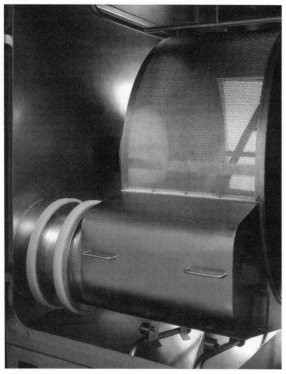

FIGURE 33.23   Exterior of the fully perforated coating drum

Coating can be performed with any of these pans if the auxiliary equipment (blowers, heater, filters, etc.) is configured properly for the physical layout, and the individual pieces are correctly specified. Some coating pan equipment includes autodischarge. The mixing baffles are configured in these pans such that, when the pan is rotated in a reverse direction, the product will be discharged out of the door. Some coating pans have a trap door on the product drum, such that the product can be discharged into product trays placed under the units. Several of the manufacturers will supply product loading chutes that will allow the product to be loaded from above the coating pan, instead of through the drum opening.

Coating pan capacities for laboratory size units range from 0.5 liters to 110 liters. Capacities for production size coating pans range from 90 liters to 1300 liters. The laboratory-size units are used to perform feasibility studies, and develop product and processes. An example of laboratory size units is shown in Figure 33.26. In general, each manufacturer makes sizes of coating pans that are comparable.

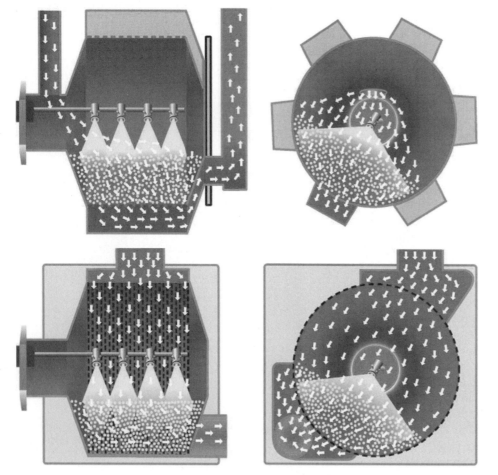

FIGURE 33.24   Air flow diagram and chamber design of a partially perforated pan

FIGURE 33.25   Air flow diagram and chamber design of a fully perforated pan

Each manufacturer will provide specifications for general operation of their coating pans. Typically, they will recommend and/or furnish the peripheral equipment required to complete a system.

33.3.3 Comparison of Continuous-coating Equipment

An example of a continuous coating unit is shown in Figure 33.27. The product is moved through a drum at a rate that allows the tablets to be completely coated as it traverses the length of the coating pan. The area where the coating occurs is in a drum which rotates. There are mixing baffles, similar to those in the batch

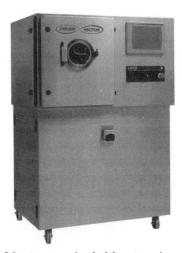

FIGURE 33.26   An example of a laboratory size coating pan

coating pans, which move the product from one end of the coating unit to the other. As the coating unit drum rotates, the product tumbles, thus allowing all sides of the product to be coated under the spray.

33.4 PROCESS AIR EQUIPMENT

All coating pan equipment, including continuous-coating equipment, requires conditioned process air to perform the coating. The process air generally should be dehumidified, cleaned, and heated. An air handler is used to perform these functions. The air handler is made up of different functional sections, as shown in Figure 33.28.

The first section will generally be composed of two filters, a bird screen followed by a prefilter. The prefilter is typically rated for 30% efficiency. The next section of the air handler is a preheat unit, followed by a dehumidification unit. The preheat section is placed before the dehumidification unit, to protect any chilled water coil (or refrigeration coil) from freezing. Three methods of dehumidification are used, chilled water, refrigeration or a desiccant dryer. The desiccant dryer is generally used to obtain lower dew points. If humidification is required (during winter time when the air is very dry), this is accomplished by injecting steam into the process air stream. A heating coil is required to heat the process air.

The air handler shown in Figure 33.28 is a face and bypass unit which will allow the unit to switch between cool air and heated air rapidly. A non-bypass type air handler will require some time to cool down,

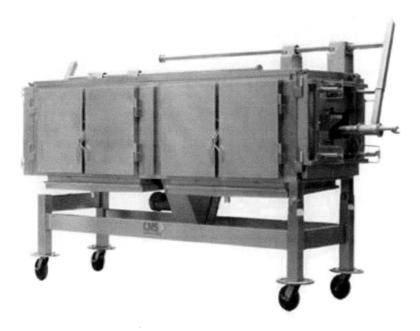

FIGURE 33.27   Example of a continuous coating pan

because the heater coils remain in the process air stream after the heat has been stopped. The product is normally cooled, before being removed from the coating pan after spraying is completed. The face and bypass unit can achieve a shorter production time, because a heating coil does not have to cool down before cooling the product. Finally, the air handler will contain a blower which must be rated for the proper quantity of process air (CFM) to provide the heat transfer into the product. The final stage of an air handler should be a HEPA filter, to provide clean air to the coating drum with 99.97% efficiency.

Figure 33.20 shows the components that may be used in a typical batch-coating pan system. The duct work between the HEPA filter and the coating pan should be stainless steel, to preserve the integrity of the clean process air. When another type of duct work is used, such as galvanized or painted duct work, chipping can occur (possibly due to rust), and allow particles to be added to the product. The quantity of process air is generally recommended by the manufacturer for the size of the equipment. It is desirable to use the maximum amount of process air possible, to achieve the maximum heat for the product. However, one must use caution when a decision is made to increase the air flow within the system, because pressure drops increase exponentially, and turbulence can be generated that will affect the spray patterns inside the coating pan. The inlet blower

should be capable of providing sufficient air pressure at the desired quantity of air to bring the pressure in the coating pan to atmospheric pressure or slightly negative (up to −100 mm of water column) when the exhaust blower is operating and product is loaded in the pan. The exhaust blower must provide a vacuum pressure at the required air flow that will overcome the losses created by the different components between the coating pan and the exhaust blower. This allows the full capability of the exhaust blower to be utilized.

The outlet process air duct should be ducted to a dust collector to collect solids that did not adhere to the product or dust that is generated when product is loaded into the coating pan. The ductwork, before and after the dust collector, and the dust collector itself, must be able to withstand the amount of vacuum that will be created by the exhaust blower. The dust collector must also be designed with an explosion vent that will relieve the pressure in case of a dust explosion. When film-coating is performed using a solvent as a carrier, the entire system must be designed to prevent or vent explosions. Typically, the manufacturer will recommend a system that will satisfy the requirements for a specific type of solvent.

As mentioned earlier, the partially-perforated coating pan will create more pressure drop, thus requiring a high pressure blower, whereas a fully-perforated coating pan requires less pressure drop, but a larger

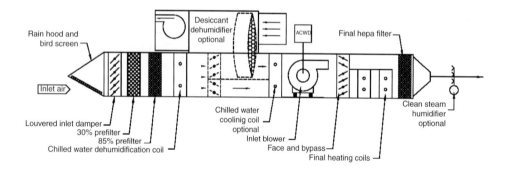

FIGURE 33.28 Example of an air handling system

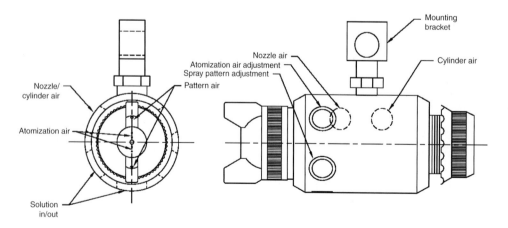

FIGURE 33.29 Example of a spray gun with separate adjustments for atomization air and pattern air

quantity of air. Finally, an exhaust blower should be used that will provide the recommended air flow for heat transfer, and be able to provide a vacuum of 25 to 100 mm of water column inside the coating pan. In areas where the noise of the blower cannot be tolerated, especially on systems that require a high pressure blower, a silencer should be used after the exhaust blower. Most manufacturers of coating pans will provide the above peripheral equipment as part of a turnkey system. Some systems will have a bypass section, which allows the process air to bypass the coating pan. This bypass section would be used where the coating pan door must be opened for several minutes, thus allowing cool air to enter the coating pan. If the temperature probe which is used for the control loop is in the exhaust duct work, the control loop will call for a higher temperature. When the coating pan door is closed, the inlet process air temperature will be considerably higher, which in turn can cause the product temperature to exceed the set limits. The bypass allows the process air temperature to remain constant. The bypass must also have a pressure drop to prevent the air flow from increasing, thus causing a temperature change during bypass conditions. Utilizing the bypass will then allow the temperature control loop to hold the process air at a constant temperature during the time the air flow is not passing through the coating pan.

33.5 SPRAY SYSTEMS

The design and operation of the spray system is critical for the coating process. In general, two types of spray systems are used, an open-loop system or a recirculation-loop arrangement. The open-loop arrangement is typically used with a hydraulic spray gun, while the recirculation-loop is used with pneumatic spray guns. The recirculation-loop provides more flexibility, but requires more equipment and tubing to configure. When the spray is off, the coating formulation is recirculated back to the solution tank, providing mixing in the tubing to prevent precipitation of solids out of solution. A separate agitator in the solution tank should be employed for coating formulations prone to precipitation. To use the recirculation-loop, a valve in the spray gun and a valve in the recirculation-loop must be provided to change from spray to recirculation. A flow measuring device is not needed for a positive displacement pump, but it is desirable. A separate pump can be provided for each spray gun or a single pump connected through a manifold can feed all spray guns. The manifold can create different pressures at each gun, due to the pressure drops in the manifold tubing, which in turn will cause different droplet sizes and distributions at each gun. Many spray systems use a multiple pump configuration, to prevent the pressure drop problem.

33.5.1 Comparison of Different Spray Guns

Two types of spray guns are typically used for coating, pneumatic and hydraulic. A third type is an ultrasonic, which has had limited success for coating processes.

33.5.2 Pneumatic Spray Gun

The pneumatic gun sprays liquid out through an orifice which is then subjected to a stream of compressed air that breaks the spray into droplets. The size of the droplets, the distribution of droplets, and the type of pattern is determined by the quantity of compressed air flow, and the physical configuration of the spray gun. An illustration of a pneumatic spray gun in Figure 33.29 shows the different ports for the air and solution. Manufacturers of spray guns are shown in Table 33.17.

Solution and air orifice sizes on the spray guns may have to be changed for different types of coating suspensions, but in general, a single orifice size will suffice for the typical coating suspensions that are used.

33.5.3 Hydraulic Spray Gun

A hydraulic spray gun uses pressure on the suspension to force it through an orifice which shears the liquid into droplets. The orifice must be changed for different types of spray patterns, and spray distributions. Hydraulic spray guns have limited use in coating pans, because the spray distribution is considerably wider than with pneumatic spray guns.

In both types of spray gun, as the spray rate is changed, the pattern, droplet size, and distribution will vary. The pneumatic gun provides more flexibility, because the atomizing air can be varied to obtain the desired spray without changing the nozzle. The ultrasonic spray gun, on the other hand, provides a small droplet size over the range of spray rate. Typically, with suspensions presently being used to coat, the small droplet size causes difficulty in the coating process, due to spray dry of the droplets and turbulence in the coating pan. The big advantage of the ultrasonic spray gun is that a large orifice is used, resulting in less plugging of the nozzle. Both the hydraulic and pneumatic spray guns are subject to plugging, causing

TABLE 33.17   Spray gun manufacturers

Manufacturer	Address	Trade name	Types of spray guns
Binks Sames Corporation	Geneseo, IL 61254	Binks Guns	Pneumatic
Freund (Vector Corp.)	Marion, IA 52302	Vector or Freund Guns	Pneumatic
Schlick	Coburg, GERMANY 96540	Schlick Guns	Pneumatic Hydraulic
Spraying Systems Co.	Wheaton, IL 60189	Spraying Systems	Pneumatic Hydraulic

disruption of the droplet size distribution, and the spray pattern. The hydraulic gun is more prone to plugging than the pneumatic gun. The pneumatic gun will not drip after the solution is turned off if the atomization air is left on for a short period of time.

33.5.4 Solution Delivery Pump

The open-loop arrangement described earlier for the spray system is generally used with a positive displacement pump, such as a gear pump, a lobe pump or a peristaltic pump. These pumps are capable of supplying pressures of 1 to 7 bar gauge pressure to the spray nozzles. Peristaltic pumps are commonly used, due to ease of cleaning and lower cost. Centrifugal pumps are normally not used, because of pressure requirements and the need for a flow measurement service, due to the characteristics of the pump.

The selection of the pump is determined by the type of spray gun to be used. The hydraulic spray gun will require 2 to 4 bar of solution pressure at the desired flow rates. The pneumatic spray gun will require 0.05 to 1.0 bar at the desired flow rate. The ultrasonic spray gun requires only pressure to supply the solution to the spray head, which will be less than 0.7 bar. Normally, pumps that operate at lower pressures create fewer problems relative to pump wear and sealing of connections to the pump and spray guns. To ensure that proper flow and pressure is provided to each spray gun, many of the spray systems incorporate a separate pump for each spray gun. A single pump or a single tubing distribution system to the spray guns will result in different pressures and flow rates at the spray guns. When selecting a pump, one must consider the solution source location. Some coating formulations may require

additional pump pressure, due to a high vacuum pressure on the inlet side of the pump. When using more than one pump, the inlet tubing must be sized for the total number of pumps, and the vacuum loss due to the size of the inlet tubing.

The connections for the spray system are very critical, and must be installed with care. If there is a leak in the tubing on the inlet side of the pump, air bubbles are created in the suspension which travel to the spray heads, and cause distortion of the spray pattern and droplet size distribution. Because all spray guns are mounted inside the coating pan over the product, any leaks in the tubing, piping or connections will result in dripping onto the product, causing twinning (tablets stuck together) or peeling (tablets stuck together and separated).

33.5.5 Delivery Control

The coating on the tablets can only be consistent if the amount of suspension being sprayed is consistent. For this reason, some type of control should be used for the flow of the suspension. In the past, assumptions have been made that if a positive displacement pump is used, then the rotational speed of the pump shaft (rpm) can be used for determining the flow rate. However, because of pressure changes in the system, and where more than one pump is used, variations in the spray gun outputs can occur. Therefore, it is advisable that some form of measurement and control be used for the suspension flow. The most common form of measurement is to use a mass flow meter. Spray systems that use a manifold for the spray guns can be configured to use a single pump, but a mass flow meter should be used at the outlet of the pump. Spray systems that use multiple pumps feeding individual guns should incorporate a mass flow meter in the common source line feeding the pumps. There are several types of mass flow meters that have been used, including vortex flow meters, coriolis mass flow meters, and turbines. Turbines, typically, are not used, because they cannot be cleaned properly without removing them from the coating suspension line. Differential pressure is not used, because this requires an orifice plate which generates more pressure drop for the spray system, thus increasing the workload for the pump. These flow devices will normally have to measure mass flow over a range of 100 to 1000 cc per minute. The second best method to measure the application of the coating is to use a weight loss system. Such a system involves putting the solution tank on load cells (weight measuring sensors) and then, knowing the density of the suspension, the amount of material applied can be determined as a reduction in the tank weight. This weighting system must be capable of having the tare weight set to zero before spray is started.

33.6 SYSTEM CONTROLS

The system controls may be one of several options, and should be chosen based on the tolerance required for the product, the operator technical knowledge level, and the amount of automation desired. There are basically three types of systems:

- Manual: all functions are selected and controlled by an operator.
- Semiautomatic: these systems use a combination of manual and automatic systems.
- Automatic: this system will require a minimal amount of operator input during the coating process.

Typically a process is developed in a manner that requires the equipment to be operated at specific conditions. The following conditions should be held constant:

- process air flow;
- process air temperature into the coating pan;
- average static pressure in the coating pan;
- humidity (or dew point) in the process air going into the coating pan;
- RPM of the coating pan;
- spray rate of the coating solution.

All three control systems mentioned earlier will require certain parameters to be measured, in order to make any coating system operate with consistent results. The manual system will have only instruments that provide local readouts, which are used by the operator to adjust the controls. Both types of automation will require outputs that can be input into a PLC or computer.

The following measurements are the minimum required for any of the coating systems to provide a consistent coating operation:

- inlet process air temperature;
- exhaust process air temperature from the coating pan;
- process air flow volume or flow rate in the inlet duct to the coating pan;
- pump speed or suspension spray rate;
- coating pan rotation (RPM).

These controls are required for each of the systems:

- power to the system;
- temperature controller of some type;

- air flow control (manual or motorized dampers or blower motor speed control);
- solution volume or rate control (mechanical or pump motor speed control);
- coating pan rotational speed (mechanical or pan motor speed control).

Each of the above items for either measurement or control will be analog in nature, either by an analog meter or an analog signal to a PLC or computer.

Other measurements that may be included on a coating pan system are as follows:

- process air temperature after the preheater;
- dew point temperature after the dehumidification or humidification;
- differential pressure across the inlet filter to the air handler;
- differential pressure across the HEPA filters in the inlet air duct;
- differential pressure across the coating pan;
- static pressure in the coating pan;
- differential pressure across the dust collector;
- static pressure after the air handler;
- static pressure at the inlet of the exhaust blower;
- product temperature;
- main compressed air pressure;
- solution tank weighing system;
- solution pressure;
- solution mass flow meter;
- compressed air flow rate to pneumatic spray guns.

33.7 GENERAL CHARACTERISTICS OF THE PHARMACEUTICAL COATING PROCESS

33.7.1 Typical Process Steps

If this is the first time that a particular product has been coated, it is a good idea to estimate the approximate batch size to use. Coating pans are usually rated for a specific brim volume capacity. Brim volume can be defined as volume capacity, if loaded to the very bottom of the pan opening. The initial pan load is usually somewhat less than brim volume. This prevents product from spilling out of the pan opening, should the product volume increase during the coating process or if the product movement should change. As a starting point, this volume capacity can be multiplied by 95%. This pan volume can then be multiplied by the product's bulk density (in g/cc) to determine the approximate maximum batch capacity. The product's bulk density can be approximated by determining the weight of a 1-liter volume of tablets. Batches of 70% to 75% of the maximum can usually be coated without any problem. For smaller batch sizes, it is necessary to examine product movement to verify that it is adequate. Reduced height baffles can be used to improve product movement with smaller pan loading. In these cases it may also be necessary to use a restrictor plate to reduce the exhaust opening. This will prevent air from being drawn around the tablet bed, rather than through it.

For continuous coating pan systems, the throughput is controlled by a combination of the pan drum angle and the pan speed (rpm). A higher throughput is achieved by increasing the drum angle or increasing the pan speed. Either one of these changes causes the product to flow more rapidly through the pan, thus increasing the potential production rate. One continuous coating pan system allows the drum to be adjusted from a $-2°$ to $6°$ angle.

33.7.2 Coating Pan Set-up

The typical coating process consists of several different steps. The first step of this process is to verify proper operation of the spray delivery system. The spray system must be calibrated to deliver a consistent gun-to-gun delivery of the coating solution. This is especially critical for systems that have solution lines that are manifold together. With this type of arrangement a restriction or difference in pressure drop between the spray guns will result in a non-uniform solution delivery. Calibration can be accomplished by individually collecting and weighing the solution from all the spray guns for a set interval of time. The calibration procedure should determine if the overall delivery of solution is accurate (if it matches the theoretical rate), and also the variation in solution flow between guns. If there is an unacceptable variation (usually $>\pm5.0$ %), then the system will need to be adjusted, so that the pressure drop between guns is the same. Most spray guns are equipped with a needle valve adjustment cap that controls the clearance between the spray needle and the liquid nozzle. If a spray gun is delivering more than its prescribed quantity of solution, then the adjustment cap should be turned clockwise to restrict the flow to that particular gun. After making an adjustment to the spray guns, the solution collection should be repeated. When uniform solution delivery has been achieved, it is necessary to calibrate the nozzle air volume to the spray guns. Some spray guns have a common line for providing atomization air and pattern air. For these

systems, the air volume is achieved by setting the desired nozzle air pressure. Other guns have separate controls for the atomization and pattern air, and a mist checker or flow meter for display of the actual air volume. For these systems, a needle valve (located on the spray gun body) is usually adjusted to set the atomization air volume. Once the atomization air volume has been set for all of the guns, then a second needle valve is adjusted to the desired volume for pattern air. After these air volumes have been set, it is possible to verify the approximate dimensions of the spray pattern by passing a hand through the air stream. This spray pattern should be checked at a distance that is equal to the distance between the tablet bed and the spray guns.

33.7.3 Loading/Charging

After proper set-up of the pan has been confirmed, the pan can be loaded with product, either through the front of the pan (pan mouth ring) or through a discharge door located on the flat of the pan (if it is so equipped). During the loading of the pan, the exhaust air is usually turned on to eliminate or minimize exposure to irritating and potentially hazardous dusts. It is a good idea to minimize the distance that the product is allowed to drop during charging, this will minimize or eliminate tablet breakage. It is usually recommended that the pan be jogged occasionally during loading, to move product towards the back of the pan.

33.7.4 Preheat/Dedusting

After loading, the next step is to preheat the product to the desired process temperature. While the product is being preheated, it is also being dedusted by the process air flow. This is a good time to circulate coating solution through the spray guns (if a recirculation system is used). Verification that the spray guns are positioned correctly can be accomplished at this time, checking both the angle to, and the distance from, the tablet bed. During the preheat step, the product should be rotated continuously at a very slow speed or jogged intermittently. This will minimize attrition, while ensuring that the product is uniformly heated. For products that are heat sensitive, it will be necessary to jog on a more frequent basis, to prevent overheating the upper surface of the tablet bed. Tablets are generally preheated to a specific product or exhaust temperature. The product and exhaust are not ordinarily at the same temperature, though during the coating process they tend be fairly close. Once the exhaust air or product has been heated to the desired starting temperature, the application of the coating can be initiated.

33.7.5 Seal/Barrier Coat

In a few rare cases, it may be necessary to apply a barrier coating subsequent to the application of the film-coating. An example of the need for a barrier/seal coat is when there is an interaction between the film polymer, and the product substrate (i.e., interaction between an enteric polymer with phthalyl groups and tablets containing an alkaline drug). This problem can be eliminated by the application of a seal coat of an inert film polymer, such as HPMC, prior to the enteric polymer coating.[i] A second example is when there is an interaction between the coating solvent and the product (i.e., an aqueous coating and an effervescent product). To remedy this type of problem, a seal coating with an alternative solvent may be used. It is possible to coat, for example, some effervescent products with aqueous solutions, if the spray rate for the initial phase of the coating is reduced, and process temperatures are substantially increased.

33.7.6 Film-coating Application

To begin the spray cycle the pan is first set at the desired rotational speed. If a frequency drive is used, it is important to allow approximately five seconds for the pan to achieve the rpm set-point. Once the product has reached the required speed, the spray can be started. The initiation of the spray will cause the product and exhaust temperatures to drop slightly, due to evaporative cooling. If these temperatures drop below the desired range, the inlet temperature will need to be increased. If the coating system has an inlet air handler with some type of humidity control, there will be a very consistent batch-to-batch correlation between the inlet temperature necessary to achieve the desired exhaust and/or product temperatures. Some systems automatically control the inlet to maintain the needed exhaust temperature. The time required for the coating cycle is determined by a number of factors that include: desired coating weight gain, coating efficiency, coating solution solids level, spray rate, and the size of the spray zone. Since these factors tend to be constant for a particular product, the end of the spray cycle is usually controlled either by time or by the application of a set quantity of coating solution. If the spray cycle is controlled by solution quantity, this

can be accomplished through the use of either a mass flow meter or a mass balance. Either of these methods will provide a totalization of the solution applied.

33.7.7 Gloss Coat

After the primary coating has been completed, a dilute overcoating may be applied, to prevent the tablets from blocking or sticking (such as with some of the aqueous dispersions that are thermoplastic) or to provide a higher film gloss. If the purpose is to provide a higher gloss, a dilute HPMC solution may be used. The process temperatures may be reduced slightly to reduce the amount of spray drying that occurs.

For some of the aqueous coating dispersions, it is recommended that the product be maintained at a slightly elevated temperature to fully cure the coating, and provide a stable release profile. After coating, the product should be cooled prior to the application of a powdered wax. Cooling the product after coating also minimizes potential problems, due to heat instability of the active. The product temperature will rise after the spray is turned off, due to loss of the evaporative cooling. Product is typically cooled to an exhaust or product temperature of 25–30°C.

33.7.8 Wax Addition

After cool down of the product, a powdered wax may be used to provide a higher tablet gloss. The waxes typically used are either a carnauba wax or a combination of carnauba and beeswax. A small quantity of wax (5–10 grams per 100 kg of tablets) is applied to the rotating tablet bed. The tablets are allowed to rotate for approximately five minutes, with no process air. After five minutes the tablets are rotated for an additional five minutes, with the process air on. This allows any excess wax to be exhausted. A canvas-lined pan is not necessary for the wax application, although it may provide a slightly higher gloss.

33.7.9 Product Discharge

At this point, the product is ready for discharge. Depending on the type of pan used, the product will be discharged through a "trap-door" on the flat of the pan or out through the front pan door. If product is discharged through the front door, a scoop may be temporarily installed inside, to convey product through the front door. In other systems, the pan may be rotated backwards or counterclockwise to discharge the product, in which case the baffles are designed to direct the product out the front door. Discharge of the entire batch usually will be achieved in 2–10 minutes,

---

[i] Aquateric® case History 2, FMC Corporation, Philadelphia, PA, 1968

depending on the pan size, and type of discharge method employed. For most cases, the coated product should not be allowed to drop more than 60 to 90 cm, otherwise tablet breakage may be experienced.

33.8 UNDERSTANDING PROCESS THERMODYNAMICS

33.8.1 Adequate Evaporative Rate

The theoretical evaporative rate for aqueous film-coating can be determined by using the following equation:

$$Rate = \frac{CMH \times C_P \times \lambda \times [(T_{IN} - T_{OUT}) - 0.10(T_{IN} - T_{OUT})]}{LHV}$$

where:

Rate = evaporative rate in kilograms of water per hour
CMH = actual process air flow in cubic meters per hour
C_P = specific heat capacity of the air (Kcal/kg°C)
λ = density of the air stream (kg/m³)
T_{IN} = inlet process temperature (°C)
T_{OUT} = exhaust process temperature (°C)
H_L = heat loss of the coating system (%)
LHV = latent heat of vaporization (Kcal/kg°C).

This equation will determine the approximate quantity of water (in pounds per hour) that can be evaporated in a coating pan system. However, it will not guarantee the quality level of the film-coating. The quality level, as stated earlier, is dependent on many other factors. If all of these other critical factors are examined and optimized, this equation can be used as a tool to determine the approximate spray rate.

Example

Assumptions:

Ambient air conditions = 21.1°C/50% RH
Air flow = 2166 m³/hr
Specific heat capacity of air = 0.241 (Kcal/kg°C)
Density of the air stream = 1.015 (kg/m³)
Inlet air temperature = 70°C (167°F)
Exhaust air temperature = 40.5°C (105°F)
Coating solution solids = 12%
Number of spray guns = 4
Heat loss = 10%
Latent heat of vaporization = 577 (Kcal/kg)

$$Rate = \frac{2166 \times 0.241 \times 1.015 \times [(75.0° - 40.5°) - 0.10(75.0° - 40.5°)]}{577}$$

= 28.51 kg/hour or 475 g/min of water evaporated. At 12% solution solids this equals 540 g/min/total or ~135 g/min/gun.

33.9 PROCESS AIR

33.9.1 Volume

In all coating pans, elevated temperatures are used in conjunction with the air flow to convert the solvent in the coating solution into a vapor, and away from the tablets being coated. In general, the amount of water vapor that can be removed is directly proportional to the air volume that passes through the coating pan, and is limited by the saturation of the air stream. Therefore, if maximum evaporative capacity is the rate-limiting factor with respect to the spray rate, it would be advantageous to use air flow as high as possible, without creating spray turbulence or air leakage. Manufacturers of the coating pans will usually specify the maximum air flow that can be used, yet still maintain an acceptable level of turbulence. As the process air stream is heated, its capacity to hold water vapor increases. Again, if maximum evaporative capacity is the rate-limiting factor, the inlet air temperature should be as high as possible. However, spray rates (per spray gun) are frequently limited, not by evaporative capacities but rather, by the diminishing quality of the spray as the spray rate is increased. The total spray rate is usually limited by the number of spray guns, but more accurately, the size of the spray zone available. Therefore, the air flow capacity between pans of different sizes should be in direct proportion to the spray zone. For example, if a coating process is developed in a pan with two spray guns (each gun possessing a 20 cm spray pattern), and a process air flow of 1000 CMH (cubic meters per hour), scale-up to a larger pan with four spray guns should have an air flow of approximately 2000 CMH. Using an air flow in direct proportion to the spray rate will also allow a closer correlation between the process temperatures in the different size pans.

33.10 HUMIDITY

The process air used in a coating pan is either conditioned or unconditioned. In either case there are day-to-day variations in the moisture present in the air stream. Humidity in the inlet air stream is usually determined by the dew point temperature. Dew point temperature provides a direct indication of humidity in the air. Relative humidity can be used, however, the temperature of the air must also be known to determine the level of moisture. In the case of conditioned air, variations are less. With unconditioned air, these variations are great, and can cause coating problems. If the air is unconditioned, the spray rate must be selected such that in the most humid conditions that might occur, the film-coating would still dry at a rate that would not result in overwetting or stability problems with the product. Since most batches would be coated at lower humidities, some level of spray drying would occur. The severity of the spray drying would be directly related to the variation in the ambient humidity. Therefore, the growing trend is to dehumidify the process air stream. Dehumidification not only provides the coating process with more consistent coating conditions, but also provides for greater evaporative capacity. This allows the system to evaporate more moisture at a given air flow and temperature than an air flow of a higher humidity. With the advent of sustained-release coatings, some companies have opted for a combination of dehumidification/ humidification. Such a system allows the process to be conducted at a consistent inlet dew point temperature, and allows the coating process to operate at a reproducible drying rate, regardless of fluctuations in ambient conditions.

33.11 TEMPERATURE

As stated earlier, the coating process can be successfully controlled by the inlet, exhaust or product temperatures. Process control based on inlet air temperature control is most common. Control based on exhaust or product temperatures will often react more slowly, because of the heat sink effect of the tablet bed. With inlet temperature control, the exhaust temperature will drop slightly after the spray is started. This temperature drop is due to evaporative cooling. This will not occur with exhaust temperature control, since the inlet temperature will be controlled to maintain the desired set point. In any event, control via any of these methods will yield the same approximate temperatures. Since the moisture from the spray droplets is dried by both convection (due to the process air) and conduction (due to the product temperature), all of these temperatures are equally important. The

desired exhaust temperature is dependent on several factors.

33.11.1 Coating Solution Characteristics

The tackier the coating as it dries, the higher the exhaust or product temperatures must be to prevent over-wetting defects during the coating process. If the film polymer is thermoplastic, the product must be kept below the temperature at which the polymer begins to soften, to prevent the tablets from blocking or sticking together.

33.11.2 Product Temperature Limits

If a product exhibits instability problems at elevated temperatures, the product must be held below these limits. This is most critical during preheating of the tablet bed since evaporative cooling of the bed is not occurring, and the product may not be uniformly heated if the pan is not being continuously rotated. The product temperature will begin to rise immediately after the spray is stopped, due to the loss of the evaporative cooling effect. Therefore, it may be necessary to begin a cool-down cycle immediately after the spray cycle.

The inlet temperature required to achieve the desired exhaust temperature will be affected by the spray rate, the percentage of solids in the coating solution, the heat loss across the pan, and the condition of the drying air.

33.11.3 Pan Speed

To effectively optimize film-coating quality, the tablets must be mixed such that each tablet has the same probability of being in the spray for an equal length of time. Therefore, it is essential that the product be examined to ensure that mixing is uniform. Mixing problems that occur include: sliding of tablets (usually seen with large capsules or oval-shaped tablets), "dead-spots" or sluggish product movement (this can be an extremely serious problem if it occurs while the tablets are in the spray zone) or product thrown into the spray zone by the mixing baffles.

If product movement is not uniform, the first course of action should be to evaluate the product flow at different pan speeds. The pan speed selected should be the lowest speed that produces a rapid and continuous product flow through the spray zone. This will allow for the uniform application of a film-coating, while subjecting the tablets to a minimal amount of abuse. In general, if tablet friability is less than 0.1%, then tablet attrition will not be a problem. A smaller tablet can be slightly softer, since these tablets produce a less abusive tumbling action. Product flow can be evaluated either subjectively or through mixing studies using tablets of various colors. Tablets of different colors can be placed in different zones (e.g., front, middle, and back) of the pan. Tablet samples are taken at set time intervals, to determine the length of time required to achieve a homogeneous mixture. A more sophisticated means of evaluation includes the use of radioactively marked tablets, and a counter mounted on the spray bar to record the number of passes through the spray zone per unit time.[ii] The product speed is generally assumed to be traveling at the same linear velocity as the inside circumference of the coating pan.

In a continuous coating pan system, the product flow is from the charge port to the discharge port. Depending on the coating level the product may pass through multiple drums (these drums may be located end to end or stacked horizontally). One continuous coating pan system currently available contains five spray guns for a 1.5 m coating drum length.

33.11.4 Understanding Spray Dynamics

Spray Rate

The selection of the proper spray rate is dependent on more than just the thermodynamic considerations. If this were not so, the ultimate coating system would offer unlimited air flow and temperature. The spray rate (per spray gun) is also dependent on the spray gun's ability to produce a consistent droplet size distribution. It has been shown that the droplet size distribution will increase as the spray rate is increased. Other factors that must be considered when determining the spray rate are:

- Solution viscosity: as solution viscosity is increased, the spray gun's ability to produce an acceptable droplet size distribution is diminished. Therefore, viscosity will limit the maximum spray rate that can be used and still produce acceptable film quality.
- Spray pattern width: if the spray pattern width is set up properly, the spray pattern will essentially be the same as the spray gun spacing. The typical gun to gun spacing is 12 to 20 cm. At spacing greater than 20 cm, the uniformity of the spray across the pattern begins to deteriorate. Spacing of less than 12 cm is an ineffective use of spray guns, and

tends to add more expense for added spray guns, solution lines, and pumps. There is a limit to how much spray that can be applied to a tablet per pass through the coating zone before the tablet begins to exhibit coating defects. Therefore, the wider the spray pattern width (without overlapping adjacent spray patterns), the greater the spray rate per gun.
- Product movement: the more consistent the product flow through the spray zone, the higher the spray rate that can be delivered, and still achieve an acceptable level of film-coating uniformity. Product movement is often dictated by the pan speed, baffle design, and tablet size and shape.

Droplet Size Distribution

One of the most critical aspects of coating concerns the manner in which solution is applied onto the tablet. The spray droplets can be almost any size if the size distribution is sufficiently narrow. If the system is set up to operate such that smaller droplets dry properly then larger droplets will stay wet, and picking or twinning will occur. If the system is set up to dry larger droplets properly, small droplets will be dry and not spread properly on the tablet, thus causing "orange-peeling," and a dull, rough, film appearance will result. Most spray guns used in the industry today have a limited range over which the spray can be varied and still retain a uniform distribution (see Figure 33.30, droplet size distribution, for examples of some typical droplet size distributions). These droplet size distributions were produced using a film solution with a viscosity of 130 cps. Ideally, a spray gun that produces a narrow droplet size distribution should be used. This distribution can vary with changes in solution viscosity, spray rate or a change in the type of solution solids, therefore, the manufacturers of the spray guns will generally not provide information

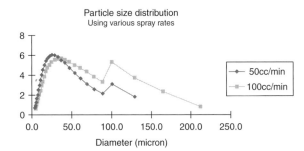

FIGURE 33.30　Droplet size distribution

[ii] Leaver, T.M. et al (1985) T. Pharm. Pharmacol. 37, 17–21.

concerning these parameters. A simple method of examining this distribution can be performed by quickly passing a sheet of paper through the spray, and subjectively analyzing the droplet size. A typical droplet distribution usually ranges from 5 to 250 microns. In general, if droplets vary in size from 5 to 1600 microns, it will be difficult to optimize the film-coating quality.

Coating Zone/Pattern

As mentioned earlier, the larger the spray zone per spray gun, the higher the maximum spray rate that can be used per spray gun. Therefore, if the gun spacing or the spray pattern is reduced, the spray rate should be reduced proportionally. Applying more spray per unit area of the tablet bed beyond a certain point will change the film-coating appearance. If the spray rate is increased above this maximum, either over-wetting or spray drying will occur, depending on whether the process is run dry or wet.

A recent trend in coating is to achieve greater production through the use of elongated or "stretch" coating pans. Lengthening the coating pan not only increases its capacity, but more importantly, the spray zone. This allows more spray guns to be used, thereby increasing the overall spray rate. An increase in pan volume achieved by increasing bed depth with no increase in spray zone does nothing to allow an increase in overall spray rate. Therefore, one means of scaling-up the process time for coating can be achieved by using the following calculations:

Spray time (large pan)

$$= \text{spray time (small pan)} \times \frac{\text{batch size (large pan)}}{\text{batch size (small pan)}}$$
$$\times \frac{\text{spray zone (small pan)}}{\text{spray zone (large pan)}}$$

These calculations assume that the coating zones for each of the pans are used efficiently.

A number of factors have an effect on the spray pattern width. As the pattern air volume for the spray gun is increased, the spray pattern is widened. An increase in the atomization air will cause a reduction in the pattern width. This is logical, since the increased volume of atomization air would make it more difficult to flatten or widen the pattern. Lastly, as the spray rate is increased, the spray pattern is widened. Therefore, if the atomization air volume or spray rates are adjusted, it is then important to re-examine the spray pattern width, to ensure that the spray zone is effectively utilized.

33.11.5 Coating Analysis

The following is a theoretical analysis of the film-coating process:

Product specification:	Tablet	8.0 mm diameter
	Weight	250.0 mg/tablet
	Density	0.73 g/cc
Coating solution specifications:	Solids	12%
	Density	1.0 g/cc
	Quantity	62.5 kg
Equipment specifications:	Pan diameter	170 cm
	Pan volume	550 L
	Pan speed	5 RPM
	4 spray guns	
Coating conditions:	Spray rate	125 g/min/gun
	Total spray rate	500 g/min
	Spray time	125 minutes

Assumptions:

Spray zone Per spray gun = spray width × spray pattern length = 7.5 cm × 20.0 cm = 150 cm^2

Total spray zone = number of spray guns × spray zone per gun = 4 × 150 cm^2 = 600 cm^2

Tablets per coating zone = total spray zone × number of tablets/cm^2

Assume 3.5 tablets/cm^2 in spray zone = 600 cm^2 × 3.5 tablets/cm^2 = 2100 tablets/coating zone

Total spray length = spray pattern width × number of spray guns = 20 cm × 4 = 80 cm

Tablet bed velocity (same as the peripheral pan velocity) = pan circumference × pan speed = 3.14 × 170 cm × 5.0 RPM = 2669 cm/min.

Tablets per minute in the spray zone Coating zone/min = tablet bed velocity × total spray length = 2669 cm/min × 80 cm = 213 520 cm/min

Tablets/min in the spray zone = coating zone/min × number of tablets/in^2 = 213 520 cm/min × 3.5 tablets/cm^2 = 747 320 tablets/min.

Coating solution per pass through the spray zone

$$\frac{\text{coating per pass}}{\text{through the spray zone}} = \frac{\text{total spray rate}}{\text{tablets per min/spray zone}}$$

$$\frac{\text{coating per pass}}{\text{through the spray zone}} = \frac{500 \text{ g/min}}{747,320 \text{ tablets/min}}$$
$$= 0.669 \text{mg/tablet}$$
$$\times (0.080 \text{mg solids}).$$

Passes through the spray zone

total passes through the spray zone

$$= \frac{\text{tablets per min/spray zone}}{\text{total number of tablets}} \times \text{spray time}$$

total passes through the spray zone

$$= \frac{747320 \text{ tablets/min}}{1700000 \text{ total tablets}} \times 125 \text{ min} = 55.0 \text{ passes}$$

Weight gain   Weight gain/tablet = coating per pass through the spray zone × number of passes

Weight gain/tablet = 0.080 mg solids/pass × 55.0 passes = 4.40 mg

$$\text{total weight gain} \approx \frac{\text{weight gain/tablet}}{\text{tablet weight}}$$

$$\text{total weight gain} \approx \frac{4.40 \text{ mg}}{225 \text{ mg/tablet}} \approx 2.0\%$$

In this analysis, each tablet would be within the spray zone approximately 55 times over the course of a 125 minute coating trial. In actuality, many of these tablets would be in the spray zone either more or less frequently, depending on the uniformity of the product movement. Additionally, failure to optimize the gun-to-gun delivery or spray distribution will have an adverse effect on the coating uniformity. Therefore, this factor should be examined to ensure a consistently high quality film-coating.

33.12 CONTROLLING COATING PROCESSES: CRITICAL FACTORS

Once all formulation requirements have been fulfilled, the following factors can be examined to optimize the coating quality and system performance. These factors can be grouped into three general areas: uniformity of spray application, uniformity of product movement, and achieving an adequate evaporative rate. These factors must all be examined and optimized, in order to optimize the coating process.

33.12.1 Uniformity of the Spray Application

Spray Gun Design

There are a variety of spray gun manufacturers. Some of the more common suppliers include Binks, Freund, Schlick, and Spraying Systems. The most common type of gun used is air atomizing or pneumatic. This type of gun allows the use of variable spray rates. In the past hydraulic gun systems were used, however, they did not allow flexibility in spray rates. The solution nozzle orifice must be sized to match the desired spray rate. In order to change the spray rate, a change in the solution nozzle was necessary. Additionally, the use of a smaller nozzle orifice made these more susceptible to plugging of the gun tip. With some types of spray guns, the air cap and spray nozzle configuration produce a predetermined ratio of atomization to pattern air at a given supply pressure. In other guns there are separate controls for adjusting the volumes of the atomization and pattern air. This allows the separate adjustment of either atomization or pattern, without having to change the air cap and/or the solution nozzle. For example, the width of the spray pattern can be changed without changing the spray droplet size. The atomization air breaks the solution stream into a fine droplet size, while the pattern air serves to flatten the spray into a fan-shaped pattern. The volume of atomization controls the mean droplet size of the spray. The pattern air volume controls the overall width of the spray.

Number of Spray Guns

The number of spray guns needs to be adequate to provide uniform coverage of the entire product bed. To maximize the uniformity and application of the coating, the spray zone should cover from the front edge to the back edge of the tablet bed. Adding more spray guns will not automatically guarantee that the overall spray rate can be increased. The use of additional guns is only justified if the current number of guns is insufficient to cover the tablet bed from the front to the back of the pan. The objective is to produce a uniform "curtain" of spray through which the tablets pass. Spray guns are usually capable of developing pattern widths of 12 to 20 cm, without adversely affecting the spray droplet distribution. At pattern widths greater than this, the volume of pattern air needed to fan out the spray can lead to a distortion of the droplet size distribution, due to recombination of spray droplets. The spray guns should be set up such that adjacent spray patterns are as wide as possible without overlapping. Overlapping of spray patterns can lead to localized over-wetting of the tablet bed.

Uniform Gun-to-gun Solution Delivery

It would seem obvious that to achieve uniformity of solution application, all spray guns must be set up to deliver the same quantity of coating solution. A recent trend in coating systems is the use of a single pump manifold to multiple spray guns. For these types of systems, it is mandatory that calibration be performed on a regular basis, to ensure that all spray guns are delivering the same quantity of solution. Furthermore, the calibration must be performed with the coating solution to be used. Calibration with water will not be satisfactory, since its viscosity is much lower than the coating formulation, and it will not be as sensitive to differences in pressure drop between the spray guns. Calibration is also recommended when using peristaltic pumps, since the tubing is subject to fatigue. Calibration is usually accomplished by adjusting a knob that controls the restriction of the spray nozzle by the spray needle.

Atomization Air Volume/Droplet Size

As stated earlier, the atomization air volume can be adjusted to control the mean droplet size of the spray. An increase in the atomization air volume can reduce the mean or average droplet size. An increase in either spray rate or solution viscosity will cause an increase in not only the droplet size distribution, but also the mean droplet size. Therefore, the droplet size should be evaluated at the exact spray rate that will be used for the coating trial. The quality of the spray, in terms of droplet size and distribution, should be evaluated at several different settings.

Spray Gun Angle

Ideally, the spray gun should be directed at the middle (midway between the leading and trailing edges of the tablet bed), and at a 90° angle to the moving tablet bed, in other words midway between the 7 and 8 o'clock positions. If the spray guns are directed higher towards the leading edge of the tablet bed, it is possible that spray could be applied to the pan or onto mixing baffles as they begin to emerge from the tablet bed. Conversely, if the spray guns are directed too low on the tablet bed, spray applied to the tablets may not have sufficient time to dry. This could result in the transfer of film from the tablets to the pan surface. If the spray guns are not directed at a 90° angle to the tablet bed, then the spray, as it exits the solution nozzle, has a tendency to build up on the wings of the air cap.

33.12.2 Uniformity of Product Movement

Pan Speed

This area was covered in an earlier section (see Section 33.11.3 Pan Speed). Product movement must be uniform if a uniform application of the coating solution is to be achieved, and the minimum pan speed necessary to achieve this objective is recommended. Once the pan speed has been determined, it can be scaled-up by duplicating the peripheral edge speed. This is done by taking the ratio of the small pan to large pan diameter times the small pan speed.

One final note is that the product movement should be continually evaluated, and adjusted as necessary, during the coating cycle. Frequently the product movement will change as a coating is applied to the tablet surface.

Tablet Size and Shape

Different tablet sizes and shapes will exhibit much different flow characteristics. In general, smaller tablets will flow better than larger tablets. Longer, less round shapes, such as capsule and oval-shaped tablets, will tend to slide and flow more poorly (more sliding) than other shapes. If the tablet shape or size is changed, the product flow properties must be re-examined. Also, if the size is too small, it will require a fine mesh to cover the perforations in the pan to prevent the exhaust of product. One other consideration is that if the product is fine (~1 mm or less), and the air flow is exhausted down through the product bed, then there will be a considerable pressure drop across the bed. This pressure drop will cause a reduction in the process air flow.

Baffle Type/Size/Number

The primary function of the mixing baffles is to transfer the product between the front and back of the coating pan. A variety of different baffle shapes and sizes exist. Coating pans are usually equipped with a standard baffle design that works well for the majority of different products. However, it may be necessary to use a different baffle design for unusual shapes and sizes. Coating pans can also be fitted with anti-slide bars. These bars are positioned on the flat of the coating pan, perpendicular to the product flow. They are used to prevent tablets with large flat surfaces from sliding inside the pan. With most coating pans it is necessary to use a reduced baffle size when working with smaller batch sizes.

Standard size baffles used with a small batch will result in sluggish product movement and/or excessive variation in the spray gun-to-product distance. As the baffle passes through the product, it will temporarily carry a portion of the tablets up out of the tablet bed, thus causing a brief increase in the gun-to-bed distance. As these tablets cascade off the baffle, the tablet bed height rises, and the gun-to-bed distance decreases. A minimum variation in the gun-to-bed distance is desired, so that the spray always travels a consistent distance, and spray droplets striking the tablets have a constant moisture level. The typical variation in gun-to-bed distance is from 2.5 to 5.0 cm. A reduced or small batch baffle is generally recommended whenever the batch size is less than 75% of the rated pan brim volume.

Batch Size

As mentioned above, the batch size/baffle combinations are critical to obtain an acceptable product movement. An acceptable batch size range for film-coating is usually from 50–95% of the rated brim volume. By using only 95% instead of 100% of the rated volume, one can eliminate spillage out of the pan mouth ring during coating. Occasionally, what appears to be an acceptable pan load initially may turn out to be excessive for those products that exhibit a change in product movement as a film is applied or with coatings of extremely high weight gain. A problem in working with smaller batches (~50%) in a perforated coating pan is that, unless part of the exhaust plenum is blocked off, the process air will preferentially pass around the tablet bed, due to less restriction or pressure drop. Batches of this size can be coated successfully, however, the drying efficiency is reduced.

33.12.3 Adequate Evaporative Capacity

Process Air Volume

The process air stream should be adjusted to the maximum volume that yields a laminar non-turbulent air flow. A turbulent air flow will distort the spray patterns, and lead to lower coating efficiency due to spray drying of the coating. It is important to periodically inspect the coating pan, to ensure that all process air passes through the tablet bed. Any air that passes around the product will result in a lowered evaporative efficiency. The inlet air volume is more important than the exhaust air volume as an indicator of the evaporative capacity, since it is this air that passes through the tablet bed and vaporizes the water from the coating, and then conveys it away from the tablets. The exhaust air volume may be slightly greater than that of the inlet, due to the addition of nozzle air from the spray guns, and also due to slight leakage that may exist. If there is a large difference between the inlet and exhaust air volumes due to leakage, this can be a problem since this air can artificially depress the exhaust temperature.

Spray Rate

The initial spray rate that is selected may be based on previous coating trials that have yielded successful results. This is an acceptable approach if the coating solution and product substrate are very similar. However, it is important to remember that changes in these factors can drastically affect the spray rate, and other parameters selected. Another method for determining an initial spray rate is to evaluate the quality of the droplet size distribution. Spray rates for aqueous film-coating vary from 6 to 30 g/min for a small 2.0 L pan, to 80 to 250 g/min/gun in a large production-scale pan. The key factors that limit the maximum spray rate per gun are the viscosity of the coating solution, the type of spray gun used, and ultimately the level of film quality that the customer deems acceptable.

Spray Gun-to-tablet-bed Distance

For small scale coating systems, the gun-to-bed distance can be as little as 2.5 to 5.0 cm. The typical gun-to-bed distance is from 20 to 25 cm for a production sized coating pan. This distance usually provides an economical trade-off between the cost of the number of guns needed to adequately cover the spray zone and the desired quality of spray. If the gun-to-bed distance is less than 20 cm, then either the spray rate must be reduced or the inlet temperature and product temperature increased, to compensate for the shortened evaporation time. If this distance is greater than 20 cm, the inlet process temperature should be reduced otherwise more spray drying will occur.

Product/Exhaust Temperature

The standard approach to the film-coating process utilizes an exhaust temperature of 38° to 44°C. Based on the desired spray rate, an inlet temperature is determined that allows the target exhaust temperature to be maintained. Coatings that develop greater tackiness upon drying will require a higher exhaust temperature to prevent over-wetting defects. For these materials, the spray droplets must be slightly drier when they strike the tablet surface to prevent over-wetting. Aqueous dispersions will require a slightly lower exhaust/product temperature, since the polymers used in these coatings are thermoplastic or become tacky when exposed to excessive heat. A typical exhaust temperature range for these coatings is 30° to 38°C.

The exhaust temperature is slightly lower (~1° to 5°C) than that of the product bed, due to heat loss between the measurement points. Usually, the greater the distance between the exhaust and product temperature probes, the greater the differential. The only time when these temperatures will vary more than this is during preheating and cool-down. A product temperature probe will display an average of the entire tablet bed. The product temperature can be determined through the use either of a probe that extends into the tablet bed or through the use of an infrared temperature probe directed just above the spray zone. Tablets in the spray zone are at a slightly lower temperature, due to evaporative cooling, and are not representative of the average product temperature.

Dew Point Temperature

The dew point temperature is a direct measure of the moisture contained in the air. Dew point temperatures can be measured using either a capacitance or a chilled mirror type dew point sensor. To accurately reproduce the drying rate from trial to trial, it is recommended to maintain the dew point within a controlled range. The more critical the coating, (i.e., sustained release coatings), the tighter the range. High dew point temperatures can be controlled through the use of dehumidification, either via chilled water coils or a desiccant dehumidification. Chilled water systems are usually specified to control the dew point at 10° to 12°C (50° to 53°F) or an absolute moisture content of 54 to 60 grains of water per pound of air. With a desiccant dehumidification system, the dew point can routinely be controlled to a temperature as low as −6°C (21°F). Dew point temperatures can be controlled on the low end by humidifying the air via the injection of clean steam into the process air. If no attempt is made to limit the variation of the inlet dew point, then fluctuations in ambient air conditions can lead to reduced coating efficiency (spray drying), longer processing times or film defects due to over-wetting.

33.12.4 Scale-up

Batch Size

The most accurate method of determining batch size is to load the coating pan to within 2.5 to 5.0 cm of the pan opening, and then rotate the pan at the desired rpm to ensure that the pan is not overfilled. However, there are two different methods for approximating the batch size. The first method is to multiply the rated brim volume times 95%, and then multiply the resultant volume by the bulk density of the product. A second method for determining the pan load size is to multiply a known ratio of batch size to pan volume for a small-scale pan times the volume of the pan being scaled to. For example:

$$\text{large pan batch size} \approx \frac{\text{small pan batch size}}{\text{small pan volume}} \times \text{large pan volume}$$

$$\text{large pan batch size} \approx \frac{65.0\,\text{kgs}}{90.0\,\text{Liters}} \times 550.0\,\text{Liters}$$
$$\approx 397.0\,\text{kgs}$$

Pan Speed (Angular Pan Velocity)

When scaling-up a coating process, it is critical that the tablet speed through the spray zone in the larger pan is comparable to that used in the smaller pan. In other words, the pan angular velocity must be the same for both coating pans. Pan velocity can be duplicated by multiplying a ratio of the small pan diameter to large pan diameter times the pan speed used for the smaller coating pan. For example:

$$\text{pan speed for large pan}$$
$$= \frac{\text{small pan diameter}}{\text{large pan diameter}} \times \text{pan speed for small pan}$$

$$\text{pan speed for large pan} = \frac{100\,\text{cm pan}}{170\,\text{cm pan}} \times 9\,\text{rpm}$$
$$= 5.3\,\text{rpm}$$

The above equation will yield a close estimation of the pan speed. However, subtle differences in the baffle design between coating pans may require a slight adjustment from this calculated pan speed.

Available Coating Zone

To scale-up the coating process with any degree of confidence, the spray rate must be determined using the same gun-to-bed distance as used in the larger coating pan. Any change in the gun-to-bed distance will change the drying time for the spray droplets, and thus alter the quality of the coating. The same spray rate used in the small-scale pan can also be used in the production-scale pan, assuming that the same spray gun spacing and spray pattern widths are used. Typically, the use of more spray guns without increasing the size of the overall spray zone will not allow an increase in either the total or the per gun sprays. Increasing the total number of spray guns will only be of value if the existing spray zone is inadequately covered with fewer spray guns. If the spray pattern width used in the larger coating pan is narrower than that used in the small pan, then the spray rate per gun should be reduced in proportion to the reduction of the spray zone width. This will allow the same density of film-coating to be applied per unit area of the tablet bed surface. Otherwise, the quantity of coating applied on the tablets per pass through the spray zone would increase. This would most likely change the quality of the coating, and could lead to over-wetting or logo bridging defects. Here is an example of scale-up using a ratio of total spray zone utilized:

	Pan #1	Pan #2
Pan volumes	90.0 L	850.0 L
Batch size	60.0 kg	566.0 kg
Coating solution	2 kg	113 kg
Number of spray guns	2	10
Spray pattern width (per gun)	20 cm	15 cm
Spray rate (per gun)	150 g/min	to be determined
Spray rate (total)	300 g/min	to be determined
Spray time	40 min	to be determined

$$\text{spray rate for large pan} = \frac{\text{pattern width for pan \#2}}{\text{pattern width for pan \#1}} \times \frac{\text{spray rate (per gun)}}{\text{for pan \#1}}$$

$$\begin{aligned}\text{spray rate for large pan} &= \frac{15 \text{ cm spray pattern}}{20 \text{ cm spray pattern}} \times 150 \text{ g/min/gun} \\ &= 113 \text{ g/min/gun}\end{aligned}$$

Total spray rate for pan #2 = per gun spray rate (pan #2) × number of spray guns (pan #2)

$$\begin{aligned}\text{total spray rate for pan \#2} &= 133 \text{ g/min/gun} \times 10 \text{ spray guns} \\ &= 1330 \text{ g/min/total}\end{aligned}$$

$$\text{Spray time} \approx \frac{\text{quantity of solution to apply}}{\text{total spray rate}}$$

$$\text{Spray time} \approx \frac{113 \text{ kgs}}{1.33 \text{ kgs/min}} \approx 85 \text{ min}$$

33.12.5 Spray Rate to Pan Speed Ratio

One factor that is quite commonly overlooked is the ratio of the spray rate to the pan speed. The ratio of spray rate to pan speed has serious implications, in both the amount of film-coating applied onto the individual tablets per pass through the spray zone, and on the overall uniformity of the film-coating itself.

Therefore, with any increase in the spray rate, one should evaluate the need for an increase in the pan speed. In some instances, the tablets may be able to withstand a greater application per pass through the spray zone without any adverse effects on film quality or the uniformity of the coating. Whenever the spray rate and pan speed are both increased, the tablets should be evaluated for signs of over-wetting or increased tablet attrition. One problem that may result if the pan speed and spray rates are too high relative to the evaporative rate is that wet film coating from the tablets may be transferred to the pan surface.

33.12.6 Air Flow to Spray Ratio

When scaling-up the film-coating process, it is recommended that the air flow used in the larger coating pan is proportional to the increase in the spray rate. If the air flow is increased in the same ratio as the increase in spray rate, and if the spray rate per unit area of the bed surface is the same, the same inlet and exhaust temperatures can be maintained. The inlet temperature must be increased to maintain the same evaporative rate if the air flow is not increased in the same proportion as the spray rate. If the spray rate per gun and the gun-to-bed distance are the same for both pans, the air flow can be scaled-up in direct proportion to the increase in spray guns. For example:

	Pan #1	Pan #2
Spray rate (per gun)	125 g/min	125 g/min
Number of spray guns	2	4
Total spray rate	250 g/min	500 g/min
Inlet air flow	660 CFM	to be determined

$$\text{airflow for pan \#2} = \frac{\text{total spray rate for pan \#2}}{\text{total spray rate for pan \#1}} \times \frac{\text{airflow for}}{\text{pan \#1}}$$

$$\begin{aligned}\text{airflow for pan \#2} &= \frac{500 \text{ g/min}}{250 \text{ g/min}} \times 1000 \text{ CMH} \\ &= 2000 \text{ CMH}\end{aligned}$$

33.13 TROUBLESHOOTING

33.13.1 Introduction to Troubleshooting

Troubleshooting is basically a "reactive" process, since it deals with something that has already gone wrong. A coating problem will usually manifest in one or more of the following ways:

- those affecting visual coated product quality;
- those affecting coated product functionality;
- those affecting coated product stability;
- those affecting processing efficiencies and costs.

When dealing with an existing, marketed product, the troubleshooting process is constrained by many regulatory issues. These problems are the most troublesome, in that the proper corrective action may require refiling with the FDA. Therefore, other less suitable remedies may be taken, which may lessen the symptoms rather than correct the actual cause of the problem.

Identifying appearance-related problems is relatively easy, because visual feedback is immediate. The magnitude of the problem is also often immediate. Identifying non-appearance related problems (such as those associated with chemical stability or drug release) is more difficult because:

- the existence of the problem is often not readily apparent;
- determination is often on the basis of some analytical procedure that evaluates only a small sample (relative to the batch size in question) of tablets;
- sampling, and the relevance of the samples selected to the characteristics of the whole batch, becomes a critical issue.

33.13.2 Up-front Approaches to Avoid Troubleshooting Issues

The best solution to "fixing problems" is to avoid them in the first place. One way in which many coating problems can be avoided is through the proper formulation of the product substrate and the film-coating solution. Before the coating process can be developed or scaled-up, the product must be evaluated to ensure that it meets the formulation requirements for film-coating. Often, problems arise because the tablet core formulation is not sufficiently robust to withstand the rigors of film-coating.

The core must be formulated such that minimal attrition occurs during the film-coating process. The deeper the product bed, the more abuse the tablets must withstand. For smaller tablets (less than 100 mg) 5–6 kp may be sufficient. For medium-sized tablets 12–16 kp may be sufficient. For larger capsule shaped tablets, such as a 1 gram capsule shape, a hardness of more than 20 kp may be necessary. A better measure of a product's suitability for coating is friability. In general, a product with a friability of 0.1% or lower

should be sufficient to avoid attrition problems during the coating process. Other core formulation issues which should be addressed prior to developing the coating process include:

- Product stability: all core ingredients must be stable at the temperatures required for the evaporative process (typically 40–45° C for aqueous based coatings).
- Product shape: the use of large flat product surfaces must be avoided, to prevent the tendency for "twinning" of product cores.
- Logo design: the core logo should be designed such that attrition and bridging of the logo do not occur.
- Resistance to dimensional changes.
- Film adhesion: the core should be sufficiently porous to allow the film to adhere properly to the surface.
- Chemical/functional robustness:
  - role of amorphous, hydrophilic materials;
  - low melting point ingredients.
- Mixing potential: smaller, rounder products will tend to flow well. Larger or longer tablet shapes will tend to exhibit "sluggish" movement.

Another issue which must be addressed before the coating process can be developed is the film solution formulation. It must be evaluated to ensure that it meets the requirements for coating. Some of the issues that must be addressed include:

- sufficient film mechanical strength to prevent cracking or edge wear;
- sufficient plasticizer to prevent the formation of a brittle film;
- sufficient pigment to mask the color of the tablet core;
- solids level that allows a coating to be applied quickly to protect the core from attrition;
- sufficient adhesion between the coating and the core surface;
- a solution viscosity that is low enough to allow the production of a uniform spray droplet size distribution;
- the coating must not exhibit stability problems, including those due to settling of suspended solids within the coating solution.

33.14 CONSIDERATION OF PRODUCT SUBSTRATE

To develop the coating process effectively the product must be evaluated to ensure that it meets the necessary criteria for a substrate.

33.14.1 Hardness/Friability

The tablet core must be capable of withstanding the rigors of tumbling in the coating pan. In a larger diameter coating pan, the bed depth will be greater, and subject the tablets to greater stress. Therefore, an acceptable tablet hardness or friability for a small coating pan may not be sufficient for a larger pan. A tablet hardness tester is used to determine the edge-to-edge (diametral) tablet hardness. Typical hardness measurement units include kilopond (Kp), Strong Cobb (Sc), and Newton (N). The kilopond is defined as the force exerted by a kilogram mass upon its support in a gravitational field of $g = 9.80665\,\text{m}/\text{sec}^2$. One kilopond is equal to 9.807 Newton units or 1.4 Strong Cobb units. Tablet hardness has traditionally been the measure of a tablet's suitability for coating. However, in many cases the tablet may be of substantial hardness, but still exhibit unacceptable capping tendencies or show excessive wear on the tablet edges or logo. Therefore, a slightly better means of determining a tablet's ability to withstand tumbling is friability. This is usually determined by tumbling a certain number or weight of tablets for a set number of rotations (usually 100 revolutions) inside a cylinder. The tablets are weighed before and after tumbling, and weight loss is expressed as the percent friability. A new innovation to the friability test is to line the inside of the friability cylinder with a mesh screen. This has been shown to provide a better correlation between the friability test, and the actual coating suitability.

33.14.2 Weight Variation

Tablet cores are usually produced to a particular weight range specification. However, sometimes these ranges are not sufficiently narrow. This usually occurs when the tablet granulation exhibits flow problems. A wide tablet weight variation will make it difficult or impossible to determine the actual tablet weight gain accurately, due to the application of the film-coating, since the weight variation in the uncoated cores can be greater than the weight of the film to be applied. Also, wide variations in tablet weight can be accompanied by variations in tablet hardness.

33.14.3 Stability

The tablets must be stable under the conditions required for coating. The product must be able to withstand the temperature and humidity of the process air flow. Product temperature is significantly less than that of the inlet air during the coating process, due to evaporative cooling. However, during the pre-heat phase the product temperature may approach that of the inlet air, if the tablets are not jogged frequently enough. Tablets should be able to handle the usual product temperature of 35 to 50°C. As mentioned earlier, it may be necessary to use drier conditions during the initial phase of the coating process, to prevent stability problems with moisture sensitive product, such as effervescent tablets.

33.14.4 Compatibility

The compatibility of the tablet core with the excipients in the film-coating solution must be verified. In some instances certain actives have exhibited an interaction with the plasticizer in the coating solution.

33.14.5 Shape

If possible, certain tablet shapes should be avoided for film-coating. Tablets with sharp edges may exhibit a greater tendency for edge wear. Cores with a large flat tablet face may result in poor product movement, due to sliding. Also, tablets with large flat surfaces will show a much greater tendency to exhibit twinning during coating. By adding a slight concavity (0.1 to 0.2 mm) to the face of the tablets, they become much less likely to agglomerate.

33.14.6 Logo Design

Sharp corners or small islands on the tablet logo can lead to logo attrition problems. If the logo is too fine or contains too much detail, the film-coating may bridge or cover the logo. A draft angle of 35° is recommended for film-coated tablets. Tooling manufacturers are usually aware of the tool design specifications for tablets that are to be film-coated.

33.14.7 Core Porosity

The tablet core must be formulated so that there is good adhesion between the film-coating and the tablet surface. If the core porosity is low, poor adhesion will result, and picking and/or peeling of the film will occur. Core porosity can be a problem with wax matrix tablets, due to poor adhesion between the tablet surface and the film-coating droplets. To remedy this, more adhesive film polymers (i.e., hydroxypropylmethylcellulose) may be used.

33.14.8 Disintegration

The disintegration of the tablet core must be sufficiently rapid, when tested prior to the addition of the film-coating. If the core does not dissolve quickly prior to coating, the addition of film-coating will only provide a further delay.

33.15 COATING SOLUTION

33.15.1 Film Mechanical Strength

The film-coating solution must be formulated such that the resultant film has adequate mechanical strength. The reasons for this are twofold. First, the film must be strong enough to protect the tablet from excessive attrition while tumbling during the coating process and, secondly, the film must be sufficiently durable to resist the erosion of the film itself. A weak film will usually exhibit wear or erosion at the tablet edges. The addition of too many non-film forming excipients will decrease the strength of the film. This may occur if a drug is added to the coating solution at a high level, or if high levels of insoluble colors or mineral fillers are added.

33.15.2 Plasticizer Level

The function of a plasticizer is to reduce the glass transition temperature (T_g) of the film, in other words, to produce a film that is not brittle at normal operating conditions. If the film is inadequately plasticized, the film will be too brittle, and more prone to cracking. If a film solution has an excessive level of plasticizer, the mechanical strength of the film will be reduced.

33.15.3 Pigment Level

If the coating solution contains insufficient pigment, it will be impossible to develop the desired color intensity. Additionally, low pigment levels can make it difficult to minimize color variation, due to poor opacity of the coating solution. Excessively high pigment levels can, as stated earlier, reduce the mechanical strength of the coating.

33.15.4 Film Solution Solids

A low solids level in the coating solution can not only needlessly increase the process time, but can also increase the time required to provide a protective film coating, thus resulting in increased tablet attrition. High solution solids levels, coupled with a low addition level, can make it difficult to achieve acceptable film-coating uniformity. High solids levels can also be a problem, if they result in a high solution viscosity. If a high solids level does not create an excessively viscous solution, it provides an excellent opportunity to reduce the volume of coating solution, and thus the coating time. The aqueous dispersions available on the market provide a solids solution at an extremely low viscosity.

33.15.5 Solution Viscosity

Solution viscosity, as stated above, is closely tied to the solution solids level. As solution viscosity is increased (above ~200–250 cps), the droplet size distribution produced by the spray guns becomes increasingly wider, due to an increase in larger droplets. Slight increases in viscosity can be compensated for by increasing the volume of atomization air. However, at higher viscosities (greater than ~350 cps) it is difficult to eliminate all of the larger droplets. To compensate for the presence of larger droplets, the operator will usually increase the inlet temperature, to prevent the larger droplets from over-wetting the product. This will result in an increase in the amount of spray drying, due to premature evaporation of water from the finer droplets. The net result is a lower coating efficiency, and a rougher film surface.

33.15.6 Stability

The coating solution must be stable for the duration of the coating time. This includes both chemical and physical stability. The most typical instability problem encountered is settling-out of solution solids. This occurs with solutions that contain an excessive percentage of solids or when the coating has insufficient suspending capacity. Settling of solids can lead to blockage of the solution lines or the spray guns.

33.15.7 Compatibility

This refers not only to the compatibility of the coating materials, but also to the compatibility between the film-coating and the tablet core. For example, the addition of color concentrates that contain ethanol has led to precipitation of some of the polymer used in aqueous dispersions. As a remedy, a propylene glycol based color was used. In another product there was an interaction between the plasticizer and the active ingredient used in the tablet core. It was necessary to reformulate the coating solution, using an alternative plasticizer.

33.15.8 Processing Issues as They Relate to Troubleshooting

Equipment Maintenance Issues

Another way in which many coating problems can be avoided is the implementation of a routine equipment maintenance program. This program must involve the periodic calibration of all analog and digital instrumentation. Poor maintenance of process monitoring equipment results in decisions being made on the basis of inaccurate information. The maintenance program should also involve the inspection of all wear items. The equipment manufacturer should be able to provide a listing of these parts, with a recommendation on the frequency of inspection.

Process Adjustment as a Troubleshooting Initiative

The dynamics associated with the spray application of the coating liquid represent perhaps one of the most under-appreciated areas of the whole film-coating process.

Key issues to be aware of include:

- Fluid flow rate through the nozzle, interaction with the driving forces for effective atomization, and the ultimate size of droplets formed.
- Droplet velocity.
- The interaction of atomized droplets with the surrounding drying environment, and the relative state of the droplets as they arrive at the tablet surface.

While the importance of many operating parameters (air flows, temperatures, spray rates, etc.) is relatively well-understood, the ultimate impact of other parameters on the issue of troubleshooting is often overlooked, such as:

- Mixing effectiveness in the pan, and the impact of, for example, baffle design.
- Pan loading, and its impact on process efficiencies and product quality.
- The potential change in tablet roll dynamics as coating is applied.

Another approach to troubleshooting involves the systematic evaluation of the film-coating process.

Film-coating issues can be classified into three objectives. These categories are as follows:

1. Achieve uniformity of the spray droplet size and application.
2. Achieve uniformity of product movement through the spray zone.
3. Achieve the proper evaporative rate for the coating process.

There are a number of issues that must be addressed with regard to each of these objectives. A partial listing of some of the factors to be considered follows.

Issues that Affect the Uniformity of the Spray Droplet Size and Application

- Can an acceptable spray droplet size distribution be produced at the desired spray rate?
- Can an acceptable spray droplet size distribution be produced using the coating solution viscosity?
- Is there adequate air volume for the atomization of the coating spray?
- Are the number and type of spray guns suitable to provide uniform coverage of the product bed?
- Are the spray guns located at the proper spacing?
- Is the spray pattern width sufficient to maximize the size of the spray zone without overlapping adjacent spray patterns?
- Is the spray gun to product bed distance correct?
- Is the solution delivery the same for all spray guns?
- Other factors.

Issues that Affect the Uniformity of the Product Movement

- Is the batch volume sufficient for the pan being used?
- Is the correct pan speed being used?
- Does the pan contain the proper baffle type, and are they in the correct position?
- Are tablets being "thrown" into the spray zone by baffles or baffle mounts?
- Is the product size and/or shape conducive to good product movement?
- Other factors.

Issues that affect the evaporative rate of the coating process

- Is the proper process air volume being used?
- Is the incoming air stream controlled to a consistent dew point?
- Are the inlet, exhaust, and product temperature correct for the tablets being coated?

- Is the proper spray rate being used?
- Other factors.

It is important that the objectives be examined in the order listed above, to effectively troubleshoot the film-coating process. One should first deal with issues affecting uniformity of spray application, then issues that affect product movement, and lastly, issues dealing with the evaporative rate of the coating process.

For example, let's assume that the product is exhibiting signs of picking, which is an over-wetting defect. Let's also assume the root cause of this defect is due to poor product movement, which causes the product to stop in the spray zone. It might be possible to eliminate this problem by increasing the process temperatures (evaporative rate factor). However, the product movement through the spray zone would still be poor, and coating uniformity would be less than optimal. A better remedy would be a corrective action which would result in improved product movement (second objective).

A second example might assume the same defect (picking), however in this case the cause of the defect is due to non-uniformity of the solution delivery through the spray guns. One of the spray guns is delivering significantly more solution that the others. One could probably reduce the spray rate to eliminate the over-wetting problem, however, this would not be the appropriate remedy. If this were done then the coating uniformity would still be less than optimal, and the corrective action would have lengthened the necessary coating process time. A more appropriate remedy would be a corrective action which resulted in an improved spray application (first objective).

33.15.9 Troubleshooting: Summary

Problems often have more than one cause.

Problem resolution is likely to be complex.

Problem resolution may encompass minor changes that have little regulatory impact.

Some problems can only be resolved by making significant (from the regulatory standpoint) changes to either formulations or processes.

The simplest approach to problem resolution is problem avoidance.

Film-coating Defects: Troubleshooting

The following table (Table 33.18) contains a brief definition of common tablet coating defects, along with typical causes and suggested remedies.

33.16 APPLICATION OF SYSTEMATIC AND STATISTICAL TOOLS FOR TROUBLESHOOTING AND PROCESS OPTIMIZATION

In the early twenty-first century, quality by design (QbD), PQRI initiatives, and risk management were introduced to allow the manufacturer and the regulator

TABLE 33.18   Tablet coating defects/corrective action

Possible cause	Remedies
1. Overwetting/picking: This condition occurs when part of the film coating is pulled off one tablet and is deposited on another. If detected early in the process it can be covered, if detected late in the process the coating will probably be unacceptable.	
Insufficient drying rate	Increase the inlet and exhaust temperatures Increase the process air volume Decrease the spray rate
Inadequate atomization	Increase the nozzle air pressure or the atomization air volume Decrease film coating viscosity
Poor product movement	Increase pan speed Switch to an alternative baffle design Adjust batch size (volume)
Poor distribution of spray	Check the uniformity of solution delivery through the spray guns (calibration)
Insufficient drying rate	Increase the inlet, exhaust, and product temperatures Increase process air volume Reduce the spray rate
Excessive variation in process air humidity	Dehumidify and/or humidify process air to maintain a constant inlet air dew point

(Continued)

TABLE 33.18   Continued

Possible cause	Remedies
2. Twinning: Twinning is a form of overwetting whereby two or more of the tablet cores are stuck together.	
May be due to any of the possible causes for overwetting	
Poor tablet core design	Change tablet design to eliminate large flat surfaces
3. Orange peel: Appears as a roughened film due to spray drying. This condition relates to the level of evaporation that occurs as the spray droplets travel from the gun to the tablet bed. If there is excessive evaporation, the droplets do not have the ability to spread and form a smooth coating. A narrow droplet size distribution is important to ensure that the majority of droplets dry at the same rate.	
Excessive evaporative rate	Reduce the inlet and exhaust air temperatures Reduce the gun-to-bed distance
Excessive atomization of the spray	Reduce the nozzle air pressure or atomization air volume
Large droplet size variation	Reduce the solution viscosity Reduce the spray rate
4. Bridging: Bridging is a condition in which the film coating lifts up out of the tablet logo.	
Poor film adhesion	Reformulate the film-coating solution to improve adhesion Reformulate the core formulation to increase porosity
Poor logo design	Redesign logo to incorporate shallower angles
5. Cracking: May occur due to internal stresses in the film.	
Brittle film-coating	Increase the addition level of the plasticizer Use a different plasticizer Use a polymer with a greater mechanical strength
Poor film adhesion	Dilute the film-coating solution Reduce the quantity of insoluble film-coating additives
6. Poor coating uniformity: Poor coating uniformity can manifest itself in either a visible variation in color from tablet to tablet or in the form of an unacceptable release profile for tablets.	
Insufficient coating	Apply a coating of 1.5 to 3.0% (for clear coating as little as 0.5%) weight gain to attain uniformity, requires higher levels if the color of the tablets and the film are of very different colors
Poor color masking	Reformulate the film-coating to a darker color and/or increase the quantity of opacifier
Poor uniformity of solution application	Increase the pan speed Reduce the spray rate/increase the coating time Increase the spray pattern width Increase the number of spray guns Check the uniformity of solution delivery through the spray guns (calibration)
7. Tablet attrition/erosion: Attrition is exhibited when some portion of the product substrate exhibits a high level of friability. This typically occurs at the tablet edge or face. Often signs of attrition will be minimal or non-existent in smaller diameter coating pans. However, when the coating process is scaled-up to a production sized pan, this problem can become more severe due to the increased batch weight and bed friction.	
Insufficient tablet friability	Reformulate the tablet core to a friability of no more than 0.1% friability
Poor film-coating formulation	Reformulate to provide coating with greater mechanical strength
Excessive pan speed	Reduce the pan speed to the minimum required to achieve a smooth and continuous bed movement
Insufficient spray rate	Increase the spray rate to provide a protective film-coating in a shorter time, this may require an adjustment in the inlet air temperature
8. Core erosion: Core erosion is another type of attrition due specifically to overwetting of the tablet core. With this type of defect excessive overwetting may cause a partial disintegration of the core surface.	
Surface overwetting	Reduce the spray rate Increase the inlet and exhaust air temperatures Increase the spray pattern width Reduce the spray droplet size/increase the atomization air volume Reformulate the core with less water sensitive excipients Improve tablet bed movementIncrease the bed to gun distance

(Continued)

TABLE 33.18 Continued

Possible cause	Remedies
9. Peeling: Peeling occurs when large pieces or flakes of the film coating fall off the tablet core.	
Poor adhesion	Reduce the amount of insoluble additives in the coating solution
	Increase the level of film former in the coating solution
	Reformulate to incorporate a film polymer with greater adhesion
	Reformulate the tablet core to increase porosity
Brittle film-coating	Increase and/or switch to an alternative plasticizer
10. Loss of logo definition: This defect occurs when the tablet logo is no longer clearly legible. It may be due to one or more of the defects previously covered: core erosion, tablet attrition, or bridging. Loss of definition can also occur when the logo is filled in with spray dried film.	
Core erosion	Reduce the spray rate
	Increase the inlet and exhaust air temperatures
	Increase the spray pattern width
	Reduce the spray droplet size/increase the atomization air volume
	Reformulate the core with less water sensitive excipients
	Improve tablet bed movement
Excessive film-coating level	Reduce the film-coating weight gain
	Improve the uniformity of the coating distribution
Tablet attrition	Reformulate the tablet core to a friability of no more than 0.1%
	Reduce the pan speed to the minimum required to achieve a smooth and continuous bed movement
	Increase the spray rate to provide a protective film-coating in a shorter time; this may require an adjustment in the inlet air temperature.
Bridging	Reformulate the coating solution to improve the film adhesion
	Reformulate the core formulation to increase porosity
	Redesign logo to incorporate shallower angles
Excessive drying rate	Reduce the inlet and exhaust air temperatures
	Reduce the gun-to-bed distance
	Reduce the nozzle air pressure or atomization air volume
11. Core stability issues: These problems may manifest as discoloration of the core or degradation of the core active.	
Moisture sensitivity	Explore the remedies for overwetting defects
	Reformulate the core with less water sensitive excipients
Heat sensitivity	Decrease the inlet and/or product temperature
Tablet component incompatibility	Investigate the compatibility of the tablet core with the coating formulation
	Determine the compatibility of the core ingredients
12. Tablet marking: Usually evident as the presence of black marking on the face of the tablets.	
Abrasion of oxide from the coating pan surface	Change to a tablet shape that tumbles rather than slides (i.e., round rather than oval/capsule)
	Reduce the level of titanium oxide in the coating
	Add baffles to reduce the sliding of tablets
	Coat the pan with coating solution to act as a barrier
	Increase the spray rate or reduce the pan speed

to better design, monitor, and control the quality of the product in US, Europe, Japan, and other countries.

Key initiatives are:

- Design space
- Quality by design (QbD)
- Risk assessment
- Design of experiments (DOE)
- Knowledge space/control space
- ICH Q8 (Development)
- ICH Q9 (Risk Management)
- ICH Q10 (Quality System)
- Key process parameter (KPP)/Critical process parameter (CPP)
- Key quality attribute (KQA)/ Critical quality attribute (CQA).

To meet these challenges, many systematic and statistical tools are being used in a sequential method to:

- identify root cause(s)
- understand the KPP/CPP and knowledge space/control space
- optimize the process
- establish the control plan.

Many pharmaceutical companies assemble a variety of systematic and statistical tools, and define the procedures of their approach. These tools include six sigma/DMAIC, design of experiment (DOE), Kepner Tregoe analysis (KT), Brightest, Pareto analysis, Gauge RR, Lean Sigma, risk assessment, and other tools.

CASE STUDY OF A COATING ISSUE USING SYSTEMATIC AND STATISTICAL TOOLS BY RIGHT-FIRST-TIME APPROACH

SHAKERS AND CONTAINERS

PFIZER METHOD 1 RIGHT-FIRST-TIME INVESTIGATION

John Z. Smith (GMS/MPS)
Michael Chen, (NPG/PPD)

DEFINE : Poor Color Uniformity and Uneven Surface of Film Coating for Product XXXXXX.

The film coating of Product XXXXXX shows a poor colour uniformity and rough surface when transfer from Site A to Site B.

MEASURE
Observation:
1) Site A:
Material: a commercial blue film coating material
Coating Pan: fully perforated
Pan Load: 45 kg
Inlet Air Temperature: 60-65°C
Bed Temperature: 40-42°C
Exhaust Temperature: 45°C
Pan Speed: 7 rpm
Number of Gun: 2
Gun to Bed Distance: 25 cm
Spray Rate: 120 g/min total

2) Site B
Material: same as Site A
Coating Pan: solid pan
Pan Load: 95 kg
Inlet Air Temperature: 45-50°C
Bed Temperature: 34-36°C
Exhaust Temperature: 40°C
Pan Speed: 10-12 rpm
Number of Gun: 3
Gun to Bed Distance: 30 cm
Spray Rate: 150-250 g/min total

The resulting tablets did not meet the Appearance Quality Limits. About 20 % of coated tablets show significant lighter shade. The rough surface appearance show some solids deposits about 500-2000 µ.

ANALYSE

Cause & Effect Analysis (Fish-Bone Analysis)

CASE STUDY   (CONTINUED)

Cause and Effect Analysis

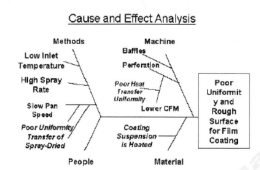

Based on the shape and size of surface defects, some coating materials are detached and transferred onto other tablets. This could due to the imbalance of heat exchange, pan speed, and spray rate,

Critical Process Parameters
1 Bed Temperature
2 Pan Speed
3 Spray Rate
4 Atomization
5 Gun to Bed Distance

IMPROVE
DOE Coating Study
.3X3 Full factorial design
Factor 1: Bed Temperature
Factor 2: Pan Speed
Factor 3: Spray Rate/Atomization

The knowledge space is identified and better understood. The optimized parameters are identified and successful full-scale batches are manufactured.

The final parameters for Site B are listed below:

Material: same as Site A
Coating Pan: solid pan
Pan Load: 95 kg
Inlet Air Temperature: 50-55°C
Bed Temperature: 40-42°C
Exhaust Temperature: 42-45°C
Pan Speed: 12 rpm
Number of Gun: 3
Gun to Bed Distance: 25 cm
Spray Rate: 180-250 g/min total

CASE STUDY   (CONTINUED)

CONTROL

The control plan is established for future manufacture.

Contact for further information: John Smith (john.z.smith@pfizer.com, 123-123-1234)

References

1. Porter, S., Bruno, C.H. & Jackson, G.J. (XXX). *Pan Coating of Tablets and Granules*. Vol. 3, Pharmaceutical Dosage Forms: Tablets.

2. Liu, L. (XXXX). The Coating Efficiency of a Film-Coating Process. Invited Speaker, Pharmaceutical Excipients Conference, June 25–27. Philadelphia, PA.

3. Liu, L., McCall, T., Tendolkar, A., Shlyankevich, A., Giambalvo, D., Baumgamer, C. & Smith, E. (2000). The Scale-Up and Process Optimization of an Ethylcellulose–Based Functional Coating and Its Impact on *In-Vitro/In-Vivo* Release of a Novel Controlled Release System. The 27th International Symposium on Controlled Release of Bioactive Materials, July 7–13. Paris, France.

4. Liu, L., Giambalvo, D., McCall, T., Labudzinski, S. & Baichwal, A. (1998). The Effect of Process Variables on Coating Efficiency of an HPMC-Based Film-coating using a Perforated Coating Pan. AAPS 1998 Annual Meeting. San Francisco, CA.

5. Freers, S., Jensen, B., Shipley, C. & Foltz, D. (XXXX). Clear Coated Tablets with High-Solids Aqueous Starch Coating and Minimal Tablet Weight Gain. Vector Corporation.

6. Liu, L., Smith, T.J., Sackett, G., Poire, E. & Sheskey, P. (2004). Comparison of Film-coating Process Using Fully Perforated and Partially Perforated Coating Pans. AAPS Annual Meeting. WHERE.

7. Bauer, K., Lehman, K., Osterwald, H. & Rothgang, G. (XXXX). *Coated Pharmaceutical Dosage Form Fundamentals, Manufacturing Techniques, Biopharmaceutical Aspects, Test Methods and Raw Materials*. CRC Press, WHERE.

8. Wade, A. & Weller, P.J. (XXXX). *Handbook of Pharmaceutical Excipients*, 2nd edn. A.Ph.A, WHERE.

9. McGinity, J.W. *Aqueous Polymeric Coatings for Pharmaceutical Dosage Form*, 2nd edn. Marcel Dekker, Inc., WHERE.

10. Rowe, R.C. & Force, S.F. (1982). Acta Pharm. Tech. 28, 207–210.

11. Russo, E.J. (1984). Typical scale-up problems and experiences. Pharm. Technol. 8(1), 46–56.

Development, Optimization, and Scale-up of Process Parameters: Wurster Coating

David Jones

34.1 INTRODUCTION

In 1959, Dr Dale Wurster, then at the University of Wisconsin, introduced an air suspension coating technique now known as the Wurster system. The Wurster process enjoys widespread use in the pharmaceutical industry for layering and film-coating of particles and pellets, as well as the emerging controlled-release tablet dosage forms. Product containers typically range in size from 3.5″ (100–500 g batch sizes) to 46″ (up to approximately 800 kg). The Wurster process is used commercially for coating particles from less than 100 microns to tablets, and for layering to produce core materials.

34.2 BASIC DESIGN

The basic design components of a commercially available Wurster system are shown in Figure 34.1 and Figure 34.2. The coating chamber is typically slightly conical, and houses a cylindrical partition (open on both ends) that is about half the diameter of the bottom of the coating chamber (in up to 24″ Wurster coaters). At the base of the chamber is an orifice plate that is divided into two regions. The open area of the plate that is under the partition is very permeable. This permits a high volume and velocity of air to pneumatically transport the substrate vertically. As they accelerate upward, particles pass a spray nozzle that is mounted in the center of this up bed orifice plate. The nozzle is referred to as a two fluid or binary type—liquid is delivered to the nozzle port at low pressure, and is

atomized by air at a preselected pressure and volume. The spray pattern is generally a solid cone of droplets, with a spray angle ranging from approximately 30–50° (Figure 34.3). The so-called "coating zone" which is formed is a narrow ellipse, and varies in volume

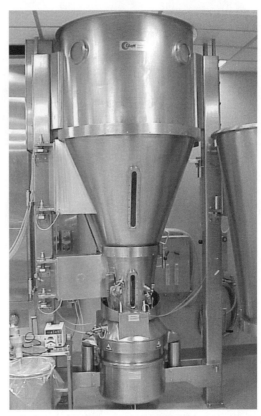

FIGURE 34.1 Glatt model GPCG-60 fluid-bed processor fitted with an 18″ HS Wurster insert. Photograph courtesy Glatt Air Techniques, Inc.

Developing Solid Oral Dosage Forms: Pharmaceutical Theory and Practice
ISBN: 978-0-444-53242-8

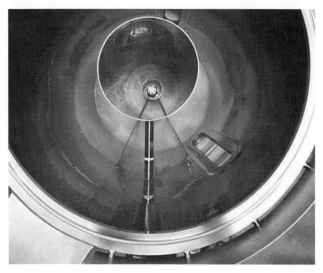

FIGURE 34.2 18″ HS Wurster coater—inside view showing spray nozzle, HS nozzle surround and partition. Photograph courtesy Glatt Air Techniques, Inc.

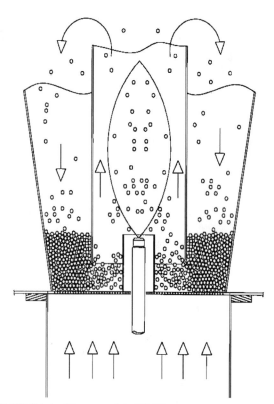

FIGURE 34.4 Diagram of the HS Wurster process

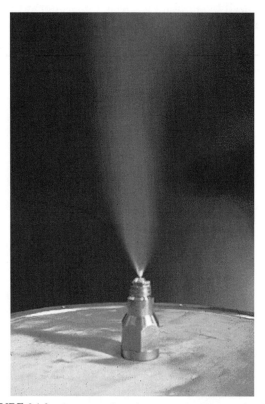

FIGURE 34.3 Spray nozzle and spray pattern (using water)

depending on the size of the substrate being sprayed and the pattern density in the partition.

The diagram in Figure 34.4 illustrates the regions of flow in the Wurster process. The region outside of the partition is referred to as the down bed. The configuration of the orifice plate in this area depends on

the size and density of the material to be processed. The purpose of the air flow in the down bed region is to keep the substrate in near-weightless suspension, irrespective of its distance to either the wall of the product container or the partition. The goal is to have it travel rapidly downward (to minimize cycling time), and then be drawn horizontally toward, and ultimately into, the gap at the base of the partition. In general, tablets require significantly more air to produce this condition than pellets or fine particles—the orifice plate must be selected accordingly (no single down bed plate can achieve good fluidization properties for all substrates). As mentioned previously, the material flow inside of the partition is controlled by the up bed or partition plate. In general, this plate is considerably more permeable than the down bed plate. In pilot and production scale Wurster systems, the up bed plates are removable, such that one or the other may be changed to "fine-tune" the behavior in these individual regions (see Figure 34.5).

A second key process variable in Wurster coating is the height that the partition sits above the orifice plate, which controls the rate of substrate flow horizontally into the coating zone. Typically, the smaller the particles to be coated, the smaller the gap will be. When the Wurster coating chamber is assembled properly, the resulting flow pattern should be relatively smooth

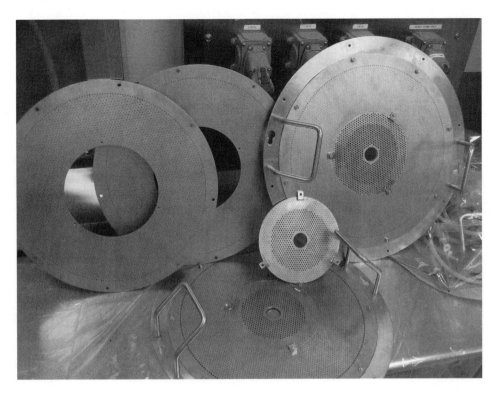

FIGURE 34.5 Up and down bed orifice plates for an 18" HS Wurster coater. Photograph courtesy Glatt Air Techniques, Inc.

and rapid in the down bed, and very dense in the up bed or partition region.

The substrate exits the partition at a high rate of speed, requiring a region to decelerate. Above the product container is the expansion area, which is typically conical to allow for decreasing air and particle velocity. Wurster machines designed for pellets and small particles employ elongated expansion chambers essentially to enhance deceleration in the air space, rather than by high velocity impact against machine components in the filter housing. By contrast, tablets do not need much expansion height and, in fact, attrition may be a severe problem. The orifice plate and partition height should be optimized so that the tablets travel upward only a very short distance out of the partition before beginning their descent. As a result, a mesh bonnet can be used in the expansion chamber, just above the product container, to keep the tablets from colliding with the expansion chamber. The coarse mesh is intended to allow the fines from the cores or some spray dried coating to exit the process area, avoiding incorporation in the layers of film. A conventional Wurster machine is not used extensively for tablet coating, due to the comparatively high stress to which the tablets may be exposed. However, it is recommended when the film quality (minimal defects), and good film or active component distribution uniformity are very important, especially for modified-release tablets. The films applied by Wurster

systems are high in quality, due to the concurrent spray and high drying efficiency of this air suspension process. There have been modifications to the Wurster process specifically for tablet coating. These include spray nozzle surrounds, partition geometry, and air flow adjustability at the interface between the wall of the product container and the down bed orifice plate (to be described in more detail later).

Pellets and small particles are layered or coated extensively via the Wurster process using water, organic solvents or even by spraying molten materials. All fluidized-bed techniques are known for high rates of heat and mass transfer, and the Wurster process is very effective in this regard. Highly water-soluble materials can be coated using water-based applications without concern for core penetration. Droplets applied to the surface spread to form a continuous film or layer, and then quickly give up their moisture to the warm, dry air. After a thin film has been applied, spray rates can be increased, since the soluble core has been isolated. Films applied with volatile organic solvents are also high in quality, because the formed droplets impinge on the substrate very quickly, minimizing the potential for spray drying of the film. Finally, there are limited applications involving the use of molten coatings. In this case, the coating or layer is applied by spraying a molten substance that subsequently congeals on the substrate surface. For a variety of reasons, the Wurster process is not the process of choice for molten coating. For a variety of reasons, especially with respect to congealing and its impact on the fluidization behavior, the Wurster is not the process of choice for molten coating. However, for coarse substrates the fluidization properties of the Wurster are preferred over other techniques in which case a molten coating may be applied reproducibly. Otherwise, top spray processing is a better choice for hot-melt coating.

34.3 HS WURSTER CONSIDERATIONS

HS Wurster technology, shown in the diagram of Figure 34.4 and the photograph of Figure 34.6, is a product of Glatt Air Techniques, Inc., in Ramsey, NJ, and involves the use of a proprietary device to influence the behavior of the substrate in proximity to the coating zone. Unfortunately, the liquid spray application rate is not controlled by the drying capacity of the fluidization air, but by the nature of the coating material (tackiness) or by the region immediately surrounding the spray nozzle (the first area of focus is this region). In all Wurster inserts, the high volume of air rushing through the partition creates suction at the partition gap. As a consequence, particles entering have a horizontal component to their flow—some travel towards the spray nozzle instead of simply making the transition from horizontal to vertical flow. The atomizing air has a very high velocity (it is likely supersonic), and creates streamlines that draw the substrate to the base of the developing spray pattern. In a standard Wurster machine, the nozzle is elevated above the orifice plate, at a position just below the confluence of fluidizing substrate particles. A portion of the developing up bed stream of product can pass the nozzle tip, either closely or at a further distance. Particles that are very close to the nozzle tip tend to be strongly over-wetted, and if they contact other particles, agglomerates are formed. To control what could otherwise be severe agglomeration, a typical response is to reduce the spray rate. This leaves a large amount of the drying capacity unused. Other commonly used agglomeration control techniques include raising the inlet (and product) temperature to increase the drying rate or raising the atomizing air pressure to shrink droplet size—options which are in conflict with producing high quality films. Even using these corrective measures, a quantity of agglomeration in traditional Wurster systems is almost inevitable.

The HS modification for the Wurster process was conceived to keep particles away from the spray nozzle until the spray pattern is more fully developed.

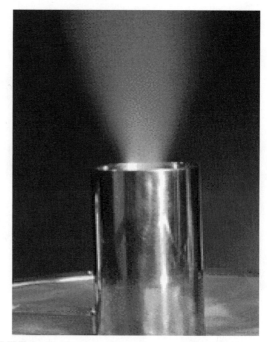

FIGURE 34.6 Spray nozzle and pattern shown with its nozzle surround (patented). Courtesy Glatt Air Techniques, Inc.

As a result, more of the excess drying capacity can be used, and the application rate increased substantially (more than doubled in many pilot-scale experiments). Because the particles are kept away from the wettest portion of the pattern (Figure 34.6), agglomeration is also substantially diminished or eliminated. An additional benefit is that the high atomizing air velocities necessary to produce very small droplets for coating of particles smaller than 100 microns may be useable without pulverizing the substrate. The velocity of this air diminishes dramatically with distance from the nozzle, and even a few centimeters are significant. Keeping the product away from the nozzle tip allows the atomization air velocity to decrease significantly before contacting the substrate, reducing the likelihood of attrition, especially during the early stages of coating.

Coating of substrates smaller than 100 microns has been achieved more frequently by using the HS Wurster coater. Success depends on many factors, both process and product related. Product considerations, such as flow properties of the substrate (generally poor in this size range, which must be improved), as well as the liquid, which must be amenable to atomizing to droplets well below 10 microns, must be addressed. The tremendous surface area of such fine particles also requires very high coating quantities, and consequently, a low potency of the final coated product (often less than 50%).

34.4 COATING AND PROCESS CHARACTERISTICS

The coating liquid is sprayed in the direction of motion of the fluidizing particles. In general, the fluidization is orderly, with very rapid, dilute phase pneumatic transport in the up bed, and relatively smooth and rapid transport in the down bed region (outside of the partition). Because the liquid is sprayed into a well-organized pattern of substrate moving relatively close to the nozzle, droplet travel distance is minimized. In this manner, droplets reach the substrate prior to any appreciable evaporation. By retaining their low viscosity they are able to spread on contact, and the resultant films are excellent, even when using organic solvents as an application medium. The drying efficiency of the fluidized-bed also minimizes the potential for core penetration, and the sample shown in Figure 34.7 clearly shows a well-defined boundary layer between the substrate and the coating material, in this case a film applied using an aqueous dispersion.

34.5 PROCESSING EXAMPLES

The Wurster process is used commercially for coating and layering (high solids build up onto a type of core material). Substrates include particles smaller than 100 microns, crystals, granules, pellets, and tablets. As mentioned previously, films may be applied using water-based solutions, aqueous dispersions or organic solvents. It is also possible to apply coatings via hot-melt (no evaporating application media), but the use of the Wurster system for this technique may be related more to the particle size of the substrate than the coating process itself. Typically, a coating applied molten will be more continuous (less porous) when it is applied at a product temperature which is as close as possible to the congealing temperature of the coating material. In this case, the viscosity of the bed is very high, and stalling outside of the partition in the Wurster process is not unexpected. The conventional top spray fluidized-bed technique has advantages in this regard. The open product container offers no impediments to flow. The process air and product temperature may be raised to slow the congealing rate to improve coating quality. The resulting increase in viscous drag in the product bed is inconsequential, because there is no partition or baffle to impede flow. However, if the substrate is coarse or dense (above 0.7 g/cc or 0.7 mm in diameter) fluidization is likely to resemble a "slugging" bed, and this is particularly significant in pilot- and production-sized equipment. This characteristic is such that a mass of material may at one instant overwhelm the spray nozzle, causing local over-wetting and agglomeration. A split second later, the mass drops a distance away from the nozzle, and droplets are spray congealed in the cooler process air, before having the opportunity to contact the substrate. Coarse, dense material is more ideal for "spouting," of which the Wurster process is essentially a hybrid. The Wurster process will offer an improvement in fluidization quality that outweighs the disadvantage of the viscous drag in the down bed, due to the nature of the coating material.

The first example of a material layered and coated using the Wurster process is shown in cross-section in Figure 34.8. The starting material is a very small nonpareil sugar seed, and it is layered to a high potency

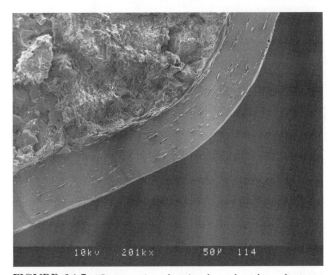

FIGURE 34.7 Cross-section showing boundary layer between coating and core material (200 × magnification)

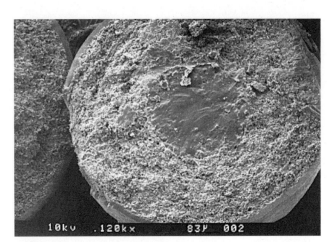

FIGURE 34.8 Cross-section of drug layered, film-coated pellet (120 × magnification)

using a suspension of drug in a dilute binder solution. Release of the drug is controlled by a film applied subsequently. All three components are clearly identifiable.

The example shown in Figure 34.9 is a tablet, film-coated (for sustained release) and layered with a loading dose, prior to drilling with a laser. Immersed in liquid, drug solute exits the laser hole in this type of dosage form. The Wurster process was selected for this product due to its abilities in film and drug distribution uniformity.

The product in Figure 34.10 is coated with a moisture barrier. The substrate contains a significant quantity of material smaller than 5 microns. Agglomeration of fine particles does occur, as seen in the scanning electron micrograph (SEM). However, the average particle size of the finished product is still less than 50 microns. The film is applied from a volatile organic solvent solution, and is typically very tacky, hence the

agglomeration "crater" where another particle has detached.

A water-soluble core, coated with a soft, heat sensitive polymer system is shown in Figure 34.11. The cross-section shows the deformable nature of the film, and these particles may be filled into capsules or compressed into tablets to be delivered. Although the product must be processed at low temperatures, core penetration was not a problem, due to the process parameters used and the drying capability of the Wurster process.

Often the economics of coating very small particles dictate whether a product ever reaches the marketplace. The drug particles shown in Figure 34.12, when coated in a standard Wurster system, proved to be too costly to produce. However, when the HS components were fitted to the pilot-scale 18″ Wurster machine, the process time was reduced by more than 50%, and the product is now commercially produced.

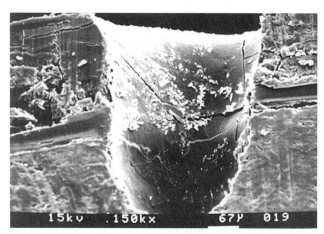

FIGURE 34.9   Cross-section of a tablet coated using the Wurster process (150 × magnification)

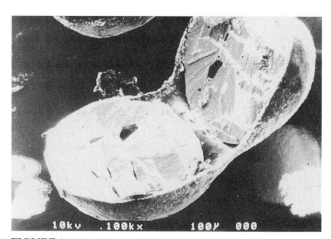

FIGURE 34.11   Water-soluble crystal coated for sustained release (100 × magnification)

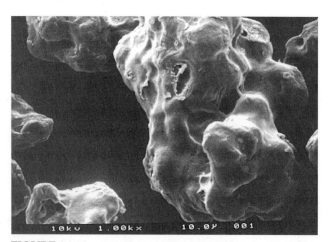

FIGURE 34.10   Very fine particles coated with a moisture barrier using the HS Wurster process (1000 × magnification)

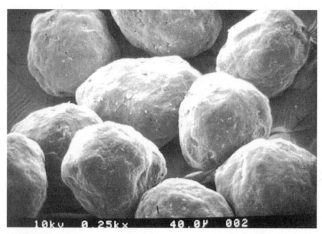

FIGURE 34.12   Drug core particles coated for taste masking, incorporation into oral suspension (250 × magnification).

The SEM shows very good morphological properties for the core, in that the particles are nearly spherical, and are not porous. In laboratory trials, this substrate was found to be very robust—attrition of the cores early in the coating process (before they were sufficiently coated to have improved surface strength) was essentially non-existent.

34.6 PROCESS VARIABLES

34.6.1 Batch Size

The working capacity for a Wurster insert of a particular size is generally defined as the volume outside of the partition, with the partition at rest on the orifice plate. Avoiding loading of product inside the partition helps to ensure that the nozzle remains clear at the beginning of the process. This is especially important for fine particle or pellet coating. For tablet coating, up to half of the volume inside the partition can also be used. As the bed becomes fluidized, the dense phase or surface of the down bed will drop, indicating that there is room for the batch to expand, as coating is applied. In some cases, it may appear that there is more than enough, and that batch size could easily be increased. The danger is that the surface of the bed is dynamic—varying in depth in response to the behavior of the up bed and surface properties of the substrate during spraying. Should substrate begin to drop down into the partition, against the desired flow, the up bed would be seriously disturbed, agglomeration would be likely, and the batch might be lost.

The minimum batch size is approximately 20–25% of working capacity. What is critical is that there must be sufficient material in the up bed region to accumulate all or most of the coating material being sprayed or "efficiency" (actual yield versus expected) will suffer. The product in the down bed "feeds" the base of the partition (entrance to the coating zone), and if its depth is insufficient, the up bed will be too sparse, favoring spray drying. In a more extreme case, coating of the inner wall of the partition may be experienced (this is more common in very small laboratory scale inserts). Use of such a small volume of the product container is recommended only if the final batch size is significantly larger than the starting volume (as in layering, for instance). Early in the process, the coating efficiency is compromised. This inefficiency diminishes as the batch size increases, improving mass flow inside the coating zone. When about half of the down bed working capacity is occupied, the efficiency will be at or near its maximum for the formulation being executed. Ultimately, the inefficiency seen

at the beginning of the process should be of little or no consequence to the finished batch.

Subsequent to the layering step, if a thin film is to be applied, it is strongly recommended that the minimum batch size be increased to about 50% of the working volume. For film-coating, inefficiency will likely impact the resultant dissolution behavior. Some amount of spray drying may result in unexpectedly rapid release of drug, particularly for a sustained-release coating.

34.6.2 Fluidization Pattern

Irrespective of the amount of substrate in the Wurster insert, the fluidization pattern is controlled by the orifice plate configuration, the partition height, and the fluidization air volume. As mentioned previously, the goal is to have a rapid and relatively smooth down bed. This is not always possible, depending somewhat on particle size (small particles are difficult, if not impossible, to fluidize without bubbling), but to a greater extent on the tackiness of the product during spraying. Some coating materials are tacky by nature or due to temperature sensitivity. If this is the case, it is more important to keep the entire bed involved by marginally over-fluidizing (turbulence or bubbling in the down bed), rather than attempting to achieve a smooth flow. This can be accomplished by raising the partition somewhat or using a more permeable down bed plate, to allow extra air to percolate through the descending product. The risk in not doing this is that the bed may stall in some region on the orifice plate, and a portion of the batch may not receive all of the desired coating.

In general, tablets require a large air volume in the down bed to keep it well-aerated. The partition region of the plate is also selected to allow only sufficient air flow to minimize the distance tablets travel out of partition to avoid attrition. By contrast, the orifice plates for pellet coating may differ significantly. The plate is permeable inside of the partition, and the down bed section is only perforated to the extent that the product flows downward in near-weightless suspension. Achieving this condition typically requires only about a quarter of the open area needed for tablet coating. Finally, plates designed for powders are even less permeable in the down bed region (and boiling may be impossible to control, due to the flow properties of fine materials).

Another critical process variable in the fluidization pattern for Wurster processing is the height of the partition above the orifice plate. The height is also substrate-dependent. For instance, tablets, a comparatively large

TABLE 34.1   Partition height as a function of substrate and Wurster coating insert size

Substrate	Partition height
Tablets	25–50 mm in small machines
	50–100 mm in 18″ Wursters and larger
Pellets	Approximately 15–25 mm small machines
	Approximately 35–60 mm in 18″ Wursters and larger
Powders	Approximately 25–50 mm in all machines

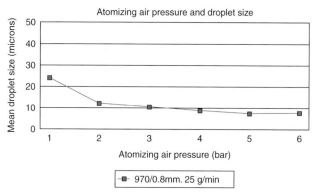

FIGURE 34.13   The relationship between atomizing air pressure and droplet size for a Schlick 970 series nozzle spraying water

substrate, would require a substantial partition height, such that a sufficient number of them could pass through the gap per unit time to absorb the maximum amount of coating being sprayed into the partition area. Pellets and intermediate particles do not need as high a partition height as tablets, and fine particles and powders need only a small gap to result in an ideal fluidization pattern. Table 34.1 profiles suggested conditions for partition height as a function of substrate and Wurster coating chamber size.

34.6.3 Atomizing Air Pressure and Volume

Droplet size should be small, relative to the particle size of product to be coated. For example, coating of tablets may need only 2 bar (30 psi) pressure. Higher pressure and air volume will result in a higher atomization air velocity, increasing kinetic energy at the interface between the spray pattern and slower moving substrate. The potential for causing attrition of the tablets by accelerating them into machine components is also enhanced. Finally, the high atomizing air velocity may distort the fluidization pattern.

When coating small particles, a somewhat higher atomization air pressure may be necessary, to achieve small droplet size and thereby avoid agglomeration. There is some risk, however, that the high shear associated with pressures in the 3–6 bar (45–90 psi) range, depending on the type and size of the spray nozzle, may cause breakage of fragile core material. The Gustav Schlick Company, in Coburg, Germany, is a supplier of spray nozzles in widespread use in Wurster processing. The 970 series nozzle is found in small (3.5″, 4″, 6″, 7″, and 9″) Wurster bottom spray coaters. With water-like materials, it is useable in a spray rate range of approximately 0–100 g/min. Figure 34.13 is a graph that shows the influence of atomization air pressure on mean droplet size for water sprayed at 25 g/min (data by Schlick). Interestingly, increasing the pressure beyond 2 bar does little to decrease the droplet size. This is, in part, due to the fact that

25 g/min is well within the nozzle's ability to atomize. What should be noted is that, if a process is being run in which agglomeration is a minor problem, if increasing the atomization air pressure seems to improve the situation, it is likely a consequence of the increased air velocity and kinetic energy, not a smaller droplet size.

Looking at the performance envelope of the Schlick 940 series nozzle (Figure 34.14), which is used in older style 12″, 18″, 24″, 32″ and 46″ Wurster coaters, it can be seen that droplet size increases with faster spray rates (at a constant atomization air pressure). In cases where the spray rate is 250 g/min or less, it is possible to increase atomization air pressure/volume/velocity to achieve droplets smaller than 20 microns. However, the data shown for the 500 g/min rate demonstrates that even at the highest practical atomization air pressure (6 bar), it is not possible to produce 20 micron droplets (spraying water). This is an important consideration in larger capacity equipment, where there may be significant drying capacity, and the rate-limiting factor is the inability of the nozzle to atomize liquid (to a satisfactory droplet size) at the rate at which the process air may remove the resultant water vapor. The only possibility for taking advantage of the increased drying capacity is to enlarge the nozzle (use more compressed air at the same pressure).

The 940 series nozzle is unable to produce droplets smaller than 20 microns at 500 g/min using water, even at very high atomization air pressures. A process that has excessive drying capacity, but is limited by droplet size (fine particle coating for example), will result in unnecessarily hindered productivity. Upgrading to the HS nozzle, which uses substantially more compressed air at the same atomization air pressures (approximately three times the volume of the 940 series nozzle), will result in a dramatic improvement in drying capacity utilization. The graph in Figure 34.14b depicts a droplet profile which is similar to the 940 series nozzle spraying

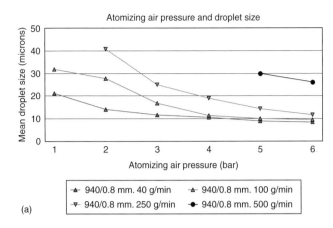

(a)

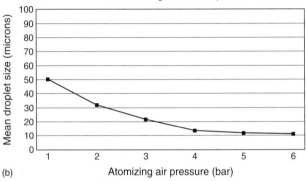

(b)

FIGURE 34.14 (a) The relationship between atomizing air pressure and droplet size for a Schlick 940 series nozzle at various spray rates using water. (b) The relationship between atomizing air pressure and droplet size for a Schlick HS Wurster nozzle at 1000 g/min spraying water

at 250 g/min, with the exception that the HS data is for 1000 g/min, a spray rate four times that of the 940 series nozzle. This permits the HS nozzle to be operated at low atomizing air volumes and pressures, limiting the potential for attrition due to high kinetic energy.

34.6.4 Nozzle Port Size

Droplet size is rarely influenced by nozzle port size. At a fixed spray rate, the velocity of the liquid into the atomization air is controlled by the nozzle port size. The lower the velocity, the more complete the atomization of the liquid will be, and the smaller the mean droplet size, as the data in Figure 34.15 for a 940 series nozzle illustrates for two different spray rates. For 100 g/min, the mean droplet size is nearly the same for all data points, with the exception of the values at 2 bar. However, this appears to be an anomaly, since the mean droplet size is the same for both port sizes at the lower pressure of 1 bar. At the higher spray rate

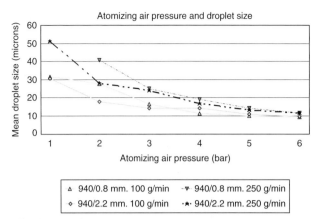

FIGURE 34.15 The relationship between atomizing air pressure and droplet size for a Schlick 940 series nozzle at 100 and 250 g/min (water) using 0.8 mm and 2.2 mm nozzle port sizes

of 250 g/min, the mean droplet sizes are the same at 3 bar and higher. Only at 2 bar is there an appreciable difference, owing to the lower liquid velocity, and longer dwell time for the liquid in the atomizing air stream. Additionally, factors such as liquid viscosity and surface tension influence this behavior and it is preferable that they both be low, to avoid the need for high atomization air pressure, regardless of the size of the substrate. If viscosity is an issue (high), nozzle port size should be selected to accommodate it (to minimize back pressure in the spray pump).

34.6.5 Evaporation Rate

Evaporation rate or drying capacity is controlled by fluidization air volume, temperature, and its absolute humidity (dew point). The temperature of the fluidization air is generally adjusted to maintain a constant product temperature. The product temperature, in turn, is influenced by spray rate and humidity of the incoming air. First, as spray rate is increased within a given batch, to take advantage of excess drying capacity, inlet temperature must be raised to keep the product temperature from dropping, due to the increase in evaporative cooling. Secondly, if the dew point of the incoming air is not controlled, the drying conditions to which the product is exposed will not be reproducible. The dew point changes seasonally, especially in northern climates, and may range from below zero during winter to more than 20°C in summer. These normal variations in weather conditions may result in some notable influences in processing.

In cold weather, static electricity during fluidization may be a problem, and in summer, high humidity conditions may result in substantially slower spray rates, due to erosion of drying capacity, especially for aqueous coatings. This phenomenon is, of course, more pronounced when product temperatures of 30°C and less are desired (thermally sensitive substrates or coating materials). Allowing the process air dew point to vary will result in a variation in the residual moisture in the applied film. This can lead to a change in the glass transition temperature for some coatings. For latex materials, residual moisture may result in "aging" effects—changes in dissolution with time (product instability). For most products, a dew point range of approximately 10–20°C throughout the year is recommended, to minimize this so-called "weather effect." If the product is very sensitive to moisture in the process air or even thermally sensitive, a desiccant dryer is suggested, and this will produce dew points well below 0°C.

34.6.6 Product Temperature

All air suspension processes are noted for their high heat and mass transfer capability. A wide range of product temperatures may be used. Values below 30°C may be used for heat sensitive materials. Values exceeding 50°C may actually be used with little or no spray drying of the applied coating. High product temperatures are especially attractive for water-based spray liquids. The rate-limiting step for most processes is related to the physical properties of the liquid being applied. The use of psychrometry is effective in determining the threshold at which moisture applied to the surface of the substrate begins to prefer to remain in the applied layer, rather than to leave with the process air. This inflection point is where agglomeration begins to take place. The surface tackiness promotes the sticking together of substrate particles. This so-called exit air relative humidity threshold is related to the product temperature. As an example, for an exit humidity threshold of 60%, the water removal rate for a product temperature of 40°C is about 100% higher than for a product temperature of 30°C. Water in air is an exponential function—for high product temperatures, the water removal rate is dramatically increased without fear of agglomeration.

34.7 CASE STUDIES FOR LAYERING AND FINE PARTICLE COATING

With an understanding of the range of application of the Wurster process, plus the process and product variables that influence its performance, it is interesting to look at some case studies. The first involves the use of an 18″ HS Wurster coater for solution layering (refer to Figure 34.16, Figure 34.17 for in-process data). A water-based solution was made, using the material in a high solids concentration. The goal of the trial was to find the maximum possible spray and production rates, avoiding agglomeration as much as possible. The starting material is very fine, requiring a reduced spray rate initially (400 g/min). However, as the particles grow larger, the spray rate can be elevated. The finished particle size is less than 200 microns, and the

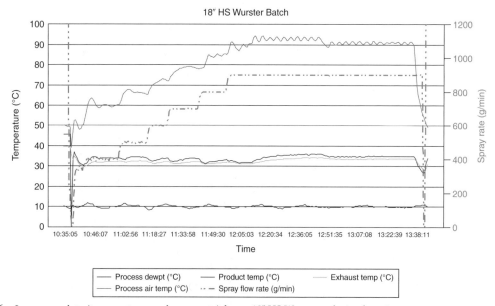

FIGURE 34.16   In-process data (temperatures and spray rate) for an 18″ HS Wurster solution layering process

18" HS Wurster Batch
Product differential pressure and process air volume

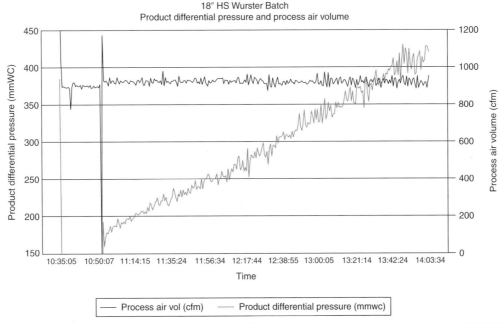

FIGURE 34.17   In-process data (process air volume and product differential pressure) for solution layering in an 18" HS Wurster coater

potential for productivity using the Wurster process is clearly in evidence here. The majority of the spray liquid is applied at 900 g/min. Heat and mass transfer rates are very high. The inlet air temperature is more than 90°C, the product temperature is approximately 35°C, and the process air volume is 900 cfm. Using psychrometry software, the exit air humidity is found to be at 85% relative humidity, indicating that the vast majority of available drying capacity is being used. An interesting tracing is that of the product differential pressure, shown in Figure 34.17, as the starting batch size is approximately one-quarter of the finished product weight. As bed depth increases in the down bed, the particles react differently to the up bed process air flow. There is a near-absence of oscillation in the early readings, because the down bed is shallow, and there is minimal coalescence of air bubbles as they enter and pass through the bed. However, as batch size increases, the down bed deepens. Small air bubbles, entering through the orifice plate and product retention screen, coalesce into larger bubbles. Back-flow or turbulence in the down bed comes in evidence. The escalating peak-to-trough values indicate bubbling air flow in the down bed. This is of no consequence to the process, provided that the down bed cycling time remains rapid, so that the mass flow in the "coating zone" continues to be high in density and velocity. A consequence of adverse fluidization properties would be agglomeration, however,

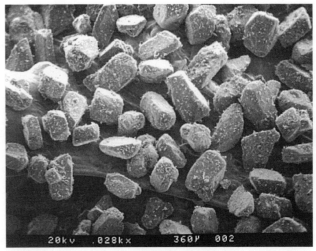

FIGURE 34.18   Uncoated acetaminophen (APAP) crystals (28 × magnification)

in this particular pilot-scale trial, this was essentially non-existent.

The second case study involved coating of fine granular acetaminophen particles for sustained release. The uncoated crystals shown in Figure 34.18 and Figure 34.19 illustrate a good substrate for coating. They are uniform in size distribution, and do not contain an appreciable amount of fines. What is not seen by SEM, however, is their fragility. As the particle

TABLE 34.2   Sieve analysis (during spraying)

Time	+30	+40	+60	+80	+100	Pan	Comments
0 min	0.0038 g	2.691 g	33.247 g	6.154 g	0.029 g	0.018 g	
	0.01%	6.39%	78.89%	14.6%	0.07%	0.04%	Starting material
3 min	0.0011 g	0.0658 g	23.441 g	4.519 g	0.327 g	0.461 g	
	0.04%	2.24%	79.69%	15.36%	1.11%	1.57%	Start spray
24 min	0.013 g	0.151 g	15.670 g	6.553 g	1.121 g	2.018 g	
	0.05%	0.59%	61.39%	25.67%	4.39%	7.91%	Pressure from 3.5 to 2.7, increased spray rate from 200 to 270 g/min
37 min	0.031 g	0.561 g	15.873 g	6.729 g	1.661 g	3.828 g	
	0.11%	1.96%	55.34%	23.46%	5.79%	13.35%	Pressure to 2.2 bar, increased spray rate from 270 to 325 g/min
58 min	0.062 g	3.322 g	17.098 g	7.166 g	1.459 g	3.852 g	
	0.19%	10.1%	51.9%	21.7%	4.4%	11.7%	325 g/min
75 min	0.074 g	3.413 g	15.903 g	6.172 g	1.366 g	3.880 g	
	0.24%	11.1%	51.6%	20.0%	4.4%	12.6%	325 g/min
87 min	0.128 g	5.604 g	14.852 g	5.331 g	1.304 g	3.289 g	
	0.42%	18.4%	48.7%	17.5%	4.3%	10.8%	325 g/min
128 min	0.563 g	9.305 g	13.806 g	5.137 g	1.305 g	2.267 g	
	1.77%	29.2%	43.3%	16.1%	4.3%	7.1%	325 g/min
178 min	2.120 g	10.63 g	11.226 g	4.124 g	0.988 g	1.067 g	
	7.0%	35.2%	37.2%	13.7%	3.3%	3.5%	28% coating

Machine configuration: 18″ Wurster coater, HS nozzle, Hi-mass flow up bed plate, no nozzle surround, initial atomizing air pressure 3.5 bar

size data shown in Table 34.2 and Table 34.3 reveals, the material is very prone to fracture. Within a few minutes of product warm-up (prior to spraying), the content of material smaller than the 80 mesh screen

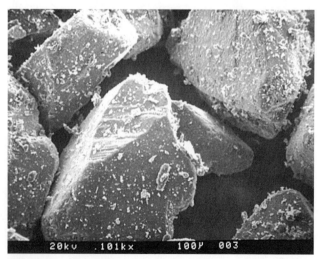

FIGURE 34.19 Uncoated acetaminophen crystals (100 × magnification)

(180 microns) escalates from nothing to more than 3%, and it continues to climb early in the spraying process until sufficient coating has been applied to improve the strength of the primary core material. It is important that the fines that exist in the initial product, plus those which are generated during the early stages of coating, are treated in one of two ways. First, using a comparatively high spray rate initially, they may be incorporated in the lower layers of film, such that the majority of the remaining film governs the coated product release properties. Secondly, an outlet filter media can be selected such that fines are permitted to exit the processor (to be collected in a remote dust collector). If attrition is serious or if fines are continually incorporated in the developing film, as was the case using the conventional 18″ Wurster coater, the release properties of the film will be affected, and in all likelihood, challenging to reproduce. In Figure 34.20 and Figure 34.21, the acetaminophen crystals have been coated to a 28% coating level (final potency of 78.1%) with AquaCoat (FMC), a pseudo-latex of ethylcellulose. The standard version 18″ Wurster equipment was used in a Glatt model GPCG-60 fluid-bed processor,

TABLE 34.3 Sieve analysis (during spraying)

Time	+30	+40	+60	+80	+100	Pan	Comments
0 min	0.0065 g	1.358 g	29.037 g	5.266 g	0.24 g	0.008 g	
	0.02%	3.8%	81.%	14.8%	0.07%	0.2%	Starting material
4 min	0.0052 g	0.094 g	26.846 g	3.747 g	0.246 g	0.787 g	
	0.02%	0.30%	84.6%	11.8%	0.8%	2.5%	Begin spray
33 min	0.0061 g	0.223 g	23.958 g	4.701 g	0.749 g	1.451 g	
	0.02%	0.72%	77.1%	15.1%	2.4%	4.67%	11.5 Kg applied
68 min	0.020 g	1.382 g	22.495 g	5.619 g	0.826 g	1.614 g	
	0.06%	4.3%	70.4%	17.6%	2.6%	5.1%	26 Kg applied
99 min	0.0359 g	3.500 g	20.138 g	4.651 g	0.749 g	1.018 g	
	0.12%	11.6%	66.9%	15.5%	2.5%	3.4%	39 Kg applied
130 min	0.0902 g	7.147 g	24.915 g	5.297 g	0.703 g	0.759 g	
	0.23%	18.4%	64.0%	13.6%	1.8%	2.0%	28% coating

Machine configuration: 18″ HS Wurster coater (with nozzle surround), "B" down bed, "G" up bed plate, atomizing air pressure 3.5 bar throughout

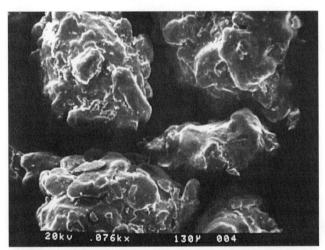

FIGURE 34.20 Acetaminophen—28% coating using standard 18″ Wurster coater (76 × magnification)

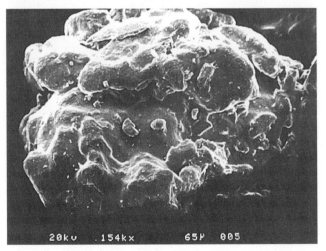

FIGURE 34.21 Acetaminophen—28% coating using standard 18″ Wurster coater (154 × magnification)

using the HS nozzle, but no HS nozzle surround, and a (then) contemporary version of an up bed plate referred to as "high mass flow." This plate may be described as having a gradient of holes (and permeability) from the outer perimeter to the spray nozzle. The highest permeability is in close proximity to the nozzle. The intent of this design was to enhance the pressure gradient at the partition gap, to increase the flow of material into the coating zone. What became apparent during these trials was that this resulted in a high concentration of substrate close to the tip of the nozzle and the developing spray pattern. Recall that this region is high in liquid content and atomizing air velocity, which can lead to attrition of fragile substrates.

The HS nozzle, for high capacity spray rates, was used so that the influence of the perforated plates and HS nozzle surround could be seen independently of a key variable such as nozzle type. In the scanning electron micrographs, at both the low and higher magnifications, the fines generated early in the spray process due to the high velocity atomization air are readily seen embedded in the film. They are present to the extent that the final particle size is substantially larger than the starting material (see Table 34.2). The resultant porous nature resulted in a faster drug release rate (Figure 34.22). This occurs in spite of the fact that the total surface area would be expected to be lower, due to the increased particle size. This type of problem should be resolved or batch-to-batch reproducibility (dissolution) will be difficult to achieve. In this example, the atomizing air pressure had to be reduced to as low as 2.2 bar to slow the generation of fines, which ultimately became embedded in the

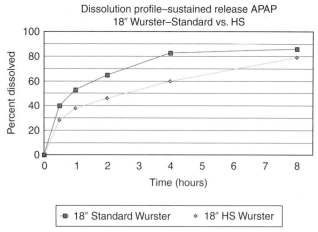

FIGURE 34.22 Dissolution profile for fine granular acetaminophen batches coated in 18" standard and HS Wursters with 28% w/w coating of AquaCoat ECD (FMC BioPolymer)

film. In Figure 34.23 and Figure 34.24, the partition plate was replaced with a more uniformly permeable type "G," and the HS nozzle surround was installed. The surround acts to keep the particles away from the highest velocity and densest droplet region of the spray pattern, as described earlier. The result is that the atomization air pressure could be maintained at 3.5 bar throughout the spraying process, with only minimal generation of fines, as evident in the SEMs. Since fewer fines were generated and embedded, the average particle size after coating was smaller than when using the standard Wurster configuration. This resulted in a less porous film, and slower drug release, as seen in the accompanying dissolution profile shown previously. An additional benefit was a reduction in process time, due to the ability to apply the coating at a higher spray rate (approximately one-third faster).

For the experiment involving the standard Wurster system, the total process time of three hours and thirty-nine minutes is not unreasonable for production. However, in the sieve analysis, the coarsest fraction disappears early in the process, and well into spraying the fraction of material defined as "fines" continues to increase to nearly 20%. Ultimately, these fines are agglomerated to the main fraction of material, and their final content is marginal. However, the average particle size shifts to the coarse side, with more than 40% retained on the 40 mesh screen in comparison to only 18% found in the batch coated using the HS components.

The process time using the HS components was reduced by 48 minutes or almost 30%. Additionally, the near absence of fines seen in the SEMs will lead to improved batch-to-batch reproducibility in the dissolution profile.

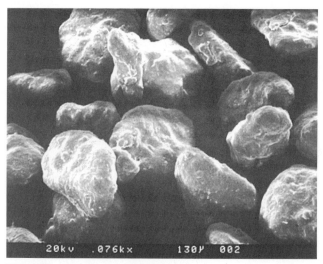

FIGURE 34.23 Acetaminophen—28% coating using 18" HS Wurster coater (76 × magnification)

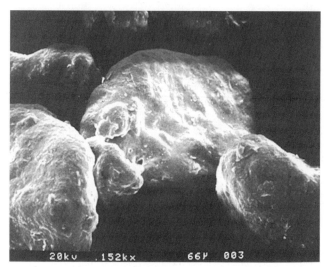

FIGURE 34.24 Acetaminophen—28% coating using 18" HS Wurster coater (152 × magnification)

34.8 SCALE-UP OF WURSTER PROCESSING

"Is the process scalable?" is a reasonable and common question. The answer typically begins "yes, but …" The ability to scale a process successfully depends on the magnitude of difference between the small and larger-sized batches. In the laboratory, development may take place with a batch size smaller than 1 kg. This size of equipment should be considered to be for screening purposes, without the expectation that the formulation that is developed will behave identically in pilot or production equipment. The batch size is small, the particle trajectory is comparatively short, the bed depth is shallow, and the spray nozzle does not use much compressed air to produce droplets. The mass of the batch is likely to be insufficient to manifest problems with attrition due to fragility of the substrate. Mass flow inside of the partition, during spraying, cannot match that of larger equipment, so the amount of coating or layer applied to the substrate will not be in the same proportion as in larger equipment.

Experience has shown that the biggest hurdles in scale-up occur when moving from a 6″ Wurster coater (or smaller) to a 7″, 9″, 12″ or 18″ Wurster coater. Usable working volumes (courtesy Glatt Air Techniques, Inc., Ramsey, NJ) are 3.6 liters (6″ Wurster coater), 8.3 liters (7″), 13.6 liters (9″), 37 liters (12″), and 102 liters (18″). In addition to the increase in volumetric capacity, the partition length increases, the partition diameter increases, bed depth and mass effects increase, particle trajectory increases, and the spray nozzle dimensions increase (in size and consumption of atomizing air volume) to accommodate the increased spray rate. High kinetic energy from the combination of high atomizing air velocity and volume may be a significant, and in many cases unpredictable, factor in scale-up.

What should be evident is that scaling from any of the laboratory-sized Wurster systems to the pilot scale 18″ Wurster coater is the true "scale-up," presenting the most significant challenges. Thereafter, production equipment typically incorporates multiples of the partitions and spray nozzles used in the 18″ Wurster. In reality, this "scale-up" should be referenced as "scale-out." Parameters such as process air volume, atomizing air pressure (and volume), spray rate, and temperatures derived for the 18″ Wurster are typically replicated on a per partition basis in the production equipment. Hardware components are also duplicated—the spray nozzle, partition diameter, and orifice plate configurations (permeability in both the up and down bed regions) are the same in both scales of equipment. Partition length is nominally longer, therefore the increase in bed depth is usually inconsequential provided that the 18″ Wurster coater is used at or near its working capacity. Examples of the pilot scale 18″, and production scale 32″ HS Wurster coaters are shown in Figure 34.2 and Figure 34.25.

Successful scale-up in Wurster processing depends on a number of factors. At a minimum, development scientists should have a good understanding of the robustness of the process in laboratory equipment. Experiments bracketing the operating ranges of key parameters should have been conducted, preferably on batch sizes exceeding 5 kg. Smaller batch sizes may be used, and the relationship of the process variables may be seen, but very small batches may not be indicative of what is seen on a somewhat larger scale. Ideally, design of experiments (DOE) should be

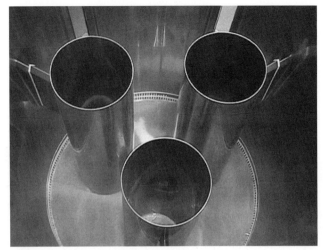

FIGURE 34.25 Inside view of 32″ HS Wurster coater. Photograph courtesy Glatt Air Techniques, Inc.

employed to quantify the magnitude of impact for the key variables.

As in any process, there is a multitude of variables to consider, including batch size, spray rate, atomizing air pressure/volume, process air volume, and temperatures (product, process air, and dew point). There are also equipment considerations—down bed and up bed orifice plate configuration, partition height above the plate, and the spray nozzle type, as mentioned previously.

Some concerns are not readily apparent. Equipment may increase in size and batch capacity, but not all components increase proportionately. For example, outlet air filter surface area actually decreases in proportion to batch size. This is problematic for products using layering or coating materials that cause filter media to blind. When a filter becomes occluded, process air volume is affected, particularly during shaking. The Wurster process requires process air flow to be continuous—it is not interrupted to shake fines back into the bed. As a consequence, when it is time to shake the filter, air flow is stopped, but only through the segment to be shaken. In contemporary machines, this means that the totality of the process air volume must now pass through the remaining half of the filter media. If the differential pressure across the filter is high, there will be a precipitous drop in process air volume. A consequence is that the velocity of substrate inside of the partition will momentarily drop, which could cause agglomeration. In an extreme case, with multiple partition production scale Wurster systems, a severe drop in total process air volume may cause one of the partitions to stop "spouting." Under this circumstance, this partition may be filled from the top by the remaining spouting partitions. Even after shaking stops, and the process air volume returns to its set point, the filled partition may not evacuate. Atomizing air from the spray nozzle inside of the partition will create a small void, into which the liquid continues to be sprayed. However, the material surrounding this void is static, and is quickly overwetted. Eventually, agglomerates and wet mass will make its way outside of the partition, and sampling will reveal a severe problem. By this time the batch is essentially lost. Ultimately, if laboratory experimentation has shown that the spray material has a propensity to cause filter blinding, even to a comparatively limited extent, filter media must be a strong consideration during scale-up activities.

Relative to the environment in which spraying takes place (the coating zone), the particle size of the substrate is becoming smaller in scale-up. This may result in a higher coating efficiency (coating material applied with respect to the theoretical or expected yield) in pilot and production equipment versus the laboratory scale. If the product is coated on a weight basis, the higher coating efficiency may lead to a change in dissolution (for sustained release coatings, it would decrease).

34.8.1 Batch Size

As mentioned previously, the maximum batch size for a Wurster process is identified as that which occupies all of the volume outside of the partitions with them at rest on the orifice plate. There is some flexibility in batch size—the process will still work when using less than the maximum working capacity. However, it has been seen in scale-up that batch size, within a given insert size, may impact finished product properties. Therefore, it is recommended that the proposed finished batch size be close to the working capacity of the larger Wurster (about 75–100% based on the finished product density).

34.8.2 Spray Rate

The spray rate for a product is typically a key variable, from several perspectives. The first is economic—long processes result in high manufacturing costs. Lengthy processes also increase the likelihood of problems during the process, particularly nozzle port clogging (there are some hardware alterations that can be made to eliminate or at least mitigate this potential problem). Spray rate also dictates the rate of accumulation of solids by the batch, and this is important for finished dosage form performance. Coated product is nearly always stronger than uncoated

core material. If the core sloughs fines, these may be incorporated in the layers of film, altering its release properties (release will be governed more by imperfection rather than by the intrinsic properties of the film). Consequently, it is a goal in scale-up to maximize the solids addition rate.

Drying capacity is a key component in scale-up. The starting point for estimating the spray rate is related to the increase in process air volume (at the same temperature as used in the laboratory scale), not the increased batch size. However, the rate-limiting factor may not be completely related to the increase in drying capacity offered by the larger Wurster system. Irrespective of the physical properties of the liquid, the application rate will more likely be strongly controlled by the interface between the accelerating core material, and the atomized droplets (coating zone). Here there may be significant benefits in using the spray nozzle surround described previously as HS Wurster equipment, which is not typically used or is of lesser benefit in small Wurster equipment. The surround prevents the flowing substrate from entering the spray pattern until it is more fully developed. This eliminates local over-wetting, preventing agglomeration in this region. A consequence is that scale-up in the Wurster process may not necessarily mean a significant increase in process time, which is a common occurrence in many types of processes.

34.8.3 Droplet Size and Nozzle Considerations

Spray conditions represent a challenge for development personnel in scale-up. Small Wurster coaters tend to use the same size nozzle (Schlick 970 series), and as the product proceeds through small increments in batch size (from 6″ to 7″ or 9″ units with batch capacities ranging from approximately 1–10 kg), only atomization air pressure need be increased to accommodate the somewhat faster spray rate. However, when shifting to the 12″ or 18″ Wurster coater, the potential increase in spray rate forces operation of this small nozzle beyond its performance envelope, and a move to a larger nozzle, with a higher atomizing air volume, is mandated. Droplet size is principally related to the air-to-liquid mass ratio, and attempting to keep this in the same range in the scale-up efforts is recommended. However, there is a caution to its use. In some calculations, the air-to-liquid mass ratio may result in atomizing air pressure values that are outside of the nozzle's recommended operating range. The spray nozzle performs two different functions. The first function is to produce droplets for the coating or layering application. The second is to attempt to prevent the nozzle from fouling. The atomizing air at the tip of the nozzle helps to clear the tip of material forming as a result of drying that occurs between the interface of the liquid and the very dry atomizing air. If the atomizing air pressure (below about 1.5 bar) and volume is too low, the velocity of the atomizing air will be insufficient to remove dried film from the nozzle tip. This material could eventually grow to a size that impacts or diverts the spray pattern, causing a sudden and severe amount of agglomeration. Additionally, the atomizing air velocity must be sufficient to permit shearing of the liquid to produce droplets. If the pressure and velocity are too low, agglomeration will be unavoidable.

At the other end of the spectrum, if the air-to-liquid mass ratio calculation yields an atomizing air pressure exceeding about 3.0 bar in the pilot-scale Wurster, attrition of the core material may be the consequence. Kinetic energy is represented as $E = 1/2\,mv^2$, where "m" is mass and "v" is velocity. Assume a scale-up from a 7″ Wurster machine (laboratory scale), with a batch size of about 5 kg, to a pilot-scale 18″ HS Wurster machine, with a batch size of about 60 kg. At 2.0 bar atomizing air pressure, the 970 series (laboratory) nozzle uses about 2.1 cfm of compressed air. At the same pressure, the HS nozzle consumes nearly 30 cfm, or about 14 times that required for the laboratory batch. The atomizing air velocities are essentially the same—both operate at supersonic speeds at this pressure. Plugging the mass numbers into the kinetic energy equation shows that the material in the pilot-scale equipment will be exposed to nearly 14 times more energy than the laboratory batch. For most applications using either water or solvent-based materials, atomizing air pressure of 1.8–3.0 bar is sufficient.

34.8.4 Process Air Volume

Process air volume is also a key factor in scale-up, providing three major functions. First, it delivers heat to the product, for evaporation and removal of the coating application medium. Secondly, and probably more significantly, it strongly affects the fluidization pattern. For scale-up, approximately the same air velocity through the partition plate for both sizes of inserts is recommended. The increase in overall air volume will then be principally related to the increase in the partition plate area through which the fluidization air will flow in the larger machine. "Scale-up" generally refers to increasing batch size and equipment geometry from small (6″, 7″, 9″, and 12″ Wurster coaters) to the pilot-scale. Partition diameter widens and its length increases, up to and including the 18″

Wurster coater. Beyond the 18″ Wurster coater the concept of "scale-out" may be more applicable, and scaling to 32″ or 46″ Wurster coaters is more direct. The larger inserts use multiples of the same diameter partition and spray nozzle found in the 18″ Wurster machine. Therefore, the increase in air flow would be a multiple of the number of partitions (700 cfm in the 18″ would lead to a target air flow of 2100 cfm in the 3 partition 32″ Wurster machine).

The final manner in which the air volume impacts the process in scale-up is also related to the fluidization pattern. In multiple partition Wurster systems (such as the 32″ and 46″ coaters), distribution of the process air across the entirety of the product container is a function of several factors. Orifice plates in both the up and down bed regions are selected based on the size, density, and surface properties of the materials being produced. As stated previously, the goal is to have the process air delivered to the product bed, such that the material in the down bed is in "near-weightless suspension" or behaving like a fluid. To achieve an essentially level surface requires a minimum of pressure across the down bed. This pressure is the result of several factors: core material quantity (initial batch size); partition height (the influence of the venturi); orifice plate configuration and finally, process air volume. As an example, if 700 cfm were used in the 18″ Wurster coater, the target value for the 3 partition 32″ Wurster coater would be 2100 cfm, as previously stated. Initial fluidization with the desired batch size may result in a tilted bed (higher in the rear of the insert than in the front), if product differential pressure was insufficient to cause the air to be uniformly distributed. Raising the partition height somewhat would increase the mass flow in the up bed region, potentially increasing overall product differential pressure. If this change were insufficient, a second approach would be to use a less permeable down bed plate. Both of these alternatives are preferred to increasing the process air volume. The consequent elevated spout height may enhance the potential for attrition, due to collision with the inside components of the filter housing.

For multiple partition production Wurster systems, it is prudent to optimize the fluidization pattern prior to actually producing a batch. A "mass flow study," which involves bracketing of process air volume and partition height for a set of orifice plates and batch size is recommended. The first step is to configure the Wurster insert with a set of up and down bed orifice plates. The initial partition height for the trial would be set at the lowest value selected for the study. Finally, the insert is positioned in the machine tower, and process air is drawn through it. The range of process air volumes to be tested should bracket the air volumes to be used for all steps of the process. At each of the selected air volumes, the product differential pressure (dP product) should be recorded. These will be the baseline contribution of the orifice plates. When the process is repeated with a batch in the insert, the difference between the total dP product and the baseline will reflect the "mass flow" in the insert. The goal is to identify the maximum product contribution, with a minimum of disruption to the fluidization pattern. An example is shown in Figure 34.26 and Figure 34.27. In Figure 34.26, the air volumes tested are 1250 cfm, 1500 cfm, 1750 cfm, 2000 cfm, 2250 cfm, and 2500 cfm. At each increase in air volume, there is a slight increase in product differential. Overall, the pressure contribution from the plates ranges from about 17 to 55 mmWC. Figure 34.27 shows the impact of putting a large batch (about 250 kg) of pellets into the insert (note: it is prudent to use a very strong substrate for these trials—they will be subjected to mechanical stress for an extended period of time). With the partition height set at 50 mm, it is evident that as air volume is increased, the quantity of product in motion (mass flow) increases. The values for 1250 cfm and 1500 cfm seem to indicate that the air volume is

insufficient to fluidize the entire batch—for certain the bed is stagnant in some region at 1250 cfm. At 1500–2000 cfm, the peak-to-trough values indicate a reasonably stable fluidization pattern. At 2250 and 2500 cfm, the enlarged peak-to-trough values reveal that some air bubble coalescence is occurring, resulting in some degree of back flow or turbulence in the down bed. This is not necessarily negative—a periodic bubble bursting through the down bed, along the wall of the product container, gives assurance that the product is not stagnant in this region. The air volume selected for this particular process was 2250 cfm. In addition to the fluidization properties, the high volume of air permits higher rates of heat and mass transfer, and this translates to faster spray rates and a shorter process time.

Higher partition heights, common for pellet coating, were also tested (60 mm and 70 mm). Interestingly, the peak-to-trough values widen at lower air volumes with higher partition heights. It is speculated that the strength of the venturi at the base of the partition, which draws product into the up bed, is either lessened or defeated, allowing air bubbles to move only vertically in the down bed.

The previous example is effective for coating or layering materials that do not exhibit tackiness in the down bed—they have a low surface coefficient of friction. Unfortunately, there are many products that display tacky behavior, and these same processing conditions may permit stalling of the batch in some region. Some users may try to counter this behavior by increasing the overall process air volume. However, it is likely that the majority of this increase will flow through the partition, and this region is not the source of the problem. It would be desirable to divert more of the process air volume to the down bed region. A method for achieving this would be to replace the up bed plates with ones that are less permeable. In this manner, at the same air volume, more of the process air is diverted through the down bed, making it more vigorous or turbulent. Figures 34.28 and 34.29 illustrate a mass flow study that is a consequence of this change. The "B" down bed plate remains, but the "G" up bed plates were replaced by the less permeable "H" plates. Once again, the partition height is set at 50 mm for the test. What can be seen is that the dP product contribution of the plates alone is now considerably higher. In this case, the range is from approximately 30 mmWC to 125 mmWC. When the same batch weight is added, stable down bed flow occurs at much lower air volumes—at somewhere between 1250 cfm and 1500 cfm. The peak-to-trough values for higher air volumes are very broad in comparison to the previous example, indicating significantly more

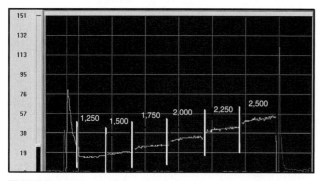

FIGURE 34.26   Product differential pressure in an empty 32" HS Wurster coater fitted with type "B" and "G" orifice plates (air volumes displayed are in cfm)

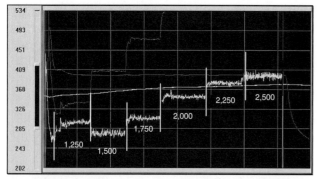

FIGURE 34.27   Product differential pressure in a 32" HS Wurster coater fitted with type "B" and "G" orifice plates, with a batch (air volumes displayed are in cfm)

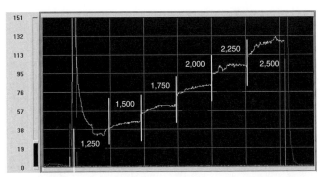

FIGURE 34.28 Product differential pressure in an empty 32″ HS Wurster coater fitted with type "B" and "H" orifice plates (air volumes displayed are in cfm)

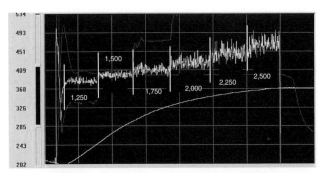

FIGURE 34.29 Product differential pressure in a 32″ HS Wurster coater fitted with type "B" and "H" orifice plates, with a batch (air volumes displayed are in cfm)

turbulence in the down bed. The selected air volume for this trial was 2000 cfm. The turbulence was sufficient to avoid regional bed stalling with the tacky coating material, and the relatively high air volume allowed for a reasonably high spray rate.

34.8.5 Process Air and Product Temperatures

As is typical of the laboratory scale, the temperature of the process air is generally adjusted to maintain a constant product temperature, and as spray rate is increased, the process air temperature is adjusted upward. If laboratory trials were conducted using a conservative or low product temperature, it may be possible to explore a higher product temperature in the production-scale equipment to improve productivity. However, it is strongly recommended that this is not done if the impact of higher product temperature on finished product attributes has not been explored, particularly for latex coating materials.

34.8.6 Mass Effects

The influence of larger batch size (or mass effects, as they are referred to), is more difficult to predict. In small-scale equipment, the product must be robust—if it must be treated cautiously in laboratory equipment, scale-up to pilot and production machinery will be nearly impossible. In Wurster processing, the big step in scale-up is from laboratory equipment (6″, 7″, 9″) to the pilot-scale 18″ Wurster machine. In small machines, bed depth rarely exceeds 200 mm, and fluidization height (substrate travel out of the partition) is principally limited by machine dimensions to 1.25 meters or less. In the 18″ unit, bed depth may range up

to 600 mm, and fluidization spout height can approach or exceed 2 meters. Product may also collide into the outlet air filters or other mechanical components of the machine. Further scale-up to the 32″ or 46″ Wurster coaters from the 18″ is somewhat simplified, since bed depth is about the same, and the objective in fluidization is to keep particle velocity similar in larger equipment to that used in the pilot-scale machine.

34.9 SUMMARY

The Wurster system is widely used for layering and coating, because of its ability to apply high quality films to a broad range of substrates. The orifice plate configuration in combination with the partition height and process air volume, organize the substrate in close proximity to the spray nozzle. Droplets of coating liquid travel only a short distance, and are applied co-current with the accelerating substrate. Productivity is related to the presentation of substrate surface area per unit time with respect to this quantity of liquid. Layering and/or film coating may be conducted using solutions or suspensions of materials in liquids comprised of organic solvents or water. The interaction between droplets and substrate is so rapid that materials applied using even the most volatile solvents are not subject to spray drying—they are high in quality, and their release is governed by their intrinsic properties, not by imperfections in the film. Also, within limits, materials can be sprayed from a molten state, congealing onto the surface of the slightly cooler substrate. As a production-scale batch processor, the Wurster has a moderate batch capacity (up to approximately 600 kg), and is efficient in terms of material balance and productivity.

CHAPTER

35

Process Analytical Technology in Solid Dosage Development and Manufacturing

Nancy E. Sever, Martin Warman, Sean Mackey, Walter Dziki and Min Jiang

35.1 INTRODUCTION

Since the late 1990s the FDA has been advocating the use of process analytical technology (PAT) in pharmaceutical development and manufacturing. The agency was interested in decreasing patient risk through improved control of pharmaceutical processes. In February 2002, the FDA formerly started the PAT initiative with the first meeting of the FDA Process Analytical Technologies Subcommittee of the Advisory Committee for Pharmaceutical Science.[1] To further promote the PAT initiative, a PAT guidance was issued in September 2004.[2] The guidance, which supports the twenty-first century cGMP, focused on using a scientific, risk-based approach in pharmaceutical development, manufacturing, and quality assurance.[3] The message was clear: increasing product and process understanding through monitoring and control of pharmaceutical processes would result in more consistent, higher quality products.

Whereas some process control and monitoring tools were already in use in the pharmaceutical industry, they did not cover all unit operations, and critical quality attributes were not necessarily measured. Implementation of new monitoring and control techniques requires high initial capital investments, more method development, operator training, validation, and qualification, and can result in internal regulatory uncertainty. This apprehension can be attributed to uncertainty of both FDA acceptance, and probability

of implementation success, since increased monitoring may identify process changes or fluctuations that were not previously observed. To quell some of the regulatory concerns, the "safe harbor" clause was added to the FDA guidance. This clause allowed pharmaceutical companies to obtain "experimental" or research data on existing processes that would not be subject to FDA inspections.[4] The goal of the "safe harbor" concept was to promote the use of PAT for process understanding, without concern for regulatory penalties.

Currently, many pharmaceutical companies have an active PAT effort within pharmaceutical development and/or manufacturing. Driving forces for this effort are to reduce production cycle time through faster release testing, to improve process consistency, to reduce batch failure or reprocessing though increased real-time sampling, and to promote real-time release. While these issues are mostly relevant in the manufacturing environment, PAT in pharmaceutical development is advocated as a tool for enhancing process understanding and reducing process development/scale-up time. Increased product and process understanding, combined with process monitoring or control, can reduce the number of experiments performed during scale-up, thereby potentially decreasing active pharmaceutical ingredients (API) usage in development and the time-to-market for new drugs. Higher production efficiency, reduced waste, consistent product quality, and faster time-to-market provide the economic incentives for the implementation of PAT in pharmaceutical development and manufacturing.

Developing Solid Oral Dosage Forms: Pharmaceutical Theory and Practice
ISBN: 978-0-444-53242-8

35.2 REGULATORY DEVELOPMENTS

The purpose of regulatory agencies, standards, and guidances is to ensure that pharmaceutical manufacturers are consistently manufacturing quality products. In order to set the stage for the implementation of PAT in pharmaceutical development and manufacturing, the Food and Drug administration (FDA), US Pharmacopeia (USP), International Conference on Harmonization of Technical Requirements for Registration of Pharmaceuticals for human use (ICH), and American Society for Testing and Materials (ASTM) international organizations have issued guidances, standards, and policies on the topic to help guide the pharmaceutical industry. The initiatives taken by these organizations are discussed below.

35.2.1 The FDA: Process Analytical Technology (PAT) Guidance

As previously mentioned, the FDA released the final guidance for the pharmaceutical industry on PAT (A Framework for Innovative Pharmaceutical Development, Manufacturing and Quality Assurance) in September of 2004. Some of the reasons cited for the initiative include the reduction of the burden on FDA resources that arise from manufacturing-related problems, such as product recalls, disruption of manufacturing operations, and shortage of essential drugs. These burdens prevent the agency from achieving the statutory biennial GMP inspections, especially for non-domestic firms. A desired goal of the PAT framework is to design and develop processes that can consistently ensure a predefined quality at the end of the manufacturing process. Such procedures would be consistent with the basic tenet of quality by design (QbD), and could reduce quality risks and regulatory concerns while improving efficiency. According to the FDA, PAT is an important factor in moving the agency forward to its cGMP "Initiative for the 21st Century," however it is only a subpart of the overall initiative at the agency.

To support process analytical technology activities, the FDA created several committees including:

1. an internal steering committee to oversee the agency's PAT activities;
2. a PAT team responsible for reviewing and inspecting PAT applications;
3. a PAT research team, to provide scientific support to policy development; and
4. an Office of Pharmaceutical Science PAT Policy Development Team to support the PAT team.

The formation of these committees solidified the agency's commitment to PAT implementation, and provide a resource for the industry to facilitate communication on new applications and PAT-containing submissions.

35.2.2 United States Pharmacopeia (USP)

The USP is the official public standards-setting authority for all prescription and over-the-counter medicines, dietary supplements, and all other healthcare products manufactured and sold in the United States. Since 2005, a USP advisory team and working groups have been working on writing or revising general information chapters on near-infrared spectroscopy, chemometrics, acoustics, definitions, rapid microbial methods, and hyperspectral imaging. These general chapters will all be numbered above 1000, in order to maintain their status as information chapters rather than test and assay chapters.

35.2.3 International Conference on Harmonization of Technical Requirements for Registration of Pharmaceuticals for Human Use (ICH)

The ICH assembles regulatory authorities from Europe, Japan, and the United States, along with experts from the pharmaceutical industry, to harmonize scientific and technical aspects of pharmaceutical submissions. Although the ICH has not issued a specific document on PAT, it is mentioned in the quality guidelines Q8 and Q9. As stated in ICH Q8 on pharmaceutical development, the purpose of pharmaceutical development is "to provide a comprehensive understanding of the product and manufacturing process," which can then be used for flexible regulatory approaches. The degree of regulatory flexibility is directly correlated to the level of relevant scientific knowledge and understanding about the product, and the manufacturing process, provided to regulatory agencies. This scientific understanding can be realized from formal experimental designs, process analytical technology (PAT), and/or prior knowledge and current knowledge gained from appropriate use of risk management tools. The ultimate regulatory goals are to facilitate risk-based regulatory decisions, to enable improvements in the manufacturing process within the design space without further regulatory review, to reduce post-approval submissions, and eventually to implement real-time quality control.

35.2.4 American Society for Testing and Materials (ASTM) Standards

The ASTM formed committee E55 on Pharmaceutical Application of Process Analytical Technology in August 2003. The scope of committee E55 was the development of standardized nomenclature and definitions of terms, recommended practices, guides, test methods, specifications, and performance standards for pharmaceutical application of process analytical technology. However in March 2007, committee E55 broadened its title and scope to include all aspects of pharmaceutical manufacturing. The new title is now committee E55 on Manufacture of Pharmaceutical Products, and the new scope is the development of standardized nomenclature and definitions of terms, recommended practices, guides, test methods, specifications and performance standards for the manufacture of pharmaceutical products. The committee brings together hundreds of technical experts from industry, academia, equiment and instrument manufacturers, and government sectors (including the FDA) to write voluntary consensus standards that will help drive new innovations in pharmaceutical manufacturing and process control. The FDAs basis of working with the ASTM, rather than the USP, is an objective of the National Technology Transfer and Advancement Act (NTTAA) of 1996 and OMB Circular A-119, which direct federal agencies to adopt private sector standards, when possible, rather than creating proprietary non-consensus standards, such as those from the USP. Thus far, the ASTM committee has issued four new standards on PAT, with at least 14 more in draft form awaiting approval.

35.3 PROCESS ANALYTICAL TECHNOLOGY (PAT) TOOLS

35.3.1 Analytical Techniques

Process analytical technology is based on the use of inline/online or atline tools to determine product quality. Ideally, test results need to be available in a timely manner to allow for feedback control. With this goal in mind, several techniques have been introduced into pharmaceutical development. These techniques include vibrational spectroscopy, acoustics, thermal effusivity, chromatography, laser diffraction, and optical techniques. A brief description of these tools is discussed below, along with common applications. The list of available tools continues to increase, as vendors of pharmaceutical equipment team-up with analytical instrumentation companies. In this discussion we focus on the more commonly-used techniques.

TABLE 35.1 Wavelength ranges for spectroscopic techniques

Spectroscopy	Wavelength range
UV-Vis	200–800 nm (50 000–12 500 cm^{-1})
Near-infrared	800–2500 nm (12 500–4000 cm^{-1})
Mid-infrared	2500–25 000 nm (4000–400 cm^{-1})
Raman	2778–1000 000 nm (3600–10 cm^{-1})

Lee, D.C. & Webb, M. (eds). (2003). *Pharmaceutical Analysis.* Blackwell Publishing CRC Press. pp. 261–267. (Reference for MIR, NIR and Raman ranges)

Vibrational Spectroscopy

Vibrational spectroscopy tools have been widely used in pharmaceutical product development and manufacturing. Vibrational spectroscopy is an optical technique that measures the vibrations of chemical bonds that result from exposure to electromagnetic energy at various frequencies. The spectra obtained are indicative of the type of chemical bonds in the sample, and when pieced together can be used to identify the chemical structure or composition of the sample. UV-Vis, mid-infrared, near-infrared, and Raman spectroscopy are among the most commonly used vibrational spectroscopy tools. The different regions of the spectrum measured by the four spectroscopic techniques are listed in Table 35.1. One advantage of these tools over other analytical chemistry techniques (i.e., HPLC, GC, etc.) is the high speed at which the measurements can be done (typically on the order of seconds). In addition, vibrational spectroscopy, with the exception of some UV-Vis applications, is usually a non-destructive analytical technique requiring minimal or no sampling preparation. Therefore, measurements can be made in-process or on a final product, without affecting the product yield or quality.

UV-Vis Spectroscopy

UV-Vis spectroscopy is typically performed on liquid solutions or suspensions. Some applications of UV-Vis include reaction monitoring,[5,6] dissolution testing,[7,8] vessel cleaning, and color determinations.[5] Developments in dissolution apparatus have increased the testing efficiency by extending a UV-Vis probe into the dissolution bath for real-time data acquisition and analysis.[8] Another important application involves using commercially available UV-Vis spectrometers to evaluate rinse water from equipment, to ensure the equipment is free of active ingredients, excipients, and detergents. This technique is mostly applied to clean-in-place systems, but can be extended to other equipment where rinse water can be collected. Analysis of rinse water is especially suited for potent manufacturing equipment that uses clean-in-place methods. Recent advances in cleaning validation have explored surface UV-Vis for cleaning inspection. In this case, equipment surfaces are analyzed for residual chemicals by reflection measurement.

Near-infrared Spectroscopy

Near-infrared (NIR) spectroscopy is one of the most versatile vibrational spectroscopy techniques in pharmaceutical analysis. With the variety of NIR instruments available on the market, new applications are continuously emerging. Some of the more common applications of NIR in solid dosage form manufacturing include:[9]

1. Chemical raw material identification;[10]
2. Polymorph identification;[11,12]
3. Crystalline versus amorphous phase identification;[13,14]
4. Blend uniformity;[53,54]
5. Wet granulation monitoring;[15]
6. Roller compaction monitoring;[16]
7. Drying end point;[65]
8. Coating end point and uniformity; and [17]
9. Potency in tablets or capsules.[18]

Several of these applications are discussed in more detail in the applications section below.

In addition to traditional NIR instrumentation, NIR chemical imaging is a more recent entry into the vibrational spectroscopy landscape. Chemical imaging technology captures a spectrum at each pixel in the image. This two-dimensional data can be used to evaluate uniformity in powder samples or tablets.[19] The technique, however, does require longer measurement time (up to ~10 min) per image. Depending on the magnification, blister packs can be imaged to identify possible counterfeiting.[20]

Mid-infrared Spectroscopy

Mid-infrared (MIR) spectroscopy is an analytical tool that has been widely used offline for decades in the pharmaceutical industry. With recent developments in fiber optics and probe designs, process MIR spectroscopy is gaining popularity. Because MIR captures the fundamental vibrations, it is highly suited for reaction monitoring in non-aqueous media.[21] However, because water has a strong absorbance in the MIR, it may overlay other smaller spectral bands in aqueous solutions. MIR can be used to analyze a wide variety of samples, including solids, gels, liquids, films, and gases. In the past, MIR was limited by the need for a short pathlength to get a useful signal. However, with the advent of attenuated total reflectance (ATR), pathlength is no

longer a restriction. Because ATR has a constant small pathlength, large and small sample sizes produce equivalent spectra. Online/inline applications of MIR in solid dosage form manufacturing include:

1. Raw material identification; and
2. Reaction monitoring.[21]

Raman Spectroscopy

Raman spectroscopy[22] is another analytical tool that has been used offline for decades, and has recently benefited from improved spectrometer designs. The advent of Fourier Transform (FT) Raman spectroscopy increased the speed and improved the safety of Raman spectroscopy. Like MIR, Raman spectra capture the fundamental vibrations of the chemical bonds. However, whereas MIR measures a change in dipole moment for polar bonds, Raman requires a change in the polarizability of symmetric/non-polar bonds. Because Raman focuses on non-polar bonds, water bands, for the most part, are absent in the Raman spectra, thereby making the technique highly suited for monitoring reactions or form changes in aqueous media. Similarly to NIR, Raman spectroscopy is versatile in accommodating various sample types, including solids, suspensions, and liquids in a non-invasive manner. Online applications of Raman spectroscopy in solid dosage form manufacturing include:[23,24]

1. Raw material identification;
2. Reaction monitoring; and
3. Polymorph screening.

Each of the spectroscopic techniques mentioned previously has advantages and disadvantages, as shown in Table 35.2. The key to selecting the appropriate technique is in understanding the needs of the process, the product attribute of interest, the specificity required, and the frequency of measurement needed.

Once the spectroscopic technique is selected, an evaluation of the instruments on the market ensues. Table 35.3 gives a list of available instruments for each spectroscopic technique. The types of instruments differ in the way light is emitted, split into the various wavelengths, and collected for analysis. These differences affect the wavelength range, intensity, and resolution of the spectra obtained. Depending on the application, the mode of installation, the sampling technique, and the location of the process, different instrument types may be more appropriate. More details on instrument selection are discussed in the Applications sections below.

In order for in/online or at/offline measurements to reflect the process in real-time, the analysis technique

TABLE 35.2 Comparison of vibrational spectroscopy techniques

Spectroscopy type	Advantages	Disadvantages
UV-Vis	Dilute liquid samples	Solid and liquid samples need to be diluted in a solvent.
Mid-infrared	High resolution, fundamental vibration band information; chemical and physical information; solid, semi-solid; liquid, film and gas samples; no sample preparation with ATR accessory; minimal data preprocessing needed.	Highly sensitive to water and some organic solvents; not suited for inline solids applications; limited use of fiber optic cables due to attenuation of signal; sample size of about 1 milligram of material may be too small to be representative of the process.
Near-infrared	No sample preparation most suited for inline and online measurements; physical and chemical information; solid and liquid samples; minimal signal attenuation across long fiber optic cables; macro sampling technique measuring hundreds of milligrams of sample.	Relies on combination bands and overtones; requires substantial data preprocessing and sophisticated multivariate analysis.
Raman	No sample preparation; not sensitive to water; suited for inline and online measurements; chemical and physical information; solid and liquid samples; minimal signal attenuation across long fiber optic cables; minimal data preprocessing needed.	Laser used requires safety precautions; sample damage can occur with FT-based NIR lasers; sample fluorescence is proportional with laser frequency; sample size of about 1 milligram of material may be too small to be representative of the process.

TABLE 35.3 Types of instruments available for different spectroscopic techniques

Spectroscopy method	Types of instruments
Mid-infrared	FT, FT-MIR microscope, FT-MIR mapping, and chemical imaging
Near-infrared	Photodiode, FT, Micro-electro mechanical system (MEMS), Acousto-optic tunable filter, dispersive, and chemical imaging
Raman	Dipsersive, FT, FT-Raman microscope, FT-Raman and dispersive mapping, and chemical imaging

needs to be fast, reliable, and the sampling needs to be representative of the entire process step. The latter point addresses the importance of proper sampling and installation location of on/inline instruments or sensors. Specific sampling techniques will be discussed in the Applications sections. Recent advances in computer speed and chemometric software have made real-time complex spectral analysis possible. More details on chemometrics and multivariate analysis are given below.

Acoustic Tools

Acoustic measurements are new to the pharmaceutical industry, but are widely used in other industries. There are two types of acoustic measurements: active and passive.

Active acoustic techniques involve sending a sound wave into a sample, and collecting the sound waves that are transmitted through the sample. The attenuation of the acoustic waves, and the change in their velocity as the waves pass through the sample, are related to the physical and thermal properties of the sample material. For example, changes between incoming and outgoing sound waves can be correlated to the density, porosity, concentration, etc., of the sample. Active acoustics relies on the ability of sound waves to travel through the sample. For this reason, most applications of active ultrasound involve liquids or suspensions that readily transmit sound. Some applications of active ultrasound include evaluation of suspensions, and fill level in bottles.

Passive acoustic techniques are based on collecting sound waves emitted during a process, and correlating those acoustic emissions to steps in the process or product attributes.[26] This technique relies on the sensitivity of the acoustic sensors, and the ability to collect sound waves at frequencies that are specific to the

TABLE 35.4 Thermal effusivities for common materials

Material	Thermal effusivity $(W \cdot s^{\frac{1}{2}}/(m^2 \cdot K))$
Static air	5
Standard pharmaceutical solids	150–800
Water	1600
Advanced composite materials	Several thousands

USP Pharmacopeial Forum 30 (4) Jul–Aug, 2004. <1072> Effusivity.

product or process monitored. The choice of frequency is important in ensuring other sounds or noises do not distort the signal. Some applications of passive acoustics include monitoring of high shear granulation,[25] fluid-bed granulations,[26] roller compaction,[27] and tablet compression.[28]

Thermal Effusivity

Thermal effusivity, the rate at which a material can absorb heat, is a material property that combines thermal conductivity, density, and heat capacity.[30] Equation 35.1 illustrates this relationship.

$$e = \sqrt{k \times \rho \times c_p} \qquad (35.1)$$

e = effusivity
k = thermal conductivity (W/m.k)
p = density (kg/m^3)
c_p = heat capacity (J/kg. K or W.S/kg. K)

Measuring effusivity can provide the user with physical information about the material that can be correlated with desired material properties. For example, increases in density will increase effusivity. Also, high variability in effusivity can be an indicator of non-uniformity. Typical thermal effusivity values are provided in Table 35.4.

Thermal effusivity is typically measured using a secondary method. The sensor is calibrated with standards of known effusivity values spanning the range of interest. Typical effusivity sensors are comprised of a heating element and temperature sensor. The sample is heated using the heating element, the rate at which its temperature changes reflects the heat capacity of the sample, and is used to calculate the effusivity according to Equation 35.1.

One of the challenges for using this technology online is sensor location. The sample must be static for a short period of time during the heating and temperature measurement (2 seconds to penetrate 0.5–1.0 mm into the powder). Because the material is continuously moving in many typical pharmaceutical processes, some

form of online sample bypass needs to be designed into the process. For an inline measurement, the process must be stopped for a short period while the measurement takes place. Atline testing is also possible if a sample can be obtained from the process. One source of variability in the data is change in the initial temperature of the sample at the time of measurement. This can be handled either by (a) using a bypass where the samples can be cooled to a constant temperature before testing or (b) measuring the initial temperature and compensating for changes in the effusivity calculation.

Because the effusivity of a material is sensitive to composition and physical properties (i.e., density, porosity, etc.), it can readily be used to monitor a number of pharmaceutical manufacturing processes, including wet granulation, blending,[30] and drying.[31,32,33] Thermal effusivity of the granulation material will change during the wet granulation process, due to the addition of binder (typically water) and densification of the granules. Using an atline technique, granulation end point can be defined as the point in time when the RSD of effusivity goes below a predefined threshold.[28] Effusivity measurements can also be used to monitor fluid-bed drying processes. Since the effusivity of water $(1600 W \cdot s^{\frac{1}{2}}/(m^2 \cdot K))$ is much greater than that of typical pharmaceutical solids $(150–800 W \cdot s^{\frac{1}{2}}/(m^2 \cdot K))$, effusivity measurements during the drying process are particularly sensitive to moisture changes. Roy et al.[30] examined both offline and atline effusivity measurements, and concluded that thermal effusivity can be correlated to the moisture content of the dried powders.

Of the potential monitoring applications for thermal effusivity, blend monitoring is probably the most mature. Effusivity measurements are taken at multiple locations during the blending process. The mean and RSD values of the measurements are calculated at various time points. As the blending process continues, the mean effusivity value will become constant, and the RSD will be minimized, indicating the blend is homogeneous.[31,32,33]

Chromatography

Chromatography, liquid or gas, has been widely employed in the pharmaceutical industry for quality assurance of in-process samples and final product. Compared to other available analytical tools, chromatography is known for its characteristics of high resolution and detection power, making it suitable for detecting multiple components in a complex mixture with high accuracy, precision, specificity, and sensitivity. Therefore, chromatography is used almost exclusively for analysis of complex mixtures, such as fermentation broths, and for trace analysis.

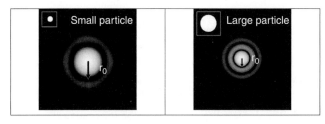

FIGURE 35.1 Example laser diffraction pattern of a small and large particle. Sympatec GmbH

Chromatography systems consist of multiple components, including a sampling system to perform sample preparation and sample injection, a mobile phase delivery system, the chromatography column itself, and one or more detectors coupled to a data processing and reporting system. Unlike laboratory systems, process chromatography systems have particular requirements including faster analysis, higher sensitivity, and wider dynamic range. The process system must be highly automated, and should require little maintenance. The system should also meet environmental requirements, such as explosion and dust resistance.

Developments in chromatography theory, chromatography materials (e.g., stationary phases, type of resin or stationary phase supporting media with defined particle and pore size), and column designs (diameter and length), as well as methods (various type of separation mechanisms), provide better separation efficiency and specificity, which makes fast online methods possible. In addition, advancements in miniaturized chromatography hardware make the systems robust, rugged, and suitable for manufacturing environments. There have been several pioneering applications of online chromatography as a PAT tool for real-time process monitoring and control. Numerous industrial applications of gas chromatography have been reported.[34] For liquid chromatography, applications in reaction monitoring for end point determination, column monitoring for product peak cut-off and collection, fermentation monitoring for nutrition addition, etc., have been reported in the literature.[35] When used for real-time quality decisions, the online chromatography measurement system needs to be time-synchronized with the process equipment, to provide efficient and accurate process control.

Laser Diffraction Tools

One of the most established tools for characterizing the physical properties of pharmaceutical products is laser diffraction. It has been applied in the characterization of aerosols, emulsions, suspensions, and sprays (including metered dose inhalers), as well as low-density powder streams (for example the outlet stream

from a mill). The measurement is based on Fraunhofer or Mie theory. The theory dictates that when a single particle interacts with laser light a simple diffraction pattern is generated, as shown in Figure 35.1.

This pattern shows a concentric ring structure, where the radius of the center globe relates to particle size. The light acquisition is performed using a semicircular multiple element photodiode.

However, rarely are individual particles found in process measurements, so it is very common to have overlapping or superimposed diffraction patterns. If the particles were static this would cause an issue, but most systems use dynamic sample presentation and because the particles are moving the effect is averaged out. Laser diffraction calculations determine mean particle diameters, and from these volume based particle size distributions are obtained. The capabilities of laser diffraction can be extended by representing the information as a population-based particle size distribution (i.e., percentage of the population with a calculated mean diameter). These data are more similar to number-based particle size distributions.

Optical Tools

In general, optical tools fall into several categories. The first utilizes the bulk properties of light interaction, such as optical density or turbidity measurements. These are perfect for determining particulate levels in liquid flows (for example to monitor filter breakthrough). There is even some evidence that they could be used to determine the presence of microbiological contamination in pharmaceutical water, and they are often used with bioprocesses.[36] The instruments use a broadband light source, with a simple photosensitive detector. The measurements are dependent on a reduction in light throughput as a function of sample property.

The next category employs a camera, instead of a detector, to obtain spatial information. The macroscale spatial information can determine the presence of a liquid layer on a filter bed, where the filter performance will be compromised if it is allowed to dry out. Other applications of macroscale optical measurement are level detection when separating multiple phase systems, where the boundary is determined by changes in optical density or by color change between the two phases.

The next class of optical tools utilizes a spatial system attached to a micro lens. These can be referred to as online optical microscopes, and have been used in many applications from packaging to API crystallization processes. Some examples include monitoring the presence of tablets/capsules in blister packs during packaging, determining the correct laser hole dimensions on controlled-release formulations, and verifying the correct print/label combination has been added on a product.

However, there are limitations to using this type of vision analysis. If the sample is moving in front of the camera during the period of the acquisition, the image will blur and generate an effect similar to a comet tail. The effect can be minimized by using fast acquisition cameras (as little as 25 ms) with increased light intensity; often laser illumination is necessary. Using a pulsed laser leads to even faster data acquisition, and allows speed and direction (vector) analysis of the particle to be made.

The biggest limitation is the compromise that must be made between field of view and number of pixels per particle (i.e., the higher the magnification, the greater the detail of information, but the lower the area covered, and the higher the likelihood of sampling bias). As the main advantage of vision analysis over alternates, such as laser diffraction, is the particle shape information obtained, the temptation is to specify the highest possible magnification. At small particle size, the greatest limitation becomes the wavelength of light used. However, the trade-off for lower magnification is lower quality of information about the shape of individual particles. Therefore, depending on the information needed from the measurement, appropriate magnification and measurement frequency should be used.

Other Tools

Other PAT tools include transformations of offline research-grade instruments to online use, e.g., NMR. When considering these types of systems, the key is to remember that they do not have the same measurement capabilities as their laboratory counterparts often their performance is reduced, because of the plant environment or because of changes needed to accommodate the online sampling system.

Some new tools involve the use of existing techniques in a novel application. One example is the use of X-ray for non-destructive monitoring of the presence of a product in an intact blister pack or to monitor the presence of foreign matter (for example contamination of API generated during drying and milling operations). X-ray is also being used as a tomography source, to obtain spatial information regarding the distribution of API within individual tablets.[37]

Spatial information can also be generated using spectroscopy with longer wavelengths in the far-infrared, such as Terahertz. Terahertz Pulsed Imaging combines imaging and Terahertz spectroscopy, resulting in 3-D information. The terahertz waves are scattered within the solid and reflect changes in the refractive index of the sample. This gives it excellent potential for monitoring coated[38] or multi-layer tablets. This technique is suitable if the thickness of the layer (or more importantly the variance in the thickness of the layers) is within the penetration capability of the technique, which is dependent on the wavelength range used.

35.3.2 Chemometrics and Multivariate Analysis

Multivariate data analysis is necessary whenever the data obtained is in more than two dimensions. Traditional two-dimensional data are obtained for a thermocouple in a process. The data are in the form of temperature versus time. These data can be analyzed readily, as temperature is presented in terms of one variable: time. In the case of spectroscopic data, absorbance is obtained as a function of wavelength. When spectroscopic data is collected in real-time, an additional time dimension is added. The data is then presented in terms of two variables: wavelength and time. The same is true for real-time acoustic, laser diffraction, and chromatography data where, in addition to time, the variables of frequency, particle size, and elution time, respectively, constitute the added dimension.

Multivariate data analysis allows for analysis of the multidimensional data, so that all significant variations are accounted for. Chemometrics can be defined as "the use of statistical and mathematical techniques to analyze chemical data."[39] As this definition implies, chemometrics was first developed for analysis of spectroscopic data, but has been applied to other types of multivariate data. There are several published text books and papers on the use of chemometrics for data analysis.[40] The type of data and the application of interest dictate the chemometric analysis required. In the Applications sections below, specific types of analysis techniques are discussed, with respect to the particular types of data sets.

35.4 PROCESS ANALYTICAL TECHNOLOGY (PAT) APPLICATIONS

In the previous section, a description of various PAT tools was given. Many of these tools have been applied to different unit operations in pharmaceutical manufacturing. The unit operations discussed include raw material identification, blending, granulation, fluid-bed drying, compression, and coating. The discussion below is not all-inclusive, and does not cover all PAT applications for all unit operations. The intent was to present examples of PAT tools applied in monitoring and controlling of select unit operations.

35.4.1 Raw material identification

The use of spectroscopic techniques for raw material identification provides two major benefits:

1. fast, accurate atline identification of the materials; and
2. the ability to use the spectroscopic data to characterize the raw materials and predict their performance in the process.

This section will focus on the first benefit, with the understanding that the second benefit could be a likely extension. NIR, MIR, and Raman spectroscopy have been used for laboratory material identification in the pharmaceutical industry. The current thrust is on developing atline methods for these spectroscopic techniques that require minimal technical expertise for operation, and can potentially be used on all raw and in-process materials in a manufacturing facility.

Near-infrared spectra contain information about the chemical and physical attributes of a material. NIR bands originate from the fundamental MIR vibrations. Overtone and combination bands for C—H, N—H, and O—H bonds provide the ability to characterize materials based on their NIR spectra in the same way as MIR fingerprinting.

NIR spectroscopy can be used to confirm sample identification and qualification. Identification is based on the chemical identity of the material. Qualification measures how well a particular sample satisfies established specifications for moisture, solid-state form particle size, residual solvents, and other chemical and physical properties.

Identification or qualification is normally achieved by comparison of the sample NIR spectrum to that of a reference library, set up using approved samples of the relevant materials as defined in the scope of the method. There are many literature references available regarding NIR library development and validation.[41,42]

The NIR bands are spectroscopically weaker, and typically less distinctive than the fundamental MIR bands, due to a degree of band overlapping. Therefore, identification by NIR is typically achieved by comparison of a mathematical/chemometric transformation of the NIR spectrum to similarly transformed spectra in a reference library. Many algorithms are available for material discrimination, including correlation methods, distance in wavelength space,[43] principle component-based analysis such as soft independent modeling of class analogy (SIMCA),[44] Mahalonobis

distance,[45] and partial least squares discriminant analysis (PLS-DA).[46] The choice of analysis technique is dependent on the user, and the scope of the library. The main advantage of an NIR identification library is the fast non-destructive nature of the test. In addition, because the NIR spectrum contains information relating to the physical attributes of the material (i.e., particle size, porosity, density, etc.), it can be used to ensure that the sample meets both chemical and physical requirements. The NIR spectrometer with a fiber optic probe also provides the ability to identify and qualify raw and in-process materials in the manufacturing facility. With more stringent requirements on raw material identification (e.g., in Europe, each drum of the active ingredient for the drug product process requires identification), a considerable saving can be obtained by using a rapid NIR identification method.

ATR MIR spectrometry can also be used for rapid atline chemical and physical identification of raw materials. It is accepted by the major pharmacopeias for identification of chemical substances, and in some instances can be used for some types of physical identification, such as differentiating between different solid-state forms.[47,48,49] Unlike NIR, ATR MIR is not sensitive to spectral effects of surface moisture and particle size. It has high specificity, and requires few reference spectra in an identification library development. Spectral data can be either visually compared to an existing spectral library or processed with discriminant analysis routines similar to those used in NIR spectroscopy. From a sampling perspective, ATR MIR does not require sample preparation, is not susceptible to variance in sample size due to its constant pathlength, requires about one minute to acquire a sample, and can generate an adequate spectrum with less than a milligram of material. These attributes make ATR MIR spectroscopy a highly suited technique for identification of potent compounds.

35.4.2 Blending

Blending is one of the most common unit operations in solid dosage manufacturing. Depending on the process, several blending steps may be needed, each requiring a uniform powder product. To ensure the blend is uniform, current industry standards require obtaining unit dose samples from either the blender or from a drum after the material has been discharged from the blender. Sampling involves using a sample thief to obtain a powder sample from different locations in the powder bed. The blend is considered uniform if the potency of the samples is between 85% and 115% of the theoretical value.[50]

Because samples obtained using a sample thief are susceptible to segregation, uniformity samples can often give misleading results.[51]

Real-time NIR[52,53,54] and Raman[55] spectroscopy have been utilized in determining blend uniformity. Depending on the location of the spectrometer, measurements can be made continuously or once per rotation. Because the powder in the blender is continuously moving, each spectra collected is from a different powder sample. The spectra obtained from the blending run can be analyzed in several ways, as discussed in a review by Blanco et al.[53] These techniques can be classified into two categories: (1) non-specific, and (2) compound-specific. The first class of analysis does not require any information on the materials in the blend, whereas the second category requires compound-specific information, such as composition, spectra of individual blend components, calibration sample set, etc. Both techniques are valid, and can be used to determine if a blend is uniform. In addition, because the measurements and analysis are done in real-time, the blend end point can be determined in real-time. This is especially beneficial for processes whose blend uniformity is sensitive to the raw materials or to upstream unit operations. The ability to ensure that each blend is uniform reduces the risk of content uniformity problems arising at later steps in the manufacturing process. In addition to blend uniformity data, physical information regarding particle size, density, moisture content or hardness of tablets has been correlated to the NIR spectra obtained during blending.[56]

Both NIR and Raman spectroscopy have been used to monitor blending processes and to determine blend end point. For tumble blenders, the following issues need to be considered when selecting the spectrometer for blend monitoring:

1. For true real-time data acquisition, the spectrometer measuring probe needs to be mounted onto the blender;
2. Wireless capability is necessary to accommodate the rotating blender;
3. Fast spectral measurement may be required to ensure that sufficient powder is in front of the measuring window or probe at the time of measurement.

In the case of continuous blenders, feedback control is possible. In that scenario, the spectrometer would be used to monitor the powder at the outlet, and depending on the uniformity obtained, the residence time or feed rate can be adjusted to result in acceptable product uniformity.

Current thief sampling methods require that the sample obtained be 1 to 3 times the dose manufactured.

To remain consistent with this rule, spectrometer sensors have been designed with a large enough surface area, such that the amount of sample contributing to the spectra is about 300 mg. This sample size falls within the 1- to 3-fold range for the majority of solid dosage forms. The location of the measurement sensor has been evaluated in the literature.[54] Depending on the size of the blender and shape (bin versus twin shell), the preferred location may be different. Studies have shown that, for twin shell blenders, the location of the measurement sensor was not critical with the four locations evaluated resulting in similar blend end point determinations.[57] However, a common practice is to place the measuring window on the lid of the blender. This location is convenient from a fabrication perspective, and requires minimal alteration to the blending equipment.

35.4.3 Granulation

Dry Granulation

Dry granulation refers to the process of densification via roller compaction, followed by gravity milling/screening to give the correct particle size distribution. Roller compaction relies on molecular forces (such as van der Waals' forces), electrostatic forces, magnetic forces, and valence forces. During compaction, the blend is compressed to the point that these forces bind all the material together to form a solid ribbon. The key attributes of a roller-compacted ribbon include API uniformity, solid fraction/porosity, lubricant uniformity, and tensile strength. The ribbons compacted in a roller compactor are milled to generate the granules to be used in subsequent unit operations (i.e., blending, compression, etc.) Typical granule attributes of interest

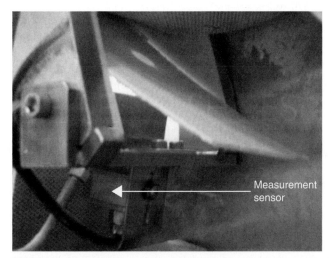

FIGURE 35.2 NIR measurement head installed in Gerteis Macropactor. Courtesy of Pfizer, Ltd

include: API uniformity, particle size distribution, density, and flowability. Uniformity in distribution of API and lubricant, as well as density (which impacts tensile strength) of roller compaction ribbons, can be monitored online, in real-time, using NIR. Specialized measuring heads (Figure 35.2) have been designed to allow installation within the roller compactor (RC), which allows measurement of API, lubricant, and density variance.[58] Whereas the concentration of API or lubricant can be monitored by tracking characteristic wavelengths, density changes are monitored by tracking the change in the baseline of the spectra. As the density increases, the pathlength for light increases resulting in an increase in light absorbance across the entire spectrum, which is presented as an upward shift in the spectrum.

Roller compaction poses an additional challenge, in that the ribbon produced may or may not be intact. In the latter case, appropriate measurement speed, geometry, and presentation are required to obtain consistent, reproducible, and meaningful information. Monitoring the quality attributes of interest real-time can alert the operator to changes in the process or environment,[59] and allow for the possible adjustments needed to return to the desired product.

Wet Granulation

The process of wet granulation has the advantage of not only enlarging particle size, and improving particle shape (making roughly spherical granulates), but also improving the hydrophilicity of the granule (promoting wetting, and consequently, disintegration and dissolution). However, there are many varieties of wet granulation including fluid-bed and high/low shear granulation. Both types can utilize a binder for granule formation. The binder can be introduced as a low or high viscosity binder solution or as a dry binder premixed in the formulation followed by the addition of a low viscosity liquid (normally water) to hydrate the binder and assist in granule growth. An additional granulation option involves either a "one-pot" processor or wet massing, followed by a different system for drying (be that tumble drying or fluidized-bed). Depending on the granulation process selected, the measurement system is chosen to match the quality attribute that is varying in that particular product.

The most common wet granulation process involves high shear mixing in the presence of an aqueous binder, followed by fluidized-bed drying. As the aqueous binder is added to the mixture, wet bridges are formed between the particles, and it is this process that is critical in defining the character of the granule produced.

The three types of bridging that can occur are pendular, funicular, and capillary as shown in Figure 35.3. In the pendular state, thin water bridges form with a high ratio of air resulting in weak capillary forces. In the funicular state, the ratio of water to air increases, and the capillary forces between the particles are maximized. In the capillary state, the intragranular space is filled completely, and the capillary forces decrease. Leuenberger[60] identified the optimal granulation point as being the initiation of the capillary state. Besides the status of the water in the granulation, dissolution of excipients or API, and particle size and density are important attributes to monitor during the granulation process.

Techniques that have been used to monitor granulation processes include power output, acoustic emission, thermal effusivity, focal beam reflectance microscopy (FBRM), and NIR spectroscopy. Power curves from a high shear granulator shaft have been used for decades to determine the end point of granulation. The power can be correlated to the quality of the granules, and provide a real-time inline tool for ensuring consistent granules are produced from batch to batch.

Near-infrared spectroscopy is suited for detecting changes in the water content, and state of the water (free versus bound), in a sample matrix. Two main NIR absorption regions describe this change. The lower absorption at about 1440 nm is the first water overtone resulting from stretching in the —OH molecular bond in water at about 3500 cm^{-1}. This band may also be produced by other compounds that contain an —OH functional group. The upper absorption at around 1940 nm is the water combination band of the —OH stretching vibration at about 3500 cm^{-1} and

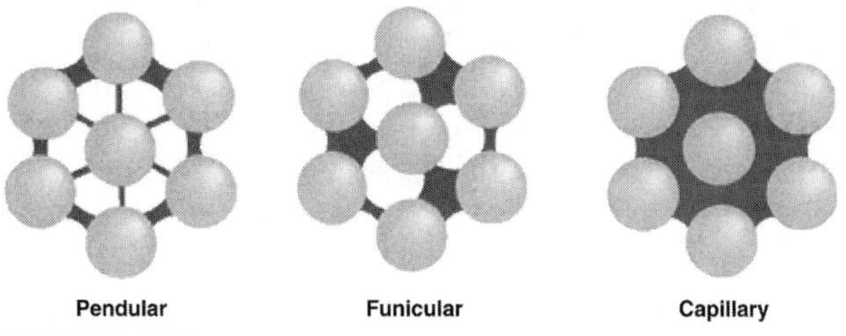

FIGURE 35.3 Mechanisms for granulate production. Courtesy of GEA Niro Inc

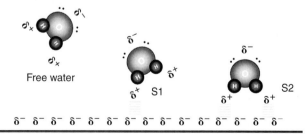

Material surface

FIGURE 35.4 Water binding modes

the corresponding deformation vibration at about $1650\,cm^{-1}$ of the water molecule. As wetting occurs, water molecules can exist in three well-defined states, as shown in Figure 35.4. In the S1 state, one hydrogen atom in the water molecule has hydrogen bonded to the material surface, in S2 both atoms have hydrogen bonded. In each case, changes in the mode of water binding result in a shift of the peak position in the NIR spectrum to a higher wavelength.

However, wet granulation is a fast process (typically around 5 mins). Therefore a high scan speed (on the order of a few seconds per scan) is a prerequisite for this application, as well as a measurement wavelength range exceeding 1940 nm. Near-infrared can also be used to monitor the distribution and dissolution of the active or excipient in the granulation, through similar trending of the signal at the appropriate wavelength.

Besides the state of water, the other quality attribute of interest is particle size. Determining the particle size distributions (both based on volume and number) are a challenge, due to the high density of the bed. Most characterization systems have an upper limit on percentage solid, and those which can cope with a high concentration of solids (for example, FBRM) can have issues with build up or coating on the probe. However these can be overcome by the optimization of installation angle, and the use of localized heating of the probe. Using the FBRM technique, the rate of granule growth can be determined and controlled.[61]

35.4.4 Near-infrared Monitoring of Fluid-bed Drying

Moisture content of powders is a perpetual concern for pharmaceutical product manufacturing. The amount of water can impact both physical (e.g., particle size, density, flowability), and chemical characteristics (e.g., dissolution, potency, degradation products) of the powder. Fluid-bed drying is commonly used to reduce the granulation moisture content to a desired level.

Typically, drying is controlled based on empirical experience, where drying is conducted for a fixed amount of time at a given set of conditions or until the exhaust temperature reaches a predetermined temperature. At the end of drying, a sample of the granulation is pulled, and tested for moisture using offline gravimetric or other instruments. If the moisture level is within the desired range the drying process is terminated, otherwise, the granulation is redried until the desired moisture level is achieved.

NIR spectroscopy provides an opportunity to make the drying process more efficient through real-time moisture monitoring. Water exhibits high absorption in the NIR spectral region, making NIR spectroscopy a viable technique for directly monitoring moisture content. In order to use NIR to monitor moisture, a calibration model must be created from spectral data collected during the drying process and/or from the laboratory, and correlated to moisture data from a referee method (e.g., Karl Fischer or loss on drying). When the calibration model is applied to NIR spectra collected during the drying process, real-time moisture values are calculated, and the drying process is continued until the desired moisture level is achieved. Terminating the drying process at the desired moisture content eliminates the need for redrying, thus reducing overall cycle time. In addition, real-time moisture monitoring allows for reducing or extending the drying time as needed, based on changes in the granulation properties to ensure the target moisture level is obtained every time.

Some factors to consider when selecting a spectrometer for a drying application include spectral resolution, spectral wavelength range, data collection speed, instrument robustness, software, and vendor experience and support. Proper installation of the spectrometer is critical to successfully using NIR to monitor the drying process. The mount should be located such that an adequate amount of material is presented to the spectrometer to ensure a suitable spectral signal to noise. Also, the mounting bracket should keep the instrument sufficiently stable to ensure consistent measurement. Finally, process controls and data management systems need to be in place, in order to upload calibration models, and handle the large amounts of spectral data generated during a run.

There are some challenges to using NIR spectroscopy to monitor moisture that should be considered during development. NIR spectra are sensitive to changes in physical (e.g., particle size, density) and chemical (e.g., composition, solid-state form) properties of the granules. Therefore, in building the calibration model, samples from various batches and campaigns need to be included. The overall reliability of the model prediction is dependent on the diversity of the samples used in developing the model. In addition, an understanding of component materials, and upstream processing parameters, needs to be established during method development. This knowledge will promote a better overall understanding of the manufacturing process, and ensure that a robust calibration model is created. A number of examples of using NIR spectroscopy to monitor moisture content during fluid-bed granulation/drying are published in the literature.[62,63,64]

35.4.5 Encapsulation

The main product quality attributes in encapsulation are content uniformity, and capsule weight. Monitoring encapsulation is challenging, due to the speed of the encapsulator and the need to monitor the powder inside the capsule before the cap is closed. Because of these challenges, vendors of encapsulation technology have led the effort of implementing online techniques. Both NIR and soft X-ray techniques have been used in real-time on commerical encapsulators to monitor content uniformity and fill weight, respectively. More simple applications involve the use of vibrational spectroscopy via a fiber optic probe to monitor the content uniformity in the hopper or powder bowl, and determine if segregation is occurring. These techniques, combined with inline capsule weight checkers, can give an indication if either the content uniformity or the weight are varying, and provide an opportunity for feedback control.

35.4.6 Compression

The main product quality attributes of the tablets are content uniformity, hardness, weight, and dissolution profile. NIR has been used to build PLS models that can predict the drug content, hardness, and dissolution profile for tablets.[65,66,67] These PLS models require substantial chemometric method development. In addition, real-time measurements of all tablets exiting a tablet press are challenging, due to the spectrometer speeds needed, and the need for modification of existing equipment. For these applications, atline instruments are often used. Commercial atline instrumentation can acquire NIR spectra and perform weight, thickness, and hardness testing, in a few minutes per tablet. The availability of this data, and the appropriate specification, can allow for parametric release. Inline force and weight instrumentation is readily available, and can be used in a feedback control-loop to adjust powder fill and force as needed, to maintain a constant weight and hardness.

35.4.7 Coating

The two most common types of tablet or particle coatings are fluid-bed and pan coating. The former typically utilizes a Wurster column within a fluidized-bed. Atomized spray from the center bottom is used to coat the fluidized tablets or particles, which are subsequently dried by hot air flow. Pan coating utilizes large rotating perforated pans that mix the tablets while they are sprayed with atomized solution and dried with heated air.

The majority of coating processes in the pharmaceutical industry are color-coating steps, where cosmetic appearance is the major concern. PAT techniques are not necessary for these types of applications. However, with the increase in functional and active coating applications, the need to determine the coating weight or thickness can be critical, as it can control both the release profile in the case of a functional coating or the potency in the case of active coating. One strategy for these processes is to assume a coating efficiency based on development work, and a certain amount of coating solution is applied. A second strategy involves weighing the tablets throughout the process, and applying coating suspension until a target weight is achieved. Neither technique is ideal, in that the former assumes a constant efficiency, which is not likely especially if the product is manufactured on different coaters, and the latter relies on the accuracy of the tablet weight, which can be unreliable in cases where the coating weight is small relative to the tablet weight.

For these reasons, real-time techniques that can monitor the amount of a particular component on a tablet are desirable. Real-time coating data can be obtained by inline or atline instrumentation. The challenges with an inline technique include installation of an instrument inside a coater, and dealing with the varying sample presentation, since most tablets are not spherical.[17] Atline techniques, which require sampling and analyzing tablets in a more controlled fashion, have been developed and demonstrated to be successful. The most common of these is the use of NIR spectrometers equipped with a tablet autosampler. Note that NIR cannot readily penetrate opacifiers such at TiO_2 found in tablet color coatings, therefore the measurements may be done prior to color coating.

Terahertz spectroscopy has also been used to determine coating thickness.[39] The technique is informative when used in development to analyze tablets with multiple coatings or bilayer tablets. Recent advances in the instrumentation make it possible to use the technique to monitor coating and compression processes real-time.

35.5 CONCLUSION

PAT is commonly used to refer to the ability to monitor a process real-time, use the data to improve process understanding, and consequently, to control the quality of the product manufactured. This chapter focused on the regulatory issues involving PAT, PAT tools, and applications of PAT in solid dosage manufacturing. There are many tools available and vendors are constantly introducing more into the market. It is important to remember that more sophisticated, and more expensive, is not necessarily better. A power curve can be just as effective as NIR or FBRM at determining the end point for granulation if sufficient development data is available to support its use. PAT is not about fancy equipment, but about monitoring the right product attribute, and using that information to control the process and manufacture a quality product.

References

1. Federal Register. (2002). February 6, Vol. 67, No. 25.
2. Guidance for Industry (2004). PAT—A Framework for Innovative Pharmaceutical Development, Manufacturing, and Quality Assurance, September. http://www.fda.gov/cder/guidance/6419fnl.pdf
3. http://www.fda.gov/cder/gmp/gmp2004/CGMP%20REPORT%20final04.pdf
4. Research data would not be subject to inspections except in certain situations as indicated in FDA/ORA Compliance Policy Guide, Sec. 130.300, FDA Access to Results of Quality Assurance Program Audits and Inspections (CPG 7151.02).
5. Brittain, H.G. (ed.). (1995). *Physical Characterization of Pharmaceutical Solids*. Chapter 2. Marcel Dekker Inc, New York.
6. Getvoldsen, G., Elander, N.E. & Stone-Elander, S.A. (2002). UV monitoring of microwave-heated reactions—a feasibility study. Chemistry: A European Journal 8(10), 2255–2260.
7. Cho, J.H., Gemperline, P.J., Salt, A. & Walker, D.S. (1995). UV/visible spectral dissolution monitoring by in-situ fiber-optic probes. Analytical Chemistry (67), 2858–2863.
8. Schatz, C., Ulmschneider, M., Alternmatt, R., Marrer, S. & Altorfer, H. (2001). Thoughts on fiber optics in dissolution testing. Dissolution Technology 12(6), 12–18.
9. Reich, G. (2005). Near-infrared spectroscopy and imaging: Basic principles and pharmaceutical applications. Advanced Drug Delivery Reviews 57, 1109–1143.
10. Blanco, M. & Romero, M.A. (2001). Near-infrared libraries in the pharmaceutical industry: A solution for identity confirmation. Analyst 126, 2212–2217.
11. Patel, A.D., Luner, P.E. & Kemper, M.S. (2001). Low-level determination of polymorph composition in physical mixtures by near-infrared reflectance spectroscopy. Journal of Pharmaceutical Sciences 90(3), 360–370.
12. Aaltonen, A., Rantanen, J., Siiriä, S., Karjalainen, M., Jørgensen, A., Laitinen, N., Savolainen, M., Seitavuopio, P., Louhi-Kultanen, M. & Yliruusi, J. (2003). Polymorph screening using near-infrared spectroscopy. Analytical Chemistry 75(19), 5267–5273.
13. Seyer, J., Luner, P.E. & Kemper, M.S. (2000). Application of diffuse reflectance near-infrared spectroscopy for determination of crystallinity. Journal of Pharmaceutical Sciences 89(10), 1305–1316.
14. Hogan, S.E. & Buckton, G. (2004). The application of near infrared spectroscopy and dynamic vapor sorption to quantify low amorphous contents of crystalline lactose. Pharmaceutical Research 18(1), 112–116.
15. Jørgensen, A.C., Luukkonen, P., Rantanen, J., Schaefer, T., Juppo, A.M. & Yliruusi, J. (2004). Comparison of torque measurements and near-infrared spectroscopy in characterization of a wet granulation process. Journal of Pharmaceutical Sciences 93(9), 2232–2243.
16. Gupta, A., Peck, G., Miller, R. & Morris, K. (2004). Nondestructive measurements of the compact strength and the particle-size distribution after milling of roller compacted powders by near-infrared spectroscopy. Journal of Pharmaceutical Sciences 93(4), 1047–1053.
17. Pérez-Ramos, J., Findlay, W., Peck, G. & Morris, K. (2005). Quantitative analysis of film coating in a pan coater based on in-line sensor measurements. AAPS PharmSciTech 6(1), E127–E136.
18. Cogdill, R.P., Anderson, C.A., Delgado-Lopez, M., Molseed, D., Chisholm, R., Bolton, R., Herkert, T., Afnán, A.M. & Drennen, J.K., III (2005). Process analytical technology case study Part I: Feasibility studies for quantitative near-infrared method development. AAPS PharmSciTech 6(2), E262–E272.
19. Lyon, R.C., Lester, D.S., Lewis, E.N., Lee, E., Yu, L.X., Jefferson, E.H. & Hussain, A.S. (2002). Near-infrared spectral imaging for quality assurance of pharmaceutical products: Analysis of tablets to assess powder blend homogeneity. AAPS PharmSciTech 3(3). Article 17.
20. Bakeev, K. (2005). *Process Analytical Technology*. Blackwell Publishing Ltd, Oxford, UK, p. 204.
21. Bakeev, K. (2005). *Process Analytical Technology*. Blackwell Publishing Ltd, Oxford, UK, p. 332.
22. Bakeev, K. (2005). *Process Analytical Technology*. Blackwell Publishing Ltd, Oxford, UK p. 147.
23. Vankeirsbilck, T., Vercauteren, A., Baeyens, W. et al. (2002). Applications of Raman spectroscopy in pharmaceutical analysis. Trends Anal. Chem. 21, 869–877.
24. Bugay, D.E., Henck, J.-O., Longmire, M.L. & Thorley, F.C. (2007). Raman analysis of pharmaceuticals. Applications of Vibrational Spectroscopy in Pharmaceutical Research and Development, 239–262.
25. Whitaker, M., Baker, G.R., Westrup, J. et al. (2000). Application of acoustic emission to the monitoring and end point determination of a high shear granulation process. International Journal of Pharmaceutics 205, 79–91.
26. Tsujimoto, H., Yhoyama, T., Huang, C. & Sekiguchi, I. (2000). Monitoring particle fluidization in a fluidized beg granulation with acoustic emission sensor. Powder Technology 113, 88–96.
27. Salonen, J., Salmi, K., Hakanen, A., Laine, E. & Linsaari, K. (1997). Monitoring the acoustic activity of a pharmaceutical powder during roller compaction. International Journal of Pharmaceutics 153, 257–261.
28. Levina, M., Rubinstein, M. & Rajabi-Siahboomi, A. (2000). Principles and application of ultrasound in pharmaceutical powder compression. Pharmaceutical Research 17(3), 257–263.
29. Fariss, G., Keintz, R. & Okoye, P. (2006). Thermal effusivity and power consumption as pat tools to monitor granulation endpoint in high shear granulators. Pharmaceutical Technology. 30(6), 60–72.
30. Roy, Y., Closs, S., Mathis, N., Nieves, E. 2004. Thermal effusibiy as a process analytical technology to optimize, monitor, and control fluid-bed drying. Pharmaceutical Technology 28(9), 21–28.
31. Léonard, G., Bertrand, F., Chaouki, J. & Gosselin, P.M. (2008). An experimental investigation of effusivity as an indicator of powder blend uniformity. Powder Technology 181(2), 149–159.
32. Mathews, L., Chandler, C., Dipali, S., Adusumilli, P., Lech, S., Daskalakis, S. & Mathis, N. (2002). Monitoring blend uniformity with effusivity. Pharmaceutical Technology 26(4), 80–84.31.
33. Roy, Y., Closs, S., Sundararajan, M., Boodram, J., Hervas, M., Larason, T., Mathis, N. & Meyer, W. (2005). A promising in-line monitoring tool for magnesium stearate blending end-point determination using thermal effusivity. Tablets and Capsules 3(2), 38–47.
34. Annino, R. & Villalobos, R. (1992). *Process Gas Chromatography*. Instrument Society of America, NC.

35. Cooley, R. & Stevenson, C. (1992). On-line HPLC as a process monitor. Biotechnology, Process Control and Quality 2, 43–53.

36. Ulber, R., Frerichs, J. & Beutel, S. (2003). Optical sensor systems for bioprocess monitoring. Analytical and Bioanalytical Chemistry 276(3), 342–348.

37. Sinka, I.C., Burch, S.F., Tweed, J.H. & Cunningham, J.C. (2004). Measurement of density variations in tablets using X-ray computed tomography. International Journal of Pharmaceutics 271(1–2) 215–224

38. Fitzgerald, A., Cole, B. & Taday, P. (2005). Nondestructive analysis of tablet coating thicknesses using terahertz pulsed imaging. Journal of Pharmaceutical Sciences 94(1), 177–183.

39. Beebe, K., Pell, R. & Seasholts, M. (1998). *Chemometrics: A Practical Guide.* John Wiley and Sons, Canada.

40. Brereton, R. (2003). *Chemometrics: Data Analysis for the Laboratory and Chemical Plant.* John Wiley and Sons, Canada.

41. Kemper, M. & Luchetta, L. (2003). A guide to raw material analysis using near infrared spectroscopy. Journal of Near Infrared Spectroscopy 11(3), 155–174.

42. Blanco, M. & Romero, M. (2001). Near-infrared libraries in the pharmaceutical industry: a solution for identity confirmation. Analyst 126, 2212.

43. Gemperline, P. & Boyer, N. (1995). Classification of near-infrared spectra using wavelength distances: Comparison to the Mahalanobis distance and residual variance methods. Analytical Chemistry 67, 160–166.

44. Gemperline, P., Webber, L. & Cox, F. (1995). Raw materials testing using soft independent modeling of class analogy analysis of near-infrared reflectance spectra. Analytical Chemistry 61, 138–144.

45. Shah, N. & Gemperline, P. (1995). Combination of the Mahalanobis distance and residual variance pattern recognition techniques for classification of near-infrared reflectance spectra. Analytical Chemistry 62, 465–470.

46. Stahle, L. & Wold, S. (1987). Partial least squares analysis with cross-validation for the two-class problem: A Monte Carlo study. Journal of Chemometrics 1, 185–196.

47. Kendal, D.N. (1953) Identification of polymorphic forms of crystals by infrared spectroscopy. Anal. Chem. 25(3), 382–389.

48. Cleverly, B. & Williams, P.P. (1959). Polymorphism in substituted barbituric acids. Tetrahedron 7, 277–288.

49. Brittain, H. (1997). Spectral methods for the characterization of polymorphs and solvates. J. Pharm. Sci. 86(4), 405–412

50. USP. General Chapter <905> Uniformity of Dosage Units.

51. Muzzio, F., Robinson, P., Wightman, C. & Brone, D. (1997). Sampling practices in powder blending. International Journal of Pharmaceutics 155, 153–178.

52. Blanco, M., Gozález Bañó, R. & Bertran, E. (2002). Talanta 56, 203–212.

53. El-Hagrasy, A., Morris, H., D'Amico, F., Lodder, R. & Drennen, J. Near-infrared spectroscopy and imaging for monitoring of powder blend homogeneity. Journal of Pharmaceutical Sciences, 90(9), 1298–1307.

54. Sekulic, S., Ward, H., II, Brannegan, D., Stanley, E., Evans, C., Sciavolino, S., Hailey, P. & Aldridge, P. (1996). On-line monitoring of powder homogeneity by near-infrared spectroscopy. Analytical Chemistry 68, 509–513.

55. Hausman, D., Cambron, R. & Sakr, A. (2005). Application of Raman spectroscopy for on-line monitoring low dose blend uniformity. International Journal of Pharmaceutics 298(1), 80–90.

56. Otsuka, M. & Yamane, I. (2006). Prediction of tablet hardness based on near infrared spectra of raw mixed powders by chemometrics. Journal of Pharmaceutical Sciences 95(7), 1425–1433.

57. Sever, N. (2004). Near Infrared Spectroscopy to Monitor Blend Uniformity. IFPAC Annual Meeting. Baltimore, MD.

58. Gupta, A., Peck, G.E., Miller, R.W. & Morris, K.R. (2005). Real-time near-infrared monitoring of content uniformity, moisture content, compact density, tensile strength, and Young's modulus of roller compacted powder blends. Journal of Pharmaceutical Sciences 94(7), 1589–1597.

59. Gupta, A., Peck, G.E., Miller, R.W. & Morris, K.R. (2005). Influence of ambient moisture on the compaction behavior of microcrystalline cellulose powder undergoing uni-axial compression and roller-compaction: A comparative study using near-infrared spectroscopy. Journal of Pharmaceutical Sciences 94(10), 2301–2313.

60. Leuenberger, H. (1994). Moist agglomeration of pharmaceutical powders (size enlargement of particulate material)—the production of granules by moist agglomeration of powders in mixers/kneaders. In: *Powder Technology and Pharmaceutical Processes, Handbook of Powder Technology*, D. Chulia, M. Deleuil, & Y. Pourcelot, (eds), Vol. 9. Elsevier, Amsterdam. pp. 377–389.

61. Hu, X., Cunningham, J. & Winstead, D. (2008). International Journal of Pharmaceutics 347(1–2), 54–61. Jan 22.

62. Findlay, W., Peck, G. & Morris, K. (2005). Determination of fluidized bed granulation end point using near-infrared spectroscopy and phenomenological modeling. Journal of Pharmaceutical Sciences 94(3), 604–612.

63. Rantanen, J., Lehtola, S., Rämjet, P., Mannermaa, J. & Yliruusi, J. (1998). On-line monitoring of moisture content in an instrumented fluidized bed granulator with a multi-channel NIR moisture sensor. Powder Technology 99, 163–170.

64. Frake, P., Greenhalgh, D., Grierson, S.M., Hempenstall, J. & Rudd, D. (1997). Process control and end-point determination of a fluid bed granulation by application of near infra-red spectrsocopy. International Journal of Pharmaceutics 151, 75–80.

65. Reich, G. (2000). Use of NIR transmission spectroscopy for non-destructive determination of tablet hardness. Proc. 3rd World Meeting APV/APGI, 3/6, April. Berlin, pp. 105–106.

66. Kirsch, J. & Drennen, J. (1995). Determination of film-coated tablet parameters by near-infrared spectroscopy. Journal of Pharmaceutical and Biomedical Analysis 13, 1273–1281.

67. Reich, G. & Frickel, H. (1999). Use of transmission spectroscopy to determine physical and functional film coat properties on tablets. Proc. Int. Symp. Control. Release Bioact. Mater, 26, 905–906.

## PART IV

SELECTED TOPICS IN PRODUCT DEVELOPMENT

The Product Development Process

Lynn Van Campen

36.1 INTRODUCTION

The selected topics in Part IV of this book provide an appropriate and important complement to the more technically-oriented chapters which precede them, providing in particular the context in which the science behind the pharmaceutical development of oral drug products is applied. Major shifts in the way the pharmaceutical industry does business today have occurred since 2000. These have resulted in large part from the globalization of industrial capability, on both the research and development fronts, of new science and technologies, and of the facilities and expertise capable of supporting them. At the same time, the costs of new drug development have soared, as also have the number and market share of generic drugs whose competition places new demands on the cost-effectiveness of the innovator's investment in new drug discovery and development programs.

In the US, a new regulatory paradigm is coming into play, which could offer significant relief from the pressure of regulations that by design have historically suppressed innovation in favor of control during all but the early stages of development. The FDAs initiative, *Pharmaceutical Quality for the 21st Century—A Risked Based Approach*, intends to enhance and modernize the regulation of pharmaceutical manufacturing and product quality, and by so doing stimulate the adoption of modern and innovative technology. The impact of integrating quality systems and risk management approaches into the latter stages of development, however, also affects earlier phases of the design and development of the physical

dosage form, chemistry, manufacturing and controls (or CMC). The concepts of "quality by design," and product "design space" encourage the pharmaceutical scientist to understand the behavior of the drug candidate from early selection and characterization, to and throughout clinical drug product formulation and process development. The higher quality of the development process and its scientific foundation leads to better knowledge of the risks involved in manufacturing the product, and how best to mitigate them, earning a flexibility from past standards of regulatory control.

Collaboration with international health and regulatory organizations has been vital to the FDAs modernization efforts. A key goal of this initiative has been to promote the assurance of drug product quality and consistency, including the application of current good manufacturing practices (cGMPs), on an international scope. To this end the FDA has participated extensively in the International Conference on Harmonization of Technical Requirements for Registration of Pharmaceuticals of Human Use (ICH) Quality (Q) topics to develop a pharmaceutical quality system based on an integrated approach to risk management and pharmaceutical science. This is part of the broader movement underway across North America, Europe, and Japan to coalesce these countries' most effective approaches to regulation into a harmonized set of requirements.

This challenge to industry comes with a price tag it should be willing to pay: a greater investment in time and resources required to achieve this level of drug substance, product and process understanding. On the premise that this approach to development

Developing Solid Oral Dosage Forms: Pharmaceutical Theory and Practice
ISBN: 978-0-444-53242-8

enables more effective decision-making, the investment is more than compensated for by higher rates of program success along the entire path of development, regulatory flexibility, and the accompanying overall cost savings. Given sufficient scientific justification, product and process adjustments can, in principle, be implemented during development, and even during production of the marketed product, without the otherwise categorical requirements for bridging studies and time-consuming regulatory submissions and review. The opportunity for continuous improvement relieves not only industry; the FDAs workload also decreases, as the responsibility for high quality is built more reliably into the sponsor's development process.

This approach to new and generic drug development is not lost on the newly emerging pharmaceutical companies in the developing nations, now able to jump into the global scene with the enlightened regulatory environment that countries with a mature industry are still struggling to refine and embrace. As the global field of pharmaceutical operations matures, some equilibration will naturally occur across all countries serving discovery, development and manufacturing; their resource and business interdependencies; the new technologies invented and incorporated into new products; and the legal systems by which their innovation and business interests are protected.

It is now unusual to find "cradle to grave" drug development capabilities within a given corporate site. Small and young pharmaceutical companies have long contracted out aspects of development outside their knowledge base or technical capability, filling in the gaps between their defined strongholds of expertise at any given time. But today it is also common to find large pharmaceutical companies which have strategically divested significant portions of their product development, and even commercial operations, to corporate subsidiaries, alliances or contract houses offshore.

36.1.1 Organizational Considerations

Regardless of where drug product development activities are conducted, they remain largely the same from product to product. As the number of development sites increases within a given program, however, strong and effective program management is critical to ensuring successful program planning, communication, and execution. A core leadership team comprised of senior, experienced members, representing the human resources who will carry out the development activities is generally appointed, providing a common

and effective means of managing a given development program. For a new drug molecule, these resources will include discovery research, pharmacology and toxicology, clinical research, development CMC, production and quality control, quality assurance, regulatory, marketing, and program management. The membership of this team will shift over time, consistent with the stage of development. It is worth noting that throughout the life of the program, with the possible exception of the earliest discovery stage, CMC will be represented.

There are challenges to organizing the core development team. First, there are usually more new compounds in development than experienced leaders available to serve as members. Dedicated resources at any level of the organization are usually a luxury, reserved for programs of only the highest priority. Secondly, choosing who leads the leaders can prove to be a good test of an organization's strength of character. Top scientists on the core team may be asked to work within the overall leadership of a less technically trained program manager carrying overall responsibility for program success. Furthermore, corporate "line function" managers will generally find that the program responsibilities of scientists, within their respective disciplinary department or division, are directed largely through the core team. The communication pathways for instilling and maintaining a level of trust between the team leadership and the line function management must remain well-oiled over the course of years. As in any organization, clear lines of responsibility and authority must be defined. Furthermore, as greater authority is given to the qualified core team, the more effective it can be.

For the typical development program whose activities are directed and conducted at multiple sites under multiple corporate banners, effective communication can prove to trump technical weaknesses in getting to market before one's competitors. Effective team leadership can eliminate two notorious causes of poor communication: the "silo effect" that limits exchange of information between different centers of expertise, and the lack of clear mechanisms for effective technology transfer throughout the course of development.

For global development operations spanning multiple companies and/or countries, counterpart individual and/or team assignments at each site are helpful to communication, enabling the identification of a "single point of contact" for a given type of development activity. Long-term exchanges of personnel, including the dedicated "man in the plant" representative often sent to a contract development facility, can engender a strong sense of collaboration between sponsor and service provider, and enable the inevitable development problems to be dealt with faster and more effectively.

36.1.2 The Target Product Profile: A Strategic Development Process Tool

The concept of a target product profile (TPP), first developed informally in the late 1990s, has been formalized in a draft FDA Guidance issued in early 2007. While not a requirement, the TPP serves several fundamental purposes: it is used to define the intended product at the start of a new program, and is updated throughout development as needed; it aligns members of the development team with regard to their planning and updating a cohesive and coherent development plan; and importantly, the TPP serves as an effective communication tool between the company sponsor and the regulatory agency.

The product criteria considered in the TPP specifically anticipate the final drug labeling. For each label claim the sponsor presents a brief commentary, including the related development plan and possible discussion topics or questions, for the reviewing agency. As milestones are achieved, review of the updated TPP enables clear discussion with the FDA regarding the ongoing suitability of the development plan in supporting the sponsor's desired label claim(s). These claims generally include the following:

- indications and usage;
- dosage and administration;
- dosage forms and strengths;
- contraindications;
- warnings and precautions;
- adverse reactions;
- drug interactions;
- use in specific populations;
- drug abuse and dependence;
- overdosage;
- description;
- clinical pharmacology;
- nonclinical toxicology;
- clinical studies;
- references;
- how supplied/storage and handling;
- patient counseling information.

While largely directed toward the clinical aspects of the target product, the TPP has much to offer those pharmaceutical scientists focusing on CMC. From these criteria, the CMC development scientist is able to narrow the choices of route of delivery and dosage form, and consider what the drug candidate's physical chemical and biopharmaceutical properties would desirably

be in order to meet the product goals. Throughout development, the TPP evolves in character and detail, changing as needed to reflect updated product goals as defined by all facets of development. Additional items that CMC might add to the above list during development include the primary target population (age, size of market, etc.), packaging configuration, production batch size, and cost. Effective use of the TPP will preclude unwelcome surprises when, for reasons of inadequate communication, marketing learns too late that R&D has developed a product they will have a hard time selling.

36.2 SUMMARY OF THE DRUG DEVELOPMENT PROCESS

In mid-2007 the FDA made available an interactive schematic of the new drug development process, given in Figure 36.1, showing the key development steps required to bring a new molecular entity (NME) from the discovery laboratory to the commercial market. During the 8–12 year course of pre-market drug development in the US, the FDA expects to meet with the company sponsor (or applicant) on a number of specific occasions, and encourages communication as needed beyond this. Additional review groups, representing both citizens and experts, are selected to participate at periodic milestones of every new development program. Their roles are fundamental to ensuring a broad ethical and technical integrity within the process. Many other countries have similar mechanisms of independent review incorporated into their regulatory processes.

The key phases of new drug product development are summarized by the following sequential activities and milestones.

Preclinical research:

- Test the NME chosen as the drug candidate, often referred to as the "development candidate," in animals to assess its *in vivo* behavior, including pharmacology, toxicology, and biopharmaceutical properties.

Clinical:

- Phase 1: test the drug candidate in a small group of healthy human volunteers to ensure it is safe to proceed to more extensive human clinical trials.
- Phase 2: test the drug candidate in a small group of patients for evidence of efficacy and determination of dose, in parallel with longer term nonclinical safety testing in animals.
- Phase 3: define the marketable dosage form of the drug candidate or "drug product," and test the

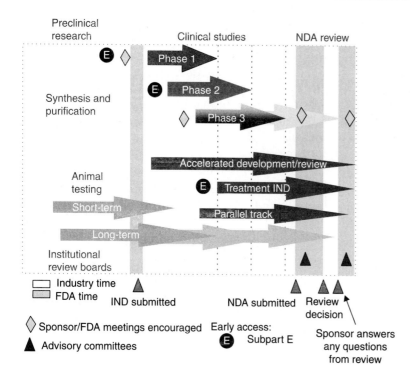

FIGURE 36.1   FDA schematic of "The New Drug Development Process: Steps from Test Tube to New Drug Application Review"

potential drug product in a large group of patients for evidence of safety and efficacy.

Regulatory review:

- Submit an application to the health agency for market approval.
- On approval, launch the drug product to market.
- Conduct phase 4 post-market surveillance as per commitment to the FDA.

The key phases of development are typically defined in terms of the clinical program, as above, and refer only implicitly to the parallel CMC development of the dosage form and its process of manufacture. In fact, over the 10–12 year course of a given development program, pharmaceutical scientists and process engineers will have developed many test "drug products" for the selected drug candidate.

These test products include preparations to satisfy the effective delivery of drug substance, in doses varying by many orders of magnitude, to one or more animal species for acute toxicology evaluation, as well as for short- and long-term safety testing. Once in the phase 1 clinic, simple preparations are needed for administering multiple dose levels to human volunteers in early safety testing. By phase 2, more sophisticated dosage forms are developed for delivering drug at multiple doses to humans by the likely route of administration to be used in the market. Desirably by late phase 2, and

definitively for phase 3, clinical drug product and packaging must represent the intended commercial product. Last but not least, the final commercial drug product must be produced in time for product launch upon regulatory approval. For every single one of these test drug products, there will be a need to establish the formulation, a defined process of manufacture and packaging, and quality control and stability testing commensurate with the stage of development.

Ideally, the development candidate will progress successfully through preclinical and clinical evaluation to market launch, with the possible modification of adjusting salt form. However, despite the diligent evaluation invested in the selection process, the probability of a given candidate's reaching the market is not high. The Pharmaceutical Research and Manufacturers of America (PhRMA) trade organization reported in 2007 that for every new drug approved for market launch, an average of five had entered clinical studies, and that these five had in effect been winnowed from hundreds of compounds that had entered preclinical development studies. Their analysis is shown in Figure 36.2. This observed rate of attrition, and the accelerating costs associated with clinical development, are the major reasons most pharmaceutical product developers call for a "fast to fail" strategy, i.e., if a compound is going to fail, it is in the best interests of its sponsor to determine its fatal flaws as early in the development process as possible.

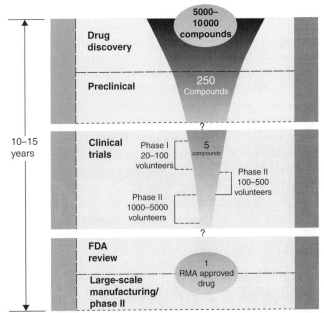

FIGURE 36.2 The R&D process: long, complex, and costly (taken from Pharmaceutical Research and Manufacturers of America (PhRMA), in Pharmaceutical Industry Profile 2007. Washington, DC: PhRMA, March 2007)

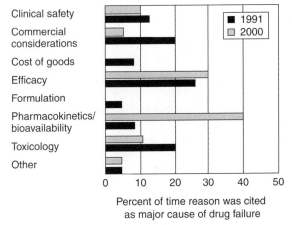

FIGURE 36.3 Causes of compound failure to reach approval to market (taken from Nature Reviews Drug Discovery 2004, 3, 711)

The reasons behind compound attrition are many. Failure to meet product objectives for any one of these development steps will lead to program delay or cancellation. Figure 36.3 shows an analysis at two different time points of why new compounds which entered preclinical testing failed to make it to market. In 1991 poor biopharmaceutical behavior (pharmacokinetics and bioavailability) was found to be the overwhelming basis for stopping a compound's development. By 2000 the major causes had shifted to toxicology and commercial considerations, reflecting in large part an increased understanding of biopharmaceutical behavior, and an ability to predict undesirable pharmacokinetic properties in a compound, before moving it forward into development. More recently, substantial research gains have also been made in rendering toxicological behavior more predictable.

Detailed descriptions of these key stages of drug development follow.

36.3 PRECLINICAL RESEARCH

36.3.1 Discovery Research

Years of discovery research may precede the initiation of preclinical research and the studies that mark the start of the new drug development program. Tailored to produce new chemical or biological entities with the potential to meet the desired therapeutic goals defined by a TPP, discovery research programs are complex, lengthy, and costly, driven by goals that may prove unachievable, and must then be modified. Generally a biochemical target is identified which relates to the disease or medical condition of interest. One or more principal *in vitro* assays involving this target are developed, for use in high throughput screening (HTS) of compounds for some measure of interaction with a suitable substrate, indicating potentially relevant pharmacological activity.

For orally administered drugs, the successful compound will likely have a molecular weight less than 1000, i.e., a "small molecule." Small molecule compound libraries are produced by synthetic or biosynthetic processes, which can yield hundreds or thousands of compounds in very short periods of time. Those compounds exhibiting a high level of response during *in vitro* testing will be selected for refinement and optimization of their respective molecular structures in order to maximize this response.

Preliminary evaluation of the optimized compounds' "developability" is generally made by predicting certain key physico-chemical properties via computational chemistry or if necessary, by measuring them in the laboratory (at greater cost). If an animal model is available for testing therapeutic efficacy, selected compounds exhibiting the best *in vitro* activity may all be tested and compared for *in vivo* activity. Finally, that compound judged to have the most suitable *in vitro* properties, and *in vivo* response profile (if available), is recommended for entry into preclinical development by a team of scientists advisedly comprised of both discovery scientists, e.g., chemists, molecular biologists, and biochemists, as well as development scientists, e.g., biopharmaceutical and formulation chemists. In addition to the identified "lead compound," additional "back-up" compounds may also be identified.

36.3.2 Preclinical Development

The primary goal of preclinical development is to ensure a reasonably safe entry into human clinical trials, by gaining a good understanding of the pharmacology and toxicity of the selected lead compound in animals. Other attributes of this compound, e.g., chemical stability, are also evaluated, in order to ensure the selection of a drug candidate that will have a high probability of success in becoming a safe and effective drug product. The CMC and biological activities that comprise this phase include the following activities, in rough chronological order:

- Synthesis and purification of milligram quantities of the lead compound.
- Development of preliminary analytical methods for assaying the compound, and its major synthetic impurities, and/or products of chemical degradation in the purified material and in formulation.
- Pharmaceutical characterization of the lead compound to evaluate developability further, as an additional component of the optimization and selection process. For compounds intended for oral delivery, the key physico-chemical properties of interest at this stage are solubility in water, partition coefficient as a rough predictor of permeability, and stability.
- Scaled-up synthesis and purification of compound in quantities needed for animal studies.
- Formulation of the lead compound for injectable and oral administration to animals.
- Evaluation of the pharmacology and toxicology of the lead compound in animals using good laboratory practices (GLPs). Every effort is made during these studies to use as few animals as possible, and to ensure their humane and proper care. Usually both rodent and non-rodent species are used in testing, because a drug may affect one species differently from another.

During the course of the above preclinical activities, and well prior to the initiation of formal GLP animal studies, there is additional opportunity to ensure that the compound taken into development is not only the "best" available from discovery, but that it is also "good enough" to survive the many development hurdles it must jump before it is launched as a new drug product. For example, new comparisons of the lead with back-up compounds can be made when data from more refined physico-chemical profiles, additional activity assay results, performance in limited *in vivo* studies, etc., become available. Additional molecular modification(s) at this stage could further improve the activity profile and developability of the lead. This "lead optimization" process is important to confirm that the compound chosen to proceed into development is indeed worthy of the substantial investment in effort and resources that will be required. The early development team will then formally designate the resulting "best compound" as the "development candidate"—a weighty decision, and the first significant milestone of the drug development program.

Pharmacology Studies

The FDA will expect to see in the Investigational New Drug application (IND), a comprehensive report on the pharmacological profile of the development candidate in animals. There are two aspects to these studies:

- Pharmacodynamic (PD) studies are designed to determine dose–response relationships, as well as the compound's primary and secondary effects on major physiological systems, its duration of effect, and mechanism of action as they relate to the proposed indication. Both desirable and undesirable pharmacodynamic or pathophysiological properties of the compound must be identified, and their relevance to human safety considered.
- Pharmacokinetic (PK) studies are designed to gain information on the extent and duration of systemic exposure to the compound, specifically its absorption, distribution, metabolism, and excretion (ADME) patterns.

Toxicology Studies

Toxicology studies offer three key pieces of information:

1. safe dose levels for the clinical program;
2. target organs affected by toxicities; and
3. the clinical parameters that should be monitored during human testing.

There are minor variations among the US, EU, and Japanese regulatory agencies with regard to their toxicology requirements and expectations around the conduct of animal studies. Reference to the FDA guidances, as well as ICH guidelines, should be consulted. While introduced here in the context of preclinical development, toxicology studies required for a typical small molecule drug candidate for market approval will continue well into phase 3, and cost upwards of $5 million.

There exists no fixed list of well-defined toxicology studies to be conducted for a given new investigational drug at specific stages of preclinical or clinical development. Rather, their timing and design depend significantly on the compound's chemical class, the intended indication and respective patient population, dosing regimen, previous relevant experience, and many other factors. Furthermore, the ethical and practical considerations of using animals as test subjects require that the testing be scientifically appropriate and necessary to establishing the safety of administering to humans the specific new drug under consideration. That stated, general expectations can be discussed.

Preliminary screening and range-finding toxicology studies are generally conducted during lead optimization, so as to provide data to help in the design of the definitive GLP toxicology studies. As with other modes of evaluation, these preliminary results will also assist in identifying the best lead compounds, prior to selection of the development candidate. Generally lasting from a few days to two weeks, these studies are valuable toward categorizing the observed toxicity, as either related to the compound's pharmacodynamics ("ON-target") or not related ("intrinsic" or "OFF-target"). Unlike ON-target toxicity, OFF-target toxicity can generally be minimized by structure-activity modification, for example, one that results in improved selectivity and/or potency.

The definitive toxicology studies will support initial dosing to humans, and are therefore required prior to filing the IND in the US. The following studies are typically required, however, for small molecules prior to the start of clinical trials, because they provide the basis for predicting and characterizing a drug's potential adverse effects in humans:

- Repeat dose toxicity (sub-acute and chronic);
- Genetic toxicology;
- Safety pharmacology.

Repeat dose toxicity studies provide a profile of activity and toxicity following the administration of a compound in at least two species, generally one rodent and one non-rodent. The route(s) of administration should include that route intended for the clinical formulation. There are two key dose targets: (1) the determination of a maximum tolerated dose (MTD), or that dose just high enough to elicit signs of minimal toxicity without significantly altering the animal's normal life span (due to effects other than

carcinogenicity); and (2) determination of a lower dose level at which no adverse effects are observed (NOAEL). At least three dose levels are tested, in order to distinguish the MTD and NOAEL doses, and to predict the shape of the dose–response curve. Of particular interest are dose dependency, extent, and duration of exposure. A control vehicle is also included. The duration of these studies should be at least equal to or greater than the duration of the proposed clinical study. For typical phase 1 studies lasting less than one week and no more than two, at least two weeks of preclinical testing is advised.

For orally delivered compounds whose solubility is poor, care must be taken to ensure that the animals attain good levels of systemic exposure, without which the determination of an MTD, and thus "safety," are at great risk of being dangerously overestimated when translated to dosing in humans. For such reasons as this, there should always be a safety factor built into translating animal toxicity to human dosing. Including a parenteral route of administration into early pharmacokinetic studies of an oral drug candidate will serve as a reference for assessing systemic exposure on oral administration.

Observations of all animals in these studies are made for up to two or more weeks post-dosing, including physical effects such as appearance, behavior, cognitive and ambulatory skills, growth, and appetite; vital signs, blood and urine chemistry; gross pathology, and microscopic examination of various tissues. Assaying compound plasma levels offers systemic exposure information, including C_{max}, half life, and exposure (AUC). Effects of the test substance on vital functions, including the cardiovascular, respiratory, and central nervous systems, are also monitored. Given the comprehensive and complex nature of the data collected, and of its reporting, it is not unusual for a one-month in-life study to require six elapsed months from start to completion of the report.

Toxicokinetic information is also important to collect in the toxicology studies. The primary objective of collecting plasma level data achieved in animals is to understand the time course of compound absorption, distribution, metabolism and excretion, and their relationships to dose level. Secondary objectives include relating compound exposure achieved in toxicity studies to the toxicological findings, and evaluating their relevance to clinical safety. These data also support species selection, dosing regimen, and protocol design in later long-term non-clinical studies.

In vitro genotoxicity and mutagenicity studies are often conducted during a preliminary stage, as a means of screening compounds prior to selection of the development candidate. Mutagenicity testing is required prior to phase 1, including the *in vitro* Ames and chromosomal aberration tests, and an *in vivo* micronucleus assay.

Also required prior to phase 1 clinical trials are safety pharmacology studies, which include an assessment of the effects on the CNS and respiratory systems (rodent), and cardiovascular system (nonrodent). These are single dose studies, and should be conducted to GLP standards.

Given the successive nature of the studies discussed to this point, as well as those which continue during clinical testing, the toxicology program to support the new drug application for a small molecule will typically require an elapsed time of about five years. It is particularly important for the planning phase to include sufficient preliminary dosing tests, e.g., dose–range finding etc., so that effective dose selection is made. Only then can longer-term studies proceed uninterrupted, and the number of animals required to serve the development program be minimized.

Recalling Figure 36.3, data available in 1991 led to the conclusion that the overwhelming basis for halting the development of NMEs during clinical evaluation was their poor pharmacokinetic profiles. There were several reasons for this. First, PK behavior has always been difficult to predict from *in vitro* studies. Secondly, combinatorial chemistry had become a predominant means of producing huge libraries of compounds by that time, and the new HTS assays by which "best leads" were identified relied largely on "ligand" properties, reflecting specific interaction with a relevant molecular or cellular target. Ligand binding can also be nonspecific, however, in which case it is strengthened as ligand hydrophobicity increases. Strategic reaction to this apparent *in vitro* "high potency" could then drive lead optimization toward higher molecular weights that accommodate this effect, while retaining the functional groups that control specificity. Such compounds notoriously exhibit poor bioavailability and significant metabolism.

By 2000 this unproductive strategy was exposed and more effectively avoided, knowledge of the role of transporters had developed, and mechanisms of metabolism had become more predictable using new *in vitro* evaluation methods. Thus, the predominant nemesis for early prediction of compound success moved to the area of toxicology. At this writing it remains a challenge to predict reliably a compound's toxicology in humans from the molecular structure or from that observed in animals. Combining the general population's inflated expectations for "total safety" with the cost of development and the increasing economic pressures on the industry, anything marginal about the toxicology profile of a new compound has become a major cause for its cancellation.

CMC Activities in Preclinical Development

While the key purpose of preclinical development studies is biological in nature, they cannot proceed without closely coordinated CMC development and support. It should be noted that the FDA encourages the "quality by design" (QbD) approach to development of the commercial product, which by definition begins in the preclinical stage. The IND will become the first formal opportunity for the CMC scientist to offer early evidence of successful implementation of QbD.

The key CMC activities which are needed for preclinical development to initiate a cycle of pharmaceutical development of the drug substance and drug product that is repeated at increasing levels of scale and refinement appropriate to each stage of development through to commercial manufacture, in roughly sequential order, include:
Drug substance (API):

- Develop a synthetic process;
- Manufacture;
- Characterize;
- Develop analytical methods;
- Set specifications;
- Release test;
- Test stability.

Drug product:

- Conduct excipient compatibility testing with drug substance;
- Develop suitable formulation(s) and characterize;
- Develop analytical methods;
- Develop manufacturing process;
- Manufacture and package;
- Set specifications;
- Release test;
- Test stability.

Control of product:

- Obtain or formulate;
- Obtain or develop analytical methods;
- Develop manufacturing process, as needed;
- Manufacture and package, as needed;
- Characterize;
- Set specifications;
- Release test;
- Test stability.

The drug substance (API) cycle will be conducted for the development candidate, and will mature in synthetic process refinement and scale, level of technical understanding and control during progression to product launch. All or most of the activities listed for the drug product cycle, however, and as needed, the control cycle, will be conducted for the development candidate many times, at every dose level of every test formulation prepared for animal studies, and of every clinical formulation tested in humans.

As stated earlier, back-up compounds may also be brought along with a lead compound for early preclinical evaluation. Desirably, the development candidate will emerge from the set of compounds early on, based on preliminary testing *in vitro* and *in vivo*. Until this occurs, however, all three cycles listed above may be initiated to some degree for each of the compounds, and geared in part to distinguishing their relative merits.

It is worth noting here that it is common, and generally reasonable, for the properties important to drug delivery to be given secondary importance in the development team's consideration of choosing the development candidate. The formulation scientist has many potential tools for dealing with undesirable properties, primarily involving manipulation of the drug substance itself or of its formulation. In contrast, the pharmacologist, toxicologist, and clinician are unable to manipulate the biology with which the drug interacts, and must weigh heavily the behavior of the compound that reflects its potential safety and efficacy in patients when supporting its candidacy for development.

Effective and efficient CMC development at the preclinical stage requires focusing on that which supports the studies at hand, and not more, until such time as the development candidate has successfully jumped the key hurdles of early toxicology testing, and is proceeding toward clinical studies in humans. For example, drug substance purity need not exceed 95–98% unless a potentially disproportionate toxicity is associated with a particular impurity. Preliminary analytical methods need not undergo full validation; rather they must be shown to assay drug content with sufficient accuracy, distinguish from and quantify major impurities in the drug substance, and be capable of detecting major degradants that appear over the time course of the intended preclinical studies.

With analytical methods in hand, laboratory characterization of the development candidate's solubility, partitioning behavior, and stability is conducted in order to confirm (or correct) earlier *in silico* predictions of *in vitro* performance. If the physico-chemical properties of the development candidate are deemed marginal for effective oral delivery, consideration should be given to modifying the compound in some way so as to improve its physico-chemical properties.

For a compound whose solubility is poor, modification could include salt preparation (if ionizable), prodrug formation, complexation or micronization.

Note that the judgment of "good solubility" is dose-dependent. The definition of good solubility given in the Biopharmaceutical Classification System[1] requires that the highest dose in humans will dissolve in 250 mL water at 37°C, and adjusted to physiological pH.

For a compound whose solid-state stability exhibits a tendency for polymorphic conversion, solvate formation or deliquescence, modification may require the discovery of an alternate crystal form of greater stability (at the risk of reducing solubility). Note here that the significant presence of impurities, common for early-stage drug substance lots, can lead to unstable behavior not otherwise intrinsic to the pure compound, and should be ruled out as a destabilizing factor prior to seeking a new solid-state form.

The new form of the compound, whether modified chemically or physically, can then be designated the "development candidate" going forward. Depending on the modification, it may be possible to develop an acceptable rationale for avoiding the repetition of preclinical studies already completed.

Formulations for administering the development candidate to animals for toxicology studies can be simple in both composition and method of preparation if solubility, stability, and dose levels allow. For the development of an oral product, oral dosing must be the primary route of administration during toxicity testing. A wide dose range will likely be needed, in order to achieve the determination of the MTD, often spanning 3–5 orders of magnitude. It may be effective to administer powdered compound for acute dosing or admix the compound into feed for longer-term dosing, if the compound remains stable and good exposure can be demonstrated. If not, oral dosing of a solution or dispersion could prove more effective, provided the stability of the preparation can be ensured throughout the dosing period.

It is useful to administer compound via intravenous injection to an additional cohort of animals, so as to provide a reference for "100% bioavailability." For poorly soluble compounds, it may be necessary to add co-solvents, complexing agents, surfactants, and/or other excipients, to achieve high doses in solution for injection. The toxicity of these excipients must be considered in such cases, and may depend on the type of injection, e.g., intravenous versus subcutaneous, versus intramuscular. The review by Strickley[2] details many approaches to formulating poorly soluble drugs for commercial product, a number of which could be useful in preparing toxicology products. It is customary to incorporate negative (vehicle) controls into the toxicology studies, especially when excipients are known to contribute some measure of toxicity.

Preliminary animal studies afford an opportunity to test formulation(s) on a small scale, to ensure suitable performance for larger-scale GLP studies. Preliminary specifications are set for both the development candidate (API), as well as the formulations, based on knowledge gained up to that point in preclinical development. Analytical controls must confirm consistency of API quality, taking special note of any changes observed in impurity profiles. Lot-to-lot comparisons of API are critical at this stage, where synthetic process and scale changes are generally unavoidable. Likewise, analytical comparisons of different formulation lots should confirm lot-to-lot homogeneity and stability from preparation through dosing, so that the target toxicity determinations in animals can be relied upon for proceeding with reasonable safety into human clinical trials.

The development candidate, as well as each of its formulations, must be tested for their respective stability under conditions of storage from manufacture to use in the toxicology laboratory. This is especially important if the toxicology laboratory is located at a distant site, requiring shipping. These studies will initiate the formal collection of API and product stability testing that will be drawn upon for insight and understanding throughout product development.

Recalling Figure 36.2, a generally understated goal of effective development is to discard a compound as soon as it exhibits a profile that shows little promise of meeting those traits required to satisfy the target product profile, even though it represents a "moving target." In this way, resources can be redirected toward a more promising candidate, minimizing the expenditure of unproductive development effort and costs.

As preclinical development proceeds, and suitable toxicology information becomes available, development of the first-in-human (FIH) clinical product can begin. Importantly, the goal of phase 1 is to evaluate the safety of the drug in humans, not to test for efficacy. As the CMC activity cycle for FIH drug product gets underway, a key consideration will therefore be the starting dose. The highest NOAEL determined in the toxicology studies provides a guide regarding the starting clinical dose by converting the NOAEL to the "human equivalent dose" or HED using established algorithms,[3] and adding a safety factor. A typical safety factor of 10 is used to reduce the HED, unless there are reasons to reduce it further because of some concern with predicted human PK, bioavailability, rate of absorption, metabolites, and clearance or with the disease state and the degree to which it is life-threatening. It is also possible that a smaller safety factor would be used to raise the calculated dose, based on previous experience.

As with toxicology formulation, it is desirable to keep the clinical formulation and process for its preparation as simple as possible, while achieving effective delivery. If the compound's PK properties allow, powder in a bottle or capsule administered with water is acceptable and straightforward to prepare. If the compound is likely to exhibit limited bioavailability at the higher dose(s) to be administered during the trial, a more complex formulation (as discussed in earlier chapters in Parts II and III) may be needed, and should then be used for all doses if vehicle effects are to be minimized. Note that any differences between the formulation used to assess toxicity in animals, and the formulation intended for first human dosing, will be questioned in terms of how they might affect the interpretation of the safety data in proceeding to the clinic. Any issue threatening the relevance of the toxicology studies to entry into the clinic will be a key topic for discussion with the FDA in the pre-IND setting.

Analytical methods will require revising and validation to support phase 1 clinical supplies preparation, given any differences in dose and excipient composition. Particularly critical is the comparison of API-derived or other drug-related impurity profiles between API and formulations used in toxicology, and those observed in the API and formulations prepared for FIH studies. Methods can be refined and validated in advance of preparing the actual clinical batches. Preliminary specifications, based on characterizing experimental formulation(s), are set for both drug substance and clinical product to provide a defined target of performance. Experimental batches are also subjected to stability testing, to demonstrate that the clinical batches will remain stable during the course of the clinical trial. While the FDA requires stability testing only over a period represented by the time from manufacture through the expected clinical trial period, it is common to extend testing to 1–3 months, especially if the formulation is likely to be used in later clinical trials.

Manufacture, packaging and labeling of the actual phase 1 clinical supplies may be scheduled so as to be released by quality control in time for shipping to the clinical site during the 30-day IND review period. The level of risk inherent in this strategy is gauged by the results of the pre-IND meeting with the FDA and the likelihood of a clinical hold, the stability of the clinical product, and the readiness of the clinical investigator to proceed immediately with patient dosing.

cGMP regulations should be followed to the degree possible and reasonable during the preparation, documentation, manufacture, and control of clinical product at this stage. The scale of manufacture will be determined by the sum of clinical protocol needs (dose levels, number of patients, etc.), and product needed for release testing, stability testing, retained samples, and that which accounts for waste. It is quite possible that for a small trial the amount of clinical product provided to the clinic is only a small proportion of the batch manufactured.

The importance of good communication and teamwork will be evident during the preclinical development stage, as it leads to the IND milestone and the start of human dosing. With good planning, organization, and execution it should be possible to prevent CMC activities from becoming a part of the critical path to clinical research and development.

The Pre-IND Meeting and IND Filing

The pre-IND meeting with the FDA is a key opportunity to review with the agency the TPP, the preclinical pharmacology, and toxicology program results, and the rationale for the early clinical program, and supportive pivotal toxicology that will run in parallel with it. Primary consideration will always be given to those aspects of the program that affect the safety of those who will be dosed with the new drug substance, including specifications and their rationale, potential safety issues associated with the formulation and its manufacturing process, and analytical data that support product quality, particularly as it concerns identity, strength, and purity. Contract facilities associated with the development program may be discussed. With regard to scheduling this meeting, it is better to meet too early than too late. Any guidance offered by the regulatory agency will clarify the development plan going forward, and ensure that the toxicology program is acceptable for supporting FIH dosing with reasonable safety for the intended indication(s).

An institutional review board (IRB) will also be asked to review the clinical program. This small group, comprised of both expert and lay people educated to the task at hand and monitored by the FDA, will review clinical protocols during the course of clinical development with the specific goal of ensuring that the safety, rights, and welfare of clinical subjects will be protected throughout the development program.

The nature of the IND filing process, and the required contents of the document, are given in the FDAs Guidance for Industry.[4] Briefly, comprehensive reports supporting all pre-IND meeting topics are included. Protocols for ongoing toxicology and intended clinical studies are presented for review. CMC information will include the composition of toxicology formulations, as well as the intended FIH drug product composition, with discussion around any differences between them that could influence the

consideration of safety in the clinic. Drug substance and drug product manufacturing processes, specifications, analytical controls, and stability are to be reported to confirm the integrity of preclinical testing completed, and ensure continued quality going forward into the clinic. Since safety is paramount, the CMC section should clearly define all product excipients, and convey a clear understanding and control of impurities and degradation products in API and drug product, for both toxicology and clinical use. The absence of such information would be the main reason for the agency to place a clinical hold on the program based on CMC.

Upon filing, the FDA Center for Drug Evaluation and Review (CDER) has 30 days to decide if there is any potential unacceptable risk to clinical study subjects (per the CMC example given above) by proceeding as planned. If the applicant receives no response from the FDA within that time frame, clinical studies may begin.

36.4 CLINICAL RESEARCH

The three phases of clinical research and development denote the rational progression of studies whose goal it is to identify an effective new drug to treat a particular disease or impairment, with absolutely minimal compromise in the safety of those people exposed to it in the process. The yin and yang of the drug development process is the struggle to move a potential life-saving new drug through development as fast as possible, without risking unnecessarily the health of volunteers and patients during the evaluation of its potential toxicities.

The clinical stages combined represent the longest portion of development, usually requiring a minimum of five years for a new molecular entity, up to 8–10 years or more for some drugs whose indications are associated with poorly quantitated or indirect clinical end points. The costs associated with development accelerate during clinical research, peaking in phase 3 in which multiple trials are conducted involving thousands of patients. In addition to these large-scale phase 3 studies, human pharmacokinetics and bioavailability studies are performed in relevant populations. Concurrently, longer-term toxicology studies in animals are conducted. With the successful conclusion and write-up of all of these multi-year studies, the New Drug Application (NDA) is submitted, in hopeful anticipation of approval and market launch within 1–2 years. However, clinical trial obligations are generally not over. It has now become routine for the FDA to require the sponsor to commit to post-approval phase 4 trial activity, during which long-term safety of the drug continues to be proactively assessed and reported back to the agency.

As clinical trials have moved to the global stage in recent years, an important observation has arisen: different cultures frequently react differently to the same pathology, and to the same drugs that are used to treat them. Clearly this, and other cross-culture healthcare anomalies, requires careful study when establishing clinical programs which depend on international collaboration.

None of the above clinical development can occur, of course, without the tailored support of CMC in every phase and facet of test product design, manufacture, and quality control. Throughout the clinical program, effective and efficient development overall will continue to depend on clear and rapid communication, and forward planning between clinical management and the CMC team, which will bridge R&D with production and quality during this phase of development.

36.4.1 Phase 1

Clinical Development

Despite the valuable insight into drug action and toxicity provided by pre- and non-clinical animal testing, humans remain the ultimate test subject. A major milestone in development, the start of phase 1 trials, enables the first exposure of an investigational new drug to a small number of human subjects, usually fewer than 100, for the primary purpose of determining the highest dose that can be administered without compromising safety. Healthy human volunteers are generally recruited for these studies, except for new oncology drugs, and for most biologics.

Specific goals of phase 1 include the evaluation of drug pharmacokinetics and pharmacodynamics, drug metabolism and mechanism of action, and gaining information about dose-related side-effects in humans. Typical study designs are single dose and/or rising dose tolerance, and short-term repeated dose studies. Results from these studies are necessary to the effective design of well-controlled and scientifically valid phase 2 studies.

The reader may wish to consult the FDA website (www.fda.gov) to learn about the opportunities for conducting FIH studies outside the guidance of the standard IND requirements via the exploratory IND application.

Toxicology

Toxicology studies conducted during phase 1 are primarily directed toward the anticipated dose regimen, for example, acute versus chronic administration. Chronic dose studies to support longer dosing periods in phase 2 and 3 may be performed in rodents over 3–6 months, and in non-rodent species for 6–9 months.

Reproduction toxicity studies will be required for those compounds which could be administered to women of childbearing age per label claim. Typically lengthy and complex in design, recommended study protocols are available for testing several species of animals, and can be found in the general and regulatory literature.

CMC Activities in Phase 1

By the time the 30-day IND review period has expired, ideally the CMC team has shipped the phase 1 clinical supplies to the test center. Packaging and labeling are straightforward in these initial studies. Following the study, the remaining supplies can be disposed of, except for a retained sample sufficient to be release tested should any question of its quality arise after the study has concluded.

As the IND filing approaches, chemical process development has been working to improve the efficiency (yield, purity, time, etc.) of the synthetic process for the API, in accordance with phase 1 GMP expectations, during the course of satisfying growing preclinical toxicology supply needs. Analytical comparison of different lots from different synthetic processes should help to identify a predictable impurity profile and its likely sources, whether drug-related or not. By phase 2, the API should be approaching a quality acceptable for marketed product, at least in qualitative impurity profile, if not quantitative. As the API process changes, specifications and analytical methods used to release and test the stability of the drug will also be updated, and revalidated.

The supply of ongoing and new toxicology studies continues, competing for API supply. While not required, toxicology supplies can be manufactured under GMP conditions, if it is more practical to do so. If there is a choice between API lots of different purity levels for toxicology, it is preferable to use the less pure material, assuming it remains qualitatively similar and within stated specifications.

Formulation development will have already begun to consider clinical drug product options for phase 2a, taking into account that the likely dose range needed for phase 2b will not be known until the conclusion of phase 2a. In keeping with the evolving TPP, and the increasing knowledge gained from pharmaceutical characterization of multiple API lots and test formulations, however, much can be defined about the QbD design space, including room for the dose range to shift up or down.

Recall that the probability of advancing the new development candidate successfully from phase 1 to market is low, therefore the commitment of resources to large formulation studies on behalf of phase 2b is risky. However, efficient excipient compatibility experiments and/or test formulation comparisons, perhaps conducted using design of experiments (DOE), would likely save considerable time during the transition to phase 2b clinical product, by which time marketing considerations may have defined the preferred oral dosage form. In any case, it is not too soon to establish a cumulative track record of test formulations prepared to date, along with their impurity profiles, API and excipient lots, purpose (experimental, toxicology or clinical), and all other pertinent preparation and performance data regarding their history. Easy reference to such a record can prove most useful toward solving the mystery of a test product's failure to meet specifications down the road.

By the time phase 1 success appears likely, the development team will have decided on the preferred dosage form, e.g., tablet or capsule, assuming the drug properties are suitable for either. The phase 2 clinical protocol and supply needs are communicated to the CMC team, and formulation development for phase 2a dosing can begin in earnest. High and low dosage strengths can be formulated and manufactured at small-scale, under varying conditions of compression, and tested to ensure that good dissolution performance, and good stability, have been achieved. If practical, administering multiple dosage units to achieve high dose levels will minimize the number of clinical products required to satisfy dose escalation. Preliminary specifications are drawn for the dosage levels requested, and confirmed once sufficient reproducibility in the quality of multiple experimental lots is attained. With good clinical development planning, and good communication of that plan at least two months in advance, the GMP manufacture and delivery of released clinical supplies to the phase 2a clinical site will occur in a timely manner.

36.4.2 Phase 2

Clinical Development

The first evaluation of efficacy is generally conducted in closely monitored phase 2 trials, involving about 100–300 patients. Often split into two stages, phase 2a trials seek evidence of short-term safety and confirmation of a therapeutic dose range. Note that the maximum tolerated dose in healthy volunteers may differ from that in patients. Clearly the development candidate is in jeopardy if there is no evidence

of efficacy at dose levels approaching the maximum tolerance. Given promising efficacy, however, somewhat larger and longer (if appropriate) studies will be conducted in phase 2b, confirming an effective dose level and regimen, and characterizing efficacy in terms of magnitude and duration of effect. Short-term side-effects and potential risks are also evaluated.

Lasting approximately 1–2 years from start of dosing to final report, phase 2 is critical to justifying the initiation of the enormous commitment of patients and resources to phase 3 studies. For this reason, it is highly desirable for the clinical supplies used in the phase 2b trials, and effectively mandatory for those used in phase 3, to be considered equivalent in process and product to the drug product intended for the market.

One of the major milestones of the overall development program is that of meeting with the FDA at the end of phase 2, to determine whether or not it is safe to begin phase 3. It provides an opportunity to review with the FDA key development progress to date, as well as the sponsor's intended phase 3 plans and objectives. The agency views this meeting as establishing a firm agreement with the sponsor regarding the phase 3 development plan.

Toxicology

Ongoing long-term toxicology studies continue. Carcinogenicity studies in rodents are generally required for any compound whose use in the clinic is expected to lead to long-term exposure from chronic administration of at least six months or accumulated exposure from intermittent use. Lasting two or more years, these studies will run in parallel to clinical testing.

By this stage of development, information will have become available regarding primary impurities and products of chemical degradation in the API and/or drug product, and metabolites. Consideration must be given to the need to test the toxicity of these compounds, prior to entering phase 3 trials involving large numbers of patients.

CMC Activities in Phase 2

The CMC team will continue to supply the toxicology laboratory on behalf of ongoing studies.

The turnaround time for manufacturing phase 2b clinical supplies may be short if the target dose(s) cannot be confirmed until phase 2a concludes. The CMC team can manufacture at risk with the consent of the development team, and at least use the batch as a "dress rehearsal" for GMP manufacture of the clinical batch most closely representative of the final drug product to that point. A 2-year stability testing program is recommended for the phase 2b supplies, as a preview for the stability of the marketed product.

The commercial process and facility for synthesis of the API should be established and used at some significant fraction of the commercial scale during the production of drug substance used in phase 3 clinical supplies. Analytical methods for quality control and specifications for significant synthetic precursors and the API product should be finalized. Effective technology transfer from R&D to production/quality should be completed. Aside from the technical challenges of completing an effective technology transfer, there are also "social" hurdles. R&D scientists and engineers are inclined and trained to design and execute staged improvements—that is, purposeful changes—in process and product at increasing scale with efficiency and effectiveness; by contrast most production and quality personnel are trained and dedicated to the challenge of maintaining a constant, consistent level of high quality of process and product at commercial scale under market pressure. Effective technology transfer will be sensitive to the necessarily different mindsets and approaches these professionals must have on both sides of the transfer. Ideally, the transfer is rich with CMC teams comprised of both types of professionals.

During phase 2, development of the phase 3 clinical supplies, including packaging, a placebo, and a likely positive comparator, must be completed. Used in the pivotal trials, which form the mainstay of support for its approval as a new drug, phase 3 clinical product should be demonstrably equivalent to the final drug product. The primary packaging (except for blinding) intended for the marketed product should also be used, and incorporated into the long-term stability testing of the supplies.

The commercial manufacturing process should be in place for manufacture of the phase 3 supplies. Given the large size and lengthy nature of these trials, multiple production lots will be needed. It is common for their GMP manufacture to occur in a pilot or production setting, in cooperation with the production/quality operations, calling for technology transfer well in advance.

Securing and blinding the comparator product may require the cooperation of a competitor corporation, taking significant lead-time to arrange. If necessary, the product can be purchased and the clinical study protocol revised to account for the unblinded control using a "double dummy" design.

As with the previous staged cycles of CMC development, any changes in API processing or clinical product manufacture will require careful evaluation of any changes in quality, and any possible revisions and

revalidation of the analytical methods used for quality control. The supply chains for API, drug product, and packaging, and their respective material vendors must be qualified and committed well in advance to phase 3 and commercial product support.

36.4.3 Phase 3

Clinical Development

Phase 3 trials may vary in design, but nearly all are large and usually multi-center in nature. Except for certain patient populations that are inherently small in number, thousands of patients will participate in various studies during the course of three or more years. These large trials are intended to gather, with statistical confidence, additional evidence of efficacy for specific indications, demonstrate short- and long-term safety on a larger scale, and to help the sponsor understand any drug-related adverse effects. In short, these trials fill in and confirm the clinical information that defines the final product label claims—the relatively short document which summarizes the results of 10–14 years of research and development.

The key pivotal trials must be adequate and well-controlled, meaning they must be randomized, double-blind, placebo-controlled trials, in order to eliminate patient or physician bias. Demonstration of efficacy, as compared to placebo, is a minimal requirement. Today, more often than not, however, demonstration of superior efficacy and benefit-to-risk ratio when compared to a positive comparator product, if available, must instead be demonstrated—clearly a much higher hurdle. Other specialized trials may be conducted in order to test efficacy in other specific indications, or to support additional label claims, e.g., the treatment of pediatric patients.

Substantial time is required to reduce the enormous clinical database collected in phase 3 to a concise argument for safety and efficacy of the new drug in the New Drug Application (NDA) and/or Common Technical Document (CTD). Improvements in electronic documentation of patient data and application filing have made this process more manageable.

Toxicology

Ongoing toxicology studies are likewise finalized and written up in preparation for the NDA and/or CTD.

CMC Activities in Phase 3

Production continues to manufacture and package multiple lots of API and clinical product as needed for phase 3, and as described under "CMC activities in phase 2" above. Their long-term stability profiles will preview and confirm an appropriate shelf life for commercial product, generally targeted at five years. Two years is considered to be a shortest acceptable shelf life, recognizing that the time required for production batch release, inventorying, shipping, and distribution via one or more points of sale all subtract time from the viable shelf life seen by the patient.

The production facilities for API and drug product will be readied for a product-specific preapproval inspection, given that the drug candidate is a new molecular entity.

The strategic and technical history of the CMC aspects of the development program, from R&D through to production/quality, is drafted for inclusion as the CMC section of the NDA and/or CTD, according to the respective guidelines accessible online. For electronic filing of the ICH-based CTD, for example, the FDA provides specific guidelines at www.fda.gov/cder/Regulatory/ersr/ectd.htm

36.4.4 Pre-new Drug Application (NDA) Meeting and the New Drug Application

The pre-NDA meeting is called to establish the presentation of data which will support the application. Discussion will include a summary of all clinical studies to be included in the NDA, and the organization and means of presenting the clinical and all other information. This is also the opportunity to discuss and resolve any problems or issues as needed, and to identify clearly the key studies the sponsor is relying on to establish the safety and effectiveness of the new drug.

The components of the NDA are consistent, but will vary from drug to drug in the quantity of information and data needed to support registration. While a new molecular entity may promise the greatest gain in therapy, it must jump the highest hurdles in establishing its benefit-to-risk profile. When the FDA Center for Drug Evaluation and Review (CDER) receives an NDA, they will screen the document for completeness prior to "filing" it. If acceptable, their review begins, prompting likely communication with the sponsor to clarify issues during the review process. At the conclusion of the CDERs review, an action letter will be sent to the sponsor signifying that the application is "Not Approvable," "Approvable," or desirably, "Approved." When nearing approval, the draft labeling for the drug will be negotiated between the sponsor and the agency, and agreed upon prior to formal approval. If not approved, the agency will meet with the sponsor to discuss the deficiencies of their application, which may or may not result ultimately in a successful approval.

In all likelihood the clinical team will discuss the phase 4 post-marketing surveillance requests of the agency. This obligation is given to the sponsor, often as a basis for approval of the NDA, in order to follow up on less common side-effects, pharmacoeconomics, expanded label studies, etc.

For the CMC team, formal process validation or its equivalent, if a QbD development approach has been taken, can be planned and executed as the NDA/CTD documents are readied for submission. Planning for the production of market launch supplies will ensure that appropriate capacity and lead time will be available as NDA approval is gauged to be forthcoming.

36.5 CONCLUDING REMARKS

The business consequences of failure at the point of NDA submission can be internally and publicly devastating to the sponsor. An unfortunate historical reality is that a significant proportion of phase 3 trials across submissions proves insufficient to support product registration. Depending on the overall deficiencies, the sponsor may choose to repeat one or more costly studies, if it is judged likely to bring the submission up to approvable standards. Among the causes for failure in phase 3 is insufficient statistical power in a pivotal trial to support a key claim regarding efficacy, especially as it compares to an established therapeutic on the market. Another notable cause involves the selection of an inappropriate dose, such that dose adjustments must be made. At the least a bridging study between the current and newly proposed dose(s), but more likely a full repeat of the phase 3 trial at the new dose, is required to validate the change as appropriate, safe, and effective. Meanwhile, significant value in the cancelled trial is lost; significant resources have been wasted; significant time in the market is lost; and significant monetary investment and corporate energy are lost when pivotal trials must be repeated. These failures all contribute to the contemporary estimate of $1.2 billion to bring one new drug successfully to market.

There are many analyses in the pharmaceutical business literature as to why drug development programs fail.[5] A credit to CMC of sorts, formulation, process development, and large-scale manufacture are not high on this list. Again, the intrinsic biological properties and performance of a drug cannot be actively controlled; by contrast, CMC scientists are very simply expected to find solutions to the inevitable development problems they will encounter.

The encouraging story of contemporary drug development is that substantial changes in CMC science and technology are in play, and enable the CMC development team to meet such high expectations. Given sufficient scientific justification, product and process adjustments can, in principle, be implemented with confidence during development, and even during production of the marketed product. This is not so much the result of industry's effective application of QbD per se, rather, it is the change in the regulatory agency's perspective, which now encourages and accepts the implications of QbD-worthy development. Their otherwise categorical requirements for bridging studies and time-consuming regulatory submissions and review will hopefully fade into history. The earned opportunity for continuous improvement relieves not only industry, but also reduces the FDAs workload, as the responsibility for high quality is built more reliably into the sponsor's development process. To quote the great Charles Darwin, "It is not the strongest of the species that survives, nor the most intelligent, but the one most responsive to change."

These changes are all a part of the broader movement underway across North America, Europe, and Japan to coalesce these countries' most effective approaches to regulation into a harmonized set of requirements. The rising tide of China and India's innovation and technological capabilities will add much to the growing international pharmaceutical presence and collaboration.

References

1. Guidance for Industry. (2000). Waiver of In Vivo Bioavailability and Bioequivalence Studies for Immediate-Release Solid Oral Dosage Forms Based on a Biopharmaceutics Classification System. US Department of Health and Human Services, Food and Drug Administration, Center for Drug Evaluation and Research (CDER), August.
2. Strickley, R.G. (2004). Review: Solubilizing excipients in oral and injectable formulations. Pharmaceutical Research 21(2). February.
3. Guidance for Industry. (2005). Estimating the Maximum Safe Starting Dose in Initial Clinical Trials for Therapeutics in Adult Healthy Volunteers. US Department of Health and Human Services, Food and Drug Administration, Center for Drug Evaluation and Research (CDER), July.
4. Guidance for Industry. (1995). Content and Format of Investigational New Drug Applications (INDs) for Phase 1 Studies of Drugs, including Well-Characterized, Therapeutic, Biotechnology-derived Products. CDER and CBER, November.
5. Bains, W. (2004). Failure rates in drug discovery and development: Will we ever get any better? Drug Discovery World, Fall.

Product Registration and Drug Approval Process in the United States

Steven F. Hoff and Yisheng Chen

37.1 BACKGROUND FOR PRODUCT REGISTRATION IN THE UNITED STATES

All new drug products must be registered and approved by the regulatory agency governing the intended market before the products can be introduced into the market. The registration process is to ensure the quality, safety, and efficacy of drug products. The requirements for the development and registration of new drug products in the United States are defined in the Federal Food, Drug, and Cosmetic Act (FD&C Act)[1] and the regulations promulgated by the Food and Drug Administration (FDA) (Figure 37.1). The FDA is an agency of the Department of Health and Human Services within the United States government.

This chapter presents an overview of the process of regulatory review and approval in two parts of (1) New Drug Applications (NDA), and (2) Abbreviated New Drug Applications (ANDA) in the United States, using the various laws enacted by Congress, the FDA regulations found in Chapter 21 of the Code of Federal Regulations (21CFR) and guidance documents issued by the FDA. References will be provided to the Internet websites for many of these documents for the reader's information.

37.2 THE NEW DRUG APPLICATION (NDA) AND REVIEW PROCESS

The FDA has a complex organization for review and approval of new drug applications (NDAs) and abbreviated new drug applications (ANDAs). When NDAs and ANDAs are submitted to the FDA, the review and approval of the applications are conducted by the Center for Drug Evaluation and Research (CDER), which reports directly to the Office of the Commissioner of the FDA, as shown in Figure 37.1. Within CDER there are a number of offices organized under the Office of the Center Director as shown in Figure 37.2. For the purposes of drug development, the majority of the industry interactions with the FDA will be with the Office of New Drugs.

During the new drug review process, the Office of Pharmaceutical Sciences is involved in the review of the Chemistry, Manufacturing and Controls (CMC) information. After approval, the Office of Surveillance and Epidemiology and the Office of Medical Policy, Division of Drug Marketing, Advertising and Communication (DDMAC) become closely involved with the post-marketing activities of new drugs.

37.2.1 Food and Drug Administration (FDA) Interactions

Generally, a sponsor (applicant, person or entity who assumes the responsibility for the marketing of a new drug, including the responsibility for compliance with the FD&C Act, and other related regulations—a sponsor can be an individual, partnership, company, government agency or institution) will have been interacting with the FDA during the new drug development process through submissions and meetings with the reviewing division. Approximately six to

Developing Solid Oral Dosage Forms: Pharmaceutical Theory and Practice
ISBN: 978-0-444-53242-8

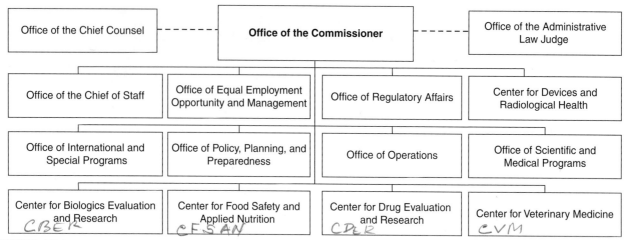

FIGURE 37.1 Food and Drug Administration organization. Source of information: http://www.fda.gov/oc/orgcharts/FDA.pdf, as of March 12, 2008

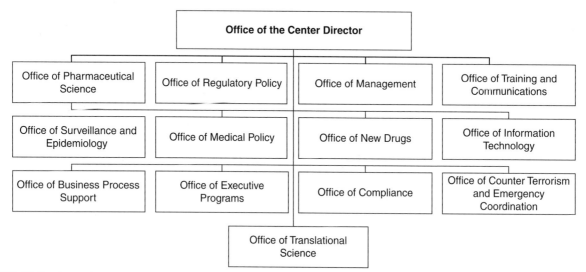

FIGURE 37.2 Center for Drug Evaluation and Research, FDA. Source of Information: http://www.fda.gov/oc/orgcharts/cder1.pdf, as of March 12, 2008

nine months prior to submitting an NDA, a sponsor should have a pre-NDA meeting with the FDA. This meeting will be scheduled by the FDA within 60 days of receipt of the request for the meeting, as discussed in the FDA Guidance, Formal Meetings with Sponsors and Applicants for PDUFA Products.[2] The procedures and information package required for scheduling and conducting the meeting are described in the above guidance. This meeting can be used for a discussion of the format and content of the NDA, including the presentation of data, types of statistical tables, types of documents to be included, electronic submission requirements, and any other questions related to the submission of the NDA.

37.2.2 New Drug Applications (NDA)

Preparation of a New Drug Applications

An NDA brings together the drug development effort by a company for the registration of a new drug product for the US market. The NDA is comprised primarily of the chemistry manufacturing and controls (CMC), non-clinical studies, clinical studies, and the proposed labeling for the new drug product. Content, format, and organization for a NDA are listed in the FDAs Conformance Review Checklist for NDAs.[3] This checklist can be used to guide the preparation of a successful NDA.

The NDA can be filed in the form of a traditional NDA (Table 37.1) or formatted as a Common Technical

TABLE 37.1 New drug application (NDA) content and regulatory source documents for drugs and biologics

1. Index
2. Labeling (*check one*) ☐ Draft Labeling ☐ Final Printed Labeling
3. Summary (21 CFR 314.50 (c))
4. Chemistry section
   A. Chemistry, manufacturing, and controls information (e.g., 21 CFR 314.50(d)(1); 21 CFR 601.2)
   B. Samples (21 CFR 314.50 (e)(1); 21 CFR 601.2 (a)) (Submit only upon FDA's request)
   C. Methods validation package (e.g., 21 CFR 314.50(e)(2)(i); 21 CFR 601.2)
5. Nonclinical pharmacology and toxicology section (e.g., 21 CFR 314.50(d)(2); 21 CFR 601.2)
6. Human pharmacokinetics and bioavailability section (e.g., 21 CFR 314.50(d)(3); 21 CFR 601.2)
7. Clinical Microbiology (e.g., 21 CFR 314.50(d)(4))
8. Clinical data section (e.g., 21 CFR 314.50(d)(5); 21 CFR 601.2)
9. Safety update report (e.g., 21 CFR 314.50(d)(5)(vi)(b); 21 CFR 601.2)
10. Statistical section (e.g., 21 CFR 314.50(d)(6); 21 CFR 601.2)
11. Case report tabulations (e.g., 21 CFR 314.50(f)(1); 21 CFR 601.2)
12. Case report forms (e.g., 21 CFR 314.50 (f)(2); 21 CFR 601.2)
13. Patent information on any patent which claims the drug (21 U.S.C. 355(b) or (c))
14. A patent certification with respect to any patent which claims the drug (21 U.S.C. 355 (b)(2) or (j)(2)(A))
15. Establishment description (21 CFR Part 600, if applicable)
16. Debarment certification (FD&C Act 306 (k)(1))
17. Field copy certification (21 CFR 314.50 (l)(3))
18. User Fee Cover Sheet (Form FDA 3397)
19. Financial Information (21 CFR Part 54)
20. OTHER (*Specify*)

Source of information: FORM FDA 356h (10/05), page 2 of 4

Document (CTD) (Figure 37.3). A combination of the two formats has also been used, using the NDA format with documents written for the CTD. This procedure can be arranged with the FDAs reviewing division. NDAs may be submitted on paper or electronically, though electronic submission is highly recommended. Paper submissions are rapidly becoming obsolete at the FDA. FDA Guidance for electronic submissions is available on the FDA website.[4]

Format and content of a New Drug Application (NDA)

The format and content of a NDA are specified in the regulations (21 CFR 314.50).[5] The NDA starts with FDA Form 356h,[6] which provides a listing of the 20 sections expected in a NDA (Table 38-1). However, this is not an absolute order of the data presentation, though highly recommended. The sections may be presented in other arrangements, but must be clearly documented in the detailed index. The Form 356h is completed and signed by the sponsor or the sponsor's authorized US agent, who resides or maintains a business site in the United States.

Index

A detailed index of the NDA is an absolute necessity, as it provides a guide through the entire application for the FDA reviewers. The index must clearly describe the contents and location of each section by volume and page number.

Labeling

Draft or final copies of the labeling for the drug product must be included in the NDA. It is recommended that the draft labeling be provided in the NDA, as the FDA will often propose alternative wording to the submitted label. This usually occurs at the end of the FDAs NDA review cycle. Labeling is now required to be submitted electronically in all cases, using structured product labeling (SPL)[8,9] formatting, and in compliance with the Physician's Labeling Rule (PLR, which was being implemented in June 2006). SPL was implemented in October 2005, and is a standard electronic format that allows the FDA to process, review, and archive the labeling.

Summary

The NDA summary provides an overview of the NDA, describing the safety and efficacy of the drug product for its proposed use. Content of the summary is listed in Table 37.2. The summary is one of the most important sections of the NDA, because every FDA reviewer receives a copy of the summary, which can provide some assurance about the quality and accuracy of the information in the application. A poorly prepared summary may raise questions about the information in the application, and cause unnecessary delays in the review process.

Chemistry

The chemistry, manufacturing and controls (CMC) section provides detailed information on the composition, manufacture, test methods, and specifications of the drug substance (active ingredient), and the final drug product. The physical and chemical characteristics are presented, as well as the stability data. Samples and method validation package are also provided in

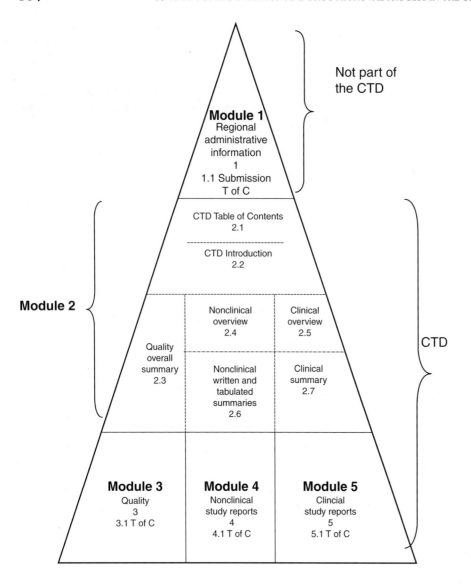

FIGURE 37.3 Graphic presentation of the common technical document. Source of information: http://www.fda.gov/cber/gdlns/m4ctd.pdf page 5[7]

the CMC section. The FDA and ICH have introduced many guidance documents regarding CMC information.[10,11] The required content of the CMC section (21 CFR 314.50(d)(1)) includes information on the drug substance, drug product, environmental impact, and the field copy certification.

The drug substance section contains information on the stability, physical and chemical characteristics of the drug substance, the name and address of the manufacturer, the method of manufacture and packaging, and the specifications, and analytical methods, for the drug substance. The drug product section provides information about the components, composition, pharmaceutical development specifications, and analytical methods of the inactive ingredients, name and address of the manufacturer(s), methods of manufacturing and packaging, specifications and analytical methods for the drug product, and stability information.

TABLE 37.2 Required content of an NDA summary (21CFR314.50(c))

- Proposed labeling with annotation to support information in the summary and technical sections of the NDA
- Pharmacological class of the drug
  - Scientific rationale for the drug
  - Intended use
  - Potential clinical benefit
- Market history (if any)
- CMC section summary
- Nonclinical pharmacology/toxicology section summary
- Human pharmacokinetics and bioavailability section summary
- Microbiology section summary (for anti-infectives only)
- Clinical data section summary
- Discussion of the risk-benefit considerations of the drug

The environmental impact analysis is required by the FDA or a claim for categorical exclusion. In 1997 the FDA issued a final regulation that stated environmental impact analysis would be required only under extraordinary circumstances.[12] Most applications are granted the categorical exclusion (i.e., exemption). A field copy certification is submitted only by US sponsors of a NDA. The applicant must certify that a field copy of the chemistry section has been provided to the sponsor's home district office.

The second part of the chemistry section is for samples. However, samples of the drug substance or drug product should not be submitted with the original NDA, but only provided upon an FDA request for these samples.

The final part of the chemistry section contains the methods validation package, which provides the FDA with all of the necessary information needed to validate all of the analytical methods for the drug substance and drug product (see ICH Guidelines, Q2A Text on Validation of Analytical Procedures and Q2B Validation of Analytical Procedures: Methodology).[13]

Nonclinical pharmacology and toxicology

The nonclinical pharmacology and toxicology section contains all of the nonclinical animal and laboratory studies conducted with the drug. The FDA looks for toxic effects of the drug that are inconsistent or have not been adequately characterized. Table 37.3 shows the expected content of the nonclinical pharmacology and toxicology section.

Details on the content of nonclinical pharmacology and toxicology can be found in the FDA and ICH guidance to industry on the same topic.[14,15]

Human pharmacokinetics and bioavailability

This section provides the data and analysis from the various pharmacokinetic and bioavailability studies

TABLE 37.3 Content of the nonclinical pharmacology and toxicology section of the NDA

- Pharmacological action and properties of the drug
- Toxic effects of the drug including acute, subacute and chronic toxicity and carcinogenicity
- Other studies of toxicity associated with administration and use of the drug
- Effects on reproduction and the development of the fetus
- ADME in animals
- Good laboratory practice (GLP) compliance statement for each study or a brief reason why a study was not conducted under GLP

conducted in human subjects, along with the analytical and statistical methods used in each study. There should also be a discussion that summarizes the pharmacokinetics and metabolism of the drug, and the bioavailability (BA) of the drug product. BA studies may need to be repeated during the drug development process, if dosage forms are reformulated during the process.

Clinical microbiology

The microbiology section is provided only for anti-infective, antiviral, special pathogens, sterile, and some nonsterile drug products. The FDA can establish effectiveness only if it has adequate information on the effects on the microbiological physiology of the targeted microorganism. Content and format for this section includes the drug action on microbial physiology, antimicrobial spectrum, resistance mechanism to the drug, and clinical microbiology laboratory methods used to evaluate the drug's use.[16]

Information regarding sterile and some nonsterile drugs, such as liquids that can support microbial growth, should be provided in the CMC section of the application.

Clinical data

The clinical data section is perhaps the most important section of the NDA, because data from human clinical trials will greatly impact the FDAs determination of safety and effectiveness for the drug product. Table 37.4 shows the content of the clinical dataset.

There is an extensive set of FDA and ICH guidance documents related to clinical studies and the presentation of the clinical data in a NDA.[10,17]

Safety update

This section is not filed with the original NDA, but is provided during the NDA review period at specific time points. Usually the first safety update report is filed as an amendment to the original NDA at four months after the original submission date, after receiving an approval letter, and at other times specified by the FDA reviewing division.

The format of the safety update report is like the ISS, and contains new safety information from ongoing studies, animal studies, and any other source. Sponsors should work with their reviewing division at the FDA on the exact content and format of these reports, in order to facilitate their review.

Statistical section

This is a key section of the NDA, closely linked to the clinical data section.[18] Applicants should work

TABLE 37.4   Content of the clinical data section

- List of investigators supplied with the drug
- List of INDs
- Other NDAs submitted for the same drug substance
- Overview of the clinical studies
- Description and analysis of
  - Clinical pharmacology studies
  - Controlled clinical studies relevant to the proposed use of the drug product
  - Uncontrolled studies
  - Other data pertaining to the evaluation of the drug product
- Integrated summary of effectiveness (ISE) including support for the dosage and administration of the drug as proposed in the product labeling
- Integrated summary of safety (ISS), which would include a discussion of the adverse events of the drug, clinical significant drug-drug interactions, pertinent animal data and other safety concerns
- Discussion and analysis of studies related to the abuse potential of the drug, if appropriate
  - This includes studies related to drug overdosage
- Integrated summary of risk-benefit (ISRB) which should clearly explain how the benefits of the drug product outweigh the risks, when used according to the approved label
- Good clinical practices (GCP) compliance statement regarding the Institutional Review Board (IRB) and informed consent (IC) regulations
  - If any study did not follow IRB regulations, then that study must be clearly identified
  - A statement regarding any transfer of obligations for the conduct of a clinical study to a third party (Contract Research Organization, CRO)
  - A listing of those studies audited or reviewed during the monitoring process by the sponsor
- The FDA is also expecting data regarding special populations such as geriatrics, pediatrics, renal and hepatic impairment patients

closely with their reviewing division at the FDA prior to the NDA submission, to come to an agreement on the format, content, tabulations, and statistical analyses to be presented. This section should be carefully addressed during the pre-NDA meeting with the review division.

Case report tabulations

Discuss with the FDA at the pre-NDA meeting about the submission of tabulations of patient data, data elements in the tables, and which case report forms (CRF) will be needed.[18]

Case report forms

The CRFs for patients who died during a clinical study, and patients who discontinued because of an adverse event, should be included in this section of the NDA. The reviewing division may require additional CRFs. This can be discussed at the pre-NDA meeting or the FDA will request the CRFs after the submission of the NDA.

Patent information

Patent information must be provided on the patent(s) for the drug or a method of use for the drug, using FDA Form 3542a.[6]

Patent certification

Patent certification is required for any relevant patents that claim the listed drug or that claim any other drug on which the investigations relied or that claim a use for the listed or other drug.

Establishment information (for biologics only)

This is to be used for certain biological product applications only.

Debarment certification

Debarment certification is required under the Generic Drug Enforcement Act of 1992, which empowered the FDA to debar individuals convicted of crimes relating to the development, approval or regulation of drugs. The individual may not provide any services to sponsors of an application.[19]

Field copy certification

Applicants based in the United States must submit a "field" copy of the CMC section, application form, and summary of the NDA to the relevant FDA district office. The information will be used during the pre-approval inspection (PAI) at the manufacturing site. Within the NDA, the applicant must certify that an exact copy of the CMC section has been sent to the district office.

User fee cover sheet

The FDA uses the information in FDA Form 3397 to determine the applicability of a user fee.[6] If one is required, this form also states that the check has been mailed to an FDA account at the same time the NDA is submitted to the FDA. More information on Form 3397 is available on line at www.fda.gov/oc/pdufa/coversheet.html

Financial information

The financial information section contains clinical investigator financial disclosures (FDA Form 3455), and certification (FDA Form 3454),[6] which provide disclosure regarding investigator financial interests and sponsor–investigator financial arrangements that could affect the reliability of the submitted data. The FDA guidance provides detailed explanations of which investigators and studies are covered under this rule.[20]

Other information

This section can be used to incorporate, by cross-reference, any information that was submitted before the NDA. A sponsor may propose other uses of this section at the pre-NDA meeting.

37.2.3 Common Technical Document (CTD)

The CTD is a major product of the international harmonization process done by the ICH. This body is composed of the pharmaceutical regulatory and industry representatives from the European Union, Japan, and the United States. The FDA highly recommends that sponsors submit their marketing applications in CTD format. This has the advantage of preparing, for the most part, a single compiled marketing application usable in all three regions. This saves time and resources during the submission process. While the CTD provides an alternative format for the marketing application, it does not alter the data or information required for a standard NDA in the US (Figure 37.3). The ICH and the FDA have issued guidance documents on CTD.[21,22]

Format and Content of a Common Technical Document (CTD)

Module 1 administrative and labeling information

Module 1 of CTD (Figure 37.3) contains the regional administrative forms and documents required by each region, as well as the proposed prescribing information (label). The content of Module 1 is determined by each region. In the US, this section contains the cover letter, form 356h, complete table of contents of the entire CTD, and other administrative documents, such as the field copy certification, debarment certification, patent information, labeling, and the annotated labeling text.

Module 2 summaries

Module 2 contains the CTD summaries for quality, nonclinical and clinical information. This module is very important, as it provides detailed summaries of the various sections of the CTD. These include:

1. a very short introduction ($\leq$1pg);
2. quality overall summary ($\leq$40 pgs);
3. nonclinical overview ($\leq$30pgs);
4. clinical overview ($\leq$30 pgs);
5. nonclinical written and tabulated summaries for pharmacology, pharmacokinetics, and toxicology;
6. clinical summary (50–400 pgs), including biopharmaceutics and associated analytical methods, clinical pharmacology studies, clinical efficacy, clinical safety, and a synopses of the individual studies.

Module 3 quality

Module 3 contains all of the quality documents for the chemistry, manufacture, and controls of the drug substance, and the drug product.

Module 4 nonclinical study reports

Module 4 contains copy of all of the final nonclinical study reports.

Module 5 clinical study reports

Module 5 contains a copy of all of the final clinical study reports.

37.2.4 User Fees

Since the implementation of the Prescription Drug User Fee Act in 1994, the FDA has been allowed to charge a fee for the review of an original NDA, and certain other NDA submissions. These fees vary according to their type, and the need to review clinical data. The fees have allowed the FDA to add new personnel and resources to the review process, and shorten the overall review time. Each year the FDA publishes the user fee schedule in the Federal Register, and these fees have been increasing each year (Table 37.5).

TABLE 37.5   User fee schedules for 2006 and 2007

Fee category	Fee 2006	Fee 2007	Fee 2008
Applications	$	$	$
Requiring clinical data	767 400	896 200	1 178 000
Not requiring clinical data	383 700	448 100	589 000
Supplements requiring clinical data	393 700	448 100	589 000
Establishments	264 000	313 100	392 700
Products	42 130	49 750	65 030

37.2.5 New Drug Application (NDA) Review Process

Background

While there is a prescribed review process within the CDER, there are some general aspects to discuss. The NDA is received by the FDAs central document room (CDR), which administratively processes the application, and gives the application a NDA number. The receipt date is also noted, and this starts the review time clock under the PDUFA guidelines. The various sections of the NDA are separated and distributed to the review division and other divisions reviewing certain technical sections.

When the NDA arrives at the review division, an acknowledgement letter is sent to the sponsor. The regulatory project manager (RPM) does an initial screening of the application, to identify any obvious deficiency in the completeness of the NDA according to the NDA checklist.[3] If the file appears to be usable, the RPM distributes the sections to the various assigned reviewers, who then do a final screening of the application. A summary of the NDA review process is shown in Figure 37.4.

Timing

Within 45 days after receipt of the NDA, the reviewing division will meet, and determine if the application is fileable. If the application is to be filed, then a review plan is established for that NDA, its review priority depending on the importance of the drug. If not fileable, a refuse to file (RTF) letter is sent to the sponsor.

Refuse to File

The refuse to file letter will explain to the sponsor the deficiencies, which make the application not reviewable unless some changes are made. Under PDUFA, the quality of market applications has increased, and the refuse to file letter rate has decreased from 26% in 1993 to 4% in 2001.

Review

The FDA reviewers conduct comprehensive scientific examination of information and data submitted in the NDA, to evaluate the quality, safety, and efficacy of the drug product, and determine the approvability of the application. During the review, questions often arise with the reviewers, necessitating communication with the sponsor. A mid-review communication may be in the form of an email, informal teleconference or a face-to-face meeting between the FDA and the sponsor. The communications usually take the form of either a discipline review (DR) letter or an information

request. The discipline review letter may include comments from one or more reviewers, who have identified potential deficiencies in a part of the NDA. The information request asks the sponsor for additional information or needed clarification that would aid in the final review of that particular section of the NDA.

Much of the FDA-sponsor communications are done by email, which provides a very rapid method of exchanging large amounts of information. Emails however, are not considered an official communication at the FDA, and so any information needed for the review and decision-making process must be officially submitted as an amendment to the NDA.

Each reviewer prepares a written evaluation of their discipline review, and usually the medical reviewer will reconcile these documents in consultation with the other reviewers (institutional decision). This may also involve the division or office director. If significant issues arise during the review process, the reviewing division can have an advisory committee meeting to evaluate any concerns.

Labeling

Final discussions about the package insert will usually take place at the end of the review period, possibly two to four weeks before the PDUFA action date. At this time, the FDA will propose any changes needed in the labeling, and engage the sponsor in bringing these negotiations to a successful close, prior to the action date. The final negotiations for the labeling are often done by email or teleconferences, until the labeling has been finalized. Once this is complete, the sponsor will submit a final version as an amendment to the NDA. This labeling must be submitted to the FDA in specific electronic formats, including SPL, and using the recently approved PRL format.[8,9]

Structured Product Labeling

Four Month Safety Update

Four months after the submission of the NDA, the regulations require the sponsor to submit a safety update report to the NDA. This will be similar to the integrated summary of safety, but contain safety information not included in the original NDA. This information will come from ongoing clinical trials, and foreign marketing information. The FDA can also request a safety update report at other times during the review process, if necessary.

Advisory Committee

During the course of a few NDA reviews, issues or controversies may arise, and the FDA may call for a consultation with one of its advisory committees. These are composed of subject matter experts in

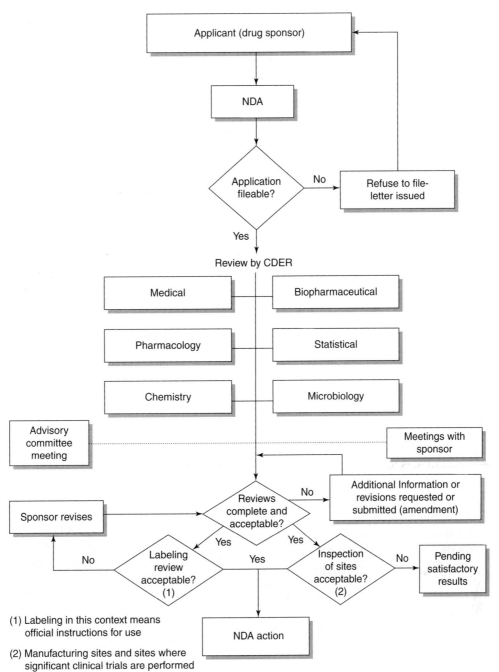

FIGURE 37.4 The new drug application (NDA) review process. Source of information http://www.fda.gov/cder/handbook/nda.htm as of March 23, 2008

various medical and scientific fields. Table 37.6 provides a listing of the advisory committees available to the CDER, and the FDA.

Food and Drug Administration (FDA) Action Letter

Final action on the NDA is taken by a review of the "institutional" decision by the division director, with

final sign-off of the action letter by the office director. The action letter can be in three forms: approval, approvable, and not approvable. An approval letter allows a product to be marketed in the US after the approval date. This assumes that the sponsor is agreeable to the negotiated labeling, and any post-marketing commitments made to the FDA. An approvable letter is sent to an applicant if the FDA believes the application can be approved, if the sponsor submits

TABLE 37.6　Center for Drug Evaluation and Research (CDER) advisory committees

Anesthetic and Life Support Drugs Advisory Committee

Anti-Infective Drugs Advisory Committee

Antiviral Drugs Advisory Committee

Arthritis Advisory Committee

Cardiovascular and Renal Drugs Advisory Committee

Dermatologic and Ophthalmic Drugs Advisory Committee

Drug Safety and Risk Management Advisory Committee

Endocrinologic and Metabolic Drugs Advisory Committee

Gastrointestinal Drugs Advisory Committee

Nonprescription Drugs Advisory Committee

Oncologic Drugs Advisory Committee

Peripheral and Central Nervous System Drugs Advisory Committee

Pharmaceutical Science, Advisory Committee for

Psychopharmacologic Drugs Advisory Committee

Pulmonary-Allergy Drugs Advisory Committee

Reproductive Health Drugs, Advisory Committee for

Source of information: http://www.fda.gov/oc/advisory/acphonecodes.html as of March 23, 2008

additional information or agrees to certain conditions. This could include labeling changes, another safety update report or additional clinical information. The sponsor has 10 days to respond to an approvable letter with a formal response or a plan to file a resubmission, a hearing request regarding the unapprovability of the NDA, a withdrawal of the application or a request for an extension of the review period to allow the sponsor time to evaluate its options. Not approvable letters mean the application did not meet FDA requirements, and the letter will describe the deficiencies in the NDA. The sponsor can take one of the above options within 10 days. If no action is taken by the sponsor, the FDA will consider the NDA to be withdrawn.

37.3 GENERIC DRUG PRODUCT REGISTRATION AND REVIEW PROCESS

37.3.1 Food and Drug Administration (FDA), Center for Drug Evaluation and Research (CDER), Office of Generic Drugs

The Office of Generic Drugs (OGD) is part of the Office of Pharmaceutical Science within the CDER, as shown in the organization chart in Figure 37.5. As indicated by the name of the office, OGD is responsible for review and approval of generic drug products.

37.3.2 Abbreviated New Drug Application (ANDA)

The Abbreviated New Drug Application (ANDA) is provided for the marketing of generic drug products after all forms of exclusivity have expired for the reference-listed drug (innovator drug). ANDAs are filed under the FD&C Act section 505(j).[1] The numbers of ANDAs submitted to the FDA has been rising steadily since 2001 (Figure 37.6), likely due to the high demand for lower cost generic products than brand products, and more companies entering the manufacture of generic products.

Generic drug products must be bioequivalent to the innovator product, though waivers of *in vivo* bioequivalence study are available in certain cases.[23] The active pharmaceutical ingredient, dosage form, dose strength, labeling, route of administration, and conditions must be the same as the reference listed drug (RLD). Also, a generic drug product must meet the same specifications as the RLD, if the RLD is listed in the USP, and meet the same cGMP requirements for manufacturing as the RLD. A sponsor of an ANDA must file a patent certification with the FDA. Table 37.7 shows the difference in the information required for the submission of an ANDA, versus a NDA.

Format and Content of an Abbreviated New Drug Application (ANDA)

The FDA strongly recommends that an ANDA be submitted in the CTD format, either paper or electronic.[24] The requirements from CFR, and the corresponding sections in the CTD for ANDAs, are summarized in Table 37.8. More information on the ANDA checklist for CTD or e-CTD can be found from the FDA website.[25]

In the FDAs *Guidance to Industry—Organization of an ANDA*, the agency provides a suggested table of contents per 21CFR314.94, as discussed below.[21]

Application form

The ANDA begins with the FDA Form 356h, as was seen with the original NDA. Table 37.7 provides a comparison of the content of a NDA, and an ANDA. A substantial amount of information is not required for the filing of an ANDA.

Basis for an ANDA submission
Patent certification and exclusivity statement

Sponsors of an ANDA must file a patent certification under one of the following paragraphs:

I. That no patent information on the drug product that is the subject of the ANDA has been submitted to the FDA;

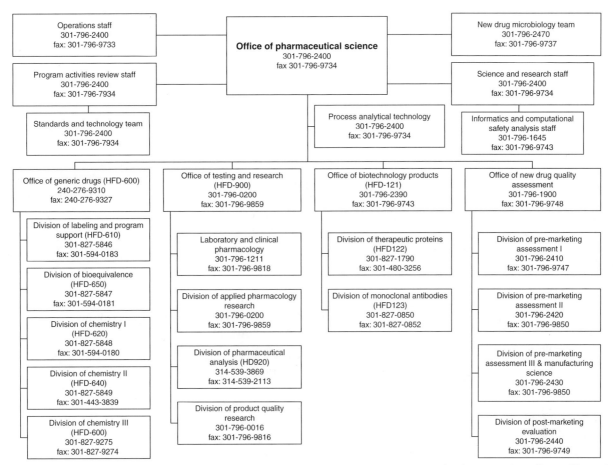

FIGURE 37.5 Office of Generic Drugs within the Office of Pharmaceutical Science. Source of information: http://www.fda.gov/cder/cderorg/ops.htm as of March 23, 2008

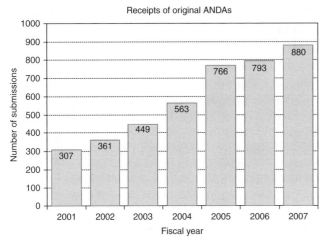

FIGURE 37.6 Increase in numbers of abbreviated new drug applications (ANDAs) filed to the Office of Generic Drugs. Source of information: GPhA Fall Technical Workshop, October 11, 2007, http://www.gphaonline.org/AM/Template.cfm?Section=Presentations1&TEMPLATE=/CM/ContentDisplay.cfm&CONTENTID=3866 as of March 2008

II. That such patent(s) has expired;

III. The date on which such patent expires; or

IV. That such patent is invalid or will not be infringed by the manufacture, use or sale of the drug product from which the ANDA is submitted.

The above are commonly referred as Paragraphs I, II, III or IV Certifications.

If the ANDA applicant files the Paragraph IV certification, the applicant must also notify the innovator within 20 days of filing of an ANDA, and the innovator has 45 days to take action upon receiving the notification. The FDA may hold the approval up to 30 months, depending on the outcome of the litigation, if any.

Comparison between generic drug and reference listed drug

This section should compare the active ingredients, as well as the route of administration, dosage form, and strength of the drug products.

TABLE 37.7   Comparison of NDA and ANDA content

NDA index	ANDA index
	Basis for submission
	Comparison between generic drug and reference listed drug
	Request for waiver for *in vivo* BA/BE studies (if applicable)
Labeling	Labeling
Summary	
Chemistry	Chemistry
Nonclinical pharmacology and toxicology	
Human pharmacokinetics and bioavailability	Human pharmacokinetics and bioavailability
Clinical microbiology (if applicable)	
Clinical data	
Safety update report	
Statistical section	
Case report tabulations	
Case report forms	Case report forms
Patent information	Patent information
Patent certification	Patent certification
Establishment description	
Debarment certification	Debarment certification
Field copy certification	Field copy certification
User fee cover sheet	
Financial information	Financial information
Other	
	References

Labeling

According to 21CFR314.94(8), differences between the applicant's proposed labeling, and labeling approved for the reference listed drug, may include differences in expiration date, formulation, bioavailability or pharmacokinetics, labeling revisions made to comply with current FDA labeling guidelines or other guidance or omission of an indication or other aspect of labeling protected by patent or accorded exclusivity under section 505 (j)(4)(D) of the act. All labeling for a generic drug product must be provided in SPL formatting, and in compliance with the Physician's Labeling Rule (PLR).

Bioavailability/bioequivalence

This section provides the key information for gaining approval of an ANDA.

Bioavailability is the rate and extent of drug available at the site of action.

Bioequivalence is the absence of a significant difference in the rate and extent of drug available at the site of action after dosing of a test product, compared to a reference product. In general, bioequivalence is evaluated by comparing the bioavailability of the test, and the reference products, in crossover clinical studies on healthy subjects. The study may include the evaluation of bioavailability of products administered with, and without, food. Recommendations of study designs and data evaluation for bioequivalence study are listed in regulatory guidance.[26,27] Bioequivalence is achieved when the 90% confidence interval (CI) for the ratio of C_{max} and AUC of the test product over the reference product on log transformed data is within 80%–125%.

CMC Information

The quality sections listed below contain very much the same information as would be submitted in a NDA. The content of the CMC for an ANDA includes the following:

- Components and composition statements;
- Raw materials;
- Description of manufacturing facility;
- Outside firms; contract testing laboratories;
- Manufacturing and processing instructions;
- In-process information;
- Packaging materials controls;
- Controls for the finished dosage form;
- Analytical methods;
- Stability of finished dosage form;
- NOTE: RESERVED;
- Samples;
- Environmental considerations;
- Generic enforcement act, and US agent letter of authorization;
- Other;
- Sterilization assurance information and data.

To modernize the CMC review for science and risk-based pharmaceutical quality assessment of ANDA applications, the FDA has developed and implemented a question-based review (QbR) approach, this includes a requirement for the sponsor to submit a quality overall summary (QoS).[28] To facilitate the QbR, the FDA has developed model quality overall summaries for immediate-release (IR) or extended-release (ER) solid oral dosage forms.[28]

37.3.3 Abbreviated New Drug Application (ANDA) Review Process

The Office of Generic Drugs (OGD) process for the review and approval of an ANDA is shown in Figure 37.7.

TABLE 37.8 Content and format of an ANDA

CFR citation source		CTD heading	
Number	Title	Module	Number
314.94(A)(1)	Application form	1	1.2
GDEA	Debarment certification	1	1.3.3
314.94(a)(2)	Table of contents	N/A	N/A
314.94(a)(3)	Basis for abbreviated new drug application submission	1	1.12.11
314.94(a)(4)	Conditions of use	1	1.11.11
314.94(a)(5)	Active ingredient	1, 2 ,3	1.11.12, 2.3S, 3.2S
314.94(a)(6)	Route of administration, dosage form and strength	1, 2 ,3	1.11.12, 2.3, 3.3
314.94(a)(7)	Bioequivalence	2, 5	2.7, 5.3.
314.94(8)(i)	Listed drug labeling	1	1.14.3.2
314.94(8)(ii)	Copies of proposed labeling	1	1.14
314.94(8)(iii)	Statement of proposed labeling	1	1.14.3.1
314.94(8)(iv)	Comparison of approved and proposed labeling	1	1.14.3.1
314.94(9)	Chemistry, manufacturing and control	2, 3	2.3, 3.2
314.94(11)	Reference to information previously submitted by sponsor	1	1.4.4
314.94(12)	Patent Information	1	1.3.5
314.95	Notice of certification of nonvalidity or noninfringement of patent	1	1.3.5.3
314.94(13)	Financial certification and disclosure	1	1.3.4
314.96	Amendment to an unapproved application: Chemistry	3	As needed
314.96	Amendment to an unapproved application: Chemistry (information no fitting under Module 3)	1	1.11.1
314.96	Amendment to an unapproved application: Clinical	5	As needed
314.96	Amendment to an unapproved application: Clinical (information not fitting under Module 5)	1	1.11.3
314.102	Communications: Meetings	1	1.6.1
314.102	Communications: Meetings	1	1.6.2
314.102	Communications: Meetings	1	1.6.3
314.103(c)	Scientific and medical disputes	1	1.10.1
314.103(c)	Scientific and medical disputes	1	1.10.2
314.150(c)	Request for withdrawal of approval	1	1.5.7
314.150(b) 314.151	Withdrawal or suspension of approval by the FDA	1	1.5.7
314.420(a)	Drug master files	1, 2, 3, 4, 5	As needed
314.420(b)	Incorporating DMF information by reference	1	1.4.1
314.420(d)	List of authorized persons to incorporate by reference	1	1.4.3

Background

The FDA recommends that an applicant file an ANDA using CTD, either paper or electronic.[24] A complete ANDA checklist for CTD or eCTD format is located on the FDA website at http://www.fda.gov/cder/ogd/anda_checklist.pdf. The order of presentation of the information in the ANDA is slightly different from that presented in the Guidance to Industry, as shown above.

As discussed earlier, the Office of Generic Drugs (OGD) has developed a question-based review (QbR) approach, including the requirement for submitting a quality overall summary (QoS) for an ANDA.[28] The QbR will transform the CMC review into a modern, science and risk-based pharmaceutical quality assessment, that incorporates and implements the concepts and principles of the FDAs "21st Century cGMP initiatives."[29]

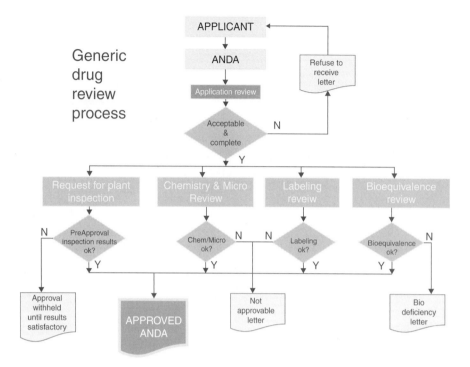

FIGURE 37.7 Abbreviated new drug application (ANDA) review process. Adapted from http://www.fda.gov/cder/handbook/anda.htm as of March 23, 2008

The QbR has two purposes:

1. To aid the reviewer's evaluation of product quality and determination of the risk level associated with the manufacture and design of drug products; and
2. To provide transparency to sponsors regarding the logic used by reviewers during the conduct of the CMC reviews.

Advantages of this new QbR approach include:

1. Stimulating the application of the quality by design (QbD) concept for product development, and the concept of developing performance-based specifications.
2. Enabling risk-based assessment to facilitate continuous improvement with minimized additional supplements.
3. Standardizing the questions for CMC evaluation in the agency for the entire pharmaceutical industry, hence improving the quality and transparency of review.
4. Increasing the CMC review efficiency, reducing the review time, shortening the time for the products to reach patients.

To facilitate the QbR, the FDA has developed a model QoS for solid oral dosage forms.[28] Some of the questions listed in the drug product sections of the model QoS are listed in the following:

- Which properties of the drug substance affect drug product development, manufacture or performance?

- How were the excipients, and their grades, selected?
- What evidence supports compatibility between the excipients and the drug substance?
- What attributes should the drug product possess?
- How was the drug product designed to have these attributes?
- Were alternative formulations or mechanisms investigated?
- How was the final formulation optimized?
- Why was the manufacturing process selected for this drug product?
- How are the manufacturing steps related to the drug product quality?
- How were the critical process parameters identified, monitored, and/or controlled?

Timing

The timing for an ANDA filing and approval depend on the exclusivity and patent status of the reference listed drug (RLD), which has been discussed in the section for patent certification and exclusivity statement in Section 37.3.2 of this chapter. If the application is of a Paragraph IV filing, the FDA may hold the approval on an ANDA for up to 30 months, depending on the outcome of the litigation between the innovator and the ANDA applicant. As more and more RLDs come off patents, and more companies engage in generic drug manufacturing, the number of

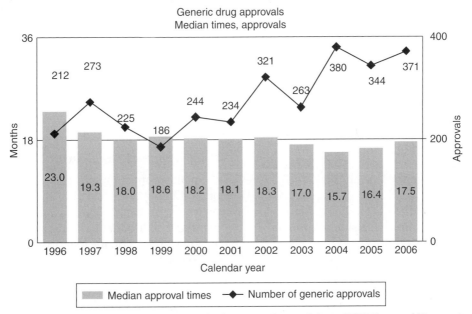

FIGURE 37.8   Approvals for generic drug products. Source of information: Steven Galson, CDER Facts and Figures. August 8, 2007

ANDA applications and approvals has been increasing over the past decade, while the mean approval time remains fairly steady at approximately18 months as shown in Figure 37.8.

Refuse to file

As with NDAs, the Office of Generic Drugs can refuse to file an ANDA application, and will provide the sponsor a listing of the deficiencies in the application.

Amendments

Amendments can be submitted to an ANDA, depending on the information requests received from the FDA. Based on past experience, information requests are most likely to involve the CMC section (stability, specifications, analytical methods) or the BE/BA section (adequate study provided in the ANDA).

Labeling

Labeling should also be provided with the ANDA application, and this should clearly correspond to the labeling of the innovator product.

Food and Drug Administration Action Letter

The FDA action letter on an ANDA can be the same type as seen with the standard NDA, as discussed in

Section 37.2.5. At this writing, the Office of Generic Drugs does not impose a user fee for ANDA applications, and does not have a PDUFA timing requirement for its review of an ANDA application.

If the Office of Generic Drugs completes the ANDA review process prior to the expiration of all exclusivity for the innovator drug product, it can issue a notice of tentative approval, which does not allow the generic drug manufacturer to enter the market. Once all exclusivity has expired for the innovator drug, then the FDA will issue an approval letter, allowing the generic product onto the market. If the ANDA applicant and the innovator are engaged in patent litigation, the FDA action may be affected, based on the outcome of the litigation. For more details, readers are referred to FD&C Act, section 505.

37.4 POST-APPROVAL ACTIVITIES FOR NEW DRUG APPLICATIONS AND ABBREVIATED NEW DRUG APPLICATIONS

37.4.1 Reports

Annual Report (21CFR314.81)

Sponsor's holding a NDA or ANDA must submit an annual report each year, within 60 days of the anniversary date of US approval of the application, to the FDA division responsible for reviewing the application. The report is required to contain in the order listed:

- Form FDA 2252 (Transmittal of Periodic Reports for Drugs for Human Use);[6]
- Summary;
- Distribution data;
- Labeling;
- CMC changes;
- Nonclinical laboratory studies;
- Clinical data;
- Status reports of post-marketing study commitments;
- Status of other post-marketing studies (CMC);
- Log of outstanding regulatory business (optional).

Annual Adverse Drug Experience Report (21CFR314.80)

A report of each adverse drug experience not reported previously during the year is reported to the FDA at quarterly intervals, for three years from the date of approval of the application, and then at annual intervals.

Adverse Event Reporting (21CFR314.80)

Sponsors must promptly review all adverse drug experience information obtained from any source, foreign or domestic, including information derived from commercial marketing experience, post-marketing clinical investigations, post-marketing epidemiological/surveillance studies, reports in the scientific literature, and unpublished scientific papers. Sponsors also need to develop written procedures for the surveillance, receipt, evaluation, and reporting of post-marketing adverse drug experiences to the FDA.

The applicant needs to report adverse drug experience information to the FDA. Post-marketing 15-day alert reports are to be submitted by the sponsor for each adverse drug experience that is both serious and unexpected, whether foreign or domestic, as soon as possible, but in no case later than 15 calendar days of initial receipt of the information by the sponsor. Follow-up reports to the post-marketing 15-day alert reports must be submitted within 15 calendar days of receipt of new information or as requested by the FDA. If additional information is not obtainable, records should be maintained of the unsuccessful steps taken to seek additional information.

37.4.2 Changes to an Approved Application (21CFR314.70)

Changes may be made to an approved NDA or ANDA.[30,31,32] Such changes may include compositions, manufacturing process, equipment, manufacturing equipment, specifications, packaging, labeling, and others. The changes can be classified as major, moderate, and minor changes, and should be reported to the FDA via prior approval supplement, changes being effected/changes being effected in 30 days, and annual report, respectively. These reporting categories are described in the following.

Prior Approval Supplement

Sponsors must submit a supplement to their NDA or ANDA for any change in the drug substance, drug product, production process, quality controls, equipment or facilities that has a substantial potential to have an adverse effect on the identity, strength, quality, purity or potency of the drug product, as these factors may relate to the safety or effectiveness of the drug product. The guidance documents[30,31,32] should be consulted for more specific examples of allowed changes, which may provide some flexibility for specific changes.

Per the regulations, these changes include, but are not limited to:

1. Changes in the qualitative or quantitative formulation of the drug product, including inactive ingredients or in the specifications provided in the approved application.
2. Changes requiring completion of studies to demonstrate the equivalence of the drug product to the drug product as manufactured without the change or to the reference listed drug.
3. Changes that may affect drug substance or drug product sterility assurance, such as changes in drug substance, drug product or component sterilization method(s) or an addition, deletion or substitution of steps in an aseptic processing operation.
4. Changes in the synthesis or manufacture of the drug substance that may affect the impurity profile and/or the physical, chemical or biological properties of the drug substance.
5. Labeling changes are also affected by this requirement and are specified in the regulations.
6. Changes in a drug product container closure system that controls the drug product delivered to a patient or changes in the type (e.g., glass to high density polyethylene (HDPE), HDPE to polyvinyl chloride, vial to syringe) or composition (e.g., one HDPE resin to another HDPE resin) of a packaging component that may affect the impurity profile of the drug product.
7. Changes solely affecting a natural product, a recombinant DNA-derived protein/polypeptide or a complex or conjugate of a drug substance with a monoclonal antibody for the

following: (a) changes in the virus or adventitious agent removal or inactivation method(s);
(b) changes in the source material or cell line; and
(c) establishment of a new master cell bank or seed.

8. Changes to a drug product under an application that is subject to a validity assessment because of significant questions regarding the integrity of the data supporting that application.

Supplement: Changes Being Effected (CBE-30)

These are changes requiring supplement submission at least 30 days prior to distribution of the drug product made using the change (moderate changes).

A supplement must be submitted for any change in the drug substance, drug product, production process, quality controls, equipment or facilities that has a moderate potential to have an adverse effect on the identity, strength, quality, purity or potency of the drug product as these factors may relate to the safety or effectiveness of the drug product. Examples of types of changes that can be reported under the CBE category can be found in the FDA guidance for industry.[30]

A supplement submitted for CBE-30 is required to give a full explanation of the basis for the change and identify the date on which the change is to be made. The supplement must be labeled "Supplement—Changes being effected in 30 days." Pending approval of the supplement by the FDA, distribution of the drug product made using the change may begin not less than 30 days after receipt of the supplement by the FDA.

The sponsor cannot distribute the drug product made using the change if the FDA informs the sponsor within 30 days following the FDAs receipt of the supplement that either: (a) the change requires approval prior to distribution of the drug; or (b) any of the required information is missing.

Supplement: Changes Being Effected (CBE)

With CBE changes, the holder of an approved application may commence distribution of the drug product involved upon receipt by the agency of a supplement for the change. Examples of changes that can be reported in this category are available in the FDA guidance on changes to approved NDAs or ANDAs.[30]

Under the CBE and CBE-30 changes, if the agency disapproves the supplemental application, it may order the manufacturer to cease distribution of the drug product(s) made with the changes.

Annual Reportable Changes

Changes that may be reported in an annual report reflect changes in the drug substance, drug product, production process, quality controls, equipment or facilities that have a minimal potential to have an adverse effect on the identity, strength, quality, purity or potency of the drug product.

These changes include, but are not limited to: (1) any change made to comply with a change to an official compendium that is consistent with the FDA statutory and regulatory requirements; (2) the deletion or reduction of an ingredient intended to affect only the color of the drug product; (3) replacement of equipment with that of the same design and operating principles, with some exceptions; (4) a change in the size and/or shape of a container containing the same number of dosage units for a nonsterile solid dosage form drug product, without a change from one container closure system to another; (5) a change within the container closure system for a nonsterile drug product, based upon a showing of equivalency to the approved system under a protocol approved in the application or published in an official compendium; (6) an extension of an expiration dating period based upon full shelf life data on production batches obtained from a protocol approved in the application; (7) the addition or revision of an alternative analytical procedure that provides the same or increased assurance of the identity, strength, quality, purity or potency of the material being tested as the analytical procedure described in the approved application or deletion of an alternative analytical procedure; (8) the addition by embossing, debossing or engraving of a code imprint to a solid oral dosage form drug product other than a modified-release dosage form, or a minor change in an existing code imprint; (9) a change in the labeling concerning the description of the drug product or in the information about how the drug product is supplied, that does not involve a change in the dosage strength or dosage form; and (10) an editorial or similar minor change in labeling, including a change to the information.

37.5 OTHER CONSIDERATIONS FOR NEW DRUG APPLICATIONS AND ABBREVIATED NEW DRUG APPLICATIONS

37.5.1 Supplemental Applications (21CFR314.71)

All procedures and actions that apply to an application under 21CFR314.50 also apply to supplements, except that the information required in the supplement is limited to that needed to support the change.

A sponsor is required to submit two copies of a supplement to the appropriate FDA reviewing division, and a field copy of the CMC information to the appropriate regional office of the FDA. Foreign applicants should submit the field copy to the OGD of the FDA. If the supplement is only for a labeling change for the product, a field copy is not required.

37.5.2 Establishment Registration and Drug Listing Requirements for Foreign Establishments (21CFR 207.40)

Foreign drug establishments whose drugs are imported or offered for import into the United States must comply with the establishment registration and drug listing requirements, unless exempt by regulation or unless the drugs enter a foreign trade zone and are re-exported from that foreign trade zone without having entered US commerce.

No drug may be imported or offered for import into the United States unless it is listed and manufactured, prepared, propagated, compounded or processed at a registered foreign drug establishment, however, this restriction does not apply to a drug imported or offered for import under the investigational use provisions in 21CFR312 part 312 or to a component of a drug imported under section 801(d)(3) of the FDC Act. Foreign drug establishments must submit all listing information, including labels and labeling, and registration information, in the English language.

Each foreign drug establishment required to register must submit the name, address, and phone number of its United States agent as part of its initial and updated registration information. Each foreign drug establishment can designate only one United States agent.

1. The United States agent must reside or maintain a place of business in the United States.
2. Upon request from the FDA, the United States agent will assist the FDA in communications with the foreign drug establishment, respond to questions concerning the foreign drug establishment's products that are imported or offered for import into the United States, and assist the FDA in scheduling inspections of the foreign drug establishment. If the FDA is unable to contact the foreign drug establishment directly or expeditiously, the FDA may provide information or documents to the United States agent, and such an action shall be considered to be equivalent to providing the same information or documents to the foreign drug establishment.

3. The foreign drug establishment or the United States agent must report changes in the United States agent's name, address or phone number to FDA within ten business days of the change.

37.6 PRE-APPROVAL INSPECTION (PAI)

37.6.1 Background and Purpose

The FDA may approve a NDA or an ANDA to enter the US market only if the drug is safe, effective, and if the methods used in, and the facilities and controls used for, the manufacture, processing, packing, and testing of the drug are found adequate to ensure and preserve its identity, strength, quality, and purity. The review and approval process include two parts: (1) scientific review based on data provided in the application, and (2) audit of the data authenticity and evaluation of cGMP compliance. Detailed scientific review of data in the application is conducted by the review scientists at the headquarters of the FDA, specifically by the Office of Pharmaceutical Science (OPS) in the CDER. The scientists review has lately been developed into a question-based review (QbR) to raise the level of scientific understanding, and for risk-assessment and management. By contrast to relying on testing of the final products to prove the quality, the FDA has been promoting new approaches to build product quality by design (QbD) in recent years, and will hence expect to review information on QbD, including the identification of critical process parameters (CPP), critical quality attributes (CQA), design space, etc., to determine if the proposed method of manufacturing and specifications meet the agency's standards on quality. In the meantime, an onsite audit, commonly referred as a pre-approval inspection (PAI), may be conducted prior to the agency's decision-making regarding the application. The purposes of the PAI are to audit the authenticity of the data submitted in the application, and to evaluate the applicant's compliance with cGMP, and the commitments made in the application for the manufacture of the product in the submission. It is the author's opinion that one of the purposes of a PAI is to determine if the applicant committed fraud in manufacturing, testing, and in clinical studies, or misrepresented data in the application.

PAI is applicable for all domestic and international firms intending to market any drug substances or products in the United States. The procedures that the FDA use to carry out PAI are described in the FDAs Compliance Program Guidance Manual (7346.832), revised March, 2005. According to this guidance manual, the FDA may determine if the PAI is necessary for each new drug application by a risk-based approach,[33] based on the most current knowledge and cGMP compliance status of a firm. If it is decided that such inspection is necessary, a request will be made by the CDER review office to the responsible ORA district office governing the area of the applicant. The ORA will then schedule the inspection, and typically give the applicant short notice or no notice for the inspection.

37.6.2 On-site Inspection

The DA may conduct on-site inspections into a firm for many reasons such as: (1) routine cGMP inspection every two years; (2) pre-approval inspection (PAI); (3) follow-up to prior warning letter(s); (4) recall effectiveness check; (5) complaints from customers, industry, etc.; and (6) any other specific causes. The PAI is conducted by the FDAs inspection team from the field or district offices under the Office of Regulatory Affairs (ORA). The inspection teams may consist of investigators, analysts, engineers, and/or computer experts, as appropriate. During the PAI, the FDA investigators conduct on-site inspection at the manufacturing and testing facilities, and clinical sites when applicable, to audit the accuracy and adequacy of information submitted in the application against the sponsor's manufacturing and clinical practices. The key tasks of the PAI include the following:

- Evaluate the manufacturer's compliance with cGMP and manufacturing-related commitments made in the application;
- Verify the authenticity, accuracy, and adequacy of data in the submission, including in-process and release testing results, bioequivalency, and bioavailability data.
- Determine whether the firm has the necessary facilities, equipment, controls, and skills to manufacture the new drug for which it has applied for approval;
- Collect a variety of drug samples for analysis by FDA field and CDER laboratories. These include samples for methods validation, methods verification, and forensic screening for substitution.

For data verification, the audit is to ensure that all data submitted in the NDA or ANDA are real, verifiable, and no fraud has been committed during the course of product manufacturing and testing.

To audit the cGMP compliance, the inspection can cover all areas related to pharmaceutical manufacturing. Since 2002, the FDA has adopted a system-based inspection approach. The systems in this include: (1) quality; (2) facilities and equipment; (3) materials;

(4) production; (5) packaging and labeling; and (6) laboratory controls. During each inspection, the inspectors may or may not have enough time to cover all the areas. The quality system will be included any time, and the inspector can decide or change other systems to inspect. For more information on what may be audited, readers are referred to the FDAs Compliance Program Guidance Manual, Program 7346.832 for Pre-approval inspections/Investigations, and ORAs internal Guide to Inspections of Drugs.[34] In recent years, the FDA has also taken a risk-based approach to inspection. More thorough inspection may be warranted if there is a higher level of risk existed in any specific system of a firm. GMP deficiencies in US domestic and foreign inspections by the FDA (Tables 37.9, 37.10, 37.11)[35] indicate that the level of risk in quality, laboratory controls, and facility/equipment systems is substantially higher than other systems. Similar results were found in Europe by European Medicines Agency (EMEA) inspections

TABLE 37.9 Most common cGMP deficiency by systems, 2004–2005 US Domestic Inspection

System	% deficiency
Quality	47.5
Laboratory controls	18.8
Facility and equipment	17.6
Production	10.6
Materials	5.5
Packaging and labeling	0

Reference 35

TABLE 37.10 GMP deficiencies for foreign dosage manufacturers in 2004

System	% deficiency
Failure/OOS investigation	11
Laboratory controls	9
Equipment/cleaning validation	8
Lack of or inadequate SOP	7
Water system	5
Production/process control	5
Materials control	5
Analytical method validation	5
Media fill	5
Environmental control	5
Others	35

Reference 35

TABLE 37.11 Top ten GMP deficiencies in European communities during 1955–2005

No	Category of GMP deficiency	Number of incidences	%
1	Documentation—quality system elements/procedures	1341	14.1
2	Design and maintenance of premises	634	6.7
3	Design and maintenance of equipment	594	6.2
4	Documentation—manufacturing	526	5.5
5	Contamination, microbiological—potential for	463	4.9
6	Documentation—specification and testing	432	4.5
7	Status labeling—work in progress, facilities and equipment	371	3.9
8	Environmental monitoring	323	3.4
9	Process validation	317	3.3
10	Sampling—procedures and facilities	297	3.1

Reference 36

during 1995–2005. According to EMEA, deficiencies in quality, facility/equipment, manufacturing, and testing are highest among different categories of deficiencies[36] (Table 37.10).

As indicated above, globally, quality system has the highest rate of cGMP deficiency among other systems. The reason for such a high deficiency rate is likely due to the complexity, and the strict regulatory expectation, of the system. The following aspects are the important components of, and questions to ask for a quality system:

- Management controls, responsibility of a leader with executive power to develop and control of an effective quality organization and system;
- Written SOPs, GMP, and technical training and documentations;
- Corrective and preventive actions (CAPA):
  - Is there a CAPA system?
  - Are failure investigation procedures followed and recorded?
  - Are the root causes of quality problems identified?
  - What are the corrective and preventive actions?
  - Are the corrective actions implemented?
  - Are the corrective actions effective?
- Design controls;

- Deviation and OOS investigations;
- Production and process controls;
- Equipment and facility controls;
- Material controls;
- Records, documents, and change controls.

Deficiencies could exist in different ways and areas in pharmaceutical manufacturing. Examples of common deficiencies observed in the past include:[35]

1. Written procedures were not followed in production and process control.
2. The responsibilities and procedures for QC unit were not written or followed.
3. There were no written procedures for production and process controls designed to ensure that the drug products have the identity, strength, quality, and purity they purport or are represented to possess.
4. Testing and release of drug products did not include appropriate laboratory determination of satisfactory conformance to specifications prior to release.
5. Batch production and control records were not prepared for each batch of drug product or did not include complete information relating to each batch.
6. Control procedures were not established to monitor and validate the manufacturing processes that could be responsible for causing variability in the characteristics of in-process material and the drug product.
7. Employees were not trained in the particular operations they performed as part of their function.
8. Laboratory controls did not include the establishment of scientifically sound and appropriate specifications, standards, sampling plans or test procedures designed to ensure that the materials/components conform to appropriate standards of identity, strength, quality, and purity.
9. Drug product production and control records were not reviewed or approved by the quality control unit to determine the compliance with all established, approved written procedures before a batch is released or distributed.
10. Procedures describing the handling of all written and oral complaints regarding a drug product were not written or followed.

The minimum cGMP requirements for other systems related to manufacturing pharmaceutical products, and hence may be audited for compliance, can be found in 21 CFR Part 210 and 211. It should be noted that although process validation of batch manufacturing is required by cGMP, it is not required prior to approval, and not required for audit during PAI. Process validation for commercial manufacturing can be conducted later, but must be completed successfully before the product is shipped for marketing.

Early product R&D activities are not required to comply with cGMP, and, in the past, R&D data were not commonly audited during inspection. This is no longer the case at the present time. With the current requirement of using the common technical document (CTD) for filing, firms are required to submit a pharmaceutical development report in Section 3.2.P.2 and in the quality overall summary (QoS) for NDAs and ANDAs. It is common for industry to use R&D data in these sections for filing. Remember that one of the objectives of PAI is to audit the authenticity of data included in the submission. It is therefore apparent that the development data can be audited in the PAI with the current regulatory requirement.

37.6.3 Preparation

Preparation for a successful PAI is not a simple task to complete at the last minute of the new drug application process. The best way to prepare is to follow cGMP (21 CFR Parts 210 and 211) in all aspects, from the beginning and throughout the product development cycle. Among others, this includes cGMP training and education of all personnel involved to understand the regulatory requirements and the prospective of the FDA for PAI, implementing a quality system, having adequate written procedures, and following the procedures in all systems, to ensure that the drug development works are done right from the beginning and consistently throughout the development cycle, and finally putting all things into order for the inspection. It would be very difficult to prepare at the last minute if the work performed does not meet cGMP requirements. For information on what may be audited in PAI, readers are referred to the ORAs Guide to Inspections of Drugs.[34]

References for PAI preparation are available in the literature.[37] In order to coordinate and facilitate the PAI, a firm should establish a knowledgeable PAI team or task force responsible for the preparation, auditing, execution, and follow-up, with observations if there are any. Team members of this task force should include empowered people from product/analytical R&D, operation, quality, and regulatory affairs, depending on the complexity of the inspection. The responsibility of each team member should be clearly defined, and be coordinated by the team leader.

Overall, the responsibility of the PAI team includes the following:

- Develop a checklist for PAI;
- Conduct a gap analysis, and identify the tasks to be completed;
- Establish a schedule for completing the tasks, and follow up on the activities;
- Identify suitable people to assume the responsibility for the inspection, including subject experts and other roles, provide training to staff;
- Gather necessary documents and organize the documents in a suitable location to facilitate the inspection;
- Review or coordinate internal audit of all the documents, and prepare corrections or explanations if necessary;
- Verify the locations and amount of samples that may be collected by inspectors;
- Develop the logistics for audit;
- Work with the FDA inspectors during audit;
- Follow up with observations if there are any.

As discussed in the above section, the FDA inspectors will audit the authenticity of data in the submission, and evaluate the compliance with cGMP in pharmaceutical manufacturing. Documents that should be readily available for audit may include, but are not limited to, the following:

- Supportive document and data for the CMC sections in the NDA or ANDA:
  - Executed batch record of the biobatches or the primary stability batches,
  - Analytical method development and validation,
  - Specifications, laboratory test results, and stability data,
  - Dissolution profiles of oral solid dosage forms,
  - Product development report,
  - Process development report.
- SOPs.
- Exceptional document and investigation report.
- Cleaning validation protocol and results.
- Master batch record for commercial manufacturing.
- Design and validation/qualification of building/facility and water system.
- Validation/qualification/calibration records for equipment.
- Organization chart.
- Employee training record.

Inspectors may also collect the following samples of finished products and raw materials. The quantity of each sample can be found in FDA Program 7346.832.

- Method validation/verification sample of the biobatch, must be collected by the FDA, *not* prepared and packaged by the firm for pick-up, and not forwarded to the FDA by the firm.
- Profile samples:
  - Sample of biobatch.
  - Sample of the biotest portion of the biobatch sent to biotest laboratory.
  - Sample of innovator product sent to biotest laboratory.
  - Samples of excipients.
- Biotest sample:
  - Biobatch and innovator's product, collected at the biotest laboratory.
- Innovator sample:
  - Collected by the FDA from the innovator firm.

For the inspection, the site being audited should establish a dedicated conference room that is close to the documentation room, and is equipped with all necessary communication tools such as telephone, fax machine, copier, and documentation aids. The company should also assign people to assume different roles during the inspection, such as administrator, escort, scribe, runner, coordinator, and subject expert. Training should be provided for these roles. During the inspection, it is expected that the requested information/document will be readily available. If the requested information cannot be delivered in the expected time frame, an explanation should be provided. It is important to be honest in answering all questions. Don't lie or fabricate any information, under any circumstance. It is acceptable to ask for clarification if any question is not clear. You can also refer the questions to other qualified persons, if you are not in the position to answer or if you do not have the answers. Do not guess or speculate when you do not have the information or say anything that will not happen in a limited time frame. It is not recommended to be confrontational or argue destructively with inspectors or make a flat refusal to a request. Professional, truthful, respectful, and collaborative approaches are helpful to facilitate the audit and the decision-making processes for the NDA or ANDA.

37.6.4 Outcome of the Pre-approval Inspection

During the audit, inspectors may record any cGMP deficiency or deviations on FDA Form-483, Inspectional Observations. At the close of the inspection, Form 483 is provided to the company. It is a formal notification of the inspection findings. Items listed on the form are the opinion of the investigators, not yet the FDAs official position at the time inspection is

completed. The company has an initial opportunity to respond to the observation during an exit discussion with the inspector. Subsequently, a formal written response to the observations should be sent to the FDA. After leaving the inspection site, the inspectors will report the observations to the district office for review. If the deficiency is confirmed as significant, and the response from the company is not satisfactory, the FDA may issue a warning letter to the company, confirming the finding of significant deficiency as the FDAs position, and providing the opportunity to the company for voluntary correction. Based on the findings of the PAI, the district office will make a recommendation to the headquarters regarding the approval of the NDA or ANDA. The recommendation can be either approval or withholding approval. No application will be recommended for approval if the company is found to have significant cGMP violation, until satisfactory correction is made. If an unsatisfactory recommendation is made to the headquarters, the FDA will issue a not approval letter to the applicant. For generic drugs, approval will not occur until a reinspection is satisfactory, and an approval recommendation is made.

The warning letter may serve three purposes: (1) to officially notify the company and the public about the finding of significant regulatory violation; (2) to stimulate voluntary corrective action promptly; and (3) to establish a background of prior warning should further regulatory action by the FDA be needed at a later date.

Both Form 483 and the warning letter are serious documents that must be responded to carefully and promptly, e.g., within a week or two. In the response:

- Address the impact of each item on product quality.
- Determine the root cause of the problems.
- Provide a plan on how, when, and who will correct each of the observations, including the preventive actions to assure a true fix of the problem.
- If corrections have been made, provide pertinent documentation in support of corrective actions.
- If you do not agree with the FDA, provide reasons and documents to support your position.

In the response, develop the corrective actions from the quality system level. It is important not to commit any unworkable plans or unrealistic timelines, and any commitment made must be carried out promptly. Any undelivered promise will damage the credibility of the company, and raise more problems in the follow-up reinspection, leading to not approval of the NDA or ANDA. Persistent and significant GMP violations may lead to enforcement actions by the FDA.

For a company with approved products on the market, enforcement actions, such as recall, injunction, seizure, consent decree, prosecution, debarment or closing plant may be taken, if the significant violation in manufacturing is not corrected adequately in a timely manner.

37.6.5 Summary

To summarize, PAI is an integral part of the NDA or ANDA approval process. The purposes of the PAI are to verify the authenticity of data submitted in the applications, and to evaluate the cGMP compliance of the applicant. Application will not be approved if the applicant is found to have significant violation of cGMP. The best way to prepare for a successful PAI is to comply with cGMP consistently throughout the product development cycle. Proper training for personnel, good organization of documents, professional presentation, and honest and cooperative interaction with inspectors will facilitate the PAI process. When Form 483 or a warning letter is received after a PAI, careful response to the FDA in a timely manner to ensure that corrective actions are taken adequately and promptly will help to obtain the approval of the application from the FDA.

References

1. Federal Food Drug and Cosmetic Act. (2008). www.fda.gov/opacom/laws/fdcact/fdctoc.htm as of March 20.
2. FDA Guidance for Industry. (2000). Formal Meetings with Sponsors and Applicants for PDUFA Products, February.
3. Conformance Review Checklist for NDAs. (1999). January. www.fda.gov/cder/regulatory/ersr/ndaconform.pdf as of March 20, 2008.
4. FDA Draft guidance for Industry. (2003). Providing Regulatory Submissions in Electronic Format—General Considerations, October.
5. Electronic Code of Federal Regulations. (2008). http://ecfr.gpoaccess.gov/cgi/t/text/text-idx?c=ecfr&tpl=%2Findex.tpl as of March 20.
6. www.fda.gov/opacom/morechoices/fdaforms/default.html as of March 23, 2008.
7. FDA Guidance for Industry. (2008). M4: Organization of the CTD, August, 2001, ICH.
8. Structured Product Labeling Resources. www.fda.gov/oc/datacouncil/spl.html as of March 23.
9. FDA Draft Guidance for Industry. (2006). Labeling for Human Prescription Drug and Biological Products—Implementing the New Content and Format Requirements, January.
10. FDA Guidance Document. (2008). website: www.fda.gov/cder/guidance/index.htm as of March 23.
11. ICH website. (2008). http://www.ich.org, as of March 23.
12. FDA Guidance for Industry. (1998). Environmental Assessment of Human Drug and Biologics Applications, July.
13. ICH Q2A Guidance. (2005). Validation of Analytical Procedures: Text and Methodology, Q2(R1).
14. FDA Guidance to Industry. (1987). Guideline for the Format and Content of the Nonclinical Pharmacology/Toxicology Section of an Application, February.
15. ICH Guideline. (2000). Maintenance of the ICH Guideline on non-clinical safety studies for the conduct of human clinical trials for pharmaceuticals. M3(R1), Step 4, November 9.
16. FDA Guidance for Industry. Guideline for the Format and Content of the Microbiology Section of an Application.
17. ICH Guidelines. (2008). http://www.ich.org/cache/compo/276-254-1.html as of March.
18. FDA Guidance for Industry. (1988). Format and Content of the Clinical and Statistics Sections of an Application, July.
19. FDA Draft Guidance for Industry. (1998). Submitting Debarment Certification Statements, September.
20. FDA Guidance for Industry. (2008). Financial Disclosure by Clinical Investigators. http://www.fda.gov/oc/guidance/financialdis.html as of March 23.
21. http://www.ich.org/cache/compo/276-254-1.html
22. FDA Guidance for Industry. (2001). M4Q-CTD-Quality, August, ICH.
23. FDA guidance for industry. (2000). Waiver of In Vivo Bioavailability and Bioequivalence Studies for Immediate-Release Solid Oral Dosage Forms Based on a Biopharmaceutics Classification System, August.
24. Yu, L.X. (2007). Question-based review: A new pharmaceutical quality assessment system, an update. GPhA Fall Technical Conference, October 11.
25. ANDA Checklist for CTD or e-CTD Format. (2008). http://www.fda.gov/CDER/ogd/anda_checklist.pdf as of March 23.
26. ICH Guidance. (1997). General Considerations for Clinical Trials, E8, Step 4, July 17.
27. FDA Guidance for Industry. (2003). Bioavailability and Bioequivalence Studies for Orally Administered Drug Products—General Considerations, March.
28. Question-Based Review for CMC Evaluation of ANDAs. (2008). http://www.fda.gov/cder/OGD/QbR.htm as of March 23.
29. FDA. (2008). Pharmaceutical cGMP for the 21st Century—A Risk-based Approach-Final Report. http://www.fda.gov/cder/gmp/gmp2004/GMP_finalreport2004.htm as of March 23.
30. FDA Guidance for Industry. (2004). Changes to an Approved NDA or ANDA, April.
31. FDA Guidance for Industry. (2001). Changes to an Approved NDA or ANDA, Questions and Answers, January.
32. FDA Guidance for Industry. (2004). Changes to an Approved NDA or ANDA, Specifications—Use of Enforcement Discretion for Compendial Changes, November.
33. FDA. (2003). Pharmaceutical cGMP for the 21st Century—A Risk-Based Approach; Second Progress Report and Implementation Plan, http://www.fda.gov/cder/gmp/2ndProgressRept_Plan.htm as of March 24.
34. FDA. (2008). Internal Guide to Inspections of Drugs: www.fda.gov/ora/inspect_ref/igs/iglist.html as of March 24.
35. FDA. (2008). Presentation: System Inspection. http://www.fda.gov/cder/about/smallbiz/Presentations/6.ppt as of March 24.
36. EMEA. (2008). Good Manufacturing Practice: An analysis of regulatory inspection findings in the centralized procedure. Doc Ref: EMEA/INS/GMP/23022/2007, www.emea.europa.eu/Inspections/docs/2302207en.pdf as of March 24.
37. DeVito, J., Vudathala, G. & Tammara, V. (2006). Preparation for a regulatory pre-approval inspection. Clinical Research and Regulatory Affairs 23, 97–123.

Modern Pharmaceutical Quality Regulations: Question-based Review

Wenlei Jiang and Lawrence X. Yu

38.1 INTRODUCTION

The Food and Drug[1] Administration (FDA) drug regulations ensure that safe and effective drugs are available to the US public. Since the first original Pure Food and Drug Act published in 1906 to forbid manufacturers from adulterating or mislabeling products,[1] the drug regulations have gone through a metamorphosis over the past century. In response to specific health events and public needs, numerous pharmaceutical regulations and practices, including proof of safety and efficacy of drug products, ethical treatment of human subjects, and labeling, were established and improved throughout the years. In 1984, the Drug Price Competition and Patent Term Restoration Act authorized the FDA to accept abbreviated new drug applications (ANDAs) for generic versions of post-1962 drugs.[2] A generic drug is a drug that is produced and distributed without patent protection. It must contain the same active ingredient(s) as the reference listed drug (RLD), be identical in the strength, dosage form, and route of administration, have the same use of indications, be bioequivalent to the RLD, meet the same batch requirements for the identity, strength,

purity, and quality, and be manufactured under the strict standards of cGMP regulations. ARLD is a FDA approved drug product listed in the orange book,[3] e.g., an RLD can be an innovator drug that is protected by patents on its chemical formulation or manufacturing process. Since generic manufacturers do not incur the cost of drug discovery and clinical trials to prove drug safety and efficacy, generic drugs are often developed at a lower cost, and therefore typically sold at substantial discounts from the branded product price. ANDA approvals by the FDA Office of Generic drugs (OGD), and successful use of generic drug products by millions of patients, have resulted in substantial savings to consumers and the US Government.

Conventional drug manufacturing was generally accomplished by using batch processing with testing conducted on raw materials, in-process and final products to assure quality, i.e., quality by testing (QbT). The FDA oversees the quality of drug products, by reviewing applications and inspecting manufacturing facilities for conformance to requirements for current good manufacturing practice (cGMP). These two programs have served to help ensure the quality of drug products available in the US, and build the US public's confidence in pharmaceuticals' safety and efficacy. However, there are rising drug recall problems.[4] Drugs are delayed from the market, due to manufacturing problems. The pharmaceutical industry, unlike the food, chemicals, and semiconductor industries, did not benefit a great deal from recent progress in manufacturing

---

*The opinions expressed in this report by the authors do not necessarily reflect the views or policies of the Food and Drug Administration (FDA)

science on improving the manufacturing process while reducing costs.[5] In addition, the regulation of pharmaceutical manufacturing and product quality has remained stagnant since 1978, when the cGMP concept was first introduced.

There are strong needs for better, and less costly, pharmaceutical development and manufacturing pathways, as well as modern pharmaceutical regulations for safe and effective drugs. In 2002, the FDA announced a significant new initiative—*Pharmaceutical cGMPs for the 21st Century: A Risk-Based Approach*.[5] This initiative intends to enhance and modernize the FDAs regulation of pharmaceutical quality, and establish a new regulatory framework based on the latest science of risk management and quality assurance. Under this initiative, the FDA steer industry further in the direction of a quality by design (QbD) approach to drug product development, to ensure consistent product quality and encourage innovations. The pharmaceutical cGMPs for the twenty-first century initiative envisions that manufacturers have the ability to link process variability to product attributes, and are capable of controlling changes, and therefore can make manufacturing changes with less restrictive oversight from the FDA.[5]

This chapter first discusses challenges and issues with QbT and the old pharmaceutical assessment system, and then introduces the concepts and understanding of QbD for generic drugs. To implement underlying QbD principles and concepts, a new quality assessment system, question-based review (QbR), was developed by the FDA OGD for the chemistry, manufacturing, and controls (CMC) evaluation of ANDAs.[6] The impacts and benefits of QbR, as well as how QbR embodies QbD are illustrated in this chapter, to demonstrate that QbR is gradually transforming the CMC review into a modern, science and risk-based pharmaceutical quality assessment.

38.2 ISSUES WITH QbT AND THE OLD PHARMACEUTICAL QUALITY ASSESSMENT SYSTEM

Traditionally, pharmaceutical quality was defined as the drug meeting its prespecified quality attributes or regulatory specifications.[7] This old quality definition emphasized the importance of specification and testing, however, places little or no emphasis on clinical performance, and provides no link between the product quality attributes and clinical performance.

In the QbT approach, the FDA ensures quality via a fixed manufacturing process, tight specifications, and testing results on raw materials, in-process materials, and finished products. All pharmaceutical products in regulatory evaluation are weighted equally, without regard to the risk to the consumer,[6,8,9] for example, CMC review assessments of complex dosage forms (modified-release products, topicals, transdermals), as well as narrow therapeutic index (NTI) drugs, differ only marginally from those of simple dosage forms (many immediate-release solid oral products). The root causes of this QbT approach are limited understanding between product quality attributes and clinical performances, poor mechanistic understanding of the product and process, and insufficient communication between the pharmaceutical industry and the FDA.

Considering the above-mentioned limitations, QbT has caused some negative impacts, on both the pharmaceutical industry and the regulatory agencies.[6,8,9] Because of very rigid and inflexible specifications, sponsors may have to discard many products that failed the release specifications, but that may have acceptable clinical performance, resulting in excessive wastage. Significant industry and FDA resources were spent on issues related to establishment of specification acceptance criteria, testing control, and acceptable variability. In addition, sponsors have to file supplements, to report any change of process parameters specified in batch records.[10,11,12,13] As a result, the FDA has been overwhelmed by the volume of CMC supplements. For example, in 2005 and 2006, the FDA OGD received over 3000 CMC supplements annually. This burdensome regulatory requirement of supplements, in turn, discourages ANDA sponsors from continuously improving manufacturing processes, and introducing new technologies and innovations into pharmaceutical manufacturing. Furthermore, lack of risk assessment puts the ANDA sponsors at risk of insufficient control on complex dosage forms and narrow therapeutic index drugs. It also leads to poor allocation of review resources in the regulatory agency.

Besides testing, many current test methods have severe limitations in the mass production environment, such as sampling problems and representativeness.[7] For example, for a finished product, testing of 10 tablets out of several millions constrains the ability of the tested sample to adequately represent the variability of the entire batch. For in-process testing, large variability may be introduced via sample thieves in the traditional offline setting.

In summary, under QbT, product quality and performance are achieved predominantly by restricting flexibility in the manufacturing process, and by end product testing. The old pharmaceutical assessment system focuses more on end product testing results, rather than on how an efficient formulation and manufacturing process are designed to ensure product quality. Severe drawbacks exist with current test methods in the mass production environment. QbT is wasteful and inefficient. The wastage caused by the QbT approach could inflate production costs by as much as 10%.[14]

38.3 QUALITY BY DESIGN

Over the last two decades, there have been an increased number of pharmaceutical products, and a greater role of medicines in healthcare. The number of foreign applications has increased, along with the globalization of the pharmaceutical industry. The rate of increase in regulatory submissions has outpaced the rate of growth of the review resources. These pharmaceutical and regulatory environment changes, *a priori* mentioned technical and regulatory issues with QbT and the old pharmaceutical assessment system, along with advancements in manufacturing sciences,[15] have accelerated the need for a modern regulatory framework that encourages risk and science-based, cost-efficient, continuously improved pharmaceutical development and regulatory quality assessment.

In 2002, the FDA announced a new initiative (*cGMPs for the 21st Century: A Risk-Based Approach*).[5] This initiative intended to modernize the FDAs regulation of pharmaceutical quality, and establish a new regulatory framework focused on quality by design (QbD), risk management, and quality systems.[5] The initiative challenged the industry to look beyond QbT for ensuring product quality and performance.

Woodcock defined pharmaceutical quality as a product that is free of contamination and reproducible, delivering the therapeutic benefit promised on the label to the consumer.[7] This definition of product quality centers on the performance of the drug product, and connects the product quality attributes with clinical performance. Furthermore, it points out that pharmaceutical quality cannot merely be derived from performance of test batches, but has to be scientifically designed in the product, to meet specific objectives.

QbD is a systematic approach to development that begins with predefined objectives, and emphasizes product and process understanding and process control, based on sound science and quality risk management.[16] QbD requires an understanding of how formulation and process variables influence product quality. For example, under QbD, the specifications for raw materials, in-process controls, and finished products are established based on mechanistic understanding of how formulation and process factors impact product and process performance, while ones under QbT are derived empirically from limited batch data.

Further, the specifications under QbD are solely used for the confirmation of product quality, not for assurance of manufacturing consistency and process control. Moreover, the in-process control in QbD can provide feedback to the system; manufacturers have the ability to effect continuous improvement and continuous "real-time" assurance of quality.

Generic and innovator drugs have the same product safety, efficacy, and quality. However, the development approach and environment of generic drug product differs slightly from those of innovator drug products. For example, innovator companies design the drug substance and drug product, whereas the ANDA sponsors design to duplicate the drug product. A generic drug must meet the same requirements for identity, purity, quality, stability, and comply with the same rigid standards of GMP regulations for manufacturing as the innovator product. Nevertheless, ANDA sponsors need not repeat costly animal and clinical research on active ingredients or dosage forms already approved for safety and effectiveness. Instead, they face the challenges of bioequivalence requirements, and the constraints of patent issues. ANDA sponsors spend much less time and resources than innovator companies to develop a drug product, usually about 12–18 months and $3 million. For the drug substances, innovator companies discover and manufacture their own active pharmaceutical ingredients (APIs), while ANDA sponsors often source them from outside firms.

Considering these specific aspects of generic drug development, Lionberger et al. proposed that a QbD development process for generics may include the following elements:[17]

- begin with a target product profile (TPP) that describes the use, safety, and efficacy of the product;
- define a target product quality profile (TPQP) that is used by formulators and process engineers as a quantitative surrogate for aspects of clinical safety and efficacy during product development;
- gather relevant prior knowledge about the drug substance, potential excipients, and process operations into a knowledge space. Use risk assessment to prioritize knowledge gaps for further investigation;
- design a formulation and identify the critical material attributes (CMA) of the final product that must be controlled to meet the target product quality profile;
- design a manufacturing process to produce a final product having these critical material attributes;
- identify critical process parameters (CPP) and input (raw) material attributes that must

be controlled to achieve the critical material attributes of the final product. Use risk assessment to prioritize process parameters and material attributes for experimental verification. Combine prior knowledge with experiments to establish a design space or other representation of process understanding;

- establish a control strategy for the entire process. The strategy may include input material controls, process controls and monitors, design spaces around individual or multiple unit operations, and final product tests. The strategy should encompass expected changes in scale;
- constantly monitor and update the process to ensure consistent quality.

Table 38.1 presents a summary of the key terminology in QbD.[16,17,18] Compared to QbD for innovator drugs, there are several unique aspects of generic QbD. First, the TPP and TPQP of generic drug products are well-defined and can be readily obtained from NDA products. Secondly, biopharmaceutical properties of APIs, such as polymorphism, absorption, and pharmacokinetic information, are often known to ANDA sponsors from innovator companies' published data or scientific literature. Some physico-chemical properties of drug substances, including solubility, impurity profile, and stability, may also be obtained from drug master file (DMF) holders. Thirdly, because of the rich generic drug product pool, ANDA sponsors have accumulated strong experiences in formulation

TABLE 38.1　Key terminologies in quality by design (QbD)[16,17,18,49]

Terminology	Definition	Notes
Target product profile (TPP)	The TPP provides a statement of the overall intent of the drug development program, and gives information about the drug at a particular time in development. TPP is organized according to the key sections in the drug labeling and links drug development activities to specific concepts intended for inclusion in the drug labeling	Route of administration, dosage form and size, maximum and minimum doses, pharmaceutical elegance (appearance), and target patient population are included in TPP
Target product quality profile (TPQP)	TPQP is a quantitative surrogate for aspects of clinical safety and efficacy that can be used to design and optimize formulation and manufacturing process. It should include quantitative targets for impurities and stability, release profiles (dissolution) and other product specific performance requirements	For IR product, TPQP includes acceptable tablet characteristics, rapid and complete dissolution, assay, stability, purity, dissolution, bioequivalence (for generic drugs)
Critical material attributes (CMA)	CMA are physical, chemical, biological or microbiological properties or characteristics of materials including drug substance, excipients, in-process materials and drug product, that need to be controlled to ensure the desired product quality	e.g., drug substance impurity, particle size, in-process material moisture content, and/or tablet hardness
Critical quality attributes (CQA)	CQAs are physical, chemical, biological or microbiological properties or characteristics that need to be controlled (directly or indirectly) or within an appropriate limit, range, or distribution to ensure the desired product quality	Elements of TPQP (e.g., dissolution) and TPP, CMA of drug substance, excipients, in-process materials and drug product and critical process parameters can be examples of CQA
Process parameter	Process parameter refers to input operating parameters and process state variables of a process or unit operation	e.g., mixing speed, flow rate, temperature, pressure
Key process parameter (KPP)	KPP are process parameters that are important and even essential to product quality. KPP may be critical or non-critical	e.g., impeller speed, KPP is usually determined via prior knowledge and experience
Critical process parameter (CPP)	A parameter is critical when a realistic change in that parameter can cause the product to fail to meet TPQP	e.g., impeller speed, CPP can be identified via process development studies, prior knowledge and experience
Design space	The multidimensional combination and interaction of input variables (e.g., material attributes) and process parameters that have been demonstrated to provide assurance of quality	A design space may be constructed for a single unit operation, multiple unit operations, or for the entire process. Design space is not a check-box requirement
Control space	The upper and/or lower limits for the critical raw material attributes and process parameters between which the parameter and material are routinely controlled during production in order to assure reproducibility	A control space should be within a design space

and manufacturing process development, especially with conventional solid dosage forms. To save development time and improve efficiency, some firms may establish an internal formulation database system or a decision tree of formulation selection, based on drug substance properties and expected product performance. Similarly to formulation selection, an internal database or a decision tree of process selection, based on formulation properties and product performance, may also exist.

ANDA sponsors should take advantage of the uniqueness of QbD for generic drug, and fully utilize their formulation and process development experiences in their drug product development process. When fully deployed, QbD means that critical quality attributes of the drug product, including critical material attributes of the finished product (elements of TPQP), critical raw material attributes (critical drug substance and excipient properties), and critical process parameters, are identified and well-understood. Further, relationships between critical material attributes and CPP are established, leading to proper control of the process or even self-control and continuous improvement of the process. Successful deployment of QbD will produce significant business benefits, including reduced batch failure rates, reduced final product testing, lower batch release costs, lower operating costs, and potentially faster regulatory approval.[19]

38.4 QUESTION-BASED REVIEW FOR GENERIC DRUGS

To gain marketing access in the US, a sponsor must submit an ANDA to the FDA OGD for review and approval of a proposed generic drug product. The ANDA must have information to show that the proposed generic product is pharmaceutically equivalent and bioequivalent, and therefore therapeutically equivalent, to the RLD. Pharmaceutical equivalence[20] means that the drug product contains the "same" active ingredient(s) as the RLD, and they are identical in strength, dosage form, route of administration, and that they meet the same or compendial or other applicable standards of strength, quality, purity, and identity. Bioequivalence[21] indicates the active drug ingredient or active moiety in the test product must exhibit the same rate and extent of absorption as the RLD. In addition, the sponsor must show that the proposed product is appropriately labeled, and that it is manufactured in compliance with good manufacturing practice (cGMP) guidelines. After ANDA approval

by the FDA OGD, the sponsor may manufacture and market the generic drug product in the US.

Figure 38.1 provides a comparison between the requirements of a NDA, and an ANDA. The main difference between the requirements of a NDA and an ANDA is that the preclinical and clinical data in the NDA that establishes the safety and efficacy of the API does not need to be repeated for the ANDA, since these trials have already been conducted by innovator companies. Nevertheless, the ANDA sponsors need to submit bioequivalence trial data for evaluation. The remaining requirements, including those for chemistry, manufacturing, controls, testing, and labeling, are similar for both an ANDA and a NDA.

The chemistry, manufacturing, and controls documentation of an ANDA consists of information on the drug substance, including characterization, method of manufacture, and controls, and information on the drug product, including composition, controls, method of manufacture, packaging, and stability. To ensure the quality of the drug product, the CMC data of an ANDA are carefully examined before approval.

In response to the FDAs Pharmaceutical cGMPs and QbD initiatives, generic sponsors are urged to implement QbD in drug product development and manufacturing. Accordingly, the FDA OGD developed a new quality assessment system that enables assessment and promotion of QbD in ANDAs, i.e., question-based review (QbR) (Figure 38.2). The QbR contains a series of scientific and regulatory questions that would appropriately assess critical quality attributes, formulation, manufacturing process parameters, and controls, to establish regulatory specifications relevant to product performance, and to prepare a consistent and comprehensive evaluation of the ANDA. Appendix A lists all the FDA QbR questions.[22]

The development of QbR follows four underlying principles:[10]

- quality built in by design, development, and manufacture, and comfirmed by testing;

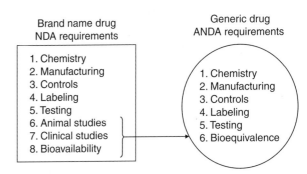

FIGURE 38.1 A new drug application (NDA) versus an abbreviated new drug application (ANDA) review process

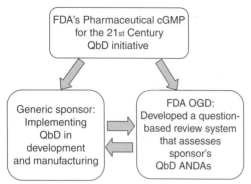

FIGURE 38.2 The Food and Drug Administration's cGMP initiative: quality by design, and question-based review

- risk-based approach to maximize economy of time, effort, and resources;
- preservation of the best practices of the old OGD review system and organization;
- best available science and open communication with stakeholders.

Under the QbR system, ANDAs are submitted in common technical document (CTD) format, and include a pharmaceutical development section, as outlined in the International Conference on Harmonisation (ICH) Q8, and a quality overall summary (QOS) that addresses all the QbR questions. QOS models for an immediate-release and an extended-release dosage form posted on the FDA OGD website give examples of the types of information expected within an ANDA submission.[23]

For CMC reviews, the sponsor-prepared QOS provides the primary reviewer with a quick overview of the entire CMC package, and reduces the review time spent on documentation. Pharmaceutical development information helps reviewers to have a better understanding of how drug substance and formulation variables affect the performance and stability of the drug product, and establishes appropriate performance-based specifications.

Due to its significant benefits, QbR was well-received by ANDA sponsors and the FDA OGD chemistry reviewers, and has both parties commitment. In July 2007, more than 90% of ANDA submissions included a quality overall summary that answered the QbR questions with every ANDA submission.[24] Details about the impact and benefits of QbR are discussed in several commentary papers[6,8,10,25] and will not be repeated here.

38.5 QbR QUESTIONS EMBODY QbD

QbR questions are designed to assess, concretely and practically, ANDA sponsors' implementation of concepts and principles of quality by design. The FDA OGD asks the following questions relevant to QbD. How these QbR questions embody the QbD is elaborated below.[8,17,26]

38.5.1 Questions Related to Desired Product Performance

What Attributes Should the Drug Product Possess?

This question requests the ANDA applicant to clearly define TPP and TPQP at the beginning of development. TPP is primarily expressed in clinical terms, such as clinical pharmacology, indications and usage, contraindications, warnings, precautions, adverse reactions, drug abuse and dependence, overdosage, etc, which can be readily obtained from the labeling section of the RLD.[8] A generic drug product is therapeutically equivalent to the RLD in terms of dosage form, strength, route of administration, quality, performance characteristics, safety, and intended use. Therefore, a generic version and its RLD would be expected to have the same TPP.

The target product quality profile (TPQP) includes the quality characteristics, e.g., identity, assay, dissolution profile, dosage form, purity, stability, and bioequivalence, that the drug product should possess in order to deliver the therapeutic benefit promised in the TPP.[8] Some of the TPQPs of a generic drug can be determined from the RLD, by reverse engineering. Reverse-engineering on the RLD includes physical, chemical, and packaging characterization. For solid tablets, physical characterization may include size, weight and shape, while chemical characterization may include dissolution profile, purity profile, stability, content uniformity, excipient grade and amount. Packaging characterization focuses on what type of desiccant or O_2 scavengers are used. Elements of TPQP are also termed as critical material attributes of the finished drug product. Along with other available information from the scientific literature and possibly the pharmacopeia, the TPQP can be used to define product specifications, to some extent, even before the product is developed. With clear TPP and TPQP defined, formulation scientists can establish strategies, and keep formulation effort focused and efficient.

Do the Differences Between this Formulation and the RLD Present Potential Concerns with Respect to Therapeutic Equivalence?

It is acceptable that an ANDA product may have different inactive ingredients or a different formulation mechanism, as long as the product performance and safety are equivalent to the RLD. Several specific dosage forms have stricter requirements with regard to inactive ingredients, as indicated in the Code of Federal Register (CFR). For example, parenteral solutions must be Q1 (the same inactive ingredients), and Q2 (the same concentration of inactive ingredients), except for preservative, buffer or antioxidant.[27] For modified-release products, if a formulation with a different release mechanism from the RLD is used, the ANDA sponsor needs to explain the differences, and provide comparative dissolution data between the RLD and the ANDA products in multiple dissolution media. In addition, it is possible for two products with very different plasma concentration profiles (such as different shapes or different T_{max}) to have equivalent AUC and C_{max}. The sponsor needs to provide justification as to why the differences in plasma concentration profiles do not affect the therapeutic equivalence. Satisfactory answers to this question demonstrate scientific understanding of the ANDA sponsor to the underlying formulation design and biopharmaceutical principles.

38.5.2 Questions Related to Product Design

How was the Drug Product Designed to have these Attributes?

By answering this question, the ANDA sponsor informs the FDA how they design their product to be bioequivalent to the RLD, and meet other aspects of TPQP. A generic drug development scientist usually starts product design with studies of innovator product intellectual property, reverse engineering of the RLD, and preformulation. After studying the intellectual property of the RLD, the generic sponsors may elect to go around the patent or follow the patent, and market the product prior to or after the patent exclusivity has expired. With the data obtained from reverse-engineering on the RLD, they may discuss the intended dissolution or drug release profile, the choice of release mechanism, and identification of critical formulation and manufacturing variables that were adjusted to yield a bioequivalent product. If a design of experiment (DOE) was used to identify which formulation variables were critical, then it should be described in this question. With preformulation data, they may identify critical material attributes of drug substance that may affect manufacturing and product performance. For example, for problematic drugs, they may include discussion on selection of formulation strategies based on prior knowledge, to overcome limitations of the drug substance such as poor solubility, poor dissolution, poor permeability, poor stability or short plasma duration.

Were Alternative Formulations or Mechanisms Investigated?

Usually, for complex formulations, the ANDA sponsor has multiple candidate formulations investigated during drug product development. This question encourages the ANDA sponsor to share formulation development information with the FDA, e.g., studies used to adjust formulation or manufacturing variables, to obtain a bioequivalent product by either DOE or a trial-and-error process. This development information may be used for purposes such as to:

- assess post-approval formulation changes;
- develop dissolution;
- set acceptance limits on raw material or drug substance properties.

How were the Excipients and their Grades Selected?

In this question, the selection of excipients and grades that provide the functionality is described. It is important to indicate when a grade of excipient has been discovered to be critical. For example, when the polymer molecular weight and particle size are found to affect the release of a sustained release tablet, the relevant information should be documented in the answer. If necessary, control of grade is established to ensure the quality of the finished drug product.

How was the Final Formulation Optimized?

An optimization study is distinguished from an early screening study that explores a large range of space. An optimization study is more like fine tuning, and evaluates relatively small variations around a target formulation. A formulation optimization will establish the robustness of the formulation, and may support a design space for the formulation composition. Formulation optimization may also be conducted to optimize the manufacturing process, such as determining the optimal lubricant level.

Which Properties or Physico-chemical Characteristics of the Drug Substance Affect Drug Product Development, Manufacture or Performance?

Typical drug substance properties include physical, chemical, biological, and mechanical properties. Details of these properties are presented in Table 38.2.[28,29] Solid understanding and characterization of drug substance properties are crucial to the successful development of a robust formulation and manufacturing process.

TABLE 38.2   Typical drug substance properties[28,29]

Physical and mechanical property	Color, odor, particle size distribution, shape, crystallinity, polymorphic form, hygroscopicity, bulk density, tapped density, true density, surface area, electrostatic charge, surface energy, elasticity, plasticity (ductility), viscoelasticity, brittleness
Chemical property	pKa, aqueous solubility as a function of pH, chemical stability in solid-state and solution state, photolytic and oxidative stability
Biological property	partition coefficient, membrane permeability, and/or oral bioavailability

Besides collecting information from literature and DMF sponsors, the generic sponsors are strongly encouraged to perform their own preformulation studies to obtain some key properties of drug substance, such as pH-solubility and stability profile, solid polymorphisms, bulk and tap density, etc. The impact of pharmaceutical solid polymorphism on product quality and performance has received much attention recently, and the findings have been presented in several review articles.[30,31,32] Decision trees that provide recommendations on monitoring and controlling polymorphs in drug substances and/or drug products can be referred to the recently published guidance.[33]

Based on the aqueous solubility, dose, and intestinal permeability of drug substance, the ANDA sponsors may want to determine its Biopharmaceutics Classification System (BCS) class.[34,35] With BCS class identified, the ANDA sponsors can understand and identify what may be the key properties or critical material attributes that affect the drug product development, and propose reasonable formulation strategies. For example, for class II drug substances (low solubility and high permeability), particle size reduction may be proposed as a formulation approach to improve delivery and manufacturability of a dissolution-limited drug substance. For a drug with $10\mu g/ml$ solubility, in order for the drug product to achieve 80% dissolution in 30 minutes, the particle size has to be reduced to about $10\mu m$ (assuming log-normal distribution, sink conditions, spheres).[36] Rohrs et al. published a paper to predict the effect of particle size distribution on content uniformity.[37] For a 1 mg dose, the particle size of drug substance, with very broad distribution (e.g., geometric standard deviation is 3.5), is predicted to be about $15\mu m$ to pass the USP 905 stage 1 content uniformity test for tablets, whereas for monodisperse particles (e.g., geometric standard deviation is 1), particles around $150\mu m$ are able to meet the content uniformity requirement. In these examples, particle size

and distribution of drug substance are critical material attributes which need to be controlled to ensure product quality, and their specifications can be set based on understanding how they affect product performance.

In another example, oxidative degradation of the drug substance may require a stabilizer to be included in the formulation. We first need to understand the oxidation mechanisms of the drug substance, and then select appropriate stabilization strategies.[38,39] If the drug substance oxidation is heavy metal catalyzed, chelators such as EDTA and citric acid should be used in the formulation. In cases where peroxides are believed to be the problem, stabilization strategies can be focused on careful selection of excipients with lower peroxide levels, lower concentrations of suspect excipients, and use of antioxidants.

What Evidence Supports Compatibility Between the Excipients and the Drug Substance?

Quality by design requires identification of mechanistic and formulation factors that affect drug product stability. Acceptable finished drug product stability cannot be accepted as evidence of excipient–drug substance compatibility, since end product testing only demonstrates that the quality was reached for the tested samples, but does not address how the product is designed to achieve the quality. Based on ICH Q8 recommendations, a drug substance/excipient compatibility study should be evaluated as a part of pharmaceutical development.[40]

Typically, a drug substance/excipient compatibility study is performed with binary mixtures which are prepared in the presence/absence of added water, stored at accelerated conditions, and then analyzed by stability-indicated methodology, such as HPLC.[39,41] The addition of water allows the pH of the drug–excipient blend and the role of moisture to be investigated. Alternatively, thermal analysis methods, including differential scanning calorimetry (DSC) and isothermal calorimetry (ITC), are used to screen binary mixtures for their compatibility. However, data obtained via DSC/ITC are sometimes difficult to interpret or even misleading.[39,42]

Binary mixture approach is simple, but time and resource intensive, and may differ completely from a multi-component system.[41] Due to these concerns, the ANDA sponsors can also perform drug–excipient compatibility studies via a prototype/trial formulation approach, with binary systems as a diagnostic back-up. In this complementary fashion, formulators may select one promising prototype formulation to move forward and identify any "culprit" excipient causing stability issues. The sponsor should use prior knowledge to justify inclusion or exclusion of certain excipients. For example, if the drug substance is a primary amine, and known to react with reducing sugar, the sponsor can include this as a rationale for not having lactose tested in the excipient compatibility studies. In addition, DOE can be applied in the compatibility study, to determine the chemical interactions among components.

When the ANDA is Q1 and Q2 the same as the RLD, in the absence of known stability problems, historical data may be acceptable in lieu of compatibility studies. However, ANDA sponsors should be cautioned that there might be incompatibilities between drug substance and excipients used in the RLD. A systemic drug–excipient compatibility study will equip the product development scientist with a mechanistic understanding of formulation factors that affect drug product stability, and reduce formulation risk, leading to a decrease in development time and costs.

TABLE 38.3 Examples of pros and cons of typical tablet manufacturing process[36]

Tablet manufacturing process	Pros	Cons
Direct compression	Simplified process, retains compactibility of materials	Segregation Flow
Dry granulation	Overcomes poor physical properties of API (particle size, shape)	Longer processing time, may compromise compactibility
Wet granulation	Improves uniformity, flow and compactibility	Physical and chemical stability
		Residual solvents (non-aqueous granulation)

What Specific Container Closure Attributes are Necessary to Ensure Product Quality?

The ANDA sponsor may give the rationale, e.g., drug product stability concerns, for selecting a particular container closure system, including light resistance, moisture protection or inert atmosphere. For example, when atmospheric oxygen is the source of drug oxidation, the formulator can select appropriatce packaging material (material with lower oxygen transmission rate) and packaging methods (packaging under inert gas) to overcome the oxidation problems.[38] Controlling the oxygen permeability and headspace oxygen in bottles is appropriate for drug product shelf stability, but cannot ensure drug stability after the consumer has opened the product. Therefore, blister packaging may need to be used for some extremely oxygen-sensitive drugs.

38.5.3 Questions Related to Process Design

What are the Unit Operations in the Drug Product Manufacturing Process?

Why was the Manufacturing Process Selected for this Drug Product?

The sponsor should list unit operations in the drug product manufacturing process, and indicate the factors considered during manufacturing process selection, including the properties of the drug substance, the desired characteristics of the drug product, the complexity and robustness of the process, in-house process expertise, facility and equipment availability.

Table 38.3 lists common tablet manufacturing processes, and their pros and cons.[36] For example, for a drug with poor flowability and high drug loading, the granulation process may be considered to overcome the potential processing issues. Once the process is selected, a sponsor should focus on the description of rationales to select a particular method when multiple alternatives are available (e.g., rationale for the selection of single pot granulation versus high shear granulation/fluid-bed drying combination). Rationales can include scalability, yield, formulation aspects, expected granule characteristics, etc.[43] For granules that need to dissolve quickly, granulation techniques with lower shear forces, e.g., spray drying, can be selected. Spray drying produces granules with a more open, porous structure, but mechanically less stable.

Depending upon the product being developed, type of process, and process knowledge the development scientists have, it may be necessary to conduct preliminary feasibility studies prior to process development.

How are the Manufacturing Steps (Unit Operations) Related to the Drug Product Quality?

This question is designed to connect the unit operations to the TPQP, and identify which unit operations are critical steps, through risk management analysis, prior knowledge, and pilot-scale studies. Once a step is identified as being critical, then the sponsor must design their process to ensure that this step succeeds or have tests in place to detect if the step fails. For example, for a formulation with low drug loading, the mixing process (a manufacturing step) is considered critical to have the desired content uniformity (a TPQP). Geometric dilution, multiple sieving, and the blending process may be selected for this formulation. In addition, blend uniformity and powder flow testing will be employed to ensure ideal blend properties, to achieve desired content uniformity. In another example, controlled-release coating is predicted to affect the product dissolution profile. Tablet weight gain, and surface roughness, may be monitored and correlate with the dissolution profile. It is suggested that the ANDA sponsor presents the relationship between unit operations and quality attributes of the drug product in the form of a matrix, as shown in Table 38.4.

38.5.4 Questions Related to Process Understanding and Control

How were the Critical Process Parameters Identified, Monitored, and/or Controlled?

First, the sponsor needs to identify all the process parameters and material attributes of the raw materials, intermediate materials, and drug product, based on prior experience and knowledge. Risk management and analysis determine the limited number of potentially critical parameters and material attributes for further investigations. Table 38.5 lists typical tablet manufacturing unit operations, potential process parameters, and material attributes of solid dosage forms.[8]

Secondly, CPP and CMA are identified by scientific investigations and controlled variations of operating parameters among potential CPP and CMA. In addition, equipment maintenance, operator training, standard of operation (SOP) related to the specific product manufacturing, and facility supporting systems may link to product quality, directly or indirectly. Therefore, risk assessment should also be employed to reduce the potential CPP and CMA to be investigated. Studies to identify CPP, CMA, and their functional relationships can be conducted at pilot- or laboratory-scale, and do not need to be conducted under cGMP.

Thirdly, CPPs, CMAs, and their functional relationships are considered during scale-up. Some CPPs may be scale-dependent, while others are not. Therefore, when scaling-up, additional experimental work may be needed to determine if the model generated at the small-scale is predictive at the large-scale. Prior knowledge can play a very significant role in this regard, as most generic companies use the same manufacturing technologies and raw materials on a regular basis. Monitoring CMA of in-process material properties makes scaling less equipment-dependent as opposed to only monitoring CPP.

Finally, after the scale-sensitivity of CPP and CMA are established, appropriate control strategies can be designed, including input material controls, process controls and monitoring, and/or final product specifications used to ensure consistent quality.

The most basic control is to have knowledge of the operating range, as well as the proven acceptable range of the process parameters. Proven acceptable range is defined as a characterized range of a process parameter for which operation within this range will result in producing a material meeting the relevant quality criteria, while keeping the other parameters constant.[44] The operating range is within the proven acceptable range, and is the routine control parameter during production in order to assure reproducibility.[44] Proven acceptable range is based on univariate experimentation, and does not take account of interaction of multiple process parameters. Proven acceptable range can provide some information about process, but limited.

In the presence of interacting critical process parameters and critical material attributes, a design space is a better approach to ensure product quality, although it is not a check-box requirement. Design space is the multidimensional combination and interaction of input variables (e.g., material attributes) and process parameters that have been demonstrated to provide assurance of quality.[16,40] For generic drugs, the design space is likely established using DOE at small-scale batches, verified at commercial scale. It is best to exploit dimensionless parameters and material attributes to define the design space, as they are scale-independent. Design space is proposed by the applicant, and is subject to regulatory assessment and approval. Working within the FDA approved design space is not considered a manufacturing change. Movement out of

TABLE 38.4   Effect of raw material and manufacturing processes on quality attributes of the drug product

	Raw material	Drug layering	CR coating	Encapsulation
Purity	High			
Assay/content uniformity		High		High
Release profile	High		High	High
Stability			High	

TABLE 38.5 Typical unit operations, key process parameters, and key quality attributes for tableting[8]

Pharmaceutical unit operation	Example key process parameter	Potential quality attributes
Mixing	• Type and geometry of mixer • Order of addition • Mixer load level • Number of rotations (time and speed) • Agitating bar (on/off pattern)	• Blend uniformity • Particle size distribution • Bulk/tapped density • Moisture content • Flow properties
Milling	Impact/cutting/screening mills • Mill type • Speed • Blade configuration and type • Screen size and type • Feeding rate Fluid energy mill • Number of grinding nozzles • Feed rate • Nozzle pressure • Classifier	• Particle size • Particle size distribution • Particle shape • Bulk/tapped density • Flow properties • Polymorphic form
Wet granulation	High shear granulation • Pre-binder addition mix time • Impeller speed, configuration, and location • Chopper speed, configuration • Spray nozzle type and location • Method of binder addition • Binder fluid temperature • Binder addition rate and time • Post-granulation mix time • Bowel temperature Fluid-bed granulations • Mixing time • Spray nozzle (type/quantity/ pattern/configuration) • Method of binder addition • Binder fluid temperature • Binder fluid addition rate and time • Inlet air flow rate, volume, temperature, and dew point • Exhaust air temperature, flow • Filter properties and size • Shaking intervals • Product temperature	• Power consumption (process control) • Blend uniformity • Flow • Moisture content • Particle size and distribution • Granule size and distribution • Granule strength and uniformity • Solid form
Drying	Fluidized-bed • Inlet air volume, temperature, dew point • Exhaust air temperature, flow • Filter properties • Shaking intervals • Product temperature • Total drying time Tray • Quantity carts and trays per chamber • Quantity of product per tray • Drying time and temperature • Air flow • Inlet dew point	• Granule size and distribution • Granule strength, and uniformity • Particle size • Flow • Bulk/tapped density • Moisture content • Residual solvents

(Continued)

TABLE 38.5   (Continued)

Pharmaceutical unit operation	Example key process parameter	Potential quality attributes
	Vacuum/microwave • Jacket temperature • Condenser temperature • Impeller speed • Vacuum strength • Microwave potency • Electric field • Energy supplied • Product temperature	
Roller compaction	• Roll speed • Gap setting • Roll pressure • Auger screw rate • Roller type	• Appearance • Ribbon/particle size and shape • Ribbon density, strength, and thickness • Solid form
Compaction	• Compression speed and force • Pre-compression force • Feed frame type and speed • Hopper design, height, and vibration • Tablet weight and thickness • Depth of fill • Punch penetration depth	• Target weight • Weight uniformity • Content uniformity • Hardness • Thickness • Tablet porosity • Friability • Visual attributes • Moisture content
Coating Fluid bed, Pan	• Product temperature • Total pre-heating time • Spray nozzle (type/quantity/ pattern/configuration) • Individual gun spray rate • Total spray rate • Pan rotation speed • Atomization air pressure • Pattern air pressure • Inlet air flow, temperature, dew point • Exhaust air temperature, air flow • Product temperature • Total coating time	• Weight of core tablets • Appearance • Visual attributes • Percentage weight gain • Film thickness • Color uniformity • Hardness • Thickness • Friability

the design space is considered to be a change, and would normally initiate a regulatory post-approval change process. Control space is within the design space, and not subject to regulatory approval. If the control space is much smaller than the design space, the process is then considered robust.

A problem with design space is that it can limit flexibility, and pursuit of a design space may move away from a flexible manufacturing process.[17] An alternative to design space-based control strategies is active control with the application of process analytical technology (PAT). PAT is a system for designing, analyzing, and controlling manufacturing through timely measurements (i.e., during processing) of critical quality and performance attributes of raw and in-process materials and processes, with the goal of ensuring final product quality.[45]

PAT can be utilized offline, atline, online, and inline, and its implementation in different solid dose unit operations is summarized in Table 38.6.[17] In the blending process, the use of online NIR can evaluate the mixing status of API and excipients, and monitor compositional variability over the entire blending time, rather than the traditional one-time end blending sampling points. This allows for the evaluation of segregation or demixing potential, and identifies the safe-zone of uniform mixing or the most appropriate mixing time. Understanding of critical processes, as well as justification of process parameters and in-process specification ranges via PAT work, provides superior control quality. Ideally, PAT can help provide feedback to the control system, and manufacturers have the ability to effect continuous improvement and continuous "real-time" assurance of quality. Nevertheless, there are some regulatory, QA, cGMP, and

TABLE 38.6 Process analytical technology (PAT) implementation in solid oral unit operation and its benefits in product development[47]

Unit operation	PAT technologies employed	Benefits in product development
Particle size reduction	NIR spectroscopy	Design/control milling process of API and in-process agglomerates
Blending/mixing	NIR spectroscopy FT-Raman spectroscopy	Identify safe-zone and the most appropriate mixing time
Granulation	NIR, Raman XPRD spectroscopy Thermal effusivity Combination of an image-process device and a fuzzy control system Acoustic emission Stress fluctuation spectroscopy	Justify granulation process parameter ranges with controlled granulation quality
Drying	NIR spectroscopy	Identifying drying curve and end point Justify moisture content specifications
Coating	NIR spectroscopy Raman spectroscopy	Determine coating rate and end point with minimized manufacturing variability; interpret coating uniformity
Unit dosing (compression or encapsulation)	NIR spectroscopy Raman spectroscopy	Detect drug distribution uniformity in finished product. Identify undesired process deviation

validation challenges associated with the adoption of PAT. Pharmaceutical industries are strongly encouraged to prepare for the challenges, and promote drug product development and process understanding via PAT efforts. The FDA has approved a number of applications that implemented PAT, including drug substance and drug product manufacturing processes for innovator products, generic products, and veterinary products, demonstrating success with this initiative.

What is the Scale-up Experience with the Unit Operations in this Process?

Under this question, the ANDA sponsor needs to summarize the scale-up plan, and the process development studies that support it. Valuable scale-up experience includes experience with most recent ANDAs, using the same unit operations, literature references/vendor scale-up factors, and the laboratory scale to exhibit batch process transfer for this product, exhibit batch production, as well as modeling and dimensional analysis. For reference to other ANDAs, similarity of dosage form, physical properties of the drug, excipients, equipment, and change of scale should be considered. Pharmaceutical development scientists can also make use of computer-aided process design (CAPD), and process simulation, such as roller compaction simulation, and tablet simulation, to support process development and optimization of manufacturing.[48] The

increased use of CAPD and process simulation in the pharmaceutical industry should promise more robust processes developed faster, and at a lower cost, resulting in higher quality products.

In the Proposed Scale-up Plan, What Operating Parameters will be Adjusted to Ensure the Product Meets all in-Process and Final Product Specifications?

OGD expects the release specifications and process description to be fixed. The specifications are set based on product performance, not derived empirically from one or more batches. The ANDA sponsor has flexibility in adjusting operating parameters (time, flow rate, temperature, etc.) to meet these constraints during scale-up. For commercial scale-up, an ANDA sponsor may either propose fixed ranges for these operating parameters in a proposed master batch record or indicate that an operating parameter will be adjusted to reach a desired endpoint. The scale-up rationale should focus on critical steps and build on experience obtained from drug development and/or the production of exhibit batch(es).

In summary, QbR questions were designed to embody QbD elements including desired product performance, product and process design, and process performance and controls. With QbR regulatory frame, QbD principles are best implemented to enhance drug product development and manufacturing.

38.6 CONCLUSIONS

QbT and QbD are different to one another fundamentally. The assertion is that quality cannot be tested into a product, but is built by design. Within QbD, formulation and manufacturing processes are understood at a mechanistic level. Design incorporates knowledge of the product and the process to ensure all critical quality parameters are adequately controlled. The adoption of QbD in the pharmaceutical industry is an evolving process. QbR, a new pharmaceutical quality assessment system, incorporates QbD principles, and focuses on critical pharmaceutical quality attributes. QbR facilitates the implementation of QbD and help transform ANDA CMC review into a modern, science and risk-based pharmaceutical quality assessment.

38.A1 Appendix:[22] QbR Questions

2.3 INTRODUCTION TO THE QUALITY OVERALL SUMMARY

- Proprietary name of drug product;
- Non-proprietary name of drug product;
- Non-proprietary name of drug substance;
- Company name;
- Dosage form;
- Strength(s);
- Route of administration;
- Proposed indication(s).

2.3.S Drug Substance

2.3.S.1 General Information

- What are the nomenclature, molecular structure, molecular formula, and molecular weight?
- What are the physico-chemical properties including physical description, pKa, polymorphism, aqueous solubility (as function of pH), hygroscopicity, melting points, and partition coefficient?

2.3.S.2 Manufacture

- Who manufactures the drug substance?
- How do the manufacturing processes and controls ensure consistent production of drug substance?

2.3.S.3 Characterization

- How was the drug substance structure elucidated and characterized?
- How were potential impurities identified and characterized?

2.3.S.4 Control of Drug Substance

- What is the drug substance specification?
- Does it include all the critical drug substance attributes that affect the manufacturing and quality of the drug product?
- For each test in the specification, is the analytical method(s) suitable for its intended use, and if necessary, validated?
- What is the justification for the acceptance criterion?

2.3.S.5 Reference Standards

- How were the primary reference standards certified?

2.3.S.6 Container Closure System

- What container closure system is used for packaging and storage of the drug substance?

2.3.S.7 Stability

- What drug substance stability studies support the retest or expiration date and storage conditions for the drug substance?

2.3.P Drug Product

2.3.P.1 Description and Composition

- What are the components and composition of the final product?
- What are the function(s) of each excipient?
- Does any excipient exceed the IIG limit for this route of administration?

- Do the differences between this formulation and the RLD present potential concerns with respect to therapeutic equivalence?

2.3.P.2 Pharmaceutical Development

2.3.P.2.1 Components of the Product

2.3.P.2.1.1 *Drug substance*
- Which properties or physical chemical characteristics of the drug substance affect drug product development, manufacture, or performance?

2.3.P.2.1.2 *Excipients*
- What evidence supports compatibility between the excipients and the drug substance?

2.3.P.2.2 Drug Product

- What attributes should the drug product possess?
- How was the drug product designed to have these attributes?
- Were alternative formulations or mechanisms investigated?
- How were the excipients and their grades selected?
- How was the final formulation optimized?

2.3.P.2.3 Manufacturing Process Development

- Why was the manufacturing process described in 2.3.P.3 selected for this drug product?
- How are the manufacturing steps (unit operations) related to the drug product quality?
- How were the critical process parameters identified, monitored, and/or controlled?
- What is the scale-up experience with the unit operations in this process?

2.3.P.2.4 Container Closure System

- What specific container closure attributes are necessary to ensure product performance?

2.3.P.3 Manufacture

- Who manufactures the drug product?
- What are the unit operations in the drug product manufacturing process?
- What is the reconciliation of the exhibit batch?
- Does the batch formula accurately reflect the drug product composition?
- If not, what are the differences and the justifications?
- What are the in-process tests and controls that ensure each step is successful?

- What is the difference in size between commercial scale and exhibit batch?
- Does the equipment use the same design and operating principles?
- In the proposed scale-up plan, what operating parameters will be adjusted to ensure the product meets all in-process and final product specifications?
- What evidence supports the plan to scale-up the process to commercial scale?

2.3.P.4 Control of Excipients

- What are the specifications for the inactive ingredients, and are they suitable for their intended function?

2.3.P.5 Control of Drug Product

- What is the drug product specification?
- Does it include all the critical drug product attributes?
- For each test in the specification, is the analytical method(s) suitable for its intended use, and if necessary, validated?
- What is the justification for the acceptance criterion?

2.3.P.6 Reference Standards and Materials

- How were the primary reference standards certified?

2.3.P.7 Container Closure System

- What container closure system(s) is proposed for packaging and storage of the drug product?
- Has the container closure system been qualified as safe for use with this dosage form?

2.3.P.8 Stability

- What are the specifications for stability studies, including justification of acceptance criteria that differ from the drug product release specifications?
- What drug product stability studies support the proposed shelf life and storage conditions?
- What is the post-approval stability protocol?

References

1. The long struggle for the 1906 law. http://www.cfsan.fda.gov/~lrd/history2.html Accessed March 8, 2008.
2. What are generic drugs? http://www.fda.gov/cder/ogd/#Introduction Accessed March 8, 2008.

3. http://www.gphaonline.org/Content/NavigationMenu/AboutGenerics/Glossary Accessed March 8, 2008.

4. Nasr, M. (2004). Risk-based CMC review paradigm. FDA Advisory Committee for Pharmaceutical Science meeting, July 20–21.

5. US Food and Drug Administration (2003). Final Report on Pharmaceutical cGMPs for the 21st Century—A Risk-Based Approach. http://www.fda.gov/cder/gmp/gmp2004/GMP_finalreport2004.htm Accessed March 8, 2008.

6. Yu, L.X., Raw, A., Lionberger, R., et al. (2007). US FDA question-based review for generic drugs: A new pharmaceutical quality assessment system. Journal of Generic Medicine 4, 239–248.

7. Woodcock, J. (2004). The concept of pharmaceutical quality. Am. Pharm. Rev. 7, 10–15.

8. Yu, L.X. (2008). Pharmaceutical quality by design: Product and process development, understanding, and control. Pharm. Res., published on line January 10th.

9. US Food and Drug Administration. (1995). Guidance for Industry: Immediate Release Solid Oral Dosage Forms Scale-Up and Postapproval Changes: Chemistry, Manufacturing, and Controls, In Vitro Dissolution Testing, and In Vivo Bioequivalence Documentation, November.

10. US Food and Drug Administration Office of Generic Drugs White Paper on Question-based Review. http://www.fda.gov/cder/OGD/QbR.htm Accessed March 8, 2008.

11. US Food and Drug Administration. (1997). Guidance for Industry: Modified Release Solid Oral Dosage Forms Scale-Up and Postapproval Changes: Chemistry, Manufacturing, and Controls, In Vitro Dissolution Testing, and In Vivo Bioequivalence Documentation, September.

12. US Food and Drug Administration. (1997). Guidance for Industry: Nonsterile Semisolid Dosage Forms Scale-Up and Postapproval Changes: Chemistry, Manufacturing, and Controls, In Vitro Dissolution Testing, and In Vivo Bioequivalence Documentation, May.

13. US Food and Drug Administration. (2004). Guidance for Industry: Changes to an Approved NDA or ANDA, April.

14. Afnan, A.M. Quality counts. Next generation pharmaceuticals http://www.ngpharma.com/currentissue/article.asp?art=25536&issue=143 Accessed March 8, 2008.

15. Gottlieb, S. New frontiers in drug development. Next generation pharmaceuticals http://www.ngpharma.com/currentissue/article.asp?art=26424&issue=159 Accessed March 8, 2008.

16. ICH. Draft consensus guideline: pharmaceutical development annex to Q8. Available at: http://www.ich.org/LOB/media/MEDIA4349.pdf Accessed March 8, 2008.

17. Lionberger, R.A., Lee, S.L., Lee, L., Raw, A. & Yu, L.X. (2008). Quality by design: Concepts for ANDAs. The AAPS Journal 10, 269–276.

18. US Food and Drug Administration (2007). Draft Guidance for Industry. Pharmaceutical Quality System July.

19. Neway, J.O. Quality by Design is essential in the new U.S. regulatory environment, Next Generation Pharmaceuticals. http://www.ngpharma.com/pastissue/article.asp?art=271746&issue=225 Accessed March 8, 2008.

20. US Food and Drug Administration. (2008). Center for Drug Evaluation and Research, Approved drug products with therapeutic equivalence evaluations, 28th edn.

21. US Food and Drug Administration. (2003). Guidance for Industry: Bioavailability and Bioequivalence Studies for Orally Administered Drug Products—General Considerations, March.

22. US Food and Drug Administration. (2006). Office of Generic Drugs, http://www.fda.gov/cder/OGD/QbR_Summary_outline.htm Accessed March 8, 2008.

23. US Food and Drug Administration. (2006). Office of Generic Drugs, www.fda.gov/cder/ogd/OGD_Model_Quality_Overall_Summary.pdf and www.fda.gov/cder/ogd/OGD_Model_QOS IR Product.pdf Accessed March 8, 2008.

24. US Food and Drug Administration. (2007). Office of Generic Drugs, http://www.fda.gov/cder/OGD/QbR/QBR_submissions_upd.htm Accessed March 8, 2008.

25. Yu, L.X., Lee, L., et al. (2007). US FDA Office of Generic Drugs' pharmaceutical quality initiative: Progress and feedback on question based review. Pharmaceutical Engineering 27, 52–60.

26. US Food and Drug Administration. (2007). FDA office of Generic Drugs, http://www.fda.gov/cder/OGD/QbR/QbR%20Frequently%20Asked%20Questions%20June2007.pdf Accessed March 8, 2008.

27. US 21 CFR 314.94(a) (9).

28. Amidon, G.E., He, X. & Hageman, M.J. (2004). Physicochemical Characterization and Principles of Oral Dosage Form Selection. In: Burgers Medicinal Chemistry and Drug Discovery, Donald J. Abraham (ed.), Vol 2. Wiley-Interscience, Chapter 18.

29. Amidon, G.E. (1995). Physical and Mechanical Property Characterization of Powders. In: Physical Characterization of Pharmaceuticals Solids, H.G. Brittain, (ed.), Marcel Dekker, Inc., New York. pp.281–320.

30. Yu, L.X., Furness, M.S., Raw, A., Woodland Outlaw, K.P., Nashed, N.E., Ramos, E., Miller, S.P.F., Adams, R.C., Fang, F., Patel, R.M., Holcombe, F.O., Jr., Chiu, Y. & Hussain, A.S. (2003). Scientific considerations of pharmaceutical solid polymorphism in abbreviated new drug applications. Pharmaceutical Research 20, 531–536.

31. Raw, A.S., Furness, M.S., Gill, D.S., Adams, R.C., Holcombe, F.O., Jr. & Yu, L.X. (2004). Regulatory considerations of pharmaceutical solid polymorphism in abbreviated new drug applications (ANDAs). Advanced Drug Delivery Reviews 56, 397–414.

32. Miller, S.P.F., Raw, A.S. & Yu, L.X. (2006). FDA Perspective on Pharmaceutical Solid Polymorphism. In: Polymorphism—In the Pharmaceutical and Fine Chemical Industry, Rolf Hilfiker (ed.) Wiley-VCH, Verlag Gmbh & Co., Weinheim, Germany. pp.385–403.

33. US Food and Drug Administration. (2007). Guidance for Industry: ANDAs: Pharmaceutical solid polymorphism Chemistry, Manufacturing, and Controls information, July.

34. Amidon, G.L., Lennernas, H., Shah, V.P. & Crison, J.R. (1995). A theoretical basis for a biopharmaceutic drug classification: the correlation of in vitro drug product dissolution and in vivo bioavailability. Pharmaceutical Research 12, 413–420.

35. US Food and Drug Administration. (2000). Guidance for industry, Waiver of In Vivo Bioavailability and Bioequivalence Studies for Immediate Release Solid Oral Dosage Forms Based on a Biopharmaceutics Classification System, August, CDER/FDA.

36. Amidon, G.E. (2006). Data driven formulation development using material sparing mehtods. 4th Annual G.E. Peck Symposium.

37. Rohrs, B.R., Amidon, G.E., Meury, R.H., Secreast, P.J., King, H.M. & Skoug, C.J. (2006). Particle size limits to meet USP content uniformity criteria for tablets and capsules. Journal of Pharmaceutical Sciences 95, 1049–1059.

38. Waterman, K.C., Adami, R.C., Alsante, K.M., Hong, J., Landis, M.S., Lombardo, F. & Roberts, C.J. (2002). Stabilization of pharmaceuticals to oxidative degradation. Pharmaceutical development and technology 7, 1–32.

39. Waterman, K.C. & Adami, R.C. (2005). Accelerated aging: Prediction of chemical stability of pharmaceuticals. International Journal of Pharmaceutics 293, 101–125.

40. US Food and Drug Administration. (2006). Guidance for Industry, Q8 Pharmaceutical Development, May.

41. Serajuddin, A.T.M., Thakur, A.B., Ghoshal, R.N., Fakes, M.G., Ranadive, S.A., Morris, K.R. & Varia, S.A. (1999). Selection of solid dosage form composition through drug-excipient compatibility testing. Journal of Pharmaceutical Sciences 88, 696–704.

42. Mura, P., Faucci, M.T., Manderioli, A., Bramanti, G. & Ceccarelli, L. (1998). Compatibility study between ibuproxam and pharmaceutical excipients using differential scanning calorimetry, hot-stage microscopy and scanning electron microscopy. Journal of Pharmaceutical and Biomedical Aanalysis 8, 151–163.

43. Stahl, H. Comparing different granulation techniques. http://www.niro.co.uk/NUK/CMSDoc.nsf/WebDoc/ndkw73yphb. Accessed March 8, 2008.

44. ISPE PQLI. Draft PQLI Summary Update Report. http://www.ispe.org/cs/pqli_product_quality_lifecycle_implementation_/draft_pqli_summary_update_report. Accessed November 21, 2007.

45. US Food and Drug Administration. (2006). Guidance for Industry, PAT—A Framework for Innovative Pharmaceutical Development, Manufacturing, and Quality Assurance, September.

46. Munson, J., Stanfield, C.F. & Gujral, B. (2006). A review of process analytical technology (PAT) in the U.S. pharmaceutical industry. Current Pharmaceutical Analysis 2(4), 405–414.

47. Zu, Y., Luo, Y. & Ahmed, S.U. (2007). PAT initiative in generic product development. Am. Pharm. Rev. 10, 10–16.

48. Petrides, D.P., Koulouris, A. & Lagonikos, P.T. (2002). The role of process simulation in pharmaceutical process development and product commercialization. Pharmaceutical Engineering 22, 1–8.

49. US Food and Drug Administration. (2007). Draft Guidance for Industry and Review Staff. Target Product Profile—A Strategic Development Process Tool, March.

Intellectual Property Law Primer

Joseph A. Fuchs

39.1 INTRODUCTION

This chapter will present an overview of intellectual property law, with a principal focus on United States Patent Law. The chapter is divided into two parts. The first part focuses on the process of filing a patent application, corresponding with a patent office to place the claims in a condition for allowance, and obtaining patent grant or issuance. This process is generally referred to as patent prosecution. The second part of this chapter will provide an overview of how patent owners enforce their patents through a lawsuit filed in a US Federal District Court. The enforcement of patents is generally referred to as patent litigation.

39.2 PATENT PROSECUTION

The term "intellectual property" is an umbrella term encompassing patents, trademarks, copyrights, trade secrets, and knowhow. Patents are used to protect inventions or discoveries of "… any new and useful process, machine, manufacture, or composition of matter or any new and useful improvement thereof…" 35 U.S.C. §101. Trademarks are used to protect words, phrases, and logos that are used in the sale of a good or service in interstate commerce, and serve to identify the source of the goods or services. Copyrights are used to protect works of authorship fixed in a tangible medium, such as written materials, visual arts, performances, sound recordings, music, and computer software to name a few. Trade secrets are used to protect formulations (such as the Coca Cola recipe),

processes or machinery that is not known to the public, and is carefully maintained in secrecy. Knowhow refers to information relating to how to do something in an efficient and reliable manner. These terms are often confused by persons who will say things such as, "you should trademark that idea" or you should "patent that saying." The misuse of these terms can be humorous to those of us who know their definition.

Because this text is focused on addressing technical issues surrounding oral dosage forms we thought it most appropriate, with the brief space available to us, to dedicate our focus on obtaining and enforcing patents.

39.2.1 Types of United States Patent Applications

There are four basic types of patent applications in the US:

- provisional,
- utility,
- plant, and
- design.

A provisional patent application allows for the filing of a patent application in a form that is less formal than other types of applications. The provisional patent application is not examined by a patent examiner, but allows an inventor to establish a date of invention for what is disclosed in the application. A utility patent application and international patent application counterparts should be filed within twelve months from the provisional filing date, to claim priority to

Developing Solid Oral Dosage Forms: Pharmaceutical Theory and Practice
ISBN: 978-0-444-53242-8

the provisional patent application filing date. 35 U.S.C. § 119 (e): Upon expiry of the twelve month period the provisional patent application lapses and no further action is taken in the provisional application.

Design patent applications cover the non-functional, ornamental features of an article of manufacture. 35 U.S.C. § 171: A design patent application includes figures showing the ornamental features from all sides. The design application will typically include a single claim such as "The ornamental design for a [insert article of manufacture] as shown and described."

Plant patent applications can be obtained by "[whoever] invents or discovers and asexually reproduces any distinct and new variety of plant, including cultivated sports, mutants, hybrids, and newly found seedlings, other than tuber propagated plant or a plant found in an uncultivated state ..." 35 U.S.C. § 161. This is all I can tell you about plant patent applications, so I will move on to utility patent applications. I apologize to the gardeners and botanists who are reading this.

39.2.2 Standards for Patentability

Utility patent applications are the most common type of patent application, and can cover a wide variety of inventions including processes, machines, and compositions of matter. For an invention to be patentable it must be novel, non-obvious, and have utility. The legal standards for determining whether these standards are met can be quite complicated, so we will limit our discussion to a brief overview, and will urge readers if they have questions relating to this matter to consult a patent attorney.

Novelty

Generally speaking, the novelty standard in the United States requires that, for an invention to be patentable, the invention has not been used in the public in the United States or disclosed in a written publication in the United States or elsewhere for more than one year prior to the filing of the subject patent application. Novelty can also be destroyed, if the invention is known or used by others in the United States or appears in a written publication anywhere in the world before the invention by the applicant. Take note that the invention date can be, and in most cases is, different from the filing date of the patent application. An invention date is the date when an inventor has conceived of an invention, and has put it into practice. The publications and public uses, referenced above, are referred to as "prior art." If a single textual prior art reference or public use discloses every element of the invention claimed, the claim is said to be "anticipated."

The US novelty standard is unique to the US. Most other countries of the world require that a patent application be on file prior to the date of any public disclosure of the invention anywhere in the world. This is known as "absolute novelty." Also, if there is a dispute between or among parties who have applied for a patent on the same invention, the party who filed first is the party who wins the dispute. This is known as "the first to file rule."

Because the United States allows inventors one year from their invention date to file a patent application, written references and public uses that occur less than one year before the filing date of an application may not necessarily be novelty-destroying. If such a reference or use is cited by a patent examiner to reject claims, it may be possible for the inventors to "swear behind" the cited reference, by providing proof in the form of a sworn statement that the inventors conceived of their invention prior to the date of the reference, and used diligence from the date of the reference to the date of reduction to practice. In the case of a patent reference, diligence must be shown from the earliest effective filing date of the application that includes claims of priority to domestic patent references, but not to foreign patent references. However, if the cited reference or public use has occurred more than one year before the filing date, the inventors cannot swear behind such reference. This type of reference is known as a "statutory bar," and can be the death knell to a patent application.

Another interesting consequence of the United States allowing inventors one year from their invention date to file their patent applications is that disputes can arise between or among individual inventors or groups of inventors over who invented first. The United States, therefore, is known as a "first to invent" country, as opposed to a "first to file" country. In order for such disputes to occur, none of the party's patent applications can be statutory bars to the other patent applications. The United States Patent Office is capable of resolving these disputes in an interference proceeding. An interference can occur between parties having pending patent applications or it can involve a patent and one or more patent applications. The United States legislators are considering amending the US patent laws to move to a first-to-file system, which would put an end to interference proceedings.

The US novelty requirements also require, you may be surprised to know, that the inventors identified in the application are the actual inventors.

Non-Obvious

A patent claim is deemed obvious, and, therefore, not patentable, "… though the invention is not identically disclosed or described … if the differences between the subject matter sought to be patented and the prior art are such that the subject matter as a whole would have been obvious at the time of the invention was made to a person of ordinary skill in the art to which such subject matter pertains." 35 U.S.C. § 103 (a): A patent examiner can cite to a single reference or a combination of prior art references to make an obviousness rejection. Obviousness rejections can be attacked in numerous ways.

For example, a patent applicant can argue that there must be a motivation within the references to combine them together. Recent case law from the United States Supreme Court has stated that the motivation to combine the references does not have to appear in the references. It is enough that one of ordinary skill facing the wide range of needs created by the developments in the field of endeavor would see the benefit in combining the references. KSR v. Teleflex, 550 U.S.____, 127 S.Ct. 1727 (2007). Thus, US patent examiners may find it easier, and less subject to a legal challenge, to combine references after this case.

A patent applicant can also argue against an obviousness rejection by proving that the claimed invention has met with commercial success, has solved a long-felt need, has provided a solution where others have failed, and that the cited reference or combination of references teaches away from the claimed invention. A patent applicant can support such arguments by providing sworn statements known as §132 Affidavits.

Utility

Article 1, § 8, of the United States Constitution, grants Congress the power to "promote the Progress of Science and Useful Arts." The patent law under Title 35 was drafted in accordance with the constitution and requires that, for an invention to be patentable, it must fall into one of four statutory categories of invention. It also requires that only one patent be granted for an invention, and that the patented invention be "useful." The four statutory categories of invention are:

1. useful process;
2. machine;
3. manufacture; or
4. composition of matter. 35 U.S.C. § 101.

To be "useful" an invention does not have to be an improvement over what is disclosed in the prior art.

It need only have to offer a practical and positive benefit to society. Applying the "useful" standard to the mechanical arts area is relatively simple. For example, an assembly for providing fluid access to a container clearly is beneficial. However, biochemical and bioscience inventions can meet with stiff resistance from the patent office, unless the patent application contains proof that the invention provides some benefit. Patent examiners seem to have shifted rejections for lack of utility to rejections based on a lack of written description or failure to provide an enabling disclosure. Regardless of the statutory construct of the examiner's rejection, such arguments can be overcome by disclosures and proof in the application of the benefit to society of the practical use of the invention. This is not as easy as it may seem in many complex bioscience patent applications, where the practical utility of the invention may be difficult to discern.

39.2.3 The United States Utility Patent Application

A US utility patent application usually has two principal parts, a specification followed by a claim or a set of claims.

The Specification

The specification must disclose in clear, concise, and exact terms to enable one of ordinary skill in the art to practice the invention. If necessary, the specification will make reference to figures. The specification must also disclose the best mode for practicing the invention. The grant of patent rights allows one to exclude others from practicing the claimed invention. These rights are granted by the US government to the inventor, as a *quid pro quo* for the inventor making a sufficiently detailed invention disclosure.

The requirement to disclose the best mode can sometimes lead to a bone of contention between a patent attorney and the inventor. Frequently, inventors are initially reluctant to disclose the best mode, as they believe they are giving away too much information. However, when inventors are advised that their patent can be invalidated by a court for failure to provide sufficient disclosure, they usually concede by providing an adequate disclosure.

The Claims

The claims portion of the patent application is where patent applicants define what they believe to be the patentable features of their inventions. Patent examiners will review the claims for clarity purposes, and determine whether the claims are allowable in view of prior art patents and publications. Patent examiners conduct a search of the prior art and then prepare an office action allowing or rejecting the pending claims. Office actions should include a detailed reason for allowing or rejecting the claims, and if the rejection is based on a prior art reference or a combination of references, the examiner needs to provide the legal basis for the rejection, and the patent number or other identifying information for the prior art, and the location within the document that discloses the invention being rejected. Applicants will file a reply to the office action, where they can amend the claims and explain why the amendments place the claims into allowable form or they submit arguments without claim amendments. When the claims are in acceptable form to the examiner and the applicant, the examiner will notify the applicant the claims are allowable. The applicant must then pay an issuance fee. Several months later the patent will issue. A US utility patent will typically have a term of twenty years from the earliest effective filing date.

Claims come in numerous different varieties including, for example: compositions of matter; formulations; processes; articles of manufacture; product by process; product by physical property; and means plus function. A claim in US format will typically have a preamble, followed by a transitional phrase or term, followed by the body of the claim. The preamble introduces the general subject matter that is to be claimed such as "an assembly" or "a device."

The transitional phrase or term can be critical to determining the scope of the claim. There are three commonly used transitional phrases or terms, "comprising" or "including," "consisting of," and "consisting essentially of." The transitional terms "comprising" and "including" are interpreted as being open-ended. This means that the claim recites the minimum elements of an invention, and that as long as a party uses the recited elements, even if they add additional elements, they will infringe the claim.

The transitional phrase "consisting of" is interpreted as being close-ended. This means that in order to infringe such a claim an accused product must include only the recited elements, and nothing more. Such a claim is typically more narrowly interpreted when compared to an open-ended claim. Close-ended claims are useful to claim inventions, such as a process, where the inventive aspect is the removal of a step required in the prior art.

The transitional phrase "consisting essentially of" is interpreted as open-ended for some purposes and close-ended for other purposes. The claim is interpreted as open-ended for accused products that include what is recited in the claim and additional components that do not materially affect the basic and novel characteristics of the invention. Say, for example, you claim a transparent film "consisting essentially of" components A, B, and C. Say a competitor produces a film having components A, B, C, and carbon black. The claim will be interpreted as close-ended because the inclusion of carbon black will destroy the transparency of the film, a basic and novel characteristic of the invention.

39.2.4 Representative Pharmaceutical Related Patent Subject Matter and Claims

Some of the first patent applications applied for by innovator drug companies will be for the compositions of matter of new drug discoveries. Because the time to obtain FDA approval for the sale and use of a new drug in the United States can be quite lengthy, the twenty-year term of the patent remaining after receiving approval may be substantially diminished. Accordingly, it is critical for competitors in the pharmaceutical industry to have a well-planned succession of patents to protect forms of the drug being developed for later use.

It is a common patent filing strategy employed by pharmaceutical companies to file what are known as patent line extension patent applications. These extension patent applications are designed to present additional hurdles to competitors to create competing drug products. The subject matter for patent line extension patent applications can include, for example, modification of the chemical structure of the patented drug, formulations to deliver the drug, new indications, delivery devices, in combination with the drug, and new routes of delivery. Patents covering modifications to chemical structures can be directed to, for example, chiral isomers of the drug, differing polymorphic forms of the claimed drug, prodrugs, metabolites, and pediatric studies.

Chiral Isomers

Patents directed to a specific chiral isomer of a drug may disclose that the specific chiral isomer of the drug provides benefits, such as improved pharmacological profiles, when compared to a racemic mixture of the drug. One example of a claim to a specific isomer of a drug is in US Patent No. 5 362 755, directed to (R)-albuterol and recites as follows:

- Claim 1. A method of treating asthma in an individual with albuterol, while reducing side effects associated with chronic administration of racemic albuterol, comprising chronically administering to the individual a quantity of an optically pure R(−) isomer of albuterol sufficient to result in bronchodilation, while simultaneously reducing undesirable side-effects, said R isomer being substantially free of its S(+) isomer.

Polymorphic Forms

Products containing varying polymorphic forms of drugs include, for example, Ranitidine (Zantac), Cedadroxil (Duricef), Tertenadine (Seldane), and Omeprazole (Prilosec). An example of a patent claim to a specific polymorphic form is found in US Patent No. 4 521 431, and specifically claims form 2 of Ranitidine.

- Claim 1. Form 2 ranitidine hydrochloride characterized by an infrared spectrum as a mull in mineral oil showing the following main peaks: 3260 3190 3100 2560 2510 2470 1620 1590 1570 1263 1230 1220 1195 1163 1075 1045 1021 1006 991 972 958 810 800 760 700 660 640 620 cm^{-1}.

Prodrugs

Patents directed to prodrugs are directed to the precursor of an active ingredient, which can be designed for targeted delivery or to reduce toxicity. For example, US Patent No. 6 486 182, provides an example of a claim to a prodrug of amlodipine and atorvastin.

- Claim 1. A compound which is a mutual prodrug of amlodipine and atorvastatin or a pharmaceutically acceptable salt thereof.

New Formulations and Delivery Technologies

There are numerous patenting opportunities pertaining to drug-containing formulations, and delivery technologies. Formulation patents are typically directed to reducing adverse effects of the drug, simplifying dosing regimen and administration, extended-release of the drug, chronotherapeutic release, improved shelf life of the drug formulation, improved dissolution and aqueous solubility (especially for parenteral administration), fast absorption, pediatric formulations, and combo-drug formulations.

Controlled-release

US Patent Application No. 2004/0131671 A1 discloses a controlled-release form of tramadol and acetaminophen having a combination of a sustained-release and an immediate-release. Allowed claim 1 recites as follows:

- Claim 1: A capsule for sustained release of drugs, including a combination of acetaminophen of

from about 100 mg to about 1000 mg, and tramadol or its salts of from about 15 mg to about 150 mg comprising:

1. an immediate-release portion comprising from about 25%–75% of the total effective amount of the acetaminophen and tramadol, in the form selected from pellets, beads, granules, and mini-tablets;
2. a sustained-release portion comprising:
   a. from about 25%–75% of the total effective amount of the acetaminophen and tramadol, in the form selected from pellets, beads, granules, and mini-tablets; and
   b. a gelling polymer in an amount by weight of the capsule of about 6% to about 50%; and
3. the capsule releases about 25%–60% of the acetaminophen and the tramadol in the first hour in a simulated gastric fluid dissolution media, about 50%–90% of the acetaminophen and the tramadol in the first four hours, and not less than 80% of the acetaminophen and the tramadol in the first 12 hours in a simulated intestinal fluid dissolution media using USP dissolution method II at 50 rpm.

Improved Shelf Life

An example of a patent disclosing an improved shelf life formulation for a premixed famotidine formulation is disclosed in US Patent No. 5 650 421. Claim 1 recites as follows:

- Claim 1. A pharmaceutical composition suitable for administration parenterally and through injection, comprising a solution having an effective amount of famotidine or at least one physiologically acceptable salt of famotidine, between about 0.1 mg/ml to about 0.8 mg/ml, the solution having a pH adjusted by an acid to be in the range of 5.7 to about 6.4.

Pediatric Formulation Claim

US Patent No. 5 698 562 is directed to a palatable formulation of trimethoprim oral solution. Claim 1 recites as follows:

- Claim 1. A palatable pharmaceutical oral solution formulation for pediatric dosing consisting of:
  - about 1.25 to 8 mg trimethoprim per mL (wt./vol.) of purified water;
  - hydrochloric acid (HCl) in sufficient concentration with purified water to permit said trimethoprim to dissolve at the appropriate concentration, wherein

the solution of dissolved trimethoprim has a pH of between 4.0 and 6.0; and

- sucrose and flavoring, other than sucrose, in an amount sufficient to overcome the bitterness of said trimethoprim.

39.3 PATENT ENFORCEMENT/ LITIGATION

An owner of a patent has the right to exclude others from practicing the claimed invention. A patent does not provide the right for the owner of a patent to practice the claimed invention. It is common for people to confuse the concepts of patentability, and freedom to operate. Whether an invention is patentable, which is discussed in some detail above, depends on what is disclosed in the prior art. Whether a party is free to practice an invention depends on what is claimed in patents that are in their enforceable term. An operating example may help clarify these two concepts. If you find yourself confusing these concepts, try to remember the following example, which should help clarify your thinking.

39.3.1 Example: Patentability Versus Freedom to Operate

Thomas Edison conceives of, and reduces to practice, a first generation light bulb. He files a patent application describing the light bulb in complete detail. He discloses in the specification that his light bulb has a sealed glass envelope surrounding an iron filament, which has opposed ends in communication with a source of electricity, and the filament provides light when electrical current is applied to the filament. Claim 1 of the Edison patent recites:

1. A light bulb comprising: a sealed glass envelope defining a chamber, a filament positioned in the chamber and having first and second ends in electrical communication with a source of electricity, wherein when current is applied to the filament it provides light, and when the current is removed it becomes dark.

The patent examiner reviewing the Edison patent application searches the prior art, and when he is unable to find any prior art to reject Claim 1 he deems the claim to be in a condition for allowance, and the patent issues. Thus, the patent examiner has determined that Edison's invention is patentable.

Continuing with this example, say a second inventor, who has seen an Edison light bulb, decides to attempt to develop an improved light bulb. After great effort the second inventor finds that when he uses a tungsten filament, instead of an iron filament, that his new light bulb lights for many days longer than the Edison light bulb. The second inventor prepares a patent application, disclosing his improved light bulb with a tungsten filament. Claim 1 of the second inventor's patent application recites as follows:

1. A light bulb comprising: a sealed glass envelope defining a chamber, a tungsten filament positioned in the chamber and having first and second ends in electrical communication with a source of electricity, wherein when current is applied to the filament it provides light, and when the current is removed it becomes dark.

The patent examiner reviews Claim 1 and he conducts a search of the prior art, and finds the Edison patent on the light bulb. The examiner reviews the specification of the Edison patent, and finds no disclosure of a tungsten filament. The examiner also concludes the use of a tungsten filament and the inclusion in a light bulb is novel, and non-obvious in view of the Edison patent, and has utility. Thus, Claim 1 reciting a light bulb with a tungsten filament is found to be in allowable form, and the second inventor's patent issues.

Now, the second inventor decides that he would like to make his improved light bulb. He consults his local patent attorney to inquire if he would be taking a business risk if he were to make the improved light bulb, and sell it in the United States. The patent attorney conducts a search of US Patents, and finds the Edison patent. Assuming, for the sake of this example, that the Edison patent is still within its enforceable life span, the patent attorney concludes that because the improved light bulb meets every limitation of Claim 1 of the Edison patent, the second inventor does not have freedom to operate. Thus, if the second inventor makes, uses, offers for sale, sells or imports the improved light bulb, he may be sued by Edison for patent infringement.

Continuing further with this example, say that Edison hears of the improved light bulb with the tungsten filament, and decides he would like to replace the light bulbs he is making and selling with iron filaments with a tungsten filament. Edison visits his patent attorney and asks him if he is taking any business risk if he makes and sells the improved light bulb with a tungsten filament. Edison's patent attorney conducts a search of US patents, and finds the second inventor's patent, which is still within its enforceable life span. Edison's patent attorney concludes that Edison would be taking a risk of being sued for patent infringement by the second inventor if he were to make the improved light bulb with the tungsten filament, because such a light bulb would include every element recited in Claim 1 of the second inventor's patent.

This may seem to be a strange outcome, but it is a common occurrence. Edison's patent is referred to as a dominating patent, and the second inventor's patent is referred to as a blocking patent. If Edison or the second inventor would like to sell the improved light bulb during the term of the two patents, they will have to enter into a cross-licensing agreement.

39.3.2 Patent Infringement Litigation

Patent infringement lawsuits must be first brought in a United States Federal District Court. All appeals from patent lawsuits on patent-related issues are taken to the United States Court of Appeals for the Federal Circuit (CAFC), located in Washington, DC.

There are several different types of infringement allegations including:

- direct,
- contributory, and
- inducement.

For the sake of brevity, we will discuss infringement in terms of a claim to a product, but it should be understood that this discussion applies equally to claimed methods. Direct infringement can be alleged against a single entity who makes, uses, offers for sale, sells or imports into the United States (infringing acts) a product that has all of the elements of a single claim of a patent. Contributory infringement can be alleged against a party who does not directly infringe a patent, but who supplies a product to another party who directly infringes a patent. Inducing infringement can be alleged against a party who does not directly infringe, but encourages another party to infringe a patent.

Patent infringement can occur by literally infringing a claim of a patent or by infringing the claim under the doctrine of equivalents. Literal infringement occurs if every element of a single claim is present in an accused product. A product that does not literally infringe upon the express terms of a patent claim may, nonetheless, be found to infringe under the doctrine of equivalents if there is "equivalence" between the elements of the accused product or process, and the claimed elements of the patented invention. The essential inquiry under the doctrine of equivalents is whether the accused product contains elements identical or equivalent to each claimed element of the patented invention.

An infringement analysis entails two steps. The first step, commonly known as claim construction or interpretation, is to determine the meaning and scope of the patent claims asserted to be infringed. Once a construction has been made, the second step is to compare the properly construed claims to the device accused of infringing. If an accused product meets all of the limitations of the claim, either literally or under the doctrine of equivalents, the product infringes the claim.

For a proper claim construction, the words of the claims are construed in light of the specification, the prosecution history, and the prior art, but independent of the accused device. Claim terms are given their ordinary and accustomed meaning, unless examination of the specification, prosecution history, and other claims indicates that the inventor intended otherwise. For claim construction purposes, the written description contained in the specification may act as a dictionary to explain the invention, and to define terms used in the claims. The interpretation of claims is a matter for a judge to decide, as opposed to a jury. A proceeding to interpret claims is conducted in what is known as a Markman hearing. During a Markman hearing, both the patent owner and accused infringer urge the court to interpret the claims in their favor. After the hearing, the court issues an order stating how the claims are to be interpreted.

During a Markman hearing, the patent owner must walk a fine line between urging a claim interpretation broad enough to read on the accused product, so that it may prove its case for infringement, while at the same time being careful not to urge such a broad reading that the claim reads on the prior art, thereby presenting an argument to the accused infringer that the claims are invalid. The accused infringer will urge either a narrow or a broad reading. The accused infringer can argue a narrow claim reading, such that the claims do not read on the accused product and, therefore, the accused product does not infringe the asserted claims. The accused infringer can also urge a broad reading, so that the asserted claims read on the prior art and, therefore, provide an argument that the claims are invalid. Patent infringement actions can be won or lost at an early stage in the proceedings if a party gets an unfavorable claim construction order from the court.

The CAFC has held that a finding of infringement under the doctrine of equivalents requires proof of insubstantial differences between the claimed and accused product or processes. The vantage point of one of ordinary skill in the relevant art provides the perspective for assessing the substantiality of the differences.

There are limitations placed on the use of the doctrine of equivalents, namely prosecution history estoppel. Prosecution history estoppel limits the range of equivalents available to a patentee by preventing recapture of subject matter surrendered during prosecution of the patent. For example, if a patent applicant amends a claim in view of prior art or for other reason pertaining to patentability, from reciting a formulation having 20–35% of component A to reciting 25–35% of component A to obtain issuance of the claim, the patentee cannot then allege that a product having 24% of component A infringes under the doctrine of equivalents. The patentee is said to be estopped from making such an allegation.

Another limitation of the application of the doctrine of equivalents can be found if a patentee is deemed to have dedicated subject matter to the public. A certain court opinion rendered by the CAFC held that subject matter disclosed by an applicant in a patent application, but that was not claimed was dedicated to the public, the applicant could not resort to the doctrine of equivalents to prove infringement, even where the specification explicitly taught the equivalence of the subject matter.

In yet another limitation, the doctrine of equivalents may not be used to expand the scope of the patentee's right to exclude, so as to encompass the prior art. This ruling, of course, makes sense since a patent applicant should not be allowed to obtain a claim reading in court that it could not obtain during the prosecution of the patent application.

39.3.3 Remedies for Patent Infringement

A party who succeeds in proving a claim for patent infringement will typically have two types of remedies available, including monetary damages and injunctive relief. There are numerous theories for calculating monetary damages, some of which include: a reasonable royalty; actual damages; lost profits from lost sales; convoyed sales; and price erosion. If an infringer is found to have willfully infringed the patent, the amount of damages can be multiplied by a factor up to three times damages. Also, in certain exceptional cases, the court can order the losing party to pay the prevailing party's attorneys' fees. This is a departure from the normal situation in the United States, where each party is responsible for paying its attorneys' fees regardless of whether a party prevails or not.

Injunctive relief can be a potent weapon against a party found to be infringing. An injunction is an order from a court that the party found to be infringing must cease all infringing acts relating to the asserted patent.

39.3.4 Defenses to Patent Infringement

Defenses to patent infringement can be divided into three categories, non-infringement, invalidity, and unenforceabilty. A defense of non-infringement will be sustained if the party asserting its patent fails to show that the accused product has every element of the asserted claim, either literally or under the doctrine of equivalents.

Patents are entitled to a presumption of validity. The courts defer to the skill and experience of the US Patent Office to issue valid patents, and will upset the grant of a patent only upon a strong showing by the party moving to prove invalidity or unenforceability. Thus, a party moving to invalidate a patent must prove its case by clear and convincing evidence. Clear and convincing evidence requires greater proof than that commonly used in most civil cases, such as breach of contract actions. The clear and convincing standard, however, requires less proof than the beyond a reasonable doubt standard required of the government in criminal cases. Using a baseball analogy, which may not mean anything to some readers, clear and convincing evidence is like hitting a baseball off an outfield wall. Beyond a reasonable doubt would be a home run, and a mere preponderance would be an infield hit.

The arguments made by the defending party that a patent is invalid are essentially the same arguments made by a patent examiner in rejecting claims. The defending party can rely on a single reference to anticipate the claims or a single reference or a combination of references, to prove the asserted claims are obvious. Invalidity defenses are usually based on prior art documents that were not before the patent office during the prosecution of the patent application that issued as the patent being asserted.

Invalidity can also be proven by showing that the patent does not provide sufficient disclosure for one of ordinary skill in the art to practice the invention. A patent can also be invalidated for failure by the patent applicant to have disclosed the best mode known to it for practicing the invention.

A defending party can also defend itself by proving the patent is unenforceable due to "inequitable conduct." Inequitable conduct usually means the patent was procured by the patent applicant using improper means, such as failing to disclose material prior art to the patent office during the prosecution of the patent application that could impact the scope of the claims, and filing an affidavit including statements known to be false.

This chapter was not intended to discuss all aspects of intellectual property in depth. Rather it was meant to expose the reader to certain fundamental concepts of intellectual property law, without getting into too much detail.

Product Lifecycle Management (LCM)

Erika A. Zannou, Ping Li and Wei-Qin (Tony) Tong

40.1 INTRODUCTION

In recent years, the challenges facing the pharmaceutical industry have been intensifying. These global challenges include patent expirations, generic competition, mounting cost of drug development, price controls, antitrust investigations, increased skepticism by both financial institutions and general public, and tougher regulatory environment. As one of the consequences, augmenting and maximizing the value of their pipelines has become one of the most important tasks facing today's pharmaceutical companies.[1]

Despite the increased investments in R&D by pharmaceutical companies, and the advancement in high throughput technologies in discovery, the industry's current R&D yield is neither optimal nor sustainable. The number of products coming off-patent in the recent years is far greater than the number of new products being approved by the regulatory authorities. Realizing this short fall, pharmaceutical companies are on the defensive, and have been looking for ways to realize financial gains and continued growth.[2,3]

Lifecycle management (LCM) is one strategy that has proven successful in the last few years. Pharmaceutical companies have been managing in an innovative and proactive way the life of those products which they invested billons of dollars in to bring to the market. Typically, the life of a pharmaceutical product begins with product launch, after securing regulatory approval and, to a significant extent, ends at the point at which a generic competitor is able to enter the market and sell the drug at a lower cost. Better LCM of their innovative products has allowed pharmaceutical companies either to delay the generic

entry into the market or to minimize the market share canibalized by the me-too products. This strategy, aimed at protecting the innovator's product, has been the key for blockbuster drugs which can account for the majority of a pharmaceutical company's revenues.

LCM is, however, a complex task and requires a multi-disciplinary approach, not only good business and legal strategies, but also good science and technologies. With so much money at stake, it is understandable that LCM should gain as much attention as developing new chemical entities. In fact, for timely implementation of the LCM strategy, activities are in most cases starting even before the innovative product is filed with Health Authorities. There are many excellent cases where a product's life has been prolonged way beyond the original patent expiration date, resulting in substantial financial returns or gains. The most commonly used LCM strategies can be grouped into four areas:

1. extension of product life by shortening development time to market;
2. brand protection strategies to extend time on the market without generic competition;
3. market expansion strategies to increase sales within the patent protected period;
4. market protection actions to defend against competitive erosion of sales.

These four categories include indication expansion, reformulation (combination products, modified release formulations, etc.), and second-generation launch. Other marketing strategies to maximize sales are also employed, such as direct to consumer advertisement, and drug pricing strategies upon patent expiration.

Developing Solid Oral Dosage Forms: Pharmaceutical Theory and Practice
ISBN: 978-0-444-53242-8

40.2 BASIC PATENT LAWS GOVERNING THE LIFE OF PHARMACEUTICAL PRODUCTS

A pharmaceutical product's lifecycle is ultimately determined by the international patent laws, and the applicable law in the country of interest. Historically, the United States, Europe, and Japan have been the largest consumers of pharmaceutical products, and thus the countries where pharmaceutical companies were focusing their efforts and strategies. The pharmaceutical companies' world is, however, evolving, with emerging markets such as China, India, and South America increasing their consumption in the global market. How these countries interpret and apply the international patent laws, and their specific laws, is becoming critical and complicates the pharmaceutical companies' global strategies.

In the United States, for example, the date of approval of generic competitors is directly tied to patent expiration for many (although not all) important pharmaceutical products.[4] The Drug price competition and patent term restoration act, also known as the Hatch–Waxman Act, that was put in place in 1984, sets forth the rules that govern the ongoing battle between brand name and generic drug manufacturers—with patents as the battleground. The FDA publication, the *Orange Book*, contains information on every innovator manufacturer's patents for their products that are submitted for approval. These usually include patents for ingredient, composition or use (but not process). Generic manufacturers must consult this published list before they can decide whether or not to challenge any patent. If they decide to challenge a patent, they have to notify the FDA, as well as the innovator manufacturer and patent holder. Typically, the patent holder will subsequently bring a patent infringement suit against the generic manufacturer, within 45 days of receipt of notice of a challenge to its patent. The FDA must then withhold approval of the generic product for a period of 30 months. Some pharmaceutical patents can be extended to recover time lost in the regulatory approval process, as defined by the patent term restoration under the Hatch–Waxman Amendments. In addition, so-called "market exclusivity"—designed by the US Congress to provide incentives for the development of new drugs—gives an extension in product life irrespective of patent protection. In addition, developing a product for the pediatric population provides the innovator's company with an additional six months exclusivity.

For the first generic company to challenge a patent listed for an innovator drug, one market exclusivity provision of the 1984 Amendments provides a 180 day head start to the market.

40.3 LIFECYCLE MANAGEMENT THROUGH SALTS, CRYSTAL FORMS AND FORMULATIONS

When the first API patent is filed, it may not cover all potential salts and polymorphs. Sometimes a new salt and/or polymorph may have some advantage that can be patented separately. These new patents may provide additional life for the specific product if they are used adequately, as illustrated in Figure 40.1.[5] The consequence of not adequately cover these crystal and salt forms may be detrimental. From the side of

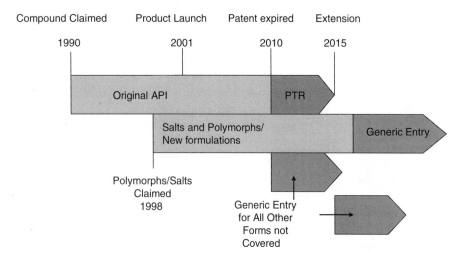

PTR: Patent Term Restoration = half of the investigational period + all of the FDA review period

FIGURE 40.1 Salts, polymorphs and new formulations can potentially provide additional patent coverage in the US

generic companies they have begun to look for, and find alternative crystalline forms of drugs, either with a view to improving them or to marketing bioequivalent versions before the original drugs have gone generic. For example, Dr. Reddy's Laboratories did in filing an NDA to market a chemical variation of the active ingredient in Pfizer Inc.'s blood pressure-lowering drug amlodipine (*Norvasc*®).[4,6]

The same applies to new formulation patents. They may also include patents on reformulated products.

40.4 EXTENSION OF PRODUCT LIFECYCLE BY SHORTENING PRODUCT DEVELOPMENT TIME

Once the API patent is filed, the clock starts ticking, leading to the patent expiration 20 years later. It is obvious that the faster the company can develop the compound into a product, the longer the product exclusivity will be.

Pharmaceutical companies and regulatory agencies are collaborating with the multiple aims of improving the development process, of gaining better understanding of the science behind drug product development, and of better following drug product quality throughout the manufacturing process. For example, one of the main initiatives between pharmaceutical companies and the Food and Drug Administration (FDA) is the quality by design (QbD) initiative, which should eventually contribute to better first-time product quality, thus shortening review time required by the FDA.

Traditionally, the drug development is a very lengthy, labor-intensive, and highly regulated process. One of the key limiting factors in developing drug product is the time required to produce the active pharmaceutical ingredient (API), with adequate quality and quantity, required for the development work. If technology advancement makes it possible to develop robust formulations with less drug substance, the pharmaceutical development may avoid being a rate-limiting step in the development process. Also, introducing to the market as fast as possible a less polished drug product when possible (such as a capsule rather than a tablet) can be of added value, specially in therapeutic areas where there is an unmet medical need, such as in the treatment of some cancers or some life-threatening but less common diseases.

The same pharmaceutical processes, such as wet granulation, tabletting or fluid-bed coating, have been in practice for the last few decades. Robustness of pharmaceutical processes upon scaling-up has also been a significant challenge in the development

process. Development of continuous pharmaceutical processing reduces the risk associated with the scale-up steps required for traditional processes. Recently, the use of melt extruder as a granulation tool has been successfully demonstrated. The advantage of melt granulation using the extruder is that it can be easily adopted into a continuous process, thus reducing scale-up risks, and time required for the process development.[7]

Leveraging the advancement in the area of IT systems, such as electronic data capturing, remote site monitoring, and computer modeling, will certainly bring significant saving and speed to drug discovery and development.

40.5 LIFECYCLE MANAGEMENT THROUGH NEW DRUG DELIVERY SYSTEMS

As one of the most important strategies for LCM, new drug delivery systems provide commercial opportunities through intellectual property, product differentiation, and recognition. By infusing the drug into an enhanced delivery system, this strategy is valuable and cost-effective in the management of overall product lifecycle resource. It improves the product's therapeutic benefits, and patient's convenience, as well as compliance. With extended product's profitable life, it also fends off generic competition, and gives back financial advantages to pharmaceutical companies.

Formulation technologies for LCM are numerous. They include modified-release for oral delivery, taste-masking, orally disintegrating tablets (ODT), depot formulations, high-strength parenterals, inhalation, emerging technologies for bioavailability enhancement, etc. Over the years, a variety of technology platforms have also emerged, many of which led to the success of marketed products.

In this section, the main focus will be placed on innovations for oral new drug delivery systems as LCM tools. Three drug delivery systems will be discussed:

1. Modified-release: to extend or delay the drug release profile in the gastro-intestinal (GI) tract for enhanced therapeutic effect;
2. Enhanced bioavailability: to increase the drug exposure by reformulating it with emerging or novel formulation technologies, which proves to be effective with many BCS class II and IV compounds (poorly water soluble compounds with moderate to very low GI permeability);
3. Alternative delivery systems and devices.

40.5.1 Modified-Release

Modified-release products are effective dosage forms, which alter the drug release characteristics (time, course, and/or location) for improved therapeutic effects, convenience, and compliance. The technology is broadly used as part of the LCM strategy of many innovator products. It can be applied to almost all administration routes, including oral, parenteral, transdermal, and nasal.

For oral modified release, an important technical approach is to extend the drug release profile. This can be achieved by formulating the drug with release-retardant excipients in a matrix core (often polymers). A variety of polymeric colloidal particles or microencapsulates, such as microparticles or microspheres, have been developed in the form of reservoir and matrix devices.[8] Hydroxypropylmethylcellulose (HPMC, also known as hypromellose) is probably the most commonly employed cellulose derivative in hydrophilic matrices. When HPMC (as a matrix) is exposed to aqueous medium (content of the stomach and/or the intestine), it undergoes rapid hydration and chain relaxation to form a viscous gelatinous layer, also referred to as "gel layer," at the surface of the tablet.[9] The rate of diffusion of the drug through the gel layer depends on the nature and properties of the matrix composition. Drug substance release is thus controlled, and extended to the desired pharmacokinetic profile. One key property of the HPMC polymers is that their hydration is not affected by natural variation in pH environment throughout the gastrointestinal (GI) tract.

A wide variety of extended-release technologies have been developed. For example, Penwest Pharmaceutical Inc., developed a series of release technology templates for a wider range of drugs. An extended-release technology, TIMERx® system, for example, is based on the synergistic interaction of heteropolysaccharide (xanthan), and galactomannam (locust bean gum), which in the presence of a sugar forms a strong binder gel in water. Drug release is controlled by the rate of water penetrating into the hydrophilic matrix, and the subsequent expansion of gel, which releases the active drug. Table 40.1 lists the drug products that are already in the market using this technology (www.penwest.com).

Geminex™ is another interesting release technology developed by Penwest. This is a dual drug delivery system that controls the release rate of each component, to maximize its individual therapeutic effect and minimize its side-effects.

Recently, Penwest also developed SyncroDose™, a hydrophilic matrix system like TIMERx®, it offers various predetermined lag times, and hence better control of the drug release.

The Oros® system (or osmotic pump system) developed by ALZA Corp (now part of Johnson & Johnson), is an extended-release technology. It controls drug release rate in the GI tract via osmotic pressure, which increases in the tablet when it encounters the aqueous environment. Drug release from the system is governed by various formulation factors, such as drug solubility, osmotic pressure of the core component(s), size of the delivery orifice (in the membrane), and nature of the rate-controlling membrane. One significant advantage of this dosage form is that drug release is mostly independent of the GI physiological factors. Hence, it is possible to develop and optimize the formulation components and process factors, and to develop an osmotic system for delivering drugs of diverse nature at a predetermined release rate. Since the early 1980s, more than ten extended-release drug products using Oros® technology have been introduced to the market. Many of these products are designed for once-daily dosing, which is critical for the patient's convenience. Examples of marketed osmotic pump systems include Concerta® (methylphenidate HCl) for attention deficit hyperactivity disorder or ADHD (by Johnson & Johnson), Procardia XL® (nifedipine) for angina and hypertension (by Pfizer), Sudafed 24 Hour® (pseudoephedrine HCl) for temporary relief of nasal congestion due to common cold, hay fever, and other respiratory allergies (by Pfizer), and Tegretol®XL (carbamazepine) for anticonvulsant therapy (by Novartis).

TABLE 40.1   Approved products using TIMERx® technology

Brand name	Generic name	Indication	Collaborative	Territory
Opana® ER	Oxymorphhone ER	Moderate to severe pain	Endo Pharmaceuticals	Worldwide
Procardia® XL	Nifedipine	Hypertension, angina	Mylan Pharmaceuticals	USA
SOlfedipine® XL	Nifedipine	Hypertension, angina	Sanofi-Synthelabo	UK and Italy
Cronodipin®	Nifedipine	Hypertension	E. Merck	Brazil
Crystrin® CR	Oxybutynin	Urinary incontinence	Leiras OY	Finland

source: www.penwest.com

Enteric coating is also an important technical approach in modified-release. The primary rationale for this technology is to minimize or eliminate drug chemical degradation in the stomach or to target drug release in specific areas of the GI tract. The same enteric coating technology may also be used to provide protection to the stomach, so as to minimize potential local drug irritation. Coating materials or polymers are required to be biocompatible, and ideally biodegradable. The literature provides ample examples. For naturally occurring polymers, Aquacoat® (developed by FMC Corp., spheronised to sub-micron sized, aqueous-based, pseudo-latex dispersions) is one of the most commonly used. For synthetic polymers, the Eudragit® series, acrylate-based polymers by Röhm Pharma have enjoyed wide popularity in pharmaceutical industry. The Eudragit® polymers contain carboxylic acid group(s) as functional moieties. These polymers remain unionized in low pH stomach, and start to ionize and consequently release the drug compounds as the pH level rises along the GI tract. For example, Eudragit® L30 D-55, L100, and LS100 ionize at pH 5, 6, and 7, respectively, effectively targeting drug delivery at different sections of GI tract. Both the Aquacoat® and Eudragit® series products are broadly used in drug product enteric coating for various therapeutic benefits.

40.5.2 Formulations with Enhanced Bioavailability

Another important aspect of the potential LCM strategy is the application of emerging formulation technologies to enhance bioavailability of the original product. Most of these technologies aim to improve drug solubility and/or dissolution, thus positively impacting bioavailability. Nanosuspension, microemulsion, and solid dispersion are the main technologies used for bioavailability enhancement.

Nanosuspensions essentially consist of nanoparticulates in solution, and are an improved version of a microparticulate or microsuspension system. Due to its consistent and stabilized small particle system, this dosage form usually provides significant dissolution and bioavailability enhancement for many poorly water-soluble drug compounds (especially those in BCS class II or those which are solubility/dissolution rate-limited). With particles in the nano-range with a narrow distribution, nanosuspensions also have an advantage for formulation physical stability, and batch-to-batch reproducibility. A variety of preparation techniques can be used for manufacturing, such as wet milling, high-pressure homogenization, spray drying,

solvent precipitation, supercritical fluid technology, etc. The Nanocrystal™ technology developed by Elan Pharmaceuticals is probably one of the best known. The technology uses a NanoMill™, wet milling process, with cross-linked polystyrene beads as the grinding material,[10] together with a selection of surfactants and polymers in the formulation. Two oral liquid products in the US market are manufactured using the Nanocrystal™ technology, Rapamune® (sirolimus) by Wyeth for immunosuppression, and Emend® (aprepitant) by Merck against nausea and vomiting.

A lipid-based system, microemulsion is a significantly improved version of the emulsion. It has a lot of potential for delivery of BCS class II and IV drug compounds. In principle, microemulsions offer many advantages, as compared to emulsions, small particles (nano-range, often <150nm), thermodynamic stability, and potential to improve bioavailability. A number of literature reviews provide extensive and detailed information on the principles, practice, and applications of lipid-based formulations as a viable dosage form for bioavailability enhancement.[11] A common version for oral microemulsion is the self-(micro)emulsifying drug delivery system (SEDDS or SMEDDS). This technology has been introduced into the market with the product Neoral® (cyclosporin A) by Novartis.

The term solid dispersion encompasses two major formulations principles:

1. where the drug is dispersed as fine particles in a carrier or polymer;
2. where the drug is molecularly dispersed in the polymer.

The latter is often referred to as solid solution formulation, since the drug is solubilized in the polymer, but exists as in a solid-state. The solid solution formulation transforms a crystalline drug into a high-energy amorphous state and, as a result, it allows the formation of a stable supersaturated solution for the poorly soluble drug compounds. This effectively increases the drug dissolution, and hence the bioavailability. Two manufacturing approaches are commonly employed, hot-melt extrusion, and spray drying. In hot-melt extrusion, drug and polymer(s) are heated in an extruder to a temperature at which the drug is dissolved in the polymer, and then extruded. The extrudate is subsequently processed via milling or other methods, before further processing and capsule-filling/tableting. In spray drying, drug and polymers(s) are dissolved in organic solvent(s). The organic solution is spray dried under pressure and hot air/nitrogen. The spray dried material often contains certain levels of solvents, and further drying (or secondary drying) is often required (via fluid-bed dryer or tray dryer).

It is worth noting that, for solid solution formulations, it is critical that the extrudate or the spray dried material retains amorphous characteristics. Current marketed products include Gris-PEG® (griseofulvin) by Novartis for anti-fungal activity, Cesamet® (nabilone) by Lilly as an antiemetic, and Kaletra® (lopinavir/ritonavir) by Abbott for HIV, all of which are oral solid dosage form (tablets).

40.5.3 Examples of Successful New Drug Delivery Systems

Ambien®CR Versus Ambien®

Zolpidem is a hypnotic drug that is administered orally. It has been sold in the US and elsewhere as immediate-release (IR) tablets containing 5 and 10 mg of zolpidem tartrate under the tradename Ambien®. The product is characterized by a rapid onset of action, as well as minimal residual and rebound effect, and hence its effect on sleep-maintenance has been less inconsistent. In addition, the product went off patent in US in April 2007, and faced severe generic competition. Sanofi-Aventis has since launched a new version of the product, under the tradename Ambian®CR. The new product is an extended-release zolpidem formulation. The tablets contain zolpidem tartrate at strengths of 6.25, and 12.5 mg. These are two-layered tablets (US Pat. No. 6 514 531), one layer contains approximately 70% of the zolpidem tartrate content, and releases the content immediately after oral ingestion, the other layer allows for slower release of the remaining drug content. The purpose of the slower release layer is to provide extended plasma concentration beyond three hours after administration. The new product Ambien®CR shows an improved absorption profile over its immediate-release version Ambien®, and has successfully fended off generic competition.

Neoral® Versus Sandimmune®

Cyclosporine A is an immunosuppressant drug widely used in post-organ-transplant to reduce the activity of the patient's immune system, and hence the risk of organ rejection. The drug is marketed by Novartis under Sandimmune®. A lipid-based formulation, this product has a number of issues, relatively low oral bioavailability, significant food effect, and substantial variability in the extent and kinetics of drug absorption from the formulation. The variability in exposure is often associated with poor efficacy. Novartis hence developed an improved version of the formulation, Neoral®. This is a self-emulsifying drug delivery system upon oral ingestion. The new product has shown advantages

in all aspects over Sandimmune®, 30% increase in relative bioavailability, minimal food effect, and significantly reduced individual variability.[12] The enhanced absorption profile has special importance to liver transplant patients, as the new product is less dependent on the presence of bile salts to aid absorption.

40.6 LIFECYCLE MANAGEMENT THROUGH FIXED COMBINATION PRODUCTS

Based on the US Code of Federal Regulations (21 CFR Part 3 Section 3.2(e)) by which the FDA abides, combination products are single articles having multiple attributes, components or articles; a product being defined as a drug, a biologic or a device. There are four definitions of combination products:

1. a product comprised of two or more regulated components that are physically, chemically or otherwise combined or mixed, and produced as a single entity;
2. two or more separate products packaged together in a single package or as a unit;
3. a product packaged separately, which according to its investigational plan or proposed labeling, is intended for use only with an approved individually specified product, where both are required to achieve the intended use, indication or effect, and where, upon approval of the proposed product, the labeling of the already approved product would need to be changed to reflect a change in intended use, dosage form, strength, route of administration or significant change in dose;
4. any product packaged separately that, according to its proposed labeling, is for use only with another individually specified investigational product, where both are required to achieve the intended use, indication or effect.

In this section, we will be discussing only combination drugs, partly described in the first definition, and composed of drug–drug combinations only (not biologics or devices). We will also mainly be discussing considerations pertaining to the US and European Health Authorities (FDA–Food and Drug Administration and EMEA–European Medicines Agency, respectively), as per their respective guideline documents on combination products. In the past few years, the number of combination therapies being introduced to the worldwide market has significantly increased (refer to Table 40.2 for a non-exhaustive list of combination products).

TABLE 40.2 Examples of some combination therapies recently introduced on the US and worldwide market

Brand name	Generic name	Indication	Manufacturer
Vytorin®	ezetimibe/simvastatin	Control of high cholesterol	Merck
Lotrel®	amlodipine besylate/benazepril HCl	Control of high blood pressure	Novartis
Co-Diovan®	valsartan/hydrochlorothiazide	Control of high blood pressure	Novartis
Exforge®	amlodipine besylate/valsartan/hydrochlorothiazide	Control of high blood pressure	Novartis
Ziac®	hydrochlorothiazide/bisoprolol	Control of high blood pressure	
Caduet®	amlodipine besylate/atorvastatin calcium	Control of high blood pressure and high cholesterol	Pfizer
Stalevo®	carbidopa/levodopa/entacapone	Treatment of Parkinson's disease	Novartis
Glucovance®	glipizide/metformin HCl	Treatment of type 2 diabetes	Bristol-Myers Squibb
Janumet®	sitagliptin/metformin HCl	Treatment of type 2 diabetes	Merck
Avandamet®	rosiglitazone maleate/metformin HCl	Treatment of type 2 diabetes	GlaxoSmithKline
Allegra D®	fexofenadine HCl/pseudoephedrine HCl	Treatment of seasonal allergies	Sanofi-Aventis
Advair®	fluticasone propionate/salmeterol xinafoate	Treatment of asthma	GlaxoSmithKline
Symbicort®	budesonide/formoterol	Treatment of asthma	AstraZeneca, Merck
Augmentin®	amoxicilline/clavulanate potassium	Antibacterial	GlaxoSmithKline
Combivir®	lamivudine/zidovudine	Antiviral against HIV	GlaxoSmithKline
Trizivir®	abacavir sulfate/lamivudine/zidovudine	Antiviral against HIV	GlaxoSmithKline
Kaletra®	lopinavir/ritonavir	Antiviral against HIV	Abbott
Atripla®	emtricibatine/tenofovir/efavirenz	Antiviral against HIV	Bristol Myers Squibb, Gilead, Merck
Symbyax®	olanzapine/fluoxetine HCl	Treatment of bipolar depression	Eli Lilly
Treximet®	sumatriptan/naproxen sodium	Acute treatment of migraine	GlaxoSmithKline

Due to the many benefits of combination products, pharmaceutical companies (innovator and generic) are currently working on multiple double or triple combinations, with actives targeting the same disease and having either a synergistic effect or acting on different targets, and with actives targeting diseases which are related in the patient population (such as high cholesterol, and high blood pressure). These combination products are of three types:

1. combining already marketed products;
2. combining already marketed product(s) with new chemical entitie(s) (NCEs); and
3. combining NCEs.

Depending on the type and scope of a specific combination product, the clinical, technical, and business challenges are numerous and various.

In addition, the business hurdles for such combination products are increasing overall. In most cases, it is not intended to extend the original patent life anymore, but rather to increase the market potential as part of a line extension or a second generation launch. The combination product needs to have a significant market potential, and to demonstrate a significant therapeutic advantage. Also, with the steady increase in the filing of combination products, regulatory agencies are reviewing these filings very critically.

40.6.1 Benefit of Fixed Combination Products

Combination products have many potential benefits which render them a very attractive strategy for drug product development. From a therapeutic standpoint, combination therapy offers better overall disease management. Combination products can provide convenience, they can significantly increase patient's compliance,[13] they can also in some cases have synergistic effects, and decrease potential resistance. Combination products, such as the multivitamins, are widely available and accepted in the health industry. Their availability is increasing in the pharmaceutical field, where their value is also continuously discussed. Wald and Law[14] have argued, based on the analysis of 750 randomized clinical trials with a total of 400000 patients, that a "polypill," acting on lowering four of the key cardiovascular key factors, could reduce cardiovascular disease by more than 80%. Combination products can also treat multiple risk factors, thus increasing overall efficacy against treatment of concomitant disease states.

From an economic standpoint, combination products offer a significant pricing advantage, with the pricing of two or more drugs at once rather than individually. From a pharmaceutical industry perspective, the development time, and thus the investment, is potentially lower, with potentially high returns. Combination products also allow a pharmaceutical company to maximize a brand value and potentially extend the patent life through innovative LCM approaches. In the context of very competitive dynamics, combination products also allow protection of the patent life of a product to its full extent, even if it does not extend it, thus preserving market share and sustaining returns.

Even in the current pharma–economic environment, with increasing pressure on reimbursement and pricing, and the overall negative perception of the pharmaceutical companies, combination therapy and associated product development are still progressing fast, mainly due to an improvement in the knowledge of the disease risk factors and how they interact, combined with better clinical markers and their use in clinical trials.

40.6.2 Clinical Challenges

Combination therapy is a very attractive concept, based on the multi-factorial causes of diseases and pharmacogenomics, a "multi-pill" would be a panacea. Combination therapy is, however, more complex compared to monotherapy drug product development. The clinical challenges and the design of clinical studies are very different, whether the combination product is intended to be a first or second line therapy (initial or replacement therapy, respectively).

As a first line therapy, the underlying principle is that the patient's exposure to two or more products instead of one will not be increasing the overall adverse effects, and will improve the therapeutic outcome, either by synergy or because of the poor clinical outcome of each of the monotherapies. Ziac®, for example, is a combination product of two actives with dose-related adverse effects. The combination therapy allows lower doses to be administered, thus decreasing adverse effects, but retaining adequate efficacy for blood pressure lowering. Stalevo® is a first line product for the treatment of Parkinson's disease, containing levodopa and carbidopa (prodrug of levodopa), as well as entacapone, which does not have any individual therapeutic effect, but significantly increases the levodopa half life, thus increasing the therapeutic window.

Clinical studies for combination products are usually bypassing Phase I studies, where safety of each of the monotherapies is demonstrated within a specific dose range. The burden on the Phase II/III fixed dose combination (FDC) trials is higher than for single component studies. The main objective is to demonstrate, in the target population, the improved benefit-to-risk ratio relative to a suitable comparator at the chosen FDC doses. Multiple factors have to be taken into consideration during the design of these studies, including the scientific and marketing rationale, the preclinical and Phase I findings, the study population, and the dosages. In addition, the health authorities' requirements may vary. Some regulatory agencies are specifically looking at non-responder populations to each of the treatments, either for proof of non-inferiority or for proof of superiority of the combination. The clinical team also has to decide whether the clinical trials should be geared towards demonstrating bioequivalence to each of the components or therapeutic non-inferiority/superiority or both.

Dose selection for each of the single components is probably the most difficult part of designing these clinical trials. One of the challenges is for therapies where the prescribers are used to adjust the dose of each component independently, depending on the patient's response. Combination products do not, in most cases, provide the flexibility to be able to titrate patients. For therapies where the dose escalation is fairly straightforward, the number of possible combinations might be very high, and all the needed combinations might not be available. Also, the two or more components may be having additive or synergistic effects. These potential drug–drug interactions need to be very well studied, both in light of efficacy, and of potential adverse events. This is particularly difficult when one of the components has a challenging pharmacokinetic profile, such as with prodrugs. In Vytorin®, for example, the pharmacokinetic parameters of ezetimibe, simvastatin, and simvastatin's active metabolite had to be followed. Also, the interactions between the two or more components may vary, depending on which doses of the spectrum are combined (for example low dose of drug 1 with high dose of drug 2 or *vice versa*).

Demonstrating improved benefit-to-risk ratio is a long and complex process, whether the combination product has an improved safety profile with similar efficacy, an improved efficacy with similar safety profile or both improved safety profile and efficacy, compared to each of the single treatments. The use of statistics at each level of the clinical study designs and interpretations is a key factor. Factorial designs for these studies are usually preferred. Clinical studies for one combination product would at least encompass:

- a Phase IIa study as a proof of concept, to demonstrate efficacy;
- a Phase IIb study, to justify the fixed combination doses;
- a Phase III studies, to confirm (superior) efficacy;
- additional studies such as long-term safety or efficacy studies, food effect studies or studies in special populations, such as the elderly, renally or hepatically impaired, etc.

40.6.3 Technical Challenges

Overall, combination products are technically challenging to develop. In addition, since the formulation principle and/or process, as well as the clinical proof of the monotherapy, are already achieved, the tendency is to assume that the development of combined already known drugs, whether they are already marketed or NCE(s), is simple and can be achieved rapidly. Moreover, since this LCM development is usually to be completed long before the expiration of the main patent, so as to maximize returns, the time pressure is great. An additional challenge is the number of doses, for two drugs with 3–4 dose levels each, 9–16 FDC would be required to cover the entire prescription spectrum. Thus, the first challenge is to define the combination product strategy, including the submission timelines, and the number of doses to be filed.

Formulation challenges are first to be tackled, demonstrating physical and chemical compatibility of the two or more drug substances. Based on the extent of compatibility or incompatibility, the formulation principles to be applied are very different. For incompatible compounds, bilayer or trilayer technologies are available. One can also protect one of the components with other excipients, before mixing them together in the same matrix. Many approaches are feasible, however, one must keep in mind the processing aspects. The tablet size needs to be reasonable, and the manufacturing process needs to be robust and easily scalable to production size. One also needs to keep in mind that any new technology which may be introduced to meet the challenges of a combination product also brings additional uncertainties and potential complications, which may have a significant time impact on the product development. Physical compatibility should not be underestimated. Matching dissolution of multiple components with different release mechanisms can be a difficult task, and may have direct implications on the bioequivalence of one or all the drugs of the combination product.

An additional complication is the dose differential between the two or more drug substances, which can lead to recovery challenges, as well as loss of potency or uniformity. In Exforge® for example, developed by Novartis for the treatment of hypertension, the largest dose differential is between the 5 mg of amlodipine besylate, and the 320 mg of valsartan. This dose differential, and the obligation of keeping the tablet size reasonable, sometimes forces the formulation principle to vary for the same combination product depending on doses, presenting an additional degree of challenges, since this could also have some bioequivalence implications.

In some instances, the formulation and process of a marketed product to be included in the combination product cannot be significantly altered for stability, processing, and/or bioequivalence reasons. The burden on the formulator is then even higher, to combine such a product with another while preserving its original performance. To minimize the technical challenges of combination product development, and to complete development activities within the business relevant timelines, multiple formulation and process approaches may need to be considered in parallel. When choosing the final formulation and process approach, attention should be given to production costs, to make sure they are in line with the expected return on the combination product.

Last but not least, analysis and quality control have to be considered. With potential interactions between various components (drugs and excipients), recovery of all actives and relevant degradation products is challenging. In addition, for time and cost reasons, single methods are also preferred for combination products, but not always achievable. Codetection might not be a problem, except if one of the drugs does not carry a chromophore. More challenging is compound separation and relative sensitivity, especially when the dose differential is high. When multiple methods are needed, robotics can be very helpful and save resources, but require a very detailed validation and comparison to the original, high resource consuming manual methods.

Stability programs for these high number of doses-multiple formulation principles-combination products can also be very tricky. However, bracketing, with the agreement of the relevant health authorities, is usually acceptable.

40.6.4 Business Challenges

From a business perspective, combination products are also challenging. Many factors need to be taken into consideration before deciding to develop a combination product, such as market potential, acceptability from the point of view of the prescriber, patient, health and reimbursing authorities, position relative to own and competitor portfolio, and foremost, timing of the introduction of this potential new product into the market.

In some rare cases, combination products give a clear competitive advantage when allowing the extension of the original indication of each of the individual components. Prozac® and Zyprexa®, compounds marketed by Eli Lilly for the treatment of depression, were successfully combined into Symbyax® for the treatment of bipolar disorder. This is, however, not the norm, and the business challenges are increasing, especially in the current climate of increasing and earlier patent challenges, and pressure by authorities on reducing the cost of pharmaceuticals.

In most cases, the introduction of a combination product allows the extension of a specific brand name, fulfilling an unmet medical need or bringing a significant therapeutic advantage. This directly delays the competition, and specifically the generic introduction into the market. The marketing strategy however, needs to be very clear and simple, and the combination product needs to be very well-positioned compared to the monotherapy products to, as much as possible, avoid unwanted cannibalization. Competitive pricing, combined with significant therapeutic advantage, is a valuable tool for combination products, if they are priced below the cost of their combined individual components.

Introducing a combination product is however, not a simple task. The pharmaceutical industry as a whole has had many failed attempts, such as the tentative by Merck and Schering-Plough to combine Singulair® and Claritin® for the treatment of seasonal allergies. The Phase III clinical trials failed to demonstrate a significant improvement, compared to the individual products administered separately.

In addition, launching of a combination product does not necessarily mean that the launch will be successful. Glucovance®, a combination of glyburide and metformin HCl, was launched by Bristol-Myers Squibb in anticipation of the loss of patent on the Glucophage® blockbuster, but only performed poorly against metformin generic competition pricing, despite demonstrated significant clinical advantage.

However, marketing of combination products is still an attractive and potentially lucrative business opportunity which pharmaceutical companies, innovators and generics alike, keep pursuing for the overall benefit of disease management.

40.7 CONCLUSIONS

Lifecycle management (LCM) is an attractive but challenging product development strategy which allows, either through salt, polymorph or formulation changes, new delivery systems or fixed combination products, improvement in overall pharmaceutical product efficacy. Beside the added benefit to the patient, this strategy allows the pharmaceutical companies to sustain or enhance the returns on investment for the innovator's drug product.

This strategy needs to be implemented early during the development of the original drug product, so as to maximize its patent life and/or brand image. However, the future fate of the various LCM options will be significantly impacted by changes in the regulatory environment of the multiple health authorities, and by changes in the international and country-specific patent law.

References

1. Rhodes, J. & Mulder, J. (2005). Challenges and opportunities converge in today's pharmaceutical industry. www.deloitte.com/us/lifesciences.
2. Capgemini. (2004). Pharmaceutical industry success dependent on better product lifecycle management. www.capgemini.com, October 6.
3. Visiongain. (2006). Product lifecycle management. Strategic report, www.piribo.com, May.
4. Slowik, H. (2003). The battle for IP. In Vivo: The Business and Medicine Report 21(6), 75–82.
5. Lucas, J. & Burgess, P. (2004). When form equals substance: The value of screening in product life-cycle management. Pharma Voice, February.
6. Tong, W.Q. (2004). Integrating business considerations into scientific approaches for salt and crystal form screening and selection, 43rd annual Eastern Pharmaceutical Technology Meeting, October 1.
7. McGinity, J.W., Zhang, F., Repka, M.A. & Koleng, J.J. (2001). *Hot-melt extrusion as a pharmaceutical process.* American Pharmaceutical Review, Russell Publishing,
8. Douglas, S.J., Davis, S.S. & Illum, L. (1987). Nanoparticles in drug delivery. CRC Critical Review Ther. Drug Carr. Syst. 3(3), 233–261.
9. Rajabi-Siahboomi, A.R., Melia, C.D., Davies, M.C., Bowtell, R.W., McJury, M., Sharp, J.C. & Mansfield, P. (1992). Imaging the internal structure of the gel layer in hydrophilic matrix systems by NMR imaging. J. Pharm. Pharmacol. 44(suppl), 1062.
10. Liversidge, G.G., Cundy, K.C., Bishop, J. & Czekai, D. (1991). Surface modified drug nanoparticles. US Patent 5145 684.
11. Charman, W.N. (2000). Lipids, lipophilic drugs, and oral drug delivery—some emerging concepts. J. Pharm. Sci. 89, 967–978.
12. Holt, D.W. et al. (1994). Trans. Proc. 26(5), 2935–2939.
13. Bangalore, S., Kamalakkannan, G. & Parkar, S. (2007). Fixed-dose combinations improve medication compliance: A meta-analysis. The American Journal of Medicine 120, 713–719.
14. Wald, N.J. & Law, M.R. (2003). A strategy to decrease cardiovascular disease by more than 80%. BMJ 326(7404), 1419.

Bibliography

AAPS (American Association of Pharmaceutical Scientists). (2006). Workshop on Challenges in developing fixed-dosed combination oral solid dose products, 13–14 September. Pharmaceutical Research 23(9), 2230–2231. Arlington, VA.

Beers, D.O. (2002). An increase in life expectancy. Legal Week Global, November, Arnold & Porter LLP.

European Medicines Agency (EMEA). (2008). Committee for Medical Products for Human Use (CHMP), Draft Guideline on fixed combination medicinal products, 21 February, http://www.emea.europa.eu/pdfs/human/ewp/024095en.pdf.

Food and Drug Administration (FDA). (2006). US Department of Health and Human Services, Guidance for Industry and FDA Staff, Early Development Considerations for Innovative Combination Products, September, http://www.emea.europa.eu/pdfs/human/ewp/024095en.pdf.

Lehman Brothers. (2007). Pharma Pipelines. Strategic Analysis and Conclusions 2007, September 19, www.lehman.com.

Lifecycle Management Strategies. (2006). Maximizing ROI through indication expansion, reformulation and Rx-to-OTC switching, Business Insights Limited, February, http://www.bioportfolio.com/cgi-bin/acatalog/info_333.html.

Pharmaceutical Law & Industry Report. (2003). Vol. 1, No.11, March 28, pp. 312–316.

Rathbone, M.J., Hadgraft, J. & Roberts, M. S. (2003). Modified release drug delivery technologies. *Drugs and Pharmaceutical Sciences*, Vol. 126. Informa Health Care.

United States Code of Federal Regulations (21 CFR).

Index

Clinical plan template
. clinical supply liason
. Lean manufacturing, requires ~~less~~ fewer resources, less
  a dynamic system,
- Fewer resources   R
- Less material   M
- Less inventory   I
- Less Labor   L
- Less Equipment   E
- Less time   T
- Less space   S

M - material
R - Resources
L - Labor
E - Equipment
T - Time
S - space
I - Inventory